THE NEUROLOGY OF EYE MOVEMENTS

FOURTH EDITION

SERIES EDITOR
Sid Gilman, M.D., F.R.C.P.
William J. Herdman Professor of Neurology
University of Michigan Medical Center

Contemporary Neurology Series

19 THE DIAGNOSIS OF STUPOR AND COMA, Third Edition
Fred Plum, M.D., and Jerome B. Posner, M.D.

53 SLEEP MEDICINE
Michael S. Aldrich, M.D.

54 BRAIN TUMORS
Harry S. Greenburg, M.D., William F. Chandler, M.D., and Howard M. Sandler, M.D.

56 MYASTHENIA GRAVIS AND MYASTHENIC DISORDERS
Andrew Engel, M.D., *Editor*

57 NEUROGENETICS
Stefan-M. Pulst, M.D., *Editor*

58 DISEASES OF THE SPINE AND SPINAL CORD
Thomas N. Byrne. M.D., Edward C. Benzel, M.D., and Stephen G. Waxman, M.D., Ph.D.

59 DIAGNOSIS AND MANAGEMENT OF PERIPHERAL NERVE DISORDERS
Jerry R. Mendell, M.D., David R. Cornblath, M.D., and John T. Kissel, M.D.

60 THE NEUROLOGY OF VISION
Jonathan D. Trobe, M.D.

61 HIV NEUROLOGY
Bruce James Brew, M.B.B.S., M.D., F.R.A.C.P.

62 ISCHEMIC CEREBROVASCULAR DISEASE
Harold P. Adams, Jr., M.D., Vladimir Hachinski, M.D., and John W. Norris, M.D., F.R.C.P.

63 CLINICAL NEUROPHYSIOLOGY OF THE VESTIBULAR SYSTEM, Third Edition
Robert W. Baloh, M.D., and Vicente Honrubia, M.D.

64 NEUROLOGICAL COMPLICATIONS OF CRITICAL ILLNESS, Second Edition
Eelco F.M. Wijdicks, M.D., Ph.D., F.A.C.P.

65 MIGRAINE: MANIFESTATIONS, PATHOGENESIS, AND MANAGEMENT, Second Edition
Robert A. Davidoff, M.D.

66 CLINICAL NEUROPHYSIOLOGY, Second Edition
Jasper R. Daube, M.D., *Editor*

67 THE CLINICAL SCIENCE OF NEUROLOGIC REHABILITATION, Second Edition
Bruce H. Dobkin, M.D.

68 NEUROLOGY OF COGNITIVE AND BEHAVIORAL DISORDERS
Orrin Devinsky, M.D., and Mark D'Esposito, M.D.

69 PALLIATIVE CARE IN NEUROLOGY
Raymond Voltz, M.D., James L. Bernat, M.D., Gian Domenico Borasio, M.D., DipPallMed, Ian Maddocks, M.D., David Oliver, F.R.C.G.P., Russell K. Portenoy, M.D.

THE NEUROLOGY OF EYE MOVEMENTS

FOURTH EDITION

R. John Leigh, M.D., F.R.C.P.

Blair-Daroff Professor of Neurology,
Professor of Neurosciences, Otolaryngology,
and Biomedical Engineering
Case Western Reserve University
Department of Veterans Affairs Medical Center
and University Hospitals
Cleveland, Ohio

David S. Zee, M.D.

Professor of Neurology, Ophthalmology,
Otolaryngology and Head and
Neck Surgery, and Neuroscience
The Johns Hopkins University School of Medicine
Baltimore, Maryland

OXFORD
UNIVERSITY PRESS
2006

OXFORD
UNIVERSITY PRESS

Oxford University Press, Inc., publishes works that further
Oxford University's objective of excellence
in research, scholarship, and education.

Oxford New York
Auckland Cape Town Dar es Salaam Hong Kong Karachi
Kuala Lumpur Madrid Melbourne Mexico City Nairobi
New Delhi Shanghai Taipei Toronto

With offices in
Argentina Austria Brazil Chile Czech Republic France Greece
Guatemala Hungary Italy Japan Poland Portugal Singapore
South Korea Switzerland Thailand Turkey Ukraine Vietnam

Published by Oxford University Press, Inc.
198 Madison Avenue, New York, New York 10016
www.oup.com

Library of Congress Cataloging-in-Publication Data

Leigh, R. John.
The neurology of eye movements / R. John Leigh, David S. Zee.— 4th ed.
p. ; cm. — (Contemporary neurology series ; 70)
Includes bibliographical references and index.
ISBN-13: 978-0-19-530090-1
ISBN-10: 0-19-530090-4
1. Eye—Movement disorders—Diagnosis. 2. Eye—Movements.
3. Diagnosis, Differential. I. Zee, David S. II. Title. III. Series.
[DNLM: 1. Eye Movements—physiology. 2. Ocular Motility Disorders.
WW 400 L529n 2006]
RE731.L44 2006
617.7′62—dc22 2005022301

The science of medicine is a rapidly changing field. As new research and clinical experience broaden our knowledge, changes in treatment and drug therapy do occur. The authors and the publisher of this work have checked with sources believed to be reliable in their efforts to provide information that is accurate and complete, and in accordance with the standards accepted at the time of publication. However, in light of the possibility of human error or changes in the practice of medicine, neither the authors, nor the publisher, nor any other party who has been involved in the preparation or publication of this work warrants that the information contained herein is in every respect accurate or complete. Readers are encouraged to confirm the information contained herein with other reliable sources, and are strongly advised to check the product information sheet provided by the pharmaceutical company for each drug they plan to administer.

9 8 7 6 5 4 3 2 1

Printed in the United States of America
on acid-free paper

Preface

In the seven years since the publication of the Third Edition of *The Neurology of Eye Movements*, thousands of new papers concerning eye movements have been published. In part this is because of a sustained interest in eye movements themselves—elucidation of the neurobiology with new techniques and development of more plausible *neuromimetic* models. A second reason for the increased popularity of eye movements is their application as experimental tools, especially the use of saccades to investigate a range of psychological topics ranging from attention and memory to visual search and reading.

Since the "big bang" of electronic publication of scientific journals in 1997, the accessibility to research papers has greatly improved, making it possible to quickly search and find information concerning any aspect of eye movements. Thus, the reader might well ask: What possible use could a monograph like *The Neurology of Eye Movements* serve when, even at the moment of its publication, new papers are appearing at such a rate? What we hope to provide is a conceptual framework that can be used to interpret current and new findings. This framework has been in evolution since the first edition of our book, and is based on a quarter-century of hypothesis testing in the laboratory and clinic. In some cases, this evolution has been an orderly refinement, but to use the term introduced by Thomas Kuhn, we have witnessed at least one scientific revolution—the discovery of pulleys that dictate the pulling directions of the extraocular muscles—necessitating a re-evaluation of basic concepts. Further seismic shifts of our concepts may well occur—the field is far from definitive, even though it leads probably every other aspect of motor control. The use of eye movements as experimental tools has also brought about important conceptual advances in other fields by using them to probe attention, memory, reward, and volition.

As in the prior edition, we have included a DVD with video clips showing examples of eye movement disorders that we think may be helpful; they are not copy-protected and can be copied and incorporated into lectures and presentations—our goal is dissemination of knowledge. In addition, we have included the videos in twenty-three video displays of clinical syndromes, which combine the clips, with legends, related figures and listed features and pathogenesis. We are indebted to our teacher and mentor, David A. Robinson, for agreeing to our including his hand-written lecture notes, "Linear Control Systems in the Oculomotor System."

During the period that we were preparing the Fourth Edition, we were both fortunate to be enjoying a sabbatical in the rich intellectual environment provided by the Laboratory of Sensorimotor Research (LSR) at the National Eye Institute of the National Institutes of Health in Bethesda Maryland. Thus, we are indebted to the scientists of the LSR, whom we list below, for their advice and comments during numerous informal discussions, and also for their reading sections of manuscript drafts. We are also grateful to Drs. Paul Sieving, Sheldon Miller, Lance Optican, and Carl Kupfer for making that sabbatical possible and agreeing to our including some of the videos made by the late David G. Cogan on the accompanying DVD.

A large number of individuals have contributed to the Fourth Edition, whom we list alphabetically, grateful for their help but acknowledging that any errors are ours, not theirs. They include: Rahila Ansari, Steven Arbogast, David and Rosemary Armington, Claudio Busettini, Jean Büttner-Ennever, Bruce Cumming, Robert Daroff, Joseph Demer, Edmund FitzGibbon, Yanning Helen Han, Okihide Hikosaka, Simon Hong,

Anja Horn, Jonathan Jacobs, Henry Kaminski, Edward Keller, Sangeeta Khanna, Michael King, Arun Kumar, Richard Leigh, Ke Liao, Susanna Martinez-Conde, Frederick Miles, Lloyd Minor, Neil Miller, Michael Mustari, Kae Nakamura, David Newman-Toker, Daniele Nuti, Lance Optican, Nick Port, John Porter, Christian Quaia, Stefano Ramat, Holger Rambold, Stephen Reich, Janet Rucker, Asim Shahid, Aasef Shaikh, Xiaoyan Shan, Mark Shelhamer, Boris Sheliga, David Solomon, William Stacey, John Stahl, Berta Steiner, Dominik Straumann, Max Tischfield, Robert Tomsak, Ronald Tusa, John van Opstal, Mark Walker, Agnes Wong, Shirley Wray, Robert Wurtz, Stacy Yaniglos, and the Cleveland Museum of Art.

Contents

PART 1

THE PROPERTIES AND NEURAL SUBSTRATE OF EYE MOVEMENTS

Chapter 1

A Survey of Eye Movements: Characteristics and Teleology

WHY STUDY EYE MOVEMENTS?

The study of eye movements is a source of valuable information to both basic scientists and clinicians. To the neurobiologist, the study of the control of eye movements provides a unique opportunity to understand the workings of the brain. To neurologists and ophthalmologists, abnormalities of ocular motility are frequently the clue to the localization of a disease process. Moreover, the visual and perceptual consequences of eye movements are important to both basic scientists and clinicians. Over the past three decades, eye movements have increasingly been applied as an experimental tool to gain insight into disorders ranging from muscular dystrophy to dementia.[40,46] Eye movements have even been used to address fundamental issues of human behavior, such as free will and conflict resolution, as subjects respond to visual targets while their frontal lobe activity is monitored by functional magnetic resonance imaging (fMRI) (see Fig. 1–7).[59] And careful clinical observations combined with genetic linkage studies have provided insights into the nature of diseases as diverse as myopathy and cerebellar ataxia.[49,82] Eye movements are also being used to identify and test new therapies for a range of genetic and degenerative disorders.[72] In fact, recent functional imaging studies in human beings and recordings of activity of single neurons in monkeys performing in sophisticated behavioral paradigms have shown that activity related to eye movements can be found in almost every corner of the brain. This should come as no surprise, because we are creatures who depend upon clear vision, and must focus our attention to make prompt, correct responses to what is happening around us. Eye movements both reflect and facilitate this central role for vision in survival.

The singular value of studying eye movements stems from certain advantages that make them easier to interpret than movements of the axial or limb musculature. The first advantage is that eye movements are essentially restricted to rotations of the globes; translations (linear displacements) are negligible. This facilitates precise measurement (Fig. 1–1 and Appendix B), which is a prerequisite for quantitative analysis. A second advantage is the apparent lack of a classic, monosynaptic stretch reflex.[41] This is not unexpected because the eye muscles move the globe against an unchanging mechanical load. Third, different classes of eye movements (Table 1–1) can be distinguished on the basis of how they aid vision, their physiological properties, and their anatomical substrates. Fourth, many abnormalities of eye movements are distinctive and often point to a specific pathophysiology, anatomical localization, or pharmacological disturbance. Finally, eye movements are readily accessible to observation and systematic examination. For this reason, we provide a DVD with Video Displays, and individual video clips, which we hope will immediately bring to life the nature of a disorder being discussed in the text. This chapter provides an overview of the normal behavior of eye movements, and introduces the reader to some current concepts of the underlying neural control. We start by examining why the eyes must move at all—the *raison d'être* of eye movements.[25,69,86a,89]

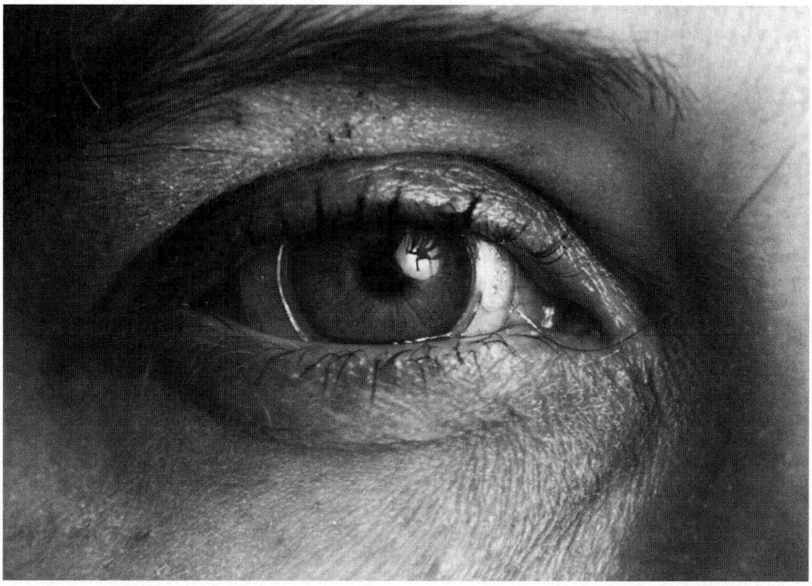

Figure 1–1. The scleral search coil method for precise measurement of horizontal, vertical, and torsional eye rotations. The subject is wearing a silastic annulus in which are embedded two coils of wire, one wound in the frontal plane (to sense horizontal and vertical movements) and the other wound in effectively the sagittal plane (to sense torsional eye movements). When the subject sits in a magnetic field, voltages are induced in these search coils that can be used to measure eye position (see Appendix B for details).

Table 1–1. **Functional Classes of Human Eye Movements**

Class of Eye Movement	Main Function
Vestibular	Holds images of the seen world steady on the retina during brief head rotations or translations
Visual Fixation	Holds the image of a stationary object on the fovea by minimizing ocular drifts
Optokinetic	Holds images of the seen world steady on the retina during sustained head rotation
Smooth Pursuit	Holds the image of a small moving target on the fovea; or holds the image of a small near target on the retina during linear self-motion; with optokinetic responses, aids gaze stabilization during sustained head rotation
Nystagmus quick phases	Reset the eyes during prolonged rotation and direct gaze towards the oncoming visual scene
Saccades	Bring images of objects of interest onto the fovea
Vergence	Moves the eyes in opposite directions so that images of a single object are placed or held simultaneously on the fovea of each eye

VISUAL REQUIREMENTS OF EYE MOVEMENTS

What visual needs must eye movements satisfy? To answer this question, we must first identify the prerequisites for a clear and stable view of the environment. Simply stated, clear vision of an object requires that its image be held fairly steadily on the central, foveal region of the retina. Otherwise visual acuity declines and patients may experience oscillopsia— illusory movement of their visual environment (see Video Display: Treatments for Nystagmus).

Just how steadily must images of the world be held on the retina for vision to remain clear and stable? The amount of retinal image motion that can be tolerated before vision deteriorates depends upon what is being viewed, and specifically, its spatial frequency. For objects with higher spatial frequencies, such as the Snellen optotypes used for conventional testing, retinal image motion should be held below about 5 degrees per second; above this threshold, visual acuity declines in a logarithmic fashion.[7,15] An exception to these general rules concerns eye rotations about the line of sight—torsional movements when the subject views a small object with the fovea; in this case, geometry dictates that horizontal and vertical components of retinal image motion will remain relatively small.

For clearest vision of a single feature of the world, its image must not only be held fairly steady on the retina, but must also be brought close to the center of the fovea, where photoreceptor density is greatest. Visual acuity declines steeply from the fovea to the retinal periphery.[15,39] For example, at 2 degrees from the center of the fovea, visual acuity has declined by about 50%. For best vision, the image of the object of regard should be within 0.5 degrees of the center of the fovea. Thus, during visual search of the environment, the fovea must be pointed at features of interest (Fig. 3–8A, Chapter 3).[91]

Under normal circumstance, the angle of gaze (which corresponds to eye position in space and the line of sight) is held steadily enough that our perception of the world is clear and stationary. The normal, small movements of the eyes that occur as we fix upon an object (Figs. 1–2A) do not interfere with clear vision, and may actually enhance it.[53,81] However, when disease causes abnormal oscillations of the eyes, such as nystagmus (Fig. 1–2B), the images of stationary objects move excessively on the retina and patients report blurring of vision and oscillopsia (see Video Display: Treatments for Nystagmus).

FUNCTIONAL CLASSES OF EYE MOVEMENTS

Since our eyes (and retinas) are attached to our heads, the greatest threat to clear vision during

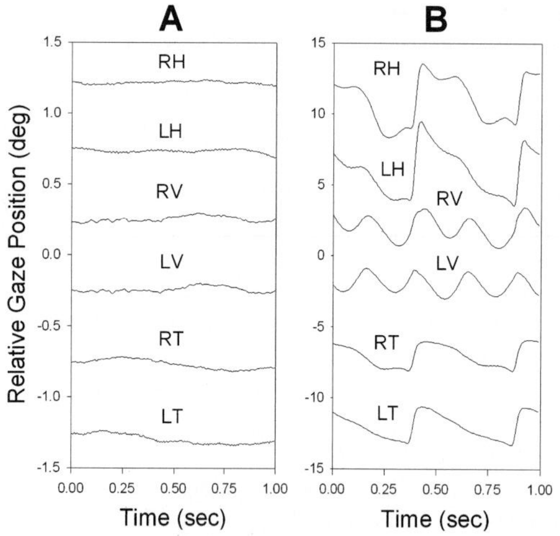

Figure 1–2. Normal and abnormal eye movements during attempted visual fixation of a stationary target. (A) One-second, representative record of the gaze of a normal subject. (B) One-second record from a 35-year-old woman with multiple sclerosis, in whom acquired pendular-jerk nystagmus (see Video Display: Treatments for Nystagmus) precluded steady fixation. Her main complaints were that she could not see clearly and that the world appeared to be moving (oscillopsia) in a direction corresponding to that of her nystagmus. Measurements were made using the magnetic search coil technique. RH: right horizontal; LH: left horizontal; RV: right vertical; LV: left vertical; RT: right torsional; LT: left torsional. Note that gaze positions are relative, having been offset to aid the clarity of the display, and that the scales differ by a factor of 10. Polarity: positive = right, up, or clockwise.

natural behavior is head perturbations, especially those that occur during locomotion (Fig. 7–1).[33,56] If we had no eye movements, images of the visual world would "slip" on the retina with every such head movement. This would cause our vision to become blurred and our ability to recognize and localize objects to be impaired whenever we moved through the environment. To this end, two distinct mechanisms evolved to stabilize images on the retina in general, and the fovea in particular, during such head perturbations. The first comprises the vestibulo-ocular reflexes, which depend on the ability of the labyrinthine mechanoreceptors to sense head accelerations. The second consists of visually-mediated reflexes (optokinetic and smooth-pursuit tracking), which depend on the ability of the brain to determine the speed of image drift on the retina. Together, these reflexes *stabilize the angle of gaze*, so that the fovea of each eye remains pointed at the object of regard whenever the head is moving.

With the evolution of the fovea, a second requirement of eye movements also arose: when a new object of interest appears in the visual periphery, we need to point this central portion of the retina so that the object can be seen best. This requires a repertoire of eye movements to *change the angle of gaze*. In animals without a fovea, such as the rabbit, eye movements are dominated by vestibular and optokinetic stabilization. When such animals choose to change their center of visual attention, they must link a rapid eye movement to a voluntary head movement and so override or cancel vestibular and optokinetic drives. With the emergence of foveal vision, it became necessary to change the line of sight independently of head movements. In this way, images of objects of interest could be brought to and held on that portion of the retina providing best visual acuity. With the evolution of frontal vision and binocularity, disjunctive or vergence eye movements also became necessary, so that images of an object of interest could be placed on the fovea of each eye simultaneously, and then held there.

Thus, eye movements are of two main types: those that stabilize gaze and so keep images steady on the retina, and those that shift gaze and so redirect the line of sight to a new object of interest.[9,16] The chief functional classes of eye movement are summarized in Table 1–1. Each functional class has properties suited to a specific purpose.[25,69,89] Moreover, as detailed in the following chapters, certain anatomical circuits make distinctive contributions to each functional class of movements. An understanding of the properties of each functional class of eye movements will guide the physical examination; knowledge of the neural substrate will aid topological diagnosis. But before discussing each of these various classes of eye movement, we must first examine the mechanical properties imposed on the eye by its surrounding tissues and muscles. The brain must deal with these mechanical factors in order to program fluent and accurate eye movements.

ORBITAL MECHANICS: PHASIC AND TONIC INNERVATION

The tissues supporting the eyeball impose mechanical constraints on the control of gaze. To move the eye, it is necessary to overcome

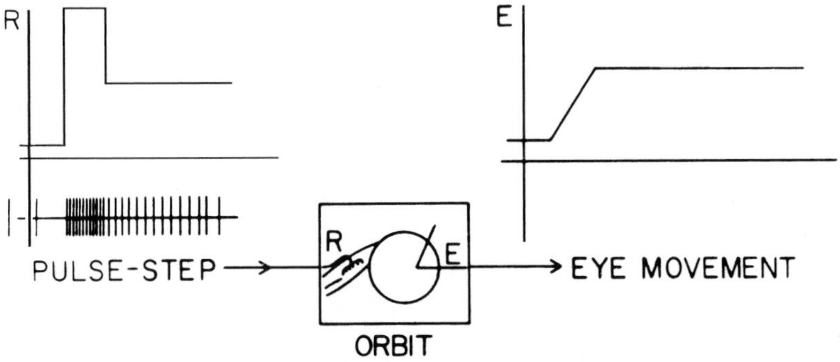

Figure 1–3. The neural signal for a saccade. At right is shown the eye movement: E is eye position in the orbit; the abscissa scale represents time. At left is shown the neural signal sent to the extraocular muscles to produce the saccade. The vertical lines indicate the occurrence of action potentials of an ocular motoneuron. The graph above is a plot of the neuron's discharge rate (R) against time (firing frequency histogram). It shows the neurally encoded pulse (velocity command) and step (position command).

viscous drag and elastic restoring forces imposed by the orbital supporting tissues. To overcome the viscous drag, a powerful contraction of the extraocular muscles is necessary. For rapid movements (e.g., a saccade), this requires a phasic increase or burst of neural activity in the ocular motor nuclei*—the pulse of innervation (Fig. 1–3). Once at its new position, the eye must be held there against elastic restoring forces that tend to return the globe to its central position. To hold the eye in an eccentric position requires a steady contraction of the extraocular muscles, arising from a new tonic level of neural activity—the step of innervation. (For a demonstration of the elastic forces acting on the eyeball, see Video Display: Disorders of Gaze Holding.) When this pulse-step of innervation is appropriately programmed, the eye is moved rapidly to its new position, and held there steadily. (For an audiovisual example of ocular motoneuron activity during saccades, see Video Display: Disorders of Saccades.) Some of the first studies of the discharge characteristics of ocular motoneurons (see Fig. 5–2, Chapter 5) in monkeys,[27,67,70,74] and of eye muscles in human beings (see Fig. 9–6, Chapter 9),[19] confirmed the presence of both the pulse and step of innervation during saccades.† Without the pulse (velocity command), the progress of the eye would be slow; without the step (position command), the eyes could never be maintained in an eccentric position in the orbit. Moreover, the pulse and step must be correctly matched to produce an accurate eye movement and steady fixation following it. These concepts are important for interpreting clinical disorders of eye movements, such as internuclear ophthalmoplegia, when there is a pulse-step mismatch that causes the adducting eye to drift slowly to the target (see Video Display: Pontine Syndromes).

Although our discussion so far has concerned the generation of saccades, the same considerations about mechanical properties of the orbit apply to the commands for all types of eye movement. Studies of the activity of ocular motor neurons in alert monkeys have shown that the neural commands for all conjugate movements (vestibular, optokinetic, saccadic, and pursuit) and for vergence movements have both velocity and position components.[57,85,87] How are the velocity and position components of the ocular motor commands synthesized?

Neurophysiological evidence indicates that the position command (e.g., for saccades, the step) is generated from the velocity command (e.g., for saccades, the pulse) by the mathematical process of integration with respect to time. A neural network integrates, in this mathematical sense, velocity-coded signals into position-coded signals; this network is

*We use the term "ocular motor" to refer to the eye movement control system as a whole, or the third, fourth, and the sixth cranial nerves or their nuclei collectively, and "oculomotor" to indicate the third nerve or its nucleus alone.

†In fact, the mechanical properties of the orbital contents dictate the need for a more complicated ocular motor command, namely a pulse-slide-step, which is discussed in Chapter 5.

referred to as the neural integrator.[2,77] When this process is faulty, the eye is carried to its new position by the pulse but cannot be held there and drifts back to the central position. This is evident clinically as gaze-evoked nystagmus (see Video Display: Disorders of Gaze Holding). Since all types of conjugate eye movements require both velocity-coded and position-coded changes in innervation, all conjugate eye movement commands need access to a common neural integrator. Experimental lesions of structures vital for neural integration affect all classes of conjugate eye movements.[2,13] Furthermore, it appears that vergence eye movements are also synthesized from velocity and position commands, the latter generated by a vergence integrator.[29]

The past decade has witnessed a revolution in our concepts of the organization of the extraocular muscles and the orbital tissues.[23] Current evidence indicates that each extraocular muscle consists of outer orbital and inner global layers, each with special fiber types that endow properties such as fatigue resistance. The outer orbital layer inserts not into the eyeball but into a fibrous pulley, which acts as the functional point of origin for the global layer that passes through and inserts onto the globe (Fig. 9–1). In Chapter 9 we discuss the functional implications of the orbital pulleys, and the contribution they make to determining the axes about which the eyes rotate.[22,32]

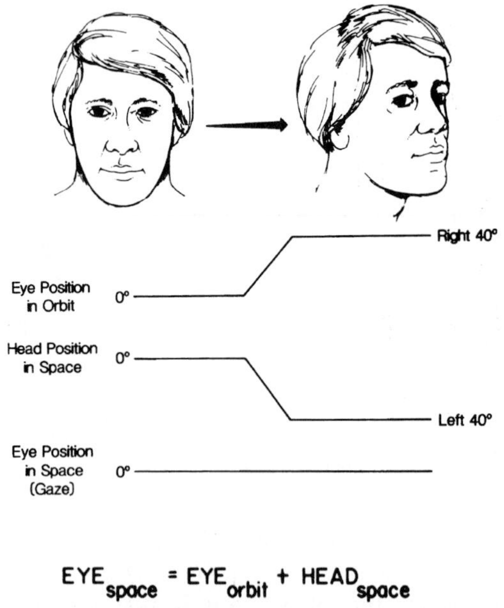

Figure 1–4. The angular vestibulo-ocular reflex (VOR). As the head is rapidly turned to the left, the eyes move by a corresponding amount in the orbit to the right. Below, head position in space and eye position in the orbit are plotted against time. Because the movements of head and eye in orbit are equal and opposite, the sum, eye position in space (the angle of gaze or "gaze"), remains zero (bottom equation). If gaze is held steady, images do not slip on the retina and vision remains clear. During viewing of targets at optical infinity, eye rotations are equal and opposite to head rotations. During viewing of near targets, eye rotations are greater than head rotation, because the eyes do not lie in the center of the head (see Chapters 2 and 7).

VESTIBULAR AND OPTOKINETIC SYSTEMS

The Vestibulo-Ocular Reflex: Responses to Brief Angular and Linear Head Movements

The vestibular system stabilizes gaze and ensures clear vision during head movements, especially those that occur during locomotion. Vestibular eye movements are generated much more promptly (i.e., at shorter latency) than are visually mediated eye movements. This is because the acceleration sensors of the labyrinth signal motion of the head much sooner than the visual system can detect motion of images on the retina. Thus, the vestibulo-ocular reflex (VOR) (Fig. 1–4) generates eye movements to compensate for head movements at a latency of less than 15 ms,[52,64,83] whereas visually mediated eye movements are initiated with latencies greater than 70 ms.[31] This difference becomes an important issue during locomotion because the head perturbations that occur with each footfall contain predominant frequencies ranging from 0.5 to 5.0 Hz.[20,33] Only the short-latency VOR is fast enough to generate eye movements to compensate for head perturbations at these frequencies. This becomes clinically evident in patients who have lost labyrinthine function, who complain, for example, that they cannot read street signs while they are in motion.[38] (For a demonstration of the visual consequences of losing the VOR see Video Display: Disorders of the Vestibular System.)

Although the VOR acts independently of visually mediated eye movements, the brain continuously monitors its performance by evaluating the clarity of vision during head movements. Thus, an appropriately sized eye movement must be generated by the VOR in order for the angle of gaze (eye position in space) to be held steady and the image of the world to remain fairly stationary upon the retina (Fig. 1–4). If it is not, then the performance of the VOR undergoes adaptive changes to restore optimal visuo-motor performance.

The vestibular system can respond to movements that have angular (rotational) or linear (translational) components.[1,20] The angular VOR (Fig. 1–4) depends on the semicircular canals, of which there are three in each inner ear (see Fig. 2–1). In health, the semicircular canals work together to sense head rotations in any plane. Thus, the angular VOR stabilizes images on the retina during head rotation. However, when disease affects an individual semicircular canal, spontaneous eye movements (nystagmus) occur in the plane of that canal, reflecting a common evolutionary relationship between individual semicircular canals and the pulling directions of the extraocular muscles.[18,76] An appreciation of this fundamental physiologic and anatomic feature of vestibulo-ocular control helps one interpret various patterns of nystagmus observed in vestibular disease. For example, in the common disorder, benign paroxysmal positional vertigo that affects the posterior semicircular canal, nystagmus consists of eye rotations in the plane of the affected canal (see Video Display: Disorders of the Vestibular System). Because the eyes are not at the center of rotation of the head, but are situated eccentrically, in the orbits, pure head rotations also produce translations, or linear displacements, of the eye. This geometry becomes important if head rotations occur during viewing of a near object, when the brain must independently adjust the size of movements of each eye so that they can remain pointed at the object of regard.

The translational VOR (Fig. 1–5) depends on otolithic organs, the utricle and the saccule (see Fig. 2–1, bottom).[1] Otolithic-ocular reflexes become important if a subject views a near object, when they generate eye rotations to compensate for translation of the head, including the orbits, which house the eyes.[56] The translational VOR is essentially a binocular foveally driven reflex. Its function is to stabilize images upon the fovea of both eyes and so must tailor its response to the point of intersection of the lines of sight of each eye in three-dimensional space. Natural head movements have both rotational and translational components; the eye rotations to compensate for them may have horizontal and vertical components, and must be appropriate for the viewing distance of the visual scene.

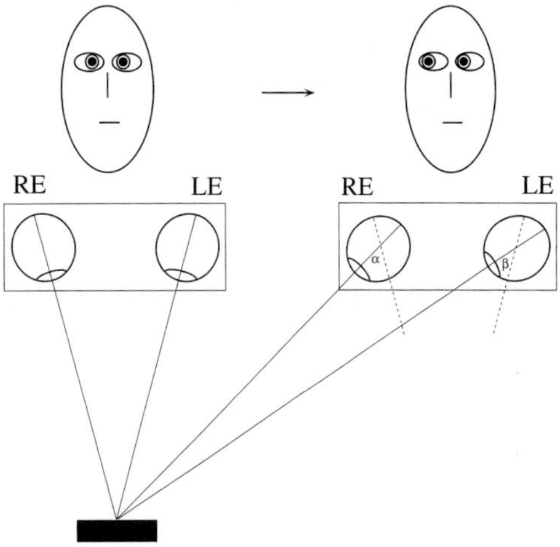

Figure 1–5. The translational VOR. Before the head movement (left panel), both the right eye (RE) and left eye (LE) fix on a stationary, near target, which requires convergence. As the subject's head translates to his left (arrow), a compensatory eye rotation movement to the right is generated. After the head movement (right panel), note that the right eye has rotated through a larger angle (α) than the left eye (β) because of the asymmetry of the geometric relationship between each eye and the target. Eye rotations are only necessary to compensate for head translations while viewing near targets.

Eye Movements in Response to Sustained Rotations: The Optokinetic System

Although the labyrinthine semicircular canals reliably signal transient head rotations, their Achilles' heel is a sustained (low frequency) rotation, which they signal progressively less accurately because of the mechanical properties of the semicircular canals. If a subject is rotated in darkness at a constant velocity, the slow phases of vestibular nystagmus, which are initially compensatory, decline in velocity and, after about 45 seconds, the eyes become stationary (Fig. 1–6). Sustained rotation may occur naturally as a component of a sustained chase, and the declining vestibular responses

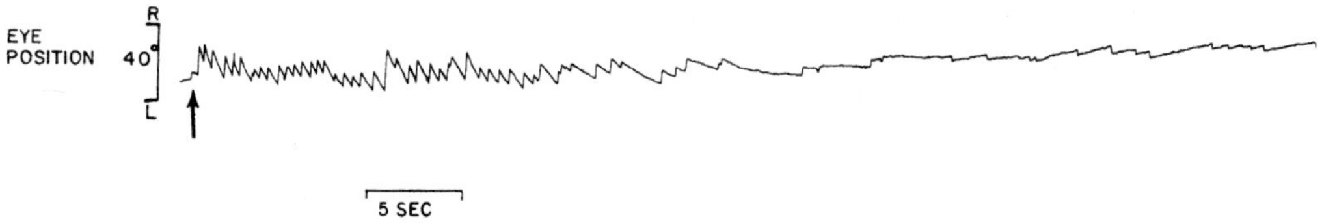

Figure 1–6. Record (D.C. electrooculography) of the vestibulo-ocular response to sustained rotation. Horizontal eye position is plotted against time. At the arrow, the subject starts to rotate clockwise, in darkness, at 50 degrees per second, and this velocity is maintained throughout the record. Initially there is a brisk nystagmus consisting of vestibular slow phases that hold gaze steady during the head rotation, and quick phases that not only reset the eyes to prevent them from lodging at the corners of the orbit but move them into the direction of head rotation. After about 30 seconds of rotation, the nystagmus (i.e., the vestibular response) dies away. Because of the mechanical limitations of the semicircular canals, the motion detectors cannot accurately inform the brain about sustained rotations. Eventually, nystagmus develops in the opposite direction (reversal phase); this represents the effect of short-term vestibular adaptation, a phenomenon discussed in Chapter 2. Upward deflections indicate rightward eye movements.

would, if acting alone, lead to degradation of vision and so threaten survival. Hence there is a need for alternative means of stabilizing retinal images to supplant the fading vestibular response. Visually mediated eye movements can serve this function, because sustained responses do not require a short latency of action. In afoveate animals, such as the rabbit, visually mediated eye movements can only be driven if the entire visual scene moves—the optokinetic response. However, in foveate, frontally eyed animals, both behavioral and neurophysiological evidence suggests that smooth-pursuit eye movements are mainly responsible for holding gaze on an object during self-motion.[56] The supplementation of the VOR by visually mediated eye movements is more than a summation of responses that are generated independently. For example, in the vestibular nuclei of the monkey, some neurons are driven by both visual (optokinetic) and vestibular stimuli (Fig. 2–5, Chapter 2), implying a "neural symbiosis."[68,87] As the labyrinthine signal declines, visual drives take over and maintain compensatory slow-phase eye movements during sustained rotation.

Visually mediated eye movements also supplement the translational VOR, when the visual scene is close to the subject.[8,88] In this case, smooth-pursuit eye movements are important, because they allow steady fixation of a small, near target, the position of which changes with respect to the background, as the subject translates. If we view distant objects, no eye movements are needed to compensate for head translations but, no matter what the viewing distance, eye movements are always needed to compensate for head rotations.

SACCADIC SYSTEM

Quick Phases

Most head movements are brief and require only small compensatory eye movements to maintain the stability of gaze. Any sustained head rotation would, however, cause the eyes to lodge at the corners of the orbit, in extreme contraversive deviation, where they no longer could make appropriate movements. This is not normally observed because of corrective quick phases (Fig. 1–6). These rapid eye movements, the evolutionary forerunners of voluntary saccades, have been likened to a resetting mechanism for the eye. In fact they do more than this because, during head rotation, quick phases move the eyes in the orbit in the same (anti-compensatory) direction as that of head rotation (Fig. 1–6) and so enable perusal of the oncoming visual scene.[55] Quick phases of nystagmus are rapid, with maximal velocities as high as 500 degrees per second, repositioning the eye in the shortest time possible.[30] The anatomic substrate of these rapid eye movements is in the paramedian reticular formation of the pons and mesencephalon (Fig. 6–3, Chapter 6), the same as that for saccades.[10] In disorders in which the quick-phase mechanism fails, the eyes hang up at the extremes of the orbit (see Video Display: Congenital Ocular Motor Apraxia).

Voluntary Saccades

Foveate animals have developed the ability to redirect the line of sight even in the absence of head movements: they have both quick phases and voluntary saccades. With the evolution of the fovea, it became important to be able to direct this specialized area of the retina at the object of interest during visual search. Saccades may be triggered in day-to-day life by objects actually seen or heard, or from memory, or as part of a natural strategy to scan the visual scene. There is usually a delay of about 200 ms from the stimulus for a saccade until its enactment, and this time presumably includes neural processing in the retina, cerebral cortex, superior colliculus, and cerebellum (see Voluntary Eye Movements, below). The final neural instruction for voluntary saccades arises from the same brainstem neurons in the paramedian reticular formation that generate the quick phases of nystagmus. Normal saccades are fast, brief, and accurate, so they do not interfere with vision. Disease may cause them to become slow, prolonged, or inaccurate, when they may cause visual disability (for example, see Video Display: Disorders of Saccades).

SMOOTH PURSUIT AND VISUAL FIXATION

Smooth Pursuit

With the evolution of a fovea has also come the need to track a moving object smoothly. This is possible to only a limited degree with saccadic movements, since once captured on the fovea by a saccade, the image of the moving target soon slides off again, with a consequent decline in visual acuity. The pursuit system, however, generates smooth tracking movements of the eyes that closely match the pace of the target. To overcome the delays inherent in the visual system (the latency of responses, which ranges between 80 ms – 120 ms), predictive mechanisms can adjust the eye movements when the motion of the target can be anticipated.[4] It seems possible that smooth-pursuit eye movements evolved in response to the need to sustain foveal fixation on a near target during self-motion (translation).[56] In this case, to compensate for movement of the head, the visual system would need to generate eye movements appropriate for the proximity of the near target, and relative motion between the near target and background.

Factors other than vision can be used to generate pursuit, because some normal subjects can follow their own fingers in darkness.[80] In fact, the brain relies on a number of sensory inputs, and its own motor efforts, to determine the motion of the target of interest. Smooth pursuit performance declines with age, and as a side effect of many drugs with effects on the nervous system, and thus, alone, impaired pursuit does not allow accurate localization of a disease process. Recent studies of visual processing in cerebral cortex, and the effects of discrete lesions, have clarified much about the neural substrate of smooth pursuit, and have suggested than some of the organization of the pursuit system has similarities with other voluntary eye movements, such as saccades.[43] Diseases that disrupt smooth pursuit do not usually cause visual disability, but they can provide valuable diagnostic information (see Video Display: Disorders of Smooth Pursuit).

Visual Fixation

Visual fixation of a stationary target may represent a special case of smooth pursuit—suppression of image motion caused by unwanted drifts of the eyes,[91] but it might also be due to an independent visual fixation system.[50] Such a mechanism would reflect the ability of the visual system to detect retinal image motion caused by unwanted drifts of the eyes and program corrective movements. Especially in the wake of a saccade, moving, large-field textured stimuli can induce ocular following at a latency of about 70 ms.[31] These ultra-short latency responses are driven by first-order visual stimuli, defined by the spatial distribution of luminance, and are not dependent on the attentive state of the subject.[17] Thus, short-latency ocular following is probably an important component of the fixation mechanism.

Another aspect of steady fixation is the ability to suppress saccadic eye movements that turn the fovea away from the object of interest. Thus, certain neurons in the frontal eye fields and superior colliculus seem important for suppressing saccades when steady fixation of a target (e.g., threading a needle) is necessary.[5,37,81] The concept of a fixation system becomes important in certain disease states. For example, following a peripheral vestibular lesion, the nystagmus is “suppressed” if visual fixation of a stationary object is possible. On the other hand, unwanted saccades may intrude on steady fixation, for example, as opsoclonus (see Video Display: Saccadic Oscillations and Intrusions).

Similarities and Differences between Fixation, Smooth-Pursuit, and Optokinetic Eye Movements

We have described three situations in which smooth, sustained eye movements may be made in response to motion of images across the retina. When such eye movements are in response to viewing the whole visual scene during sustained self-rotation, we have referred to them as optokinetic. When they oppose drifts of the eyes directed away from a stationary target, we have called them fixation. And when they are used to smoothly follow a moving object, or maintain fixation on a near, stationary target during self-motion, we have used the term smooth pursuit. In each of these cases, areas of cerebral cortex extract information about the direction and speed of retinal image slip from each eye, so that brainstem and cerebellar circuits can program an eye movement. The overlap and interaction between these types of eye movements are discussed in later chapters. Here, however, we have presented them as three different functional classes of eye movements because of their different purposes and properties, which lead to distinct methods of testing during clinical and laboratory examinations.

COMBINED MOVEMENTS OF THE EYES AND HEAD

The study of eye movements with the head held stationary is useful for investigative purposes but is artificial because, during natural behavior, humans usually move their eyes and head together. We have already indicated how vestibular responses compensate for the head perturbations due to locomotion. Such vestibular drives, however, may become an encumbrance when voluntary changes of the angle of gaze (eye position in space), using the eyes and head, are required. For example, if we are *smoothly* tracking a target moving to the right with a combined movement of the eyes and head, the eyes would continually be taken off target to the left if the VOR went unchecked. In fact, however, the eyes remain relatively stationary in the orbit as if the VOR were turned off. This implies an ability to override those vestibular drives invoked by voluntary head movements made to track a moving target. Current evidence suggests that two mechanisms contribute: (1) the VOR signal is canceled by an oppositely directed smooth-pursuit signal; (2) there is a parametric adjustment of the magnitude (gain) of the VOR response itself.[21] Thus, disorders that disrupt smooth pursuit often also interfere with smooth eye-head tracking (see Video Display: Disorders of Smooth Pursuit).

During *rapid* gaze changes, achieved with the eyes and head, saccadic and vestibular signals are appropriately combined so that gaze is accurately redirected toward the desired target; this may be achieved by either adding the two oppositely directed signals or by effectively "disconnecting" the VOR.[45] Which process takes place may depend partly upon the size of the gaze change.[84] Especially for larger movements that exceed the ocular motor range, disconnecting the VOR may be the major strategy.[54,83] Patients who have difficulty generating saccades with their eyes alone often make a combined eye-head movement to generate a gaze-shift (see Video Display: Acquired Ocular Motor Apraxia).

VERGENCE EYE MOVEMENTS

With the development of frontal vision it became possible to direct the fovea of both eyes at one object of interest. This requires disjunctive or vergence movements that, in contrast to conjugate or visional movements, move the eyes in opposite directions. Two principal types of stimulus drive vergence eye movements: image disparity and image blur. *Disparity or fusional vergence* movements occur in response to disparity between the locations of images of a single target on the retina of each eye. This type of vergence eye movement may be elicited at the bedside by placing a wedge prism before one eye. *Accommodative vergence* is stimulated by loss of focus of images (blur) on the retina and occurs in association with accommodation of the lens and pupillary constriction, as part of the near triad. Accommodative effort alone can produce vergence movements. Thus, if one eye is covered and the other eye suddenly changes fixation from a distant to a near target, then the eye under cover responds by converging. A similar effect may be induced by placing a negative diopter (minus) lens in front of the viewing eye. Other stimuli are also important inputs for vergence, including the sense of nearness of the object of interest and a sense of motion of the target away from or towards oneself ("looming").

When vergence eye movements are performed alone, they are characteristically slow. During natural visual search, however, vergence movements are invariably accompanied by saccades, because the position of most objects in our environment differs in both direction (horizontal and vertical) and in distance (depth). When vergence movements are accompanied by near-synchronous saccades, they are speeded up, whereas the saccadic component is slowed down.[92] Since vertical saccades can speed up horizontal vergence, it seems most likely that these interactions between saccades and vergence occur centrally. Abnormalities of the vergence are responsible for many symptomatic ocular motor disorders, ranging from childhood strabismus to psychological spasm of convergence, to specific defects of vergence eye movements following brainstem strokes (see Video Display: Disorders of Vergence).[65]

THREE-DIMENSIONAL ASPECTS OF EYE MOVEMENTS

The eyes can rotate about any combination of three axes, which conventionally are described as X (parasagittal), Y (transverse), and Z (vertical) and intersect at the center of the globe (Fig. 9–3, Chapter 3). The orientation of the eye (i.e., the amount of torsion), at a given eye position, however, is governed by Listing's law, which confines the axes of eye rotation that describe eye position to a single plane—Listing's plane, which approximates the frontal plane (Fig. 9–3). The term "primary position" is now defined with reference to Listing's law. It is the unique position at which the line of sight is perpendicular to Listing's plane and the position from which purely horizontal or purely vertical rotations of the eye to a new position are unassociated with any torsion. Primary position is usually close to but not necessarily exactly straight ahead. In this book, we use the term "central position" simply to denote that the eye is pointing straight ahead (visual axis is parallel to the midsagittal plane of the head). Measurements, using reliable methodology to measure 3-D rotations,[26] have confirmed that Listing's law is approximately obeyed for saccades and pursuit, but less so for vestibular movements in response to head rotations [58] On the other hand, the eye movement responses to head translations do obey Listing's law, which probably reflects their close relationship to other foveally driven reflexes such as saccades and smooth pursuit.[88] These properties of eye rotations have been used to identify the pathogenesis of abnormal eye movements. For example, a form of nystagmus that obeys Listing's law would be more likely to arise from an abnormality within the pursuit system or translational VOR than from within the rotational VOR. In Chapter 9, we discuss further aspects of 3-D eye rotations, Listing's law and Donder's law, and the possible role of the extraocular muscle pulleys in enforcing it.

ADAPTIVE CONTROL OF EYE MOVEMENTS

To achieve clear, stable, single vision, the control of eye movements must be accurate. One of the most impressive aspects of ocular motor control is the way in which the brain constantly monitors its performance and, in the face of disease and aging, adjusts its strategies accordingly. For example, the performance of the VOR can be appropriately modified to new visual circumstances (e.g., a change in spectacle lens correction).[12,62] Furthermore, inaccurate saccades and deficient smooth pursuit caused, for example, by abducens nerve palsy can be corrected (see Video Display: Disorders of Smooth Pursuit).[60] Even the yoking of conjugate eye movements is under some degree of adaptive control.[3] The cerebellum plays a central role in recalibrating ocular motor reflexes for optimal visual performance,[66] using cues from cerebral cortical areas that process visual motion.[14] Within the cerebellum are a variety of neurons that influence eye movements. The vestibulocerebellum (flocculus, paraflocculus, and nodulus) is particularly important in the control of smooth pursuit, in vestibular eye movements, and in holding positions of gaze.[6] The dorsal vermis (lobules V–VII) and underlying fastigial nucleus enable both saccades and pursuit to be accurate.[71] Thus, disease affecting the cerebellum may not only disrupt the control of eye movements, but also impair the individual's ability to correct them.

The adaptive repertoire consists of many levels of response to disease, from relatively low-level adjustments in innervation, to higher-level strategies that may depend upon the context in which they are elicited, such as reward in animal experiments.[24,42] So patients may develop different adaptive states that, based upon the context in which they must be elicited, allow for different innervational commands for the same type of eye movement.[75]

VOLUNTARY CONTROL OF EYE MOVEMENTS

The control of eye movements ranges from the most reflexive responses (e.g., a quick-phase of vestibular nystagmus) to eye movements that are willed without a sensory stimulus (e.g., a saccade made to a remembered or imagined location). Voluntary control of gaze depends upon a number of areas in cerebral cortex; their separate contributions have been elucidated by electrophysiological and lesion studies in monkeys. Homologous areas have been suggested in humans, based upon studies of either the behavioral effects of discrete lesions or functional imaging (see Fig. 6–8).

As a generalization, the anterior areas of cerebral cortex contribute more to the generation of voluntary, internally generated behaviors whereas posterior cortical areas play a more important role in more externally triggered reflexive behaviors. There is evidence that each cortical eye field may coordinate the components of more complex responses, for example, combined vergence-pursuit movements to targets moving smoothly in depth and direction.[28] From these cortical areas, parallel projections descend via the basal ganglion and superior colliculus to the brainstem and cerebellar circuits that fashion premotor eye movement commands.[36] Certain neurons in these pathways may encode mismatches between eye and target positions, which can be used to program more than one type of eye movement.[44] There is some redundancy of these pathways, so that lesions affecting one cortical area tend not to produce a permanent defect of voluntary gaze. Thus, independent lesions of either the frontal or parietal eye fields in monkeys produce subtle, chronic defects of saccadic eye movement control. However, combined lesions of these structures cause more severe and enduring limitation of ocular motility (see Video Display: Acquired Ocular Motor Apraxia).[51]

An important issue in the control of voluntary eye movements is the way that the brain transforms sensory signals into motor commands. Thus, visual stimuli are encoded in a place code, such as the topographic map of the visual fields in primary visual cortex. On the other hand, the ocular motoneurons encode the properties of an eye movement in their temporal discharge characteristics (Fig. 1–3). Thus, a spatial-temporal transformation of neural signals is required if, for example, a saccade is to be made in response to a visual target. The site and mechanism by which this transformation is achieved are subjects of present research, but cortical areas, the superior colliculus, cerebellum, and brainstem reticular formation may all contribute.

A recent trend has been to use eye movements to probe the highest cognitive functions such as conflict resolution and free will. By applying ingenious stimulus paradigms that provide visual stimuli with instructions that vary from trial to trial (such as a countermand after the stimulus is presented),[73] or by changing subsequent stimuli based upon eye movement responses, it has been possible to identify functional activation in parts of human pre-supplementary motor area (pre-SMA) and supplementary eye fields corresponding to volition, conflict, and registration of success or failure (Fig. 1–7).[59]

EYE MOVEMENTS AND SPATIAL LOCALIZATION

Since the eyes, head, and body can all move with respect to each other, the retinal location of an image cannot specify the position of the object in space. For this, information is required concerning the direction of gaze (eye

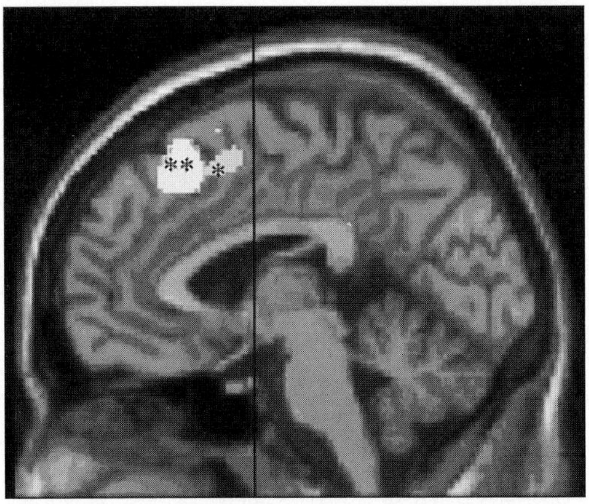

Figure 1–7. Pre-supplementary motor area (pre-SMA) activation associated with changing volitional plans (two asterisks or yellow) and free choice (one asterisk or cyan) in an ocular motor task. The black line corresponds to the position of the anterior commissure (VCA line). (Reprinted from Nachev P, Rees G, Parton A, Kennard C, Husain M. Volition and conflict in human medial frontal cortex. Curr Biol 15, 122–128, with permission from Elsevier.)

in space), and this in turn must be computed from information about the position of the eye in the orbit, and the direction in which the head and body point. Neurophysiological studies of the parietal lobe have demonstrated populations of neurons with visual responses that are influenced by the direction of gaze, and take into account the direction in which the head points.[90] Such neuronal behavior is a prerequisite for encoding the location of objects in head- and body-centered frames of reference.

How the brain determines the position of the eyes in the head is not settled. The most widely accepted mechanism is that the brain internally monitors its own motor commands (efference copy or corollary discharge),[79,86] and inactivation of pathways from brainstem to cerebral cortex interfere with this mechanism and cause eye movements to become inaccurate.[78] Another possibility is proprioceptive information from the extraocular muscles. Although there appears to be no stretch reflex in the extraocular muscles, proprioceptors do exist in extraocular muscle,[11] and they project to the brainstem via the ophthalmic division of the trigeminal nerve.[61] However, if the trigeminal nerve is cut, eye movement control is not acutely affected, and adaptation to novel visual demands is still possible.[34,48] Other studies suggest that extraocular proprioception may contribute to recovery from extraocular ocular muscle palsy,[47] and could account for suppressive effects of eye muscle surgery on infantile forms of nystagmus.[35] Finally, there is evidence that the brain may also estimate the direction of gaze based upon visual cues. Thus, when normal subjects make saccades to the remembered locations of targets, their eye movements are influenced by the position on a moving visual background at which a target light was previously flashed.[93] Clearly, the brain tries to use every source of information available—efference copy, proprioception, and visual inputs—to determine what might be the correct relation of the eyes and the body to the outside world when these inputs become incongruent as in disease, and symptoms arise.

THE SCIENTIFIC METHOD APPLIED TO THE STUDY OF EYE MOVEMENTS

Our understanding of the way that the brain controls eye movements has advanced conceptually because of the scientific method of formulating and testing hypotheses, an approach championed in this field by D. A. Robinson. Robinson's lecture notes "Linear Control Systems in the Oculomotor System" can be found on the compact disk that accompanies this book. A wealth of information concerning the neural mechanisms for control of eye movements has been provided by electrophysiological and lesion studies in trained monkeys; this information can be readily applied to understanding the effects of human disease by developing testable hypotheses. Conversely, the careful study of patients with disorders of eye movements, with these hypotheses in mind, has led to a better understanding of how the normal brain functions. In this regard, the study of eye movements offers a further advantage because it is relatively easy to construct hypotheses that are quantitative (mathematical models). A most useful approach has been the application of control systems analysis to understanding the effects of feedback and oscillations. A more recent trend has been the application of neural networks to account for the behavior of populations of neurons, with the goal of making more realistic "neuromimetic" representations of how the brain works. Such an approach, for example, has been applied to understand better saccadic oscillations such as opsoclonus.[63]

Not all clinicians will want to attempt quantitative mathematical descriptions of disturbed forms of eye movement, but an understanding of certain simple principles of control systems analysis may help in the bedside interpretation of clinical signs. For example, a mismatch of the pulse and step is the cause of the adduction lag encountered in internuclear ophthalmoplegia (see Video Display: Pontine Syndromes). Furthermore, qualitative tests of hypotheses concerning the control of eye movements are often possible using careful clinical observations. Throughout the remaining chapters, we will refer to certain relatively basic principles of control systems analysis that have direct clinical implications.

Finally, the study of eye movements has afforded clinicians a chance to make important contributions to basic neuroscience using bedside observations of eye movement abnormalities in patients from their own clinical practices. Even without fancy instruments or precise quantification, eye movements are so accessible to observation that much is still to be learned at the bedside.

SUMMARY

1. Normal eye movements are a prerequisite for clear, stable, single vision. For best vision of objects such as the words of a book, the images must be brought to the fovea of the retina and held there with image drift less than about 5 degrees per second.
2. Eye movements can be best understood by considering their functions. Of the conjugate types of eye movements, vestibular, optokinetic, and visual fixation systems act to hold images of the seen world steady on the retina; their function is to hold gaze steady. Saccades, smooth pursuit, and vergence eye movements, working together, acquire and hold images of objects of interest on the fovea; their function is to shift gaze. Vergence movements have both gaze-holding and gaze-shifting properties.
3. To move the eyes conjugately (for example, as a saccade) requires a phasic-tonic or pulse-step of innervation (Fig. 1–3). The pulse moves the eyes rapidly against viscous forces and the step holds the eyes steady against elastic restoring forces. The pulse is a velocity command; the step is a position command. All eye movement commands have velocity and position components. Position components are created from velocity components by a process of mathematical integration, performed by the nervous system. Fibrous pulleys guide the pulling directions of the extraocular muscles.
4. Vestibular and visually mediated eye movements work together to maintain clear vision during head movements—both rotations (Fig. 1–4) and translations (Fig. 1–5). The vestibulo-ocular reflex promptly produces eye movements to compensate for the brief head perturbations that occur during most natural activities. During sustained head rotations and translations, visually mediated eye movements supplement the vestibular response. If one fixes upon a near object there must also be an adjustment for the translational components of head motion.
5. With the evolution of the fovea and frontal vision, saccadic, smooth pursuit, fixation, and vergence systems became necessary. These gaze-shifting movements are under voluntary control so that it is possible to choose which part of the visual scene one wants to scrutinize using the fovea.
6. The performance of the ocular motor system is undergoing constant recalibration and readjustment to assure optimal visual capabilities. The cerebellum plays an important role in this adaptive control of eye movements.
7. An understanding of the properties of each functional class of eye movements (Table 1–1) will guide the physical examination. Knowledge of the neural substrate of each class of eye movements will aid topological diagnosis. Knowledge of current hypotheses of the control of eye movements aid the interpretation of disorders of ocular motility and may advance understanding of how the brain controls movements of the eyes in normal human beings.

REFERENCES

1. Angelaki DE. Eyes on target: what neurons must do for the vestibuloocular reflex during linear motion. J Neurophysiol 92, 20–35, 2004.
2. Arnold DB, Robinson DA. The oculomotor integrator: testing of a neural network model. Exp Brain Res 113, 57–74, 1997.
3. Averbuch-Heller L, Lewis RF, Zee DS. Disconjugate adaptation of saccades: contribution of binocular and monocular mechanisms. Vision Res 39, 341–352, 1999.
4. Barnes GR, Schmid AM, Jarrett CB. The role of expectancy and volition in smooth pursuit eye movements. Prog Brain Res 140, 239–254, 2002.
5. Basso MA, Krauzlis RJ, Wurtz RH. Activation and inactivation of rostral superior colliculus neurons during smooth-pursuit eye movements in monkeys. J Neurophysiol 84, 892–908, 2000.
6. Belton T, Mccrea RA. Role of the cerebellar flocculus region in the coordination of eye and head movements during gaze pursuit. J Neurophysiol 84, 1614–1626, 2000.
7. Burr DC, Ross J. Contrast sensitivity at high velocities. Vision Res 22, 479–484, 1982.
8. Busettini C, Miles FA, Schwarz U. Ocular responses to translation and their dependence on viewing distance. II. Motion of the scene. J Neurophysiol 66, 865–878, 1991.
9. Büttner U, Büttner-Ennever JA. Present concepts of oculomotor organization. In Büttner-Ennever JA (ed). Neuroanatomy of the Oculomotor System. Prog Brain Res 151, 1–42, 2006.
10. Büttner-Ennever JA, Büttner U. The reticular formation. In Büttner-Enever JA (ed). Neuroanatomy of the Oculomotor System. Elsevier, New York, 1988, pp 119–176.
11. Büttner-Ennever JA, Horn A, Graf W, Ugolini G. Modern concepts of brainstem anatomy: from extraocular motoneurons to proprioceptive pathways. Ann N Y Acad Sci 956, 75–84, 2005.
12. Cannon SC, Leigh RJ, Zee DS, Abel LA. The effect of the rotational magnification of corrective spectacles on the quantitative evaluation of the VOR. Acta Otolaryngol (Stockh) 100, 81–88, 1985.
13. Cannon SC, Robinson DA. Loss of the neural integrator of the oculomotor system from brain stem lesions in monkey. J Neurophysiol 57, 1383–1409, 1987.
14. Carey MR, Medina JF, Lisberger SG. Instructive signals for motor learning from visual cortical area MT. Nat Neurosci 6, 813–819, 2005.
15. Carpenter RHS. Vision and visual function. In Cronly-Dillon JR (ed). Eye Movements. Vol. 8. MacMillan Press, London,1991, pp 1–10.
16. Carpenter RHS. Movements of the Eyes. Pion, London, 1988.
17. Chen KJ, Sheliga BM, FitzGibbon EJ, Miles FA. Initial ocular following in humans depends critically on the Fourier components of the motion stimulus. Ann N Y Acad Sci 1039, 260–271, 2005.
18. Cohen B. Vestibular system. In Kornhuber HH (ed). Handbook of Sensory Physiology, Vol. VI/1. Springer, New York,1974, pp 477–540.
19. Collins CC. In Lennerstrand G, Bach-y-Rita P (eds). Basic Mechanisms of Ocular Motility and their Clinical Implications. Pergamon, Oxford,1977, pp 145–180.
20. Crane BT, Demer JL. Human gaze stabilization during natural activities: translation, rotation, magnification, and target distance effects. J Neurophysiol 78, 2129–2144, 1997.
21. Cullen KE, Roy JE. Signal processing in the vestibular system during active versus passive head movements. J Neurophysiol 91, 1919–1933, 2004.
22. Demer JL. Pivotal role of orbital connective tissues in binocular alignment and strabismus. Invest Ophthalmol Vis Sci 45, 729–738, 2004.
23. Demer JL, Miller J, Poukens V, Vinters HV, Glasgow BJ. Evidence for fibromuscular pulleys of the recti extraocular muscles. Invest Ophthalmol Vis Sci 36, 1125, 1995.
24. Deubel H. Separate adaptive mechanisms for the control of reactive and volitional saccadic eye movements. Vision Res 35, 3529–3540, 1995.
25. Dodge R. Five types of eye movement in the horizontal meridian plane of the field of regard. Am J Physiol 8, 307–329, 1903.
26. Ferman L, Collewijn H, Jansen TC, Van Den Berg A. Human gaze stability in the horizontal, vertical and torsional direction during voluntary head movements, evaluated with a three dimensional scleral induction coil technique. Vision Res 27, 811–828, 1987.
27. Fuchs AF, Luschei ES. Firing patterns of abducens neurons of alert monkeys in relationship to horizontal eye movement. J Neurophysiol 33, 382–392, 1970.
28. Fukushima K, Yamanobe T, Shinmei Y, Fukushima J, Kurkin S. Role of the frontal eye fields in smooth-gaze tracking. Prog Brain Res 143, 391–401, 2004.
29. Gamlin PDR, Clarke RJ. Single-unit activity in the primate nucleus reticularis tegmenti pontis related to vergence and ocular accommodation. J Neurophysiol 73, 2115–2119, 1995.
30. Garbutt S, Han Y, Kumar AN, et al. Vertical optokinetic nystagmus and saccades in normal human subjects. Invest Ophthalmol Vis Sci 44, 3833–3841, 2003.
31. Gellman RS, Carl JR, Miles FA. Short latency ocular-following responses in man. Visual Neuroscience 5, 107–122, 1990.
32. Ghasia FF, Angelaki DE. Do motoneurons encode the noncommutativity of ocular rotations? Neuron 47, 1–13, 2005.
33. Grossman GE, Leigh RJ, Abel LA, Lanska DJ, Thurston SE. Frequency and velocity of rotational head perturbations during locomotion. Exp Brain Res 70, 470–476, 1988.
34. Guthrie BL, Porter JD, Sparks DL. Corollary discharge provides accurate eye position information to the oculomotor system. Science 221, 1193–1195, 1983.
35. Hertle RW, Dell'Osso LF, FitzGibbon EJ, et al. Horizontal rectus tenotomy in patients with congenital nystagmus. Ophthalmology 110, 2097–2105, 2003.
36. Hikosaka O, Takikawa Y, Kawagoe R. Role of the basal ganglia in the control of purposive saccadic eye movements. Physiol Rev 80, 953–978, 2000.
37. Izawa Y, Suzuki H, Shinoda Y. Initiation and suppression of saccades by the frontal eye field in the monkey. Ann N Y Acad Sci 1039, 220–231, 2005.
38. JC. Living without a balancing mechanism. N Engl J Med 246, 458–460, 1952.
39. Jacobs RJ. Visual resolution and contour interaction in the fovea and periphery. Vision Res 19, 1187–1195, 1979.
40. Kaminski HJ, Leigh RJ (eds). Neurobiology of eye

movements. From molecules to behavior. Ann N Y Acad Sci 956, 1–619, 2002.
41. Keller EL, Robinson DA. Absence of a stretch reflex in extraocular muscles of the monkey. J Neurophysiol 34, 908–919, 1971.
42. Kobayashi S, Lauwereyns J, Koizumi M, Sakagami M, Hikosaka O. Influence of reward expectation on visuospatial processing in macaque lateral prefrontal cortex. J Neurophysiol 87, 1488–1498, 2002.
43. Krauzlis RJ. Recasting the smooth pursuit eye movement system. J Neurophysiol 91, 591–603, 2004.
44. Krauzlis RJ, Basso MA, Wurtz RH. Shared motor error for multiple eye movements. Science 276, 1693–1695, 1997.
45. Laurutis VP, Robinson DA. The vestibulo-ocular reflex during human saccadic eye movements. J Physiol (Lond) 373, 209–233, 1986.
46. Leigh RJ, Kennard C. Using saccades as a research tool in the clinical neurosciences. Brain 127, 460–477, 2004.
47. Lewis RF, Zee DS, Gaymard B, Guthrie B. Extraocular muscle proprioception functions in the control of ocular alignment and eye movement conjugacy. J Neurophysiol 71, 1028–1031, 1994.
48. Lewis RF, Zee DS, Hayman MR, Tamargo RJ. Oculomotor function in the rhesus monkey after deafferentation of the extraocular muscles. Exp Brain Res 141, 349–358, 2001.
49. Lossos A, Baala L, Soffer D, Averbuch-Heller L, et al. A novel autosomal recessive myopathy with external ophthalmoplegia linked to chromosome 17p13.1-p12. Brain 128, 42–51, 2005.
50. Luebke AE, Robinson DA. Transition dynamics between pursuit and fixation suggest different systems. Vision Res 28, 941–946, 1988.
51. Lynch JC. Saccade initiation and latency deficits after combined lesions of the frontal and posterior eye fields in monkeys. J Neurophysiol 68, 1913–1916, 1992.
52. Maas EF, Huebner WP, Seidman SH, Leigh RJ. Behavior of human horizontal vestibulo-ocular reflex in response to high-acceleration stimuli. Brain Res 499, 153–156, 1989.
53. Martinez-Conde S, Macknik SL, Hubel DH. Microsaccadic eye movements and firing of single cells in the striate cortex of macaque monkeys. Nat Neurosci 3, 251–258, 2000.
54. Mccrea RA, Gdowski GT. Firing behaviour of squirrel monkey eye movement-related vestibular nucleus neurons during gaze saccades. J Physiol 546, 207–224, 2003.
55. Melvill Jones G. Predominance of anticompensatory oculomotor response during rapid head rotation. Aerospace Med 35, 965–968, 1964.
56. Miles FA. The neural processing of 3-D visual information: evidence from eye movements. Eur J Neurosci, 10, 811–822, 1998.
57. Miles FA, Fuller JH. Visual tracking and the primate flocculus. Science 189, 1000–1002, 1975.
58. Misslisch H, Tweed D, Fetter M, Sievering D, Koenig E. Rotational kinematics of the human vestibuloocular reflex. III. Listing's law. J Neurophysiol 72, 2490–2502, 1994.
59. Nachev P, Rees G, Parton A, Kennard C, Husain M. Volition and conflict in human medial frontal cortex. Curr Biol 15, 122–128, 2005.
60. Optican LM, Zee DS, Chu FC. Adaptive response to ocular muscle weakness in human pursuit and saccadic eye movements. J Neurophysiol 54, 110–122, 1985.
61. Porter JD. Brainstem terminations of extraocular muscle primary afferent neurons in the monkey. J Comp Neurol 247, 133–143, 1986.
62. Ramachandran R, Lisberger SG. Normal performance and expression of learning in the vestibulo-ocular reflex (VOR) at high frequencies. J Neurophysiol 93, 2028–2038, 2005.
63. Ramat S, Leigh RJ, Zee DS, Optican LM. Ocular oscillations generated by coupling of brainstem excitatory and inhibitory saccadic burst neurons. Exp Brain Res 160, 89–106, 2005.
64. Ramat S, Straumann D, Zee DS. The interaural translational VOR: suppression, enhancement and cognitive control. J Neurophysiol 94, 2391–2402, 2005.
65. Rambold H, Sander T, Neumann G, Helmchen C. Palsy of "fast" and "slow" vergence by pontine lesions. Neurology 64, 338–340, 2005.
66. Raymond JL, Lisberger SG, Mauk MD. The cerebellum: a neuronal learning machine? Science 272, 1126–1131, 1996.
67. Robinson DA. Oculomotor unit behavior in the monkey. J Neurophysiol 33, 393–404, 1970.
68. Robinson DA. Linear addition of optokinetic and vestibular signals in the vestibular nucleus. Exp Brain Res 30, 447–450, 1977.
69. Robinson DA. The purpose of eye movements. Invest Ophthalmol Vis Sci 17, 835–837, 1978.
70. Robinson DA, Keller EL. The behavior of eye movement motoneurons in the alert monkey. Bibl Ophthalmol 82, 7–16, 1972.
71. Robinson FR, Fuchs AF. The role of the cerebellum in voluntary eye movements. Annu Rev Neurosci 24, 981–1004, 2001.
72. Rucker JC, Shapiro BE, Han YH, et al. Neuro-ophthalmology of late-onset Tay-Sachs disease (LOTS). Neurology 63, 1918–1926, 2004.
73. Schall JD. The neural selection and control of saccades by the frontal eye field. Philos Trans. R Soc Lond B Biol Sci 357, 1073–1082, 2002.
74. Schiller PH. The discharge characteristics of single units in the oculomotor and abducens nuclei of the unanesthetized monkey. Exp Brain Res 10, 347–362, 1970.
75. Shelhamer M, Zee DS. Context-specific adaptation and its significance for neurovestibular problems of space flight. J Vestib Res 13, 345–362, 2003.
76. Simpson JI, Graf W. In Berthoz A, Melvill Jones G (eds). Adaptive Mechanisms in Gaze Control. Elsevier, Amsterdam,1985, pp 3–16.
77. Skavenski AA, Robinson DA. Role of abducens neurons in the vestibuloocular reflex. J Neurophysiol 36, 724–738, 1973.
78. Sommer MA, Wurtz RH. A pathway in primate brain for internal monitoring of movements. Science 296, 1480–1482, 2002.
79. Sperry RW. Neural basis of the spontaneous optokinetic response produced by visual inversion. J Comp Physiol Psychol 43, 482–489, 1950.
80. Steinbach MJ. Eye tracking of self-moved targets: the role of efference. J Exp Psychol 82, 366–376, 1969.

81. Steinman RM, Haddad GM, Skavenski AA. Miniature eye movement. Science 181, 810–819, 1973.
82. Swartz BE, Li S, Bespalova I, et al. Pathogenesis of clinical signs in recessive ataxia with saccadic intrusions. Ann Neurol 54, 824–828, 2003.
83. Tabak S, Smeets JBJ, Collewijn H. Modulation of the human vestibuloocular reflex during saccades: probing by high-frequency oscillation and torque pulses of the head. J Neurophysiol 76, 3249–3263, 1996.
84. Tomlinson RD. Combined eye-head gaze shifts in the primate. III. Contributions to the accuracy of gaze saccades. J Neurophysiol 56, 1558–1570, 1990.
85. Van Gisbergen JAM, Robinson DA, Gielen S. A quantitative analysis of the generation of saccadic eye movements by burst neurons. J Neurophysiol 45, 417–442, 1981.
86. Von Holst E, Mittelstaedt H. Das Reafferenzprinzip. Wechselwirkung zwischen Zentralnervensystem und Peripherie. Naturwissenschaften 37, 464–476, 1950.
86a. Wade NJ, Tatler BW. The Moving Tablet of the Eye. Oxford University Press, Oxford, 2005.
87. Waespe W, Henn V. Neuronal activity in the vestibular nuclei of the alert monkey during vestibular and optokinetic stimulation. Exp Brain Res 27, 523–538, 1977.
88. Walker MF, Shelhamer M, Zee DS. Eye-position dependence of torsional velocity during interaural translation, horizontal pursuit, and yaw-axis rotation in humans. Vision Res 44, 613–620, 2004.
89. Walls G. The evolutionary history of eye movements. Vision Res 2, 69-80, 1962.
90. Xing J, Andersen RA. Models of the posterior parietal cortex which perform multimodal integration and represent space in several coordinate frames. J Cogn Neurosci 12, 601–614, 2000.
91. Yarbus AL. Eye Movements and Vision. Plenum, New York, 1967.
92. Zee DS, FitzGibbon EJ, Optican LM. Saccade-vergence interactions in humans. J Neurophysiol 68, 1624–1641, 1992.
93. Zivotofsky AZ, Rottach KJ, Averbuch-Heller L, et al. Saccades to remembered targets: the effects of smooth pursuit and illusory stimulus-motion. J Neurophysiol 76, 3617–3632, 1996.

Chapter 2

The Vestibular-Optokinetic System

This chapter deals with the ocular motor subsystems that hold images steady upon the retina during motion of the head. This ocular gyroscopic function guarantees clear and stable vision during natural activities that induce head perturbations, such as locomotion (Fig. 7–1). To hold gaze steady, the brain primarily uses labyrinthine and visual cues, though in disease, information from muscle spindles and joint receptors may also substitute for deficient vestibular signals.

Historically, quantitative descriptions of vestibular and optokinetic behavior long preceded any knowledge of the substrate for these reflexes. The labyrinth itself received its name from Galen in the second century AD when he first peered into the inner ear and noted the similarity to the Cretin 'labyrinthos'.[388] In 1796, Erasmus Darwin described how body rotation induced movement of the eyes [183] and, in 1819, Purkinje reported how optokinetic nystagmus and sensations of movement were produced while watching a cavalry parade.[359] The mechanisms for these phenomena were unknown and the prevailing notion was that sensations of movement emanated from cutaneous receptors that detected displacement of the body fluids. The important role of the vestibular organ in initiating eye movements that compensate for head movements was first demonstrated by Flourens [289] and later elaborated upon by Ewald.[271] These pioneers noted that opening or applying pressure to the lumen of the semicircular canals of animals produced movements of the head or eyes in the plane of the canal being stimulated. Ewald also first emphasized that there must be resting tone in the vestibular nuclei even when the head was still. This discovery of the significance of the vestibular organ led to systematic clinical study of vestibular function. Bárány[68] formalized aspects of rotational testing and introduced positional and caloric stimulation of the vestibular labyrinth. Mach[394] and Ter Braak[795] predicted, based upon human and animal studies, that vestibular and visual information must interact centrally, a notion that was confirmed by modern neurophysiologic research. Steinhausen[772] developed the mathematical equations to describe how the cupula is able to transduce head motion. In more recent years, pioneers in vestibular physiology including among others, Geoffrey Melvill Jones and Victor Wilson,[551,552,879] Jay Goldberg and César Fernández,[12] and Bernard Cohen,[185,186,189] have made vestibular research a major focus of both basic and clinical neuroscience.

In this chapter, we will (1) identify the functional demands made of the vestibular-optokinetic system during natural activities; (2) discuss its inner workings; (3) summarize the quantitative performance of this system in response to natural and laboratory stimuli; (4) describe testing of patients with vestibular disease; and (5) apply these principles to understand the pathophysiology of vestibular disorders. A glossary of commonly used terms and abbreviations appears in Table 2–1. Throughout the chapter, we refer to Video Displays on the accompanying DVD, which illustrate tests of the vestibular system and important physical findings.

Table 2–1. **The Vestibulo-Optokinetic System: A Glossary of Terms and Abbreviations**

Circularvection	Illusion of self-rotation induced during optokinetic stimulation
Eccentric rotation	Rotation around an earth-vertical axis with the head located away from the usual head-centered axis of rotation
Gain	Ratio of output (e.g., eye velocity) to input (e.g., head velocity)
Ocular counterrolling	Torsional rotations of the eyes induced by rolling the head, ear to shoulder. During rotation the response is generated by the rotational vestibulo-ocular reflex (r-VOR). When the head is kept in the tilted position, the torsional response is driven by a static otolith-ocular reflex
OKN	Optokinetic nystagmus
OKAN	Optokinetic after-nystagmus (usually measured in darkness), which follows a period of optokinetic stimulation

(Continued on following page)

Table 2–1. *(continued)*

Oscillopsia	Illusory, to-and-fro movements of the environment
OVAR	Off-vertical axis rotation. Rotation about an axis tilted away from earth-vertical
Phase	Measure of the temporal synchrony between input (e.g., head velocity) and output (e.g., eye velocity)
Time constant	Time taken for slow-phase eye velocity to decline to 37% of its initial value after the onset of a velocity-step stimulus
Velocity step stimulus	Sudden acceleration ("impulse") to a constant velocity rotation
Velocity storage	Central vestibular mechanism whereby the peripheral labyrinthine response is prolonged or perseverated. Optokinetic after-nystagmus (OKAN) is also generated by this mechanism
Vertigo	Illusion of movement (usually turning) of self or environment
VOR	Vestibulo-ocular reflex
r-VOR	Rotational VOR, compensatory slow phase driven by the semicircular canals in response to angular motion of the head
t-VOR	Translational VOR, compensatory slow phase driven by the otolith organs in response to linear motion of the head

FUNCTION OF THE VESTIBULAR-OPTOKINETIC SYSTEM

Head Rotations and Translations

The vestibular system must respond to both the angular (rotational) and linear (translational) components of head motion. To be more precise, rotations of the eyes must compensate for movements of the orbits. Angular and linear motions of the head are sensed by different structures. The semicircular canals respond to angular acceleration and the otolith organs respond to linear acceleration. Together, they provide the inputs for the vestibulo-ocular reflex or VOR. The response to the *rotational* (angular) component of head motion is called the r-VOR, and the response to the *translational* (linear) component of head motion is called the t-VOR. A third type of VOR—ocular counterroll—also is mediated by the otolith organs and reflects a response to linear acceleration, but, in this case, the stimulus is a change in the static orientation of the head with respect to the pull of gravity. There is a small change in static torsion (counterrolling) of the eyes in the opposite direction to a sustained head tilt.

The r-VOR responds to the three possible directions of head rotation, producing horizontal (around the rostral-caudal, yaw, or z-axis), vertical (around the interaural, pitch, or y-axis), and torsional (around the naso-occipital, roll, or x-axis) eye movements. The t-VOR responds to the three possible directions of head translation, producing horizontal (heave or side to side, along the interaural axis), vertical (bob or up and down, along the dorso-ventral axis), and vergence (surge or fore and aft, along the naso-occipital axis) eye movements, though the exact pattern of eye movements also depends upon where they are in the orbit.[347] Since the eyes are horizontally separated and the axis of rotation of the head is usually behind the eyes, rotational head movements almost invariably produce translations, or linear displacements, of the orbits. Even if the axis of rotation is centered on one orbit, the other eye will still be translated during rotation of the head with the only exception being pitch rotation around an axis passing though the center of both orbits. The ocular compensation required for translation of the orbits—during both rotations and translations of the head—is, of necessity, a function of the location of the point of regard. For rotations in yaw and pitch, the closer the object of interest, the larger must be the compensatory response to prevent unwanted motion of images on the retina. Furthermore, depending upon the location of the axis of rotation of the head relative to each of the two eyes (e.g., closer to one eye than the other), and the location of the object of interest relative to each of the two eyes (e.g., on the midline or off to one side), the brain must adjust the movements of each eye independently, so that they can both remain pointed at the object of regard during any pattern of head motion. For a more detailed analysis of the relationships among these variables, see Laboratory Evaluation of Eye-Head Movements, in Chapter 7.

Most naturally occurring rotational head perturbations are of high frequency (0.5 to 5.0 cycles/second), commonly due to vibrations from heel strike, which are transmitted through the body to the head during walking (see Figure 7–1). These head movements are compensated for, at least in part, by an oligosynaptic pathway consisting of three or four neurons. This pathway, the elementary VOR,[783] extends from the labyrinth to the extraocular muscles. The r-VOR has a latency of action (i.e., time from start of head turn to initiation of compensatory eye rotation) in the range of 7 ms to 15 ms largely depending upon the nature of the stimulus but also on the sensitivity of the recording system.[196] There is also a slight difference between the two eyes, possibly due to the additional abducens internuclear neuron in the horizontal VOR pathway to the medial rectus.[196] No other sensory mechanism that contributes to the generation of eye movements that compensate for head movements is so prompt in its action. If the VOR fails owing to disease, then vision during walking is impaired. The effects of "living without a balancing mechanism" were reported vividly by a physician who had lost labyrinthine function after receiving streptomycin.[437] When walking in the street, he could not recognize faces or read signs unless he stood still (see Video Display: Disorders of the Vestibular System). These symptoms indicate that visual-following reflexes, because of slow retinal processing, cannot adequately substitute for the VOR during natural head movements. Indeed, the latency of visual-mediated eye movements in humans is at least 75 ms.[323]

Head rotations in roll (around the naso-occipital axis of the head) place different demands upon the VOR than do head rotations in yaw (horizontally) or in pitch (vertically). This difference is because head movements in roll displace images away from the fovea much less than do head rotations in yaw or pitch; only in the periphery of the retina will appreciable slip of images occur. The torsional compensatory responses to head rotations in the roll plane need not be increased for near viewing since translation of the orbits during roll does not alter the needs for image stabilization for rotations of the globe around its line of sight. In this case, however, horizontal and vertical eye movements must be larger because of the increased requirements for compensation from the horizontal and vertical translation of the orbits. During roll head rotation the eyes can become misaligned vertically (producing a skew deviation) due to *translation of the orbits,* one up and the other down. Another cause for vertical misalignment during head roll is that the eyes rotate around an axis *parallel to the axis of head rotation* even when they are converged; thus one fovea moves up and the other down. Depending upon exactly where the eyes are in the orbit and how much the vertical t-VOR can compensate for the relative up and down motion of the two orbits, there can be varying degrees of vertical ocular misalignment. In essence, there are two competing needs during and after rotation of the head around the roll axis. First, there is a response to the need for full-field stabilization of the image on the retina during rotation, which when the head is rotating within a plane perpendicular to the ground (i.e., upright), also keeps the retinal meridians aligned with earth horizontal. Secondly, vertical misalignment and foveal disparity must be minimized to maintain single vision and stereopsis. Indeed some investigators have found suppression of the static and of the dynamic torsional VOR during near viewing, which would help prevent vertical diplopia[84,443,588] though other mechanisms such as torsional quick phases also help maintain eye alignment.[572]

Head Tilt

The otolith organs respond to linear accelerations. During translation of the head, its signals are transformed into the t-VOR. But the otoliths also respond to the pull of gravity, the most pervasive form of linear acceleration. Hence, when the attitude of the otoliths is altered relative to gravity, a tilt of the head is signaled and a compensatory reorientation of the eyes occurs. The action of this static otolith-ocular reflex can be seen clearly in afoveate, lateral-eyed animals such as the rabbit.[186] When the head is tilted laterally and kept there, the eyes are moved and held in a compensatory position relative to earth horizontal (one up in the orbit and the other down, in a physiological skew deviation). When the head is pitched forwards or backwards, the eyes counterroll and are then held in their new position to keep the retinas aligned with the horizontal meridian. In human beings, if the head is pitched forward (chin to chest), the object of interest can be fixed upon using saccades, so that static compensatory eye movements to keep the retina aligned along the horizontal meridian are unnecessary. When the head is tilted laterally, a dynamic component, primarily mediated by the semicircular canals, preserves vision during the head movement. During sustained lateral head tilts, however, we still rely on the static otolith-ocular reflex that produces ocular counterrolling, because our ability to make voluntary torsional movements is limited. Counterrolling of the eyes in humans is vestigial and compensates for only about 10% of the head tilt.[39,103,197,628,641,645]

The relatively feeble ocular counterrolling to static head tilt does not seem disadvantageous for vision because changes in the torsional orientation of the retina have little effect on foveal acuity. Indeed for viewing near objects it may even be advantageous to have a lower gain of counterrolling to minimize any potential vertical misalignment (see Head Rotations and Translations). Nevertheless, a fundamental question in vestibular physiology is how, and to what degree, the vestibular system resolves the inherent ambiguity between translation and tilt.[13,14,557] The otolith organs respond in the same way to linear accelerations of any type, and their afferent discharge in itself does not allow for a distinction between tilt and translation. Recent experimental evidence suggests that information from the semicircular canals allows the brain to 'decide', through an internal model of the relationship of the head to the pull of gravity, if the change in otolith activity is due to a tilt or to a translation of the head.[14,34,35,73,564,565,910,912] Single-unit recordings in monkeys have revealed neurons within the brainstem and cerebellum that could represent internal models of the "physical equations of motion", and thus help resolve the inherent ambiguity in tilt versus translation, which is discussed below.[34,743,744] At the level of perception there appears to be a representation of the pull of gravity in the areas of cerebral cortex that receive vestibular inputs within which the motion of visual objects can be deciphered.[425] Furthermore, in response to otolith stimulation, subjective sensations and compensatory ocular motor responses may be dissociated, each meeting the specific functional needs for perception of self-motion and orientation and for stabilization of gaze and effective binocular vision.[559,560]

Vestibular-Visual Symbiosis

Both the t-VOR and r-VOR perform optimally in response to brief, high-frequency motion of the head. The ability of the r-VOR to transduce reliably the motion of the head fades during sustained, low-frequency head rotation. Consequently, other mechanisms must substitute for the declining vestibular response, and visual-following reflexes assume the burden of maintaining stability of images on the retina during prolonged (low-frequency) rotation of the head.[185,577,730] Specifically, the optokinetic system appears to have evolved to supplement the r-VOR. Its action is easily appreciated in lateral-eyed animals (such as the rabbit) that do not have foveae, and in which other forms of visual tracking such as smooth pursuit and vergence are rudimentary. Consider the rabbit as it moves in a large circle for 30 or 40 seconds, a typical response while the animal is being chased by predators. The rotational component of this movement will have a low frequency. Because of the mechanical properties of the semicircular canals, the r-VOR, by itself, can only hold the eyes steady during the first few seconds of turning (the cupula slowly returns toward its initial position during a sustained rotation). As the animal moves around the circle, vestibulo-ocular compensation declines and visual images of the world increasingly slip across the retina. This is the stimulus to the optokinetic system. Consequently, vestibular compensation is replaced by optokinetic visual following during sustained self-rotation.

When the optokinetic system is tested artificially in the rabbit, in isolation (for example, using a drum rotating around the animal to produce a sudden movement of the visual surround at a constant velocity), the optokinetic response slowly builds (charges) over time until it reaches a velocity close to that of the stimulus.[194] Then, if the lights are turned off, the optokinetic system slowly discharges, producing an optokinetic after-nystagmus (OKAN). This charging and discharging behavior is just the backup that is needed to substitute for the fading vestibular response during rotation in the light and to help suppress the unwanted post-rotatory vestibular nystagmus that occurs when the rabbit suddenly stops its sustained rotation. These optokinetic responses are mediated centrally by the Velocity-Storage Mechanism (see below).

The t-VOR has similar limitations in its ability to transduce low-frequency stimuli, in this case in response to linear motion of the head. Pure translations of low frequency are partially misinterpreted as tilts of the head with respect to gravity. They elicit both ocular counterroll and compensatory slow phases of vertical or horizontal nystagmus.[14,559,560,794] These low-frequency isolated translational stimuli, however, are unlikely to occur naturally. The actions of the t-VOR are best seen in foveate animals under more natural conditions, in which case translations are usually of higher frequency and commonly combined with rotations of the head. In lateral-eyed animals, the t-VOR and visual-following responses are rudimentary; a robust translational response in a lateral-eyed animal could actually become a hindrance during forward motion in the environment by pinning the eyes onto the visual scene behind the animal. The inherently poor optokinetic response of lateral-eyed animals to nasal-temporal directed motion could reflect the need to avoid inappropriate visual stabilization during forward locomotion.[858]

Once animals became frontal-eyed and developed foveae, they evolved systems to focus their lines of sight in a particular depth plane, necessitating compensatory responses for head translation that depended upon viewing distance.[577] Likewise, the visual-driven compensatory response for translation of the head depends upon the distance of the target of interest. To maintain fixation of objects of interest moving in a particular depth plane, two mechanisms are required. First, there must be a disjunctive mechanism—vergence—for maintaining the alignment of eyes for the desired depth plane, and second, a conjugate mechanism—pursuit—for keeping the line of sight on the particular target of interest within the desired depth plane. As might be predicted, the frequency ranges in which the t-VOR and pursuit function optimally are complementary.[794] The t-VOR and pursuit also behave similarly with respect to associated torsion. They obey Listing's law (discussed in Chapter 9) rather well in contrast to the r-VOR, which does not.[2,850]

With the evolution of binocular, foveate vision, circumstances arise when there might be a conflict between the needs for stabilization of images on the fovea and for stabilization of images on the rest of the retina. This might occur, for example, when fixing upon a small object relatively close to oneself, while walking. The more distant background would move on the retina in the opposite direction. In these circumstances, the pursuit system, with its attentional focus, dominates visual following. A similar response can be seen when foveate animals are subject to artificial movement of the visual environment, such as within an optokinetic drum or with a visual scene projected onto a tangent screen. There is an immediate, almost involuntary pre-attentive response, variously called the direct, early, rapid, or immediate component of optokinetic nystagmus (OKN) or, more simply, the ocular-following response.[577] This response is likely mediated by pursuit pathways, though with a shorter latency than seen with the onset of pursuit tracking of a small target.[2,790] Perhaps with a full-field stimulus, the time for the attentional decision-making processes that are associated with voluntary pursuit of small objects can be bypassed. In humans, optokinetic nystagmus is dominated by smooth pursuit, blurring the distinction.

Vestibulo-ocular reflex suppression or cancellation of the VOR refers to modulation of VOR responses during combined eye-head tracking, when the object of interest is not stationary but moves in the direction of the head. The mechanism is related to smooth pursuit and is discussed in Chapter 7.

ANATOMY AND PHYSIOLOGY OF THE PERIPHERAL VESTIBULAR SYSTEM

The Structure of the Labyrinth

The membranous labyrinth lies within its bony counterpart in the temporal bone, cushioned by perilymph (Fig. 2–1, top left).[523,879] It contains the cristae of the semicircular canals,

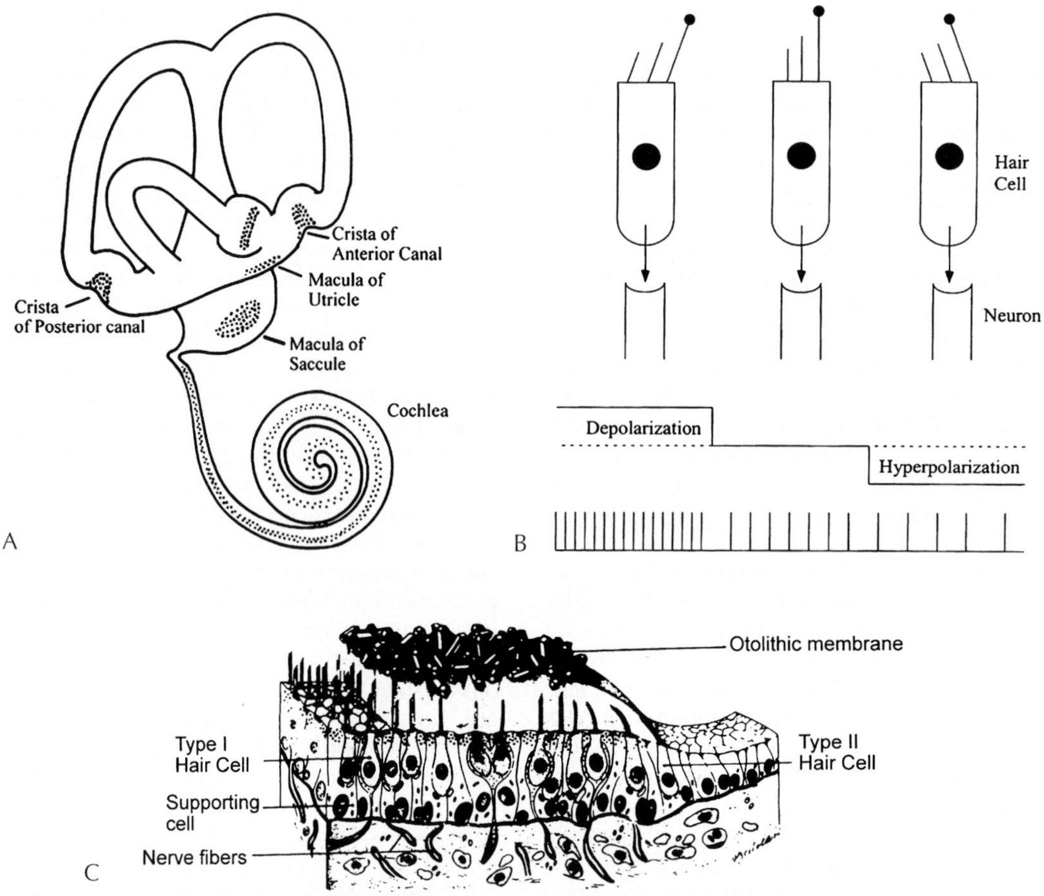

Figure 2–1. (A) Schematic of the mammalian labyrinth. The crista of the lateral semicircular canal is shown but not labeled. (B) Motion transduction by the vestibular hair cells. At rest there is a resting rate of action potential discharge in the primary vestibular afferents (center). Shearing forces on the hair cells cause depolarization (right) if the stereocilia are deflected toward the kinocilium (indicated by longest cilium, with beaded end), or hyperpolarization (left) if the stereocilia are deflected away from the kinocilium. This modulates the discharge rate in the vestibular nerve (neuron). (C) Schematic drawing of a macula, showing how the cilia of the hair cells are embedded in the gelatinous otolith membrane, to which are attached calcium carbonate crystals—otoconia. (A redrawn from Wersall DJ, Bagger-Sjoback D. Morphology of the vestibular sense organs. In Kornhuber HH (ed): Handbook of Sensory Physiology, Vol. VI/1, Vestibular System. Springer, New York, 1974, pp 123–170, with permission. B from Precht W,[669] with permission. C adapted from Iurato S. Submicroscopic Structure of the Inner Ear, Pergamon Press, Oxford, 1967.)

which sense head rotation, and the maculae of the utricle and saccule, which sense linear motion and static tilt of the head. Both cristae and maculae contain specialized hair cells of two forms (Type I and Type II, defined by the presence or absence of a calyx or chalice) that transduce mechanical shearing forces into neural impulses. The processes of each hair cell consist of many stereocilia and one kinocilium. The cilia are aligned so that they react best to shearing forces applied in a specific orientation. Deflection of the stereocilia toward the kinocilium causes depolarization (stimulation) of the hair cell; deflection in the opposite direction causes hyperpolarization (inhibition) (Fig. 2–1, top right).[530] The processes of the hair cells of the cristae are embedded in a gelatinous, sail-like structure, called the cupula. One cupula lies in each of the ampullae (regions of enlargement) of the three semicircular canals. Each turning movement of the head causes the endolymph within the semicircular canals to lag behind and to bend the cupula and so change the discharge of the hair cells that lie at its base.

The hair cells of the maculae also have their

processes embedded in a gelatinous membrane, but attached to this are calcium carbonate crystals called otoconia (Fig. 2–1, bottom). The main stimulus to the macula is linear acceleration of the head, including the gravitational pull on the otoconia. The arrangement of the hair cells on the macula, which is more complex than that of the cristae, enables detection of any linear motion permitted by 3-D space. Hair cells of opposite polarization tend to be aligned on either side of a central stripe of hair cells called the striola. The macula of the utricle lies approximately in the horizontal plane and the macula of the saccule approximately in the parasagittal plane. They respond best to linear accelerations in these planes, though both are curved structures like ellipsoids and respond, to some degree, to linear acceleration in any direction.[438,439,601,602] It has been suggested that the lateral portion of the utricle may respond best to translations and the medial portion to the pull of gravity.[503] This idea, coupled with the phenomenon of 'cross-striolar inhibition' in which activation of hair cells on one side of the striola can inhibit activity in hair cells on the other (discussed below), would account for the seeming paradox that patients with a unilateral loss of labyrinthine function have a deficit in the t-VOR when translated toward the side of the lesion, and a deficit in ocular torsion when tilted toward the side of the lesion.[354] Neurophysiologic evidence for this hypothesis is awaited.

The Blood Supply and Innervation of the Labyrinth

The **blood supply** of the membranous labyrinth is from the internal auditory or labyrinthine artery.[537,876] The labyrinthine artery usually arises from the anterior inferior cerebellar artery (AICA), but sometimes arises directly from the basilar artery. After giving a branch to the eighth nerve in the cerebellopontine angle, the internal auditory artery traverses the internal auditory meatus. When it reaches the labyrinth, it branches into (1) the anterior vestibular artery, which supplies the anterior and lateral semicircular canals and most of the utricular macula and a small portion of the sacculus; (2) the vestibulo-cochlear artery, with two rami—cochlear and vestibular (the latter is also called the posterior vestibular artery, and supplies primarily the posterior semicircular canal and the saccular macula); and (3) the main (proper) cochlear artery. The internal auditory artery is an end artery; when it or its source, the AICA, is occluded, inner ear function is lost (see Video Display: Cerebellar Syndromes). Selective occlusion of branches of the internal auditory artery, such as the anterior vestibular artery, may cause selective loss of labyrinthine function.[287,339,620]

Nerves from the cristae and maculae pass through the perforations of the lamina cribrosa to reach Scarpa's ganglion at the lateral aspect of the internal auditory canal. The vestibular nerve is divided into two branches: (1) the superior division, which innervates the anterior and lateral semicircular canals and the utricle, and (2) the inferior division branch, which innervates the posterior semicircular canal and most of the saccule. This anatomical separation has important clinical implications with respect to a predilection for viral infections to involve the superior division (see Chapter 11). A small branch from the superior vestibular nerve (Voit's anastomosis) innervates the anterosuperior part of the saccule. The superior branch runs with the facial nerve, and the inferior branch runs with the cochlear nerve. A small number of vestibular fibers may also run in the cochlear division. The anterior vestibular artery supplies the structures innervated by the superior branches of the vestibular nerve, and the posterior vestibular artery supplies structures innervated by the inferior branches. From Scarpa's ganglion, the vestibular nerve passes medially, traversing the cerebellopontine angle. It then lies posterior to the cochlear nerve and below the facial nerve, entering the brain stem between the inferior cerebellar peduncle and the spinal trigeminal tract, to synapse in the vestibular nuclei.[607]

The Mechanical Properties of the Semicircular Canals and Otolith Organs

The physical properties of the labyrinthine motion sensors are important determinants of the overall vestibular responses. The crista ampullaris is most sensitive to brief head turns, because of the physical properties of the cupula and surrounding endolymph, which have been likened to those of an overdamped torsion pendulum.[163,772,879] The internal diameter of the semicircular canals is small relative to their radius of curvature, so, given the hydrodynamic properties of the endolymph, the motion of endolymph—and hence the change in the position of the cupula—caused by a head rotation is approximately proportional to head velocity.[225,879] Thus, the semicircular canals mechanically integrate the angular head acceleration that they sense, allowing them to provide the brain with a head-velocity signal. This has been confirmed electrophysiologically by recording from semicircular canal afferents in the vestibular nerve.[276,332] Another consequence of these mechanical features is that only a small amount of endolymph displacement occurs, even with high-acceleration head turns, and the cupula is not in danger of being excessively displaced. With sustained head rotations, the elastic properties of the cupula become important and cause it to return to its resting position with an exponentially decaying time course. The time constant of return of the cupula cannot be directly measured in humans, but has been estimated to be about 6 seconds.[185,303,592]

The return of the cupula to its resting position can be related to the decline in nystagmus during velocity-step rotations (an impulse of acceleration to some constant velocity). This per-rotational nystagmus is greatest at the onset of the stimulus, but then slow-phase velocity shows an approximately exponential decline. If the subject is suddenly stopped after a sustained, constant-velocity rotation, post-rotational nystagmus will be produced. This reflects displacement of the cupula in the direction opposite to that when the rotation began. In animals, and probably humans, per-rotational nystagmus lasts considerably longer than the time required for the cupula to drift back to its starting position. This suggests that the brain manipulates the canal signal so as to prolong the time that motion of the head can be perceived. This phenomenon is mediated by the velocity-storage mechanism, and is common to both vestibular and optokinetic responses.

Flow of endolymph within each canal, in one direction, produces excitation in its ampullary nerve (increasing its discharge rate) and, in the other direction, produces inhibition. For the lateral (or horizontal) canals, flow toward the ampulla (ampullopetal flow) is excitatory. For the vertical canals, flow away from the ampulla (ampullofugal flow) is excitatory. The semicircular canals are arranged so that each canal on one side of the head is paired with another on the opposite side, both lying in nearly the same plane. Careful measurements have shown that the relative planes of the three canals vary among individuals,[224] however, and complementary canals on opposite sides of the skull may not be precisely aligned.[241,787] Clearly the brain must make adjustments for such individual variations. Despite these small differences, the semicircular canals can be thought of as working in pairs. Thus, an ampullofugal flow of endolymph within the right anterior semicircular canal will be accompanied by an ampullopetal flow in the left posterior semicircular canal. This push-pull arrangement stands the organism in good stead in the event that disease should destroy one labyrinth, since the brain can then still use a (normal) decrease in activity from the intact labyrinth to detect head rotation toward the side of the lesion. The effects of stimulating individual semicircular canals are summarized in Figure 2–2A. Each canal produces movements of the eyes in the plane of that canal (described by Flourens for head movements (Flourens' law) and Ewald for eye movements (Ewald's first law)).[211,212,629] These findings have important clinical significance, which is discussed later in this chapter in the section on disorders of the vestibular-optokinetic system.

The physical properties of the otolith maculae are more difficult to analyze than those of the semicircular canals, in part because they are curved structures, and so sense linear acceleration in many different directions.[220,439] The utricular macula lies on the floor of the utricle, approximately in the plane of the lateral semicircular canals. The saccular macula lies on the medial wall of the saccule, nearly parasagittal with respect to the head (i.e., in a plane approximately orthogonal to the utricular macula). The utricle is oriented to respond best to lateral or fore-and-aft tilts, and side-to-side translations of the head. The saccule is oriented to respond best to up-and-down translations of the head. Hence these two otolith organs serve complementary roles in sensing gravitational and other linear forces applied to the head. Because the maculae are located eccentric to the axes of rotation of the head, they are able to sense both tangential and centrifugal forces during head rotations.

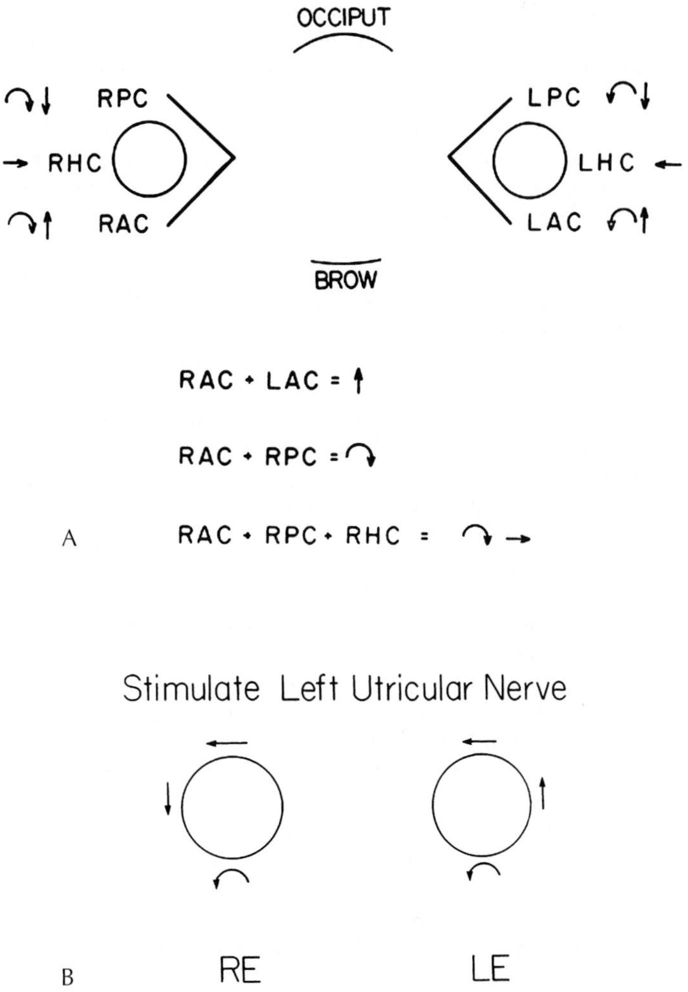

Figure 2–2. (A) Schematic summary of the ocular motor effects of stimulating individual semicircular canals and combinations of canals. Stimulation of a single canal produces slow-phase movements of the eyes in a plane parallel to one in which the canal lies. As shown by the equations at the bottom, purely vertical nystagmus can only be induced by simultaneous stimulation of the same canal on both sides. Purely torsional nystagmus can only be produced by stimulation of both vertical canals, but not the lateral canal, on one side. Thus, disease of the labyrinth seldom produces purely vertical or purely torsional nystagmus. Combined involvement of all three canals on one side causes a mixed horizontal-torsional nystagmus. (B) The effects of left utricular stimulation. Besides torsional eye movements, there is a vertical deviation of the optic axes (skew deviation) and horizontal deviation away from the side of stimulation.

The mechanism of action of the otoliths is an inertia-generated shearing movement of the otoconial layer, parallel to the underlying surface of the sensory epithelium. In this way, the otoliths can sense both translational head movements (i.e., linear accelerations) and static tilts of the head (with respect to the pull of gravity). Electrical stimulation of the utricle and saccule produces various patterns of eye movements including upward movement of the ipsilateral eye and downward movement of the contralateral eye with torsion.[219,337,338] Similar results are produced by stimulation of the utricular nerve, although there is also a horizontal component. (Fig. 2–2B)[780] The results of these stimulation studies must be interpreted cautiously because of issues such as current spread, effects of anesthesia, and the differences in responses depending upon which particular part of the macula is stimulated. Behavioral studies also suggest that the saccule can contribute to ocular torsion, and perhaps to disconjugate torsion.[237] It must be reiterated that the otolith maculae are curved structures, not flat, and that both the saccule and utricle can respond, to some extent, to linear accelerations in any direction.

Neural Activity in Vestibular Afferents

The discharge properties of the vestibular nerve are distinguished by continuous spontaneous activity or resting vestibular tone.[331,332,403] For the semicircular canal afferents this resting discharge frequency is modulated up or down during rotation of the head. The modulation of vestibular activity by rotational stimuli has been extensively studied in many species. For the physiologic range of head movements, the signal from the semicircular canals is a representation of rotational head velocity, though head acceleration is the stimulus that leads to excitation of the hair-cell receptors. The integration from acceleration to velocity is largely a mechanical one, related to the physical properties of the endolymph and semicircular canals, but the information about head motion carried by the afferents is also affected by the dynamics of transfer of information at the connection between the hair cell and its afferent nerve fiber. Thus, a transduction of the acceleration of the actual movement of the head to a signal proportional to the rotational velocity of the head carried on individual vestibular afferents is an oversimplification.[403,679] Rather it is the central processing of the ensemble of different types of peripheral afferent information that leads to the correct eye movement response to the motion of the head. Furthermore, adaptation to sustained (low-frequency) head rotations, in particular, seems to reflect a number of processes beginning from the hair cell itself, to the vestibular afferents and eventually, to the central networks within the vestibular nuclei and possibly the cerebellum. Again, the final, calibrated and optimized eye movement response to head motion must reflect the entire cascade of physiological processing of information within the complex anatomical organization that underlies the VOR.

Vestibular stimuli that are outside the natural range of head motion, for example, at especially high velocities or accelerations, or at especially low or high frequencies, present particular challenges to the ability of the vestibular periphery to reliably transduce head motion. For example, at high head velocities, when the discharge of one set of canal afferents is fully inhibited, the VOR will depend upon the excitatory response from one labyrinth alone. This asymmetry in response at high velocities leads to one form of Ewald's second law that, in its generic form, states that excitation is a relatively better vestibular stimulus than is inhibition. Ewald's second law becomes particularly evident when there is a loss of the function of the labyrinth on one side. Another equally important form of Ewald's second law may apply to the acceleration and frequency characteristics of head rotation (see Clinical Findings with Dynamic Vestibular Imbalance, below).

The nonlinear effects of Ewald's second law have important implications even in normal behavior. The r-VOR has a gain—ratio of output (eye velocity) to input (head velocity) —of 1.0 in normals for rotational velocities up to 350° per second– 400° per second,[675,705] even though vestibular afferents are presumably driven into inhibitory cutoff at velocities well below 200° per second.[276,276] Therefore, for high speeds of head rotation there must be a mechanism to compensate for the loss of the contribution of the afferents (disinhibition) on the side opposite to rotation (when these afferents are driven into inhibitory cutoff). Several suggestions have been made as to how central mechanisms ensure such a wide range of linear responses. One hypothesis is that when activity no longer comes from the inhibited labyrinth, there is a central disinhibition that increases the sensitivity of the response to afferent activity emanating from the excited labyrinth.[897] Alternatively, the presence of quick phases may prevent vestibular neurons from being driven into inhibitory cutoff and so improve their linear range of response.[313,759] Just as for the slow phases, the timing and amplitude of quick phases are also affected during vestibular compensation.[170,217,326] Finally, the combined effects of irregularly and regularly discharging afferents (see below) may help to make the reflex linear and enable it to respond to a wide range of frequencies and accelerations.[331,419]

DIFFERENT CLASSES OF VESTIBULAR AFFERENTS

Vestibular nerve fibers have been classified as regular afferents or irregular afferents, depending upon the regularity of their discharge rate, and both project to neurons within the vestibular nuclei that discharge in relation to the VOR.[120,331,333,383,581] The exact functional differences between irregular and regular afferents are uncertain, though theories abound. Regular afferents have tonic response dynamics, resembling the displacement of the cupula or of the otolith membrane, and have a low sensitivity to head rotations or linear forces. The caliber of their axons is medium to small and they end as dimorphic units and bouton units in intermediate and peripheral zones of the cupula or macula. Irregular afferents have phasic-tonic response dynamics, including sensitivity to the velocity of cupula and otolith membrane displacement, and hence show acceleration sensitivity in the case of afferents from the semicircular canals, and 'jerk', the derivative of acceleration, in the case of afferents from the otolith organs. Their axons are medium to large.

Irregular afferents in the central zone of the cristae have low rotational sensitivities and terminate as calyx endings onto Type I hair cells. Irregular afferents located away from the center have high rotational sensitivities and terminate as dimorphic endings onto both Type I and Type II hair cells. The irregular canal afferents have been posited to play a role in VOR adaptation including the compensatory response to unilateral labyrinthine loss and especially for high-frequency and high-velocity rotational stimuli toward the side opposite the lesion. On the other hand, regular afferents may be involved in the compensatory response to unilateral labyrinthine loss for lower velocity stimuli for rotations to either side. Irregular afferents have also been posited to play a role in modulation of the VOR during eccentric rotation and for near viewing, in cancellation of the VOR, in the generation of the low-frequency, velocity-storage component of the VOR; and perhaps in extending the linear range of the VOR at high speeds of head rotation.[32,181,251,339,383,418,493,542,544] The inputs to the VOR from irregular afferents from the semicircular canals can be modulated at the vestibular nuclei according to context that we will discuss below.[172,216,544] The irregular otolith afferents may play a role in the generation of off-vertical axis rotation (OVAR), possibly through the velocity-storage mechanism.[33]. Both irregular and regular otolith afferents appear to contribute to the high-frequency, high-amplitude t-VOR.[27] It has also been suggested that the vestibular system compares activity between irregular and regular otolith afferents to distinguish tilt and translation.[911]

The neurotransmitter used by vestibular afferents appears to be glutamate,[231,239,546] though GABA may also play a role at the hair cell synapse.[413] Recent work has detailed specific involvement of the metabotropic glutamate, N-methyl-D-aspartate and the kainate/AMPA excitatory amino acid receptors.[761] Other transmitters including nitric oxide synthetase (NOS), opiode peptides, and purines may also have a role in modulation of peripheral vestibular transmission.

Not all fibers within the vestibular nerve are afferent. Some vestibular efferents carry impulses to the labyrinth, but their function in mammals is unknown.[331] They do not suppress unwanted vestibular responses during passively evoked combined movements of head and eyes[158] and do not appear to modulate activity in active versus passive head movements.[215] Perhaps they play some role in VOR adaptation as axon collaterals of vestibular efferents project to the cerebellar flocculus.[676,755]

BRAINSTEM ELABORATION OF THE VESTIBULO-OCULAR REFLEX

Anatomic Organization of the Vestibulo-Ocular Reflex

How the brain stem fashions the precise compensatory eye movements from the raw vestibular signals has been extensively investigated since Adrian first recorded the activity of neurons within the vestibular nucleus.[3,70,159,523] Of prime importance has been the study of the three-neuron arc: vestibular ganglion, vestibular nuclei, and ocular motor nuclei. Although this elementary vestibulo-ocular reflex arc[783] is readily equated with the notion of a rapidly acting reflex, parallel polysynaptic projections are equally important for generation of an appropriate, compensatory eye movement.[519] The direct neuronal pathways include both excitatory and inhibitory contributions.

Each semicircular canal directly influences a pair of extraocular muscles that move the eyes approximately in the plane of that canal, regardless of the initial position of the eye in the orbit. Important to the clinician is that disease selectively affecting one semicircular canal may produce nystagmus that rotates the globe in a plane parallel to that in which the canal lies (see, for example, benign paroxysmal positional vertigo (BPPV) or the syndrome of superior canal dehiscence, in Chapter 11). In summarizing pathways that mediate the r-VOR (Table 2–2 and Fig. 2–3), we have drawn largely on studies of central vestibular connections in primates,[159,165,214,543] but also mention pathways reported in other species.[70,167,523,823-825]

Table 2–2. **Direct Vestibulo-Ocular Projections as Determined by Electrophysiologic and Anatomic Studies in Monkey, Cat, and Rabbit**

Receptor	Effect	Muscle	Relay Nucleus	Pathway	Motor Nucleus
LC	Excitation	c-LR	M/LVN	MLF	c-VI
		i-MR	M/LVN	ATD	i-III
	Inhibition	i-LR	MVN	MLF	i-VI
		c-MR	—	Poly	c-III
AC	Excitation	i-SR	M/LVN*	MLF*	c-III
		c-IO	M/LVN*	MLF*	c-III
	Inhibition	i-IR	SVN	MLF	i-III
		c-SO	SVN	MLF	i-IV
PC	Excitation	c-IR	M/LVN	MLF	c-III
		i-SO	M/LVN	MLF	c-IV
	Inhibition	c-SR	SVN	extra	i-III
		i-IO	SVN	extra	i-III
U	Excitation	i-SO	LVN	MLF	c-IV
		i-SR	LVN	MLF	c-III
		i-MR	LVN	ATD	i-III
		c-IO	LVN	MLF	c-III
		c-IR	LVN	MLF	c-III
		c-LR	LVN	MLF	c-VI
S	Excitation		y-group	BC	

Muscles: LR: lateral rectus muscle; MR: medial rectus muscle; SR: superior rectus muscle; IO: inferior oblique muscle; IR: inferior rectus muscle; SO: superior oblique muscle; Relay Nucleus: M/LVN: medial and adjacent lateral vestibular nucleus (*: other nuclei and pathways such at the ventral tegmental tract, are also probably involved; see Figure 2–3); MVN: medial vestibular nucleus; SVN: superior vestibular nucleus; LVN: lateral vestibular nucleus; Pathway: MLF: medial longitudinal fasciculus; ATD: ascending tract of Deiters; poly: polysynaptic pathway lying outside MLF; extra: extra-MLF pathway; Motor Nucleus: VI: abducens nucleus; III: oculomotor nucleus; IV: trochlear nucleus; c-: contralateral; i-: ipsilateral. References: [340,541,543,669-671,780]

The anatomy of the vestibular nuclei in humans has been well characterized,[778] and most features are similar to those of nonhuman primates and other mammalian species.[159,399a,607] In humans, the volume of the vestibular nuclei is about 67 mm^3 and it contains over 200,000 neurons. Vestibular nuclei neurons receive projections from the vestibular nerve that contains about 14,000 to 18,000 axons. As a generalization, larger neurons in the vestibular nuclei receive labyrinthine input from axons of a larger caliber with an irregular discharge rate (perhaps type B vestibular nucleus neurons, see below); smaller neurons receive input from smaller-caliber axons, with a regular discharge rate (perhaps type A).[715] There are four major vestibular nuclei: medial vestibular nucleus of Schwalbe (MVN), lateral vestibular nucleus of Deiters (LVN), inferior or descending vestibular nucleus (DVN), and superior vestibular nucleus of Bechterew (SVN). In addition, there are several smaller accessory subgroups, including the interstitial nucleus (IN), with its cells distributed among the vestibular rootlets as they enter the brainstem, and the y-group, near the superior cerebellar peduncle. The MVN has the greatest volume and is the longest vestibular nucleus. Its rostral portion is a major receiving area for afferents from the semicircular canals and its cells project to the III, IV, and VI cranial nuclei, which mediate the vestibulo-ocular reflexes. Its caudal portionis reciprocally connected to the cervical region of the spinal cord, presumably mediating vestibulo-collic reflexes. The caudal MVN is also reciprocally connected to the cerebellum.

The rostroventral portion of the LVN receives afferents from the cristae of the semicircular canals and the macula of the utricle. Like the rostral MVN, it participates in vestibulo-ocular reflexes, in part through the

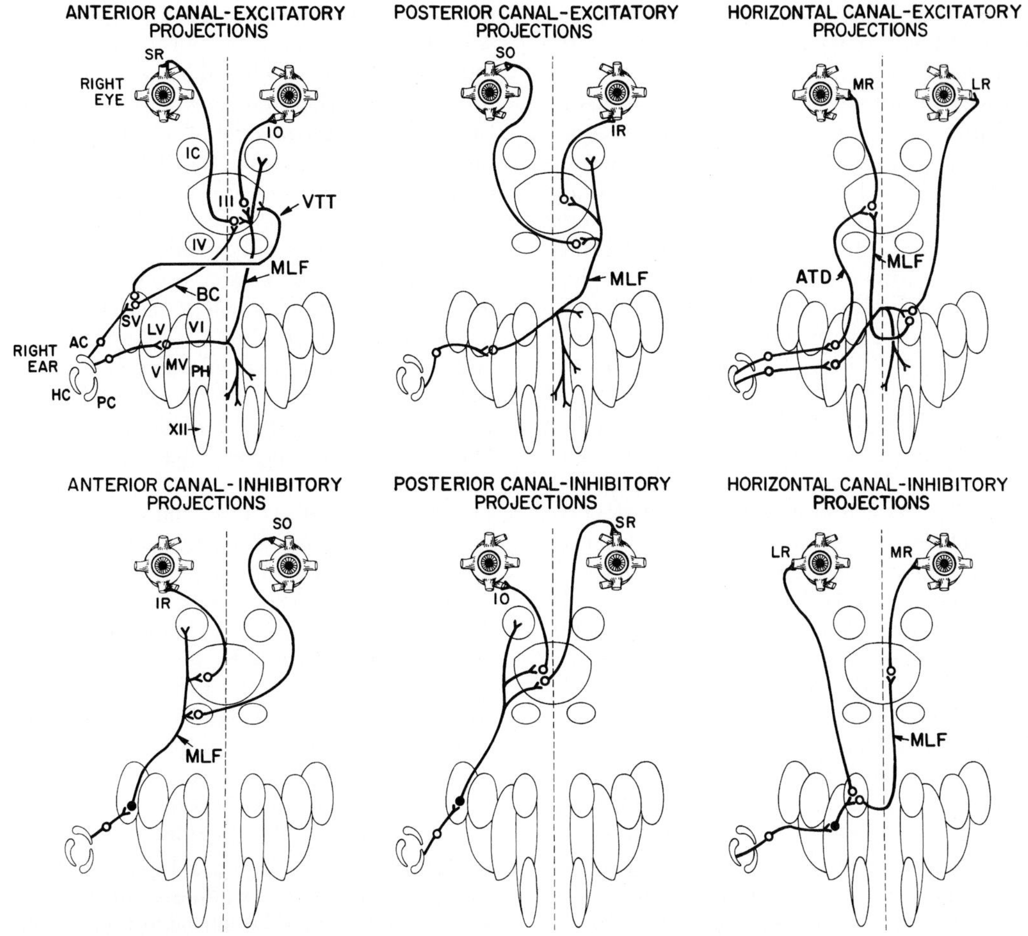

Figure 2–3. Summary of probable direct connections of vestibulo-ocular reflex, based upon findings from a number of species.[53,159,165,166,340,400,433,542,543,622,669–671,691] Excitatory neurons are indicated by open circles, inhibitory neurons by filled circles. III: oculomotor nuclear complex; IV: trochlear nucleus; VI: abducens nucleus; XII: hypoglossal nucleus; AC: anterior semicircular canal; ATD: ascending tract of Deiters; BC: brachium conjunctivum; HC: "horizontal" or lateral semicircular canal; IC: interstitial nucleus of Cajal; IO: inferior oblique muscle; IR: inferior rectus muscle; LR: lateral rectus muscle; LV: lateral vestibular nucleus; MLF: medial longitudinal fasciculus; MR: medial rectus muscle; MV: medial vestibular nucleus; PC: posterior semicircular canal; PH: prepositus nucleus; SV: superior vestibular nucleus; SO: superior oblique muscle; SR: superior rectus muscle; V: inferior vestibular nucleus; VTP: ventral tegmental pathway.

ascending tract of Deiters to the oculomotor nucleus. The LVN also has projections to the spinal cord, mainly via the ipsilateral lateral vestibulospinal tract but also through the contralateral medial vestibulospinal tract. In its most rostral aspect, the DVN also projects to the ocular motor nuclei.

There is considerable divergence of single primary afferents within the vestibular nuclei (about 15 neurons per axon). A single axon from a lateral semicircular canal can impinge upon neurons in the central part of the SVN, the rostral half of the MVN, the medial-rostral part of the DVN, and the ventromedial part of the LVN.

The primary vestibular afferents enter the medulla at the level of the lateral vestibular nucleus. Almost all afferents bifurcate, giving a descending branch to terminate in MVN and DVN and an ascending branch to the SVN, with a final destination in the cerebellum, especially the anterior vermis and the nodulus and uvula.[159,523,778] All canals and otoliths project to zone 1, which lies around the borders of ventromedial LVN, medial MVN, and dorsomedial DVN. All canals also converge on a small patch in the ventromedial SVN. These two areas contain the secondary vestibulo-ocular neurons that project to the abducens, oculomotor, and trochlear nuclei. Canal afferents also converge on the interstitial nucleus of the vestibular nerve, which projects to the flocculus.

Utricular afferents project to the rostral MVN and saccular afferents project to the y-group. Some projections from the utricle overlap with those from the lateral semicircular canal, presumably reflecting their common roles in detecting horizontal motion; and some projections from the saccule, which is involved in detecting vertical motion, overlap with those from the vertical semicircular canals.[23,252,464,556,614,822,823,906,907] Recently, utricle and saccule projections were reinvestigated in the monkey.[614] Both project to the caudal descending vestibular nucleus presumably related to spinal mechanisms. The principal ocular motor areas within the brainstem to which saccular nerve terminated were the lateral portion of the superior vestibular nucleus and ventral nucleus y. The principal cerebellar projection was to the uvula with a less dense projection to the nodulus. Principle ocular motor brainstem areas of termination of the utricular nerve were the lateral/dorsal medial vestibular nucleus, and the ventral and lateral portions of the superior vestibular nucleus. In the cerebellum, a strong projection was observed to the nodulus and weak projections were present in the flocculus, ventral paraflocculus, bilateral fastigial nuclei, and uvula. Many of the central vestibular neurons that receive otolith afferents also project to the vestibulocerebellum.[626]

For both the horizontal and vertical r-VOR, many neurons in the vestibular nuclei that receive inputs from primary vestibular afferents encode not only head velocity, but also eye position, and varying amounts of smooth pursuit and saccadic signals.[13,15,16,213,216,541,544,555,706-708,731] A common and important cell type is the position-vestibular-pause (PVP) neuron. It encodes head velocity and eye position and becomes silent (pauses) during saccades. It appears to change its activity, depending upon whether vestibular stimulation is passive, as during steady fixation, or active, as part of a gaze change.[706,708]

Another cell type is the floccular target neuron (FTN), which receives inputs from both the labyrinth and the cerebellar flocculus and may be important in VOR adaptation.[96a,99,402,510] Additional cell types include those that show a sensitivity to eye and head velocity (EH, eye–head neurons), to head movement alone (VO, vestibular-only neurons), and to eye velocity and eye position burst-position (BP) neurons.[13,731] These secondary vestibular neurons may also show changes depending upon the particular combination of stimuli, including during cancellation of the r-VOR, during eccentric rotation, and comparing active versus passive head motion.[213,216,540,544,814] Vestibular nuclei neurons not only project to motoneurons; they also send axon collaterals to the nucleus prepositus hypoglossi (NPH) and the nucleus of Roller (see Table 5–1, and to the cell groups of the paramedian tracts (PMT) (see Box 6–4 in Chapter 6).[160,161] The NPH and adjacent medial vestibular nucleus (the NPH-MVN region, see Chapter 5) have a crucial role in holding gaze steady (neural integration). The cell groups of the PMT may be important for relaying an internal or efference copy of eye movement signals to the flocculus of the cerebellum.[161,609] In addition, certain cells in NPH that receive vestibular inputs project to burst neurons in the PPRF to trigger quick phases of nystagmus.[170,217,299,326,624] Finally, many secondary vestibular axons have dual projections, both rostrally as VOR neurons and caudally as vestibulo-collic neurons.[584]

Neurons within the vestibular nucleus also can be classified by their membrane properties as Type A (tonic firing rates, responding linearly) and Type B (phasic firing rates, responding nonlinearly) although there probably is a continuum.[701,740,835] Whether or not these different properties relate to the segregation of afferent activity into regular and irregular, or the so-called linear and nonlinear VOR pathways (see below) remains to be shown. Following unilateral labyrinthectomy, however, there are different patterns of change on the ipsilateral and contralateral sides in the Type A and Type B cell types suggesting they play separate roles in the mechanisms of adaptation to a unilateral loss of function (probably related to restoration of tone and increase of responsiveness to contralateral inputs).[82,83,700]

The main vestibulo-ocular projection neurons lie in zone 1 and the center of SVN. Zone 1 predominantly carries excitatory PVP cells, and is also the origin of the ascending tract of Deiters, which runs laterally to the medial longitudinal fasciculus (MLF) to impinge upon the medial rectus subdivision of the oculomotor nucleus (Fig. 2–3). Zone 1 is under little direct cerebellar influence. Inhibitory PVP cells also lie in rostral MVN. The center zone in SVN contains predominantly burst-position cells (neurons that discharge with eye velocity and eye position); most are related to vertical canal inputs. These neurons, along with those in the dorsal y-group, the marginal zone (between MVN and nucleus prepositus), and the rostral MVN, are under the influence of the flocculus. In general, the peripheral areas of the vestibular complex are the source of intrinsic interconnections and commissural connections. They also receive projections from the cerebellar nodulus and the accessory optic nuclei. Taken together, this pattern of connectivity suggests that they play a role in the velocity-storage mechanism. The interstitial nucleus of Cajal (INC) receives axon collaterals from all secondary vestibular afferents that supply the oculomotor nucleus, and sends reciprocal projections, predominantly ipsilateral, to the vestibular nuclei (see Box 6–6, in Chapter 6).

VERTICAL SEMICIRCULAR CANAL PROJECTIONS

For the vertical semicircular canals, several important principles may be summarized. First, the excitation of the anterior semicircular canals produces upward and torsional eye movements (with the primary projections being to the ipsilateral superior rectus and contralateral inferior oblique muscles), and excitation of the posterior semicircular canals produces downward and torsional eye movements (with the primary projections being to the ipsilateral superior oblique and contralateral inferior rectus muscles).[211,212,629] Second, each vestibular nucleus neuron concerned with the vertical VOR contacts two motoneuron pools, one for each eye.[896] Third, excitatory projections from the vestibular nuclei cross the midline, but inhibitory connections do not. Fourth, the pathways taken by axons conveying the upward and downward VOR differ.[665]

For the *anterior canal system*, there may be three excitatory pathways by which information is carried rostrally for the vertical VOR. *Excitatory* PVP cells in the MVN or adjacent ventral lateral vestibular nucleus (VLVN) project medially and dorsally, crossing the midline caudally, differing with the projections of the posterior-canal PVP cells. After crossing, they ascend in or just below the MLF to contact the superior rectus and inferior oblique subdivisions of the oculomotor complex. Axon collaterals of these fibers project to the INC, the cell groups of the PMT, and the perihypoglossal nuclei, including NPH. Recall that the projections of the superior rectus subnucleus are crossed but those of the inferior oblique subnucleus are uncrossed. Thus, this excitatory pathway connects the anterior semicircular canal to the ipsilateral superior rectus and contralateral inferior oblique muscles (Fig. 2–3).

Another cell group, described in the cat, which may contribute excitatory inputs to the anterior canal system, lies in the SVN. Their axons cross the midline in the ventral tegmental tract, close to the medial lemniscus at the rostral pole of the nucleus reticularis tegmenti pontis (NRTP), and then abruptly turn rostrally, passing through the decussation of the superior cerebellar peduncle, to terminate mainly on the superior rectus and inferior oblique subdivisions of the oculomotor complex.[166] Also, in some species, the SVN projects rostrally, just near the brachium conjunctivum, to the oculomotor nuclei. Thus, three pathways may contribute to the generation of eye movements during stimulation of the anterior semicircular canal; the projections in primates have not yet been completely described.

Inhibitory neurons for the anterior canal system lie in the SVN. Their axons exit from the rostromedial aspect of this nucleus and course medially and rostrally in the lateral wing of the ipsilateral MLF, to contact superior oblique motoneurons in the trochlear nucleus, and inferior rectus neurons in the oculomotor nucleus. Axon collaterals project to NPH and to cell groups of the PMT. The neurotransmitter of these inhibitory vestibular neurons may be Gamma-aminobutyric acid (GABA).[230,239,546]

For the *posterior canal system*, PVP cells are also found at the junction of the MVN and VLVN. These *excitatory* neurons project rostrally, medially, and dorsally through MVN until, at the level of the caudal abducens nucleus, they turn medially and cross the midline beneath the NPH and abducens nucleus, ventral to the MLF. After crossing the midline, they enter the MLF and project rostrally to the trochlear nucleus and inferior rectus subdivision of the oculomotor complex. Axon collaterals also pass, via the MLF, to the NPH and PMT cell groups, and to the INC. The projections of the trochlear motoneurons are contralateral, but those of the inferior rectus are ipsilateral. Thus, this excitatory pathway connects the posterior semicircular canal to the ipsilateral superior oblique and contralateral inferior rectus (Fig. 2–3). In addition, the posterior semicircular canal also projects to the contralateral abducens nucleus. This projection for horizontal eye movements perhaps reflects the somewhat tilted orientation of the posterior canals in the labyrinth so they are stimulated during rotation around the yaw axis and might make a contribution to the horizontal VOR.

Inhibitory neurons subserving the posterior semicircular canals are found in the SVN and rostral MVN. Their axons project through the pontine reticular formation to reach the ipsilateral MLF and then contact the superior rectus and inferior oblique subdivisions of the oculomotor complex. These neurons also contact PMT cell groups and the INC. Like the inhibitory neurons of the anterior canal system, these cells also may use GABA as an inhibitory neurotransmitter.[239,414,546]

HORIZONTAL SEMICIRCULAR CANAL PROJECTIONS

For the *lateral (or horizontal) canals*, PVP neurons are located in the ventral part of the MVN and adjacent VLVN. Most of these *excitatory* neurons course rostrally and medially through MVN, pass through or beneath the ipsilateral abducens or rostral NPH, and cross the midline at the level of the abducens nucleus or slightly rostral to it. Soon after crossing the midline, these axons give collaterals that either terminate in the abducens nucleus or project to the NPH and PMT cell groups. Some PVP neurons project rostromedially, passing through the abducens nucleus, and run in the ascending tract of Deiters (ATD) to terminate in the medial rectus subdivision of the ipsilateral oculomotor complex; some of these axons send collaterals to PMT cell groups. Thus, these excitatory pathways connect the lateral semicircular canal to the ipsilateral medial rectus and contralateral lateral rectus muscles (Fig. 2–3). The functional significance of the pathway through the ATD is uncertain, but it may relate to VORs associated with translation or near viewing.

Inhibitory pathways for the lateral canals pass from the MVN to the adjacent abducens nucleus; these neurons may use glycine as a neurotransmitter.[546] The medial rectus neurons are peculiar in having no known disynaptic inhibitory input, although a multisynaptic, extra-MLF pathway may play a role.[53,400]

OTOLITH PROJECTIONS

Central otolith projections for the t-VOR have been less well studied than those concerned with the r-VOR; current concepts are summarized in Figure 2–4. As discussed previously, in the monkey,[51,614] the principal projections from the saccule are to the ventral portion of the y-group, lateral SVN, and to the uvula and nodulus. The principal projections from the utricle are to the laterodorsal MVN, and ventrolateral SVN. There are also projections to the nodulus, flocculus, ventral paraflocculus, fastigial nuclei, and uvula. Based upon anatomy, saccule projections seem more important for vestibulospinal mechanisms. Experimental stimulation of the utricular nerve causes eye movements that suggest contraction of the ipsilateral superior oblique, superior rectus, and medial rectus, and the contralateral inferior oblique, inferior rectus, and lateral rectus muscles,[780] though under different conditions of anesthesia and different parameters of electrical stimulation primarily ipsilateral-directed horizontal eye movements can be elicited.[219,337] Experimental stimulation of the saccular nerve causes vertical eye movements with a preponderance for downward-directed slow phases.[219,338]

The interpretation of these results of experimental stimulation of the otoliths is confounded by the fact that all the hair cells are not oriented in the same direction on the macula (and hence with stimulation are not all excited in one direction and inhibited in the other) as is the case for the cupula and the semicircular canals.[439] Thus, artificial stimulation might elicit different directions of eye motion depending upon the location of the electrical stimulus. The level of anesthesia may also play a role in the nature of the response. Presumably central vestibular mechanisms are able to extract the needed information about head motion elicited in natural circumstances using 1) commissural pathways and so-called cross-striolar inhibition in which afferent inputs from one side of the macula influence activity from afferents on the other[621,823,826] and 2) concurrent signals from the vertical semicircular canals, which help to

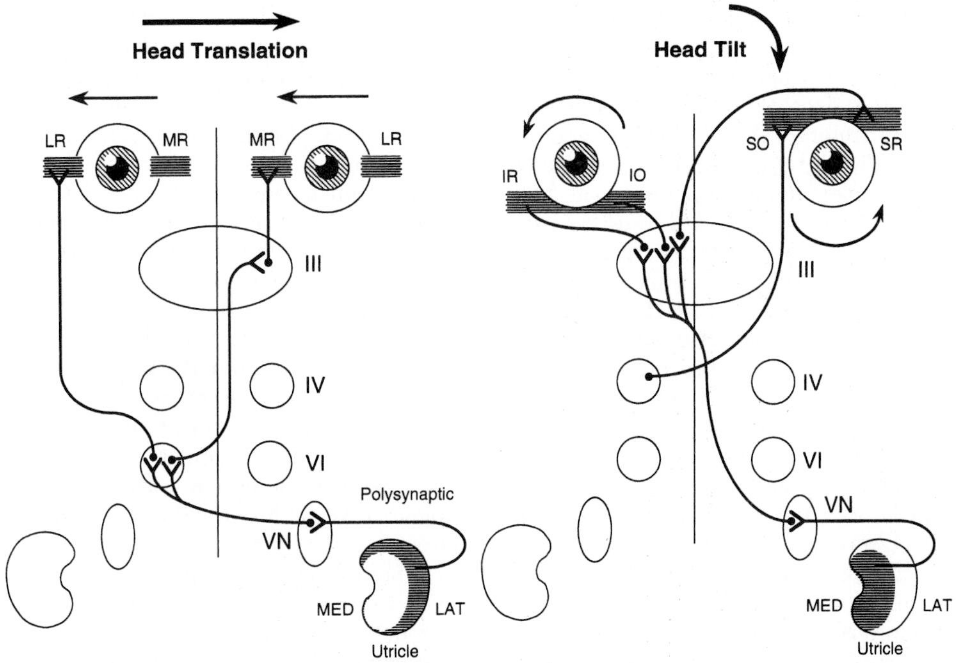

Figure 2–4. Hypothetical otolith pathways for tilt and translation. The medial portion of the utricle would be excited by ipsilateral head tilt and would lead to counterolling of the eyes by connections to the vertical torsional muscles. The lateral portion of the utricle would be excited by ipsilateral head translation and would lead to an oppositely directed horizontal slow phase presumably via polysynaptic connections, possibly through the cerebellum, to the horizontal muscles.

distinguish tilt from translation (see The Velocity-Storage Mechanism). Indeed, for generating the horizontal t-VOR, polysynaptic connections might arise from the lateral portion of the utricle, and reach the vestibular nuclei on the opposite side of the brain stem, possibly via the cerebellum, and are probably more important for the horizontal compensatory eye movements of the t-VOR than the direct projections to the ipsilateral vestibular nuclei.[13] On the other hand, projections from the medial portion of the utricle may be more important for signaling head tilt and lead to compensatory counterrolling using vertical torsional eye muscles.[354,503] Figure 2–4 shows such a scheme. Table 2–2 summarizes some of the direct anatomic pathways involved.

The vestibular nuclei also receive projections from a number of areas apart from the vestibular periphery. They include, of course, other brain stem nuclei, the cerebellum, and the cerebral hemispheres. As discussed below, vestibular neurons carry sensory information from the visual system as well as from proprioceptors and other somatosensory receptors in the neck and body. There are also large inputs from many areas in the cerebral hemispheres, reflecting the central role that the vestibular nuclei have in generating compensatory motor responses—during passive perturbations as well as self-generated movement, using information about spatial orientation and motion from all available sources (see Vestibular Sensation below).

A number of neurotransmitters have been implicated in synaptic transmission within and between the vestibular nuclei.[761] Glutamate, glycine, NOS, and GABA (especially related to commissural inhibition) are important. Hormonal receptors such as arginine-vasopressin, cannaboid receptors, and opioid-related receptors such as nociceptin, likely modulate synaptic transmission centrally.

Basic Neurophysiology of the Vestibulo-Ocular Reflex

The functional organization of the vestibulo-ocular responses is more complicated than the elementary anatomic connections suggest. For horizontal rotations, neurons in the vestibular nuclei that encode head velocity can be divided into two main types. Type-I neurons increase their discharge rate for ipsilateral rotations and decrease their discharge rate during contralateral rotations; type-II neurons show the converse. Thus, each vestibular nuclear complex monitors rotation in both directions. This facility is aided by a vestibular commissure,[165] whereby ipsilateral type-I vestibular neurons drive contralateral type-II neurons. The organization of this vestibular commissure is specific, so that neurons in the right vestibular nucleus that receive input from the right lateral semicircular canal project to neurons in the left vestibular nucleus that are driven by the left lateral semicircular canal. A similar reciprocal connection is found for vertical canals (e.g., the right anterior canal and the left posterior canal). The vestibular commissure probably contributes to the velocity-storage mechanism (see next section).[189,345,461,863] Its precise role in vestibular compensation is unclear.[153,284,461]

A role for the vestibular commissure is less clear for otolith-ocular reflexes, being more certain for utricular than for saccular responses.[823,826] As described above, it has been shown that the equivalent of a push-pull relationship for saccular (and probably utricular) reflexes can be created on just one side of the brainstem.[825,826] This can be achieved by combining on the same vestibular nucleus neuron, monosynaptic excitatory inputs from one population of hair cells on one side of the striola, and disynaptic inhibitory inputs from another population of hair cells on the other side of the striola. This is called cross-striolar inhibition.

As described previously, vestibular nucleus neurons encode a range of sensory and motor signals: vestibular, ocular motor, visual, and somatosensory. Head velocity, the primary vestibular signal, is still present, but eye position is also encoded neurally. The presence of eye position signals on vestibular nucleus neurons reflects the crucial role played by the NPH-MVN region in gaze holding (neural integration of velocity-coded to position-coded signals); this role is discussed further in Chapter 5.

One must ask why there are so many different cell types within the vestibular nuclei, and why they each may carry multiple signals in varying proportions. Part of the answer relates to the complexity of the processing within the vestibular nuclei: inputs from the otoliths and semicircular canals are combined with visual and other sensory inputs within the brainstem to create a 'best estimate', using all available information, as to the orientation of the body and its motion within the environment. One part of this task is to decipher the source of any imposed linear acceleration: Am I translating or am I tilted? And the correct response must then be elaborated based upon where the eyes are in the orbit and the depth and location of the point of regard relative to each orbit. Indeed, much of the complexity arises from requirements related to the t-VOR. In the past few years, some order has emerged, based upon combining the results from single unit recordings in the vestibular nuclei during different patterns of motion, with novel computational models of how the different signals must interact.[34,344,345,692,911]

A neural network approach also has been used to account for the diversity of signals encountered in the vestibular nuclei.[9] The essence of this idea is that the central nervous system adjusts the activity of an ensemble of neurons for optimal vestibular performance even though there can be considerable variability amongst individual neurons as to exactly what signals they carry and to which head rotations they respond optimally.[8] The attractive feature of such a model is that it is able to predict and account for the seemingly paradoxical finding of individual neurons that carry velocity signals for movement in one direction, and position signals for movement in another.

The Velocity-Storage Mechanism

Vestibular neurons respond to sustained rotational stimuli with an initial increment in discharge rate that declines exponentially with the same time constant as the r-VOR (15 seconds), not as the cupula or vestibular nerve (6 seconds). So, as early in the pathway as the vestibular nucleus, the performance of the r-VOR has been improved. This central phenomenon, by which the raw vestibular signal is prolonged or perseverated, is accomplished by the velocity-storage mechanism. It improves the ability of the r-VOR to transduce the low-frequency components of head rotation.[693] During sustained (low-frequency) rotations, the velocity-storage mechanisms also function to realign the axis of eye velocity with the direction of gravito-inertial acceleration (which usually calls for slow phases in a plane close to earth-horizontal). This effect, while seen in humans for small angles of lateral head tilt, is much more pronounced in monkeys.[18,21,226,280,282,327,692,694] Another related, and perhaps more fundamental, role for the velocity-storage mechanism may be in distinguishing tilt from translation so that the vestibular system can generate an appropriate t-VOR. Angelaki and Green have proposed a model for processing of linear acceleration signals, which has as a key component a head-velocity to head-position integrator used in distinguishing tilt from translation. It has been suggested that this integrator is identical to the velocity-storage integrator that determines the time constant of the r-VOR, though this remains to be proven.[13,34,344,345]

As noted above the vestibular commissure seems to be important for velocity storage. If it is sectioned, velocity storage is abolished.[412,461] Presumably interruption of pathways connecting the central portions of both MVN—the putative site for the generation of velocity storage—is responsible. Optokinetic after-nystagmus (OKAN), the decaying after response that is seen when a subject is placed in darkness following sustained optokinetic stimulation; the bias component of off-vertical axis rotation (OVAR), discussed in the next paragraph; and the modulation of the direction and time constant of the r-VOR with changes in head orientation, are also lost after section of the vestibular commissure.[863] Thus, without velocity storage, the r-VOR generates slow phases in a head-coordinate system, regardless of the direction of gravito-inertial acceleration. Presumably, the ability to distinguish tilt from translation would also be lost after interruption of the vestibular commissure. Although achieved by central vestibular connections, velocity storage depends upon the tonic discharge of the vestibular nerves;[187] section of one vestibular nerve shortens the time constant of the r-VOR. Because optokinetic signals also are processed in this same velocity-storage mechanism, bilateral vestibular nerve section abolishes OKAN.[188,904] Visual fixation of a full-field, earth-stationary surround for even a few seconds largely discharges or nullifies activity within the velocity-storage mechanism.[185,849] Ablation of the cerebellar nodulus and uvula (see Box 12–3 in Chapter 12) maximizes velocity storage, except perhaps when torsion is stimulated.[17,846] Stimulation of the nodulus and parts of the ventral uvula discharge velocity storage, sometimes asymmetrically.[769] The velocity-storage mechanism can also be influenced by cervical inputs.[456] The velocity-storage mechanism is suppressed by baclofen; presumably it mimicks the inhibitory, GABAergic actions of Purkinje cells from the nodulus on to the vestibular nuclei.[184,226a,410-412,846]

Off-vertical axis rotation is the compensatory response induced when a subject's body is rotated around its own axis when it is tilted away from the vertical. During a constant-velocity rotation, there is an initial response from stimulation of the semicircular canals due to the r-VOR. As the response from the semicircular canals dies away, it is replaced by an otolith-mediated response consisting of a steady-state velocity (bias component of OVAR) and a component that changes with the gravity vector (modulation component of OVAR). The bias component derives from the velocity-storage mechanism, and the modulation component from the direct otolith signal.[232,304,306,307,386,397,486,694,856] A similar pattern of response to OVAR can be obtained during constant velocity rotation about a vertical axis when combined with sinusoidal translation.[532] Because the changing orientation of the head with respect to gravity imposes a changing linear acceleration along the naso-occipital axis, not only is there the modulation component of slow-phase velocity, but also a sinusoidal modulation of the vergence angle as a function of head position with respect to gravity.[227] Bilateral lesions of vestibular nerve afferents abolish continuous nystagmus during OVAR.[187] Unilateral lesions lead to asymmetries in the modulation component.[451] Lesions of the nodulus affect the bias component of OVAR by virtue of its influence on the velocity-storage mechanism.[19,864] Patients with cerebellar ataxia may have an increased modulation component but an abnormal bias response.[11] Patients with brain stem lesions, too, may show different patterns of OVAR, with abnormalities in the bias component with caudal lesions and abnormalities in the modulation component with more rostral lesions.[811] Finally, age also has an effect on OVAR with a relative increase in the modulation component and relative decrease in the bias component.[304-306]

NEURAL SUBSTRATE FOR OPTOKINETIC RESPONSES

Both smooth pursuit and optokinetic systems contribute to the stabilization of images of stationary objects during head rotations. In humans, the optokinetic response to a full-field, moving visual stimulus has two stages: first, the prompt generation of nystagmus within 1 to 2 seconds of stimulus onset, with slow-phase velocity approximating stimulus velocity. This initial response mainly reflects smooth pursuit. Second, there is a slower buildup of "stored" neural activity. This activity is revealed as OKAN when the subject is placed in darkness.

In monkeys, vestibular nucleus neurons that respond to head rotation also are driven by optokinetic stimuli (Fig. 2–5).[395,848] Moreover, when the lights are turned off after a period of optokinetic stimulation, the vestibular nucleus neurons continue discharging for some seconds;[847] this is the neurophysiological correlate for OKAN. Vestibular nucleus neurons only respond well to low-frequency visual stimuli, in agreement with the demands made of the optokinetic system in replacing the r-VOR during sustained rotation.[119] Thus, during combined vestibular and optokinetic stimulation—which occurs during the natural situation of self-rotation—as the vestibular drive declines, the optokinetic input takes over and maintains a steady vestibular discharge that continues to generate compensatory eye movements (Fig. 2–5B). Thus the importance of testing OKAN is that it allows one to assay activity within the vestibular nuclei without employing any motion of the head. The neural substrate for OKN, and especially the nucleus of the optic tract (NOT) and accessory optic nuclei (AON), are discussed further in Chapter 4.

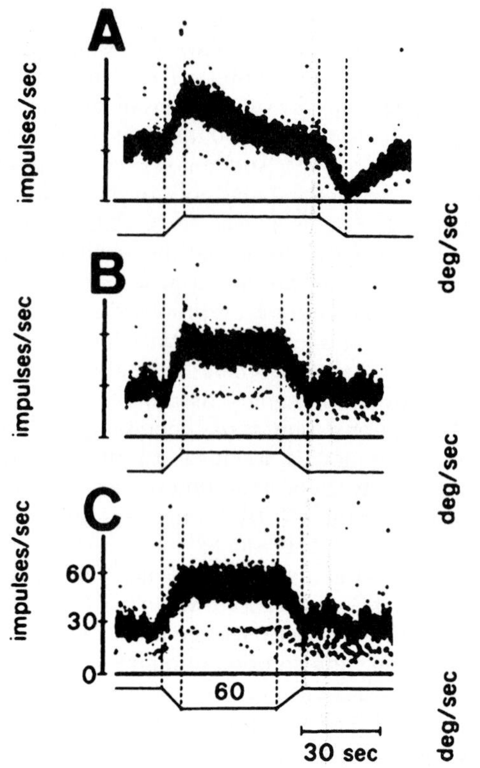

Figure 2–5. The response of a type I vestibular nucleus neuron of the alert rhesus monkey to vestibular and optokinetic stimulation. In each panel, instantaneous discharge rate (ordinate) is plotted against time (abscissa). Below each panel, the direction and magnitude of the stimulus is indicated (60 degrees per second). (A) The monkey is rotated in darkness. The initial vestibular response declines (to parallel the decline of per-rotatory nystagmus; see Figs. 1–4 and 2–7). (B) The monkey is rotated in the light. This time the neuron's response is sustained during the period of rotation. (C) The monkey sits stationary within a rotating optokinetic drum. This visual stimulus causes a sustained response of the same vestibular nucleus. (From Waespe and Henn,[848] with kind permission of Springer Science and Business Media.)

QUANTITATIVE ASPECTS OF THE VESTIBULAR-OPTOKINETIC SYSTEM

A quantitative description of any type of control system compares the output with a known input. Here we compare induced eye movements with head movements, using three important characteristics: (1) the ratio of amplitudes of the output and input (VOR gain); (2) the angle between the axis of head rotation and the axis of eye rotation (VOR direction); and (3) the temporal synchrony between the output and input (described by VOR phase or VOR time constant). We assume here that, to a first approximation, the VOR can be treated as a linear control system. In this case, transient and sinusoidal stimuli give rise to responses that are equivalent in terms of the mathematical information they reveal about the dynamic characteristics of a particular system. There are, however, important nonlinearities in the VOR, especially at high velocities, high accelerations, and at frequencies outside the usual range of natural head movements. These nonlinearities have important clinical and physiological implications.

Vestibulo-Ocular Reflex Gain, Direction, and Phase: General Characteristics

For the r-VOR, gain is given by the ratio of amplitude of eye rotation to amplitude of head rotation. For sine-wave stimuli (i.e., sinusoidal rotation of a subject in darkness, Fig. 2–6A), gain is usually calculated from peak slow-phase eye velocity/peak head velocity (Fig. 2–6B). The temporal difference between output and input is described by phase. Using sine-wave stimuli, the phase of eye and head movements may be compared (Fig. 2–6B); the difference (or phase shift) is expressed in degrees. For the frequencies of head rotation that correspond to most natural head rotations (0.5 cycles/second – 5.0 cycles/second), gain is close to 1.0 and phase shift is close to 180 degrees: equal-sized eye movements and head movements occur synchronously in opposite directions. By convention, the gain of the r-VOR that perfectly compensates for head rotations is assigned a value of 1.0, and the phase that perfectly compensates for head rotations is assigned a value of 0 degrees. For lower frequencies of rotation (less than 0.01 cycle/second), a shift in phase occurs and gain falls; this reflects the inability of the r-VOR to compensate for more sustained head rotations that contain low-frequency components. The ways that gain and phase change with different stimulus frequencies can be represented graphically, as a Bode plot (Fig. 2–6C).

Recent studies in the squirrel monkey have suggested that the phase and gain characteristics of the r-VOR can be best modeled with parallel linear (tonic) and nonlinear (phasic) pathways.[583] At higher frequencies of head rotation the gain of the r-VOR rises when velocity is above 20 degrees/second and this has been attributed to the actions of the nonlinear pathway. Likewise, the nonlinear pathway may mediate changes in the r-VOR for near viewing [575] and in adaptive changes in the r-VOR for higher frequency and higher velocity stimuli.[181,182,491,492,643] In the rhesus monkey, however, while there are also parallel phasic and tonic pathways, there is no evidence for a comparable nonlinearity to that of the squirrel monkey.[421] There is other evidence for parallel r-VOR pathways based upon studies of adaptation of the VOR.[681] The r-VOR in humans has also been modeled with parallel phasic and

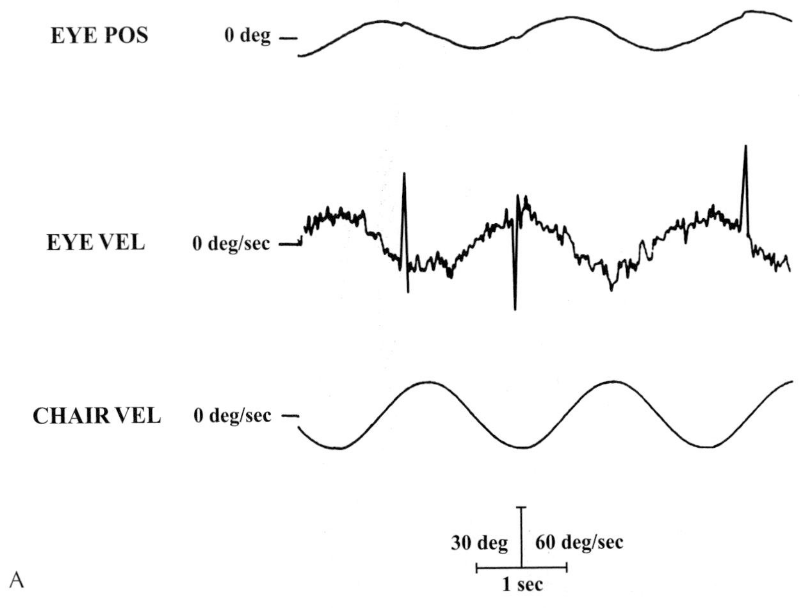

Figure 2–6. Quantitative evaluation of the vestibulo-ocular reflex using sinusoidal rotation in darkness. (A) A typical record of the VOR during sinusoidal rotation at 0.5 Hz. The subject is imagining the location of an earth-fixed target.

(Continued on following page)

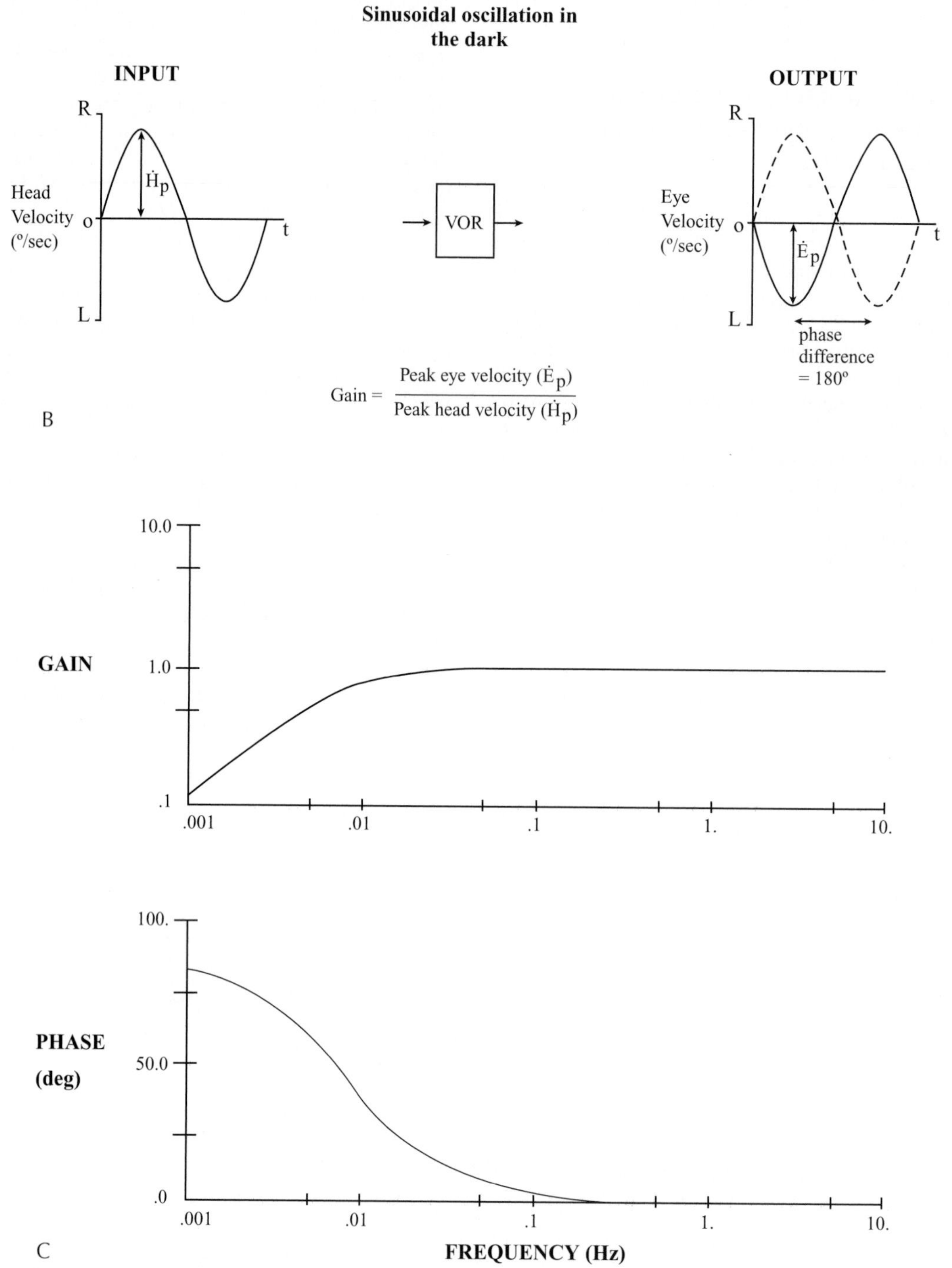

Figure 2–6. *(Continued)* (B) Schematic summary of vestibulo-ocular reflex during sinusoidal stimulation, as shown in (A). The graph on the left shows characteristics of the stimulus (head velocity) and the graph on the right shows the response (slow-phase eye velocity, quick-phases having been disregarded). R = right; L = left; t = time. In this case, vestibulo-ocular reflex gain is 1.0 and the phase difference between eye velocity and head velocity is 180° (by convention, this is referred to as "zero phase shift"). The dashed curve on the right represents head velocity. (C) A Bode diagram of the vestibulo-ocular reflex showing the idealized behavior of gain and phase with varying stimulus frequencies. Note that for the frequency range of most natural head rotations (0.5–5.0 Hz), gain is 1.0 and phase shift is zero degrees.

tonic pathways though the nature of any nonlinearity in the phasic pathway is as yet unclear.[493,643] An attractive, but not yet proven hypothesis is that the tonic (linear) and phasic (possibly with a nonlinearity) pathways correspond, at least in part, to the regular (tonic) and irregular (phasic) afferents, and to the type A and type B neurons within the vestibular nuclei, respectively (see above).

For sustained, constant velocity rotation (also called velocity steps or impulsive stimuli (i.e., an impulse of acceleration)), gain is usually calculated from initial eye velocity/head velocity. With such sustained rotations in darkness, vestibular eye movements (slow phases of nystagmus) progressively decline in velocity, and after about 30 to 45 seconds, the eye movements cease (see Fig. 1–6). The time course of the decline of slow-phase velocity is similar to a decaying exponential curve that can be defined by a time constant (Fig. 2–7). After one time constant, eye velocity has declined to 37% of its initial value; after three time constants, eye movements have nearly stopped. The time constant is mathematically related to the phase of the r-VOR observed during low-frequency sinusoidal stimulation: the larger the time constant, the less the dif-

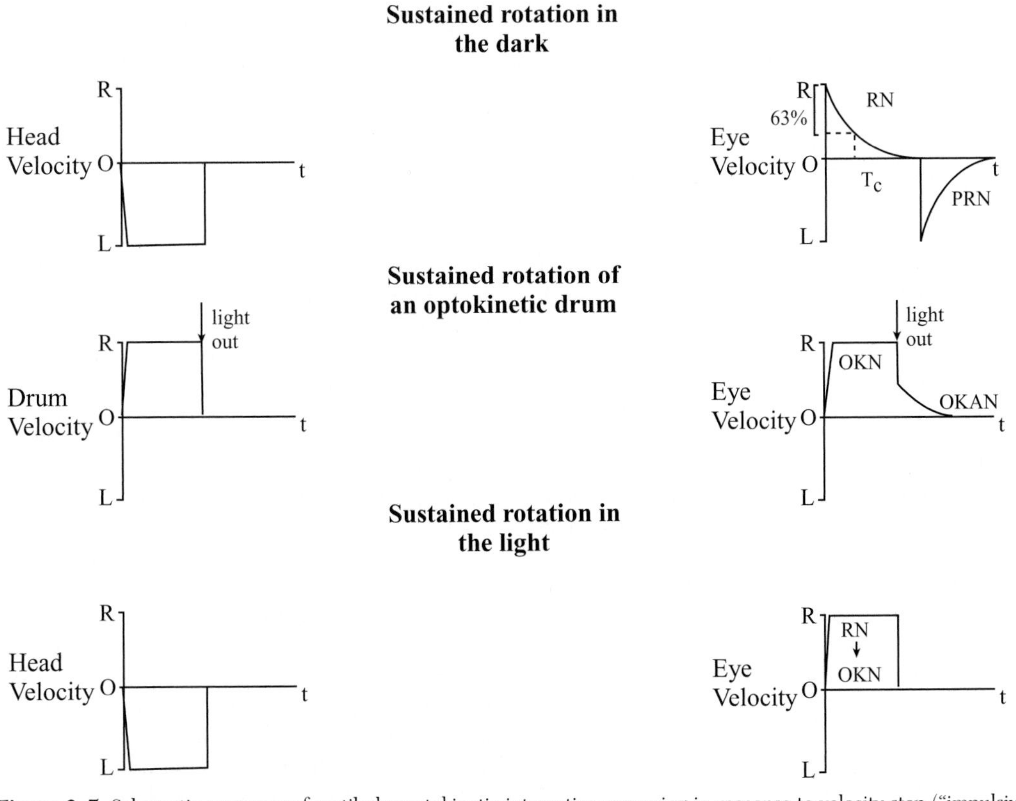

Figure 2–7. Schematic summary of vestibular-optokinetic interaction occurring in response to velocity-step ("impulsive" or constant velocity) rotations. Graphs on the left show characteristics of the stimulus (head velocity during rotation or drum velocity during optokinetic stimulation); graphs on the right show the responses (slow-phase eye velocity, quick-phases having been removed). R = right; L = left; t = time. In the top panel, constant-velocity rotation to the left in the dark produces slow-phase movements to the right (per-rotatory nystagmus, RN) with initial eye velocities equal to head velocity (VOR gain = 1.0). Slow-phase velocity subsequently declines. This decline may be approximated by a negative exponential with a time constant, T_C, given by the time taken for a 63% decline in eye velocity. When rotation stops, nystagmus starts in the opposite direction (post-rotatory nystagmus, PRN). In the middle panel, an optokinetic stimulus (drum rotation to the right) causes a sustained optokinetic nystagmus (OKN), with slow-phases to the right during the entire period of stimulation. When the lights are turned off during stimulation, eye movements do not stop immediately but persist as optokinetic after-nystagmus (OKAN). In the lower panel, the subject is rotated in the light (natural situation of self-rotation). This gives a combined vestibular and optokinetic stimulus. The response is a sustained nystagmus. When the chair stops rotating, eye movements stop nearly completely: post-rotatory nystagmus is suppressed by the oppositely directed optokinetic after-nystagmus and by visual fixation of the stationary world.

ference in phase between the head and eye at a given frequency and, hence, the better the compensation. The latency of the r-VOR is about 7 to 15 ms.

DETERMINANTS OF VESTIBULO-OCULAR REFLEX GAIN: ROTATIONAL VESTIBULO-OCULAR REFLEX

The gain and time constant of the human r-VOR are influenced by many factors, so normal ranges vary considerably. The torsional VOR, in response to roll rotation, has a lower mean gain value, typically 0.5, than the horizontal or vertical VOR to yaw or pitch rotations and can be influenced by the relative position of the roll axis and the gravity vector.[76,104,355,572,575a,658,658,720,721,735,736,819,821] The r-VOR measured in the light—the natural circumstance—may be more accurate (gain and axis of eye rotation) in the light than the dark, even at high frequencies of head rotation when visual following mechanisms are thought to be ineffective.[235,281,381,550]

During natural activities such as locomotion, the frequencies of rotational head perturbations may be greater than 5.0 Hz.[357] Measurements of the gain of the r-VOR with high frequency or brief, high acceleration stimuli have suggested that gain of the r-VOR is slightly less than 1.0 until frequencies of about 2 to 4 Hz and then rises to values of 1.0 or even higher at higher frequencies.[524,784] In response to transient stimuli the acceleration and velocity gains approach 1.0 early on, though there is a confounding effect of translation of the globe in the orbit, which may lead to a brief 'zero' latency anticompensatory response.[196] There is also a slight difference in latency between the two eyes with the adducting eye lagging the abducting eye by about 1 ms. This difference presumably reflects the presence of an extra neuron (the abducens internuclear neuron) in the pathway to the medial rectus.

Target Proximity

One important factor is that the gain of the VOR during head motion is affected by the proximity of the target (or imagined target) of interest. During viewing of a near target, the brain must compensate not only for the rotation of the head but also for the lateral or vertical displacement (translation) of the orbits (Fig. 7–7, Chapter 7). Consequently, the gain of the VOR for yaw or pitch axis rotation increases during viewing of a near object.[200,202,381,405,572,575,638,836] The perception of distance may be more important than the fixation distance based on vergence angle or on the actual target distance itself;[179,381,747] this is another piece of evidence for the relatively strong influence of higher-level cognitive control of adjustment of the gain of the t-VOR for translation of the head.[682] The exception to an adjustment for near viewing is the gain of the roll VOR, which elicits torsion and hence requires no change for near viewing. In fact, as discussed previously, there is some evidence that the gain of the roll VOR decreases at near to eliminate problems related to potential vertical misalignment of the eyes.[84,243a,443,572]

Mental Set

A second important determinant of the gain of the VOR, particularly when measured during rotation in darkness, is the mental set or imagined percept that the subject chooses during rotation.[74,381,446,590,591,638] If the subject imagines fixation of an earth-fixed visual scene during low-amplitude and low-frequency sinusoidal rotation, the gain of the r-VOR increases to approximately 1.0. On the other hand, if the subject imagines a visual stimulus that moves with the head, then the gain of the r-VOR declines to about 0.1. Finally, if the subject makes no attempt to imagine a visual stimulus but is distracted by performing mental arithmetic, the gain of the r-VOR is intermediate between these two extremes.[74] This voluntary control of the gain of the r-VOR is most effective during lower-frequency head rotations. If the subject daydreams or closes the eyes, the gain of the r-VOR is variable and low; thus it is important to keep the subject alert, such as by asking the subject to vocalize during vestibular testing.[536,872]

Active Versus Passive Head Rotation

While the passively induced r-VOR is close to compensatory over a relatively wide range of frequencies and velocities, active head rotations around the pitch and yaw axes still lead to a more faithful response, taking into account viewing distance and the different needs of both eyes related to translation of the orbits relative to the point of regard.[96,550] On the other hand, active head rotation around the roll axis still leads to an undercompensatory torsional VOR response. This might be due to a relative lack of exposure to pure roll rotations during natural behavior, the relative unimportance of torsional retinal slip in the retinal periphery, and the need to prevent vertical misalignment during rotation in roll when the eyes are converged.[586] The gain of the r-VOR is also enhanced by a prior eye movement,[234] light, *per se*,[235] and by predictive mechanisms during sinusoidal rotation.[381,877] Clearly, many factors can confound the interpretation of whether or not the gain of the VOR in a given subject under a given set of circumstances is normal.

Changes with Age

The VOR also changes with age. The elderly show a decrease in gain, predominantly at low frequencies of stimulation and high speeds of rotation. This is associated with increasing phase lead (i.e., a lower r-VOR time constant).[57,65,631,659,660] These changes in the r-VOR are probably related to the senescence of the velocity-storage mechanism and age-related loss of neurons within the vestibular system.[518,791] There are also age-related changes in OVAR.[304] Higher gains of the r-VOR have been reported in normal children, though OKN gains were equivalent to those for adults.[712] With head impulses in the elderly there are also changes in the r-VOR; initially the response is normal but it fades quickly.[800]

DETERMINANTS OF VESTIBULO-OCULAR REFLEX GAIN: TRANSLATIONAL VESTIBULO-OCULAR REFLEX

A number of investigators have measured the t-VOR response of human subjects to lateral motion.[49,67,144,203,323,324,638,682,683,728,750] The results are largely in accord with findings in monkeys.[28,547,577,639,640,728,794] All studies show that compensatory slow phases are a linear function of the reciprocal of the viewing distance, though humans tend to have a lower gain than monkeys (i.e., the movements are not truly compensatory). One possible explanation for the difference in the gain between the two species is that the various cues used to estimate the distance of the target of interest are weighted differently by monkeys and humans. Vergence and accommodation may be relatively more important for monkeys; size and other cognitive cues to distance may be more important for humans.[54,154,179,201,747,794,870] Another reason for an undercompensatory response of the human t-VOR is that the compensatory response to a given head translation depends critically upon the relationship of the position of the eyes in the orbit relative to the location and motion of the target relative to the head (see below). For example, during surge (fore and aft) translations the eye movement response is very different depending upon whether one is looking straight ahead (when vergence is called for) or when one is looking eccentrically (when there must be a large, nearly conjugate, horizontal or vertical component). Thus, it may be advantageous to keep the baseline t-VOR relatively low so the reflex can be adjusted up or down more easily depending upon viewing requirements.[682,683] Vergence cues may also be more important for adjusting the t-VOR gain for distance when the frequency of the stimulus is higher.[635,794] Mental set and context probably play important roles in "preparing" the anticipated response to head translation.[682] Indeed without the knowledge of whether the fixation point is going to be head fixed or space fixed, the t-VOR behaves differently than with the usual space-fixed target in which the t-VOR is traditionally tested. Because of the general undercompensatory nature of the t-VOR saccades become an important part of the response, being triggered automatically and scaling in a similar way to the slow-phase response. Thus, as is the case for the r-VOR when it is made undercompensatory by disease, the vestibular system uses the full ocular motor repertoire in the attempt to optimize vision during head motion. Finally, the gain of the actively generated t-VOR is much closer to ideal than is the response to passive translations, even in normal subjects.[549]

Influences of Direction of Gaze

As indicated above the response of the t-VOR critically depends on where the eyes are pointing (i.e., their positions in the orbit). The correct axis of eye rotation for a given direction of head translation must be calculated, so, for example, during naso-occipital motion, if the eyes are pointing upward, a vertical eye rotation is called for, but if the eyes are pointing to the side a horizontal eye rotation is called for. Depending upon whether gaze is up or down, or right or left, the direction of the eye movement will reverse. In addition, disconjugate eye movements may be needed (for example, during horizontal translation when the target of interest is off to the side), and even disjunctive eye movements—convergence and divergence—are required during naso-occipital translation when looking straight ahead.[547,639,684,765,803,813] The latency of the t-VOR in humans may be influenced by mental set, context, and viewing distance, especially at lower frequencies. For abrupt, high acceleration stimuli the latency is less than 20 ms.[682,683] The compensatory responses to vertical (bob, up-down) linear accelerations are subject to viewing distance in a way similar to the horizontal t-VOR.[634] In monkeys, the latencies of the vertical and horizontal t-VOR are about 12 to 18 ms.[25,155,728]

Several important questions about how otolith signals are processed to produce responses to linear acceleration are unanswered. First, the brain must distinguish linear acceleration associated with lateral tilt of the head, which calls for a static change in torsion or ocular counterroll, from linear acceleration associated with translation of the head, which calls for horizontal (to interaural translation) or vertical (to dorsal-ventral translation) slow phases. Inappropriate torsion occurs during interaural translation,[509] especially at low frequencies of translation.[794] Thus, the frequency of the stimulus may be one important cue, because in natural circumstances, relatively high-frequency stimulation of the otoliths is usually associated with translation, and relatively low-frequency stimulation with head tilt.[20,637,640,794] A model incorporating this idea is presented in Figure 2–8. There are other important factors, however. The static orientation of the head relative to gravity, on which an additional (translational) linear acceleration is imposed, can also influence whether inappropriate torsion occurs in response to translation, and whether it is conjugate.[558,561,562]

Recent work, using both intact and canal-plugged animals, with patterns of canal and otolith stimulation (roll-tilt and translation) that allow one to isolate the canal and otolith inputs to the t-VOR, has emphasized the importance of contextual cues from simultaneous semicircular canal activation during otolith stimulation.[26,344] For example, the activation of the vertical canals in association with activation of the otoliths during lateral head tilt and not in association with activation of the otoliths

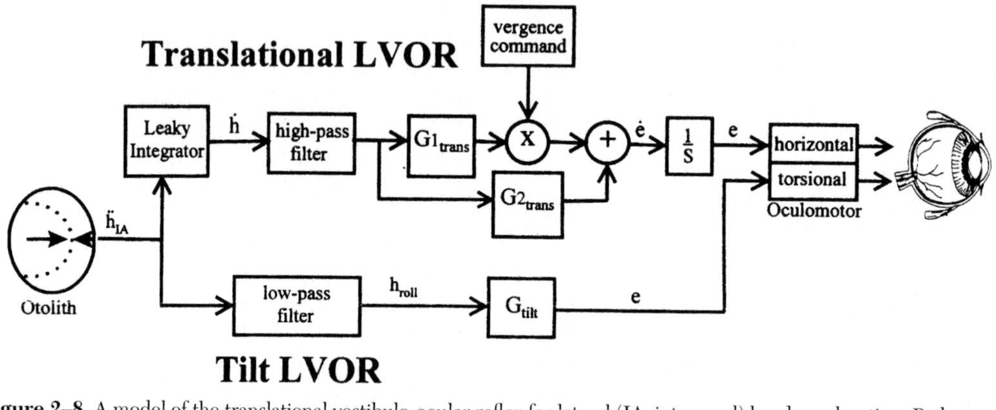

Figure 2–8. A model of the translational vestibulo-ocular reflex for lateral (IA, interaural) head acceleration. Pathways for the L-VOR (linear VOR) are shown. The tilt pathway contains a low-pass filter and scaling (G_{tilt}) to produce ocular counterroll. The translational pathway includes a mathematical integration (acceleration-to-velocity) and a high-pass filter before splitting into two subpathways, one with a gain element ($G2_{trans}$) that accounts for the response at zero vergence (an offset term, since theoretically no t-VOR is required when viewing is at optical infinity and vergence is zero), and another with a gain element ($G1_{trans}$) and a multiplier by which a "vergence command" signal is used to modulate response amplitude (which accounts for the slope of t-VOR gain as a function of vergence (i.e., viewing distance)). The summed output of these two subpathways (which is a velocity signal) is passed to a second integrator (the classic velocity-to-position integrator for conjugate eye movements) that generates the signal to control eye position. S is the Laplace transform operator. (Reproduced with permission of the American Physiological Society from Telford, Seidman, and Paige.[794])

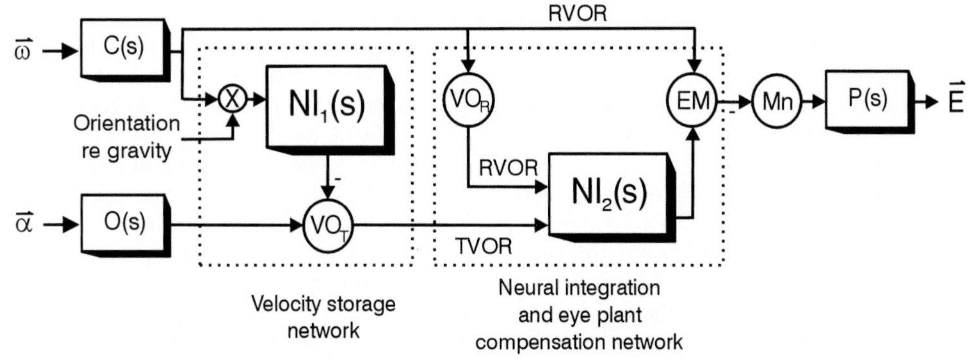

Figure 2–9. A model of the vestibulo-ocular reflex using an orientation detector based upon signals from the semicircular canals to resolve tilt and translation. Inputs to the model are angular head velocity $\{\vec{\omega}\}$, sensed by the semicircular canals C(s) and linear acceleration $\{\vec{\alpha}\}$, sensed by the otolith organs O(s). Output of the model is eye position $\vec{E}$. Boxes in the schematic are dynamic elements that represent either a sensor [C(s) and O(s)], the motor plant [P(s)], or a neural filtering process [NI_1(s), NI_2(s)]. Two central filtering processes include the "oculomotor integrator" [NI_1(s)] and an integrative network for the canal signals [NI_1(s)] that could be the velocity-storage integrator. Circles are summing junctions used to represent particular cell populations including vestibular-only (VO) cells, VO_r and VO_t, that mediate sensory signal flow in the RVOR and TVOR pathways, respectively, premotor eye-movement-sensitive (EM) neurons and motoneurons (Mn). Circle labeled with an X in the schematic indicates a proposed head-orientation-dependent modulation in the coupling between semicircular canal sensory signals and the integrative network NI_1. (Reproduced with permission from Green and Angelaki with permission of the American Physiological Society.[345])

during translation can help the brain to distinguish head translation from tilt.[14,26,34,35,345,911]

Based upon the above observations several groups have proposed new models for the organization of the central neural circuits underlying the generation of the t-VOR.[16,30,34,35,344-346,564-566,599,637,743a,911] One new idea relates to the processing of otolith signals by central vestibular pathways, and the other idea to distinguishing tilt from translation. These ideas are summarized in a recent model of the generation of the r-VOR and t-VOR (Fig. 2–9).[13,345]

There are two key points. First, at least in part, otolith and canal signals are processed differently within central vestibular pathways. While both are integrated centrally to produce an eye position signal, the canal signals have a strong direct projection to ocular motor neurons (which compensates for the filtering properties of the ocular motor plant), while otolith signals have a weaker direct projection to the ocular motor neurons so that at high frequencies of stimulation a second integration is provided by the ocular motor plant. These two integrations allow the t-VOR to transform the original otolith signals conveying information about linear acceleration into the appropriate position-coded signals for the eyes to compensate for head motion. The second point relates to how tilt and translation are distinguished. The crucial circuit here is an orientation network into which both canal and otolith signals project. They are then multiplied and integrated by a head velocity to head position integrator. The output of the integrator within this orientation network is then compared—possibly on vestibular only (VO) cells—with the net gravitoinertial acceleration as detected by the otoliths. Using these two signals the vestibular system can compute an internal estimate of head translation, which then drives the t-VOR. This model has many attractive features and the behavior of a number of neurons within the brain stem and cerebellum (including the fastigial nuclei) fit the requirements of the model.[34,345,743]

The following issues are still to be sorted out:

1. The effects of stimulation of the medial versus lateral portions of the utricle on which compensatory response is elicited, tilt or translation
2. The relative importance of the primary and of the polysynaptic projections of otolith-ocular reflexes
3. The possible role of irregular versus regular otolith afferents in distinguishing tilt from translation
4. The specific circuits that mediate

responses to tilt (which induces counterroll and must activate the vertical rectus and oblique muscles) and translation (which requires horizontal eye motion and must activate the horizontal rectus muscles)

5. The specific circuits that calculate and implement the necessary adjustments to the t-VOR response based upon the location of the eyes in the orbit relative to the direction of translation of the head.

Another issue relates to the role of the smooth pursuit system in the generation of the t-VOR.[54,144,638,752] Recall that functionally, pursuit and the t-VOR are complementary in the same way as OKN and the r-VOR. It may be that pursuit plays some role in generating the slow phases in response to low-frequency translations; the usual response to a natural low-frequency linear acceleration (tilt of the head) is ocular counterroll. High-frequency responses to linear acceleration (translation) probably occur independently of pursuit, as is the case for the r-VOR during high frequencies of head rotation.

DETERMINANTS OF VESTIBULO-OCULAR REFLEX GAIN: ECCENTRIC ROTATION

Transient responses to linear acceleration have also been investigated using a paradigm in which the axis of head rotation is placed eccentrically, combining linear and angular components. Both the viewing distance and the location of the axis of rotation relative to the orbits must be taken into account. Results in monkeys[561,639,766-768,836] are similar to those in humans.[10,201,208,561,738]

Studies in the monkey of the compensatory response to an abrupt rotation, with the head positioned eccentrically to the axis of rotation, have shown three sequential adjustments for viewing distance and the linear motion of the orbits that follow the initial response.[767] The first 20 ms of the slow-phase response is independent of viewing distance and the location of the rotation axis. In the next 20 ms, an adjustment is made for viewing distance. The next adjustment is for translation of the otoliths and occurs within 30 ms. The final adjustment—within 100 ms—is for eye translation relative to the visual target and compensates for the difference in the relative anatomic locations of the otoliths and the orbits. Coincident with these adjustments is an imposed disconjugacy of the VOR, which does not become evident until at least 10 ms after the VOR has begun. The adjustment of the VOR for vergence angle appears to be on the basis of an efference copy signal of vergence or some other internal measure of target distance, since the change in r-VOR anticipates the vergence change by about 50 ms.[768] The substrate for the modulation of the r-VOR during eccentric rotation may be, at least in part, in the flocculus of the cerebellum.[766] Patients with cerebellar disease also have difficulty adjusting the r-VOR for near viewing.[205]

In humans, the pattern of response to eccentric rotation appears roughly similar,[208,738] though recent work has emphasized the importance of cognitive set and prior knowledge of to where the line of sight must point.[682] In the first 40 ms after the onset of rotation there is an adjustment for target distance that is independent of translation. In the next 60 ms, an otolith-related adjustment (relative to target distance and the eccentricity of the head from the axis of rotation), appears and eventually masks the initial canal-related adjustment. The VOR during eccentric rotation is also adjusted during sinusoidal rotation.[207,351,738,838]

How are the various signals from the labyrinth during eccentric rotation combined centrally? In the monkey, the interaction between the angular and the linear VOR has been studied using combinations of linear and angular accelerations, at different frequencies, amplitudes, and head orientations.[637,792,793] By placing the head in front of or behind the center of rotation, the t-VOR can be made to add or subtract from the r-VOR. Overall, these data are compatible with the idea that the VOR during eccentric rotation is accounted for by summation of the isolated response to a comparable pure translation stimulus on a linear sled, and the isolated response to rotation with the head centered on the axis of rotation.

In humans, the linear and angular components of the VOR during eccentric rotation interact in a similar way, though there is some disagreement as to how well the interactions can be accounted for by simple summation of the t-VOR and r-VOR. In one study, the linear response associated with rotation was reported to be higher than would be predicted from simple linear summation of the t-VOR induced during pure translation and the r-VOR induced during head-centered rotation.[10] Likewise, the response to stimulation of the semicircular canals may inappropriately dominate the linear response and the effect of viewing distance.[145] In other studies of eccentric rotation during yaw (horizontal) and pitch (vertical) rotation, a linear model of canal and otolith interaction could account for the findings.[199,199,637,738] The specifics of the neuronal processing underlying these canal-otolith interactions remain to be demonstrated. As discussed above several models have been presented recently that emphasize building an internal model of head orientation using signals from the otoliths and the concomitant excitation of the semicircular canals to determine whether linear acceleration signals reflect tilt or translation.[34,73,563,692,694,911]

DETERMINANTS OF VESTIBULO-OCULAR REFLEX GAIN: DIRECTION AND THE AXIS OF EYE ROTATION

The direction of the r-VOR is determined by the angle between the axes of head and eye rotation. Not only must the amplitude of the VOR be equal (and opposite) to that of head rotation, but the axis of eye rotation must be parallel to that of head rotation. If this is not the case, there will be a misalignment of the axes around which the eyes and head rotate leading to inappropriately directed slow-phase eye movements. In the past this has been called 'perverted" nystagmus when, for example, caloric stimulation or horizontal head-shaking elicits a vertical nystagmus.[579,815] Such vestibular axis shifts arise in several circumstances. One example is when the VOR produces a normal amplitude and correctly directed response along the axis of stimulation but with an additional inappropriately directed component (e.g., a vertical component during yaw axis rotation). Another example is when the gain of one component of the VOR is different from that of the other during a rotation of the head around an axis that calls for two compensatory responses (e.g., a mixed vertical-torsional response during rotation around an axis perpendicular to the coplanar vertical canals on each side, for example, right anterior—left posterior (RALP), or left anterior—right posterior (LARP)). The gain of the torsional VOR is normally less than the gains of the vertical and horizontal VOR, so rotation of the head around any axis that calls for a mixed vertical-torsional or mixed horizontal-torsional response will lead to misalignment of the axes of head and eye rotation.[48,384,572,587,770,821]

Another source of axis misalignment for the horizontal and vertical VOR occurs when the position of the eye is moved in a direction orthogonal to the plane of eye rotation (e.g., positioning the eye up or down and then measuring the horizontal VOR for rotation around the yaw axis). If the axis of eye rotation remains head-fixed (and does not obey Listing's law—see Chapter 9) there should be no axis shift. Indeed this non-Listing's law strategy is optimal for the r-VOR as one would want the eye to rotate around an axis exactly parallel to that of the axis around which the head is rotating. If Listing's law is obeyed, however, there will be a torsional eye velocity component that, in the case of the horizontal VOR, is related to the degree of vertical eccentricity in the orbit, or in the case of the vertical VOR, to the degree of horizontal eccentricity in the orbit. The amount is dictated by the so-called half-angle rule for Listing's Law (the axis tilts by half the angle of eccentricity). The r-VOR actually obeys approximately a quarter-angle rule (producing a small amount of axis misalignment) though during the initiation of the VOR during rapid head impulses there is controversy as to whether or not the axis of eye rotation changes as the head rotation continues.[204,644,799,802]

Axis shifts also occur during sustained head rotations (i.e., low-frequency stimuli), and relate to the velocity-storage mechanism and the orientation of head with respect to gravity.[692] The cerebellar nodulus plays a key role in determining the axis shifts related to the velocity-storage mechanism.[189]

For the t-VOR, slightly more than the half-angle rule is obeyed (which is close to obeying Listing's law and similar to that of pursuit or saccades), as would be expected from a reflex that primarily serves the needs of foveal stabilization and binocular vision.[36,587,642,850] Another important determinant of the axis of eye rotation during the t-VOR is the location of the target of interest relative to the head (i.e., eye position in the orbit). For example, during surge (fore and aft) translations of the head, if the eyes are looking up, rotation around the pitch axis is desired; if looking laterally, rotation around the yaw axis; if looking straight ahead, a vergence movement is required. Because the calculation of the correct axis of eye rotation during translation of the head is so complex, one might expect that inappropriately directed eye movements during head translation would be common in both peripheral and central vestibular disorders. This may be true but has been looked at only in a few circumstances, with cerebellar lesions and after experimental unilateral labyrinthectomy, for example.[633,901]

One other issue related to the function of the VOR and Listing's plane is how the eyes get back into Listing's plane after a torsional slow-phase response to roll VOR or roll OKN stimulation. One strategy, of course, is to keep the gain of the torsional VOR relatively low, and this is the case.[586] Vestibular-induced saccades (i.e., quick phases) also help reset the torsional orientation of the eyes.[494,572,820]

Axis shifts become even more complicated with near viewing because Listing's plane undergoes a temporal shift when the eyes converge.[528,573,585] Another source of axis shift and disconjugacy in the horizontal VOR may relate to the changes in the position of the horizontal rectus connective tissues pulleys within the orbit. These pulleys determine the axis of eye rotation and they may change their positions on up and down gaze.[244] Pulley shifts also occur during static ocular counter-rolling and alter the pulling directions of the vertical torsional muscles.[243a]Axis shifts commonly occur with unilateral peripheral lesions[40,164,209,211,212] and with central, and especially cerebellar, lesions. In the latter there often is an inappropriately directed upward component during yaw axis rotation, which may also be different in the two eyes.[852,853,901] This 'cross-axis' abnormality has been attributed to 1) a loss of normal cerebellar inhibition on anterior canal VOR pathways and 2) a loss of the mechanism that adjusts for the differences in pulling directions of the oblique and rectus muscles that are innervated by the primary connections of the VOR.

DETERMINANTS OF VESTIBULO-OCULAR REFLEX PHASE AND TIME CONSTANT

The time constant of the human r-VOR, using velocity-step rotations, shows considerable inter-subject variation, with a range typically between 10 and 15 seconds.[61,185,659] As indicated above, these values are greater than predicted from the mechanical properties of the semicircular canals. Thus, the nystagmus outlasts the duration of the signal recorded from the vestibular nerve. The difference represents a prolongation or perseveration of the raw vestibular signal by the brain, and is accomplished by the velocity-storage mechanism. Factors that may cause the time constant of the r-VOR to decline include repeated testing (habituation),[4,59] peripheral vestibular disease,[136,279] and visual deprivation in early life.[754] Newborn babies have a time constant of the VOR that is about 6 seconds, but adult values are attained during the first few months of life. This change probably reflects maturation of visual pathways, which are important for calibration of the VOR, including the development of velocity storage.[756,873]

Static head position can also influence the time constant of the r-VOR though these effects are weaker in humans than in monkeys. Tilting of the head, forward or laterally, immediately following a head rotation, reduces the duration of post-rotational nystagmus, probably by disengaging or dumping activity in the velocity-storage mechanism.[105,189,282,283,692] During rotation around an earth-vertical axis, if the head is held in a tilted position, the time constant of the r-VOR measured in the earth-horizontal plane decreases in proportion to the degree of head tilt. The compensatory response has both horizontal and vertical components of rotation with respect to the orbit. The time constant of the two components may differ, leading to a change in the axis of eye rotation.[363,819]

Vertical vestibular responses may be asymmetric, often (but not always) favoring upward rather than downward slow phases.[55,56,107,468,535,819] Some of these asymmetries probably arise in the vertical velocity-storage mechanism (although this is relatively weak compared to the horizontal r-VOR), so they may appear or change direction during low-frequency stimulation (the later part of a constant-velocity rotation).[140,385,819,821] Circularvection—an illusory sensation of self motion induced by purely visual inputs—also shows an up-down asymmetry during pitch optokinetic stimulation.[311] In monkeys and cats, there is a spontaneous downbeat nystagmus in darkness; it may increase as the head is tilted away from the upright.[709] In humans, there is commonly a vertical drift in the dark, too, though in the head-upright position, it can be either up or down.[334] When the head is placed prone, an upward bias is added to the spontaneous drift present in the upright position. In the upside-down position normal subjects have a 'chin-beating' nystagmus.[466] These findings may be related to biases in the processing of information from the saccules (which are optimized to detect up-down linear acceleration of the head). Clinically, pathologic vertical nystagmus is more commonly down-beating, perhaps because of an inherent upward bias in the otolith system. Alternatively, there may be an inherent upward bias in canal pathways mediating the vertical r-VOR, either at a peripheral or central level,[111,433] though asymmetries in vestibulocerebellar pathways may also lead to an upward slow-phase bias.[531,665] The pathogenesis of downbeat nystagmus is discussed further in Chapter 10.

The time constant of the torsional VOR during rotation about an earth-vertical axis, with the subject's face supine or prone, is typically 4 to 5 seconds, suggesting that there is little velocity storage for the roll VOR.[735,819]

To sum up, the amplitude and direction of compensatory VOR responses around all three axes of rotation must be adjusted according to the rotational and translational components of the head movement, the point of regard (i.e., the target of interest), the position of the eye in the orbit, and a knowledge of the anatomic locations of the otolith organs relative to both orbits. Finally, any imposed linear acceleration must be separated into its gravitational and translational components. In addition, a number of cognitive factors come into play, depending upon context and anticipation. Thus, the VOR is subject to a variety of influences, making it a far more complicated reflex than previously thought.

Optokinetic Nystagmus

Optokinetic stimulation occurs naturally during sustained self-rotation in the light. In the laboratory, the optokinetic system is usually stimulated by rotating a large patterned drum around the stationary subject. The subject experiences a compelling sensation of self-rotation called *circularvection*, even though there is no peripheral vestibular stimulation.[77,125,569] During optokinetic stimulation in humans (e.g., the drum rotating at 60 degrees per second for 60 seconds, see Fig. 2–7), both the smooth pursuit and optokinetic systems contribute to this response. The ocular-following reflex—a rapid full-field visual following response that is closely allied to the mechanisms generating smooth pursuit—also contributes to the early phase of optokinetic tracking.[790] At the onset of the stimulus, the smooth pursuit system is most important and causes eye velocity to reach its maximum within a second or two. Typically, for stimulus velocities less than 60 degrees per second, the gain (eye velocity/stimulus velocity) is about 0.8.[66,288,831] Vertical optokinetic responses tend to be of lower gain than horizontal responses, and most subjects show a greater gain for upward stimulus motion than for downward.[107,317,535,595] A number of possibilities might explain this difference including asymmetry in otolith (saccular) inputs, vertical semicircular canal inputs, and central processing of up and down slow-phase eye movements.[665] If the subject actively looks at the moving stimulus, greater eye velocities can be achieved than if the subject passively stares at the surround. This difference may represent greater activation of smooth pursuit during the former condition. The luminance of the target is also an important factor.[859] Attention to the stimulus may be as important as the area of retina being stimulated in determining the optokinetic response.[1,1a,156,173] The gain of vertical optokinetic nystagmus (OKN) is influenced by binocular disparity. This finding supports the view that the optokinetic response is optimized for viewing of objects in the plane of regard.[416,576] The effects of attention and prediction on visual tracking are discussed further in Chapter 4. Like pursuit, OKN gain declines with age, due to a loss at both high frequencies and high velocities.[287,630] Curiously, circularvection may become enhanced with age, perhaps reflecting greater dependence on visual cues for orientation in the elderly, as labyrinthine and proprioceptive sensations become blunted.[631]

Torsional OKN can be induced by a roll stimulus. For example, watching a revolving disk directly in front of oneself elicits such a response. The gain and range of torsional OKN responses are low and depend upon size of field, speed, and disparity.[174,175,197,272,417,

[424,593,843,860] Torsional OKN may be asymmetrical in unilateral vestibular loss, showing a better response when the torsional slow phases are such that the top pole rotates toward the impaired side.[517]

Optokinetic After-Nystagmus

An important property of the optokinetic system is a persistence of the response after the stimulus has ceased. During the stimulation period, the optokinetic system effectively acts through the velocity-storage mechanism. After the lights are turned out, nystagmus continues in the same direction for some seconds, with a declining slow-phase velocity; this is called optokinetic after-nystagmus (OKAN). The velocity-storage mechanism that causes OKAN is probably the same one that causes the time constant of the r-VOR to be 2 to 3 times greater than the time constant of the cupula of the semicircular canals.

As can be seen in Figure 2–7, the optokinetic and vestibular systems temporally complement each other during and following sustained rotation in the light. Thus, during rotation, as the r-VOR declines, optokinetic responses, supplemented by the pursuit system, take over. When the period of self-rotation ends, OKAN is a mechanism by which post-rotational nystagmus can be counteracted.[75] Overall, however, in foveate animals, visual fixation (and smooth pursuit) are more important in nullifying post-rotational nystagmus.

In humans and monkeys, the properties of the optokinetic system can only be separated from those of smooth pursuit by studying OKAN. Four separate measures of OKAN are initial eye velocity, time constant of slow-phase decline, cumulative slow-phase eye position, and symmetry. If all lights are turned out after a period of optokinetic stimulation (e.g., 60 degrees per second or 150 degrees per second for 60 seconds), initial eye velocity reflects the persisting action of smooth pursuit, but this is largely gone within a second, and subsequently the initial value of OKAN can be measured. (Typically it is 10 degrees per second.)[734,808] Maximal amounts of OKAN are produced by relatively large values of retinal slip, in the range of 30 to 100 degrees per second.[288] By measuring the rate of decline of slow-phase velocity, and fitting this with a negative exponential curve, the time constant of OKAN can be determined; reported values range considerably, from 5 seconds to nearly 50 seconds. [288,488,734,808] Cumulative slow-phase eye position (the sum in degrees of all the slow phases) is another, less variable measure of OKAN.[368] Most normal subjects show less than a 6 degrees per second difference between rightward and leftward initial OKAN velocities.

Because of considerable intra-subject variability in measurements of initial OKAN eye velocity and time constant, it is necessary to make as many as a dozen separate measurements to obtain reliable results.[808] One way of achieving this, and avoiding prolonged and tedious testing, is to monitor the buildup of slow-phase velocity of OKAN during stimulation, by briefly turning out the lights at intervals.[734] This procedure is detailed further in the section below.

Optokinetic after-nystagmus declines with age.[757] OKAN may be more prominent in women.[808] With the head upright, OKAN in the vertical plane is usually absent and, when present, only occurs following upward stimulus motion.[107,502,535,595] These asymmetries are affected by head tilt[198] and space flight.[177,180] They are also modified in the altered-gravity period during parabolic flight, implicating otolith (saccule) inputs in their genesis.[177,867] There are asymmetries in the illusions of motion in response to vertically moving optokinetic stimuli that correspond to asymmetries in vertical optokinetic eye movement responses.[520] Similar to vestibular testing, repeated optokinetic stimulation can lead to reduced duration of OKAN.[444] Tilting the head forward, backward, or laterally shortens the duration of OKAN, an effect similar to that of head tilt on post-rotational nystagmus.[868] Fixation of a small, stationary target during optokinetic stimulation suppresses subsequent OKAN,[125,288] though a reversal phase of OKAN may appear if the period of stimulation is relatively long.[484] On the other hand, a brief period of fixation of a stationary target following optokinetic stimulation has little effect on OKAN.[288] These results suggest that fixation of a small target may act to "switch off" visual inputs to the velocity-storage mechanism, but once the mechanism is "charged", fixation has little influence on the course of OKAN.

Cervico-Ocular Reflex

The cervico-ocular reflex (COR), when tested in darkness using rotation of the body underneath the stationary head, has a low gain at frequencies corresponding to most natural head rotations for normal human subjects.[448,716,723] Only in some infants may a higher gain be seen,[458,697] and the gain may increase again in old age.[462] If labyrinthine function is lost due to disease, however, the COR may increase in gain and assume greater importance in generating compensatory eye rotations during natural head movements.[148,148,393,458,723] In patients with bilateral loss of vestibular function, isolated stimulation of cervical afferents during body rotation produces both slow phases and catch-up saccades in the same direction (i.e., opposite to relative head motion) to aid gaze stabilization (see Table 7–1). If labyrinthine function recovers, the cervico-ocular reflex may revert to its previous low gain.[147] In labyrinthine-defective patients, and even in normal subjects, the COR can be enhanced when subjects are instructed to attempt to fix upon a part of their trunk that is moving relative to the stationary head, rather than just to keep their eyes focused on a stationary position in space.[423] The latter instruction could act to cancel compensatory slow phases, unless there was a perception of the head moving in space. The COR can be actively trained in labyrinthine-deficient patients using magnifying and reducing lenses in a similar way to adaptation of the gain of the r-VOR.[423] Indeed adaptive changes in the COR can be induced in normal subjects.[698] Again, the mental set and the perception of the subject of the context in which the neck afferents are being stimulated are critical in determining whether the COR should be enhanced (if the head is perceived to be moving) or decreased (if the head is perceived to be still).[393,729] Cervico-ocular reflexes contribute little to ocular counterroll (with lateral tilt of the head relative to the body) in normal subjects, but in patients with bilateral labyrinthine loss, their contribution can be considerable.[101,458,666] Patients with bilateral labyrinthine loss and coincident cerebellar disease may not show enhancement of the COR, suggesting a role for the cerebellum in this aspect of vestibular adaptation.[148] Cervical afferents may influence the velocity-storage mechanism; OKAN is made asymmetric during optokinetic stimulation with the head kept turned relative to the body.[456] The COR is mediated by the same neurons in the vestibular nuclei that underlie the VOR, and the flocculus, too, may influence the COR.[321,322] The issue of cervical vertigo is discussed in Chapter 11.[122]

ADAPTIVE PROPERTIES OF THE VESTIBULO-OCULAR REFLEX

The brain shows a remarkable ability to adapt* the VOR to prevailing environmental circumstances. The VOR can compensate for the effects of disease and trauma and the changes that occur with growth and aging. From a profound loss of labyrinthine function on one or both sides to wearing a new spectacle prescription, the VOR must detect errors in performance and correct for them. Mechanisms exist to maintain balanced levels of tonic activity—to prevent spontaneous nystagmus—and to ensure calibrated compensatory responses to head motion, so that slow phases are of the correct amplitude, direction, and timing (phase). Other mechanisms and strategies also help stabilize the line of sight during head movement; they become especially evident when there is a loss of the peripheral vestibular signal. In this section we will discuss habituation, the short-term adaptation that produces the reversal phases of nystagmus, calibration of the VOR in response to imposed visual-vestibular mismatches, and then recovery from loss of labyrinthine function.

Vestibulo-Ocular Reflex Habituation

Although impaired vision during head movements is the basis for many adaptive changes in the performance of the VOR, the VOR shows

* We will not make a rigid distinction here between the terms "adaptation" and "compensation." Usually, "adaptation" is used in a more restricted sense, to imply adjustment in the basic vestibulo-ocular reflex, whereas "compensation" is used in a larger sense, to include the entire repertoire of ways, including substitution, prediction, and other cognitive strategies, by which patients recover from, and learn to live with, vestibular disorders. Habituation (see below) is the phenomenon in which there is a gradual diminution in the response to repetitions of an identical stimulus.

habituation (i.e., a reduction of time constant and gain) to repetitive stimuli in complete darkness. Habituation is most evident after repeated constant-velocity rotations or low-frequency continuous oscillations (stimuli outside the frequency range of most natural head rotations).[4,59,178] Analogous to other sensory systems, it may contribute to eliminating the persistent spontaneous nystagmus that follows a unilateral labyrinthine lesion. The vestibulocerebellum is involved in habituation as removal of the nodulus prevents it.[190] Functional imaging shows widespread changes in activation or deactivation in cerebral cortex and subcortical structures during habituation, which may relate to changes in the nystagmus pattern.[608] The relevance of habituation to clinical testing is that patients previously subjected to repetitive stimuli that contain a low-frequency component (for example, ice skaters who do long, high-speed spins), may have unusually low time constants of the r-VOR.

Short-Term Vestibulo-Ocular Reflex Adaptation that Produces Reversal Phases of Nystagmus

Adaptive mechanisms are also engaged by the presence of a persistent, unchanging vestibular stimulus. Such a stimulus almost never occurs in natural circumstances except when there is a lesion that creates an imbalance in vestibular tone between the two sides. This results in a spontaneous nystagmus. For example, with a constant-velocity rotation, after the original nystagmus dies out, a reversal phase of nystagmus may develop with slow phases in the opposite direction (i.e., the same direction as head rotation) (see Fig 1–6). This phenomenon probably reflects an adaptive mechanism, residing in both the brain stem and the peripheral vestibular apparatus, which has been activated by a persistent vestibular stimulus.[309,500] It has a time constant of action of about 80 seconds, so that its effect is completed in minutes. One natural cause of such a persisting vestibular signal is an imbalance in the tonic levels of activity due to a peripheral labyrinthine disturbance; the adaptation mechanism could help to nullify the pathologic spontaneous nystagmus. Such a mechanism, however, probably works best only for small degrees of imbalance; after a unilateral loss of labyrinthine function, it may take days for vestibular tone to be brought back into balance, eliminating the spontaneous nystagmus. Prolonged optokinetic stimulation also may cause ocular motor and perceptual aftereffects that are manifestations of motion habituation.[124] Like per-rotatory or post-rotatory nystagmus, optokinetic after-nystagmus may be followed by a reversal phase (OKAN II).

The adaptation mechanism producing the reversal phases of nystagmus is particularly prominent in infants.[873] Its action may become particularly obvious in patients with cerebellar lesions; it is responsible for the change in the direction of the slow phase that characterizes periodic alternating nystagmus (see Video Display: Periodic Alternating Nystagmus).[500] The reversal phase of head-shaking–induced nystagmus is another manifestation of this same mechanism.[364]

Visually Induced Adaptation of the Vestibulo-Ocular Reflex

The VOR functions in an inherently "open-loop" manner. Because of the brief periods and short latencies within which it must operate, immediate visual inputs cannot correct for most imperfections, because of the time taken in retinal processing. Consequently, the brain must continuously monitor the effectiveness of its VOR and adjust it accordingly when it malfunctions. Longer-term adaptive capabilities, based upon visual error signals during head motion, must be used.

ADAPTATION TO REVERSING PRISMS AND SPECTACLE LENSES

A dramatic example of the effects of changed visual demands upon the VOR are the consequences of viewing the world through head-fixed optical devices such as mirrors or prisms that laterally invert the world, left to right.[335,336,551] While wearing such devices, head turns cause the environment to appear to move in the same direction as head turning. After just a few minutes of head rotation during reversed vision, the gain of the r-VOR (measured during rotation in darkness) declines. Subjects also adopt strategies such as altering the pattern of head motion or using saccades to help stabilize gaze in this altered visual environment.[86,553] After removal of the optical device, gain rapidly returns to its previous value. With longer periods of exposure to visual inversion, changes in the VOR are retained for a longer period, such as overnight. In subjects who wear reversing prisms for 3 to 4 weeks, large changes of gain and phase occur that actually reverse their VOR; head rotations cause eye movements in the same direction. Thus, the gain and phase of the r-VOR are changed so that images are once again stable upon the retina during head movements. While these adaptive changes are taking place, subjects report symptoms of motion sickness, reflecting the conflict between vestibular and visual cues.[554]

A less extreme and more common visual demand on the VOR is wearing a spectacle correction. Spectacle lenses have a prismatic effect that is called rotational magnification, to distinguish it from the linear magnification that produces clearly focused images. This means, for example, that individuals who wear high-positive lenses (e.g., for aphakic correction or hyperopia) must rotate their eyes more when they attempt to change their line of sight, compared to when they are not wearing their glasses. Similarly, they will be required to rotate their eyes proportionally more during rotations and translations of the head in order to hold images steady upon the retina, compared to when they are not wearing glasses. Nearsighted (myopic) individuals who habitually wear negative spectacle lenses have lower values for the gain of the r-VOR than far-sighted (hyperopic) individuals, or patients who have had their lenses removed and habitually wear positive spectacle lenses.[162] Individuals who habitually wear contact lenses show no such changes in the gain of the r-VOR; because the contact lenses rotate with the subject's eyes, there is no rotational magnification effect. Adaptation of the r-VOR to spectacle correction occurs rapidly in normal subjects. More than 50% of subjects show significant changes in the gain of the r-VOR after wearing telescope lenses for 15 minutes.[245] Older subjects are capable of developing such short-term adaptation, but the response is diminished.[631] Theoretically, habitually wearing a spectacle correction should lead to changes in the t-VOR but this has not been examined experimentally.

Changes in the gain of the r-VOR occur over a broad frequency range and not just at the testing frequency. With prolonged training at one frequency of rotation, however, adaptive gain changes are greatest at the training frequency.[512] If subjects wear '2X' magnifying lenses for several days during natural behavior, then an increase of the gain of the r-VOR is most evident for testing frequencies of rotation of the head greater than 2 cycles/second.[429] With shorter periods of wearing the lenses, however, adaptation may be greater for lower frequencies.[636] Amplitude nonlinearities, with less adaptation at higher velocities, may become apparent.[636] There are also differences in adaptive capabilities that can be frequency (high or low) or direction (up or down) dependent.[408,533] Critical to understanding why there are such differences in adaptive responses is consideration of an important principle of VOR, and presumably many other types of motor adaptation: the adaptive response is tailored to the context of the adaptive stimulus. Differences in how subjects move their heads under natural circumstances may influence the adapted response.

In addition to using optical devices, VOR adaptation can be studied by prolonged rotation of subjects while artificially manipulating the visual surround, either across the visual field,[479] or even in depth.[5] One can use an optokinetic drum that surrounds the subject, and rotate it in phase—in the same direction as chair rotation—to produce a decrease in the gain of the VOR, or out of phase—opposite the direction of chair rotation—to produce an increase in the gain of the VOR. If the amplitude of drum rotation is exactly equal to that of the chair, the required VOR gain would be 0.0 for in-phase viewing (so-called $\times$ 0 viewing) and 2.0 for out-of-phase viewing (so-called $\times$ 2 viewing). The usual duration for VOR training in these types of paradigms is an hour or two, although adaptation of the VOR can probably be detected within minutes of the onset of the change in the relationship between the visual and vestibular stimuli.[195] These relatively short-term adaptation experiments probably test only one type of vestibular adaptation, because the learned response is not sustained in the absence of continued stimulation. There is also a long-term adaptive process, taking days to weeks, rather than just minutes to hours, which gradually supervenes and leads to a more enduring, resilient adaptive change.[401,406,407,458a,485] Thus, one must be cautious when extrapolating results from these short-term experiments to the long-term problems of patients adapting to chronic vestibular deficits.

Adaptive capabilities have been investigated in elderly subjects[631] and at higher frequencies (above about 0.75 Hz); their ability to increase the gain of the r-VOR adaptively is significantly diminished. Because the r-VOR is most needed to compensate for the high-frequency components of head rotation, a loss of adaptive capability in elderly patients could account for their more disabling and persistent symptoms after a vestibular loss. Furthermore, with aging, patients with deficient vestibular responses lose some ability to substitute corrective saccades for hypometric slow phases.[804,805]

CROSS-AXIS ADAPTATION OF THE VESTIBULO-OCULAR REFLEX

A variety of paradigms have been used to demonstrate the wide repertoire of VOR adaptive responses, including the ability to change the direction, phase (timing), and amplitude of the VOR. For example, if the head is rotated horizontally (in yaw) while the visual display is synchronously rotated vertically, after a training period, horizontal rotations in darkness will produce eye movements that have a vertical component.[24,298,465,651,727,851] Similar adaptation occurs with head rotation in pitch and horizontal pursuit eye tracking,[300] or head rotation in yaw and torsional optokinetic stimulation.[816] This *cross-axis plasticity* accords with electrophysiological evidence that secondary neurons in the vestibular nucleus receive inputs from one, two, or all three pairs of semicircular canals.[52] Furthermore, during cross-axis training, neurons in the vestibular nuclei that are normally maximally sensitive to pitch axis (vertical) stimulation increase their sensitivity to yaw axis (horizontal) rotation,[678] providing a neurophysiologic substrate for the change in direction of the VOR. Similar considerations apply to the fact that wearing left-right reversing prisms calls for a change in the torsional (roll) but not vertical (pitch) VOR gain. Such a selective change in the VOR takes place even though both torsional and vertical signals are carried on the same vestibular afferents.[78,90,91]

A matrix analysis of the problem of producing slow phases in a direction orthogonal to head motion, or producing a change in torsional gain alone has been presented by D.A. Robinson.[703,703] Thus, one matrix represents the vectors of the semicircular canals, a second matrix represents the pulling actions of the extraocular muscles, and a third matrix represents the strength of central connections between vestibular neurons and ocular motoneurons. The third matrix—the brain stem matrix—makes the necessary adjustments both for the contributions of the different semicircular canals to the detection of the axis of head rotation and for the different pulling directions of the extraocular muscles that are innervated by the primary VOR reflex pathways. When head movements are artificially dissociated from apparent motion of the visual environment, as described above, then a change in the central, brain stem matrix must occur so that, for example, vertical eye rotations are coupled to horizontal head rotations, or the torsional VOR gain is selectively enhanced or depressed. A similar matrix analysis has been developed for binocular responses to the VOR.[839]

OTHER FORMS OF VESTIBULO-OCULAR REFLEX ADAPTATION

Other examples of VOR adaptive capabilities include changes in dynamic characteristics such as the phase (timing) of the VOR.[391,480,481,667,695,696] Adaptation of the phase of the VOR also leads to a change in the time constant of the ocular motor velocity-to-position integrator (either making it less reliable ('leaky') or unstable), emphasizing the important role of the neural gaze-holding integrator in assuring that compensatory slow phases have the correct phase relationships during motion of the head.[171,391,481,758] Disconjugate adaptation of the r-VOR may occur in response to a unilateral muscle palsy,[837,880,881] for example, or to wearing prisms in front of one eye.[627] Such a capability is especially important for a correct compensation to the translational component of head (orbit) motion, because the eyes must rotate by different amounts whenever the point of regard is near to the subject. The vertical and torsional VOR undergo similar adaptive adjustments as does the horizontal

VOR though in the case of torsion the mechanisms may be somewhat different.[90,91,771,816]

Otolith-ocular reflexes are also subject to adaptive control. VOR learning acquired with training during upright (yaw axis) rotation is transferred to the otolith-derived modulation component of OVAR.[477,857] Similarly, there is (inappropriate) transfer to otolith-mediated slow-phase compensation during orthogonally directed rotations (head-over-heels).[664] Prolonged centrifugation can lead to changes in the roll (torsional) r-VOR,[356] though 2 hours of static lateral head tilt (up to 34°) in monkeys induced no change in ocular counterrolling.[782] The response of the VOR to translation of the head is also under adaptive control.[391,476,682,737,857,869,909] In the absence of canal-driven responses, otolith-ocular responses to a changing gravity vector (which can occur when rotation is around an axis tilted away from the vertical) are potentiated, leading to improved stabilization of gaze during off-axis rotation of the head.[30]

Cognitive Control of Vestibulo-Ocular Reflex Adaptation

Although a visual stimulus (motion of images on the retina) is the main determinant of the pattern of these adaptive changes of the VOR, even imagination of a visual stimulus can be enough to bring about plastic changes in the gain of the r-VOR, although at about half the rate that occurs when visual stimuli are used.[552] Indeed, simply imagining body rotation can lead to compensatory slow-phase eye movements.[704] Along these lines,[266] it has been shown that just paying attention to, without even looking at, the new location of a target after a head rotation (i.e., using a position rather than a retinal image motion error), leads to adaptive modification of the VOR. Thus, what are usually called psychological factors—motivation, attention, effort, and interest—may actually play a more specific role in promoting adaptive recovery. Even an afterimage placed on the retina or strobe illumination, neither of which allow for retinal image motion, can stimulate adaptation of the r-VOR.[300,529,749] There are perceptual concomitants of adaptation of the VOR that accord nicely with the ocular motor responses that are measured in darkness.[102]

Context-Specific Vestibulo-Ocular Adaptation

Probably one of the more critical aspects of successful vestibular compensation in natural circumstances is a capability for VOR adaptive responses to be expressed on the basis of context. The attitude of the head relative to gravity, the position of the eye in the orbit including the vergence angle, and the frequency content and pattern of the head movement are potent contextual cues for the gating of different vestibular responses.[480,505,668,748,753,809,866,886,888,889] For example, the horizontal r-VOR can be made to have an increased gain when the vertical eye position is up in the orbit, and a decreased gain when the eye is down in the orbit,[751] or the horizontal r-VOR can be adapted selectively for different viewing distances.[505] In other words, the brain has mechanisms to enlist different learned vestibular responses depending upon the circumstances in which they must occur. This type of adaptive capability has important clinical implications for the programs of physical therapy that are prescribed for patients with vestibular deficits. The specific exercises should be close to the type of stimuli that are encountered naturally and produce symptoms if the VOR is not working correctly.

Mechanisms of Recovery from Lesions in the Labyrinth

Thus far, we have discussed adaptive responses that affect the gain of the VOR symmetrically. But a common and important clinical problem is how the brain compensates for unilateral labyrinthine lesions (see Box 11–1, Chapter 11). What factors influence the rate and pattern of recovery from a peripheral vestibular lesion?[222,223,230,612,762,763] Here we will highlight some key features based upon a study of experimental, unilateral labyrinthectomy in monkeys, which illustrates how different parts of the recovery process depend upon visual or non-visual factors.[286,897] In the first 24 hours following labyrinthectomy in the monkey, there is a head tilt and turn towards the side of the lesion. With the head stationary, spontaneous nystagmus, with slow phases directed towards the side of the lesion, is present in light and darkness. The nystagmus indicates a static vestibular imbalance. The slow-phase velocity in the dark (20 degrees per second to 60 degrees per second) is much greater than in the light (up to 4 degrees per second), illustrating that visual fixation suppresses this nystagmus. The velocity of the slow phases of nystagmus declines during the next few days, irrespective of whether the monkeys are kept in a dark or an illuminated environment. Moreover, in monkeys that have previously undergone bilateral occipital lobectomy, resolution of spontaneous nystagmus occurs at a similar rate. Thus, recovery from the static imbalance that follows a unilateral labyrinthine lesion does not depend upon vision. Recovery of static balance from unilateral labyrinthine loss in humans may never be complete; in darkness, some patients show spontaneous nystagmus years after their lesion. The basis of the resolution of the spontaneous nystagmus after a unilateral loss of function is largely a restoration of activity on the side of the lesion.[762]

Other factors may supervene early in the compensation process, including, for example, suppression of activity on the intact side.[538,699] Later during compensation, subjects may employ strategies apart from changing the gain of the slow-phase response, especially the use of saccades to substitute for hypometric slow phases.[87,96,652,653,732,771a,801] An additional finding after recovery from labyrinthectomy in monkeys is an increased response to cold caloric stimulation of the normal ear. Similar findings have been reported in humans.[422] The change in caloric responses may represent an adaptive increase in vestibular nucleus sensitivity on the intact side.

Recovery from the dynamic vestibular imbalance that follows unilateral labyrinthectomy depends on *visual inputs*; the gain of the VOR does not increase in monkeys kept in darkness. Moreover, monkeys that have undergone bilateral occipital lobectomy before labyrinthectomy show only a partial recovery, with little compensation for high-velocity stimuli. This finding suggests that both striate and extrastriate visual pathways play a role in the recovery of dynamic vestibular responses following unilateral labyrinthectomy. These findings contrast with the recovery from static vestibular imbalance, which does not depend upon visual factors.

Presumably, the contribution of the occipital lobes is that they transmit information about slippage of images on the retina during head movements to the more caudal structures that, in turn, use this error information to readjust the dynamic performance of the VOR. The nucleus of the optic tract (NOT) in the pretectal region of the midbrain is one such structure shown to be important in VOR adaptation. The NOT receives visual information from the cerebral cortex as well as directly from the retina. It has a strong projection to the inferior olive and to other brainstem nuclei that also project to the cerebellum. Lesions in the NOT interfere with compensation to unilateral labyrinthectomy,[773] and VOR adaptation in general.[887] But the NOT does more than simply relay visual information for adaptive changes in the VOR since lesions in the NOT also lead to change in the baseline VOR gain. Whether or not the NOT is important for maintaining long-term adaptive changes is not known but presumably that is the case. The NOT may be the anatomical substrate by which a patient with cortical blindness and monkeys following bilateral occipital lobectomy still showed at least some VOR adaptive capability.[286,625] The cerebellum must be constantly appraised of the need for adaptive recalibration and visual inputs are critical. Even if a patient can "see" in the usual sense, if lesions in the brainstem interfere with the transmission of visual information to the cerebellum, the VOR can still become uncalibrated.[320] The role of the NOT in smooth pursuit is discussed further in Chapter 4.

Recent studies have shown that recovery following unilateral labyrinthine lesions is less complete when stimuli are comprised of high accelerations or high frequencies because of Ewald's second law.[223] Certainly some adaptation does take place, requiring a recalibration of peripheral activity coming from the intact labyrinth. This process may use information from irregular afferents that are part of a phasic (and possibly nonlinear) pathway, which runs in parallel with a tonic, linear pathway to mediate the VOR.[181,182,491,492,643]

Recovery from peripheral vestibular lesions depends in part upon the degree to which peripheral function is spared. Plugging of individual semicircular canals has shown that compensation can be partly restored by using information from the remaining intact canals though residual function in the plugged semicircular canal may be important, too.[885] The spatial tuning of information from the intact canal (as a function of the plane of rotation) is readjusted centrally so that it can provide a better signal of rotation in a plane close to that of the plugged canal.[22,108,112,398]

Vestibulo-ocular reflex adaptation and compensation depend upon the integrity of a number of structures, including the cerebellum and perhaps the vestibular commissure. After destruction of one labyrinth, vestibular nucleus neurons ipsilateral to the lesion are driven exclusively by the contralateral vestibular nucleus, through the vestibular commissure; this finding led to the suggestion that this structure is important in compensation from peripheral vestibular lesions.[341] A change of neural tone in the vestibular nucleus, however, independent of changes in commissural gain, could also be important.[169,273,284] Such a change of neural tone might be achieved by the deep cerebellar nuclei or by intrinsic factors within the vestibular nuclei. Changes in the membrane properties of vestibular neurons, and in intrinsic pacemaker activity also may be important in the recovery after unilateral labyrinthine loss.[82,83,229,341,360a,506,700] A number of biochemical changes accompany adaptation; whether they are primary or secondary is largely unknown.[38,167a,229,230,329,330,341,360a,415,469,471,472,506,521,526,714,760,761,764,905] Compensation for a bilateral loss of labyrinthine function includes a number of compensatory responses and strategies, which are further discussed below (Pathopysiology of Bilateral Loss of Vestibular Function).

VESTIBULOCEREBELLAR INFLUENCES ON THE VESTIBULO-OCULAR REFLEX

Anatomical Pathways by Which the Vestibulocerebellum Influences the Vestibulo-Ocular Reflex

The vestibulocerebellum consists of the flocculus, nodulus, ventral uvula, and ventral paraflocculus.[841,842] The flocculi and adjacent paraflocculi share anatomic connections and physiologic properties. The flocculus receives bilateral, mossy fiber inputs, primarily from the vestibular nuclei and nucleus prepositus hypoglossi (NPH), but also from the pontine nuclei and nucleus reticularis tegmenti pontis. The climbing fiber inputs to the flocculus are from the dorsal cap of the contralateral inferior olivary nucleus.[490,890] Another input to the flocculus is from the cell groups of the paramedian tracts (PMT), which may relay an efference copy of eye movement.[161] Thus, the flocculus receives vestibular, visual, and ocular motor signals. In primates, the flocculus probably receives relatively few direct vestibular nerve afferents, though the nodulus is more richly innervated directly from the vestibular nerve.[70,490,604] The flocculus projects to the ipsilateral vestibular nuclei, y-group, and the basal interstitial nucleus of the cerebellum.[489] Particularly important are the floccular target neurons (FTN) in the vestibular nuclei, which probably play a role in vestibular adaptation.[96a,97,402] These anatomical connections are summarized in Box 6–10, in Chapter 6.

Electrophysiological Aspects of Vestibulocerebellum Control of the Vestibulo-Ocular Reflex

Recordings from the flocculus of alert, trained monkeys have revealed a particular group of Purkinje cells that do not modulate their discharge during vestibular eye movements in darkness, nor during head rotation while fixating a stationary target. Their discharge modulates in relation to *gaze velocity* (velocity of the eye in space) during pursuit of a moving target with the head still nor during combined eye-head tracking.[483] The role of these gaze-velocity Purkinje cells in the control of eye movements is not settled; they may play a role both in the on-line modulation of the VOR using visual-following reflexes, and in the long-term changes in the VOR related to adaptation partly via the y-group (see Box 6–8).[96a,98,118,152,190,401,402,432,482,513,514,606,647,686,884] The flocculus also plays a role in recovery of function after unilateral labyrinthine loss. Although restoration of relatively small degrees of imbalance between the vestibular nuclei can probably take place independently of the flocculus,[361] large amounts of spontaneous nystagmus and the recovery of amplitude and symmetry of gain during head movement probably require the flocculus.[50,470,473,594] The Purkinje cells in the flocculus may also participate in adjusting the gain of the r-VOR or the t-VOR, when subjects view targets that are close to the head.[766] Another role for the flocculus may be in modulating the cervico-ocular reflex, especially in suppressing the reflex when it would lead to image motion on the retina.[321] The flocculus appears to have a more prominent role in adjusting the passive, gaze-stabilizing VOR rather than in adjusting the VOR during active combined eye-head changes of gaze.[79] Still unknown is what role the vestibulocerebellum plays in the control of the VOR in response to linear accelerations, both static counterrolling and the t-VOR.

Patients with cerebellar disorders may show deficits in the t-VOR but whether this arises from involvement of the vestibulo-cerebellum or other parts of the cerebellum including the dorsal vermis is unknown. Patients with cerebellar deficits also show a disorder of eye alignment—skew deviation that changes sense with right and left lateral gaze—which has been interpreted as a manifestation of disturbed processing of otolith information for static head tilt in pitch similar to the ocular tilt reaction (OTR) for static head tilt in roll.[894] It is possible that that the nodulus, which is important for orienting the vector of the slow phase of nystagmus relative to gravity during low-frequency angular VOR responses, also contributes to low-frequency linear VOR responses such as head tilt. Thus eye alignment with head tilt might become abnormal with nodulus lesions. Clearly our knowledge of the role of the cerebellum in the control of static and dynamic responses to linear acceleration is meager and demands further investigation both in experimental models and human patients with cerebellar disturbances.

Effects of Vestibulocerebellar Lesions on the Vestibulo-Ocular Reflex

Experimental lesions of the primate flocculus and paraflocculus produce relatively small changes in rotational vestibular responses; the gain of the r-VOR may be slightly higher or lower.[190,845,903] On the other hand, the ability to adapt the gain of the r-VOR in response to visual demands is abolished.[513,727] Human patients with cerebellar disease may show abnormalities in adaptation of the r-VOR;[301,710,883] these deficits are likely due to involvement of the flocculus. Optokinetic nystagmus and the velocity-storage mechanism are relatively preserved after flocculectomy, but smooth tracking, either with the head still or moving, is impaired.[845,903] The output of the gaze-holding integrator—the step of innervation—cannot be maintained when the eye is put into an eccentric position, producing gaze-evoked nystagmus. The step is also not matched correctly to the amplitude of the velocity command that moved the eye to its new position, producing postsaccadic drift (glissades). Little is known about the effects of vestibulocerebellar lesions on the t-VOR. Since pursuit is impaired, however, and there is a close functional symbiosis between pursuit and the t-VOR, one might expect severe deficits in the t-VOR with vestibulocerebellar lesions, but this remains to be shown. The known deficits with vestibulocerebellar lesions are summarized in Box 12–2.

Experimental lesions of the nodulus and ventral uvula of monkeys (Box 12–3, Chapter 12) maximize horizontal velocity storage, which increases the time constant of the horizontal VOR. The lesion also prevents habituation of the VOR, impairs tilt-suppression of post-rotatory nystagmus, disturbs the reorientation of the velocity-storage mechanism to earth-horizontal with head tilt, alters vertical OKAN, and causes periodic alternating nystagmus in darkness.[404,846,862,865] In monkeys, but presumably not in humans (who show little torsional velocity storage),[735,735,736] ablation of the nodulus and ventral uvula decreases the time constant of the roll (torsional) VOR.[17]

Role of Cerebellum in Vestibulo-Ocular Reflex Adaptation

The exact sites and specific mechanisms underlying the cerebellar contribution to learning in the VOR are still uncertain.[7,50,98,99,118,152,167a,382,432,458a,485,545,606,686] Ito proposed that the error signal for an inadequate VOR—drift of images on the retina—is relayed, via the inferior olivary nucleus and climbing fibers, to Purkinje cells in the flocculus.[430,432] Based upon this visual information, and vestibular inputs relayed by mossy fibers and then onto the parallel fibers of granule cells, Purkinje cells would be able to make appropriate changes in the VOR via their projections to

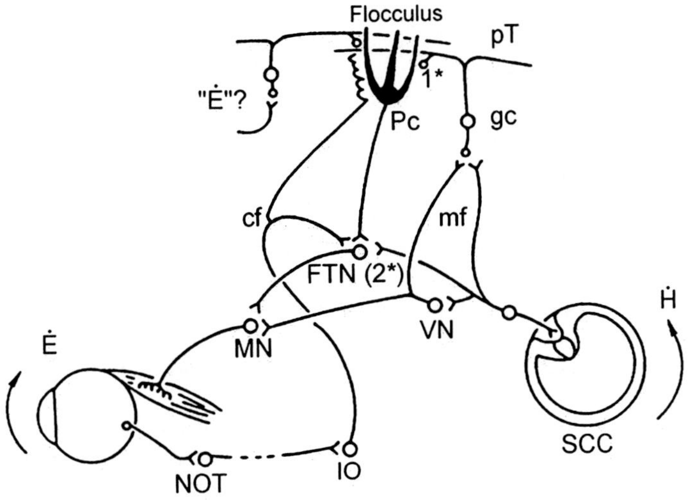

Figure 2–10. Hypothetical scheme to account for vestibulo-ocular adaptation. Head velocity (Ḣ) is transduced by the semicircular canals (SCC) and sent to the vestibular nuclei (VN) to be relayed, via a three neuron arc, to the motoneurons (MN), to create an equal but opposite eye velocity (Ė). The canal signal is relayed to the flocculus (Floc) on mossy fibers (mf) that are axon collaterals of either first- or second-order vestibular neurons, via granule cells (gc) and their parallel-T fibers to Purkinje cells (Pc). Retinal image motion is sensed by direction-selective cells in the retina, relayed through the nucleus of the optic tract (NOT), to the inferior olivary nucleus (IO), and thence to the Pcs on climbing fibers (cf). The Pc project to a subset of second- or third-order cells in the VN called floccular target neurons (FTN), which also receive an axon collateral from the cfs. The Pc's are also thought to receive a copy of the eye velocity signal (Ė). According to Ito, the error signal is carried by cfs, and the modifiable synapses are on Pc dendrites at site 1*. According to Lisberger and colleagues, the Pc carry the error signal and the main modifiable synapses are on FTNs at site 2*. (From Luebke and Robinson,[522] with kind permission of Springer Science and Business Media.)

the vestibular nucleus (Fig. 2–10). Thus, it was proposed that the vestibulocerebellum is the site of a form of motor learning, due to modifiable synapses between parallel fibers and Purkinje cells. Ito has proposed that this learning is due to a long-term depression (LTD) of synaptic transmission from parallel fibers to the Purkinje cell.[431,432] This synaptic change depends upon calcium ions and glutamate receptors, and is induced by the nearly simultaneous arrival of signals from climbing fibers and parallel fibers on Purkinje cells.

Although Ito's flocculus hypothesis has many attractive features, it does not account for all the experimental data in primates, including the behavior of the so-called gaze-velocity Purkinje cells previously discussed.[511,578,696] The "flocculus hypothesis" does not completely account for the effects on VOR adaptation of silencing the climbing fibers of the inferior olivary nucleus with a local anesthetic, or experimentally stimulating climbing fibers to produce "floccular shutdown."[246,522] Furthermore, a critical issue in VOR learning is how the correct relative timing between the arrival of signals conveying information about motion of the head, and motion of images on the retina (the error signal), is deciphered by floccular Purkinje cells.[511,696] Likewise there is evidence for differential regulation of the gain of the VOR and its dynamic properties. Low-frequency training stimuli tend to produce frequency-specific changes in gain; high-frequency training stimuli tend to produce changes in gain that are relatively frequency-independent.[695] It has been suggested that the frequency-specific changes are mediated by calcium channels, and the frequency-independent changes by calcium-activated potassium channels.[264] One source of the discrepancy between Ito's work and the results described in primates may be disagreement about what the flocculus is. Parts of what has traditionally been called the flocculus are probably part of the ventral paraflocculus, which may be more associated with pursuit rather than with VOR adaptation.[431,603,605,606,686,842]

An alternative explanation is that the flocculus, rather than being the sole site of VOR learning, serves other functions in VOR adaptation.[99,118,152,510,511,606,648] It could provide an error correction signal to the neurons in the vestibular nucleus, called the flocculus target neurons (FTN), which would be one site of motor learning for VOR adaptation (Figure 2–10). Perhaps adaptive changes in the amplitude of the VOR would be mediated by this mechanism. The flocculus, however, could still be a site of learning for other types of vestibular adaptation (e.g., the response to low-frequency training stimuli, the responses that require a change in the timing or dynamic response of the VOR, or in context-driven VOR learning). The cerebellar flocculus, with its rich sources of afferent information and internal copies of motor commands, would be ideally poised to gate different VOR responses based upon the circumstances in which they are needed.

As discussed above the flocculus plays a role in recovery of function after unilateral labyrinthine loss. The inferior olive, which presumably relays critical error signals to the flocculus, shows unilateral changes in mRNA expression of brain-derived neurotrophic factor following unilateral loss of labyrinthine function.[508]

Of course, a number of other adaptive strategies are used to compensate for a vestibular loss, apart from adjusting the gain of slow phase of the VOR. They include preprogramming of compensatory eye movements.[458] Whether or not the cerebellum is involved in these "higher level" strategies is not known. It has been shown, however, that when a rabbit is exposed to sustained sinusoidal oscillation of the head, some climbing fibers in the nodulus of the rabbit discharge in a sinusoidal fashion after the animal stops rotating.[71] This finding is compatible with the idea that the cerebellum can learn patterns of vestibular stimulation and generate them even after the actual stimulus has ceased.

As discussed above, many neurotransmitters and neuropeptides have been implicated in the process of vestibular adaptation. In the vestibulocerebellum, nitric oxide, NMDA receptors, acetylcholine, and catecholamines appear to be important.[230] Long-term depression (LTD) has been implicated in the cerebellar contribution to VOR adaptation and long-term potentiation (LTP) may also be important.[275,342,432,485,830] Specific transmitters may relate to the direction (increase versus decrease) or the frequency spectra (high versus low) of a particular adaptive response,[167a,458a,507,673] which, at least hypothetically, may relate to the behavioral differences in adaptation related to frequency content or direction of response (e.g., up versus down in direction, or increase versus decrease in amplitude).[408,673]

Numerous computational models have been proposed to account for many aspects of VOR learning including adaptation of the phase and gain of the VOR, and restoration of dynamic balance after unilateral lesions. Many such models include a potential role for the cerebellum.[98,118,315,343,407,432,511,663,677,696,786,871,892] But often lacking from these models are correlations between behavior and neural activity.

VESTIBULAR SENSATION AND THE ROLE OF THE CEREBRAL HEMISPHERES IN THE VESTIBULO-OCULAR REFLEX

Inputs from the labyrinth constitute the basis for a "sixth sense".[128] Thus, rotation in the dark at a constant velocity produces a sensation of turning that declines, as do the induced eye movements. Similarly, one can detect and identify static tilts of the head and body. Vestibular sensations are usually accompanied by congruent visual and somatosensory inputs; when conflict arises, discomfort and motion sickness can result.[100,114] During natural activities, it is necessary to distinguish between sensations due to self-motion and those due to movement of objects in the environment. One insight into how this is achieved is the observation that real or perceived thresholds for detecting motion of objects in the environment are elevated during locomotion.[674] Such a change in perceptual thresholds may contribute to the ability to maintain a sense of a stable world during locomotion, and act as an adaptive strategy in patients with vestibular loss and oscillopsia.[95,142,151,349,452,570,610,745]

The vestibular system also plays an important role in the perception of the position of the head on the body, the body in space, and how sensory conflicts might be resolved.[457,487,567,568] Evaluation of perception, including the sense of where the head is pointing in darkness, and the attitude of the visual or body vertical may be valuable in detecting lesions in various parts of the vestibular system, from the labyrinth to the cerebral cortex.[95,128,296,426,427,452,610,729,828]

A number of cerebral cortical areas receive vestibular inputs and/or project to the vestibular nuclei.[88,115,116,296,360,498,796] Much has been learned from functional brain imaging and cortical stimulation, which have supplemented the more traditional studies that use anatomical techniques, single-unit recordings from awake behaving animals, and clinical studies of the effects of lesions or seizures.[80,81,133,238,256,262,268a,269,390,449,474,475,515,608,722a]

The vestibular nuclei project diffusely to the lateral and inferior portion of the ventroposterior lateral thalamic nucleus (VPL), where activity related to head rotation in darkness can be recorded.[157] Thalamic neurons appear to receive their major inputs from excitatory rather than inhibitory secondary vestibular neurons, though the inhibitory neurons are clearly important for the VOR itself.[534] Stimulation of the human thalamus during operations for intractable pain or movement disorders can produce sensations of movement[389] and lesions there can produce changes in cerebral cortex activation, as reflected in functional imaging, during vestibular stimulation.[255] In monkeys, projections from the VPL pass rostrally to parietal, parieto-insular, and frontal cortex.[6] These several regions of vestibular cortex include area 2v at the anterior tip of the intraparietal sulcus, area 3av in the lateral sulcus, the medial superior temporal visual area (MST), and the parieto-insular-vestibular cortex (PIVC) deep in the Sylvian sulcus posterior to the insular cortex. In this last area, most of the cells are multi-modal, often responding to labyrinthine, visual (optokinetic), proprioceptive (usually from the neck), or somatosensory inputs from the skin. Neurons can be excited for ipsilateral (type I) or contralateral (type II) rotation, as is the case for neurons in the vestibular nuclei. Optokinetic and labyrinthine inputs can be synergistic (excited for opposite directions, as occurs during natural head rotation) or antagonistic (excited for the same direction). Neurons that carry inputs from the neck and labyrinth also may be synergistic or antagonistic. The three aforementioned cortical vestibular areas—2v, 3a, PIVC—are strongly interconnected with each other and with the opposite hemisphere. Area PIVC, in particular, seems to be a nexus for spatial orientation, as it also receives projections from areas 3aH (hand), 6pa, 7a,b, 8a, cingulate gyrus, and the visual temporal Sylvian area. Recent studies have defined further the roles of VIP (the ventral-intraparietal area) and periarcuate cortex in the frontal lobes in this cortical vestibular circuit.[138,139,717,718,779]

The vestibular projections to the cerebral cortex presumably carry information for spatial orientation, but they could also be involved in other aspects of vestibulo-ocular control, including carrying information for cerebral influences on vestibular adaptation, and in gating different vestibular responses, related to context or anticipation of an upcoming required motor response.[487,832] Indeed there are strong descending projections to the vestibular nuclei—both ipsilateral and contralateral—that could mediate these effects,[296,360] and there are widespread descending projections from the cerebral cortex to the vestibulocerebellum that could be important in higher-level modulation of the VOR.

In humans, multiple cortical areas receive vestibular signals.[80,131,133,238,256,262,269,274,449,474,475,515,589,608,781] Functional imaging has shown that optokinetic stimuli activate many of these same areas, again emphasizing the symbiosis between vision and labyrinthine stimulation in the processing of information about motion and spatial orientation.[248,249,258,453,478] Vection—the illusory sense of motion induced by purely visual stimuli—is likely mediated by these same areas though there may be some segregation between areas that mediate sensations of rotation and of translation.[249] The temporal lobes have been thought to mediate a vestibular sense, based on Penfield's observation that stimulation of the superior temporal gyrus of awake patients caused sensations of bodily displacement.[650] He and others also reported focal seizures—vestibular or "tornado" epilepsy—starting in this area, with auras consisting of sensations of rotation. Similar seizures, sometimes with epileptic nystagmus (see Video Display: Disorders of Gaze Holding), and even skew deviation, have subsequently been reported in association with focal discharges in frontal, parietal, or temporal lobes.[308,316,454,774] PET and fMRI studies have identified cortical areas responding to caloric stimulation in humans. The results largely agree with the anatomic and physiological studies described above (see Fig. 6–8).[116,117,294,840] Ice water produces predominantly contralateral activation. In addition to the "vestibular" cortical areas described above, the anterior cingulate cortex, insula, and putamen are activated during caloric stimulation. Patients with vestibular neuritis show a similar pattern of activation,[80,269] though patients with more central vestibular nucleus lesions, such as Wallenberg's syndrome show different patterns.[257] Humans with lesions in cerebral cortex (probably in a region homologous to PIVC and nearby parietal cortex) show altered perceptions of the subjective visual vertical.[128,128,390,711a] and disturbances of circularvection.[392,775] They may occasionally have rotational vertigo.[113,135,240] Lesions in PIVC also produce deficits in generating memory-guided saccades to a previously seen target, after the head is displaced to a new position in the dark.[428] Sensations of linear motion can be induced artificially with electrical stimulation, and naturally during seizures, in the paramedian area of precuneus cortex.[878]

Several important principles have emerged from the many recent functional imaging studies of the vestibular system.[80,123,133,255,262] First, activation with unilateral vestibular stimulation is asymmetric, greater in the hemisphere ipsilateral to the stimulated ear. Second, there is an overall predominance in the non-dominant hemisphere, which is related to handedness. This finding agrees with greater asymmetries of vestibulo-ocular function in patients with right hemisphere lesions,[833] and the general importance of the non-dominant hemisphere in spatial orientation and attention and neglect. Thirdly, there is a directional dependence; the hemisphere ipsilateral to the fast phase of nystagmus is activated more strongly. Fourthly, vestibular stimulation not only leads to activation in some areas of cortex (e.g., parietal-insular vestibular cortex), but also relative deactivation in other areas of the cortex (e.g., bilateral occipital visual cortex). Visual stimulation alone leads to a reciprocal pattern with activation in occipital cortex and deactivation in parietal-insular cortex. These findings support the idea of a reciprocal visual-vestibular interaction used for spatial orientation and motion perception, and for resolving conflicts between incongruent sensory inputs. Finally, there is considerable 'cross-talk' between the two cerebral hemispheres, which could be used to resolve sensory conflicts (e.g., when one hemisphere 'sees' a moving visual world and the other 'sees' a stationary visual world) by adjusting the relative weights of the two conflicting sensory inputs depending upon the task at hand.

The large amount of new information about the contributions of the cerebral cortex to vestibular perception and to the control of the VOR itself indicates that the new approaches using functional imaging and other types of stimulation and recording techniques are rich and promising areas for clinical investigation.

CLINICAL EXAMINATION OF VESTIBULAR AND OPTOKINETIC FUNCTION

General Principles for Evaluating Vestibular Disorders

Here we apply the basic principles already discussed to the clinical and laboratory evaluation of the patient with vestibular disease (see Appendix A for a summary, and Video Displays: Disorders of the Vestibular System and Positional Nystagmus). A more systematic treatment of specific vestibular disorders is given in Chapter 11. The reader is referred to neurootologic texts for details on otoscopy, audiometry, and vestibulospinal testing.[58,420] We will begin by recapitulating certain important physiologic properties that will guide the examination.[163]

First, to maintain steady gaze during head rotation, the r-VOR produces eye movements that compensate for head rotations. VOR gain (eye velocity/head velocity) and phase (temporal relationship between input and output during sinusoidal stimuli) are used to quantify this reflex. Phase relationships during sinusoidal rotations, and measurements of the time course of decay of the response to constant-velocity stimuli (velocity steps), provide a measure of the time constant of the r-VOR. The time constant is a function of both peripheral vestibular properties and central velocity storage.

Second, when the head of a healthy subject is stationary, the left and right vestibular nerves and nuclei show resting discharge rates (vestibular tone) that are balanced. It is around this level of tone that compensatory slow phases are generated in response to head motion, either rotations or translations. This is accomplished by a 'push-pull' system in which motion in one direction causes one side (the side ipsilateral to head motion) to be excited and the other side inhibited. If disease causes a static imbalance of vestibular tone, a spontaneous nystagmus results (see Box 10–1, in Chapter 10). This imbalance causes slow phases with horizontal components directed toward the side with lower tonic activity (quick phases away from the side of the lesion).

Third, disease can also lead to a dynamic imbalance during head rotation and translation. This is similar to the directional preponderance of caloric testing (discussed later) and causes, for example, an r-VOR gain greater for head turns away from the side of the lesion than for head turns toward it.

Fourth, vestibular deficits are more easily appreciated with high acceleration, high velocity, and high frequency stimuli because Ewald's second law (excitatory stimuli are more effective than inhibitory stimuli) is most evident when the vestibulo-ocular reflex must operate under conditions that exceed the range in which the normal 'push-pull' mechanism can operate effectively.

Static otolith-ocular reflexes are relatively vestigial in human beings but disturbances of otolith pathways cause characteristic symptoms and signs including disturbances of the subjective visual vertical, and skew deviation, ocular counterroll, and head tilt.[126,127,149,268,352,362,455,633] With acute unilateral vestibular loss, the translational VOR elicited by side-to-side stimulation and the rotational VOR elicited with head impulses, are both abnormal for ipsilaterally directed head motion.[617]

Both the optokinetic and smooth pursuit systems supplement the VOR during sustained rotations in the light so that compensatory eye movements can be maintained as vestibular input decays. To evaluate the optokinetic system alone, relatively independent of pursuit, it is necessary to study optokinetic afternystagmus (OKAN) in darkness.

History-Taking in Patients with Vestibular Disorders

Patients with vestibular disease may complain of disequilibrium, unsteadiness, or vertigo, which often reflect imbalance of vestibular tone. Vertigo is a distressing, illusory sensation of motion (literally, turning) of self or of the environment.[142] As distinct from one's perception of self-motion during natural locomotion, vertigo is linked to impaired perception of a stationary environment. The mismatch between the actual sensory inputs and the expected pattern of sensory stimulation with the head stationary causes vertigo. The nature of the vertigo may distinguish between disturbances of the semicircular canals and the otoliths. Rotational vertigo connotes disturbance of the semicircular canals or their central projections, whereas sensations of body tilt or impulsion (e.g., lateropulsion, levitation, translation) imply a disturbance in the otolith system.

Patients with rotational vertigo due to acute, peripheral vestibular lesions are often uncertain of the direction of their vertiginous illusions. This is because their vestibular sense indicates self-rotation in one direction, but their eye movements (the slow phases of vestibular nystagmus) cause visual image movements that, when self-referred, connote self-rotation to the opposite side. It is worthwhile to evaluate the vestibular sense alone by asking specifically about the perceived direction of self-rotation with the eyes closed, thus eliminating possible confounding visual stimuli. On the other hand, with the eyes open, one should ask about the direction of image motion, from which one can deduce the direction of the nystagmus. The direction of the slow phase of nystagmus is usually reported to be opposite to the direction of apparent motion of the visual world.

Complaints of tilts of the perceived world or body are often encountered in patients who have suffered Wallenberg's Syndrome (Lateral Medullary Infarction). Such patients may describe, for example, a 180-degree rotation of the environment, so that they see the floor where the ceiling should be; these complaints should not be dismissed as fanciful. Again, one should also eliminate conflicting visual stimuli by asking about the perception of the body when the eyes are closed.

Oscillopsia is an illusory, side-to-side or up-and-down movement of the seen environment. When brought on or accentuated by head movement, it is usually of vestibular origin and reflects an inappropriate VOR gain, direction or phase. Vision becomes blurred so that, for example, fine print on grocery items can only be detected if the patient stands still in the store aisle. In the most severe cases, even the transmitted pulsations of the heart may interfere with vision.[437]

The Clinical Examination of Patients with Vestibular Disorders

Our strategy will be (1) to determine if any static or dynamic vestibular imbalance is present; (2) to determine if a change in head position or other maneuvers will induce an imbalance; (3) to estimate the gain and direction of the VOR. In certain circumstances we will elicit vestibular nystagmus by rotating the patient, and perform bedside caloric testing. The bedside clinical tests of the vestibular system are summarized in Table 2–3.[132,134,143,236,254,268,277,370,420]

CLINICAL FINDINGS WITH STATIC VESTIBULAR IMBALANCE

Initially inspect the eyes as the patient keeps the head stationary and fixes upon a distant point. Nystagmus may be present, particularly with acute vestibular imbalance. The hallmark of vestibular nystagmus is that it is initiated or accentuated when fixation is removed (see Box 10–1, in Chapter 10). (The effect of removal of fixation upon nystagmus is analogous to the Romberg test for postural instability in which case sway of the body increases on removal of vision.) During gentle eye closure, nystagmus may be seen as the lid ripples with each quick phase, or it may be palpated through the lids. A steady-state deviation of the eyes under closed lids may be inferred from the appearance of a corrective saccade back to primary position when the eyes are opened (see Video Display: Medullary Syndromes). Sometimes, horizontal vestibular nystagmus is induced during vertical smooth pursuit, perhaps because a separate fixation mechanism is turned off. In some patients, vestibular nystagmus is most apparent on upward gaze, perhaps because steady fixation is more difficult.

The effect of *fixation* on nystagmus also can be observed during ophthalmoscopy.[895] First, the patient fixes on a distant target with one eye while the examiner observes the optic disc of the other. Any drift of the optic nerve head is noted; then the fixing eye is covered for a few seconds in order to compare drift velocity with and without fixation. In interpreting the findings during ophthalmoscopy, it is sometimes easier to detect nystagmus by observing the slow-phase drifts, because the quick phases may be infrequent. Also, because the retina is behind the center of rotation of the eye, the direction of horizontal and vertical movement is the opposite of the direction seen when viewing the front of the eye. Torsional nystag-

Table 2–3. **Clinical Tests of Vestibular Function**

TESTS OF VESTIBULAR BALANCE	
Static imbalance	
Gaze stability	—during fixation —during ophthalmoscopy —behind Frenzel goggles
Dynamic imbalance	
Nystagmus following head-shaking	
Gaze stability with rapid head turns (impulses) or translations (heaves)	
Positional-induced imbalance	
Positional nystagmus	
Imbalance induced by other measures	
Tragal pressure	
Valsalva maneuvers	
Hyperventilation	
Mastoid vibration	
Sounds	
TESTS FOR ABNORMALITIES OF VESTIBULO-OCULAR GAIN	
Comparison of visual acuity with head stationary and during head shaking at above 2 Hz	
Ophthalmoscopic examination during head shaking at about 2 Hz	
TESTING FOR VESTIBULAR NYSTAGMUS	
After sustained rotation for about 45 seconds, observation of post-rotational nystagmus, behind Frenzel goggles	
BEDSIDE CALORIC TESTING	
Minimal ice water caloric stimulation, with Frenzel goggles	

mus may be detected during ophthalmoscopy if movement of the vessels around both sides of the macula is observed; on one side, quick phases will be directed upward and, on the other, downward. Likewise, laterally directed quick phases will appear that change direction when one looks above and below the macula. A beat of torsional nystagmus may also be elicited in patients with a unilateral loss of function asking them to blink—the top pole of the slow phase rotates towards the paretic ear.[722]

Frenzel goggles also are used to study eye movements in the absence of fixation. The commercially available illuminated goggles are best, but expensive; an alternative is +20 diopter lenses mounted in a spectacle frame and fitted with side-blinkers. The room lights should be turned off and the lights of the goggles or a pen light (illuminating one eye behind the goggles) used to illuminate the eyes. The patient should not fix on the illuminating light bulbs, lest nystagmus be spuriously created by the retinal afterimages that they produce.[94] Fixation can also be removed by having the patient look at a blank white sheet of paper while the examiner peeks in from the side to see the effect of removal of fixation.

CLINICAL FINDINGS WITH DYNAMIC VESTIBULAR IMBALANCE

In patients with vestibular symptoms, a dynamic vestibular imbalance can be elicited relatively easily using three maneuvers: single, rapid head turns or head 'impulses', sustained head shaking, and mastoid vibration. We will also discuss a variant of the head impulse test, the head 'heave' test, to assess the function of the utricle and the translational VOR. Examples of these tests may be viewed in the Video Display: Disorders of the Vestibular System.

A single rapid head turn—the head impulse maneuver or head impulse test—is perhaps the most effective method for detecting a complete loss of labyrinthine function at the bedside (see Video Displays: Cerebellar Syndromes and Disorders of the Vestibular System).[370,374] Ask the patient to fix upon a target, usually the examiner's nose, while you briskly turn the head from one position to another, horizontally or vertically. The hands of the examiner are applied over the side of the patient's head with the force largely being transmitted through the bottom of the palms over the patient's temples. The rotation should not be large (less than 15°), but should be abrupt and of high acceleration. If the r-VOR is working normally, gaze will be held steady; if not, a corrective saccade will be needed at the end of the head movement to bring the image of the target back to the fovea. An abnormal test result is another manifestation of Ewald's second law. In this case, high-acceleration and/or high-frequency head motion are not transduced as well when the nerve is being inhibited as when it is being excited. Hence, in the absence of one-half of a push-pull pair of canals, the response is defective when the head is rotated toward the side of a unilateral loss of function.

The head impulse test can also be used to evaluate individual coplanar pairs of the vertical semicircular canals using a combined vertical-roll motion,[42,209,371,497] or by turning the head (but not the trunk) to the right or left by 45° and then rotating the head in the pitch plane relative to the body (i.e., up and down). Just as for the horizontal canals, an Ewald's law for high-frequency, high-acceleration stimuli can be used to identify loss of function of a single vertical canal. Take for example, a complete unilateral loss of labyrinthine function on the left side. With the head turned to the right on the body, the left anterior and right posterior semicircular canals (SCC) will be maximally excited with a pitch (relative to the body) stimulus. A corrective saccade will be present with rapid rotation of the head downwards (impaired function of the left anterior canal). Conversely, if the head is turned to the left on the body, the left posterior and right anterior SCC will be maximally excited with the pitch stimulus and a corrective saccade will be present with rapid rotation of the head upwards (impaired function of the left posterior canal).

The head impulse test is best performed in the planes of a pair of canals: right anterior, left posterior (RALP), left anterior, right posterior (LARP), or in the case of the lateral canals, with the head down about 30°.[726] Defects are probably best appreciated if the stimulus direction and amplitude is unpredictable.[726] The head impulse test is most consistently positive when there is a complete loss of labyrinthine function involving the lateral canal. Frequently, however, the test can be positive with a partial loss of function, and rarely, even in the absence of any abnormality on caloric testing.[672] When performed as an active test by patients who have a unilateral loss of function, the head impulse test may not be positive because the slow-phase gain is higher and also the corrective saccades occur earlier. The corrective saccades can become embedded in the earliest part of the response and are completed before the head stops moving. These early, embedded saccades are difficult to discern at the bedside.[96,652] Even with passive rotations the corrective saccades sometimes may be hard to see (see Video Display: Disorders of the Vestibular System). This is especially true in young subjects and subjects who have acquired their vestibular loss slowly.

The head *heave* test is used to evaluate the t-VOR. It is a variant of the head impulse test though in this case is used to evaluate the function of the utricle (see Video Display: Disorders of the Vestibular System). As with the head impulse test, the hands of the examiner are applied over the side of the patient's head with the force largely being transmitted through the bottom of the palms over the patient's temples. An abrupt, high-acceleration lateral movement of the head is imposed while the subject is instructed to look at the examiner's nose. A corrective catch-up saccade is looked for, which indicates the t-VOR is hypoactive. Because normal individuals usually show a hypoactive t-VOR and may require a corrective saccade, the finding of an asymmetrical response (as occurs in the first days after a unilateral loss of function) is most helpful.

Clinical testing for *head-shaking nystagmus* is a useful method for detecting an induced asymmetry of velocity storage that occurs after peripheral vestibular lesions, or an actual asymmetry in velocity storage that occurs with central lesions.[37,285,366,436,460,467,657] While wearing Frenzel goggles, the patient is instructed to vigorously shake the head for 10 to 15 seconds side to side though a large excursion is not necessary. Immediately afterwards an induced nystagmus is sought (see Video Display: Disorders of the Vestibular System). The procedure is then repeated for vertical head shaking. With unilateral, peripheral, vestibular lesions, asymmetry of velocity storage is induced because there is a greater peripheral input when the head rotates toward the intact side. (One form of Ewald's second law dictates that at high speeds the intact labyrinth will not be able to decrease its discharge below zero for head rotations toward the paretic side.) After horizontal head shaking, patients with unilateral peripheral lesions may show horizontal nystagmus, initially with slow phases directed toward the side of the lesion (contralateral quick phases). The pattern of nystagmus is influenced by head orientation relative to gravity,[642] as are other manifestations of the velocity-storage mechanism such as the VOR time constant and OKAN. After vertical head shaking, patients with unilateral loss of labyrinthine function may show a relatively less prominent nystagmus with horizontal slow phases directed away from the side of the lesion (ipsilateral quick phases). This "cross-coupled" response probably reflects an asymmetry in the contribution that the posterior semicircular canal normally makes to the horizontal VOR during vertical head shaking.[364] It is important to remember that with a loss of labyrinthine function on one side, a head-shaking induced nystagmus will only occur when there is an intact velocity-storage mechanism. Velocity storage may be so impaired in some patients with an acute complete loss of vestibular function on one side, or with additional involvement on the other side, that they do not show head-shaking nystagmus.[285] Following circular head shaking (the patient rotates the head in a circle, up and left, then down and right), normal subjects produce a predominantly torsional nystagmus, which is probably a post-rotatory nystagmus rather than a nystagmus arising from the velocity-storage mechanism.[366,387] Hence the absence of circular head-shaking nystagmus can be used to infer bilateral loss of vertical canal function. Torsional OKN may be quite asymmetrical in unilateral vestibular loss with a better response with the top poles of the eyes rotating toward the paretic labyrinth.[517]

Central vestibular lesions may cause inappropriate cross-coupling of nystagmus, usually a prominent vertical nystagmus (especially downbeat) after horizontal head shaking (see Video Display: Disorders of the Vestibular System).[467,579,853] This is likely related to storage of inappropriate upward slow-phase activity during horizontal head shaking,which is discharged when the head shaking stops producing a transient down beating nystagmus. An alternative explanation would be activation of the vertical velocity-storage mechanism (which has an inherent upward bias) by the horizontal inputs *per se*, which would then discharge after head shaking. In either case, baclofen, which abolishes velocity storage,[184] should prevent vertical nystagmus after horizontal head shaking. Central lesions also may produce an asymmetry in the horizontal velocity-storage mechanism, which itself can produce horizontal head-shaking nystagmus even though the peripheral vestibular inputs are balanced. (In this case, the asymmetry of velocity storage might be revealed by finding different time constants for vestibular rotations in opposite directions.)

Some patients with peripheral lesions may show head-shaking nystagmus with ipsilateral quick phases. The mechanism may be related to recovery nystagmus,[539] which usually refers to a change in direction of spontaneous nystagmus when prior adaptive rebalancing suddenly becomes inappropriately excessive, as peripheral function recovers (see below). Similarly, a recovery in dynamic function could make prior adaptive changes inappropriate, thus causing an asymmetry in inputs to the velocity-storage mechanism during head shaking. This would cause head-shaking nystagmus in an opposite direction to that usually seen with a peripheral lesion. Relating the direction of head-shaking nystagmus to the affected ear can be particularly confusing in Ménière's syndrome in which the direction can be related to excitation, paresis, or recovery.[37,450]

Vibration applied to the mastoid tip may also bring out nystagmus in patients with unilateral loss of function and occasionally in other conditions such as superior canal dehiscence or other types of fistulae.[265,380,455,571,623,654,776] In the case of a unilateral loss of function, vibration of either mastoid (because the vibration impulses are transmitted relatively symmetrically through the skull to both labyrinths) elicits a nystagmus with a slow phase toward the paretic ear, in essence acting like a hot water caloric stimulus to the intact labyrinth. Vibration of the neck muscles can also produce changes in the subjective visual vertical, which can be asymmetrical in patients with unilateral loss of labyrinthine function.[92,548] When vibration brings out a vertical nystagmus a central lesion should be sought (see Video Display: Disorders of the Vestibular System).

POSITIONAL TESTING IN PATIENTS WITH VESTIBULAR DISORDERS

Positional testing is a key part of the vestibular examination in all patients who complain of vestibular symptoms, since benign paroxysmal positional vertigo (BPPV) is such a common cause of dizziness and imbalance, especially when induced by postural changes or turning over in bed.[141] A distinction should be made between a paroxysm of nystagmus induced by rapidly placing the patient in specific head-hanging positions (positioning nystagmus), and nystagmus that persists while the patient is held in a static position (positional nystagmus).

First, perform the Dix-Hallpike maneuver. With the patient sitting, the head is turned (not tilted) about 45° toward one side. The examiner stands in front of the patient and holds the head at the temples. After informing and reassuring the patient of the nature of the test, the head, neck, and trunk are moved en bloc to a head-hanging position (see Fig. 11–4, Chapter 11), about 30° below the horizontal. After the initial positioning of the head in the upright position, there need be little change in the position of the head on the body, apart from making sure the head gets below earth horizontal. A variant ("side-lying") in which the patient turns to the side with the nose 45° away from the tested side may be easier to tolerate for older individuals, especially if they have neck problems.[191] Note the eye movements in primary position and on left and right gaze. After about 45 seconds or earlier if any induced nystagmus has stopped, return the patient to the upright position and observe the eye movements again. Repeat the whole procedure with the head rotated 45° toward the other shoulder. Transient mixed vertical-torsional nystagmus induced by these maneuvers is usually diagnostic of BPPV emanating from the posterior semicircular canal (see Video Display: Positional Nystagmus).

Testing for nystagmus with static changes in head position (e.g., with the subject lying supine, with the head turned to the right, and with the head turned to the left) is useful in eliciting the horizontal nystagmus associated with the lateral canal variant of BPPV. This nystagmus usually changes direction with lateral head turn (direction-changing nystagmus), such that it is either always beating toward the earth (geotropic) or always beating away from the earth (apogeotropic). When there is a question of a positional nystagmus being caused by vertebral artery compression one can compare nystagmus induced with changing the orientation of the head with respect to the body with nystagmus induced during en bloc rotation of the body. Direction-changing nystagmus can occur with either peripheral or central vestibular lesions,[60,63,861] but the lateral canal variant of BPPV is probably the most common cause. Some normal subjects show a weak horizontal nystagmus with positional testing in darkness. It is usually in the same direction with respect to the head (direction-fixed nystagmus), whether the head is turned to the left or to the right. The clinical features of BPPV and other forms of positional nystagmus are discussed in detail in Chapter 11.

OTHER TECHNIQUES FOR TESTING PATIENTS WITH VESTIBULAR SYMPTOMS

Several other clinical maneuvers may be used to induce an inappropriate nystagmus. Tragal compression can be used to test for a fistula, or for abnormalities of the ossicular chain and its connection to the oval window. A pneumatic otoscope is a better way to apply pressure to the tympanic membrane. The Valsalva maneuver (tested against both the closed glottis and against pinched nostrils) may produce symptoms and signs in patients with craniocervical junction anomalies such as the Arnold–Chiari malformations or with perilymph fistula or canal dehiscence syndromes.[687] A change in direction of the nystagmus during a Valsalva performed with pinched nostrils, versus with a closed glottis, is characteristic of the superior canal dehiscence syndrome. Hyperventilation may precipitate nystagmus in patients with a variety of lesions including compensated peripheral lesions,[713] fistulas, and compressive lesions on the vestibular nerve[582] including tumors (see Chapter 12, Case History: Hyperventilation-Induced Nystagmus, and Video Display: Disorders of the Vestibular System). Central lesions such as abnormalities at the craniocervical junction or demyelination may also produce hyperventilation-induced nystagmus. Hyperventilation may, of course, bring out manifestations of an anxiety syndrome, but without any nystagmus. An audiometer can also be used to look for sound-induced nystagmus (the Tullio phenomenon, see Video Display: Disorders of the Vestibular System).[580]

The ability to perform VOR suppression using visual fixation, either during caloric stimulation or combined eye-head tracking of a moving target (cancellation of the VOR), is a test of smooth pursuit (see Chapter 7). Note that patients who have intact VOR cancellation but impaired smooth pursuit may have a decreased VOR response (and hence have nothing to cancel when they track a target moving with their head).[574]

Vestibular nystagmus can be elicited by rotating the patient in a swivel chair at an approximately constant velocity (per-rotatory nystagmus). The head can be positioned to induce nystagmus that is horizontal (head upright), vertical (head turned to one shoulder), torsional (looking up at the ceiling), or mixed vertical-torsional from a push-pull pair of vertical canals (head turned 45° to the right and then pitched back by 90°). If rotation is maintained for about 45 seconds, at one revolution every 3 seconds, and the chair is then suddenly brought to a halt, post-rotational nystagmus will be induced. If the patient wears Frenzel goggles to abolish visual references, the duration of post-rotational nystagmus can be estimated, in each plane. The normal presence of quick phases also can be confirmed.

CLINICAL TESTS OF VESTIBULAR GAIN

Disturbances of visual acuity due to abnormalities of vestibular gain are most satisfactorily tested by quantitative methods.[806] Nevertheless, a simple assessment is possible by measuring dynamic visual acuity during head rotations. Ask the patient to read the optotypes of a visual acuity card while you passively rotate the head (horizontally, vertically, and then in roll (ear to shoulder)) at a frequency of about 2 cycles per second. Dynamic visual acuity is more degraded by head motion when viewing at near than at far,[662] and may diminish with age, especially in the vertical plane.[724] Encourage the patient not to stop at the turnaround points to prevent vision of the chart as the head slows down. If vestibular gain is abnormal, visual acuity will deteriorate by several lines compared with what the patient can read with the head still. Note that roll movements of the head do not usually lead to a significant decrease in visual acuity when labyrinthine function is lost, because foveal acuity is relatively independent of rotation of the eye around its visual axis. Thus, patients with factitious symptoms may report a marked decrease in visual acuity during roll as well as horizontal and vertical rotation of the head.

In some patients who have an abnormal gain of the r-VOR, it may be possible to detect corrective saccades during sinusoidal head rotation at a variety of frequencies (e.g., 0.5–2.0 Hz) during attempted fixation upon a target (see Video Display: Disorders of the Vestibular System); these saccades may be more apparent during fixation of a near target (e.g., at 15 cm). If the gain is too low, saccades will be directed opposite to the movement of the head; if the gain is too high, the converse occurs.

A more sensitive bedside assessment of the gain of the r-VOR can be made using the ophthalmoscope.[895] While the examiner views one optic nerve head and vessels, the patient is asked to view a distant target and shake the head from side to side. At frequencies greater than about 2 cycles per second, the pursuit system alone is unable to hold images stable upon the retina; consequently at this frequency gaze stability depends solely upon the VOR. The fixing eye can also be covered during head shaking to eliminate visual cues to pursuit. Recall that because the retina is behind the center of rotation of the eye, the direction of horizontal or vertical movement is the opposite of what is seen when viewing the front of the eye. If the gain of the VOR is unity, then the position of the eye with respect to the observer (eye in space) is stable, since eye movement in the orbit is equal and opposite to head movement in space: the optic nerve head and retinal vessels appear stationary. If the vessels or disc appear to move opposite to the direction of the head, then the reflex is hypoactive (gain less than 1.0); if they move in the same direction, then the reflex is hyperactive (gain greater than 1.0). If the nerve head drifts in the same direction regardless of the direction of head movement, there is a directional preponderance caused by vestibular imbalance. In the unconscious patient, visual systems are in abeyance, and once again the vestibular system can be studied in isolation, using rapid head turns or the ophthalmoscope test (see also Chapter 12). Recall that patients who habitually wear a spectacle correction may adaptively change the gain of their VOR. The results of the ophthalmoscope test must be interpreted accordingly: the gain goes up with a hyperopic correction, and down with a myopic correction. Finally, patients with essential head tremor and vestibular failure may show abnormal oscillations during ophthalmoscopy,[146] and decreased visual acuity.[891]

BEDSIDE CALORIC TESTING

Caloric testing is often valuable in determining the side of a peripheral vestibular lesion. After verifying that the tympanic membrane is intact and that wax is absent, the minimal ice water caloric test may be performed.[611] The patient's head should be elevated 30° relative to earth-horizontal, to place the lateral semicircular canal in a vertical position. This ensures that thermally induced changes in the density of the endolymph lead to a maximal deflection of the cupula. Ideally, eye movements should be observed behind Frenzel goggles or recorded in darkness, to avoid the effects of visual fixation. A normal response can be elicited with as little as 0.2 mL of ice-cold water. Being essentially a low-frequency stimulus, caloric testing can detect vestibular impairment that may not be apparent during higher-frequency head rotation.[61] Conversely caloric testing may be in the normal range when head rotations are abnormal.[672]

LABORATORY EVALUATION OF VESTIBULAR AND OPTOKINETIC FUNCTION

By recording movements of the eyes, it is possible to quantify the vestibulo-ocular and optokinetic responses. Some methods available for testing vestibular and optokinetic responses are listed in Table 2–4; methods for recording eye movements are summarized in Appendix B.

In quantifying the performance of the VOR, the goals of testing are to determine VOR gain, phase, and imbalance. A static vestibular imbalance is manifest by spontaneous nystagmus and is best detected by recording eye movements in the absence of fixation (see Box 10–1, in Chapter 10). Such nystagmus may

Table 2–4. **Laboratory Evaluation of Vestibular Function**

VESTIBULO-OCULAR REFLEX (SEMICIRCULAR CANALS)	
Quantitative Caloric Testing	
Rotational Testing	
Passive rotation:	Sinusoidal Velocity steps Pseudo-random Accuracy of "gaze-adjusting" saccades
Active head shaking: sinusoidal or sudden head turns (position steps)	
OPTOKINETIC SYSTEM	
Measurement of OKAN, in darkness, following varying periods of full-field optokinetic stimulation	
OTOLITHIC-OCULAR REFLEXES	
Linear acceleration on moving platform, sometimes combined with rotations, giving six degrees of freedom	
Human centrifuge	
Passive change in tilt (roll) (up to 360 degrees)	
Rotation about an axis tilted from earth-vertical (e.g., OVAR or "barbecue-spit")	
Rotation of body about earth-vertical axis with head positioned eccentrically (e.g., forward or to side of the axis of rotation)	
Parallel swing	
Linear carts	
Subjective visual vertical (and horizontal)	

follow Alexander's law and can be classified as first degree (present only when looking in the direction of quick phases), second degree (also present in primary position), and third degree (present in all directions of gaze). In some patients, the nystagmus may reverse direction between right and left gaze. The effects of different gaze positions upon vestibular nystagmus probably relate to interactions between a vestibular imbalance and the gaze-holding network (neural integrator) (see Chapters 5 and 10).

Quantitative Caloric Testing

Laboratory caloric testing[168,373,656] is useful for detecting loss of peripheral vestibular function.[302] Introduced by Bárány, the method was standardized and popularized by Fitzgerald and Hallpike. The caloric response is due to two separate effects of the thermal stimulus: convection currents induced in the endolymph, and a direct effect of the temperature change on the discharge rate of the vestibular nerve; the convection currents are more important.[632]

Caloric responses are best tested with the subject in complete darkness or wearing Frenzel goggles in a dark room. It is important to maintain the state of arousal of the subject with an alerting stimulus such as vocalization.[855,872] The head of the supine subject is tilted upwards by 30°; thermal gradients then principally stimulate the lateral semicircular canals, since the canals are approximately vertical in this head position. Traditionally, water is infused into the external auditory meatus at temperatures of 30° and 44°C, although air also may be used. After checking that the tympanic membranes are intact, the procedure typically consists of first infusing 250 mL of water at 44°C for 40 seconds into one ear and recording the ensuing nystagmus. After a recovery period of 5 minutes, the same stimulus is repeated for the opposite ear. Then each ear is stimulated, in turn, with water at 30°C. Shorter versions of the test have been advocated, often using simultaneous bilateral stimulation, or bithermal stimulation (hot immediately followed by cold or vice versa).[72] In analyzing the nystagmus induced by caloric stimulation, maximum horizontal slow-phase velocity is considered the most reliable index of peripheral vestibular function. Each laboratory should establish its own range of normal values because the conditions of testing are partly responsible for the variability of results. Curiously, age has been reported to have little impact on caloric responses, though rotational testing results are affected by age (see above).[527]

If both warm and cold stimuli produce less response in one ear than in the other, and this asymmetry is 25% or greater, then a unilateral peripheral vestibular disturbance (often called canal paresis) is likely. When caloric stimuli cause a greater ocular response in one direction (e.g., greater slow-phase velocities—to the left—from warm water in the right ear and cold water in the left ear, than slow-phase velocities—to the right—produced by the opposite stimuli), there is a directional preponderance of the vestibular system. If the asymmetry of leftward and rightward slow phases exceeds 30%, then the directional preponderance is likely to be significant. Directional preponderance occurs with both peripheral and central vestibular lesions; by itself, it has no localizing value.[373] Some normal subjects and patients with vestibular symptoms may show a vertical (usually downbeating) component to their caloric-induced nystagmus. Provided that there is a horizontal component (so that the nystagmus is oblique), this appearance is not necessarily abnormal.[69]

In a few laboratories more sophisticated caloric testing is performed. Caloric testing can be modified to simulate a rotational stimulus and information about the time constant of the VOR and any adaptive responses can also be obtained.[291] Furthermore a three-dimensional analysis of caloric nystagmus with the head in different orientations can be used to evaluate the function of each of the semicircular canals and to infer interactions between the otoliths and the semicircular canals.[46,47,661]

Quantitative Rotational Testing

Rotational tests give more accurate and reproducible results than do caloric tests, though, of course, they have the disadvantage of not being able to stimulate a single labyrinth alone.[302] The alertness and mental state of the patient while in darkness may influence the results. Testing should be performed with the eyes open, in darkness;[855] if this is not possible, patients should gently vocalize (e.g., count aloud) while their eyes are closed.[536,872] VOR gain may be obtained by measuring the peak eye velocity in response to a velocity step (e.g., sudden sustained rotation at 50 or 100 degrees per second). The gain of the VOR also can be measured during sinusoidal rotation; consideration should be given to the distance at which a visual (or remembered) target is fixated, since this will affect gain (see Laboratory Evaluation of Eye-Head Movements, in Chapter 7). Rotational testing also can reveal asymmetry (or directional preponderance), in which the gain of the VOR is greater in one direction than in the other.[314]

The time constant of the r-VOR can be estimated from the phase shift at low frequencies of sinusoidal rotation. When the phase shift is 45°, the time constant is equal to the reciprocal of the frequency, expressed in radians per second. For velocity-step stimuli, the time constant can be estimated in several ways, assuming the decay is a simple exponential. One method is to use the logarithm of slow-phase velocity as a function of time. As a rough approximation, the time constant of the VOR can be estimated from the time that it takes slow-phase velocity to drop to 37% of its initial value (Fig. 2–7). Alternatively, one can measure cumulative slow-phase eye position (by adding up all the slow phases of the response) and then compute the time constant of the VOR from the ratio of cumulative slow-phase eye position to the initial value of slow-phase velocity (at the onset of the response).

At low frequencies (less than 0.01 Hz) of passive rotation in a vestibular chair, gain and phase relationships reveal information about peripheral vestibular disease. The time constant is often decreased in such patients (to values less than 10 seconds), but repetitive low-frequency stimuli can themselves shorten the VOR time constant because they habituate the response. Nevertheless, low-frequency stimuli are useful for revealing peripheral vestibular loss.[61,600]

An asymmetry of the vestibular responses due to unilateral labyrinthine disease (even involving just one semicircular canal) is more easily demonstrated with either head accelerations exceeding 2000 degrees per second,[42,43,370,371] or head velocities exceeding 100 degrees per second.[64,705] It is generally easier to apply such stimuli with a manual head turn than with a vestibular chair. Deficits in function of the lateral canals can also be demonstrated if high-speed rotations of the chair are applied with the head pitched forward 30°, so as to stimulate maximally the lateral semicircular canals. In this way rotation toward the paretic side is more likely to reveal an abnormality.[818] By recording the rotation of the eye around all three axes (horizontal, vertical, and torsional), in response to different patterns of head rotation that maximally stimulate different pairs of canals, the function of individual canals can be evaluated and pathology can be more precisely localized to an individual semicircular canal or a combination of canals.[45,209,280,292,370,882] Pseudorandom (white noise) chair rotations offer a broad bandwidth of stimulus frequencies and short testing time and negate effects of prediction on the VOR. They require substantial instrumentation and analysis programs, however.

Another simple way to test the VOR uses the presence of corrective saccades and does not require precise measurement of slow-phase eye movements.[733] The patient views an earth-stationary target; then the lights are turned off and the chair is briefly turned. The patient is required to keep looking at the remembered target location. Normal subjects show a combination of a vestibular slow phase and usually a small gaze-adjusting saccade. The lights are then turned on and any inadequacy of the combined vestibular-saccadic response that occurred in darkness is revealed by a corrective saccade that brings the fovea to the target. Although the response during this test is the sum of a slow phase and a saccade, vestibular and other sensory inputs are essential in programming the size of the saccade. The test may be a sensitive way of detecting vestibular imbalance.[732] A similar strategy can be used to assay otolith function during translation of the body,[89] though this has not yet been applied clinically.

Active head rotation is a convenient way to test for unilateral labyrinthine lesions.[242,616] Caution is required, however, in equating eye movements generated during active head rotation with the passively induced VOR.[499] Especially in patients with bilateral vestibular loss, active head rotation tests not only the VOR but also preprogrammed eye movements and the contribution of the cervico-ocular reflex (see Video Display: Disorders of the Vestibular System). Abnormalities of gain and phase during high-frequency (2 Hz–6 Hz), active head movements have been reported to be at least as sensitive as caloric testing in detecting unilateral vestibular hypofunction,[619,711] or abnormalities in Ménière's syndrome.[409,615] Active pitch head rotations may not be as effective in detecting disturbances of individual vertical semicircular canals;[325] canal plane stimulation using non-predictable passively imposed head impulses is probably the best way.[242,243] Active head rotations have also been used to monitor the progress of patients undergoing physical therapy for vestibular loss due to ototoxicity, for example.[96,618]

Other ways to test the VOR, and especially to distinguish end organ from nerve involvement, or canal from otolith involvement, include galvanic stimulation[263,295,440,441,525,597,742] and recording of vestibular-evoked and sound-evoked potentials.[192,375,378,447,463,516,597,598,742,812,874,908] With the exception of recording sound-induced myogenic potentials in the neck muscles as a measure of saccule function (vestibular evoked myogenic response (VEMPs)), which is useful in the diagnosis of superior canal dehiscence or large vestibular aqueduct syndrome, these galvanic stimulation and evoked potential methods are rarely used in a routine clinical setting.

Optokinetic Testing

Optokinetic testing requires a stimulus that fills the field of vision. A common method is for the patient to sit inside a large, patterned optokinetic drum. Virtual reality (VR) technology has been used to overcome the cumbersome nature of large mechanical rotating drums.[479] Another method is to rotate the patient at a constant velocity for more than a minute with the eyes open in an illuminated room; as the labyrinthine signal dies away, the sustained nystagmus is due to purely visual drives. Small hand-held optokinetic drums or tapes primarily test the pursuit system. The optokinetic response is judged by both the nystagmus during visual stimulation (which in primates consists of pursuit and optokinetic components), and the optokinetic after-nystagmus (OKAN) that occurs after the lights are turned out (Fig. 2–7). The instructions to the patient influence the pattern of nystagmus quick phases during optokinetic stimulation.[817] If the patient is asked to follow the stripes, there are prolonged slow phases with large corrective saccades (look nystagmus). If the patient is asked to stare straight ahead as the stripes pass by, quick phases are smaller and more frequent (stare nystagmus).

The velocity-storage component of the optokinetic system is best evaluated by measuring

OKAN, though this can be a somewhat feeble and variable response in many subjects. The initial slow-phase velocity of OKAN, after a 60-second period of stimulation, ranges from 6 degress per second to 20 degrees per second, and right-left asymmetry does not exceed about 6 degrees per second.[808] As previously discussed, the initial velocity of OKAN and its time constant vary considerably, so several measurements should be made for each patient. A convenient method is to sample the buildup of the slow-phase velocity of OKAN during frequent, 2-second periods of darkness during stimulation.[288,734] These periods are too short to discharge the velocity-storage mechanism. It is important to discard data from the first second of each of these 2-second epochs, to prevent contamination by the influences of the pursuit system.

Testing Otolith-Ocular Responses

Testing of otolith-ocular function in humans has traditionally been relegated to a few sophisticated laboratories because it usually requires elaborate equipment such as moving platforms or parallel swings that impose linear acceleration, human centrifuges, or special chairs that rotate the subject around the roll axis (to test ocular counterroll).[348,350,633,649] Recently, however, several more practical tests of otolith function have been introduced.[134,370,685] Measures of the subjective visual vertical or subjective visual horizontal can be used to infer the torsional position of the eye, and hence imbalance in otolith-ocular reflexes,[85,110,259,362,844] and can be carried out in the clinic with a hand-held laser fitted with inexpensive line-generating optics.[741] The functional integrity of the saccule and of its afferents carried in the inferior division of the vestibular nerve, can be tested using clicks or head vibration (with a reflex hammer) as the stimulus, and measuring the response in the surface EMG activity of the sternocleidomastoid—which is a sacculo-collic reflex.[193,370,379,596,702,875] For example, patients with vestibular neurolabyrinthitis who develop BPPV have a normal click-evoked neck EMG, confirming sparing of the inferior division of the vestibular nerve.[596] Conversely, these potentials are abnormal in inferior vestibular neuritis.[372]

Tilt-suppression of post-rotatory nystagmus (the subject's static head position is reoriented with respect to gravity at the beginning of post-rotatory nystagmus) is a test of the ability of the nodulus to modulate the velocity-storage mechanism. It uses a change in otolith activity to signal a change in orientation of the head with respect to gravity.[282] Tilt-suppression is abnormal with nodulus lesions (Box 12–3, Chapter 12).[369]

It may be possible to identify the side of an acute utricular lesion by measurement of the asymmetry of torsional eye movements (ocular counterrolling) during lateral head tilt,[250] or changes in torsion or in the perception of tilt of a light-bar (oculogravic illusion) during imposed linear acceleration in a human centrifuge.[221,228] During yaw axis rotation one can look for an asymmetry in utricular function by placing the axis of head rotation first though one labyrinth and then the other, and measuring ocular counterroll or displacement of the subjective visual vertical.[176]

The translational VOR (t-VOR) , as measured during an abrupt, high-acceleration lateral movement of the head (head 'heave') may be asymmetrical with an acute unilateral lesion with a lesser response when the head is moved toward the side of the lesion (probably reflecting a form of Ewald's second law for the otoliths).[29,31,503,504,617,685] The t-VOR also shows a loss of modulation with viewing distance. Chronically, asymmetries are much less in the t-VOR than r-VOR, though the t-VOR gain may be reduced bilaterally.[49,206,504,685] In monkeys, abnormalities of the tVOR following unilateral loss of function are more prominent and enduring during fore-aft stimulation with abnormally directed slow phases when the eyes are directed toward the side of the lesion.[31] The effect of otolith stimulation also can be measured during sustained rotation about an axis tilted from earth vertical (OVAR), which in the extreme case is about an earth-horizontal axis and is called barbecue-spit rotation (see OVAR above). Another method is to rotate the subject about an earth-vertical axis with the head positioned in front of the center of rotation of the chair in which the subject sits (eccentric rotation);[49,207,354,738] such a stimulus causes the gain of compensatory eye movements to increase, especially if the subject views or imagines a near target. In some patients, this enhancement of gain with eccentric head position has been found to be absent; in others, asymmetries appeared that were not evident with the head centered. The practical role of these types of rotational testing in evaluating otolith dysfunction is not yet established.

PATHOPHYSIOLOGY OF DISORDERS OF THE VESTIBULAR SYSTEM

Disorders of the peripheral or central vestibular system disrupt eye movements, following the pathophysiological principles summarized in Table 2–5. In Chapter 11, we discuss these abnormalities from a viewpoint of topological diagnosis.

Pathophysiology of Acute Unilateral Disease of the Labyrinth or Vestibular Nerve

Acute, unilateral vestibulopathy causes a static imbalance of vestibular tone; the difference in neural activity of the left and right vestibular nuclei causes spontaneous nystagmus (Box 10-1, Chapter 10). For example, unilateral loss of an entire labyrinth or destruction of the vestibular nerve causes a mixed horizontal-torsional nystagmus, with slow phases directed toward the side of the lesion. The pattern of nystagmus reflects the summed influence of individual semicircular canals on one side (Fig. 2–2A). Disease restricted to a single canal or its immediate projections causes nystagmus in the plane of that canal, independent of the position of the eye in the orbit. So, for example, disease of the left posterior semicircular canal causes a nystagmus that appears more vertical

Table 2–5. **Disorders of the Vestibular-Optokinetic System**

Type of Disorder	Features
Unilateral peripheral vestibular disorders	Static imbalance of canal inputs causing spontaneous nystagmus
	Dynamic imbalance with lower gain for horizontal head rotations or head translations, at high velocity or high accelerations, towards the side of the lesion
	Loss of velocity storage causing reduced r-VOR time constant
	Imbalance of otolith inputs causing skew deviation; positional nystagmus
Bilateral peripheral vestibular disorders	Severest impairment of gain is usually for low-frequency stimuli
	VOR time constant shortened to less than 6 seconds
	Loss of OKAN
	Loss of response to circular head shaking
Central vestibular disorders	Imbalance of canal connections causing nystagmus that is often purely vertical or purely torsional
	Imbalance of otolith connections causing skew deviation
	Increased or decreased r-VOR gain
	Prolonged or shortened r-VOR time constant
	Decreased t-VOR gain
Optokinetic disorders	Loss of OKAN with peripheral vestibular lesions
	Slow buildup of OKN with lesion affecting various parts of the visual pathways
	Asymmetric, monocular OKN in individuals who have not developed binocularity

OKAN, optokinetic afternystagmus; VOR, vestibulo-ocular reflex; r-VOR, rotational VOR; t-VOR, translational VOR.

on looking to the right and more torsional on looking to the left; the eyeball rotates approximately in the same plane in the head, irrespective of the direction of the line of sight. This pattern of nystagmus is commonly encountered in benign paroxysmal positional vertigo (see Video Display: Positional Nystagmus).[211]

Disease of the *superior division* of the vestibular nerve—which is usually due to viral infections—also produces a distinctive pattern of nystagmus. Patients show a mixture of horizontal, vertical (slow phase downward), and torsional nystagmus that is compatible with involvement of the anterior and lateral semicircular canals.[41,278] Similarly, selective involvement of the *inferior division* of the vestibular nerve can be identified, often with an accompanying loss of hearing, due to involvement of the cochlea, and abnormal sound-induced VEMP due to involvement of the sacculus.[40,372,596] Rarely, the slow phases of spontaneous nystagmus are directed away from the side of the lesion; in some cases, this may represent a compensatory mechanism and has been called recovery nystagmus (discussed above).

A *dynamic vestibular imbalance* the VOR, affecting gain and time constant, is also produced by a unilateral loss of labyrinthine function. In labyrinthectomized monkeys, the VOR gain initially falls from a preoperative value of about 1.0 to approximately 0.5 and the time constant of the VOR declines from 35 seconds to about 7 seconds.[282] The decline in the time constant represents loss of velocity storage, which is also evident from a loss of OKAN, particularly following optokinetic drum rotations toward the side of the intact ear. In addition, the VOR is asymmetric (directional preponderance), partly owing to the spontaneous nystagmus. When correction is made for the spontaneous nystagmus, however, VOR gain is still lower for high-speed head rotations toward the side of the lesion. This finding is consistent with Ewald's second law. Similar changes are found in humans with unilateral labyrinthine loss,[136,365,367,789] although even at lower head velocities there may be some asymmetry of response.[315] Some recovery of these dynamic disturbances occurs if monkeys are kept in an illuminated environment: VOR gain increases towards a value of 1.0 and the time constant of the VOR rises slightly (to about 9 seconds). At higher head velocities, however, VOR gain remains lower than preoperatively (approximately 0.8) and is asymmetric, being lower for head rotations toward the side of the lesion. A similar course of recovery has been reported in humans who suffer unilateral labyrinthine loss,[62,150,279,285,353,399,445,655] although with high accelerations the recovery of the rotational VOR is considerably more limited.[44,45,209,719,807] Another finding with unilateral loss is hypometria of gaze-adjusting saccades following ipsilateral head turns.[732]

If the other labyrinth is destroyed after recovery from a unilateral labyrinthine lesion, a deficit occurs as if the original damaged labyrinth were intact. This *Bechterew's phenomenon* reflects the rebalancing of central vestibular tone following the first lesion. The second lesion then creates a new imbalance and reflects the actions of *adaptive mechanisms* in a similar way to the adaptive rebalancing mechanism that underlies the appearance of *recovery nystagmus*.[459,899]

Unilateral disease of the vestibular organ also may cause imbalance of otolith function.[134,176,352,354] Sometimes there is a prominent ipsilateral head tilt, and an ocular skew deviation in which the eye ipsilateral to the lesion is lower and extorted; the contralateral eye is higher and intorted. This is the ocular tilt reaction (OTR).[126,129,312,376,725] The torsion can also be detected objectively, or by measurements of the subjective visual vertical or horizontal.[85,109,110,218,221,362,435,785,834] This pathological skew and torsion is quite different from that produced physiologically by static head tilt in normals.[93,197,844] Pathological skew resembles the otolith imbalance produced by experimental stimulation of the utricle in lower animals (Fig. 2–2B). In lateral-eyed animals, a skew deviation of the eyes is the appropriate response to a lateral head tilt. Even in normal human subjects,[384,442,572,646] and in monkeys,[739] a small amount of dynamic skewing may be associated with rolling the head. The amount of skewing is influenced by the location of the point of regard. There may also be a pathological ocular torsion with a presumed lesion of a vertical semicircular canal alone, but in this case there is no displacement of the subjective visual vertical, implying that a perception of tilt requires a veridical signal from the otoliths about the orientation of gravity relative to the head.[777]

Otolith inputs also may interact centrally with the connections of the semicircular canals. For example, it has been suggested that the reason that patients with an acute labyrinthine lesion often lie with the affected ear up is to use otolith inputs to decrease the imbalance between the canals, and so reduce nystagmus and discomfort.[290] A possible reason for this effect is that the change in the attitude of the head with respect to gravity (which calls for ocular counterroll) may be misinterpreted as a translation of the head away from the ground (which calls for a horizontal nystagmus with slow phases directed toward the intact labyrinth), which in turn could nullify the spontaneous nystagmus. As discussed earlier in this chapter, recent physiological studies emphasize the importance of semicircular canal signals in allowing a distinction between utricular activation by linear acceleration during lateral head tilt (which calls for ocular torsion) and utricular activation by lateral head translation (which calls for horizontal eye motion).[345,911] One can envision that if signals about head translation and head tilt are misinterpreted, as might be the case with a unilateral vestibular imbalance, there could be a diminution or enhancement of any spontaneous nystagmus depending upon the particular pattern of canal-utricular imbalance. In support of this idea is the finding that head-shaking nystagmus in patients with a unilateral peripheral neuritis is modulated by the static attitude of the head, being worse with the affected ear down.[642]

A dynamic otolith imbalance, following experimental unilateral otolith lesions, has been demonstrated in monkeys.[788] Acutely, the increase in gain of the VOR that is normally produced if the animal's head is positioned in front of the axis of rotation is no longer present. Recovery occurs in weeks. In humans with unilateral lesions, during off-vertical axis rotation (OVAR), with the body and axis of rotation tilted together away from upright (including earth-horizontal or barbecue-spit rotation), there is an abnormally low-amplitude or even inappropriately directed bias component when the head is rotated toward the lesioned side.[233,310,649] The modulation component is intact. Patients with a recent (one week) unilateral loss of labyrinthine function show a decreased response when their head is translated toward the abnormal side.[503,504,617] This may reflect the equivalent of an Ewald's law for the otolith response. Patients with more chronic lesions, however, usually show little asymmetry in the translational VOR though the responses to linear accelerations as high as 1g have not usually been investigated.[49,206,504] As discussed previously it has been suggested that the lateral portion of the utricle may respond best to translations (perhaps high-frequency linear acceleration stimuli that produce horizontal eye rotations) and the medial portion to the pull of gravity (perhaps low-frequency linear acceleration stimuli that produce torsion). This would account for the seeming paradox that patients with a unilateral loss of labyrinthine function have a deficit in the translational VOR when moving toward the lesioned side, and abnormal ocular counterroll when tilted toward the side of the lesion.[354]

In sum, there are a number of ways to diagnose unilateral labyrinthine hypofunction, and using the latest physiological understanding of vestibular function with important technical advances now allow for testing each of the individual components of the rotational and translational VOR. Head impulse and head heave testing in the correct planes of motion probe the function of each of the semicircular canals and of the utricle, while vestibular evoked myogenic potentials probe the function of the saccule.

Pathophysiology of Bilateral Loss of Vestibular Function

Bilateral labyrinthine loss presents a sensory deficit to which the brain cannot so readily adapt. In the acute phase of loss of labyrinthine function, the inadequate VOR causes visual images to move on the retina with every head movement; this causes oscillopsia and impairment of vision (see Video Display: Disorders of the Vestibular System). Some clinical causes of bilateral vestibular loss are included in Table 11–3, Chapter 11. Patients with partial, bilateral vestibular loss may show preferential sparing of the r-VOR for high-frequency stimuli;[61] testing with lower-frequency rotations or caloric stimuli are more likely to demonstrate the deficit though the converse is occasionally true.[672] With time, a number of strategies may be developed to compensate for this deficit (see Table 7–1, Chapter 7).[458] These include potentiation of the cervico-ocular reflex, preprogramming of compensatory eye movements, substitution of small saccades and quick phases in the direction opposite head rotation to augment inadequate vestibular slow phases, improvement of smooth pursuit, restriction of head movement, and perceptual threshold changes to ignore oscillopsia.[96,106,134,142,358,377,396,570,613,652,653,801] Because of these adaptive mechanisms, the gain of compensatory eye movements may be near normal during active head rotation. During less predictable head motions, however, such as those occurring during walking, it is harder to compensate for the deficit, and gaze instability causes impaired vision and sometimes oscillopsia. Like unilateral vestibular lesions, bilateral disease causes loss of velocity storage with a consequent shortening of the time constant of the r-VOR,[61] and of OKAN.[188,367,904]

Pathophysiology of Lesions of Central Vestibular Connections

Disturbance within central vestibular structures also may produce disturbances of balance, gain, direction and phase (time constant) of the VOR.[267,688] One way to approach these central disorders is to divide them into those that affect the different planes of rotation (roll, yaw, and pitch), which in turn have topographical diagnostic use.[130,253] Imbalance of otolith inputs and disturbance of optokinetic nystagmus may occur. Moreover, disturbance of gaze-holding function may be impaired because the medial vestibular nucleus is an important contributor to the neural substrate for gaze-holding (see Chapter 5). Central lesions may occasionally mimic isolated peripheral vestibular lesions, for example, infarction of the cerebellar nodulus[495,496] or pontine lesions.[797]

Imbalance of central vestibular tone leads to spontaneous nystagmus that is usually present in primary position. Examples discussed further in Chapter 10 are downbeat (Box 10–2), upbeat (Box 10–3), and torsional nystagmus (Box 10–4). Some cases of horizontal nystagmus also may represent imbalance of central vestibular connections. A number of hypotheses have been proposed to explain the pathogenesis of central vestibular nystagmus; these are discussed in Chapter 10. Experimental ablation of the flocculus and paraflocculus (Box 12–2, Chapter 12) invariably produces downbeat nystagmus, perhaps because these structures inhibit the VOR in an asymmetric pattern.[531,903] Purkinje cells from the flocculus send inhibitory projections to the central connections of the anterior canal but not to those of the posterior canal.[434] Downbeat nystagmus (see Video Display: Downbeat, Upbeat, Torsional Nystagmus) is commonly present in patients with the Arnold–Chiari malformation and other abnormalities at the craniocervical junction.

Experimental ablation of the nodulus and uvula in monkeys (Box 12–3, Chapter 12) causes prolongation of velocity storage and a loss of the normal ability to reduce post-rotational nystagmus by pitching the head forward when post-rotational nystagmus begins.[846] Humans with midline cerebellar tumors show a similar pattern of abnormality.[369] In addition, monkeys with nodulus lesions show downbeat nystagmus and defects in generating the bias component of OVAR.[19] They also develop periodic alternating nystagmus when in darkness (Box 10–5, Chapter 10);[846] this nystagmus is discussed in Chapter 10 (see Video Display: Periodic Alternating Nystagmus). A patient with a new uvula lesion superimposed on a lesion in the vestibular nucleus developed a paroxysmal alternating skew deviation and spontaneous nystagmus, presumably due to a loss of inhibition upon the vestibular nuclei.[680]

Experimental unilateral lesions of the vestibular nuclei in monkeys do not produce purely vertical or horizontal nystagmus; it is mixed horizontal-torsional, mixed vertical-torsional, or pure torsional.[827] With lesions of the vestibular nerve root and caudal lateral parts of the vestibular nucleus, the horizontal component of slow phases is directed toward the lesion. When the superior vestibular or rostral medial vestibular nuclei are lesioned, the horizontal component of the slow phases is directed away from the lesion. Nystagmus with vestibular nucleus lesions is more persistent than that caused by labyrinthectomy. Some patients with central vestibular lesions, however, may manifest nystagmus that corresponds to the effects of stimulating one semicircular canal.[688] Wallenberg's syndrome (lateral medullary infarction) may cause mixed horizontal-torsional nystagmus with slow phases directed towards the side of the lesion. Experimental lesions of the medial vestibular nuclei and nucleus prepositus hypoglossi, which are essential elements of the gaze-holding mechanism (neural integrator), cause a combination of deficits of gaze holding and vestibular imbalance. These interactions and their relationship to Alexander's law of nystagmus are discussed in Chapter 5.

Lesions of the cerebral hemispheres, such as hemidecortication, cause some dynamic imbalance of the r-VOR.[270,832] During rotation in darkness, a mild asymmetry of r-VOR gain is present, with greater values being obtained for eye movements away from the side of the lesion. This asymmetry is greater if the patient either imagines or views a stationary target,[746] but is absent for higher-frequency rotations (see Chapter 12). Central lesions may affect the vestibular nerve as it courses through the brainstem or in the medial vestibular nuclei itself, causing a unilateral caloric paresis, but not usually a complete paralysis.[293]

The gain of the VOR is variably decreased or increased with central lesions. For example, disease affecting the vestibular nucleus at the root entry zone may cause loss of vestibular function similar to that from a more peripheral lesion in the labyrinth. Thus, with an occlusion of the anterior inferior cerebellar artery (AICA), the vestibular disturbance can be due to a combination of central vestibular and peripheral labyrinthine dysfunction (see Video Display: Cerebellar Syndromes). Lesions involving the flocculus and paraflocculus may cause either an increase or decrease in vestibular gain.[903] Patients with cerebellar disease may show vestibular hyper-responsiveness (VOR gain greater than 1.0), often with an upward predominance, as well as inappropriately directed slow phases commonly with an upward component.[246,328,798,852-854,898,901] Lesions of the vestibulocerebellum cause an inability to adapt the gain of the VOR in response to new visual demands.[513,686]

Disturbances of the phase and the time constant of the r-VOR may occur with disease affecting a variety of central structures. Bilateral lesions of the medial longitudinal fasciculus (MLF) (bilateral internuclear ophthalmoplegia (INO)) cause reduced gain of the vertical r-VOR; in addition, slow-phase eye velocity lags head velocity.[690] The torsional and vertical VOR may be affected in unilateral INO by virtue of greater involvement of posterior versus anterior semicircular canal pathways owing to their anatomical separation.[210] Lesions of the MLF also impair the horizontal VOR because of weakness of the ipsilateral medial rectus muscle. The consequence of these disturbances of phase and gain are impaired vision and oscillopsia with head movements. The interstitial nucleus of Cajal may influence the phase relationships of both the vertical and torsional r-VOR,[297,689] but quantitative studies of the effects of restricted lesions of this nucleus on the VOR in humans are lacking.

Unilateral lesions of central otolith connections cause skew deviation and the ocular tilt reaction.[253,259,725] With lateral medullary lesions affecting the vestibular nuclei, such as Wallenberg's syndrome (lateral medullary infarction) (Box 12–1, Chapter 12), the head is typically tilted (i.e., rolled ear-to-shoulder) toward the side of the lesion, and there is a skew deviation with hypotropia and excyclotropia of the ipsilateral eye (see Video Display: Medullary Syndromes).[260,810] Certain complaints of these patients, such as perceived tilts of the environment, probably also represent central disturbance of otolith inputs. Unilateral MLF or midbrain lesions may cause a contralateral head tilt and ipsilateral hypertropia,[259,261] consistent with interruption of the crossed pathways that subserve otolith inputs (Table 2–2).

Disturbance of visual inputs, whether due to immaturity of the visual pathways,[873] albinism,[247] or blindness,[754] may affect the time constant and gain of the r-VOR. It seems likely that such visual information is passed to the cerebellum, because cerebellar lesions cause similar deficits of ocular motility.[501,900,902]

Pathophysiology of Disorders of the Optokinetic System

Abnormalities of the optokinetic responses (Table 2–5) are caused by peripheral and central vestibular disease and by both developmental and acquired lesions affecting the visual pathways.[66,318,319,829] In primates, optokinetic nystagmus (OKN) represents the responses of both smooth pursuit and optokinetic systems. The performance of the velocity-storage component of the optokinetic response is most reliably evaluated by studying optokinetic after-nystagmus (OKAN) in the dark.

Unilateral peripheral vestibular disease (see Box 11–1, in Chapter 11), particularly during the acute phase, may also cause a directional preponderance of OKN, with increased slow-phase velocity toward the side of the lesion.[121] Unilateral labyrinthine lesions reduce OKAN to both sides but more so with visual stimuli moving toward the intact side.[137] Torsional OKN is also asymmetrical after vestibular loss with relative perseveration of slow phases with top poles rotating toward the lesioned side.[517] Patients who have bilateral labyrinthine loss show normal nystagmus during the period of optokinetic stimulation, but afterward show no OKAN in darkness.[893,904] This finding supports the notion that OKAN in humans, as in other species, depends on normal central vestibular tone. Disease of central vestibular connections that impairs velocity storage may abolish OKAN as well as affect the VOR time constant, and the ability to distinguish tilt from translation.

SUMMARY

1. During head perturbations, such as those caused by natural activities, the vestibulo-ocular, optokinetic, and smooth pursuit systems work together to generate compensatory eye movements and so maintain clear vision of the environment. The rotational vestibulo-ocular reflex (r-VOR), relying on inputs from the semicircular canals, generates compensatory slow-phase eye movements, at short latency, during brief (high-frequency) head turns (Fig. 1–4). The translational vestibulo-ocular reflex (t-VOR), relying on inputs from the otolith organs, generates compensatory slow-phase eye movements, at short latency, during brief (high-frequency) head translations (Fig. 1–5). During translation and horizontal and vertical rotation, the VOR must be adjusted for the viewing distance of the target of interest; the gain (amplitude) of the VOR must increase for viewing near targets.
2. The VOR functions less well at lower frequencies of stimulation so that the optokinetic system and smooth pursuit supplement the VOR during sustained rotations (Fig. 2–7) or translations.
3. Otolith inputs—responding to the pull of gravity—also generate a change in the static torsional alignment of the eyes (ocular counterrolling) in response to sustained lateral tilt of the head.
4. Inputs from the semicircular canals, otolith organs, visual system, and somatosensors are combined centrally, in the vestibular nuclei, to give the brain's best estimate of the orientation and the motion of the head.
5. Stimulation of any one semicircular canal causes compensatory eye movements in the plane of that canal (Fig. 2–2). The semicircular canals are arranged in three pairs, one from each pair on either side. The vestibular nerve shows a resting discharge rate that is modulated up or down according to head motion. This organization maximizes vestibular sensitivity and provides the system with an opportunity to cope with the effects of unilateral disease.
6. The VOR is capable of considerable adaptation of its properties in response to visual demands. This is a form of motor learning that depends upon the vestibulocerebellum and its projection sites within the vestibular nuclei (Fig. 2–10). There are, however, limitations on adaptive capabilities, imposed by Ewald's second law, that are the basis for useful diagnostic maneuvers for clinical vestibular testing. There are also significant cognitive contributions to VOR adaptation implying important cerebral hemisphere inputs to lower-level vestibular adaptive mechanisms.
7. Testing of the VOR requires measurement of symmetry (balance), gain (ratio of eye movement to head rotation), direction of the eye movement relative to the head movement, and the temporal synchrony between head and eye movements (reflected by phase or time constant). A number of factors influence the gain of the VOR. These include mental set, viewing distance of a target, and habitual wearing of a spectacle refraction as well as the nature of the stimulus. Testing of the optokinetic system entails

measurement of optokinetic after-nystagmus (OKAN). Testing of otolith function requires linear acceleration of the subject's head, rotation about an axis tilted from the gravitational vertical, or measurement of ocular counterroll to sustained head tilt. A useful clinical test of static otolith function is measurement of the percept of subjective visual vertical.

8. Disorders of the VOR cause changes in gain, phase, direction, and balance. Abnormalities in the VOR are best elicited with motion of the head that exceeds the usual range of frequency, velocity, or acceleration to which we are subject in everyday life. Disorders of the optokinetic system are characterized by abnormalities of OKAN; they occur in diseases that affect the peripheral or central vestibular system. Otolith disorders produce static tilts of the head, ocular torsion, and skew deviation—the ocular tilt reaction.

REFERENCES

1. Abadi RV, Pantazidou M. Monocular optokinetic nystagmus in humans with age-related maculopathy. Br J Ophthalmol 81, 123–129, 1997.

1a. Abadi RV, Howard IP, Ohmi M, Lee EE. The effect of central and peripheral field stimulation on the rise time and gain of human optokinetic nystagmus. Perception 34, 1015-1024, 2005.

2. Adeyemo B, Angelaki DE. Similar kinematic properties for ocular following and smooth pursuit eye movements. J Neurophysiol 93, 1710–1717, 2005.

3. Adrian ED. Discharges from vestibular receptors in the cat. J Physiol (Lond) 101, 389–407, 1943.

4. Ahn SC, Lee CY, Kim DW, Lee MH. Short-term vestibular responses to repeated rotations. J Vestib Res 10, 17–23, 2000.

5. Akao T, Kurkin S, Fukushima K. Latency of adaptive vergence eye movements induced by vergence-vestibular interaction training in monkeys. Exp Brain Res 158, 129–132, 2004.

6. Akbarian S, Grüsser O-J, Guldin WO. Thalamic connections of the vestibular cortical fields in the squirrel monkey (Saimiri sciureus). J Comp Neurol 326, 423–441, 1992.

7. Anastasio TJ. Input minimization: a model of cerebellar learning without climbing fiber error signals. NeuroReport 12, 3825–3831, 2001.

8. Anastasio TJ, Robinson DA. Distributed parallel processing in the vestibulo-oculomotor system. Neural Computation 1, 230–241, 1989.

9. Anastasio TJ, Robinson DA. The distributed representation of vestibulo-oculomotor signals by brainstem neurons. Biol Cybern 61, 79–88, 1989.

10. Anastasopoulos D, Gianna CC, Bronstein AM, Gresty MA. Interaction of linear and angular vestibulo-ocular reflexes of human subjects in response to transient motion. Exp Brain Res 110, 465–472, 1996.

11. Anastasopoulos D, Haslwanter T, Fetter M, Dichgans J. Smooth pursuit eye movements and otolith-ocular responses are differently impaired in cerebellar ataxia. Brain 121, 1497–1505, 1998.

12. Angelaki DE. The physiology of the peripheral vestibular system: the birth of a field. J Neurophysiol 93, 3032–3033, 2005.

13. Angelaki DE. Eyes on target: what neurons must do for the vestibuloocular reflex during linear motion. J Neurophysiol 92, 20–35, 2004.

14. Angelaki DE, Dickman JD. Gravity or translation: central processing of vestibular signals to detect motion or tilt. J Vestib Res 13, 245–253, 2003.

15. Angelaki DE, Dickman JD. Premotor neurons encode torsional eye velocity during smooth-pursuit eye movements. J Neurosci 23, 2971–2979, 2003.

16. Angelaki DE, Green AM, Dickman JD. Differential sensorimotor processing of vestibulo-ocular signals during rotation and translation. J Neurosci 21, 3968–3985, 2001.

17. Angelaki DE, Hess BJ. The cerebellar nodulus and ventral uvula control the torsional vestibulo-ocular reflex. J Neurophysiol 72, 1443–1447, 1994.

18. Angelaki DE, Hess BJ. Inertial representation of angular motion in the vestibular system of rhesus monkeys. II. Otolith-controlled transformation that depends on an intact cerebellar nodulus. J Neurophysiol 73, 1729–1751, 1995.

19. Angelaki DE, Hess BJ. Lesion of the nodulus and ventral uvula abolish steady-state off-vertical axis otolith response. J Neurophysiol 73, 1716–1720, 1995.

20. Angelaki DE, Hess BJ. Three-dimensional organization of otolith-ocular reflexes in rhesus monkeys. I. Linear acceleration responses during off-vertical axis rotation. J Neurophysiol 75, 2405–2424, 1996.

21. Angelaki DE, Hess BJM. Inertial representation of angular motion in the vestibular system of rhesus monkeys. I. Vestibuloocular reflex. J Neurophysiol 71, 1222–1249, 1994.

22. Angelaki DE, Hess BJM. Adaptation of primate vestibuloocular reflex to altered peripheral vestibular inputs. II. Spatiotemporal properties of the adapted slow-phase eye velocity. J Neurophysiol 76, 2954–2971, 1996.

23. Angelaki DE, Hess BJM. Organizational principals of otolith- and semicircular canal-ocular reflexes in rhesus monkeys. Ann N Y Acad Sci 781, 332–347, 1996.

24. Angelaki DE, Hess BJM. Visually induced adaptation in three-dimensional organization of primate vestibulo-ocular reflex. J Neurophysiol 79, 791–807, 1998.

25. Angelaki DE, McHenry MQ. Short-latency primate vestibuloocular responses during translation. J Neurophysiol 82, 1651–1654, 1999.

26. Angelaki DE, McHenry MQ, Dickman DJ, Newlands SD, Hess BJ. Computation of inertial motion: neural strategies to resolve ambiguous otolith information. J Neurosci 19, 316–327, 1999.

27. Angelaki DE, McHenry MQ, Dickman JD, Perachio AA. Primate translational vestibuloocular reflexes.

III. Effects of bilateral labyrinthine stimulation. J Neurophysiol 83, 1662–1676, 2000.
28. Angelaki DE, McHenry MQ, Hess BJ. Primate translational vestibuloocular reflexes. I. High-frequency dynamics and three-dimensional properties during lateral motion. J Neurophysiol 83, 1637–1647, 2000.
29. Angelaki DE, McHenry MQ, Newlands SD, Dickman JD. Functional organization of primate translational vestibulo-ocular reflexes and effects of unilateral labyrinthectomy. Ann N Y Acad Sci 871, 136–147, 1999.
30. Angelaki DE, Newlands SD, Dickman JD. Inactivation of semicircular canals causes adaptive increases in otolith-driven tilt responses. J Neurophysiol 87, 1635–1640, 2002.
31. Angelaki DE, Newlands SD, Dickman JD. Primate translational vestibuloocular reflexes. IV. Changes after unilateral labyrinthectomy. J Neurophysiol 83, 3005–3018, 2000.
32. Angelaki DE, Perachio AA. Contribution of irregular semicircular canal afferents to the horizontal vestibuloocular response during constant velocity rotation. J Neurophysiol 69, 996–999, 1993.
33. Angelaki DE, Perachio AA, Mustari MJ, Strunk CL. Role of irregular otolith afferents in the steady-state nystagmus during off-vertical axis rotation. J Neurophysiol 68, 1895–1900, 1992.
34. Angelaki DE, Shaikh AG, Green AM, Dickman JD. Neurons compute internal models of the physical laws of motion. Nature 430, 560–564, 2004.
35. Angelaki DE, Wei M, Merfeld DM. Vestibular discrimination of gravity and translational acceleration. Ann N Y Acad Sci 942, 114–127, 2001.
36. Angelaki DE, Zhou HH, Wei M. Foveal versus full-field visual stabilization strategies for translational and rotational head movements. J Neurosci 23, 1104–1108, 2003.
37. Asawavichiangianda S, Fujimoto M, Mai M, Desroches H, Rutka J. Significance of head-shaking nystagmus in the evaluation of the dizzy patient. Acta Otolaryngol Suppl 540, 27–33, 1999.
38. Ashton JC, Zheng Y, Liu P, Darlington CL, Smith PF. Immunohistochemical characterisation and localisation of cannabinoid CB1 receptor protein in the rat vestibular nucleus complex and the effects of unilateral vestibular deafferentation. Brain Res 1021, 264–271, 2004.
39. Averbuch-Heller L, Rottach KG, Zitovsky AZ, et al. Torsional eye movements in patients with skew deviation and spasmodic torticollis: responses to static and dynamic head roll. Neurology 48, 506–514, 1997.
40. Aw ST, Fetter M, Cremer PD, Karlberg M, Halmagyi GM. Individual semicircular canal function in superior and inferior vestibular neuritis. Neurology 57, 768–774, 2001.
41. Aw ST, Fetter M, Cremer PD, Karlberg M, Halmagyi GM. Individual semicircular canal function in superior and inferior vestibular neuritis. Neurology 57, 768–774, 2001.
42. Aw ST, Halmagyi GM, Black RA, et al. Head impulses reveal loss of individual semicircular canal function. J Vestib Res 9, 173–180, 1999.
43. Aw ST, Halmagyi GM, Curthoys IS, Todd MJ, Yavor RA. Unilateral vestibular deafferentation causes permanent impairment of the human vertical vestibulo-ocular reflex in the pitch plane. Exp Brain Res 102, 121–130, 1994.
44. Aw ST, Halmagyi GM, Curthoys IS, Todd MJ, Yavor RA. Unilateral vestibular deafferentation causes permanent impairment of the human vertical vestibulo-ocular reflex in the pitch plane. Exp Brain Res 102, 121–130, 1994.
45. Aw ST, Halmagyi GM, Haslwanter T, et al. Three-dimensional vector analysis of the human vestibuloocular reflex in response to high-acceleration head rotations. II. Responses in subjects with unilateral vestibular loss and selective semicircular canal occlusion. J Neurophysiol 76, 4021–4030, 1996.
46. Aw ST, Haslwanter T, Fetter M, Dichgans J. Three-dimensional spatial characteristics of caloric nystagmus. Exp Brain Res 134, 289–294, 2000.
47. Aw ST, Haslwanter T, Fetter M, Heimberger J, Todd MJ. Contribution of the vertical semicircular canals to the caloric nystagmus. Acta Otolaryngol 118, 618–627, 1998.
48. Aw ST, Halmagyi GM, Haslwanter T, et al. Three-dimensional vector analysis of the human vestibuloocular reflex in response to high-acceleration head rotations. I. Responses in normal subjects. J Neurophysiol 76, 4009–4020, 1996.
49. Aw ST, Todd MJ, Mcgarvie LA, Migliaccio AA, Halmagyi GM. Effects of unilateral vestibular deafferentation on the linear vestibulo-ocular reflex evoked by impulsive eccentric roll rotation. J Neurophysiol 89, 969–978, 2003.
50. Babalian AL, Vidal PP. Floccular modulation of vestibuloocular pathways and cerebellum-related plasticity: an in vitro whole brain study. J Neurophysiol 84, 2514–2528, 2000.
51. Bai R, Meng H, Sato H, et al. Properties of utricular-activated vestibular neurons that project to the contralateral vestibular nuclei in the cat. Exp Brain Res 147, 419–425, 2002.
52. Baker J, Goldberg J, Hermann G, Peterson BW. Optimal response planes and canal convergence in secondary neurons in vestibular nuclei of alert cats. Brain Res 294, 133–137, 1984.
53. Baker R, Highstein SM. Vestibular projections to medial rectus subdivision of oculomotor nucleus. J Neurophysiol 41, 1629–1646, 1978.
54. Baloh RW, Beykirch K, Honrubia V, Yee RD. Eye movements induced by linear acceleration on a parallel swing. J Neurophysiol 60, 2000–2013, 1988.
55. Baloh RW, Demer JL. Gravity and the vertical vestibulo-ocular reflex. Exp Brain Res 83, 427–433, 1991.
56. Baloh RW, Demer JL. Optokinetic-vestibular interaction in patients with increased gain of the vestibulo-ocular reflex. Exp Brain Res 97, 334–342, 1993.
57. Baloh RW, Enrietto J, Jacobson KM, Lin A. Age-related changes in vestibular function: a longitudinal study. Ann N Y Acad Sci 942, 210–219, 2001.
58. Baloh RW, Halmagyi GM. Disorders of the Vestibular System. Oxford Press, Oxford, 1996.
59. Baloh RW, Henn V, Jäger J. Habituation of the human vestibulo-ocular reflex with low-frequency harmonic acceleration. Am J Otolaryngol 3, 235–241, 1982.
60. Baloh RW, Honrubia V, Jacobson K. Benign positional vertigo: clinical and oculographic features in 240 cases. Neurology 37, 371–378, 1987.

61. Baloh RW, Honrubia V, Yee RD, Hess K. Changes in the human vestibulo-ocular reflex after loss of peripheral sensitivity. Ann Neurol 16, 222–228, 1984.
62. Baloh RW, Honrubia V, Yee RD, Langhofer L, Minser K. Recovery from unilateral vestibular lesions. In Keller EL, Zee DS (eds). Adaptive Processes in Visual and Oculomotor Systems. Pergamon Press, Oxford, 1986, pp 349–356.
63. Baloh RW, Jacobson K, Honrubia V. Horizontal semicircular canal variant of benign positional vertigo. Neurology 43, 2542–2549, 1993.
64. Baloh RW, Jacobson KM, Beykirch K, Honrubia V. Horizontal vestibulo-ocular reflex after acute peripheral lesions. Acta Otolaryngol (Stockh) Suppl 468, 323–327, 1989.
65. Baloh RW, Jacobson KM, Socotch TM. The effect of aging on visual-vestibuloocular responses. Exp Brain Res 95, 509–516, 1993.
66. Baloh RW, Yee RD, Honrubia V. Clinical abnormalities of optokinetic nystagmus. In Lennerstrand G, Zee DS, Keller EL (eds). Functional Basis of Ocular Motility Disorders. Pergamon, Oxford,1982, pp 311–320.
67. Baloh RW, Yue Q, Demer JL. The linear vestibulo-ocular reflex in normal subjects and patients with vestibular and cerebellar lesions. J Vestib Res 5, 349–361, 1995.
68. Bárány R. Physiologie und Pathologie des Bogengangsapparates biem Menschen. Deuticke, Vienna, 1907.
69. Barber HO, Stoyanoff S. Vertical nystagmus in routine caloric testing. Otolaryngol Head Neck Surg 95, 574–580, 1984.
70. Barmack NH. Central vestibular system: vestibular nuclei and posterior cerebellum. Brain Res Bull 60, 511–541, 2003.
71. Barmack NH, Shojaku H. Vestibularly-induced slow phase oscillations in climbing fiber responses of Purkinje cells in the cerebellar nodulus. Neuroscience 50, 1–5 (1992).
72. Barnes G. Adaptation in the oculomotor response to caloric irrigation and the merits of bithermal stimulation. Br J Audiol 29, 95–106, 1995.
73. Barnett-Cowan M, Dyde RT, Harris LR. Is an internal model of head orientation necessary for oculomotor control? Ann N Y Acad Sci 1039, 314–324, 2005.
74. Barr CC, Schultheis LW, Robinson DA. Voluntary, nonvisual control of the human vestibuloocular reflex. Acta Otolaryngol (Stockh) 81, 365–375, 1976.
75. Barratt HJ, Hood JD. Transfer of optokinetic activity to vestibular nystagmus. Acta Otolaryngol (Stockh) 105, 318–327, 1988.
76. Bartl K, Schneider E, Glasauer S. Dependence of the torsional vestibulo-ocular reflex on the direction of gravity. Ann N Y Acad Sci 1039, 455–458, 2005.
77. Becker W, Raab S, Jurgens R. Circular vection during voluntary suppression of optokinetic reflex. Exp Brain Res 144, 554–557, 2002.
78. Bello S, Paige GD, Highstein SM. The squirrel monkey vestibulo-ocular reflex and adaptive plasticity in yaw, pitch, and roll. Exp Brain Res 87, 57–66, 1991.
79. Belton T, McCrea RA. Context contingent signal processing in the cerebellar flocculus and ventral paraflocculus during gaze saccades. J Neurophysiol 92, 797–807, 2004.
80. Bense S, Bartenstein P, Lochmann M, et al. Metabolic changes in vestibular and visual cortices in acute vestibular neuritis. Ann Neurol 56, 624–630, 2004.
81. Bense S, Deutschlander A, Stephan T, et al. Preserved visual-vestibular interaction in patients with bilateral vestibular failure. Neurology 63, 122–128, 2004.
82. Beraneck M, Hachemaoui M, Idoux E, et al. Long-term plasticity of ipsilesional medial vestibular nucleus neurons after unilateral labyrinthectomy. J Neurophysiol 90, 184–203, 2003.
83. Beraneck M, Idoux E, Uno A, et al. Unilateral labyrinthectomy modifies the membrane properties of contralesional vestibular neurons. J Neurophysiol 92, 1668–1684, 2004.
84. Bergamin O, Straumann D. Three-dimensional binocular kinematics of torsional vestibular nystagmus during convergence on head-fixed targets in humans. J Neurophysiol 86, 113–122, 2001.
85. Bergenius J, Tribukait A, Brantberg K. The subjective horizontal at different angles of roll-tilt in patients with unilateral vestibular impairment. Brain Res Bull 40, 385–391, 1996.
86. Berthoz A. Adaptive mechanisms in eye-head coordination. In Berthoz A, Melvill Jones G (eds). Adaptive Mechanisms in Gaze Control. Elsevier, Amsterdam,1985, pp 177–201.
87. Berthoz A. The role of gaze in compensation of vestibular dysfunction: the gaze substitution hypothesis. Progr Brain Res 76, 411–420, 1988.
88. Berthoz A. How does the cerebral cortex process and utilize vestibular signals? In Baloh RW, Halmagyi GM (eds). Disorders of the Vestibular System. Oxford Press, Oxford, 1996, pp 113–125.
89. Berthoz A, Israël I, Vieville T, Zee DS. Linear head displacement measured by the otoliths can be reproduced through the saccadic system. Neurosci Lett 82, 285–290, 1987.
90. Berthoz A, Melvill Jones G. Differential visual adaptation of vertical canal-dependent vestibulo-ocular reflexes. Exp Brain Res 44, 19–26, 1981.
91. Berthoz A, Melvill Jones G. Long-term effects of dove prism vision on torsional VOR and head-eye coordination. Exp Brain Res 44, 277–283, 1981.
92. Betts GA, Barone M, Karlberg M, MacDougall H, Curthoys IS. Neck muscle vibration alters visually-perceived roll after unilateral vestibular loss. NeuroReport 11, 2659–2662, 2000.
93. Betts GA, Curthoys IS, Todd MJ. The effect of roll-tilt on ocular skew deviation. Acta Otolaryngol (Stockh) Suppl 520, 304–306, 1995.
94. Biessing R, Kommerell G. Pseudo-spontannystagmus unter der Frenzel-Brille. Laryngol Rhinol Otol (Stuttg) 67, 453–456, 1988.
95. Bisdorff AR, Wolsley CJ, Anastasopoulos D, Bronstein AM, Gresty M A. Subjective postural vertical in peripheral and central vestibular disorders. Brain 119, 1523–1534, 1996.
96. Black RA, Halmagyi GM, Thurtell MJ, Todd MJ, Curthoys IS. The active head-impulse test in unilateral peripheral vestibulopathy. Arch Neurol 62, 290–293, 2005.
96a. Blazquez PM, Hirata Y, Highstein SM. Chronic changes in inputs to dorsal Y neurons accompany VOR motor learning. J Neurophysiol published online, 2005.
97. Blazquez P, Partsalis A, Gerrits NM, Highstein SM.

Input of anterior and posterior semicircular canal interneurons encoding head-velocity to the dorsal Y group of the vestibular nuclei. J Neurophysiol 83, 2891–2904, 2000.
98. Blazquez PM, Hirata Y, Heiney SA, Green AM, Highstein SM. Cerebellar signatures of vestibulo-ocular reflex motor learning. J Neurosci 23, 9742–9751, 2003.
99. Blazquez PM, Hirata Y, Highstein SM. The vestibulo-ocular reflex as a model system for motor learning: what is the role of the cerebellum? Cerebellum 3, 188–192, 2004.
100. Bles W, Bos JE, Kruit H. Motion sickness. Curr Opin Neurol 13, 19–25, 2000.
101. Bles W, de Graaf B. Ocular rotation and perception of the horizontal under static tilt conditions in patients without labyrinthine function. Acta Otolaryngol 111, 456–462, 1991.
102. Bloomberg J, Melvill Jones G, Segal B. Adaptive modification of vestibularly perceived rotation. Exp Brain Res 84, 47–56, 1991.
103. Bockisch CJ, Haslwanter T. Three-dimensional eye position during static roll and pitch in humans. Vision Res 41, 2127–2137, 2001.
104. Bockisch CJ, Straumann D, Haslwanter T. Human 3-D aVOR with and without otolith stimulation. Exp Brain Res 161, 358–367, 2005.
105. Bockisch CJ, Straumann D, Haslwanter T. Eye movements during multi-axis whole-body rotations. J Neurophysiol 89, 355–366, 2003.
106. Bockisch CJ, Straumann D, Hess K, Haslwanter T. Enhanced smooth pursuit eye movements in patients with bilateral vestibular deficits. NeuroReport 15, 2617–2620 2004.
107. Böhmer A, Baloh RW. Vertical optokinetic nystagmus and optokinetic afternystagmus in humans. J Vestib Res 1, 309–315, 1990.
108. Böhmer A, Henn V, Suzuki J-I. Vestibulo-ocular reflexes after selective plugging of the semicircular canals in the monkey—response plane determination. Brain Res 326, 291–298, 1985.
109. Böhmer A, Mast F, Jarchow T. Can a unilateral loss of otolithic function be clinically detected by assessment of the subjective visual vertical? Brain Res Bull 40, 423–429, 1996.
110. Böhmer A, Rickenmann J. The subjective visual vertical as a clinical parameter of vestibular function in peripheral vestibular diseases. J Vestib Res 5, 35–45, 1995.
111. Böhmer A, Straumann D. Pathomechanism of downbeat nystagmus: a simple hypothesis. Neurosci Lett 250, 127–130, 1998.
112. Böhmer A, Straumann D, Suzuki J-I, Hess BJM, Henn V. Contributions of single semicircular canals to caloric nystagmus as revealed by canal plugging in rhesus monkeys. Acta Otolaryngol (Stockh) 116, 513–520, 1996.
113. Boiten J, Wilmink J, Kingma H. Acute rotatory vertigo caused by a small haemorrhage of the vestibular cortex. J Neurol Neurosurg Psychiatry 74, 388, 2003.
114. Bos JE, Bles W, de Graaf B. Eye movements to yaw, pitch, and roll about vertical and horizontal axes: adaptation and motion sickness. Aviat Space Environ Med 73, 436–444, 2002.
115. Bottini G, Karnath HO, Vallar G et al. Cerebral representations for egocentric space: Functional-anatomical evidence from caloric vestibular stimulation and neck vibration. Brain 124, 1182–1196, 2001.
116. Bottini G, Paulesu E, Frith CD, Frackowiak RSJ. Functional Anatomy of the Vestibular Cortex In Collard M, Jeannerod M, Christen Y (eds). Le Cortex Vestibulaire. Editions IRVINN, Paris, 1996, pp 27–48.
117. Bottini G, Sterzi R, Paulesu E, et al. Identification of the central vestibular projections in man: a positron emission tomography activation study. Exp Brain Res 99, 164–169, 1994.
118. Boyden ES, Katoh A, Raymond JL. Cerebellum-dependent learning: the role of multiple plasticity mechanisms. Annu Rev Neurosci 27, 581–609, 2004.
119. Boyle R, Büttner U, Markert G. Vestibular nuclei activity and eye movements in the alert monkey during sinusoidal optokinetic stimulation. Exp Brain Res 57, 362–369, 1985.
120. Boyle R, Goldberg JM, Highstein SM. Inputs from regularly and irregularly discharging vestibular nerve afferents to secondary neurons in squirrel monkey vestibular nuclei. III. Correlation with vestibulospinal and vestibuloocular output pathways. J Neurophysiol 68, 471–484, 1992.
121. Brandt T, Allum JHJ, Dichgans J. Computer analysis of optokinetic nystagmus in patients with spontaneous nystagmus of peripheral vestibular origin. Acta Otolaryngol (Stockh) 57, 362–369, 1978.
122. Brandt T, Bronstein AM. Cervical vertigo. J Neurol Neurosurg Psychiatry 71, 8–12, 2001.
123. Brandt T, Deutschlander A, Glasauer S, et al. Expectation of sensory stimulation modulates brain activation during visual motion stimulation. Ann N Y Acad Sci 1039, 325–336, 2005.
124. Brandt T, Dichgans J, Büchele W. Motion habituation: inverted self-motion perception and optokinetic after-nystagmus. Exp Brain Res 21, 337–352, 1974.
125. Brandt T, Dichgans J, Koenig E. Differential effects of central versus peripheral vision on egocentric and exocentric motion perception. Exp Brain Res 16, 476–491, 1973.
126. Brandt T, Dieterich M. Skew deviation with ocular torsion: a vestibular sign of topographic diagnostic value. Ann Neurol 33, 528–534, 1993.
127. Brandt T, Dieterich M. Vestibular syndromes in the roll plane: topographic diagnosis from brain stem to cortex. Ann Neurol 36, 337–347, 1994.
128. Brandt T, Dieterich M. Why do vestibular disorders affect spatial orientation and motion perception? In Baloh RW, Halmagyi GM (eds). Disorders of the Vestibular System. Oxford Press, Oxford, 1996, pp 126–139.
129. Brandt T, Dieterich M. Vestibular syndromes in the roll plane: topographic diagnosis from brain stem to cortex. Ann Neurol 36, 337–347, 1994.
130. Brandt T, Dieterich M. Central vestibular syndromes in roll, pitch and yaw. Neuro-ophthalmol 15, 291–303, 1995.
131. Brandt T, Dieterich M. The vestibular cortex. Its locations, functions, and disorders. Ann N Y Acad Sci 871, 293–312, 1999.
132. Brandt T, Dieterich M, Strupp M. Vertigo and Dizziness: Common Complaints. Springer, London, 2005.
133. Brandt T, Glasauer S, Stephan T, et al. Visual-vestibular and visuovisual cortical interaction: new insights from fMRI and pet. Ann N Y Acad Sci 956, 230–241, 2002.

134. Brandt T, Strupp M. General vestibular testing. Clin Neurophysiol 116, 406–426, 2005.
135. Brandt TH, Botzel K, Yousry T, Dieterich M, Schulze S. Rotational vertigo in embolic stroke of the vestibular and auditory cortices. Neurology 45, 42–44, 1995.
136. Brantberg K, Fransson P-A, Magnusson M, Johansson R, Bergenius J. Short vestibulo-ocular reflex time-constant in complete unilateral vestibular lesions. Am J Otol 16, 787–792, 1995.
137. Brantberg K, Magnusson M. Asymmetric optokinetic afterresponse in patients with vestibular neuritis. J Vestib Res 1, 279–289, 1990.
138. Bremmer F. Navigation in space—the role of the macaque ventral intraparietal area (VIP). J Physiol 566, 29–35, 2005.
139. Bremmer F, Klam F, Duhamel JR, Ben HS, Graf W. Visual-vestibular interactive responses in the macaque ventral intraparietal area (VIP). Eur J Neurosci 16, 1569–1586, 2002.
140. Brettler SC, Baker JF. Timing of low frequency responses of anterior and posterior canal vestibulo-ocular neurons in alert cats. Exp Brain Res 149, 167–173, 2003.
141. Bronstein AM. Vestibular reflexes and positional manoeuvres. J Neurol Neurosurg Psychiatry 74, 289–293, 2003.
142. Bronstein AM. Vision and vertigo: some visual aspects of vestibular disorders. J Neurol 251, 381–387, 2004.
143. Bronstein AM. Vestibular reflexes and positional manoeuvres. J Neurol Neurosurg Psychiatry 74, 289–293, 2003.
144. Bronstein AM, Gresty MA. Short latency compensatory eye movement responses to transient linear head acceleration: a specific function of the otolith-ocular reflex. Exp Brain Res 71, 406–410, 1988.
145. Bronstein AM, Gresty MA. Compensatory eye movements in the presence of conflicting canal and otolith signals. Exp Brain Res 85, 697–700, 1991.
146. Bronstein AM, Gresty MA, Mossman SS. Pendular pseudonystagmus arising as a combination of head tremor and vestibular failure. Neurology 42, 1527–1531, 1992.
147. Bronstein AM, Morland AB, Ruddock KH, Gresty MA. Recovery from bilateral vestibular failure: Implications for visual and cervico-ocular function. Acta Otolaryngol (Stockh) Suppl 520, 405–407, 1995.
148. Bronstein AM, Mossman S, Luxon LM. The neck-eye reflex in patients with reduced vestibular and optokinetic function. Brain 114, 1–11, 1991.
149. Bronstein AM, Perennou DA, Guerraz M, Playford D, Rudge P. Dissociation of visual and haptic vertical in two patients with vestibular nuclear lesions. Neurology 61, 1260–1262, 2003.
150. Brookes GB, Faldon M, Kanayama R, Nakamura T, Gresty MA. Recovery from unilateral vestibular nerve section in human subjects evaluated by physiological, psychological and questionnaire assessments. Acta Otolaryngol (Stockh) Suppl 513, 40–48, 1994.
151. Brookes GB, Gresty MA, Nakamura T, Metcalfe T. Sensing and controlling rotational orientation in normal subjects and patients with loss of labyrinthine function. Am J Otol 14, 349–351, 1993.
152. Broussard DM, Kassardjian CD. Learning in a simple motor system. Learn Mem 11, 127–136, 2004.
153. Broussard DM, Priesol AJ, Tan YF. Asymmetric responses to rotation at high frequencies in central vestibular neurons of the alert cat. Brain Res 1005, 137–153, 2004.
154. Busettini C, Miles FA, Schwarz U, Carl JR. Human ocular responses to translation of the observer and of the scene: dependence on viewing distance. Exp Brain Res 100, 484–494, 1994.
155. Bush GA, Miles FA. Short-latency compensatory eye movements associated with a brief period of free fall. Exp Brain Res 108, 337–340, 1996.
156. Büttner U, Meienberg O, Schimmelpfennig B. The effect of central retinal lesions on optokinetic nystagmus in the monkey. Exp Brain Res 52, 248–256, 1983.
157. Büttner U, Henn V, Oswald HP. Vestibular related neuronal activity in the thalamus of the alert monkey during natural vestibular stimulation. Exp Brain Res 30, 435–444, 1977.
158. Büttner U, Waespe W. Vestibular nerve activity in the alert monkey during vestibular and optokinetic nystagmus. Exp Brain Res 41, 310–315, 1981.
159. Büttner-Ennever JA. Patterns of connectivity in the vestibular nuclei. Ann NY Acad Sci 656, 363–378, 1992.
160. Büttner-Ennever JA, Horn A, Schmidtke K. Cell groups of the medial longitudinal fasciculus and paramedian tracts. Rev Neurol (Paris) 145, 533–539, 1989.
161. Büttner-Ennever JA, Horn AKE. Pathways from cell groups of the paramedian tracts to the floccular region. Ann N Y Acad Sci 781, 532–540, 1996.
162. Cannon SC, Leigh RJ, Zee DS, Abel L. The effect of the rotational magnification of corrective spectacles on the quantitative evaluation of the VOR. Acta Otolaryngol (Stockh) 100, 81–88, 1985.
163. Carey JP, Della Santina CC. Principles of applied vestibular physiology. In Cummings CC (ed). Otolaryngology Head & Neck Surgery. Elsevier Mosby, Philadephia, 2005, pp 3115–3159.
164. Carey JP, Minor LB, Peng CG, et al. Changes in the three-dimensional angular vestibulo-ocular reflex following intratympanic gentamicin for Meniere's disease. J Assoc Res Otolaryngol 3, 430–443, 2002.
165. Carleton SC, Carpenter MB. Afferent and efferent connections of the medial, inferior and lateral vestibular nuclei in the cat and monkey. Brain Res 278, 29–51, 1983.
166. Carpenter M, Cowie R. Connections and oculomotor projections of the superior vestibular nucleus and cell group 'y'. Brain Res 336, 265–287, 1985.
167. Carpenter MB. Vestibular nuclei: afferent and efferent projections. Progr Brain Res 76, 5–15, 1988.
167a. Carter TL, McElligott JG. Cerebellar AMPA/KA receptor antagonism by CNQX inhibits vestibulo-ocular reflex adapation. Exp Brain Res 166, 157–169, 2005.
168. Cartwright AD, Cremer PD, Halmagyi GM, Curthoys IS. Isolated directional preponderance of caloric nystagmus: II. A neural network model. Am J Otol 21, 568–572, 2000.
169. Cartwright AD, Curthoys IS. A neural network simulation of the vestibular system: implications on the role of intervestibular nuclear coupling during vestibular compensation. Biol Cybern 75, 485–493, 1996.

170. Cartwright AD, Gilchrist DP, Burgess AM, Curthoys IS. A realistic neural-network simulation of both slow and quick phase components of the guinea pig VOR. Exp Brain Res 149, 299–311, 2003.
171. Chan WW, Galiana HL. Integrator function in the oculomotor system is dependent on sensory context. J Neurophysiol 93, 3709–3717, 2005.
172. Chen-Huang C, McCrea R, Goldberg JM. Contributions of regularly and irregularly discharging vestibular-nerve inputs to the discharge of central vestibular neurons in the alert squirrel monkey. Exp Brain Res 114, 405–422, 1997.
173. Cheng M, Outerbridge JS. Optokinetic nystagmus during selective retinal stimulation. Exp Brain Res 23, 129–139, 1975.
174. Cheung BS, Howard IP. Optokinetic torsion: dynamics and relation to circularvection. Vision Res 31, 1327–1335, 1991.
175. Cheung BS, Money KE, Howard IP. Dynamics of torsional optokinetic nystagmus under altered gravitoinertial forces. Exp Brain Res 102, 511–518, 1995.
176. Clarke AH, Schonfeld U, Helling K. Unilateral examination of utricle and saccule function. J Vestib Res 13, 215–225, 2003.
177. Clement G. A review of the effects of space flight on the asymmetry of vertical optokinetic and vestibulo-ocular reflexes. J Vestib Res 13, 255–263, 2003.
178. Clement G, Flandrin JM, Courjon JH. Comparison between habituation of the cat vestibulo-ocular reflex by velocity steps and sinusoidal vestibular stimulation in the dark. Exp Brain Res 142, 259–267, 2002.
179. Clement G, Maciel F. Adjustment of the vestibulo-ocular reflex gain as a function of perceived target distance in humans. Neurosci Lett 366, 115–119, 2004.
180. Clément G, Popov KE, Berthoz A. Effects of prolonged weightlessness on horizontal and vertical optokinetic nystagmus and optokinetic after-nystagmus in humans. Exp Brain Res 94, 456–462, 1993.
181. Clendaniel RA, Lasker DM, Minor LB. Differential adaptation of the linear and nonlinear components of the horizontal vestibuloocular reflex in squirrel monkeys. J Neurophysiol 88, 3534–3540, 2002.
182. Clendaniel RA, Lasker DM, Minor LB. Horizontal vestibuloocular reflex evoked by high-acceleration rotations in the squirrel monkey. IV. Responses after spectacle-induced adaptation. J Neurophysiol 86, 1594–1611, 2001.
183. Cohen B. Erasmus Darwin's observations on rotation and vertigo. Human Neurobiol 3, 121–128, 1984.
184. Cohen B, Helwig D, Raphan T. Baclofen and velocity storage: a model of the effects of the drug on the vestibulo-ocular reflex in the rhesus monkey. J Physiol (Lond) 393, 703–725, 1987.
185. Cohen B, Henn V, Raphan T, Dennett D. Velocity storage, nystagmus, and visual-vestibular interactions in humans. Ann N Y Acad Sci 374, 421–433, 1981.
186. Cohen B, Maruta J, Raphan T. Orientation of the eyes to gravitoinertial acceleration. Ann N Y Acad Sci 942, 241–258, 2001.
187. Cohen B, Suzuki J-I, Raphan T. Role of the otolith organs in generation of horizontal nystagmus: effect of selective labyrinthine lesions. Brain Res 276, 159–164, 1983.
188. Cohen B, Uemura T, Takemori S. Effects of labyrinthectomy on optokinetic nystagmus (OKN) and optokinetic after-nystagmus (OKAN). Int J Equilib Res 3, 88–93, 1973.
189. Cohen B, Wearne S, Dai M, Raphan T. Spatial orientation of the angular vestibulo-ocular reflex. J Vestib Res 9, 163–172, 1999.
190. Cohen H, Cohen B, Raphan T, Waespe W. Habituation and adaptation of the vestibulo-ocular reflex; a model of differential control by the vestibulo-cerebellum. Exp Brain Res 110, 110–120, 1993.
191. Cohen HS. Side-lying as an alternative to the Dix-Hallpike test of the posterior canal. Otol Neurotol 25, 130–134, 2004.
192. Colebatch JG. Vestibular evoked potentials. Curr Opin Neurol 14, 21–26, 2001.
193. Colebatch JG, Halmagyi GM. Vestibular evoked potentials in human neck muscles before and after unilateral vestibular deafferentation. Neurology 42, 1992.
194. Collewijn H. The Oculomotor System of the Rabbit and its Plasticity. Springer, New York, 1981.
195. Collewijn H, Martins AJ, Steinman RB. Compensatory eye movements during active and passive head movements: fast adaptation to changes in visual magnification. J Physiol (Lond) 340, 259–286, 1983.
196. Collewijn H, Smeets JB. Early components of the human vestibulo-ocular response to head rotation: latency and gain. J Neurophysiol 84, 376–389, 2000.
197. Collewijn H, Van der Steen J, Ferman L, Jansen TC. Human ocular counterroll: assessment of static and dynamic properties from electromagnetic scleral coil recordings. Exp Brain Res 59, 185–196, 1985.
198. Correia MJ, Kolev OI, Rupert AH, Guedry FE. Vertical optokinetic nystagmus and after-responses during backward tilt. Aviat Space Environ Med 68, 289–295, 1997.
199. Crane BT, Demer JL. A linear canal-otolith interaction model to describe the human vestibulo-ocular reflex. Biol Cybern 81, 109–118, 1999.
200. Crane BT, Demer JL. Human gaze stabilization during natural activities: translation, rotation, magnification, and target distance effects. J Neurophysiol 78, 2129–2144, 1997.
201. Crane BT, Demer JL. Human gaze stabilization during natural activities: translation, rotation, magnification, and target distance effects. J Neurophysiol 78, 2129–2144, 1997.
202. Crane BT, Demer JL. Human horizontal vestibulo-ocular reflex initiation: effects of acceleration, target distance, and unilateral deafferentation. J Neurophysiol 80, 1151–1166, 1998.
203. Crane BT, Tian J, Wiest G, Demer JL. Initiation of the human heave linear vestibulo-ocular reflex. Exp Brain Res 148, 247–255, 2003.
204. Crane BT, Tian JR, Demer JL. Human angular vestibulo-ocular reflex initiation: relationship to Listing's Law. Ann N Y Acad Sci 1039, 26–35, 2005.
205. Crane BT, Tian JR, Demer JL. Initial vestibulo-ocular reflex during transient angular and linear acceleration in human cerebellar dysfunction. Exp Brain Res 130, 486–496, 2000.
206. Crane BT, Tian JR, Ishiyama A, Demer JL. Initiation and cancellation of the human heave linear vestibulo-ocular reflex after unilateral vestibular deafferentation. Exp Brain Res. 161, 519–526, 2005.

207. Crane BT, Viirre ES, Demer JL. The human horizontal vestibulo-ocular reflex during combined linear and angular acceleration. Exp Brain Res 114, 304–320, 1997.
208. Crane BT, Viirre ES, Demer JL. The human horizontal vestibulo-ocular reflex during combined linear and angular acceleration. Exp. Brain Res. 114, 304–320, 1997.
209. Cremer PD, Halmagyi GM, Aw ST, et al. Semicircular canal plane head impulses detect absent function of individual semicircular canals. Brain 121, 699–716, 1998.
210. Cremer PD, Migliaccio AA, Halmagyi GM, Curthoys IS. Vestibulo-ocular reflex pathways in internuclear ophthalmoplegia. Ann Neurol 45, 529–533, 1999.
211. Cremer PD, Migliaccio AA, Pohl DV, et al. Posterior semicircular canal nystagmus is conjugate and its axis is parallel to that of the canal. Neurology 54, 2016–2020, 2000.
212. Cremer PD, Minor LB, Carey JP, Della Santina CC. Eye movements in patients with superior canal dehiscence syndrome align with the abnormal canal. Neurology 55, 1833–1841, 2000.
213. Cullen KE. Sensory signals during active versus passive movement. Curr Opin Neurobiol 14, 698–706, 2004.
214. Cullen KE, Chen-Huang C, McCrea R. Firing behavior of brain stem neurons during voluntary cancellation of the horizontal vestibuloocular reflex. II. Eye movement related neurons. J Neurophysiol 70, 844–856, 1993.
215. Cullen KE, Minor LB. Semicircular canal afferents similarly encode active and passive head-on-body rotations: implications for the role of vestibular efference. J Neurosci 22, RC226, 2002.
216. Cullen KE, Roy JE. Signal processing in the vestibular system during active versus passive head movements. J Neurophysiol 91, 1919–1933, 2004.
217. Curthoys IS. Generation of the quick phase of horizontal vestibular nystagmus. Exp Brain Res 143, 397–405, 2002.
218. Curthoys IS. The role of ocular torsion in visual measures of vestibular function. Brain Res Bull 40, 399–405, 1996.
219. Curthoys IS. Eye movements produced by utricular and saccular stimulation. Aviat Space Environ Med Suppl S8, A192–A197, 1987.
220. Curthoys IS, Betts GA, Burgess AM, et al. The planes of the utricular and saccular maculae of the guinea pig. Ann N Y Acad Sci 871, 27–34, 1999.
221. Curthoys IS, Dai MJ, Halmagyi GM. Human ocular torsional position before and after unilateral vestibular neurectomy. Exp Brain Res 85, 218–225, 1991.
222. Curthoys IS, Halmagyi GM. Vestibular compensation: a review of the oculomotor, neural, and clinical consequences of unilateral vestibular loss. J Vestib Res 5, 67–107, 1995.
223. Curthoys IS, Halmagyi GM. Vestibular compensation. Adv Otorhinolaryngol 55, 82–110, 1999.
224. Curthoys IS, Markham CH. Planar relationships of the semicircular canals in man. Acta Otolaryngol (Stockh) 80, 185–196, 1975.
225. Curthoys IS, Oman CM. Dimensions of the horizontal semicircular duct. ampulla and utricle in the human. Acta Otolaryngol (Stockh) 103, 254–261, 1987.
226. Dai M, Raphan T, Cohen B. Spatial orientation of the vestibular system: dependence of optokinetic after-nystagmus on gravity. J Neurophysiol 66, 1422–1439, 1991.
226a. Dai M, Raphan T, Cohen B. Effects of baclofen on the angular vestibulo-ocular reflex. Exp Brain Res published online, 2005.
227. Dai M, Raphan T, Kozlovskaya I, Cohen B. Modulation of vergence by off-vertical yaw axis rotation in the monkey: normal characteristics and effects of space flight. Exp Brain Res 111, 21–29, 1996.
228. Dai MJ, Curthoys IS, Halmagyi GM. Linear acceleration perception in the roll plane before and after unilateral vestibular neurectomy. Exp Brain Res 77, 315–328, 1989.
229. Darlington CL, Dutia MB, Smith PF. The contribution of the intrinsic excitability of vestibular nucleus neurons to recovery from vestibular damage. Eur J Neurosci 15, 1719–1727, 2002.
230. Darlington CL, Smith PF. Molecular mechanisms of recovery from vestibular damage in mammals: recent advances. Prog Neurobiol 62, 313–325, 2000.
231. Darlington CL, Smith PF. What neurotransmitters are important in the vestibular system. In Baloh RW, Halmagyi GM (eds). Disorders of the Vestibular System. Oxford, Oxford, 1996, pp 140–144.
232. Darlot C, Denise P, Droulez J, Cohen B, Berthoz A. Eye movements induced by off-vertical axis rotation (OVAR) at small angles of tilt. Exp Brain Res 73, 91–105, 1989.
233. Darlot C, Toupet M, Denise P. Unilateral vestibular neuritis with otolithic signs and off-vertical axis rotation. Acta Otolaryngol (Stockh) 117, 7–12, 1997.
234. Das VE, Dell'Osso LF, Leigh RJ. Enhancement of the vestibulo-ocular reflex by prior eye movements. J Neurophysiol 81, 2884–2892, 1999.
235. Das VE, Yaniglos S, Leigh RJ. The influence of light on modulation of the human vestibulo-ocular reflex. J Vestib Res 10, 51–55, 2000.
236. Davies R. Bedside neuro-otological examination and interpretation of commonly used investigations. J Neurol Neurosurg Psychiatry 75 Suppl 4, iv32–iv44, 2004.
237. de Graaf B, Bos JE, Groen E. Saccular impact on ocular torsion. Brain Res Bull 40, 321–330, 1996.
238. De Waele C, Baudonniere PM, Lepecq JC, Tran Ba HP, Vidal PP. Vestibular projections in the human cortex. Exp Brain Res 141, 541–551, 2001.
239. de Waele C, Mühlethaler M, Vidal P-P. Neurochemistry of the central vestibular pathways. Brain Res Bull 20, 24–46, 1995.
240. Debette S, Michelin E, Henon H, Leys D. Transient rotational vertigo as the initial symptom of a middle cerebral artery territory infarct involving the insula. Cerebrovasc. Dis. 16, 97–98, 2003.
241. Della Santina CC, Potyagaylo V, Migliaccio AA, Minor LB, Carey JP. Orientation of human semicircular canals measured by three-dimensional multiplanar CT reconstruction. J Assoc Res Otolaryngol, published online, 2005.
242. Della Santina CC, Cremer PD, Carey JP, Minor LB. Comparison of head thrust test with head autorotation test reveals that the vestibulo-ocular reflex is enhanced during voluntary head movements. Arch Otolaryngol Head Neck Surg 128, 1044–1054, 2002.

243. Della Santina CC, Cremer PD, Carey JP, Minor LB. The vestibulo-ocular reflex during self-generated head movements by human subjects with unilateral vestibular hypofunction: improved gain, latency, and alignment provide evidence for preprogramming. Ann N Y Acad Sci 942, 465–466, 2001.
243a. Demer JL, Clark RA. Magnetic resonance imaging of human extraocular muscles during static ocular counter-rolling. J Neurophysiol 94, 3292–3302, 2005.
244. Demer JL, Crane BT, Tian JR. Human angular vestibulo-ocular reflex axis disconjugacy: relationship to magnetic resonance imaging evidence of globe translation. Ann N Y Acad Sci 1039, 15–25, 2005.
245. Demer JL, Porter FI, Goldberg J, Jenkins JA, Schmidt K. Adaptation to telescopic spectacles: vestibulo-ocular reflex plasticity. Invest Ophthalmol Vis Sci 30, 159–170, 1989.
246. Demer JL, Robinson DA. Effects of reversible lesions and stimulation of olivocerebellar system on vestibuloocular reflex plasticity. J Neurophysiol 47, 1084–1107, 1982.
247. Demer JL, Zee DS. Vestibulo-ocular and optokinetic deficits in albinos with congenital nystagmus. Invest Ophthalmol Vis Sci 25, 74–78, 1984.
248. Deutschlander A, Bense S, Stephan T, et al. Sensory system interactions during simultaneous vestibular and visual stimulation in PET. Hum Brain Mapp 16, 92–103, 2002.
249. Deutschlander A, Bense S, Stephan T, et al. Rollvection versus linearvection: comparison of brain activations in PET. Hum Brain Mapp 21, 143–153, 2004.
250. Diamond SG, Markham CH. Ocular counterrolling as an indicator of vestibular otolith function. Neurology 33, 1460–1469, 1983.
251. Dickman JD, Angelaki DE. Dynamics of vestibular neurons during rotational motion in alert rhesus monkeys. Exp Brain Res 155, 91–101, 2004.
252. Dickman JD, Fang Q. Differential central projections of vestibular afferents in pigeons. J Comp Neurol 367, 110–131, 1996.
253. Dieterich M. The topographic diagnosis of acquired nystagmus in brainstem disorders. Strabismus 10, 137–145, 2002.
254. Dieterich M. Dizziness. Neurologist 10, 154–164, 2004.
255. Dieterich M, Bartenstein P, Spiegel S, et al. Thalamic infarctions cause side-specific suppression of vestibular cortex activations. Brain 128, 2052–2067, 2005.
256. Dieterich M, Bense S, Lutz S, et al. Dominance for vestibular cortical function in the non-dominant hemisphere. Cereb Cortex 13, 994–1007, 2003.
257. Dieterich M, Bense S, Stephan T, et al. Medial vestibular nucleus lesions in Wallenberg's syndrome cause decreased activity of the contralateral vestibular cortex. Ann N Y Acad Sci 1039, 368–383, 2005.
258. Dieterich M, Bense S, Stephan T, Yousry TA, Brandt T. fMRI signal increases and decreases in cortical areas during small-field optokinetic stimulation and central fixation. Exp Brain Res 148, 117–127, 2003.
259. Dieterich M, Brandt T. Ocular torsion and tilt of subjective visual vertical are sensitive brainstem signs. Ann Neurol 33, 292–299, 1993.
260. Dieterich M, Brandt T. Wallenberg's syndrome: lateropulsion, cyclorotation, and subjective visual vertical in thirty-six patients. Ann Neurol 31, 399–408, 1992.
261. Dieterich M, Brandt T. Thalamic infarctions: differential effects on vestibular function in the roll plane (35 patients). Neurology 43, 1732–1740, 1993.
262. Dieterich M, Brandt T. Vestibular system: anatomy and functional magnetic resonance imaging. Neuroimaging Clin N Am 11, 263–273, 2001.
263. Dieterich M, Zink R, Weiss A, Brandt T. Galvanic stimulation in bilateral vestibular failure: 3-D ocular motor effects. NeuroReport 10, 3283–3287, 1999.
264. du Lac S. Candidate cellular mechanisms of vestibulo-ocular reflex plasticity. Ann N Y Acad Sci 781, 489–498, 1996.
265. Dumas G, Lavieille JP, Schmerber S. Vibratory test and head shaking test and caloric test: a series of 87 patients. Ann Otolaryngol Chir Cervicofac 121, 22–32, 2004.
266. Eggers SD, De Pennington N, Walker MF, Shelhamer M, Zee DS. Short-term adaptation of the VOR: non-retinal-slip error signals and saccade substitution. Ann N Y Acad Sci 1004, 94–110, 2003.
267. Eggers SD, Zee DS. Central vestibular disorders. In Cummings CC (ed). Otolaryngology Head & Neck Surgery. Elsevier Mosby, Philadelphia, 2005, pp 3254–3290.
268. Eggers SD, Zee DS. Evaluating the dizzy patient: bedside examination and laboratory assessment of the vestibular system. Semin Neurol 23, 47–58, 2003.
268a. Eickhoff SB, Weiss PH, Amunts K, Fink GR, Zilles K. Identifying human parieto-insular vestibular cortex using fMRI and cytoarchitectonic mapping. Hum Brain Mapp, Published online, 2005.
269. Emri M, et al. Cortical projection of peripheral vestibular signaling. J Neurophysiol 89, 2639–2646, 2003.
270. Estanol B, Romero R, De Viteri MS, Mateos JH, Corvera J. Oculomotor and oculovestibular function in a hemispherectomy patient. Arch Neurol 37, 365–368, 1980.
271. Ewald JR. Physiologishe Untersuchungen über das Endorgan des Nervus Octavus. Bergmann, Wiesbaden, 1892.
272. Farooq SJ, Proudlock FA, Gottlob I. Torsional optokinetic nystagmus: normal response characteristics. Br J Ophthalmol 88, 796–802, 2004.
273. Farrow K, Broussard DM. Commissural inputs to secondary vestibular neurons in alert cats after canal plugs. J Neurophysiol 89, 3351–3353, 2003.
274. Fasold O, von Brevern M, Kuhberg M, et al. Human vestibular cortex as identified with caloric stimulation in functional magnetic resonance imaging. Neuroimage 17, 1384–1393, 2002.
275. Feil R, Hartmann J, Luo C, et al. Impairment of LTD and cerebellar learning by Purkinje cell-specific ablation of cGMP-dependent protein kinase I. J Cell Biol 163, 295–302, 2003.
276. Fernandez C, Goldberg J. Physiology of peripheral neurons innervating semicircular canals of the squirrel monkey. II. Response to sinusoidal stimulation and dynamics of peripheral vestibular system. J Neurophysiol 34, 661–675, 1971.
277. Fetter M. Assessing vestibular function: which tests, when? J Neurol 247, 335–342, 2000.

278. Fetter M, Dichgans J. Vestibular neuritis spares the inferior division of the vestibular nerve. Brain 119, 755–763, 1996.
279. Fetter M, Dichgans J. Adaptive mechanisms of vor compensation after unilateral peripheral vestibular lesions in humans. J Vestib Res 1, 9–22, 1990.
280. Fetter M, Hain TC, Zee DS. Influence of eye and head position on the vestibulo-ocular reflex. Exp Brain Res 64, 208–216, 1986.
281. Fetter M, Misslisch, H, Sievering D, Tweed D. Effects of full-field visual input on the three-dimensional properties of the human vestibuloocular reflex. J Vestib Res 5, 201–209, 1995.
282. Fetter M, Tweed D, Hermann W, Wohland-Braun B, Koenig E. The influence of head position and head reorientation on the axis of eye rotation and the vestibular time constant during postrotatory nystagmus. Exp Brain Res 91, 121–128, 1992.
283. Fetter M, Heimberger J, Black R, Hermann W, Sievering F, Dichgans J. Otolith semicircular canal interaction during postrotatory nystagmus in humans. Exp Brain Res 108, 463–472, 1996.
284. Fetter M, Zee DS. Recovery from unilateral labyrinthectomy in rhesus monkey. J. Neurophysiol 59, 370–393, 1988.
285. Fetter M, Zee DS, Koenig E, Dichgans J. Head-shaking nystagmus during vestibular compensation in humans and rhesus monkeys. Acta Otolaryngol (Stockh) 110, 175–181, 1990.
286. Fetter M, Zee DS, Proctor LR. Effect of lack of vision and of occipital lobectomy upon recovery from unilateral labyrinthectomy in rhesus monkey. J Neurophysiol 59, 394–407, 1988.
287. Fife TD, Baloh RW, Duckwiler GR. Isolated dizziness in vertebrobasilar insufficiency. clinical features, angiography, and follow-up. J Stroke Cerebrovasc Dis 4, 4–12, 1994.
288. Fletcher WA, Hain TC, Zee DS. Optokinetic nystagmus and after-nystagmus in human beings: relationship to nonlinear processing of information about retinal slip. Exp Brain Res 81, 46–52, 1990.
289. Flourens, P. Recherches Experimentales sur les Proprietes et les Fonetions du Systeme Nerveux dans Ies Animaux Vertebres. Crevot, Paris, 1824.
290. Fluur E. Interaction between the utricles and the horizontal semicircular canals. Acta Otolaryngol (Stockh) 76, 349–352, 1973.
291. Formby C, Robinson DA. Measurement of vestibular ocular reflex (VOR) time constants with a caloric step stimulus. J Vestib Res 10, 25–39, 2000.
292. Foster CA, Demer JL, Morrow MJ, Baloh RW. Deficits of gaze stability in multiple axes following unilateral vestibular lesions. Exp Brain Res 116, 501–509, 1997.
293. Francis DA, Bronstein AM, Rudge P, du Boulay EP. The site of brainstem lesions causing semicircular canal paresis: an MRI study. J Neurol Neurosurg Psychiatry 55, 446–449, 1992.
294. Friberg L, Olsen T, Roland P, Paulson O, Lassen N. Focal increase of blood flow in the cerebral cortex of man during vestibular stimulation. Brain 108, 609–623, 1985.
295. Fujimoto C, Iwasaki S, Matsuzaki M, Murofushi T. Lesion site in idiopathic bilateral vestibulopathy: a galvanic vestibular-evoked myogenic potential study. Acta Otolaryngol 125, 430–432, 2005.
296. Fukushima K. Corticovestibular interactions: anatomy, electrophysiology, and functional considerations. Exp Brain Res 117, 1–16, 1997.
297. Fukushima K. The interstitial nucleus of Cajal in the midbrain reticular formation and vertical eye movement. Neurosci Res 10, 159–187, 1991.
298. Fukushima K, Fukushima J, Chin S, Tsunekawa H, Kaneko CRS. Cross axis vestibulo-ocular reflex induced by pursuit training in alert monkeys. Neurosci Res 25, 255–265, 1996.
299. Fukushima K, Fukushima J, Ohashi T, Kase M. Possible downward burster-driving neurons related to the anterior semicircular canal in the region of the interstitial nucleus of Cajal in alert cats. Neurosci Res 12, 536–544, 1991.
300. Fukushima K, Fukushima J, Yamanobe T, Shinmei Y, Kurkin, S. Adaptive eye movements induced by cross-axis pursuit—vestibular interactions in trained monkeys. Acta Otolaryngol Suppl 545, 73–79, 2001.
301. Furman JM, Balaban CD, Pollack IF. Vestibular compensation in a patient with a cerebellar infarction. Neurology 48, 916–920, 1997.
302. Furman JM, Cass SP. Laboratory evaluation 1. Electro nystagmography and rotational testing. In Baloh RW, Halmagyi GM (eds). Disorders of the Vestibular System. Oxford, Oxford, 1996, pp 191–210.
303. Furman JM, Muller ML, Redfern MS, Jennings JR. Visual-vestibular stimulation interferes with information processing in young and older humans. Exp Brain Res 152, 383–392, 2003.
304. Furman JM, Redfern MS. Effect of aging on the otolith-ocular reflex. J Vestib Res 11, 91–103, 2001.
305. Furman JM, Redfern MS. Visual-vestibular interaction during OVAR in the elderly. J Vestib Res 11, 365–370, 2001.
306. Furman JM, Schor RH. Semicircular canal-otolith organ interaction during off-vertical axis rotation in humans. J Assoc Res Otolaryngol 2, 22–30, 2001.
307. Furman JM, Whitney SL. Central causes of dizziness. Phys Ther 80, 179–187, 2000.
308. Furman JMR, Crumrime PK, Reinmuth OM. Epileptic nystagmus. Ann Neurol 27, 686–688, 1990.
309. Furman JMR, Hain TC, Paige GD. Central adaptation models of the vestibuloocular and optokinetic systems. Biol Cybern 61, 255–264, 1989.
310. Furman JMR, Schor RH, Kamerer DB. Off-vertical axis rotational responses in patients with unilateral peripheral vestibular lesions. Ann Otol Rhinol Laryngol 102, 137–143, 1993.
311. Fushiki H, Takata S, Yasuda K, Watanabe Y. Directional preponderance in pitch circular vection. J Vestib Res 10, 93–98, 2000.
312. Galetta SL, Liu GT, Raps EC, Solomon D, Volpe NJ. Cyclodeviation in skew deviation. Am J Ophthalmol 118, 509–514, 1994.
313. Galiana HL. A nystagmus strategy to linearize the vestibulo-ocular reflex. IEEE Trans Biomed Engineering 38, 532–543, 1991.
314. Galiana HL, Smith HL, Katsarkas A. Comparison of linear vs. non-linear methods for analyzing the vestibulo-ocular reflex (VOR). Acta Otolaryngol (Stockh) 115, 585–596, 1995.
315. Galiana HL, Smith HL, Katsarkas A. Modelling non-linearities in the vestibulo-ocular reflex (VOR) after unilateral or bilateral loss of peripheral vestibular function. Exp Brain Res 137, 369–386, 2001.

316. Galimberti CA, Versino M, Sertori I, et al. Epileptic skew deviation. Neurology 50, 1469–1472, 1998.
317. Garbutt S, Han Y, Kumar AN, et al. Vertical optokinetic nystagmus and saccades in normal human subjects. Invest Ophthalmol Vis Sci 44, 3833–3841, 2003.
318. Garbutt S, Han Y, Kumar AN, et al. Disorders of vertical optokinetic nystagmus in patients with ocular misalignment. Vision Res 43, 347–357, 2003.
319. Garbutt S, Harris CM. Abnormal vertical optokinetic nystagmus in infants and children. Br J Ophthalmol 84, 451–455, 2000.
320. Garbutt S, Thakore N, Rucker J, et al. Effects of visual fixation and convergence on periodic alternating nystagmus due to MS. Neuro-ophthalmology 28, 221–229, 2004.
321. Gdowski GT, Belton T, McCrea RA. The neurophysiological substrate for the cervico-ocular reflex in the squirrel monkey. Exp Brain Res 140, 253–264, 2001.
322. Gdowski GT, McCrea RA. Neck proprioceptive inputs to primate vestibular nucleus neurons. Exp Brain Res 135, 511–526, 2000.
323. Gellman RS, Carl JR, Miles FA. Short latency ocular-following responses in man. Vis Neurosci 5, 107–122, 1990.
324. Gianna CC, Gresty MA, Bronstein AM. The human linear vestibulo-ocular reflex to transient accelerations: visual modulation of suppression and enhancement. J Vestib Res 10, 227–238, 2000.
325. Gianna-Poulin CC, Stallings V, Black FO. Eye movement responses to active, high-frequency pitch and yaw head rotations in subjects with unilateral vestibular loss or posterior semicircular canal occlusion. J Vestib Res 13, 131–141, 2003.
326. Gilchrist DP, Cartwright AD, Burgess AM, Curthoys IS. Behavioural characteristics of the quick phase of vestibular nystagmus before and after unilateral labyrinthectomy in guinea pig. Exp Brain Res 149, 289–298, 2003.
327. Gizzi M, Raphan T, Rudolph S, Cohen B. Orientation of human optokinetic nystagmus to gravity: a model-based approach. Exp Brain Res 99, 347–360, 1994.
328. Glasauer S, von LH, Siebold C, Buttner U. Vertical vestibular responses to head impulses are symmetric in downbeat nystagmus. Neurology 63, 621–625, 2004.
329. Gliddon CM, Darlington CL, Smith PF. GABAergic systems in the vestibular nucleus and their contribution to vestibular compensation. Prog Neurobiol 75, 53–81, 2005.
330. Godfrey DA, Xu J, Godfrey MA, Li H, Rubin AM. Effects of unilateral vestibular ganglionectomy on glutaminase activity in the vestibular nerve root and vestibular nuclear complex of the rat. J Neurosci Res 77, 603–612, 2004.
331. Goldberg JM. Afferent diversity and the organization of central vestibular pathways. Exp. Brain Res 130, 277–297, 2000.
332. Goldberg JM, Fernandez C. Physiology of peripheral neurons innervating semicircular canals of the squirrel monkey. 1. Resting discharge and response to constant angular accelerations. J Neurophysiol 34, 635–660, 1971.
333. Goldberg JM, Lysakowski A, Fernández C. Structure and function of vestibular nerve fibers in the chinchilla and squirrel monkey. Ann N Y Acad Sci 656, 92–107, 1992.
334. Goltz HC, Irving EL, Steinbach M, Eizenman M. Vertical eye position control in darkness: orbital position and body orientation interact to modulate drift velocity. Vision Res 37, 789–798, 1997.
335. Gonshor A, Melvill Jones G. Extreme vestibuloocular adaptation induced by prolonged optical reversal of vision. J Physiol (Lond) 256, 381–414, 1976.
336. Gonshor A, Melvill Jones G. Short-term adaptive changes in the human vestibulo-ocular reflex. J Physiol (Lond) 256, 361–379, 1976.
337. Goto F, Meng H, Bai R, et al. Eye movements evoked by the selective stimulation of the utricular nerve in cats. Auris Nasus Larynx 30, 341–348, 2003.
338. Goto F, Meng H, Bai R, et al. Eye movements evoked by selective saccular nerve stimulation in cats. Auris Nasus Larynx 31, 220–225, 2004.
339. Grad A, Baloh RW. Vertigo of vascular origin. Clinical and electronystagmographic features in 84 cases. Arch Neurol 46, 281–284, 1989.
340. Graf W, Ezure K. Morphology of vertical canal related second order vestibular neurons in the cat. Exp Brain Res 63, 35–48, 1986.
341. Graham BP, Dutia MB. Cellular basis of vestibular compensation: analysis and modelling of the role of the commissural inhibitory system. Exp Brain Res 137, 387–396, 2001.
342. Grassi S, Pettorossi VE. Synaptic plasticity in the medial vestibular nuclei: role of glutamate receptors and retrograde messengers in rat brainstem slices. Prog Neurobiol 64, 527–553, 2001.
343. Green A, Galiana HL. Exploring sites for short-term VOR modulation using a bilateral model. Ann N Y Acad Sci 781, 625–628, 1996.
344. Green AM, Angelaki DE. Resolution of sensory ambiguities for gaze stabilization requires a second neural integrator. J Neurosci 23, 9265–9275, 2003.
345. Green AM, Angelaki DE. An integrative neural network for detecting inertial motion and head orientation. J Neurophysiol 92, 905–925, 2004.
346. Green AM, Galiana HL. Hypothesis for shared central processing of canal and otolith signals. J Neurophysiol 80, 2222–2228, 1998.
347. Gresty M, Barratt H, Bronstein A, Page NG. Clinical aspects of otolith-oculomotor relationships. In Keller EL, Zee DS (eds). Adaptive Processes in Visual and Oculomotor Systems. Pergamon Press, 1986, pp 357–365.
348. Gresty MA. Vestibular tests in evolution. 1. Otolith testing. In Baloh RW, Halmagyi GM (eds). Disorders of the Vestibular System. Oxford, New York,1997, pp 243–255.
349. Gresty MA, Barratt HJ, Page NG, Ell JJ. Assessment of vestibulo-ocular reflexes in congenital nystagmus. Ann Neurol 17, 129–136, 1985.
350. Gresty MA, Bronstein AM. Testing otolith function. Br J Audiol 26, 125–136, 1992.
351. Gresty MA, Bronstein AM, Barratt H. Eye movement responses to combined linear and angular head movement. Exp Brain Res 65, 377–384, 1987.
352. Gresty MA, Bronstein AM, Brandt T, Dieterich M. Neurology of otolith function: peripheral and central disorders. Brain 115, 647–673, 1992.
353. Gresty MA, Hess K, Leech J. Disorders of the vestibuloocular reflex producing oscillopsia and

mechanisms compensating for loss of labyrinthine function. Brain 100, 693–716 1977.
354. Gresty MA, Lempert T. Pathophysiology and clinical testing of otolith dysfunction. Adv Otorhinolaryngol 58, 15–33, 2001.
355. Groen E, Bos JE, de Graaf B. Contribution of the otoliths to the human torsional vestibulo-ocular reflex. J Vestib Res 9, 27–36, 1999.
356. Groen E, de Graaf B, Bles W, Bos JE. Ocular torsion before and after 1 hour centrifugation. Brain Res Bull 40, 331–335, 1996.
357. Grossman GE, Leigh RJ, Abel LA, Lanska DJ, Thurston SE. Frequency and velocity of rotational head perturbations during locomotion. Exp Brain Res 70, 470–476, 1988.
358. Grunfeld EA, Morland AB, Bronstein AM, Gresty MA. Adaptation to oscillopsia: a psychophysical and questionnaire investigation. Brain 123, 277–290, 2000.
359. Grüsser O-J. Purkyne's contribution to the physiology of the visual, the vestibular and the oculomotor systems. Human Neurobiol 3, 129–144, 1984.
360. Guldin WO, Grusser OJ. Is there a vestibular cortex? Trends Neurosci 21, 254–259, 1998.
360a. Guilding C, Dutia MB. Early and late changes in vestibular neuronal excitability after deafferentation. Neuroreport 16, 1415–1418, 2005.
361. Haddad GM, Friendlich AR, Robinson DA. Compensation of nystagmus after VIIIth nerve lesions in vestibulo-cerebellectomized cats. Brain Res 135, 192–196 1977.
362. Hafstrom A, Fransson PA, Karlberg M, Magnusson M. Idiosyncratic compensation of the subjective visual horizontal and vertical in 60 patients after unilateral vestibular deafferentation. Acta Otolaryngol 124, 165–171, 2004.
363. Hain TC, Buettner UW. Static roll and the vestibulo-ocular reflex (VOR). Exp Brain Res 83, 463–471, 1990.
364. Hain TC, Fetter M, Zee DS. Head-shaking nystagmus in patients with unilateral peripheral vestibular lesions. Am J Otolaryngol 8, 36–47, 1987.
365. Hain TC, Heroman SJ, Holliday M, et al. Localizing value of optokinetic afternystagmus. Ann Otol Rhinol Laryngol 103, 806–811, 1994.
366. Hain TC, Spindler J. Head-sharing nystagmus. In Sharpe JA, Barber HO (eds). The Vestibulo-Ocular Reflex and Vertigo. Raven Press, New York,1993, pp 217–228.
367. Hain TC, Zee DS. Velocity storage in labyrinthine disorders. Ann N Y Acad Sci 656, 297–304, 1992.
368. Hain TC, Zee DS. Abolition of optokinetic afternystagmus by aminoglycoside ototoxicity. Ann Otol Rhinol Laryngol 100, 580–583, 1991.
369. Hain TC, Zee DS, Maria B. Tilt-suppression of the vestibulo-ocular reflex in patients with cerebellar lesions. Acta Otolaryngol (Stockh) 105, 13–20, 1988.
370. Halmagyi GM. New clinical tests of unilateral vestibular dysfunction. J Laryngol Otol 118, 589–600, 2004.
371. Halmagyi GM, Aw ST, Cremer PD, Curthoys IS, Todd MJ. Impulsive testing of individual semicircular canal function. Ann N Y Acad Sci 942, 192–200, 2001.
372. Halmagyi GM, Aw ST, Karlberg M, Curthoys IS, Todd M. J. Inferior vestibular neuritis. Ann N Y Acad Sci 956, 306–313, 2002.
373. Halmagyi GM, Cremer PD, Anderson J, Murofushi T, Curthoys IS. Isolated directional preponderance of caloric nystagmus: I. Clinical significance. Am J Otol 21, 559–567, 2000.
374. Halmagyi GM, Curthoys IS. A clinical sign of canal paresis. Arch Neurol 45, 737–739, 1988.
375. Halmagyi GM, Curthoys IS, Colebatch JG, Aw ST. Vestibular responses to sound. Ann N Y Acad Sci 1039, 54–67, 2005.
376. Halmagyi GM, Gresty MA, Gibson WPR. Ocular tilt reaction with peripheral vestibular lesion. Ann Neurol 6, 80–83, 1979.
377. Halmagyi GM, Henderson CJ. Visual symptoms of vestibular disease. Aust N Zealand J Ophthalmol 16, 177–179, 1988.
378. Halmagyi GM, Mcgarvie LA, Aw ST, Yavor RA, Todd MJ. The click-evoked vestibulo-ocular reflex in superior semicircular canal dehiscence. Neurology 60, 1172–1175, 2003.
379. Halmagyi GM, Yavor RA, Colebatch JG. Tapping the head activates the vestibular system: a new use for the clinical reflex hammer. Neurology 45, 1927–1929, 1995.
380. Hamann KF, Schuster EM. Vibration-induced nystagmus—A sign of unilateral vestibular deficit. ORL J Otorhinolaryngol Relat Spec 61, 74–79, 1999.
381. Han YH, Kumar AN, Reschke AF, et al. Vestibular and non-vestibular contributions to eye movements that compensate for head rotations during viewing of near targets. Exp Brain Res 165, 294–304, 2005.
382. Hansel C, Linden DJ, D'Angelo E. Beyond parallel fiber LTD: the diversity of synaptic and non-synaptic plasticity in the cerebellum. Nat Neurosci 4, 467–475, 2001.
383. Haque A, Angelaki DE, Dickman JD. Spatial tuning and dynamics of vestibular semicircular canal afferents in rhesus monkeys. Exp Brain Res 155, 81–90, 2004.
384. Harris L, Beykirch K, Fetter M. The visual consequences of deviations in the orientation of the axis of rotation of the human vestibulo-ocular reflex. Vision Res 41, 3271–3281, 2001.
385. Haslwanter T, Curthoys IS, Black RA, Topple AN, Halmagyi GM. The three-dimensional human vestibulo-ocular reflex: response to long-duration yaw angular accelerations. Exp Brain Res 109, 303–311, 1996.
386. Haslwanter T, Jaeger R, Mayr S, Fetter M. Three-dimensional eye-movement responses to off-vertical axis rotations in humans. Exp Brain Res 134, 96–106, 2000.
387. Haslwanter T, Minor LB. Nystagmus induced by circular head shaking in normal human subjects. Exp Brain Res 124, 25–32, 1999.
388. Hawkins JE, Schacht J. Sketches of otohistory. Audiol Neurootol 10, 185–190, 2005.
389. Hawrylyshyn PA, Rubin PA, Tasker RR, Organ LW, Fredrickson JM. Vestibulothalamic projections in man—a sixth primary sensory pathway. J Neurophysiol 41, 394–401, 1978.
390. Hegemann S, Fitzek S, Fitzek C, Fetter M. Cortical vestibular representation in the superior temporal gyrus. J Vestib Res 14, 33–35, 2004.

391. Hegemann S, Shelhamer M, Kramer PD, Zee DS. Adaptation of the phase of the human linear vestibulo-ocular reflex (LVOR) and effects on the oculomotor neural integrator. J. Vestib Res 10, 239–247, 2000.
392. Heide W, Blossfeldt TP, Koenig E, Dichgans J. Optokinetic nystagmus, self-motion sensation and their aftereffects in patients with long-lasting peripheral visual field defects. Clin Vision Sci 5, 133–143, 1990.
393. Heimbrand S, Bronstein AM, Gresty MA, Faldon ME. Optically induced plasticity of the cervicoocular reflex in patients with bilateral absence of vestibular function. Exp Brain Res 112, 372–380, 1996.
394. Henn V. Mach on the analysis of motion sensation. Human Neurobiol 3, 145–148, 1984.
395. Henn V, Young LR, Finley C. Vestibular nucleus units in alert monkeys are also influenced by moving visual fields. Brain Res 71, 144–149, 1974.
396. Herdman SJ, Schubert MC, Das VE, Tusa RJ. Recovery of dynamic visual acuity in unilateral vestibular hypofunction. Arch Otolaryngol Head Neck Surg 129, 819–824, 2003.
397. Hess BJ, Jaggi-Schwarz K, Misslisch H. Canal-otolith interactions after off-vertical axis rotations. II. Spatiotemporal properties of roll and pitch postrotatory vestibuloocular reflexes. J Neurophysiol 93, 1633–1646, 2005.
398. Hess BJ, Lysakowski A, Minor LB, Angelaki DE. Central versus peripheral origin of vestibuloocular reflex recovery following semicircular canal plugging in rhesus monkeys. J Neurophysiol 84, 3078–3082, 2000.
399. Hess K, Dürsteler M, Reisine H. Analysis of slow phase eye velocity during the course of an acute vestibulopathy. Acta Otolaryngol (Stockh) Suppl 406, 227–230, 1984.
399a. Highstein SM, Holstein GR. The anatomy of the vestibular nuclei. Prog Brain Res 151, 157–203, 2005.
400. Highstein SM, Baker R. Excitatory termination of abducens internuclear neurons on medial rectus motoneurons: relationship to syndrome of internuclear ophthalmoplegia. J Neurophysiol 41, 1647–1661, 1987.
401. Highstein SM, Blazquez PM, Hirata Y. Responses of floccular purkinje cells following chronic adaptation of the vertical VOR [abstract]. Soc Neurosci Abstr 27, 2001.
402. Highstein SM, Partsalis A, Arikan R. Role of the Y-group of the vestibular nuclei and flocculus of the cerebellum in motor learning of the vertical vestibulo-ocular reflex. Progr Brain Res 114, 383–397, 1997.
403. Highstein SM, Rabbitt RD, Holstein GR, Boyle RD. Determinants of spatial and temporal coding by semicircular canal afferents. J Neurophysiol 93, 2359–2370, 2005.
404. Himi T, Igarashi M, Takeda N. Effect of vestibulocerebellar lesions on asymmetry of vertical optokinetic functions in the squirrel monkey. Acta Otolaryngol (Stockh) 109, 188–194 1990.
405. Hine T. Effects of asymmetric vergence on compensatory eye movements during active head rotation. J Vestib Res 1, 357–371, 1991.
406. Hirata Y, Highstein SM. Acute adaptation of the vestibuloocular reflex: signal processing by floccular and ventral parafloccular Purkinje cells. J Neurophysiol 85, 2267–2288, 2001.
407. Hirata Y, Highstein SM. Plasticity of the vertical VOR: a system identification approach to localizing the adaptive sites. Ann N Y Acad Sci 978, 480–495, 2002.
408. Hirata Y, Lockard JM, Highstein SM. Capacity of vertical VOR adaptation in squirrel monkey. J Neurophysiol 88, 3194–3207, 2002.
409. Hirvonen TP, Aalto H, Pyykkö I, Juhola, M. Phase difference of vestibulo-ocular reflex in head autorotation test. Acta Otolaryngol (Stockh) Suppl 529, 98–100, 1997.
410. Holstein GR, Martinelli GP, Cohen B. The ultrastructure of GABA-immunoreactive vestibular commissural neurons related to velocity storage in the monkey. Neuroscience 93, 171–181, 1999.
411. Holstein GR, Martinelli GP, Cohen B. Ultrastructural features of non-commissural GABAergic neurons in the medial vestibular nucleus of the monkey. Neuroscience 93, 183–193, 1999.
412. Holstein GR, Martinelli GP, Wearne S, Cohen B. Ultrastructure of vestibular commissural neurons related to velocity storage in the monkey. Neuroscience 93, 155–170, 1999.
413. Holstein GR, Rabbitt RD, Martinelli GP, et al. Convergence of excitatory and inhibitory hair cell transmitters shapes vestibular afferent responses. Proc Natl Acad Sci U S A 101, 15766–15771, 2004.
414. Horii A, Kitahara T, Smith PF, et al. Effects of unilateral labyrinthectomy on GAD, GAT1 and GABA receptor gene expression in the rat vestibular nucleus. NeuroReport 14, 2359–2363, 2003.
415. Horii A, Masumura C, Smith PF, et al. Microarray analysis of gene expression in the rat vestibular nucleus complex following unilateral vestibular deafferentation. J Neurochem 91, 975–982, 2004.
416. Howard IP, Simpson WA. Human optokinetic nystagmus is linked to the stereoscopic system. Exp Brain Res 78, 309–314, 1989.
417. Howard IP, Sun L, Shen X. Cycloversion and cyclovergence: the effects of the area and the position of the visual display. Exp Brain Res 100, 509–514, 1994.
418. Hullar TE, Della Santina CC, Hirvonen T, et al. Responses of irregularly discharging chinchilla semicircular canal vestibular-nerve afferents during high-frequency head rotations. J Neurophysiol 93, 2777–2786, 2005.
419. Hullar TE, Minor LB. High-frequency dynamics of regularly discharging canal afferents provide a linear signal for angular vestibuloocular reflexes. J Neurophysiol, 82, 2000–2005, 1999.
420. Hullar TE, Minor LB, Zee DS. Evaluation of the patient with dizziness. In Cummings CC (ed). Otolaryngology Head & Neck Surgery. Elsevier Mosby, Philadelphia, 2005, pp 3160–3199.
421. Huterer M, Cullen KE. Vestibuloocular reflex dynamics during high-frequency and high-acceleration rotations of the head on body in rhesus monkey. J Neurophysiol 88, 13–28, 2002.
422. Huygen PLM, Nicolasen MGM, Verhagen WIM, Theunissen EJJM. Contralateral hyperactive caloric

responses in unilateral labyrinthine weakness. Acta Otolaryngol (Stockh) 107, 1–4, 1989.
423. Huygen PLM, Verhagen WIM, Nicolasen MGM. Cervico-ocular reflex enhancement in labyrinthine-defective and normal subjects. Exp Brain Res 87, 457–464, 1991.
424. Ibbotson MR, Price NS, Das VE, Hietanen MA, Mustari MJ. Torsional eye movements during psychophysical testing with rotating patterns. Exp Brain Res 160, 264–267, 2005.
425. Indovina I, Maffei V, Bosco G, et al. Representation of visual gravitational motion in the human vestibular cortex. Science 308, 416–419, 2005.
426. Israël I, Bronstein AM, Kanayama R, Faldon M, Gresty MA. Visual and vestibular factors influencing vestibular "navigation". Exp Brain Res 112, 411–419, 1996.
427. Israël I, Fetter M, Koenig E. Vestibular perception of passive whole-body rotation about horizontal and vertical axes in humans: goal-directed vestibulo-ocular reflex and vestibular memory-contingent saccades. Exp Brain Res 96, 335–346, 1993.
428. Israël I, Rivaud S, Gaymard B, Berthoz A, Pierrot-Deseilligny C. Cortical control of vestibular-guided saccades. Brain 118, 1169–1184, 1995.
429. Istl-Lenz Y, Hydén D, Schwartz DWF. Response of the human vestibulo-ocular response following long-term 2x magnified visual input. Exp Brain Res 57, 448–455, 1985.
430. Ito M. Cerebellar flocculus hypothesis. Nature 363, 24–25, 1993.
431. Ito M. Long-term depression. Annu Rev Neurosci 12, 85–102, 1989.
432. Ito M. Historical review of the significance of the cerebellum and the role of Purkinje cells in motor learning. Ann N Y Acad Sci 978, 273–288, 2002.
433. Ito M, Nisimaru N, Yamamoto M. Pathways for the vestibulo-ocular reflex excitation arising from semicircular canals of rabbits. Exp Brain Res 24, 257–271, 1976.
434. Ito M, Nisimaru N, Yamamoto M. Specific patterns of neuronal connexions involved in the control of the rabbit's vestibulo-ocular reflexes by the cerebellar flocculus. J Physiol (Lond) 265, 833–854, 1977.
435. Ito Y, Gresty MA. Shift of subjective reference and visual orientation during slow pitch tilt for the seated human subject. Brain Res Bull 40, 417–421, 1996.
436. Iwasaki S, Ito K, Abbey K, Murofushi T. Prediction of canal paresis using head-shaking nystagmus test. Acta Otolaryngol 124, 803–806, 2004.
437. Living without a balancing mechanism. N Engl J Med 246, 458–460, 1952.
438. Jaeger R, Haslwanter T. Otolith responses to dynamical stimuli: results of a numerical investigation. Biol Cybern 90, 165–175, 2004.
439. Jaeger R, Takagi A, Haslwanter T. Modeling the relation between head orientations and otolith responses in humans. Hear Res 173, 29–42, 2002.
440. Jahn K, Naessl A, Schneider E, et al. Inverse U-shaped curve for age dependency of torsional eye movement responses to galvanic vestibular stimulation. Brain 126, 1579–1589, 2003.
441. Jahn K, Naessl A, Strupp M, et al. Torsional eye movement responses to monaural and binaural galvanic vestibular stimulation: side-to-side asymmetries. Ann N Y Acad Sci 1004, 485–489, 2003.
442. Jáuregui-Renaud K, Faldon M, Clarke A, Bronstein AM, Gresty MA. Skew deviation of the eyes in normal human subjects induced by semicircular canal stimulation. Neurosci Lett 235, 135–137, 1996.
443. Jauregui-Renaud K, Faldon ME, Gresty MA, Bronstein AM. Horizontal ocular vergence and the three-dimensional response to whole-body roll motion. Exp Brain Res 136, 79–92, 2001.
444. Jell RM, Ireland DJ, Lafortune S. Human optokinetic afternystagmus: effects of repeated stimulation. Acta Otolaryngol (Stockh) 99, 95–101, 1985.
445. Jenkins HA, Cohen HS, Kimball KT. Long-term vestibulo-ocular reflex changes in patients with vestibular ablation. Acta Otolaryngol 120, 187–191, 2000.
446. Johnston JL, Sharpe JA. The initial vestibulo-ocular reflex and its visual enhancement and cancellation in humans. Exp Brain Res 99, 302–308, 1994.
447. Jombik P, Bahyl V. Short latency responses in the averaged electro-oculogram elicited by vibrational impulse stimuli applied to the skull: could they reflect vestibulo-ocular reflex function? J Neurol Neurosurg Psychiatry 76, 222–228, 2005.
448. Jürgens R, Mergner T. Interaction between cervico-ocular and vestibulo-ocular reflexes in normal adults. Exp Brain Res 77, 381–390, 1989.
449. Kahane P, Hoffmann D, Minotti L, Berthoz A. Reappraisal of the human vestibular cortex by cortical electrical stimulation study. Ann Neurol 54, 615–624, 2003.
450. Kamei T, Iizuka T. Prediction of vertigo recurrences in Meniere's disease by the head-shaking test. Int Tinnitus J 5, 47–49, 1999.
451. Kamura E, Yagi T. Three-dimensional analysis of eye movements during off vertical axis rotation in patients with unilateral labyrinthine loss. Acta Otolaryngol 121, 225–228, 2001.
452. Kanayama R, Bronstein AM, Gresty MA, et al. Perceptual studies in patients with vestibular neurectomy. Acta Otolaryngol (Stockh) Suppl 520, 408–411, 1995.
453. Kansaku K, Hashimoto K, Muraki S, et al. Retinotopic hemodynamic activation of the human V5/MT area during optokinetic responses. NeuroReport 12, 3891–3895, 2001.
454. Kaplan PW, Tusa RJ. Neurophysiologic and clinical correlations of epileptic nystagmus. Neurology 43, 2508–2514, 1993.
455. Karlberg M, AW ST, Black RA, et al. Vibration-induced ocular torsion and nystagmus after unilateral vestibular deafferentation. Brain 126, 956–964, 2003.
456. Karlberg M, Magnusson M. Asymmetric optokinetic after-nystagmus induced by active or passive sustained head rotations. Acta Otolaryngol (Stockh) 116, 647–651, 1996.
457. Karnath H-O, Sievering D, Fetter M. The interactive contribution of neck muscle proprioception and vestibular stimulation to subjective "straight ahead" orientation in man. Exp Brain Res 101, 140–146, 1994.
458. Kasai T, Zee DS. Eye-head coordination in labyrinthine-defective human beings. Brain Res 144, 123–141, 1978.
458a. Kassardjian CD, Tan YF, Chung JY, Heskin R, Peterson MJ, Broussard DM. The site of a motor

memory shift with consolidation. J Neurosci 25, 7979–7985, 2005.
459. Katsarkas A, Galiana HL. Bechterew's phenomenon in human. Acta Otolaryngol (Stockh) Suppl 406, 95–100, 1984.
460. Katsarkas A, Smith H, Galiana H. Head-shaking nystagmus (HSN): the theoretical explanation and the experimental proof. Acta Otolaryngol 120, 177–181, 2000.
461. Katz E, Vianney de Jong JMB, Buettner-Ennever J, Cohen B. Effects of midline medullary lesions on velocity storage and the vestibulo-ocular reflex. Exp Brain Res 87, 505–520, 1991.
462. Kelders WP, Kleinrensink GJ, van der Geest JN, et al. Compensatory increase of the cervico-ocular reflex with age in healthy humans. J Physiol 553, 311–317, 2003.
463. Kenmochi M, Ohashi T, Nishino H, Sato S. Cortical potentials evoked by horizontal rotatory stimulation: the effects of angular acceleration. Acta Otolaryngol 123, 923–927, 2003.
464. Kevetter GA, Leonard RB, Newlands SD, Perachio AA. Central distribution of vestibular afferents that innervate the anterior or lateral semicircular canal in the mongolian gerbil. J Vestib Res 14, 1–15, 2004.
465. Khater TT, Baker JF, Peterson BW. Dynamics of adaptive change in human vestibulo-ocular reflex direction. J Vestib Res 1, 23–29, 1990.
466. Kim JI, Somers JT, Stahl JS, Bhidayasiri R, Leigh RJ. Vertical nystagmus in normal subjects: effects of head position, nicotine and scopolamine. J Vestib Res 10, 291–300, 2000.
467. Kim JS, Ahn KW, Moon SY, et al. Isolated perverted head-shaking nystagmus in focal cerebellar infarction. Neurology 64, 575–576, 2005.
468. Kim JS, Sharpe JA. The vertical vestibulo-ocular reflex, and its interaction with vision during active head motion: effects of aging. J Vestib Res 11, 3–12, 2001.
469. King J, Zheng Y, Liu P, Darlington CL, Smith PF. NMDA and AMPA receptor subunit protein expression in the rat vestibular nucleus following unilateral labyrinthectomy. NeuroReport 13, 1541–1545, 2002.
470. Kitahara T, Fukushima M, Takeda N, Saika T, Kubo T. Effects of pre-flocculectomy on Fos expression and NMDA receptor-mediated neural circuits in the central vestibular system after unilateral labyrinthectomy. Acta Otolaryngol 120, 866–871, 2000.
471. Kitahara T, Fukushima M, Takeda N, et al. Role of cholinergic mossy fibers in vestibular nuclei in the development of vestibular compensation. Acta Otolaryngol Suppl 545, 101–104, 2001.
472. Kitahara T, Kondoh K, Morihana T, et al. Steroid effects on vestibular compensation in human. Neurol Res 25, 287–291, 2003.
473. Kitahara T, Takeda N, Saika T, Kubo T, Kiyama H. Role of the flocculus in the development of vestibular compensation: immunohistochemical studies with retrograde tracing and flocculectomy using fos expression as a marker in the rat brainstem. Neuroscience 76, 571–580, 1997.
474. Klam F, Graf W. Vestibular signals of posterior parietal cortex neurons during active and passive head movements in macaque monkeys. Ann N Y Acad Sci 1004, 271–282, 2003.
475. Kluge M, Beyenburg S, Fernandez G, Elger CE. Epileptic vertigo: evidence for vestibular representation in human frontal cortex. Neurology 55, 1906–1908, 2000.
476. Koizuka I. Adaptive plasticity in the otolith-ocular reflex. Auris Nasus Larynx 30 Suppl, S3–S6, 2003.
477. Koizuka I, Furman JM, Mendoza JC. Plasticity of responses to off-vertical axis rotation. Acta Otolaryngol (Stockh) 117, 321–324, 1997.
478. Konen CS, Kleiser R, Seitz RJ, Bremmer F. An fMRI study of optokinetic nystagmus and smooth-pursuit eye movements in humans. Exp Brain Res 165, 203–216, 2005.
479. Kramer PD, Roberts DC, Shelhamer M, Zee DS. A versatile stereoscopic visual display system for vestibular and oculomotor research. J Vestib Res 8, 363–380, 1998.
480. Kramer PD, Shelhamer M, Peng GCY, Zee DS. Context-specific short-term adaptation of the phase of the vestibulo-ocular reflex. Exp Brain Res 120, 184–192, 1998.
481. Kramer PD, Shelhamer M, Zee DS. Short-term adaptation of the phase of the vestibulo-ocular reflex (VOR) in normal human subjects. Exp Brain Res 106, 318–326, 1995.
482. Krauzlis RJ, Lisberger SG. Simple spike responses of gaze velocity Purkinje cells in the floccular lobe of the monkey during the onset and offset of pursuit eye movements. J Neurophysiol 72, 2045–2050, 1994.
483. Krauzlis RJ, Lisberger SJ. Directional organization of eye movement and visual signals in the floccular lobe of the monkey cerebellum. Exp Brain Res 109, 289–302, 1996.
484. Kudo K, Yoshida M, Makishima K. Reverse optokinetic after-nystagmus generated by gaze fixation during optokinetic stimulation. Acta Otolaryngol 122, 37–42, 2002.
485. Kuki Y, Hirata Y, Blazquez PM, Heiney SA, Highstein SM. Memory retention of vestibuloocular reflex motor learning in squirrel monkeys. NeuroReport 15, 1007–1011, 2004.
486. Kushiro K, Dai M, Kunin M, et al. Compensatory and orienting eye movements induced by off-vertical axis rotation (OVAR) in monkeys. J Neurophysiol 88, 2445–2462, 2002.
487. Lackner JR, DiZio P. Vestibular, proprioceptive, and haptic contributions to spatial orientation. Annu Rev Psychol 56, 115–147, 2005.
488. Lafortune SH, Ireland DJ, Jell RM, DuVal L. Human optokinetic nystagmus. Stimulus velocity dependence of the two-component decay model and involvement of pursuit. Acta Otolaryngol (Stockh) 101, 183–192, 1986.
489. Langer T, Fuchs A, Chubb M, Scudder C, Lisberger S. Floccular efferents in the rhesus macaque as revealed by autoradiography and horseradish peroxidase. J Comp Neurol 235, 26–37, 1985.
490. Langer T, Fuchs A, Scudder C, Chubb M. Afferents to the flocculus of the cerebellum in the rhesus macaque as revealed by retrograde transport of horseradish peroxidase. J Comp Neurol 235, 1–25, 1985.
491. Lasker DM, Backous DD, Lysakowski A, Davis GL, Minor LB. Horizontal vestibuloocular reflex evoked by high-acceleration rotations in the squirrel monkey. II. Responses after canal plugging. J Neurophysiol 82, 1271–1285, 1999.

492. Lasker DM, Hullar TE, Minor LB. Horizontal vestibuloocular reflex evoked by high-acceleration rotations in the squirrel monkey. III. Responses after labyrinthectomy. J. Neurophysiol. 83, 2482–2496, 2000.
493. Lasker DM, Ramat S, Carey JP, Minor LB. Vergence-mediated modulation of the human horizontal angular VOR provides evidence of pathway-specific changes in VOR dynamics. Ann N Y Acad Sci 956, 324–337, 2002.
494. Lee C, Zee DS, Straumann D. Saccades from torsional offset positions back to listing's plane. J Neurophysiol 83, 3241–3253, 2000.
495. Lee H, Cho YW. A case of isolated nodulus infarction presenting as a vestibular neuritis. J Neurol Sci 221, 117–119, 2004.
496. Lee H, Yi HA, Cho YW, et al. Nodulus infarction mimicking acute peripheral vestibulopathy. Neurology 60, 1700–1702, 2003.
497. Lehnen N, Aw ST, Todd MJ, Halmagyi GM. Head impulse test reveals residual semicircular canal function after vestibular neurectomy. Neurology 62, 2294–2296 ,2004.
498. Leigh RJ. Human vestibular cortex. Ann Neurol 35, 383–384, 1994.
499. Leigh RJ, Brandt T. A reevaluation of the vestibulo-ocular reflex: new ideas of its purpose, properties, neural substrate, and disorders. Neurology 43, 1288–1295, 1993.
500. Leigh RJ, Robinson DA, Zee DS. A hypothetical explanation for periodic alternating nystagmus: instability in the optokinetic-vestibular system. Ann N Y Acad Sci 374, 619–635, 1981.
501. Leigh RJ, Zee DS. Eye movements of the blind. Invest Ophthalmol Vis Sci 19, 328–331, 1980.
502. LeLiever WC, Correia MJ. Further observations on the effects of head position on vertical OKN and OKAN in normal subjects. Otolaryngol Head Neck Surg 97, 275–281, 1987.
503. Lempert T, Gianna C, Brookes G, Bronstein A, Gresty M. Horizontal otolith-ocular responses in humans after unilateral vestibular deafferentation. Exp Brain Res 118, 533–540, 1998.
504. Lempert T, Gresty MA, Bronstein AM. Horizontal linear vestibulo-ocular reflex testing in patients with peripheral vestibular disorders. Ann N Y Acad Sci 871, 232–247, 1999.
505. Lewis RF, Clendaniel RA, Zee DS. Vergence-dependent adaptation of the vestibulo-ocular reflex. Exp Brain Res 152, 335–340, 2003.
506. Li H, Dokas LA, Godfrey DA, Rubin AM. Remodeling of synaptic connections in the deafferented vestibular nuclear complex. J Vestib Res 12, 167–183, 2002.
507. Li J, Smith SS, McElligott JG. Cerebellar nitric oxide is necessary for vestibulo-ocular reflex adaptation, a sensorimotor model of learning. J Neurophysiol 74, 489–494, 1995.
508. Li YX, Hashimoto T, Tokuyama W, Miyashita Y, Okuno H. Spatiotemporal dynamics of brain-derived neurotrophic factor mRNA induction in the vestibulo-olivary network during vestibular compensation. J Neurosci 21, 2738–2748, 2001.
509. Lichtenberg BK, Young LR, Arrott AP. Human ocular counterrolling induced by varying linear accelerations. Exp Brain Res 48, 127–136, 1982.
510. Lisberger SG. Neural basis for motor learning in the vestibulo-ocular reflex of primates. III. Computational and behavioral analysis of the sites of learning. J Neurophysiol 72, 974–999, 1994.
511. Lisberger SG. Motor learning and memory in the vestibulo-ocular reflex: the dark side. Ann N Y Acad Sci 781, 525–531, 1996.
512. Lisberger SG, Miles FA, Optican LM. Frequency-selective adaptation: evidence for channels in the vestibulo-ocular reflex. J Neuroscience 3, 1234–1244, 1983.
513. Lisberger SG, Miles FA, Zee DS. Signals used to computer errors in the monkey vestibuloocular reflex: possible role of the flocculus. J Neurophysiol 52, 1140–1153, 1984.
514. Lisberger SG, Pavelko TA, Brontë-Stewart HM, Stone LS. Neural basis for motor learning in the vestibuloocular reflex of primates. II. Changes in the responses of horizontal gaze-velocity Purkinje cells in the cerebellar flocculus and ventral paraflocculus. J Neurophysiol 72, 954–973, 1994.
515. Lobel E, Kleine JF, Leroy-Willig A, et al. Cortical areas activated by bilateral galvanic vestibular stimulation. Ann N Y Acad Sci 871, 313–323, 1999.
516. Loose R, Probst T, Tucha O, et al. Vestibular evoked potentials from the vertical semicircular canals in humans evoked by roll-axis rotation in microgravity and under 1-G. Behav Brain Res 134, 131–137, 2002.
517. Lopez C, Borel L, Magnan J, Lacour M. Torsional optokinetic nystagmus after unilateral vestibular loss: asymmetry and compensation. Brain 128, 1511–1524, 2005.
518. Lopez I, Honrubia V, Baloh RW. Aging and the human vestibular nucleus. J Vestib Res 7, 77–85, 1997.
519. Lorente de Nó R. Vestibulo-ocular reflex arc. Arch Neurol Psychiatr 30, 245–291, 1933.
520. Lott LA, Post RB. Up-down asymmetry in vertical induced motion. Perception 22, 527–535, 1993.
521. Lozada AF, Aarnisalo AA, Karlstedt K, Stark H, Panula P. Plasticity of histamine H3 receptor expression and binding in the vestibular nuclei after labyrinthectomy in rat. BMC Neurosci 5, 32, 2004.
522. Luebke AE, Robinson DA. Gain changes of the cat's vestibulo-ocular reflex after flocculus deactivation. Exp Brain Res 98, 379–390, 1994.
523. Lysakowski A. In Cummings CC (ed). Otolaryngology Head & Neck Surgery. Elsevier Mosby, Phildelphia, 2005, pp 3089–3114.
524. Maas EF, Huebner WP, Seidman SH, Leigh RJ. Behavior of human horizontal vestibulo-ocular reflex in response to high-acceleration stimuli. Brain Res 499, 153–156, 1989.
525. MacDougall HG, Brizuela AE, Burgess AM, Curthoys IS, Halmagyi GM. Patient and normal three-dimensional eye-movement responses to maintained (DC) surface galvanic vestibular stimulation. Otol Neurotol 26, 500–511, 2005.
526. Magnusson AK, Tham R. Vestibulo-oculomotor behaviour in rats following a transient unilateral vestibular loss induced by lidocaine. Neuroscience 120, 1105–1114, 2003.
527. Mallinson AI, Longridge NS. Caloric response does not decline with age. J Vestib Res 14, 393–396, 2004.
528. Mandelli MJ, Misslisch H, Hess BJ. Static and dynamic properties of vergence-induced reduction

of ocular counter-roll in near vision. Eur J Neurosci 21, 549–555, 2005.
529. Mandl G, Jones GM. Rapid visual vestibular interaction during visual tracking in strobe light. Brain Res 165, 133–138, 1979.
530. Markin VS, Hudspeth AJ. Gating-spring models of mechanoelectrical transduction by hair cells of the internal ear. Annu Rev Biophys Biomol Struct 24, 59–82, 1995.
531. Marti S, Straumann D, Glasauer S. The origin of downbeat nystagmus: an asymmetry in the distribution of on-directions of vertical gaze-velocity purkinje cells. Ann N Y Acad Sci 1039, 548–553, 2005.
532. Maruta J, Simpson JI, Raphan T, Cohen B. Orienting eye movements and nystagmus produced by translation while rotating (TWR). Exp Brain Res 163, 273–283, 2005.
533. Maruyama M, Fushiki H, Yasuda K, Watanabe Y. Asymmetric adaptive gain changes of the vertical vestibulo-ocular reflex in cats. Brain Res 1023, 302–308, 2004.
534. Matsuo S, Hosogai M, Nakao S. Ascending projections of posterior canal-activated excitatory and inhibitory secondary vestibular neurons to the mesodiencephalon in cats. Exp Brain Res 100, 7–17, 1994.
535. Matsuo V, Cohen B. Vertical optokinetic nystagmus and vestibular nystagmus in the monkey: up-down asymmetry and effects of gravity. Exp Brain Res 53, 197–216, 1984.
536. Matta FV, Enticott JC. The effects of state of alertness on the vestibulo-ocular reflex in normal subjects using the vestibular rotational chair. J Vestib Res 14, 387–391, 2004.
537. Mazzoni A. Internal auditory artery supply to the petrous bone. Arch Otolaryngol Head Neck Surg 81, 13–21, 1972.
538. McCabe BF, Ryu JH. Further experiments on vestibular compensation. Laryngoscope 82, 381–396, 1972.
539. McClure JA, Copp CC, Lycett P. Recovery nystagmus in Meniere's disease. Laryngoscope 91, 1727–1737, 1981.
540. McConville KM, Tomlinson RD, Na E. Behavior of eye-movement-related cells in the vestibular nuclei during combined rotational and translational stimuli. J Neurophysiol 76, 3136–3148, 1996.
541. McCrea R, Chen-Huang C, Belton T, Gdowski GT. Behavior contingent processing of vestibular sensory signals in the vestibular nuclei. Ann N Y Acad Sci 781, 292–303, 1996.
542. McCrea R, Gdowski G, Luan H. Current concepts of vestibular nucleus function: transformation of vestibular signals in the vestibular nuclei. Ann N Y Acad Sci 942, 328–344, 2001.
543. McCrea R, Strassman A, May E, Highstein S. Anatomical and physiological characteristics of vestibular neurons mediating the horizontal vestibulo-ocular reflex of the squirrel monkey. J Comp Neurol 264, 547–570, 1987.
544. McCrea RA, Luan H. Signal processing of semicircular canal and otolith signals in the vestibular nuclei during passive and active head movements. Ann N Y Acad Sci 1004 169–182, 2003.
545. McElligott JG, Beeton P, Polk J. Effect of cerebellar inactivation by lidocaine microdialysis on the vestibuloocular reflex in goldfish. J Neurophysiol 79, 1286–1294, 1998.
546. McElligott JG, Spencer RF. Neuropharmacological aspects of the vestibulo-ocular reflex. In Anderson JH, Beitz AJ (eds). Neurochemistry of the Vestibular System. CRC Press, Boca Raton, 2000, pp 199–222.
547. McHenry MQ, Angelaki DE. Primate translational vestibuloocular reflexes. II. Version and vergence responses to fore-aft motion. J Neurophysiol 83, 1648–1661, 2000.
548. McKenna GJ, Peng GC, Zee DS. Neck muscle vibration alters visually perceived roll in normals. J Assoc Res Otolaryngol 5, 25–31, 2004.
549. Medendorp WP, Van Gisbergen JA, Gielen CC. Human gaze stabilization during active head translations. J Neurophysiol 87, 295–304, 2002.
550. Medendorp WP, Van Gisbergen JA, Van PS, Gielen CC. Context compensation in the vestibuloocular reflex during active head rotations. J Neurophysiol 84, 2904–2917, 2000.
551. Melvill Jones, G. Adaptive modulation of VOR parameters by vision. In Berthoz A, Melvill Jones G (eds). Adaptive Mechanisms in Gaze Control. Elsevier, Amsterdam,1985, pp 21–50.
552. Melvill Jones G, Berthoz A, Segal B. Adaptive modification of the vestibulo-ocular reflex by mental effort in darkness. Exp Brain Res 56, 149–153, 1984.
553. Melvill Jones G, Guitton D, Berthoz A. Changing patterns of eye-head coordination during 6 h of optically reversed vision. Exp Brain Res 69, 531–544, 1988.
554. Melvill Jones G, Mandl G. Motion sickness due to vision reversal: its absence in stroboscopic light. Ann N Y Acad Sci 374, 303–311, 1981.
555. Meng H, Green AM, Dickman JD, Angelaki DE. Pursuit-vestibular interactions in brainstem neurons during rotation and translation. J Neurophysiol, 2005.
556. Meng H, et al. Morphology of physiologically identified otolith-related vestibular neurons in cats. Neurosci Lett 331, 37–40, 2002.
557. Merfeld DM. Rotation otolith tilt-translation reinterpretation (ROTTR) hypothesis: a new hypothesis to explain neurovestibular spaceflight adaptation. J Vestib Res 13, 309–320, 2003.
558. Merfeld DM. Modeling human vestibular responses during eccentric rotation and off vertical axis rotation. Acta Otolaryngol (Stockh) 520, 354–359, 1995.
559. Merfeld DM, Park S, Gianna-Poulin C, Black FO, Wood S. Vestibular perception and action employ qualitatively different mechanisms: I. Frequency response of VOR and perceptual responses during translation and tilt. J Neurophysiol 94, 186–198, 2005.
560. Merfeld DM, Park S, Gianna-Poulin C, Black FO, Wood S. Vestibular perception and action employ qualitatively different mechanisms: II. VOR and perceptual responses during combined tilt and translation. J Neurophysiol 94, 199–205, 2005.
561. Merfeld DM, Young LR. The vestibulo-ocular reflex of the squirrel monkey during eccentric rotation and roll tilt. Exp Brain Res 106, 111–122, 1995.
562. Merfeld DM, Young LR, Oman CM, Shelhamer MJ. A multdimensional model of the effect of gravity on the spatial orientation of the monkey. J Vestib Res 3, 141–161, 1993.

563. Merfeld DM, Zupan L, Peterka RJ. Humans use internal models to estimate gravity and linear acceleration. Nature 398, 615–618, 1999.
564. Merfeld DM, Zupan LH. Neural processing of gravitoinertial cues in humans. III. Modeling tilt and translation responses. J Neurophysiol 87, 819–833, 2002.
565. Merfeld DM, Zupan LH, Gifford CA. Neural processing of gravito-inertial cues in humans. II. Influence of the semicircular canals during eccentric rotation. J Neurophysiol 85, 1648–1660, 2001.
566. Mergner T, Glasauer S. A simple model of vestibular canal-otolith signal fusion. Ann N Y Acad Sci 871, 430–434, 1999.
567. Mergner T, Huber W, Becker W. Vestibular-neck interaction and transformation of sensory coordinates. J Vestib Res 7, 347–367, 1997.
568. Mergner T, Schweigart G, Muller M, Hlavacka F, Becker W. Visual contributions to human self-motion perception during horizontal body rotation. Arch Ital Biol 138, 139–166, 2000.
569. Mergner T, Wertheim A, Rumberger A. Which retinal and extra-retinal information is crucial for circular vection? Arch Ital Biol 138, 123–138, 2000.
570. Mesland BS, Finlay AL, Wertheim AH, et al. Object motion perception during ego-motion: patients with a complete loss of vestibular function vs. normals. Brain Res Bull 40, 459–465, 1996.
571. Michel J, Dumas G, Lavieille JP, Charachon R. Diagnostic value of vibration-induced nystagmus obtained by combined vibratory stimulation applied to the neck muscles and skull of 300 vertiginous patients. Rev Laryngol Otol Rhinol (Bord) 122, 89–94, 2001.
572. Migliaccio AA, Della Santina CC, Carey JP, Minor LB, Zee DS. The effect of binocular eye position and head rotation plane on the human torsional vestibuloocular reflex. Vision Res, 2006.
573. Migliaccio AA, Cremer PD, Aw ST, et al. Vergence-mediated changes in the axis of eye rotation during the human vestibulo-ocular reflex can occur independent of eye position. Exp Brain Res 151, 238–248, 2003.
574. Migliaccio AA, Halmagyi GM, Mcgarvie LA, Cremer PD. Cerebellar ataxia with bilateral vestibulopathy: description of a syndrome and its characteristic clinical sign. Brain 127, 280–293, 2004.
575. Migliaccio AA, Minor LB, Carey JP. Vergence-mediated modulation of the human horizontal vestibulo-ocular reflex is eliminated by a partial peripheral gentamicin lesion. Exp Brain Res 159, 92–98, 2004.
575a. Migliaccio AA, Schubert MC, Clendaniel R, Carey JP, Della Santina CC, Minor LB, Zee DS. Axis of eye rotation changes with head-pitch orientation during head impulses about Earth-vertical. J Assoc Res Otolaryngol 2006.
576. Miles FA. The sensing of rotational and translational optic flow by the primate optokinetic system. In Miles FA, Wallman J (eds). Visual Motion and its Role in the Stabilization of Gaze. Elsevier, Amsterdam, 1993, pp 393–403.
577. Miles FA. The neural processing of 3-D visual information: evidence from eye movements. Eur J Neurosci 10, 811–822, 1998.
578. Miles FA, Braitman DJ, Dow BA. Long-term adaptive changes in primate vestibuloocular reflex. IV. Electrophysiological observations in flocculus of adapted monkeys. J Neurophysiol 43, 1477–1493, 1980.
579. Minagar A, Sheremata WA, Tusa RJ. Perverted head-shaking nystagmus: a possible mechanism. Neurology 57, 887–889, 2001.
580. Minor LB. Labyrinthine fistulae: pathobiology and management. Curr Opin Otolaryngol Head Neck Surg 11, 340–346, 2003.
581. Minor LB, Goldberg JM. Vestibular-nerve inputs to the vestibulo-ocular reflex: a functional ablation study in the squirrel monkey. J Neurosci 11, 1636–1648, 1991.
582. Minor LB, Haslwanter T, Straumann D, Zee DS. Hyperventilation-induced nystagmus in patients with vestibular schwannoma. Acta Otolaryngol (Stockh), 1998.
583. Minor LB, Lasker DM, Backous DD, Hullar TE. Horizontal vestibuloocular reflex evoked by high-acceleration rotations in the squirrel monkey. I. Normal responses. J Neurophysiol 82, 1254–1270, 1999.
584. Minor LB, McCrea R, Goldberg JM. Dual projections of secondary vestibular axons in the medial longitudinal fasciculus to extraocular motor nuclei and the spinal cord of the squirrel monkey. Exp Brain Res 83, 9–21, 1990.
585. Misslisch H, Hess BJ. Combined influence of vergence and eye position on three-dimensional vestibulo-ocular reflex in the monkey. J Neurophysiol 88, 2368–2376, 2002.
586. Misslisch H, Tweed D. Torsional dynamics and cross-coupling in the human vestibulo-ocular reflex during active head rotation. J Vestib Res 10, 119–125, 2000.
587. Misslisch H, Tweed D, Fetter M, Sievering D, Koenig E. Rotational kinematics of the human vestibuloocular reflex. III. Listing's law. J Neurophysiol 72, 2490–2502, 1994.
588. Misslisch H, Tweed D, Hess BJ. Stereopsis outweighs gravity in the control of the eyes. J Neurosci 21, RC126, 2001.
589. Miyamoto T, Fukushima K, Takada T, DE Waele C, Vidal PP. Saccular projections in the human cerebral cortex. Ann N Y Acad Sci 1039, 124–131, 2005.
590. Moller C, Odkvist LM, White V, Cyr D. The plasticity of compensatory eye movements in rotatory tests. I. The effects of alertness and eye closure. Acta Otolaryngol (Stockh) 109, 15–24, 1990.
591. Moller C, White V, Odkvist L. Plasticity of compensatory eye movements in rotatory tests. II. The effects of voluntary, visual, imaginary, auditory and proprioceptive mechanisms. Acta Otolaryngol (Stockh) 109, 168–178, 1990.
592. Morita M, Imai T, Kazunori S, et al. A new rotational test for vertical semicircular canal function. Auris Nasus Larynx 30, 233–237, 2003.
593. Morrow MJ, Sharpe JA. The effects of head and trunk position on torsional vestibular and optokinetic eye movements in humans. Exp Brain Res 95, 144–150, 1993.
594. Murai N, Tsuji J, Ito J, Mishina M, Hirano T. Vestibular compensation in glutamate receptor delta-2 subunit knockout mice: dynamic property of vestibulo-ocular reflex. Eur Arch Otorhinolaryngol 261, 82–86, 2004.

595. Murasugi CM, Howard IP. Up-down asymmetry in human vertical optokinetic nystagmus and afternystagmus: contributions of the central and peripheral retinae. Exp Brain Res 77, 183–192, 1989.
596. Murofushi T, Halmagyi GM, Yavor RA, Colebatch JG. Absent vestibular evoked myogenic potentials in vestibular neurolabyrinthitis. An indicator of inferior vestibular nerve involvement? Arch Otolaryngol Head Neck Surg 122, 845–848, 1996.
597. Murofushi T, Monobe H, Ochiai A, Ozeki H. The site of lesion in "vestibular neuritis": study by galvanic VEMP. Neurology 61, 417–418, 2003.
598. Murofushi T, Takai Y, Iwasaki S, Matsuzaki M. VEMP recording by binaural simultaneous stimulation in subjects with vestibulo-cochlear disorders. Eur Arch Otorhinolaryngol, 2005.
599. Musallam WS, Tomlinson RD. Model for the translational vestibuloocular reflex (VOR). J Neurophysiol 82, 2010–2014, 1999.
600. Myers SF. Patterns of low-frequency rotational responses in bilateral caloric weakness patients. J Vestib Res 2, 123–131, 1992.
601. Naganuma H, Tokumasu K, Okamoto M, Hashimoto S, Yamashina S. Three-dimensional analysis of morphological aspects of the human saccular macula. Ann Otol Rhinol Laryngol 110, 1017–1024, 2001.
602. Naganuma H, Tokumasu K, Okamoto M, Hashimoto S, Yamashina S. Three-dimensional analysis of morphological aspects of the human utricular macula. Ann Otol Rhinol Laryngol 112, 419–424, 2003.
603. Nagao S. Different roles of flocculus and ventral paraflocculus for oculomotor control in the primate. NeuroReport 3, 13–16, 1992.
604. Nagao S, Kitamura T, Nakamura N, Hiramatsu T, Yamada J. Differences of the primate flocculus and ventral paraflocculus in the mossy and climbing fiber input organization. J Comp Neurol 382, 480–498, 1997.
605. Nagao S, Kitamura T, Nakamura N, Hiramatsu T, Yamada J. Location of efferent terminals of the primate flocculus and ventral paraflocculus revealed by anterograde axonal transport methods. Neurosci Res 27, 257–269, 1997.
606. Nagao S, Kitazawa H. Effects of reversible shutdown of the monkey flocculus on the retention of adaptation of the horizontal vestibulo-ocular reflex. Neuroscience 118, 563–570, 2003.
607. Naito Y, Newman A, Lee WS, Beykirch K, Honrubia V. Projections of the individual vestibular end-organs in the brain stem of the squirrel monkey. Hearing Res 87, 141–155, 1995.
608. Naito Y, Tateya I, Hirano S, et al. Cortical correlates of vestibulo-ocular reflex modulation: a PET study. Brain 126, 1562–1578, 2003.
609. Nakamagoe K, Iwamoto Y, Yoshida K. Evidence for brainstem structures participating in oculomotor integration. Science 288, 857–859, 2000.
610. Nakamura T, Bronstein AM. The perception of head and neck angular displacement in normal and labyrinthine-defective subjects—A quantitative study using a 'remembered saccade' technique. Brain 118, 1157–1168, 1995.
611. Nelson JR. The minimal ice water caloric test. Neurology 19, 577–585, 1969.
612. Newlands SD, Dara S, Kaufman GD. Relationship of static and dynamic mechanisms in vestibuloocular reflex compensation. Laryngoscope 115, 191–204, 2005.
613. Newlands SD, Hesse SV, Haque A, Angelaki DE. Head unrestrained horizontal gaze shifts after unilateral labyrinthectomy in the rhesus monkey. Exp Brain Res 140, 25–33, 2001.
614. Newlands SD, Vrabec JT, Purcell IM, et al. Central projections of the saccular and utricular nerves in macaques. J Comp Neurol 466, 31–47, 2003.
615. Ng M, Davis LL, O'Leary DP. Autorotation test of the horizontal vestibulo-ocular reflex in Meniere's disease. Otolaryngol Head Neck Surg 109, 399–412, 1993.
616. Nogami K, Uemura T, Iwamoto M. VOR gain and phase in active head rotation tests of normal subjects and patients with peripheral labyrinthine lesions. Acta Otolaryngol (Stockh) 107, 333–337, 1989.
617. Nuti D, Mandala M, Broman AT, Zee DS. Acute vestibular neuritis: prognosis based upon bedside clinical tests (thrusts and heaves). Ann N Y Acad Sci 1039, 359–367, 2005.
618. O'Leary DP, Davis LL, Li SA. Predictive monitoring of high-frequency vestibulo-ocular reflex rehabilitation following gentamicin ototoxicity. Acta Otolaryngol (Stockh) 202–204, 1995.
619. O'Leary DP, Davis LL, Maceri DR. Vestibular autorotation test asymmetry analysis of acoustic neuromas. Otolaryngol Head Neck Surg 104, 102–109, 1991.
620. Oas J, Baloh RW. Vertigo and the anterior inferior cerebellar artery syndrome. Neurology 42, 2274–2279, 1992.
621. Ogawa Y, Kushiro K, Zakir M, Sato H, Uchino Y. Neuronal organization of the utricular macula concerned with innervation of single vestibular neurons in the cat. Neurosci Lett 278, 89–92, 2000.
622. Ohgaki T, Curthoys IS, Markham CH. Morphology of physiologically identified second-order vestibular neurons in the cat, with intracellularly injected HRP. J Comp Neurol 276, 387–411, 1988.
623. Ohki M, Murofushi T, Nakahara H, Sugasawa K. Vibration-induced nystagmus in patients with vestibular disorders. Otolaryngol Head Neck Surg 129, 255–258, 2003.
624. Ohki Y, Shimazu H, Suzuki I. Excitatory input to burst neurons from the labyrinth and its mediating pathway in the cat: location and functional characteristics of burster-driving neurons. Exp Brain Res 72, 457–472, 1988.
625. Okiyama R, Shimizu N. Optokinetic response and adaptation of the vestibulo-ocular reflex (VOR) in a patient with chronic cortical blindness. Acta Otolaryngol Suppl 481, 556–558, 1991.
626. Ono S, Kushiro A, Zakir M, et al. Properties of utricular and saccular nerve-activated vestibulocerebellar neurons in cats. Exp Brain Res 134, 1–8, 2000.
627. Oohira A, Zee DS. Disconjugate ocular motor adaptation in rhesus monkey. Vision Res 32, 489–497, 1992.
628. Ooi D, Cornell ED, Curthoys IS, Burgess AM, MacDougall HG. Convergence reduces ocular counterroll (OCR) during static roll-tilt. Vision Res 44, 2825–2833, 2004.
629. Ostrowski VB, Byskosh A, Hain TC. Tullio phenomenon with dehiscence of the superior semicircular canal. Otol Neurotol 22, 61–65, 2001.

630. Paige GD. Senescence of human visual-vestibular interactions: smooth pursuit, optokinetic, and vestibular control of eye movements with aging. Exp Brain Res 98, 355–372, 1994.
631. Paige GD. Senescence of human visual-vestibular interactions. 1. Vestibulo-ocular reflex and adaptive plasticity with aging. J Vestib Res 2, 133–151, 1992.
632. Paige GD. Caloric responses after horizontal canal inactivation. Acta Otolaryngol (Stockh) 100, 321–327, 1981.
633. Paige GD. Otolith function: basis for modern testing. Ann N Y Acad Sci 956, 314–323, 2002.
634. Paige GD. The influence of target distance on eye movement responses during vertical linear motion. Exp Brain Res 77, 585–593, 1989.
635. Paige GD, Barnes GR, Telford L, Seidman SH. The influence of sensori-motor context on the linear vestibulo-ocular reflex. Ann N Y Acad Sci 781, 322–331, 1996.
636. Paige GD, Sargent EW. Visually-induced adaptive plasticity in the human vestibulo-ocular reflex. Exp Brain Res 84, 25–34, 1991.
637. Paige GD, Seidman SH. Characteristics of the VOR in response to linear acceleration. Ann N Y Acad Sci 871, 123–135, 1999.
638. Paige GD, Telford L, Seidman SH, Barnes GR. Human vestibuloocular reflex and its interactions with vision and fixation distance during linear and angular head movement. J Neurophysiol 80, 2391–2404, 1998.
639. Paige GD, Tomko DL. Eye movement responses to linear head motion in the squirrel monkey. I. Basic characteristics. J Neurophysiol 65, 1170–1182, 1991.
640. Paige GD, Tomko DL. Eye movement responses to linear head motion in the squirrel monkey. II. Visual-vestibular interactions and kinematic considerations. J Neurophysiol 65, 1183–1196, 1991.
641. Palla A, Bockisch CJ, Bergamin O, Straumann D. Residual torsion following ocular counterroll. Ann N Y Acad Sci 1039, 81–87, 2005.
642. Palla A, Marti S, Straumann D. Head-shaking nystagmus depends on gravity. J Assoc Res Otolaryngol 6, 1–8, 2005.
643. Palla A, Straumann D. Recovery of the high-acceleration vestibulo-ocular reflex after vestibular neuritis. J Assoc Res Otolaryngol 5, 427–435, 2004.
644. Palla A, Straumann D, Obzina H. Eye-position dependence of three-dimensional ocular rotation-axis orientation during head impulses in humans. Exp Brain Res 129, 127–133 1999.
645. Pansell T, Tribukait A, Bolzani R, Schworm HD, Ygge J. Drift in ocular counterrolling during static head tilt. Ann N Y Acad Sci 1039, 554–557, 2005.
646. Pansell T, Ygge J, Schworm HD. Conjugacy of torsional eye movements in response to a head tilt paradigm. Invest Ophthalmol Vis Sci 44, 2557–2564, 2003.
647. Partsalis AM, Highstein SM. Role of the Y group of the vestibular nuclei in motor learning or plasticity of the vestibulo-ocular reflex in the squirrel monkey. Ann N Y Acad Sci 781, 489–498, 1996.
648. Pastor AM, De La Cruz RR, Baker R. Cerebellar role in adaptation of the goldfish vestibuloocular reflex. J Neurophysiol 72, 1383–1394, 1994.
649. Payman RN, Wall C, Ashbernal R. Otolith function tests in patients with unilateral vestibular lesions. Acta Otolaryngol (Stockh) 115, 715–724, 1995.
650. Penfield W. Vestibular sensation and the cerebral cortex. Ann Otol Rhinol Laryngol 66, 691–698, 1957.
651. Peng GC, Baker JF, Peterson BW. Dynamics of directional plasticity in the human vertical vestibulo-ocular reflex. J Vestib Res 4, 453–460, 1994.
652. Peng GC, Minor LB, Zee DS. Gaze position corrective eye movements in normal subjects and in patients with vestibular deficits. Ann N Y Acad Sci 1039, 337–348, 2005.
653. Peng GC, Zee DS, Minor LB. Phase-plane analysis of gaze stabilization to high acceleration head thrusts: a continuum across normal subjects and patients with loss of vestibular function. J Neurophysiol 91, 1763–1781, 2004.
654. Perez N. Vibration induced nystagmus in normal subjects and in patients with dizziness. A videonystagmography study. Rev Laryngol Otol Rhinol (Bord) 124, 85–90, 2003.
655. Perez N, Martin E, Romero MD, Garcia-Tapia R. Influence of canal paresis and compensation on gain and time constant of nystagmus slow-phase velocity to yaw-axis rotation. Acta Otolaryngol 121, 715–723, 2001.
656. Perez N, Rama-Lopez J. Head-impulse and caloric tests in patients with dizziness. Otol Neurotol 24, 913–917, 2003.
657. Perez P, Lorente JL, Gomez JR, et al. Functional significance of peripheral head-shaking nystagmus. Laryngoscope 114, 1078–1084, 2004.
658. Peterka RJ. Response characteristics of the human torsional vestibuloocular reflex. J Vestib Res 3, 877–879, 1992.
659. Peterka RJ, Black FO, Schoenhoff MB. Age-related changes in human vestibulo-ocular and optokinetic reflexes: pseudorandom rotation tests. J Vestib Res 1, 61–71, 1990.
660. Peterka RJ, Black FO, Schoenhoff MB. Age-related changes in human vestibulo-ocular reflex: sinusoidal rotation and caloric tests. J Vestib Res 1, 49–59, 1990.
661. Peterka RJ, Gianna-Poulin CC, Zupan LH, Merfeld DM. Origin of orientation-dependent asymmetries in vestibulo-ocular reflexes evoked by caloric stimulation. J Neurophysiol 92, 2333–2345, 2004.
662. Peters B, Bloomberg J. Dynamic visual acuity using "far" and "near" targets. Acta Otolaryngol 125, 353–357, 2005.
663. Peterson BW, Kinney GA, Quinn KJ, Slater NT. Potential mechanisms of plastic adaptive changes in the vestibulo-ocular reflex. Ann N Y Acad Sci 781, 499–512, 1996.
664. Petropoulos AE, Wall C, III Oman CM. Yaw sensory rearrangement alters pitch vestibulo-ocular reflex responses. Acta Otolaryngol (Stockh) 117, 647–656, 1997.
665. Pierrot-Deseilligny C, Milea D. Vertical nystagmus: clinical facts and hypotheses. Brain 148, 1237–1246, 2005.
666. Popov KE, Lekhel H, Faldon M, Bronstein AM, Gresty MA. Visual and oculomotor responses induced by neck vibration in normal subjects and labyrinthine-defective patients. Exp Brain Res 128, 343–352, 1999.
667. Powell KD, Peterson BW, Baker JF. Phase-shifted direction adaptation of the vestibulo-ocular reflex in cat. J Vestib Res 6, 277–293, 1996.
668. Powell KD, Quinn KJ, Rude SA, Peterson BW, Baker JF. Frequency dependence of cat vestibulo-ocular

reflex direction adaptation: single frequency and multifrequency rotations. Brain Res 550, 137–141, 1991.
669. Precht W. Neuronal Operations in the Vestibular System. Springer, New York, 1978.
670. Precht W. Vestibular mechanisms. Annu Rev Neurosci 2, 265–289, 1979.
671. Precht W. In Lennerstrand G, Zee DS, Keller EL (eds). Functional Basis of Ocular Motility Disorders. Pergamon Press, Oxford, 1982, pp 297–302.
672. Prepageran N, Kisilevsky V, Tomlinson D, Ranalli P, Rutka J. Symptomatic high frequency/acceleration vestibular loss: consideration of a new clinical syndrome of vestibular dysfunction. Acta Otolaryngol 125, 48–54, 2005.
673. Priesol AJ, Jones GE, Tomlinson RD, Broussard DM. Frequency-dependent effects of glutamate antagonists on the vestibulo-ocular reflex of the cat. Brain Res 857, 252–264, 2000.
674. Probst T, Brandt T, Degner D. Object-motion detection affected by concurrent self-motion perception: psychophysics of a new phenomenon. Behav Brain Sci 22, 1–11, 1986.
675. Pulaski PD, Zee DS, Robinson DA. The behavior of the vestibuloocular reflex at high velocities of head movement. Brain Res 22, 159–161, 1981.
676. Purcell IM, Kaufman GD, Shinder ME, Perachio AA. Retrograde double-labeling studies of vestibular efferent neurons projecting to the flocculus [abstract]. Soc Neurosci Abstr 27, 1290, 1997.
677. Quinn KJ, Didier AJ, Baker JF, Peterson BW. Modeling learning in brain stem and cerebellar sites responsible for VOR plasticity. Brain Res Bull 46, 333–346, 1998.
678. Quinn KJ, Helminski JO, Didier AJ, Baker JF, Peterson BW. Changes in sensitivity of vestibular nucleus neurons induced by cross-axis adaptation of the vestibulo-ocular reflex in the cat. Brain Res 718, 176–180, 1996.
679. Rabbitt RD, Boyle R, Holstein GR, Highstein SM. Hair-cell versus afferent adaptation in the semicircular canals. J Neurophysiol 93, 424–436, 2005.
680. Radtke A, Bronstein AM, Gresty MA, et al. Paroxysmal alternating skew deviation and nystagmus after partial destruction of the uvula. J Neurol Neurosurg Psychiatry 70, 790–793, 2001.
681. Ramachandran R, Lisberger SG. Normal performance and expression of learning in the vestibulo-ocular reflex (VOR) at high frequencies. J Neurophysiol 93, 2028–2038, 2005.
682. Ramat S, Straumann D, Zee DS. The interaural translation VOR: suppression, enhancement and cognitive control. J Neurophysiol 94, 2391–2402, 2005.
683. Ramat S, Zee DS. Ocular motor responses to abrupt interaural head translation in normal humans. J Neurophysiol 90, 887–902, 2003.
684. Ramat S, Zee DS. Binocular coordination in fore/aft motion. Ann N Y Acad Sci 1039, 36–53, 2005.
685. Ramat S, Zee DS, Minor LB. Translational vestibulo-ocular reflex evoked by a "head heave" stimulus. Ann N Y Acad Sci 942, 95–113, 2001.
686. Rambold H, Churchland A, Selig Y, Jasmin L, Lisberger SG. Partial ablations of the flocculus and ventral paraflocculus in monkeys cause linked deficits in smooth pursuit eye movements and adaptive modification of the VOR. J Neurophysiol 87, 912–924, 2002.
687. Rambold H, Heide W, Sprenger A, Haendler G, Helmchen C. Perilymph fistula associated with pulse-synchronous eye oscillations. Neurology 56, 1769–1771, 2001.
688. Rambold H, Helmchen C. Spontaneous nystagmus in dorsolateral medullary infarction indicates vestibular semicircular canal imbalance. J Neurol Neurosurg Psychiatry 76, 88–94, 2005.
689. Rambold H, Helmchen C, Buttner U. Vestibular influence on the binocular control of verticaltorsional nystagmus after lesions in the interstitial nucleus of Cajal. NeuroReport 11, 779–784, 2000.
690. Ranalli PJ, Sharpe JA. Vertical vestibulo-ocular reflex, smooth pursuit and eye-head tracking dysfunction in internuclear ophthalmoplegia. Brain 111, 1299–1317, 1988.
691. Ranalli PJ, Sharpe JA. Upbeat nystagmus and the ventral tegmental pathway of the upward vestibulo-ocular reflex. Neurology 38, 1329–1330, 198.
692. Raphan T, Cohen B. The vestibulo-ocular reflex in three dimensions. Exp Brain Res 145, 1–27, 2002.
693. Raphan T, Matsuo V, Cohen B. Velocity storage in the vestibulo-ocular reflex arc (VOR). Exp Brain Res 35, 229–248, 1979.
694. Raphan T, Wearne SL, Cohen B. Modeling the organization of the linear and angular vestibulo-ocular reflexes. Ann N Y Acad Sci 781, 348–363, 1996.
695. Raymond JL, Lisberger SG. Behavioral analysis of signals that guide learned changes in the amplitude and dynamics of the vestibulo-ocular reflex. J Neurosci 16, 7791–7802, 1996.
696. Raymond JL, Lisberger SG. Neural learning rules for the vestibulo-ocular reflex. J Neurosci 18, 9112–9129, 1998.
697. Reisman JE, Anderson JH. Compensatory eye movements during head and body rotation in infants. Brain Res 484, 119–129, 1989.
698. Rijkaart DC, van der Geest JN, Kelders WP, De Zeeuw CI, Frens MA. Short-term adaptation of the cervico-ocular reflex. Exp Brain Res 156, 124–128, 2004.
699. Ris L, Capron B, de Waele C, Vidal P-P, Godaux E. Dissociations between behavioral recovery and restoration of vestibular activity in the unilabyrinthectomized guinea-pig. J Physiol (Lond) 500, 509–522, 1997.
700. Ris L, Capron B, Vibert N, Vidal P-P, Godaux E. Modification of the pacemaker activity of vestibular neurons in brainstem slices during vestibular compensation in the guinea pig. Eur J Neurosci 13, 2234–2240, 2001.
701. Ris L, Hachemaoui M, Vibert N, et al. Resonance of spike discharge modulation in neurons of the guinea pig medial vestibular nucleus. J Neurophysiol 86, 703–716, 2001.
702. Robertson DD, Ireland DJ. Vestibular evoked myogenic potentials. J Otolaryngol 24, 3–8, 1995.
703. Robinson DA. The use of matrices in analyzing the three-dimensional behavior of the vestibulo-ocular reflex. Biol Cybern 46, 53–66, 1982.
704. Rodionov V, Zislin J, Elidan J. Imagination of body rotation can induce eye movements. Acta Otolaryngol 124, 684–689, 2004.
705. Roy FD, Tomlinson RD. Characterization of the vestibulo-ocular reflex evoked by high-velocity movements. Laryngoscope 114, 1190–1193, 2004.

706. Roy JE, Cullen KE. Vestibuloocular reflex signal modulation during voluntary and passive head movements. J Neurophysiol 87, 2337–2357, 2002.
707. Roy JE, Cullen KE. Brain stem pursuit pathways: dissociating visual, vestibular, and proprioceptive inputs during combined eye-head gaze tracking. J Neurophysiol 90, 271–290, 2003.
708. Roy JE, Cullen KE. Dissociating self-generated from passively applied head motion: neural mechanisms in the vestibular nuclei. J Neurosci 24, 2102–2111, 2004.
709. Rude SA, Baker JF. Otolith orientation and downbeat nystagmus in the normal cat. Exp Brain Res 111, 144–148, 1996.
710. Rudge P, Chambers BR. Physiological basis for enduring vestibular symptoms. J Neurol Neurosurg Psychiatry 45, 126–130, 1982.
711. Saadat D, O'Leary DP, Pulec JL, Kitano H. Comparison of vestibular autorotation and caloric testing. Otolaryngol Head Neck Surg 113, 215–222, 1995.
711a. Saj A, Honore J, Bernati T, Coello Y, Rousseaux M. Subjective visual vertical in pitch and roll in right hemispheric stroke. Stroke 36, 588–591, 2005.
712. Sakaguchi M, Taguchi K, Sato K, et al. Vestibulo-ocular reflex and visual vestibulo-ocular reflex during sinusoidal rotation in children. Acta Otolaryngol (Stockh) Suppl 528, 70–73, 1997.
713. Sakellari V, Bronstein AM, Corna S, et al. The effects of hyperventilation on postural control mechanisms. Brain 120, 1659–1673, 1997.
714. Sansom AJ, Smith PF, Darlington CL, Laverty R. Vestibular nucleus N-methyl-D-aspartate receptors contribute to spontaneous nystagmus generation following unilateral labyrinthectomy in guinea pigs. Neurosci Lett 283, 117–120, 2000.
715. Sato F, Sasaki H. Morphological correlations between spontaneously discharging primary vestibular afferents and vestibular nucleus neurons in the cat. J Comp Neurol 333, 554–566, 1993.
716. Sawyer RN, Thurston SE, Becker KR, et al. The cervico-ocular reflex of normal human subjects in response to transient and sinusoidal trunk rotations. J Vestib Res 4, 245–249, 1994.
717. Schlack A, Hoffmann KP, Bremmer F. Interaction of linear vestibular and visual stimulation in the macaque ventral intraparietal area (VIP). Eur J Neurosci 16, 1877–1886, 2002.
718. Schlack A, Sterbing-D'Angelo SJ, Hartung K, Hoffmann KP, Bremmer F. Multisensory space representations in the macaque ventral intraparietal area. J Neurosci 25, 4616–4625, 2005.
719. Schmid-Priscoveanu A, Bohmer A, Obzina H, Straumann D. Caloric and search-coil head-impulse testing in patients after vestibular neuritis. J Assoc Res Otolaryngol 2, 72–78, 2001.
720. Schmid-Priscoveanu A, Kori AA, Straumann D. Torsional vestibulo-ocular reflex during whole-body oscillation in the upright and the supine position: II. Responses in patients after vestibular neuritis. J Vestib Res 14, 353–359, 2004.
721. Schmid-Priscoveanu A, Straumann D, Kori AA. Torsional vestibulo-ocular reflex during whole-body oscillation in the upright and the supine position. I. Responses in healthy human subjects. Exp Brain Res 134, 212–219, 2000.
722. Schneider E, Glasauer S, Dieterich M, Kalla R, Brandt T. Diagnosis of vestibular imbalance in the blink of an eye. Neurology 63, 1209–1216, 2004.
722a. Schneider JP, Reinohs M, Prothmann S, et al. Subcortical right parietal AVM rotational vertigo and caloric stimulation fMRI support a parietal representation of vestibular input. J Neurol, published online, 2005.
723. Schubert MC, Das V, Tusa RJ, Herdman SJ. Cervico-ocular reflex in normal subjects and patients with unilateral vestibular hypofunction. Otol Neurotol 25, 65–71, 2004.
724. Schubert MC, Herdman SJ, Tusa RJ. Vertical dynamic visual acuity in normal subjects and patients with vestibular hypofunction. Otol Neurotol 23, 372–377, 2002.
725. Schubert MC, Minor LB. Vestibulo-ocular physiology underlying vestibular hypofunction. Phys Ther 84, 373–385, 2004.
726. Schubert MC, Tusa RJ, Grine LE, Herdman SJ. Optimizing the sensitivity of the head thrust test for identifying vestibular hypofunction. Phys Ther 84, 151–158, 2004.
727. Schultheis LW, Robinson DA. Directional plasticity of the vestibulo-ocular reflex in the cat. Ann N Y Acad Sci 374, 504–512, 1981.
728. Schwarz U, Miles FA. Ocular responses to translation and their dependence on viewing distance. I. Motion of the observer. J Neurophysiol 66, 851–864, 1991.
729. Schweigart G, Heimbrand S, Mergner T, Becker W. Perception of horizontal head and trunk rotation: modification of neck input following loss of vestibular function. Exp Brain Res 95, 533–546, 1993.
730. Schweigart G, Mergner T, Evdokimidis I, Morand S, Becker W. Gaze stabilization by optokinetic reflex (okr) and vestibulo-ocular reflex (vor) during active head rotation in man. Vision Res 12, 1643–1652, 1997.
731. Scudder C, Fuchs AF. Physiological and behavioral identification of vestibular nucleus neurons mediating the horizontal vestibuloocular reflex in trained rhesus monkeys. J Neurophysiol 68, 244–264, 1992.
732. Segal BN, Katsarkas A. Long-term deficits of goal-directed vestibulo-ocular function following total unilateral loss of peripheral vestibular function. Acta Otolaryngol (Stockh) 106, 102–110, 1988.
733. Segal BN, Katsarkas A. Goal-directed vestibulo-ocular function in man: gaze stabilization by slow-phase and saccadic eye movements. Exp Brain Res 70, 26–32, 1988.
734. Segal BN, Liben S. Modification of human velocity storage sampled during intermittently-illuminated optokinetic stimulation. Exp Brain Res 59, 515–523, 1985.
735. Seidman SH, Leigh RJ. The human torsional vestibulo-ocular reflex during rotation about an earth-vertical axis. Brain Res 504, 264–268, 1989.
736. Seidman SH, Leigh RJ, Tomsak RL, Grant MP, Dell'Osso LF. Dynamic properties of the human vestibulo-ocular reflex during head rotations in roll. Vision Res 35, 679–689, 1995.
737. Seidman SH, Paige GD, Tomko DL. Adaptive plasticity in the naso-occipital linear vestibulo-ocular reflex. Exp Brain Res 125, 485–494, 1999.
738. Seidman SH, Paige GD, Tomlinson RD, Schmitt

N. Linearity of canal-otolith interaction during eccentric rotation in humans. Exp Brain Res 147, 29–37, 2002.
739. Seidman SH, Telford L, Paige GD. Vertical, torsional and horizontal eye movement responses to head roll in the squirrel monkey. Exp Brain Res 104, 218–226, 1995.
740. Sekirnjak C, Du LS. Intrinsic firing dynamics of vestibular nucleus neurons. J Neurosci 22, 2083–2095, 2002.
741. Serra A, Derwenskus J, Downey DL, Leigh RJ. Role of eye movement examination and subjective visual vertical in clinical evaluation of multiple sclerosis. J Neurol 250, 569–575, 2003.
742. Severac CA, Faldon M, Popov K, Day BL, Bronstein AM. Short-latency eye movements evoked by near-threshold galvanic vestibular stimulation. Exp Brain Res 148, 414–418, 2003.
743. Shaikh AG, Ghasia FF, Dickman JD, Angelaki DE. Properties of cerebellar fastigial neurons during translation, rotation, and eye movements. J Neurophysiol 93, 853–863, 2005.
743a. Shaikh AG, Green AM, Ghasia FF, Newlands SD, Dickman JD, Angelaki DE. Sensory convergence solves a motion ambiguity problem. Curr Biol 15, 1657–1662, 2005.
744. Shaikh AG, Meng H, Angelaki DE. Multiple reference frames for motion in the primate cerebellum. J Neurosci 24, 4491–4497, 2004.
745. Shallo-Hoffmann J, Bronstein AM. Visual motion detection in patients with absent vestibular function. Vision Res 43, 1589–1594, 2003.
746. Sharpe J, Lo A. Voluntary and visual control of the vestibuloocular reflex after cerebral hemidecortication. Ann Neurol 10, 164–172, 1981.
747. Shelhamer M, Merfeld DM, Mendoza JC. Vergence can be controlled by audio feedback, and induces downward ocular deviation. Exp Brain Res, 1994.
748. Shelhamer M, Peng GC, Ramat S, Patel V. Context-specific adaptation of the gain of the oculomotor response to lateral translation using roll and pitch head tilts as contexts. Exp Brain Res 146, 388–393, 2002.
749. Shelhamer M, Ravina B, Kramer PD. Adaptation of the gain of the angular vestibulo-ocular reflex when retinal slip is zero. Soc Neurosci Abstr 21, 518, 1995.
750. Shelhamer M, Roberts DC, Zee DS. Dynamics of the human linear vestibulo-ocular reflex at medium frequency and modification by short-term training. J Vestib Res 10, 271–282, 2000.
751. Shelhamer M, Robinson DA, Tan HS. Context-specific adaptation of the gain of the vestibulo-ocular reflex in humans. J Vestib Res 2, 89–96, 1992.
752. Shelhamer M, Young LR. The interaction of otolith organ stimulation and smooth pursuit tracking. J Vestib Res 4, 1–15, 1994.
753. Shelhamer M, Zee DS. Context-specific adaptation and its significance for neurovestibular problems of space flight. J Vestib Res 13, 345–362, 2003.
754. Sherman KR, Keller EL. Vestibulo-ocular reflexes of adventitiously and congenitally blind adults. Invest Ophthalmol Vis Sci 27, 1154–1159, 1986.
755. Shinder ME, Purcell IM, Kaufman GD, Perachio AA. Vestibular efferent neurons project to the flocculus. Brain Res 889, 288–294, 2001.
756. Shupert C, Fuchs AF. Development of conjugate human eye movements. Vision Res 28, 585–596, 1988.
757. Simons B, Büttner U. The influence of age on optokinetic nystagmus. Eur Arch Psychiatry Neurol Sci 234, 369–373, 1986.
758. Skavenski AA, Robinson DA. Role of abducens neurons in vestibuloocular reflex. J Neurophysiol 36, 724–738, 1973.
759. Smith HL, Galiana HL. The role of structural symmetry in linearizing ocular reflexes. Biol Cybern 65, 11–22, 1991.
760. Smith MR, Nelson AB, Du Lac S. Regulation of firing response gain by calcium-dependent mechanisms in vestibular nucleus neurons. J Neurophysiol 87, 2031–2042, 2002.
761. Smith PF. Pharmacology of the vestibular system. Curr Opin Neurol 13, 31–37, 2000.
762. Smith PF, Curthoys IS. Mechanisms of recovery following unilateral labyrinthectomy: a review. Brain Res Rev 14, 155–180, 1989.
763. Smith PF, Darlington CL. Can vestibular compensation be enhanced by drug treatment? A review of recent evidence. J Vestib Res 4, 169–180, 1994.
764. Smith PF, Zheng Y, Paterson S, Darlington CL. The contribution of nitric oxide to vestibular compensation: are there species differences? Acta Otolaryngol. Suppl 545, 57–60, 2001.
765. Smith R. Vergence eye-movement response to whole-body linear acceleration stimuli in man. Ophthal Physiol Opt 5, 303–311, 1985.
766. Snyder LH, King WM. Behavior and physiology of the macaque vestibulo-ocular reflex response to sudden off-axis rotation: computing eye translation. Brain Res Bull 40, 293–301, 1996.
767. Snyder LH, King WM. The effect of viewing distance and the location of the axis of rotation on the monkey's vestibulo-ocular reflex (VOR). I. Eye movement responses. J Neurophysiol 67, 861–874, 1992.
768. Snyder LH, Lawrence DW, King WM. Changes in vestibulo-ocular reflex (VOR) anticipate changes in vergence angle in monkey. Vision Res 32, 569–575, 1992.
769. Solomon D, Cohen B. Stimulation of the nodulus and uvula discharges velocity storage in the vestibuloocular reflex. Exp Brain Res 102, 57–68, 1994.
770. Solomon D, Straumann D, Zee DS. Three-dimensional eye movement during vertical axis rotation: Effects of visual suppression, orbital eye position and head position. In Fetter M, Haslwanter T, Misslisch H, Tweed D (eds). Three-dimensional Kinematics of Eye, Head and Limb Movement. Harwood Academic Publishers, Amsterdam,1997, pp 197–208.
771. Solomon D, Zee DS, Straumann D. Torsional and horizontal vestibular ocular reflex adaptation: three-dimensional eye movement analysis. Exp Brain Res 152, 150–155, 2003.
771a. Sprenger A, Zils E, Stritzke G, Kruger A, Rambold H, Helmchen C. Do predictive mechanisms improve the angular vestibulo-ocular reflex in vestibular neuritis? Audiol Neurootol 11, 53–58, 2005.
772. Steinhausen W. Über die Beobachtung der Cupula in den Bogengängsampullen des Labyrinthes bei

des lebenden Hechts. Pflügers Archiv für die Gesante Physiologie des Meschen und der Tierre 232, 500–512, 1933.
773. Stewart CM, Mustari MJ, Perachio AA. Visual-vestibular interactions during vestibular compensation: role of the pretectal NOT in horizontal VOR recovery after hemilabyrinthectomy in rhesus monkey. J Neurophysiol 94, 2653–2666, 2005.
774. Stodieck SRG, Brandt T, Büttner U. Visual and vestibular epileptic seizures. Electroencephalogr Clin Neurophysiol 75, 65–66, 1990.
775. Straube A, Brandt T. Importance of the visual and vestibular cortex for self-motion perception in man (circularvection). Human Neurobiol 6, 211–218, 1987.
776. Strupp M, Arbusow V, Dieterich M, Sautier W, Brandt T. Perceptual and oculomotor effects of neck muscle vibration in vestibular neuritis—ipsilateral somatosensory substitution of vestibular function. Brain 121, 677–685, 1998.
777. Strupp M, Glasauer S, Schneider E, et al. Anterior canal failure: ocular torsion without perceptual tilt due to preserved otolith function. J Neurol Neurosurg Psychiatry 74, 1336–1338, 2003.
778. Suárez C, Diaz C, Tolivia J, et al. Morphometric analysis of the human vestibular nuclei. Anat Rec 247, 271–288, 1997.
779. Sugiuchi Y, Izawa Y, Ebata S, Shinoda Y. Vestibular cortical area in the periarcuate cortex: its afferent and efferent projections. Ann N Y Acad Sci 1039, 111–123, 2005.
780. Suzuki J-I, Tokumasu K, Goto K. Eye movements from single utricular nerve stimulation in the cat. Acta Otolaryngol (Stockh) 68, 350–362, 1969.
781. Suzuki M, Kitano H, Ito R, et al. Cortical and subcortical vestibular response to caloric stimulation detected by functional magnetic resonance imaging. Brain Res Cogn Brain Res 12, 441–449, 2001.
782. Suzuki Y, Kase M, Kato H, Fukushima K. Stability of ocular counterrolling and Listing's plane during static roll-tilts. Invest Ophthalmol Vis Sci 38, 2103–2111, 1997.
783. Szentágothai J. The elementary vestibuloocular reflex. J Neurophysiol 13, 395–407, 1950.
784. Tabak S, Collewijn H. Human vestibulo-ocular responses to rapid, helmet-driven head movements. Exp Brain Res 102, 367–378, 1994.
785. Tabak S, Collewijn H, Boumans LJJM. Deviation of the subjective vertical in long-standing unilateral vestibular loss. Acta Otolaryngol (Stockh) 117, 1–16, 1997.
786. Tabata H, Yamamoto K, Kawato M. Computational study on monkey VOR adaptation and smooth pursuit based on the parallel control-pathway theory. J Neurophysiol 87, 2176–2189, 2002.
787. Takagi A, Sando I, Takahashi H. Computer-aided three-dimensional reconstruction and measurement of semicircular canals and their cristae in man. Acta Otolaryngol (Stockh) 107, 362–365, 1989.
788. Takeda N, Igarashi M, Koizuka I, Chae S, Matsunaga T. Recovery of the otolith-ocular reflex after unilateral deafferentation of the otolith organs in squirrel monkeys. Acta Otolaryngol (Stockh) 110, 25–30, 1990.
789. Takemori S. Compensation after sudden loss of unilateral vestibular function and optokinetic afternystagmus. Acta Otolaryngol (Stockh) Suppl 528, 103–108, 1997.
790. Takemura A, Kawano K. Sensory-to-motor processing of the ocular-following response. Neurosci Res 43, 201–206, 2002.
791. Tang Y, Lopez I, Baloh RW. Age-related change of the neuronal number in the human medial vestibular nucleus: a stereological investigation. J Vestib Res 11, 357–363, 2001.
792. Telford L, Seidman SH, Paige GD. Canal-otolith interactions in the squirrel monkey vestibulo-ocular reflex and the influence of fixation distance. Exp Brain Res 118, 115–125, 1998.
793. Telford L, Seidman SH, Paige GD. Canal-otolith interactions driving vertical and horizontal eye movements in the squirrel monkey. Exp Brain Res 109, 407–418, 1996.
794. Telford L, Seidman SH, Paige GD. Dynamics of squirrel monkey linear vestibuloocular reflex and interactions with fixation distance. J Neurophysiol 78, 1775–1790, 1997.
795. Ter Braak JWG. Untersuchungen über optokinetischen nystagmus. Archives Neerlandaises de Physiologie de l'homme et des animaux 21, 309–376, 1936.
796. Thier P, Erickson RG. Vestibular inputs to visual-tracking neurons in area MST of awake rhesus monkeys. Ann N Y Acad Sci 656, 960–963, 1992.
797. Thomke F, Hopf HC. Pontine lesions mimicking acute peripheral vestibulopathy. J Neurol Neurosurg Psychiatry 66, 340–349, 1999.
798. Thurston SE, Leigh RJ, Abel LA, Dell'Osso LF. Hyperactive vestibuloocular reflex in cerebellar degeneration: pathogenesis and treatment. Neurology 37, 53–57, 1987.
799. Thurtell MJ, Black RA, Halmagyi GM, Curthoys IS, Aw ST. Vertical eye position-dependence of the human vestibuloocular reflex during passive and active yaw head rotations. J Neurophysiol 81, 2415–2428, 1999.
800. Tian J-R, Shubayev I, Demer JL. Impairments in the initial horizontal vestibulo-ocular reflex of older humans. Exp Brain Res 137, 309–322, 2001.
801. Tian J, Crane BT, Demer JL. Vestibular catch-up saccades in labyrinthine deficiency. Exp. Brain Res 131, 448–457, 2000.
802. Tian J, Zee DS, Walker MF. Eye-position dependence of torsional velocity during step-ramp pursuit and transient yaw rotation in humans. Exp Brain Res, published online, 2005.
803. Tian JR, Crane BT, Demer JL. Human surge linear vestibulo-ocular reflex during tertiary gaze viewing. Ann N Y Acad Sci 1039, 489–493, 2005.
804. Tian JR, Crane BT, Wiest G, Demer JL. Effect of aging on the human initial interaural linear vestibulo-ocular reflex. Exp Brain Res 145, 142–149, 2002.
805. Tian JR, Shubayev I, Baloh RW, Demer JL. Impairments in the initial horizontal vestibulo-ocular reflex of older humans. Exp Brain Res 137, 309–322, 2001.
806. Tian JR, Shubayev I, Demer JL. Dynamic visual acuity during transient and sinusoidal yaw rotation in normal and unilaterally vestibulopathic humans. Exp Brain Res 137, 12–25, 2001.
807. Tian J-R, Crane BT, Demer JL. Vestibular catch-up saccades in labyrinthine deficiency. Exp Brain Res 131, 448–457, 2000.

808. Tijssen MAJ, Straathof CSM, Hain TC, Zee DS. Optokinetic afternystagmus in humans: normal values of amplitude, time constant and asymmetry. Ann Otol Rhinol Laryngol 98, 741–746, 1989.
809. Tiliket C, Shelhamer M, Tan HS, Zee DS. Adaptation of the vestibulo-ocular reflex with the head in different orientations and positions relative to the axis of body rotation. J Vestib Res 3, 181–196, 1993.
810. Tilikete C, Rode G, Nighoghossian N, Boisson D, Vighetto A. Otolith manifestations in Wallenberg syndrome. Rev Neurol (Paris) 157, 198–208, 2001.
811. Tilikete C, Ventre-Domine J, Denise P, Nighoghossian N, Vighetto A. Otolith dysfunction in skew deviation after brain stem lesions. Abnormalities of eye movements induced by off-vertical-axis rotation (OVAR). J Vestib Res 10, 179–192, 2000.
812. Todd NP, Rosengren SM, Colebatch JG. A short latency vestibular evoked potential (VsEP) produced by bone-conducted acoustic stimulation. J Acoust Soc Am 114, 3264–3272, 2003.
813. Tomlinson RD, Cheung R, Blakeman A. Naso-occipital vestibulo-ocular reflex responses in normal subjects. IEEE Eng Med Biol Mag 19, 43–47, 2000.
814. Tomlinson RD, McConville KMV, Na E-Q. Behavior of cells without eye movement sensitivity in the vestibular nuclei during combined rotational and translational stimuli. J Vestib Res 6, 145–158, 1996.
815. Toupet M, Pialoux P. The perverted nystagmus. Ann Otolaryngol Chir Cervicofac 98, 319–338, 1981.
816. Trillenberg P, Shelhamer M, Roberts DC, Zee DS. Cross-axis adaptation of torsional components in the yaw-axis vestibulo-ocular reflex. Exp Brain Res 148, 158–165, 2003.
817. Trillenberg P, Zee DS, Shelhamer M. On the distribution of fast-phase intervals in optokinetic and vestibular nystagmus. Biol Cybern 87, 68–78, 2002.
818. Tusa RJ, Grant MP, Buettner U, Herdman S, Zee DS. Influence of head pitch on high-velocity horizontal VOR in normal subjects and patients with unilateral vestibular nerve section. Acta Otolaryngol (Stockh) 116, 507–512, 1998.
819. Tweed D, Fetter M, Sievering D, Misslisch H, Koenig E. Rotational kinematics of the human vestibuloocular reflex. II. Velocity steps. J Neurophysiol 72, 2480–2489, 1994.
820. Tweed D, Haslwanter T, Fetter M. Optimizing gaze control in three dimensions. Science 281, 1363–1366, 1998.
821. Tweed D, Fetter M, Sievering D, et al. Rotational kinematics of the human vestibuloocular reflex. I. Gain matrices. J Neurophysiol 72, 2467–2479, 1994.
822. Uchino Y. Otolith and semicircular canal inputs to single vestibular neurons in cats. Biol Sci Space 15, 375–381, 2001.
823. Uchino Y, Sasaki M, Sato H, Bai R, Kawamoto E. Otolith and canal integration on single vestibular neurons in cats. Exp Brain Res 64, 271–285, 2005.
824. Uchino Y, Sasaki M, Sato H, et al. Utriculoocular reflex arc of the cat. J Neurophysiol 76, 1896–1903, 1996.
825. Uchino Y, Sato H, Suwa H. Excitatory and inhibitory inputs from saccular afferents to single vestibular neurons in the cat. J Neurophysiol 78, 2186–2192, 1997.
826. Uchino Y, Sato H, Zakir M, et al. Commissural effects in the otolith system. Exp Brain Res 136, 421–430, 2001.
827. Uemura T, Cohen B. Effects of vestibular nuclei lesions on vestibulo-ocular reflexes and posture in monkeys. Acta Otolaryngol (Stockh) Suppl 315, 1–71, 1973.
828. Valmaggia C, Gottlob I. Optokinetic nystagmus elicited by filling-in in adults with central scotoma. Invest Ophthalmol Vis Sci 43, 1804–1808, 2002.
829. Valmaggia C, Proudlock F, Gottlob I. Optokinetic nystagmus in strabismus: are asymmetries related to binocularity? Invest Ophthalmol Vis Sci 44, 5142–5150, 2003.
830. van Alphen AM, De Zeeuw CI. Cerebellar LTD facilitates but is not essential for long-term adaptation of the vestibulo-ocular reflex. Eur J Neurosci 16, 486–490, 2002.
831. Van Den Berg AV, Collewijn H. Directional asymmetries of human optokinetic nystagmus. Exp Brain Res 70, 597–604, 1988.
832. Ventre-Dominey J, Nighoghossian N, Denise P. Evidence for interacting cortical control of vestibular function and spatial representation in man. Neuropsychologia 41, 1884–1898, 2003.
833. Ventre-Dominey J, Nighoghossian N, Denise P. Interaction between cortical control of vestibular function and spatial representation in man. Ann N Y Acad Sci 1039, 494–497, 2005.
834. Vibert D, Hausler R, Safran AB. Subjective visual vertical in peripheral unilateral vestibular diseases. J Vestib Res 9, 145–152, 1999.
835. Vidal PP, Vibert N, Serafin M, et al. Intrinsic physiological and pharmacological properties of central vestibular neurons. Adv Otorhinolaryngol 55, 26–81, 1999.
836. Viirre E, Tweed D, Milner K, Vilis T. A reexamination of the gain of the vestibuloocular reflex. J Neurophysiol 56, 439–450, 1986.
837. Viirre ES, Cadera W, Vilis T. Monocular adaptation of the saccadic system and vestibuloocular reflex. Invest Ophthalmol Vis Sci 29, 1339–1347, 1988.
838. Viirre ES, Demer JL. The human vertical vestibulo-ocular reflex during combined linear and angular acceleration with near-target fixation. Exp Brain Res 112, 313–324, 1996.
839. Vilis T, Tweed D. A matrix analysis for a conjugate vestibulo-ocular reflex. Biol Cybern 59, 237–245, 1988.
840. Vitte E, Derosier C, Caritu Y, et al. Activation of the hippocampal formation by vestibular stimulation: a functional magnetic resonance imaging study. Exp Brain Res 112, 523–526, 1996.
841. Voogd J, Gerrits NM, Ruigrok NM. Organization of the vestibulo-cerebellum. In Highstein S, Cohen B, Büttner-Ennever JA (eds). New Directions in Vestibular Research. The New York Academy of Sciences, New York,1996, pp 553–579.
842. Voogd J, Wylie DR. Functional and anatomical organization of floccular zones: a preserved feature in vertebrates. J Comp Neurol 470, 107–112, 2004.
843. Wade NJ, Swanston MT, Howard IP, Ono H, Shen X. Induced rotary motion and ocular torsion. Vision Res 31, 1979–1983, 1991.
844. Wade SW, Curthoys IS. The effect of ocular torsional

position on perception of the roll-tilt of visual stimuli. Vision Res 37, 1071–1078, 1997.

845. Waespe W, Cohen B, Raphan T. Role of the flocculus and paraflocculus in optokinetic nystagmus and visual-vestibular interactions: effects of lesions. Exp Brain Res 50, 9–33, 1983.
846. Waespe W, Cohen B, Raphan T. Dynamic modification of the vestibulo-ocular reflex by nodulus and uvula. Science 228, 199–202, 1985.
847. Waespe W, Henn V. Vestibular nuclei activity during optokinetic after-nystagmus (OKAN) in the alert monkey. Exp Brain Res 30, 323–330, 1977.
848. Waespe W, Henn V. Neuronal activity in the vestibular nuclei of the alert monkey during vestibular and optokinetic stimulation. Exp Brain Res 27, 523–538, 1977.
849. Waespe W, Schwartz U. Characteristics of eye velocity storage during periods of suppression and reversal of eye velocity in monkeys. Exp Brain Res 65, 49–58, 1986.
850. Walker MF, Shelhamer M, Zee DS. Eye-position dependence of torsional velocity during interaural translation, horizontal pursuit, and yaw-axis rotation in humans. Vision Res 44, 613–620, 2004.
851. Walker MF, Zee DS. Rectified cross-axis adaptation of the vestibulo-ocular reflex in rhesus monkey. Ann N Y Acad Sci 956, 543–545, 2002.
852. Walker MF, Zee DS. Cerebellar disease alters the axis of the high-acceleration vestibulo-ocular reflex. J Neurophysiol 94, 3417–3429, 2005.
853. Walker MF, Zee DS. Directional abnormalities of vestibular and optokinetic responses in cerebellar disease. Ann N Y Acad Sci 871, 205–220, 1999.
854. Walker MF, Zee DS. Asymmetry of the pitch vestibulo-ocular reflex in patients with cerebellar disease. Ann N Y Acad Sci 1039, 349–358, 2005.
855. Wall C III, Furman JMR. Eyes open versus eyes closed: effects on human rotational responses. Acta Otolaryngol (Stockh) 98, 548–550, 1989.
856. Wall C III, Furman JMR. Nystagmus responses in a group of normal humans during earth-horizontal axis rotation. Acta Otolaryngol (Stockh) 108, 327–335, 1989.
857. Wall C III, Smith TR, Furman JM. Plasticity of the human otolith-ocular reflex. Acta Otolaryngol (Stockh) 112, 413–420, 1992.
858. Wallman J. Subcortical optokinetic mechanisms. In Miles FA, Wallman J (eds). Visual Motion and its Role in the Stabilization of Gaze. Elsevier, Amsterdam,1993, pp 321–342.
859. Wang L, Soderberg PG, Tengroth B. Influence of target direction, luminance and velocity on monocular horizontal optokinetic nystagmus. Acta Ophthalmologica 71, 578–585, 1993.
860. Washio N, Suzuki Y, Sawa M, Ohtsuka K. Gain of human torsional optokinetic nystagmus depends on horizontal disparity. Invest Ophthalmol Vis Sci 46, 133–136, 2005.
861. Watson P, Barber HO, Deck J, Terbrugge, K. Positional vertigo and nystagmus of central origin. Can J Neurol Sci 8, 133–137, 1981.
862. Wearne S, Raphan T, Cohen B. Control of spatial orientation of the angular vestibuloocular reflex by the nodulus and uvula. J Neurophysiol 79, 2690–2715, 1998.
863. Wearne S, Raphan T, Cohen B. Contribution of vestibular commissural pathways to spatial orientation of the angular vestibuloocular reflex. J Neurophysiol 78, 1193–1197, 1997.
864. Wearne S, Raphan T, Cohen B. Nodulo-uvular control of central vestibular dynamics determines spatial orientation of the angular vestibulo-ocular reflex. Ann N Y Acad Sci 781, 364–384, 1996.
865. Wearne S, Raphan T, Waespe W, Cohen B. Control of the three-dimensional dynamic characteristics of the angular vestibulo-ocular reflex by the nodulus and uvula. Progr Brain Res 114, 321–334, 1997.
866. Weber KD, Fletcher WA, Melvill JG, Block EW. Podokinetic after-rotation in patients with compensated unilateral vestibular ablation. Exp Brain Res 147, 554–557, 2002.
867. Wei G, Lafortune SH, Ireland DJ, Jell RM. Modification of vertical OKN and vertical OKAN asymmetry in humans during parabolic flight. J Vestib Res 7, 21–34, 1997.
868. Wei G, Lafortune SH, Ireland DJ, Jell RM. Human vertical optokinetic nystagmus and after-response, and their dependence upon head orientation with respect to gravity. J Vestib Res 4, 37–47, 1994.
869. Wei M, Angelaki DE. Cross-axis adaptation of the translational vestibulo-ocular reflex. Exp Brain Res 138, 304–312, 2001.
870. Wei M, DeAngelis GC, Angelaki DE. Do visual cues contribute to the neural estimate of viewing distance used by the oculomotor system? J Neurosci 23, 8340–8350, 2003.
871. Weissenstein L, Ratnam R, Anastasio TJ. Vestibular compensation in the horizontal vestibulo-ocular reflex of the goldfish. Behav Brain Sci 75, 127–137, 1996.
872. Weissman BM, DiScenna AO, Ekelman BL, Leigh RJ. The effect of eyelid closure and vocalization upon the vestibuloocular reflex during rotational testing. Ann Otol Rhinol Laryngol 95, 548–550, 1989.
873. Weissman BM, DiScenna AO, Leigh RJ. Maturation of the vestibuloocular reflex in normal infants during the first 2 months of life. Neurology 39, 534–538, 1989.
874. Welgampola MS, Colebatch JG. Characteristics and clinical applications of vestibular-evoked myogenic potentials. Neurology 64, 1682–1688, 2005.
875. Welgampola MS, Rosengren SM, Halmagyi GM, Colebatch JG. Vestibular activation by bone conducted sound. J Neurol Neurosurg Psychiatry 74, 771–778, 2003.
876. Wende S, Nakayama N, Schwerdtfeger P. The internal auditory artery: (embryology, anatomy, angiography, pathology). J Neurol 210, 21–31, 1975.
877. Wiest G, Demer JL, Tian J, Crane BT, Baloh RW. Vestibular function in severe bilateral vestibulopathy. J Neurol Neurosurg Psychiatry 71, 53–57, 2001.
878. Wiest G, Zimprich F, Prayer D, et al. Vestibular processing in human paramedian precuneus as shown by electrical cortical stimulation. Neurology 62, 473–475, 2004.
879. Wilson VJ, Melvill Jones G. Mammalian Vestibular Physiology. Plenum Press, New York, 1979.
880. Wong AM, Sharpe JA, Tweed D. The vestibulo-ocular reflex in fourth nerve palsy: deficits and adaptation. Vision Res. 42, 2205–2218, 2002.
881. Wong AM, Tweed D, Sharpe JA. Adaptations and deficits in the vestibulo-ocular reflex after sixth

nerve palsy. Invest Ophthalmol Vis Sci 43, 99–111, 2002.
882. Yagi T, Ohyama Y, Suzuki K, Kamura E, Kokawa T. 3D analysis of nystagmus in peripheral vertigo. Acta Otolaryngol (Stockh) 117, 135–138, 1997.
883. Yagi T, Shimizu M, Sekine S, Kamio T. New neurootological test for detecting cerebellar dysfunction. Vestibulo-ocular reflex changes with horizontal vision-reversal prisms. Ann Otorhinolaryngol 90, 276–280, 1981.
884. Yakushin SB, Bukharina SE, Raphan T, Buttner-Ennever J, Cohen B. Adaptive changes in the angular VOR: duration of gain changes and lack of effect of nodulo-uvulectomy. Ann N Y Acad Sci 1004, 78–93, 2003.
885. Yakushin SB, Dai M, Raphan T, et al. Changes in the vestibulo-ocular reflex after plugging of the semicircular canals. Ann N Y Acad Sci 942, 287–299, 2001.
886. Yakushin SB, Raphan T, Cohen B. Gravity-specific adaptation of the angular vestibuloocular reflex: dependence on head orientation with regard to gravity. J Neurophysiol 89, 571–586, 2003.
887. Yakushin SB, Reisine H, Buttner-Ennever J, Raphan T, Cohen B. Functions of the nucleus of the optic tract (NOT). I. Adaptation of the gain of the horizontal vestibulo-ocular reflex. Exp Brain Res 131, 416–432, 2000.
888. Yakushin SB, Xiang Y, Raphan T, Cohen B. Spatial distribution of gravity dependent gain changes in the vestibulo-ocular reflex. J Neurophysiol 93, 3693–3698, 2005.
889. Yakushin SB, Xiang Y, Raphan T, Cohen B. The role of gravity in adaptation of the vertical angular vestibulo-ocular reflex. Ann N Y Acad Sci 1039, 97–110, 2005.
890. Yamamoto K, Takemura A, Kawano K, Kawato M. A computational simulation of the adaptation of ocular following responses. Soc Neurosci Abstr 24, 1405, 1998.
891. Yen MT, Herdman SJ, Tusa RJ. Oscillopsia and pseudonystagmus in kidney transplant patients. Am J Ophthalmol 128, 768–770, 1999.
892. Young LR. Models for neurovestibular adaptation. J Vestib Res 13, 297–307, 2003.
893. Zasorin NL, Baloh RW, Myers LB. Acetazolamide-responsive episodic ataxia syndrome. Neurology 33, 1212–1214, 1983.
894. Zee DS. Considerations on the mechanisms of alternating skew deviation in patients with cerebellar lesions. J Vestib Res 6, 395–401, 1996.
895. Zee DS. Ophthalmoscopy in examination of patients with vestibular disorders. Ann Neurol 3, 373–374, 1978.
896. Zee DS. The organization of the brainstem ocular motor subnuclei. Ann Neurol 4, 384–385, 1978.
897. Zee DS, Fetter M, Proctor L. Recovery from unilateral labyrnthectomy in primate: Effects of usual inputs and considerations upon Ewald's second law. In Huang JC, Daunton NGWVJ (eds). Basic and Applied Aspects of Vestibular Function. University of Hong Kong Press, Hong Kong, 1988, pp 125–132.
898. Zee DS, Friendlich AR, Robinson DA. The mechanism of downbeat nystagmus. Arch Neurol 30, 227–237, 1974.
899. Zee DS, Preziosi TJ, Proctor LR. Bechterew's phenomenon in a human. Ann Neurol 12, 495–496, 1982.
900. Zee DS, Tusa R, Herdman S, Butler P, Gücer G. Effects of occipital lobectomy upon eye movements in primate. J Neurophysiol 58, 883–907, 1987.
901. Zee DS, Walker MF, Ramat S. The cerebellar contribution to eye movements based upon lesions: binocular three-axis control and the translational vestibulo-ocular reflex. Ann N Y Acad Sci 956, 178–189, 2002.
902. Zee DS, Walker MF. In Chalupa LM, Werner JS (eds). Cerebellar Control of Eye Movements in the Visual Neurosciences. MIT Press, Cambridge, MA, 2003, pp 1485–1498.
903. Zee DS, Yamazaki A, Butler PH, Gücer G. Effects of ablation of the flocculus and paraflocculus on eye movements in primate. J Neurophysiol 46, 878–899, 1981.
904. Zee DS, Yee RD, Robinson DA. Optokinetic responses in labyrinthine-defective human beings. Brain Res 113, 423–428, 1976.
905. Zhang R, Ashton J, Horii A, Darlington CL, Smith PF. Immunocytochemical and stereological analysis of GABA(B) receptor subunit expression in the rat vestibular nucleus following unilateral vestibular deafferentation. Brain Res 1037, 107–113, 2005.
906. Zhang X, et al. Convergence of the anterior semicircular canal and otolith afferents on cat single vestibular neurons. Exp Brain Res 147, 407–417, 2002.
907. Zhang X, Zakir M, Meng H, Sato H, Uchino Y. Convergence of the horizontal semicircular canal and otolith afferents on cat single vestibular neurons. Exp Brain Res 140, 1–11, 2001.
908. Zhou G, Cox LC. Vestibular evoked myogenic potentials: history and overview. Am J Audiol 13, 135–143, 2004.
909. Zhou W, Weldon P, Tang B, King WM. Rapid motor learning in the translational vestibulo-ocular reflex. J Neurosci 23, 4288–4298, 2003.
910. Zupan LH, Merfeld DM. Neural processing of gravito-inertial cues in humans. IV. Influence of visual rotational cues during roll optokinetic stimuli. J Neurophysiol 89, 390–400, 2003.
911. Zupan LH, Merfeld DM, Darlot C. Using sensory weighting to model the influence of canal, otolith and visual cues on spatial orientation and eye movements. Biol Cybern 86, 209–230, 2002.
912. Zupan LH, Peterka RJ, Merfeld DM. Neural processing of gravito-inertial cues in humans. I. Influence of the semicircular canals following post-rotatory tilt. J Neurophysiol 84, 2001–2015, 2000.

Chapter 3

The Saccadic System

THE PURPOSE OF SACCADES

Saccades are rapid eye movements that shift the line of sight between successive points of fixation (Fig. 3–1). The term saccade is French in origin, referring to the jerking of a horse's head by a tug on the reins or to the flicking of a sail in a gust of wind. Javal[334] and Landolt[378] first used the word saccade to describe the rapid eye movements associated with reading or voluntary changes of gaze. Saccades include a range of behaviors that encompass voluntary and involuntary shifts of fixation, quick phases of vestibular and optokinetic nystagmus, and the rapid eye movements that occur during REM sleep.[782] Abnormalities of saccades are often distinctive and point to disorders of specific mechanisms. Thus, saccades have become an important research tool to study a wide range of issues in the neurosciences.[392]

Dodge,[157] working with J.J. Cogan, the father of David G. Cogan, in the early 20th century, was the first to distinguish saccades clearly from other types of eye movements. He explicitly stated their function: "to move the eyes so that the point of interest will be seen with the visual center of the retina". Yarbus[769] emphasized the importance of saccades in visual search. The function of voluntary saccades in primates is directly linked to the pres-

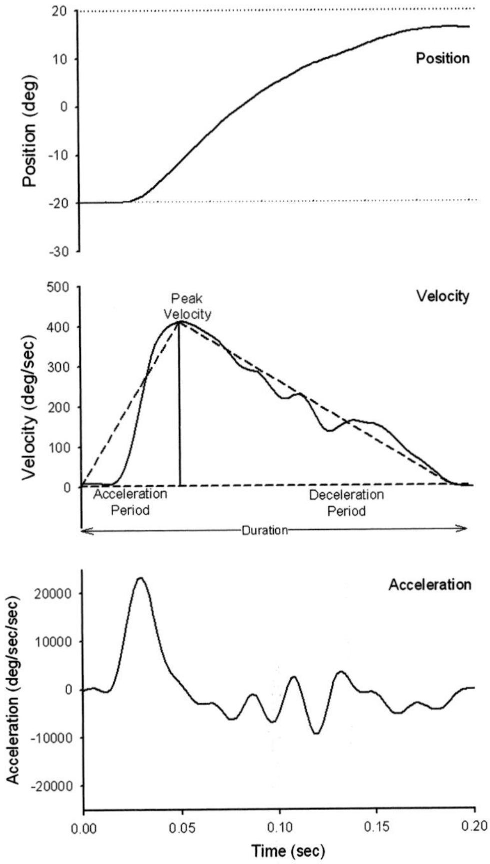

Figure 3–1. Representative record of a 36-degree horizontal saccade made by a normal subject in response to a 40-degree target jump (dotted lines in top panel). Corresponding position, velocity, and acceleration records for this saccade are shown. In the middle panel, components of the velocity waveform are shown, including the acceleration period and total duration, the ratio of which gives a measure of the skewing of the velocity waveform. Positive values correspond to rightward movements.

ence of a fovea, because images are best seen if located there. Animals without a fovea, such as the rabbit, only make voluntary saccades in association with head movements.[121,122] Afoveate animals also produce quick phases of nystagmus during passive head movements so that the slow phases of vestibular and optokinetic nystagmus do not drive the eyes into an extreme orbital position and the oncoming visual scene can be perused.

Saccadic eye movements consist of a hierarchy of behavior, from the most rudimentary of all saccades—quick phases of vestibular nystagmus during passive rotation in darkness—through reflexive saccades made in response to the sudden appearance of a novel visual stimulus, to higher-level volitional behavior such as saccades directed toward the remembered location of a visual target (Table 3–1). This organization can be applied in the clinical neuro-ophthalmologic examination. For example, if voluntary saccades cannot be generated, then it is useful to test progressively more reflexive types of saccades down to the quick phases of nystagmus. A comparable approach is used in the neurologic localization of motor disorders of all types.

BEHAVIOR OF THE SACCADIC SYSTEM

We will discuss in turn the main characteristics of saccades: velocity and duration, waveform and trajectory, reaction time or latency, and accuracy. A number of ingenious paradigms have been developed to test aspects of saccadic responses to visual stimuli (Fig. 3–2).

Table 3–1. **Classification of Saccades**

Classification	Definition
VOLITIONAL SACCADES	Elective saccades made as part of purposeful behavior
PREDICTIVE, ANTICIPATORY	Saccades generated in anticipation of or in search of the appearance of a target at a particular location.
MEMORY-GUIDED	Saccades generated to a location in which a target has been previously present (Fig. 3–2C).
ANTISACCADES	Saccades generated in the opposite direction to the sudden appearance of a target (after being instructed to do so; Fig. 3–2D).
TO COMMAND	Saccades generated on cue.

(Continued on following page)

Table 3–1. *(continued)*

Classification	Definition
REFLEXIVE SACCADES	Saccades generated to novel stimuli (visual, auditory or tactile) that unexpecedly occur within the environment.
EXPRESS SACCADES	Very short latency saccades that can be elicited when the novel stimulus is presented after the fixation stimulus has disappeared (gap stimulus; Fig. 3–2B)
SPONTANEOUS SACCADES	Seemingly random saccades that occur when the subject is not required to perform any particular behavioral task.
QUICK PHASES	Quick phases of nystagmus generated during vestibular or optokinetic stimulation or as automatic resetting movements in the presence of spontaneous drift of the eyes.

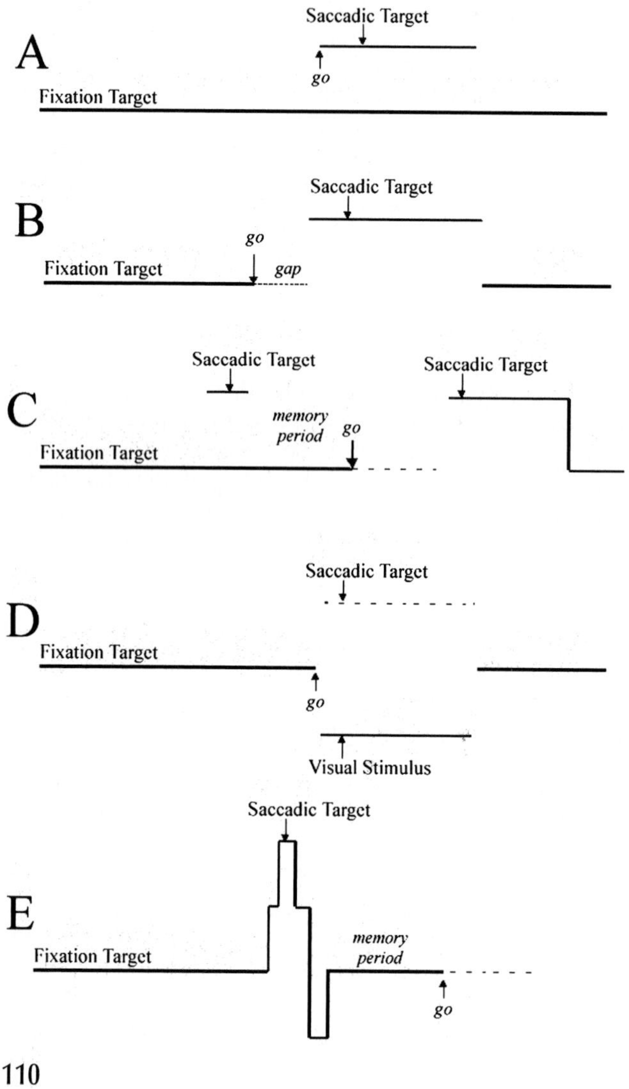

Figure 3–2. Schematic of laboratory stimulus paradigms commonly used to test saccades. In each case "go" indicates the signal for the subject to look toward the "saccadic target." (A) Overlap paradigm, in which the central fixation target stays on throughout. (B) Gap paradigm, in which fixation target is switched off before visual target is switched on. (C) Memory target task. The subject views the fixation target during the time that the visual target is flashed and after several seconds (the memory period), the fixation light is switched off and the subject looks towards the remembered location of the target. (D) The antisaccade task. The subject is required to look in the opposite direction when the visual stimulus is presented. (E) Sequence of saccades task. A series of targets at several locations are turned on in turn. After a memory period, the fixation light goes out as a signal for the subject to make a series of saccades towards the remembered series of target locations.

Saccadic Velocity and Duration

Saccades show consistent relationships among their size, speed, and duration. Thus, the larger the saccade, the greater its top speed and the longer its duration. However, even large saccades (Fig. 3–1) do not last much longer than 100 ms, which is the response time of the visual system. This means that visual feedback cannot be used to change the size of a saccade once started. Rather, the brain must monitor accuracy at the end of each saccade and make an appropriate adjustment to ensure long-term accuracy. Representative plots of peak velocity or duration as a function of amplitude are shown in Figure 3–3, and are often referred to as *main sequence relationships*,[38,80] a term borrowed from the classification of stars by astronomers. These relationships are consistent enough that they can be used to define ranges for normal saccades; deviations of measured eye movements from these intervals indicate either abnormal saccades or non-saccadic eye movements. For saccades that are smaller than about 20 degrees, there is a linear relationship between amplitude and *peak velocity*; above 20 degrees, peak velocity shows a progressive "soft" saturation with asymptotic values of about 500 degrees per second. Main-sequence relationships also apply to the smallest saccades (microsaccades);[417] these relationships are discussed under Visual Fixation in Chapter 4. A commonly used equation to describe the main sequence relationship is:

$$\text{Peak velocity} = \text{Vmax} \times (1 - e^{-\text{Amplitude}/C})$$

where Vmax is the asymptotic peak velocity and C is a constant. Other equations, such as power functions, have been used to describe the relationship between amplitude and peak velocity for smaller saccades.[225,385] The application of this and other equations describing the main sequence relationships during the laboratory evaluation of saccades is discussed below (Measurement of Saccadic Eye Movements).

The *duration* of saccades are approximately linearly related to their amplitudes for movements from 1 to 50 degrees. Power functions can be used to describe the relationship between amplitude and duration for saccades of all sizes (Fig. 3–3B).[223,225,385,769] Acceleration and its derivative, jerk, are greater than for other types of eye movement and can be used to identify saccades.[764] Saccadic speed and duration cannot be voluntarily controlled. However, a number of factors may cause variability in the peak velocity and duration of saccades of similar size, even for the same individual, from day to day.[81] For example, saccades are slower when made in darkness, to the remembered locations of visual stimuli, in anticipation of target jumps,[724] and when made in the opposite direction to a visual stimulus

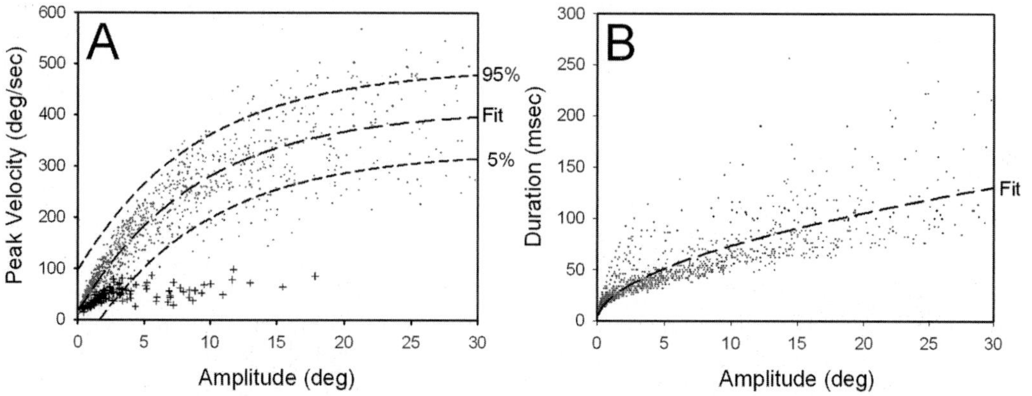

Figure 3–3. Dynamic properties of saccades. (A) Plot of peak velocity versus amplitude of vertical saccades. Data points (dots) are saccades from 10 normal subjects. These normal data are fit with an exponential equation of the form Peak Velocity = Vmax × (1 - $e^{-\text{Amplitude}/C}$), where Vmax is the asymptotic peak velocity, and C is a constant defining the exponential rise is shown. Also plotted are the 5% and 95% prediction intervals. The crossed points indicate vertical saccades from a patient with Niemann-Pick type C disease (see Fig. 5B), which lie outside the prediction intervals for normals. (B) Plot of duration versus amplitude. The data from 10 normal subjects are fit with a power equation of the form: Duration = D_1*Amplitude^n, where D_1 is the duration of a 1 degree saccade, and n is the parameter to be determined.

(the antisaccade task; Fig. 3–2D).[55,87,657,658] Saccades made between visual targets alternating position at a higher frequency (e.g., >1 Hz) are faster than to targets alternating at a lower frequency (e.g., <0.2 Hz).[405] Saccades are also faster when made in association with manual tasks,[184] or if the fixation target is turned off before the stimulus for the saccade appears ("gap" stimulus; Fig. 3–2B).[547] Saccade velocity also depends upon the direction of the movement and the initial and final orbital position.[4,121,122,523] Centripetal saccades (directed toward the center) tend to be faster than centrifugal saccades. Upward saccades made in the upper portion of the ocular motor range are slower than upward saccades made in the lower portion of the ocular motor range.[121] It is not settled whether saccadic velocity declines with age.[317,539,640,642,668,317] Saccades of normal velocity can be made by young infants if they are suitably aroused.[653] Thus, all of these factors, as well as the measurement technique, must be considered when comparing saccadic behavior in different subjects or in patients with neurological disease (see Measurement of Saccadic Eye Movements).

Saccadic Waveform

The shape of the temporal waveform of the saccade, especially its velocity profile, is another useful way to characterize saccades (Fig. 3–1). The *skewness*, or asymmetry, of the waveform can be estimated simply from the ratio of the time to reach maximum velocity (the acceleration phase) to the total duration of the saccade (middle panel of Fig. 3–1); other mathematic functions have also been used to measure skewness.[731] The skewness ratio is about 0.5 for small saccades (acceleration and deceleration phases are equal in duration) and falls to values of about 0.2 for the largest saccades (peak velocity is reached earlier relative to the end of the saccade). Skewness also increases for antisaccades, saccades made to remembered targets, and saccades made under fatigue or decreased vigilance.[658]

Another measurement of saccades, which is related to the velocity waveform, can be calculated from the ratio: *peak velocity/mean velocity (Q)*.[45,276,277,323,374] In humans, Q is about 1.6 and holds even for slow saccades made by fatigued subjects and some disorders of saccades. The value of Q is related to the velocity waveform (Fig. 3–1). A triangular velocity waveform gives a value of 2.0, whereas a rectangular waveform yields a value of 1.0; saccadic velocity profiles yield an intermediate value.[374,731] Saccades with Q values exceeding 2.0 usually have a velocity waveform interrupted by a transient, discrete deceleration (see Disorders of Saccadic Waveform).[374]

Another useful approach for analyzing saccades is by examining *phase-plane plots* of eye position versus eye velocity or acceleration (Fig. 3–11B); such plots have proven useful in investigation of abnormal saccades, saccades made with vergence movements, and corrective saccades in patients with vestibular hypofunction.[526]

During saccades, the eyes do not move perfectly together.[121,122] For horizontal refixations, saccades of the abducting eye tend to be larger, faster, and more skewed than concomitant saccades of the adducting eye. This disconjugacy between the two eyes leads to a transient intrasaccadic divergence. For vertical refixations, the eyes are better yoked, although idiosyncratic horizontal vergence movements may occur (often transient divergence with upward saccades, and convergence with downward saccades).[179,728,774] The interaction of saccades and vergence is discussed further in Chapter 8.

Following a horizontal saccade there is usually a brief drift of the eyes that has both disjunctive (vergence) and conjugate (version) components. The disjunctive component of this post-saccadic drift is convergent and may compensate for divergence during saccades. The conjugate component is in the direction of the prior movement, and may compensate for the tendency for most saccades to slightly undershoot the target. Such *post-saccadic drift* has been called a *glissade*,[753] and has been attributed to a mismatch between the sizes of the phasic (pulse) and tonic (step) components of the innervation generating saccades (see Fig. 1–3, Chapter 1). The eye drifts in a glissade because orbital elastic forces pull the eye to a position in the orbit corresponding to the new step level of innervation. Glissades occur more frequently in fatigued subjects.[40]

At the end of a saccade, an oppositely directed, post-saccadic movement occasionally occurs and appears to be as fast as a small saccade (1/4 to 1/2 degree). Such small saccades have been called *dynamic overshoots*.

Dynamic overshoots can occur after saccades of all sizes, but are more conspicuous after small saccades, including square-wave jerks (saccadic intrusions).[2] They may be conjugate or more prominent in the abducting eye;[82,343,725] they also occur with large saccades or if subjects blink with the eye movement. The origin of dynamic overshoots is debated. On the one hand, they might arise from the mechanical properties of orbital tissues rather than a central reversal of innervation;[573] measurements of the forces generated by extraocular muscles support this interpretation.[443] On the other hand, dynamic overshoots have been attributed to brief reversals of the central saccadic command.[37] Such a reversal of saccadic innervation would normally bring the eye to an abrupt stop but, if too large, would lead to a dynamic overshoot. Large dynamic overshoots occur in patients who show saccadic oscillations such as ocular flutter (Fig. 3–4).

Saccadic Trajectory

When humans make saccades in oblique directions, the horizontal and vertical components show minor slowing compared with purely vertical or purely horizontal saccades of similar size.[57,590] For diagonal saccades (45-degree inclination), the horizontal and the vertical components are similar and the trajectory is nearly straight (Fig. 3–5A). For oblique saccades made at angles other than 45-degree inclination, a smaller component that stays on the main sequence for velocity and duration does not last as long as the larger component,[39,57,258] and the trajectory of the saccade, at least in humans, tends to be curved. When the brainstem mechanism generating either the horizontal or vertical components of oblique saccades is impaired, oblique saccades have strongly curved trajectories that are evident at the bedside (see Fig. 3–5B and Video Display: Disorders of Saccades). The significance of the trajectories of oblique saccades is discussed further under Models for Saccade Generation, Pathophysiology of Saccadic Abnormalities, and Three-Dimensional Aspects of Eye Rotations (Chapter 9).

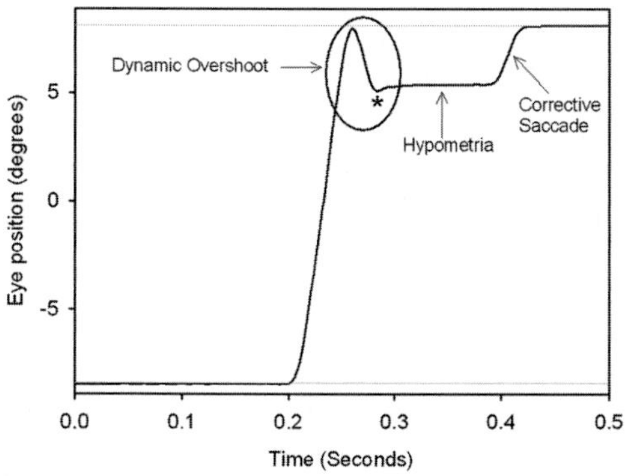

Figure 3–4. Example of a large "dynamic overshoot" in a patient recovering from brainstem encephalitis causing ocular flutter. A small oppositely directed dynamic overshoot (indicated by an asterisk) also occurs. The patient is making horizontal saccades between a stationary target (gray lines). Note that after the initial movement is over, the eye is not on target (it is hypometric) and a subsequent corrective saccade is made. Positive values correspond to rightward movements.

Saccadic Reaction Time (Latency)

The interval between target presentation and when the eye starts to move in a saccade (conventionally identified by when eye speed exceeds some threshold, such as 30 degrees per second) has received intensive study because it reflects various aspects of visual processing, target selection, and motor programming. Saccadic reaction time depends upon the nature of the stimulus—both its modality and the temporal properties of target presentation. Factors such as the amount of information available and the urgency to make a decision influence saccade latency.[107a,562]

SACCADES MADE TO DISPLACEMENTS OF A VISIBLE TARGET

When a visual target jumps from one point to another, normal subjects generate a saccade within about 200 ms. Individual latency values for a number of such trials are not distributed normally (in the statistical sense), but are skewed, with more values having higher latencies. If, however, the reciprocal of latency is plotted, as a measure of "promptness," the distribution of values is closer to a normal one.[108] It has been suggested that the variability in saccadic initiation time shown by any subject reflects the time needed to decide whether a target is in fact present.[108] Studies using a larger number of potential stimuli have shown

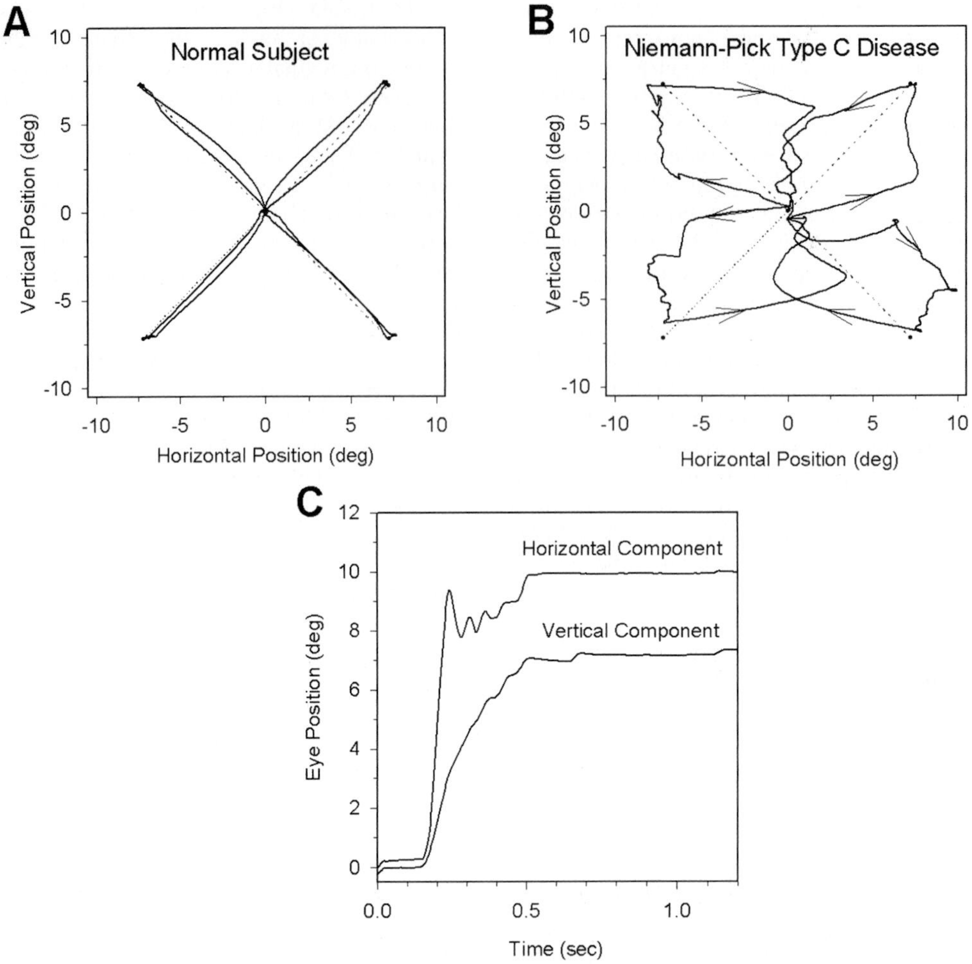

Figure 3–5. Trajectories of oblique saccades. (A) Comparison of trajectories of oblique saccades made to and from four target positions starting at primary position in a normal subject and (B) in a patient with Niemann-Pick type C disease,[590] who showed a selective slowing of vertical saccades. Arrowheads in (B) indicate the direction of eye movement. The trajectory of the target jump is shown as a dotted line. The trajectories of the patient's saccades are strongly curved, reflecting the initial, faster, horizontal component and the later, slower, vertical component. (C) Time plot comparing horizontal and vertical components of an oblique saccade made by the patient with Niemann-Pick type C disease. Horizontal oscillations occurred after the horizontal component had ended, but while the vertical component was still going on. Amplitude-peak velocity plots of vertical saccades made by this patient are shown in Fig. 3–3A.

that saccadic programming obeys Hick's law—a logarithmic relationship exists between response time and the number of alternative choices.[388]

Aside from the motivational and attentive state of the subject,[254] a number of properties of the stimulus influence saccadic initiation time. These include luminance, size, contrast, and complexity;[20,146,159,160,254,514,747,786] the nature of the visual task;[450a] whether the target is visual or auditory;[772] the size of the intended eye movement and the orbital position from which it starts;[216] the predictability of the target's motion;[588,617,646] the specific instructions given to the subject (i.e., cognitive set);[326] the presence of distracting stimuli;[133a,308a,746] the laterality of the target;[308] and the patient's age.[96,109,317,465,539,593a,642,653]

GAP AND OVERLAP STIMULI

Often, the stimulus for a saccade is the appearance of a novel object in the visual scene. In the laboratory, this type of stimulus is conveniently created by turning on a peripherally located, small "target light" in a darkened room, and turning off the "fixation light," which the subject is currently viewing with the fovea. The temporal relationship between when the fixation light is extinguished and the target light is illuminated also influences saccade latency. Reaction time is smaller when the fixation light is turned off 100 to 400 ms before the peripheral target appears ("gap" stimulus) and greater when the fixation light remains illuminated after the peripheral target appears (the "overlap" stimulus; Fig. 3–2A).[338,564,565] In the gap paradigm (Fig. 3–2B), human subjects generate some saccades with short reaction times—*express saccades*; latencies are as low as 100 ms.[197,201,202,424] Children make express saccades more easily than adults.[358] The facility improves with practice,[203] and is performed best for the target positions (saccadic vectors) used during training,[517,603a] suggesting that express saccades reflect a predictive mechanism. However, express saccades are still generated even if gap and overlap stimuli are randomly presented in a block of trials.[751] A cautionary note is that a factor contributing to the generation of express saccades concerns the direction of the recentering saccade from the prior trial; a short latency response is more likely if this recentering saccade is in the same direction as the upcoming target jump.[107] Express saccades are probably a laboratory phenomenon, being unlikely to occur in natural viewing conditions, in which a number of visual stimuli are simultaneously present.[603]

Express saccades can be generated equally well if the gap stimulus is used during fixation or smooth pursuit;[372] this implies that, in the case of the gap stimulus, "fixation" may be defined more in terms of keeping the fovea pointed towards a visual object than suppression of an eye movement. However, the shortened latency achieved with the gap stimulus applies much more to saccades than to pursuit or vergence.[371,694] Thus, it appears that the gap stimulus mainly releases an attentional fixation mechanism for saccadic gaze shifts. No equivalent change in latency can be achieved in response to auditory stimuli.[638]

Evidence reviewed below suggests that the rostral pole of the superior colliculus plays an important role in such release of fixation.[164,165,483] In monkeys, express saccades are completely eliminated with lesions of the superior colliculus but not with lesions of the frontal lobes.[271,605] Thus, express saccades provide a way of testing collicular function in humans. So-called spasm of fixation, in which a patient cannot change gaze until the fixation target is removed, may be an extreme case of the retarding influence of a persistent fixation target (overlap paradigm) upon saccade latency. Caution is required, however, in interpreting increased saccadic latency as being purely collicular in origin, since it may also be due to defects in the ability to disengage, shift, and reengage visual attention.[254,478,552] Overall, the ability to generate express saccades is probably related to an ability to turn off the fixation mechanism, a process that is influenced by directed visual attention.[752]

ANTISACCADES

To investigate the control of voluntary (as opposed to reflexive) saccades, a special test paradigm called the antisaccade task has been developed (Fig. 3–2D and Fig. 12–14, Chapter 12).[265,467] In this task, the subject is required to suppress a saccade (the "prosaccade") toward a stimulus that appears in the periphery of vision and generate instead a voluntary saccade of equal size towards the opposite side—the mirror location (the "antisaccade"). These two separate components depend on independent mechanisms,[199] which appear to compete with each other.[373] After time for the antisaccade to be made, a target light is turned on at the correct location, to check the accuracy of the movement. The simplest measure of errors of the response to this test concerns the direction of the initial saccade, expressed as the ratio of prosaccades to antisaccades; this can be tested at the bedside.[135] Normal subjects initially make frequent errors on this task, but with a brief period of practice, error rates are typically about 25%, being greater in subjects with shorted prosaccade latencies, with less eccentric target positions, and with shorter fixation periods.[187,660] Antisaccades may be less accurate, slower,[173a] and made at longer latency than prosaccades.

When the fixation point is turned off before the peripheral target is presented (gap stimulus), antisaccades are generated at a latency of about 175 ms and with errors on about 15% of trials; error rates increase if targets are more eccentric.[198] Children develop the ability to make antisaccades by adolescence.[215] In adults, the latency of antisaccades increases with age.[96,504] Patients with a variety of cerebral lesions, especially those involving the frontal lobes, show abnormalities on the antisaccade task. They are unable to suppress a reflexive saccade towards the visual target and have difficulty generating a voluntary saccade towards an imagined location. In addition, individuals who make unusually frequent express saccades, such as those with developmental dyslexia, tend to make greater numbers of prosaccade errors on the antisaccade task.[72] Such a deficit could be due to an impaired ability by the rostral pole of the superior colliculus to suppress reflexive saccades. Study of the properties of antisaccades and prosaccades made in response to more complex stimuli may provide further insights into the mechanisms of normal and abnormal saccadic programming, and they are being used to probe a range of disorders including schizophrenia (see Chapter 12).[50,659]

A related behavior is the countermanding task, in which subjects are required to make visually guided saccades on most trials but, on some, to withhold a saccade if a stop signal (such as reappearance of the fixation cue) is presented.[269,270,270] The reaction time to the stop signal is about 135 ms and is not influenced by its luminance. The stop signal may be located in the central or peripheral part of the visual field,[30] and auditory cues may also be used to stop the planned saccade.[102,124] The behavior of subjects on the countermanding task has been successfully predicted by a model in which the target initiates a response preparation signal that races against the signal initiated by the cue to inhibit the saccade.[269] The countermanding task has proven useful in understanding the contributions of frontal cortical areas to the voluntary control of saccades,[600] and has also motivated related studies of patients with frontal lobe lesions.[319]

Saccadic Accuracy

ACCURACY OF VISUALLY GUIDED SACCADES

The ideal ocular motor response to the sudden appearance of a target of interest in the visual periphery is an eye movement that rapidly reaches, and abruptly stops at, the target. Such saccades must be accurate whether the target is stationary or moving.[176,586] Saccades may be inaccurate or dysmetric in two general ways: according to whether or not the size of the rapid, pulse portion of the saccade is inappropriate (called saccadic pulse dysmetria); and whether or not the eyes drift at the end of the saccade (called post-saccadic drift or a glissade). Postsaccadic drift is often attributed to a mismatch between the two major components of saccadic innervation—the pulse and the step—producing pulse-step mismatch dysmetria. Eye movement records are usually necessary to determine whether the postsaccadic drift is conjugate or disjunctive. However, disjunctive drifts are often evident in internuclear ophthalmoplegia, when the slow adducting saccade results from the inability of the demyelinated medial longitudinal fasciculus to conduct the high-frequency discharge of the pulse; thus it is the step that mainly carries the eye, in a glissade, towards the target (see Video Display: Pontine Syndromes). In this section, we will mainly deal with features of pulse dysmetria. Saccadic step dysmetria will be discussed in the section on Adaptive Control of Saccadic Accuracy.

Normal individuals frequently show small degrees of *saccadic pulse dysmetria*—most commonly undershooting (hypometria) of the target (Fig. 3–6). The degree of dysmetria is usually relatively small, typically 10% of the amplitude of the saccade for non-predictable visual targets,[55,715] and is even less for small saccades.[370] For oblique saccades, the net trajectory of the movement is more accurate than the initial direction.[185] Hypometria is usually more prominent for centrifugally directed saccades (that is, those directed toward the periphery) and for saccades of larger amplitude. Normal individuals occasionally make hypermetric (overshooting) saccades when the saccade is small or directed centripetally (toward the center) and especially downward.[121] Fatigue and age may also influence saccade accuracy. Tired subjects may make two small, closely spaced saccades rather than a single saccade, and elderly subjects tend to make more hypometric saccades.[6,317] Infants frequently make several small saccades, instead of one large saccade, to an eccentric target.[653]

The amount of saccadic pulse dysmetria is also influenced by the particular task. Saccades to targets already present are considerably

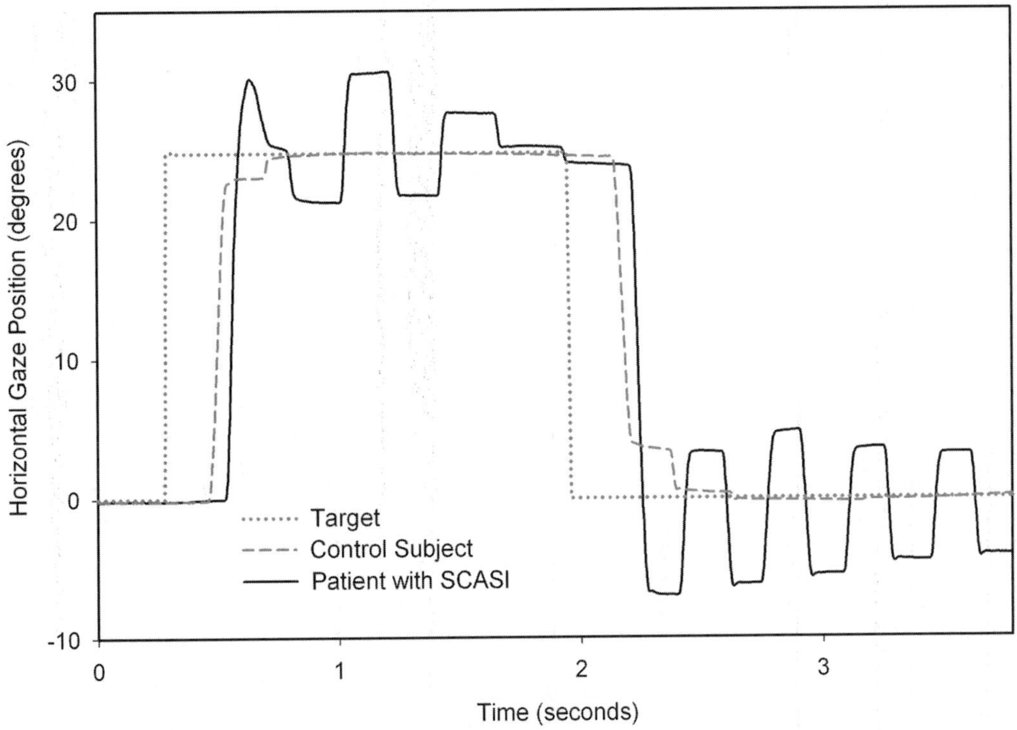

Figure 3–6. Examples of horizontal saccades made by a normal subject (gray, dashed line) and a patient with a spinocerebellar degeneration (solid line) in response to a 25-degree target jump (dotted line) from center position to right 25 degrees. After a reaction time, the normal subject makes an initial saccade that is hypometric, followed by a subsequent correction. A similar pattern occurs after the target returns to center. The patient shows hypermetria, overshooting the target when it jumps to the right, and especially when it jumps back to center, following which there are macrosaccadic oscillations about the point of fixation.[691] Positive values correspond to rightward movements.

more accurate than saccades to suddenly appearing targets.[394] Dysmetria at the end of the primary saccade is greater along the axis between the two targets (so-called amplitude dysmetria) than away from the axis between the two targets (direction dysmetria).[732] If targets appear in a set of positions, saccades overshoot the near positions and undershoot the far; this is referred to as the range effect, and it is established after only a few trials.[340,342] It may be one example of a general strategy that the brain uses to predict which motor movement will be required to achieve its goal.

Saccadic accuracy is also influenced by the background on which the target sits (the "global" effect). Moreover, if two targets are presented simultaneously and not too far apart, the saccade will often take the eye to a position between them—*averaging saccades*.[177,196,466,514] Such saccades often show variable, curved trajectories.[27,168,404] As the distance between the targets increases, the proportion of averaging saccades decreases and the eye more commonly lands on one of the two targets. If the target consists of a word, the eye usually lands close to its center;[54] (see Saccades during Visual Search and Reading, below). Changing the size or luminance of one of two targets will cause the saccade to bring the eye closer to the larger or brighter target.[146]

ACCURACY OF MEMORY-GUIDED SACCADES

When normal subjects attempt to make saccades to the remembered location of a target that they viewed a few seconds before, they do so with a little more variability than if the target were visible.[42,55,757,787] The accuracy of memory-guided saccades is generally similar whether normal subjects maintain steady fixation or shift gaze using smooth pursuit or an eye-head or body movement during the memory period (i.e., from the time of target presentation until they are required to make the memory-guided saccade, in darkness).[78,327,360a,369,399a,501,613,787] This implies that the brain takes into account the gaze shift that has occurred during the memory period. Although the brain might monitor such gaze shifts by monitoring neural signals of eye movements—efference copy or corollary discharge,[236,667,700b] visual estimates of the direction of gaze assume greater importance, when they are available.[787] The accuracy of memory-guided saccades is affected by lesions at a variety of sites, but especially with those located in the dorsolateral prefrontal cortex (see Box 12–21, Chapter 12).

CORRECTIVE SACCADES

When normal individuals undershoot the target, they usually make a corrective saccade with a latency of 100 ms to 130 ms (Fig. 3–6).[55] Such corrective movements can occur even when the target is extinguished before the initial saccade is completed. Therefore, a nonvisual or "extraretinal" signal can provide information about whether the first movement is accurate, so that a corrective saccade can be triggered if necessary. Such nonvisual information is most likely based upon monitoring of efferent ocular motor commands or efference copy ("effort of will"; see Chapter 1). Nonvisual mechanisms for generating corrective saccades are also apparent when subjects make saccades in complete darkness to remembered locations of targets.[787] If a saccade made in darkness brings the eye to a position more than about 5 degrees away from the location of the previously seen target, an accurate corrective saccade is usually made.[503] Vision, however, is still important for getting the eye on target. The probability of occurrence of a corrective saccade and its accuracy increase, and the latency to the corrective saccade decreases, if a visual signal is available at the end of the initial saccade.[151,546] Furthermore, visual information may be used during the deceleration phase of a saccade to trigger a corrective movement.[175]

Quantitative Aspects of Quick Phases of Nystagmus

The quick phases of vestibular and optokinetic nystagmus can also be characterized by their velocity, amplitude, and timing.[641] Over 95% of quick phases are less than 10 degrees in amplitude; they tend to be slightly slower than similar-sized voluntary saccades.[223] The amplitude-peak velocity relationships and amplitude-duration relationships of upward and downward quick phases are similar, but tend to be slower than horizontal quick phases.[223,224] The size and frequency of quick phases are such that they tend to bring the eye into the anticompensatory direction (i.e., the direction opposite to that of the slow phase).[438] An exception occurs when a subject, sitting inside a revolving, striped, optokinetic drum, is specifically instructed to follow a stripe, as it moves from one side to the other, and then to make a saccade in the other direction to acquire another stripe (look nystagmus). On the other hand, if the subject is asked to stare straight ahead as the stripes pass by, quick phases are smaller and more frequent (stare nystagmus). Quick phases of nystagmus have a randomness to them,[643] and probably defy the use of common statistical models to summarize their behavior.[714] Saccades that "catch-up" during smooth pursuit are also somewhat stochastic; both position and velocity information concerning the tracking error are used to trigger these movements in normals.[138,621a] During vestibular nystagmus generated by active head movements quick phase landing is programmed using information provided by the vestibular system.[554] Braking saccades, which are encountered in individuals with congenital nystagmus, also show similar dynamic properties to other types of saccade.[333]

In patients with saccadic palsies, quick phases may be absent, and gaze is a tonically deviated in the direction of the stimulus (see Video Display: Disorders of Saccades).[226] In some patients, the timing and amplitude of quick phases may be abnormal, just as the latency and amplitude of voluntary saccades may be abnormal. Thus, in patients with Wallenberg's syndrome, the amplitude of quick phases towards the side of the lesion is greater than in the other direction, a similar pattern to their ipsipulsion of voluntary saccades (see Video Display: Medullary Syndromes). Patients with congenital ocular motor apraxia may show a defect in the initiation of quick phases during passive head rotation; the eyes intermittently deviate tonically in the compensatory (slow phase) direction (see Video Display: Congenital Ocular Motor Apraxia).[780]

Ballistic Nature of Saccadic Movements

The duration of most saccades is less than 100 ms, so visual information does not have time to influence these movements once they begin. Saccades are not truly ballistic, however, because they can be modified in mid-flight by factors presented just before the eye starts to move. The first ideas on how the central nervous system processes visual information for saccades were developed by Westheimer,[754] who showed that if a target jumped to a new location and then promptly (less than 100 ms) returned to the origin—a double-step stimulus motion—the subject would still make a saccade away from the current location of the target (Fig. 3–7). Then, after a fairly constant interval (150 ms– 200 ms), the subject would make another saccade back to the original position of the target. The interval between saccades was relatively independent of the interval between the target jumps away from and back to the initial position. These findings suggested that the saccadic system can react to only one stimulus at a time, and there is a refractory period, during which a second saccade cannot be initiated after the first.

Young and Stark[771] recognized that the type of behavior shown in Westheimer's experiments was compatible with what control systems engineers call a sampled data system. They hypothesized that a "snapshot" of the visual information, at a given instant, is "sampled" by the saccadic system. If an object of interest is observed in the periphery of this "snapshot," a decision is made to generate a saccade that will bring the image of the target onto the fovea. Based on the retinal error (the distance between the retinal location of an image and the fovea), the size, direction, and duration of the upcoming saccade are calculated and an irrevocable decision to generate the saccade is made. A preprogrammed saccadic command is then generated, based upon the visual information that was acquired during the initial "snapshot." Once the saccade is completed, the visual world is again "sampled" to determine if another saccade is still needed to bring the target of interest onto the fovea. Westheimer's results could then be interpreted by assuming that the return of the target to its initial position was not actually "seen" by the saccadic system until after the first saccade was made. Therefore, a normal saccadic latency, determined by the interval between "snapshots," was required before making a second saccade to bring the eyes back to the target.

Although the sampled-data model accounts for many aspects of saccadic eye tracking, such a scheme does not explain all of the responses that normal individuals make. If Westheimer's experimental paradigm is expanded to include target jumps of different sizes and directions,

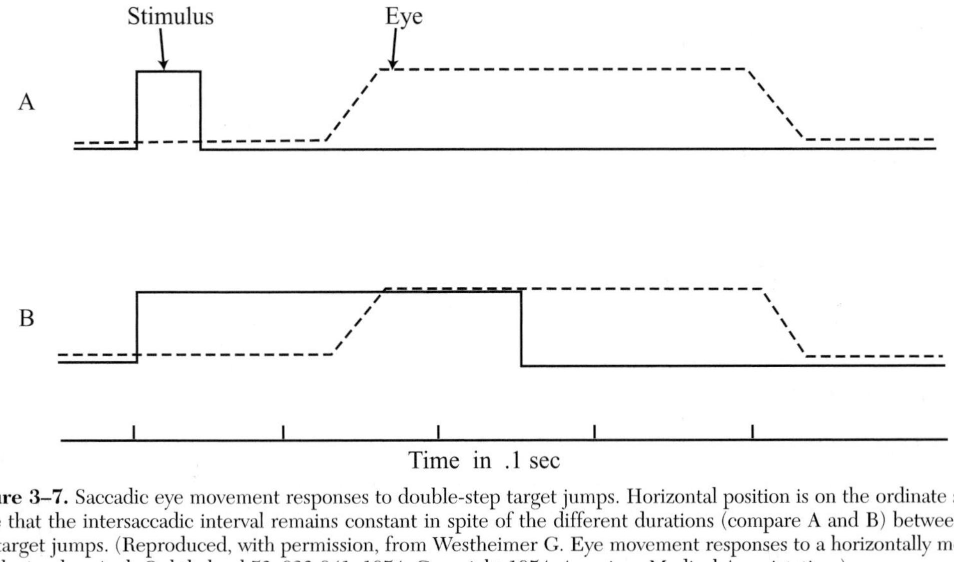

Figure 3–7. Saccadic eye movement responses to double-step target jumps. Horizontal position is on the ordinate scale. Note that the intersaccadic interval remains constant in spite of the different durations (compare A and B) between the two target jumps. (Reproduced, with permission, from Westheimer G. Eye movement responses to a horizontally moving visual stimulus. Arch Ophthalmol 52, 932-941, 1954. Copyright 1954, American Medical Associatation.)

and if a large number of responses are analyzed, it can be shown that visual information can be continuously acquired and used to modify the initial saccadic response until about 70 ms before the movement begins.[29,41] This is approximately the time it takes visual information to traverse the retina and central visual pathways and reach the brain stem ocular motor mechanisms.

Furthermore, the saccadic system does not have an obligatory refractory period; two saccades may occur with virtually no intersaccadic interval in response to the appropriate sequence of double-step motion of the stimulus.[56,249,432] Slow saccades (see Video Display: Disorders of Saccades), which occur in certain neurological diseases, can be interrupted in mid-flight when the target position is changed, even after the eye has already begun to move.[411,777] When presented with two-dimensional, double-step stimuli, normal subjects may make a single curved saccade, rather than two successive straight saccades, indicating that the saccade trajectory has been modified in-flight.[726] The earliest responses to such two-dimensional, double-step stimuli suggest that direction and amplitude may be programmed separately.[238,557a] If both targets are visible (double-cue paradigm) differences of saccadic responses from the classic double-step paradigm can be mainly attributed to the visual stimuli rather than any change in motor programming of eye movements.[648] When voluntary prosaccades or antisaccades are pitted against quick phases of vestibular nystagmus induced by rotational stimulation, an interaction between these two different types of rapid eye movement occurs that suggests parallel programming of each followed by convergence of components.[721,722] In sum, the central nervous system appears able to change saccades throughout their programming. Normal saccades only appear to be ballistic because of their high velocities and brief durations.

Saccades during Visual Search and Reading

One important function of saccades is for visual search of the environment. Since best vision corresponds to the fovea of the retina, it behooves us to point the fovea at features of interest. Yarbus[769] first systematically studied visual search by recording subjects' eye movements as they scanned pictures of faces and scenes. The idiosyncratic pattern of eye movements made when viewing a pictorial display is called a scan path (Fig. 3–8A).[196a,196b,353,401,492]

Saccades made during visual search for targets embedded in an array of stimuli are not random and such behavior can be quantified and used to study visual attention.[416,462] It is suggested that during visual search, the scan path minimizes the cognitive and attentional load.[28] During manual tasks such as copying a design, frequent eye movements are used to scan the display for information, rather than committing that information to working memory.[44,183] A factor influencing scan paths is the phenomenon referred to as *inhibition of return*, whereby search for novel features will take precedence over those recently inspected. Thus, saccades to features recently inspected show longer reaction times.[570] Electrophysiological and clinical studies have suggested that the cerebral cortex, possibly the orbitofrontal lobes, contribute to this behavior.[163,306]

Patients suffering from *hemispatial neglect* show an inability to attend to the contralateral half of space, which biases their attention towards the ipsilesional side, and so impairs their ability to search contralesional space. Furthermore, search behavior in patients with hemispatial neglect combines a spatial bias with loss of working memory for locations previously searched.[318,407,569,650]

Interpretation of ocular motor behavior during *reading* remains controversial and is difficult to interpret in the context of the known control of saccades.[427a,679] For example, there is disagreement as to whether the spaces between words, or the words themselves, serve to guide saccades.[180–182,559,738] In this regard, different languages presents different visual challenges.[337] However, it seems probable that cognitive processes are more important for driving the eyes through the text than the visual features of the text itself.[561] Similarly, it has been suggested that when subjects read music, the pattern of saccades reflects not the visual stimulus or the manual response, but the flow of information from the musical score to performances.[357]

Eye movements have been widely used as an experimental tool to investigate mechanisms underlying *developmental dyslexia*. There has even been a research effort to determine

A

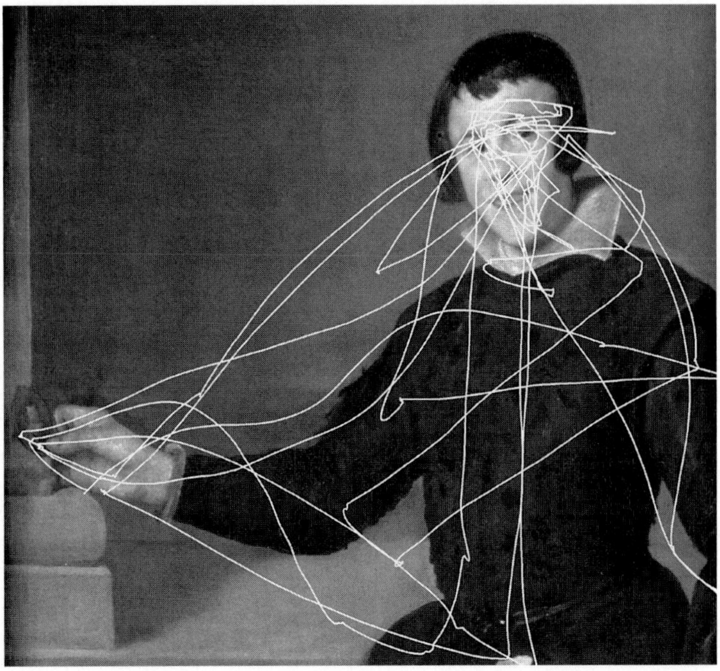

B

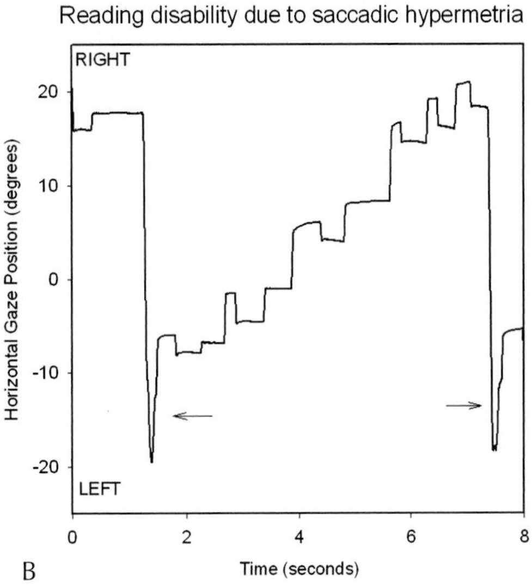

Figure 3–8. (A) Example of normal saccadic scan path during visual search of a painting. (Portrait of the jester Calabazas by Diego Velázquez is reproduced with permission of the Cleveland Museum of Art.) Each line represents a saccade as the subject moves his fixation point from one feature of interest to the next. (B) Reading in a patient with a form of spinocerebellar degeneration.[691] He moves his fixation point along the line from left to right is a series of small saccades, which often overshoot the target (word), requiring a corrective saccade. When he makes a saccade to the left to begin the next line, he overshoots the target (arrows) and often loses his place; these abnormal saccades made reading difficult and tiring.

whether developmental dyslexia is actually caused by abnormal control of saccadic eye movements;[91a] lack of consensus may, in part, reflect the heterogeneity of patients with dyslexia.[140] Thus, for example, in some patients, the underlying cause of the reading disability may be auditory-linguistic defects,[139] whereas in others, it is due to defects of dynamic visual perception.[200] Specifically, it has been suggested that some individuals with developmental dyslexia have motion-processing disorders leading to a less stable visual percept.[680] Two defects have been identified on psychophysical testing: a deficit in detecting coherent motion and a deficit in discriminating velocities.[759] Further studies may clarify whether such individuals have impaired ocular-tracking responses to first and second-order motion stimuli, a subject discussed in Chapter 4.

One reproducible finding is that dyslexic children often show impairment of steady fixation,[71,72,174] with excessive numbers of square-wave jerks.[134] The presence of this fixation abnormality in dyslexics during non-reading tasks suggests that the underlying abnormality may not be caused by language problems alone.[174] Similarly, children with attention deficit hyperactivity disorder show difficulty suppressing saccades and deficits on spatial working memory tasks when they are unmedicated.[104,359,461,464] When presented with two targets at different eccentricities, normal readers make an averaging saccade to an intermediate location ("center of gravity"), but dyslexics generate saccades that land closer to the less eccentric target, suggesting a deficit in processing of global spatial information for eye movements.[133] Dyslexic subjects show a greater reaction time for saccade made back to words just read—a variant of inhibition of return.[560]

Although the relationship between eye movement abnormalities and childhood dyslexia is not clear, patients with certain types of *acquired saccadic abnormalities* do have difficulty reading.[116] This effect is seen in patients with slow saccades or saccadic palsy due to brainstem lesions; with acquired ocular motor apraxia due to bihemispheric disease; with large saccadic intrusions or oscillations (Fig. 3–8B), and various forms of nystagmus.[274] Homonymous hemianopia may disrupt reading eye movements, especially when it is due to damage of the occipital white matter.[784] Patients with Alzheimer's disease show longer fixation periods and more saccades per line that may correspond with difficulties in reading.[406]

Visual Consequences of Saccades

An important perceptual problem is how the brain can correctly interpret motion of images on the retina as being due to movement of the eyes rather than of the visual scene. It is possible to identify two components of this problem: the perception of motion during the eye movement, and correct localization of an object in space following a gaze shift.

VISUAL STABLITY DURING SACCADES

We appear not to see during saccadic eye movements. Even though the seen world is rapidly sweeping across the retina, there is no sense of motion or a blurred image. One proposed explanation for this is that the clear perceptions before and after a saccade would mask the "gray-out" due to image motion on the retina at speeds up to 500 degrees per second.[105] Another hypothesis is that, since it is still possible to see lower spatial frequencies in an image when it moves across the retina at speeds of up to 800 degrees per second, there must be selective suppression of vision for lower spatial frequencies during saccades.[94,153] Current evidence indicates that both mechanisms—visual masking and saccadic suppression—contribute to an uninterrupted view of the world despite making several saccades per second.

Thus, on the one hand, some visual stimuli, such as fast-drifting gratings, can only be seen during saccades,[227] arguing against saccadic suppression of vision. Furthermore, magnocellular neurons in the lateral geniculate nucleus show only a weak suppression followed by strong enhancement of visual activity during saccades.[557,563] When stationary gratings of low spatial frequency (0.18 cycles per degree) are presented briefly during saccades, they may appear to move opposite to the direction of the eye movement.[110] This perception of motion is strongest if the gratings are presented during the first part of saccades, and is absent if they are visible at the end of the saccade. Thus, visual masking seems to account, at least partly, for not seeing during saccades.

On the other hand, it is still possible that an efference copy of saccades affects the magnocellular pathway and cortical visual areas concerned with motion vision, inducing a form of saccadic suppression.[705] Thus, functional imaging studies have demonstrated decreased regional cerebral blood flow in the lateral geniculate nucleus, and striate cortex during repetitive saccades made in darkness,[522,693] and evoked potentials induced by visual stimuli presented during saccades are reduced.[21] Moreover, phosphenes—small illusory visual perceptions—due to retinal simulation are suppressed during saccades, but phosphenes induced by transcranial magnetic stimulation

(TMS) to the occiput remain visible, suggesting that a suppressive process takes place between retina and visual cortex.[709]

Another line of evidence comes from patients who make pathologically slow saccades.[777] One such individual was able to modify saccades in mid-flight in response to target jumps, but was unable to detect the target's motion, suggesting that saccadic programming occurred without conscious awareness of the visual stimulus.[411] Similarly, normal subjects appear to adjust their saccades in response to targets presented at the onset of the movement, when they are not consciously perceived.[229] Only rarely do pathologically increased numbers of saccades, either intrusions or oscillations, disrupt vision and this probably occurs when the intersaccadic interval falls below 50 ms.[153] Thus, more studies are required to clarify a classic problem for visual physiology—why we do not see during saccades.

SPATIAL CONSTANCY FOLLOWING SACCADIC GAZE SHIFTS

While every saccadic eye movement causes the entire visual world to be shifted upon the retina, we are still able to maintain an appropriate sense of straight ahead with a 3-D spatial component.[756] How do we ensure such spatial constancy? The classic explanation is that our central nervous system monitors the "effort of will" and then sends this motor information, referred to as efference copy or corollary discharge, to sensory systems.[284] In this way, our perceptual sense knows and adjusts for the shift of images upon the retina using an egocentric frame of reference. It is also possible that extraocular proprioception could serve this function, but the current view is that such inputs are more important for long-term adaptive changes in the ocular motor systems,[228,263,396,397] or perhaps during mechanical hindrance of eye movements.[361]

Other evidence suggests that the brain estimates the location of objects in space with reference to other objects in the visual scene —exocentric cues.[137,524,524] For example, if visual targets are flashed just before, or during, a saccade, they are incorrectly localized as judged by subsequent saccades or finger pointing.[103,137,307,442,520,543,663] If efference copy were the mechanism by which spatial constancy was maintained, then there should be no difference in spatial localization of targets presented just before or after a saccade. The changes in visual responses to targets flashed just before a saccade may reflect changes in apparent visual direction and an apparent compression of visual space and time that is dependent on the post-saccadic visual references.[380,420,452a,587] This visual compression tends to occur at the intended target of a saccade and may last for hundreds of milliseconds.[34]

If subjects are trained on a saccadic adaptation task, they perceive separated targets, flashed before and after the saccade, as being in the same place.[35] This finding has been interpreted as showing that perception uses a signal based upon the intended saccade before adaptation, and that such a signal is used to prompt comparisons of percepts before and after saccades. Thus, efference copy could be used by the brain, not as a precise record of gaze commands, but rather as a cue to re-evaluate the visual consequences of eye movements, as suggested by MacKay.[415]

The situation may differ, however, if visual cues are lacking. Thus, a classic line of evidence to support the role of efference copy in spatial localization is that, in darkness, normal subjects perceive a small after-image, induced by a photoflash, as moving with the eye.[419] The afterimage is stationary on the retina, and its movement in space is probably due to efference copy signaling movement of the eye. However, if a large after-image of a complex scene is induced, it does not seem to move as the eye drifts in darkness.[524] Thus, a large visual after-image appears to override non-visual cues about eye movements.

Other experiments have shown that visual estimates of the direction of gaze are given preference over efference copy, even if the visual information is corrupted by illusory stimuli. For example, if a target is flashed on a moving background, a memory-guided saccade made a few seconds later is consistently inaccurate in manner determined by movement of the background. [664,787] This finding suggests that, during saccades, visual inputs become less reliable, but the brain still puts more reliance on visual than on extraretinal information. Thus, if a visual target is displaced during a saccadic eye movement, its movement may go unnoticed,[149] even if the saccade was pathologically slow.[411] If, however, the target is only shown in its new position 100 ms after the saccade ends, then its displacement to a new position is detected,[150] as if the lack of an immediate post-saccadic visual cue breaks the assumption of a stationary world. It seems that the brain weighs visual and extraretinal estimates of the direction of gaze,[344] putting more reliance on the visual estimates except when visual factors are not available. Although the visual system provides flawed information during each saccade, theoretical explanations have been offered to account for how the brain is able to piece together the puzzle.[486]

NEUROPHYSIOLOGY OF SACCADIC EYE MOVEMENTS

In this section we review the neural machinery by which saccades shift the line of sight so that an image detected in the retinal periphery is brought to the fovea, where it can be seen best. In primary visual cortex (V1, Brodmann area 17), the location of a visual stimulus is represented by the distribution of activity on the surface of the cortex: different parts of this cortical map correspond to different locations on the retina. The neural representation of the motor command for the saccadic response by brainstem neurons is quite different. The ocular motoneurons encode the characteristics of the saccade in terms of their temporal discharge; the size of the saccade is proportional to the total number of discharge spikes. The ocular motoneurons lie in the third, fourth, and sixth cranial nerves and cause the extraocular muscles to move the eyes with respect to the head (that is, in craniotopic coordinates). This means that the brain must transform the stimulus, which is encoded in terms of the location of active neurons within visual cortex (i.e., "place-coded"), into the saccadic command on ocular motoneurons, which is encoded in terms of discharge frequency and duration (i.e., "temporally coded"). Furthermore, a transformation from retinal coordinates into craniotopic coordinates is necessary. The retinal coordinates are two-dimensional, whereas the eye rotates about three axes.[132] We will return to these issues as we discuss the Brainstem Pathways for Saccades, and the cortical and subcortical structures that project to them. After reviewing the electrophysiological findings, a synthesis in the form of models for saccade generation will be presented.

Brainstem Pathways for Saccades

FINAL SACCADIC COMMAND FROM OCULAR MOTONEURONS

Electrophysiological studies of the behavior of ocular motoneurons in monkeys have delineated the changes in innervation that accompany saccades (see Fig. 1–3, Chapter 1 and Video Display: Disorders of Saccades). During a saccade, a high-frequency burst of phasic activity can be recorded from the agonist ocular muscle and, as shown in experimental animals, from the corresponding ocular motoneurons. This burst of activity, the saccadic pulse of innervation, starts about 8 ms before the eye starts to move,[725] and generates the forces necessary to overcome orbital viscous drag so that the eye will quickly move from one position to another. Following a saccade, the agonist eye muscle and its ocular motoneurons assume a new, higher level of tonic innervation, the saccadic step of innervation, which holds the eye in its new position against orbital elastic restoring forces. The transition between the end of the pulse of innervation and the beginning of the step of innervation is not abrupt but gradual, taking up to several hundred milliseconds. This is the slide of innervation. Hence the change in innervation accounting for saccades is actually a pulse-slide-step (Fig. 5–3B).[510,573]

If one records from the antagonist muscle or its motoneurons, one finds reciprocal innervational changes.[656] The antagonist muscle is silenced during the saccade by an inhibitory, off-pulse of innervation; at the end of the saccade, the antagonist assumes a new, lower level of tonic innervation, the off-step. Measurement of muscle forces generated by extraocular muscles indicates that the eye comes to rest at the end of a saccade owing to the viscous forces of the orbital tissues rather to than any "active braking" by the antagonist muscle.[443]

BRAINSTEM SACCADIC PULSE GENERATOR

Two types of neurons are critical components of the brainstem network that generates premotor commands for saccades: burst neurons and omnipause neurons, which are schematized in Figure 3–9 and Table 3–2.[98] Following the saccade, the eye is held in position by a

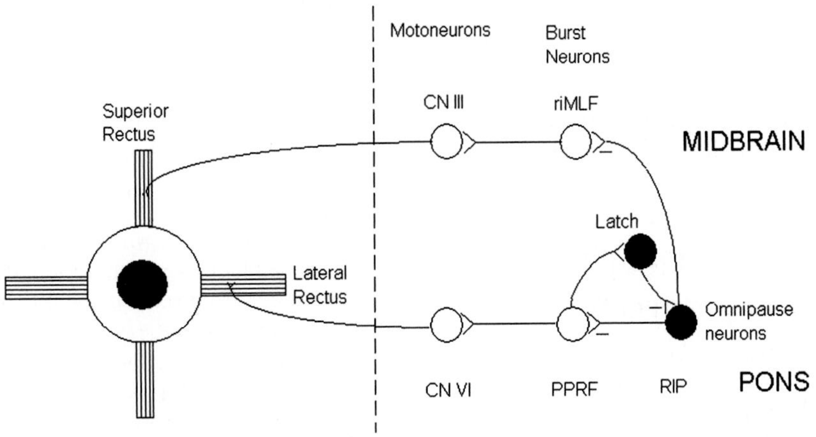

Figure 3–9. Schematic of brainstem network for saccade generation. Motoneurons innervating horizontally acting extraocular muscles receive saccadic commands from burst neurons in the paramedian pontine reticular formation (PPRF). Motoneurons innervating vertically acting motoneurons receive saccadic commands from burst neurons in the midbrain rostral interstitial nucleus of the medial longitudinal fasciculus (riMLF). Both sets of burst neurons are inhibited by omnipause neurons that lie in the pontine nucleus raphe interpositus (RIP). A saccade is initiated by a trigger signal that inhibits omnipause neurons; subsequently, hypothetical latch neurons, which receive input from burst neurons, inhibit omnipause neurons until the saccade is complete.

tonic, step-command that is generated by the neural integrator (see Chapter 5 and Fig. 1–3, Chapter 1). Classic basic and clinical studies have demonstrated that the caudal pons is important for horizontal saccades and the rostral mesencephalon for vertical saccades.[206,675] For horizontal saccades, burst neurons within the paramedian pontine reticular formation (PPRF) are essential (see Box 6–3, Fig. 6–1, and Fig. 6–2).[311] For vertical and torsional sac-

Table 3–2. **Brainstem Neurons Contributing to Saccade Generation**

Name	Properties
Premotor (medium-lead) burst neurons	Discharge ~ 12 ms prior to saccade onset
	Project monosynaptically to ocular motoneurons
Excitatory (EBN)	Horizontal EBN: Paramedian pontine reticular formation (PPRF)
	Vertical EBN: Rostral interstitial nucleus of medial longitudinal fasciculus (riMLF)
Inhibitory (IBN)	Horizontal IBN: Medullary reticular formation (MedRF)
	Vertical IBN: Interstitial nucleus of Cajal and riMLF
Long-lead burst neurons (LLBN)	Discharge > 40 ms prior to saccade onset
	Project to premotor burst neurons
	Located throughout brainstem reticular formation including nucleus reticularis tegmenti pontis (NRTP)
Collicular burst neurons	Discharge > 50 ms prior to saccade onset; location on superior colliculus related to size and direction
Omnipause neurons (OPN)	Tonic discharge that ceases ~ 16 ms before saccade onset
	Project to premotor burst neurons
	Located in nucleus raphe interpositus (rip)
Latch-circuit neurons	Reticular formation neurons that carry saccadic and smooth-pursuit signals
	Presumed to receive input from EBN and project to OPN

cades, burst neurons within the rostral interstitial nucleus of the medial longitudinal fasciculus (riMLF) play the equivalent role (see Box 6–5, Fig. 6–3, and Fig. 6–4). Omnipause neurons lie in the nucleus raphe interpositus, in the midline of the pons (see Box 6–3 and Fig. 6–2).

PREMOTOR BURST NEURONS

Pontomedullary Burst Cells

In humans, *excitatory burst neurons* (EBN) lie in the PPRF, rostral to the abducens nucleus, corresponding to the medial part of the nucleus reticularis pontis caudalis.[316,681] The EBN begin discharging at a high frequency, about 12 ms prior to, and time-locked with, the horizontal component of all types of saccades and quick phases.[286,725] Electrophysiological evidence suggests that some individual EBN in the PPRF encode saccades monocularly (i.e., for movements of one eye or the other).[783] EBN discharge preferentially for ipsilateral saccades and they appear to create the immediate premotor command that generates the pulse of activity for horizontal saccades. Three pieces of evidence support this hypothesis. First, during saccades, the instantaneous burst cell firing rate of EBN is closely correlated with instantaneous eye velocity,[288,725] and the total number of spikes in the burst of activity (the integral of the discharge rate) is proportional to the amplitude of the ipsilateral, horizontal component of the saccades. Second, stimulation of the PPRF elicits ipsilateral saccades.[118] Third, a unilateral lesion within the PPRF abolishes the ability to generate ipsilateral saccades.[287] Note, however, that EBN in the PPRF also discharge during vertical and oblique saccades,[725] and bilateral PPRF lesions not only abolish horizontal saccades but also cause slowing of vertical saccades.[273,287]

The EBN project directly to the ipsilateral abducens nucleus, where they contact both abducens motoneurons and internuclear neurons. Abducens internuclear neurons project up the contralateral MLF, to contact the medial rectus subgroup of the contralateral oculomotor nucleus (Fig. 6–1, Chapter 6). Thus, for example, during rightward horizontal saccades, the excitatory pulse reaches the ocular motoneurons from EBN in the right PPRF. The EBN also project to the perihypoglossal and vestibular nuclei, which are important for integrating the saccadic pulse into a step, to hold the eye steady at the end of the saccade. In addition, EBN also project to cell groups of the paramedian tracts (see Box 6–4, Chapter 6), which relay a copy of all ocular motor commands to the cerebellum. Finally, EBN project to ipsilateral inhibitory burst neurons, which we discuss next.

Inhibitory burst neurons (IBN) for horizontal saccades have been identified just caudal to the abducens nucleus in the nucleus paragigantocellularis dorsalis of the dorsomedial portion of the rostral medulla.[315,682] The IBN receive inhibitory inputs from omnipause neurons and contralateral IBN; they receive contralateral excitatory inputs from the superior colliculus.[689] The IBN send their axons across the midline to the contralateral abducens nucleus to inhibit contralateral abducens motoneurons and interneurons during ipsilateral saccades. Like EBN, IBN also project to the vestibular nuclei, nucleus prepositus (neural integrator), and to cell groups of the paramedian tracts.[682] One role of IBN is to silence activity in the antagonist muscle during horizontal saccades, which is an example of Sherrington's law of reciprocal innervation. A second role may be to help end the saccade when the eye is on target.[549] The synaptic connections between EBN and IBN in the pons and medulla is postulated to form a neuronal network (Fig. 3–10), in which IBN inhibits IBN, thereby forming positive feedback loops that are potentially unstable, leading to high-frequency saccadic oscillations, such as ocular flutter (discussed further under Pathophysiology of Saccadic Abnormalities).[553]

Midbrain Burst Cells

The EBN in the riMLF encode the vertical and the torsional components of saccades, just as EBN in the PPRF encode the horizontal component.[97,314,356,736] Excitatory EBN for upward and for downward saccades appear to be intermingled in the riMLF, although their projection pathways show some differences.[459,460] Thus, it appears that upward EBN in the riMLF project bilaterally to motoneurons, but downward EBN project only ipsilaterally (Fig. 6–5, Chapter 6). Electrophysiological studies have shown that EBN discharge most vigorously for rapid eye movements that rotate the eyeball in a plane parallel to that of a pair of reciprocally acting vertical semicircular canals

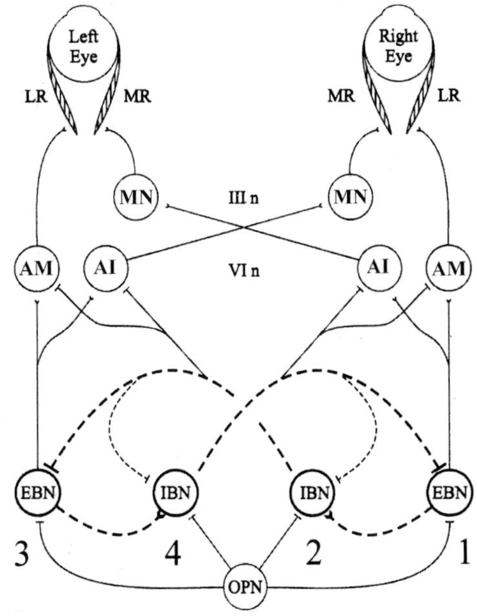

Figure 3–10. A brainstem neural network model for generation of horizontal saccades. Projections with flat ending are inhibitory, the others excitatory. Saccades require reciprocal innervation to the medial rectus (MR) and lateral rectus (LR) of both eyes. The LR is driven by the ipsilateral abducens nucleus (VI n) motoneurons (AM). The VI n also contains abducens internuclear neurons (AI) that send their axons to the contralateral oculomotor nucleus (III n), which drive the MR of the other eye. Excitatory burst neurons (EBN) provide the saccadic drive to ipsilateral AM and AI. EBN also project to inhibitory burst neurons (IBN). IBN provide inhibition to the contralateral AM and AI. Thus, an EBN/IBN pair provides reciprocal innervation. IBN also provide inhibition to the contralateral EBN and IBN. A consequence of this cross-coupling is that the EBN/IBN pairs form a short-latency, positive feedback loop. When omnipause neurons (OPN) are active, they prevent this loop from oscillating. At the beginning of a saccade, OPN neurons cease discharge allowing one set of EBN (1) to start firing and activate ipsilateral IBN (2). During IBN (2) firing, contralateral EBN (3) receive a hyperpolarizing input that keeps them silent. At the end of the saccade, when the IBN (2) cease firing, the EBN (3) start to discharge because of rebound depolarization, which stimulates ipsilateral IBN (4), which, in turn, inhibit the original EBN (1) that fired. Thus, the EBN-IBN pairs tend to spontaneously oscillate whenever the omnipause neurons are inhibited and there is no specified saccadic command. (Adapted from Ramat S, Leigh RJ, Zee DS, Opticon LM. Ocular oscillations generated by coupling of brainstem excitatory and inhibitory saccadic burst neurons. Exp Brain Res 160, 89–106, 2005, with kind permission of Spinger Science and Business Media.)

(e.g., right anterior and left posterior canals).[736] For example, EBN in the right riMLF increase their discharge when the right eye extorts and the left eye intorts. While the direction of torsion is fixed for EBN on each side, the direction of vertical rotation is upward in some and downward in others. Therefore, unilateral lesions have only mild effects on vertical saccades, but abolish ipsilateral torsional saccades. For example, with a lesion of the right riMLF, torsional quick phases, clockwise from the point of view of the subject (extorsion of the right eye and intorsion of the left eye) are lost.[690] Bilateral lesions in riMLF abolish all vertical and torsional saccades.[690]

Recent studies suggest that in monkey, the riMLF does not contain inhibitory burst neurons. Instead, the adjacent interstitial nucleus of Cajal, and surrounding reticular formation, contains neurons that send GABAergic projections to contralateral ocular motoneurons in CN III and IV and could turn out to be the vertical IBN.[311] Reciprocal connections between vertical EBN and IBN seem possible, so that a neural network similar to that postulated for horizontal saccades could account for vertical saccadic oscillations (discussed further below in Pathophysiology of Saccadic Abnormalities).

In addition to their projections to ocular motoneurons in the CN III and CN IV nuclei, vertical EBN also send axon collaterals to the interstitial nucleus of Cajal (see Fig. 6–4, and Box 6–6).[459,460] The latter structure appears to contain not only vertical IBN, but also burst-tonic neurons, thus contributing to the velocity-to-position integrator for vertical and torsional eye movements. This scheme is supported by the results of pharmacologically inactivating the interstitial nucleus of Cajal; vertical and torsional saccades can still be made, but there is centripetal post-saccadic drift, indicating impaired vertical gaze-holding.[131]

OMNIPAUSE NEURONS

Omnipause cells lie in the nucleus raphe interpositus, which is located in the midline between the rootlets of the abducens nerves (see Fig. 6–2, Chapter 6).[99,379] Omnipause neurons are medium-sized with prominent dendrites that extend horizontally across the midline. These neurons utilize glycine as their neurotransmitter,[313] consistent with their inhibitory function. An important crossed projection to the omnipause cell region arises from the rostral pole ("fixation zone") of the superior colliculus.[101,220,221] Additional projections to the omnipause neurons are from the frontal eye fields,[677] the supplementary eye fields,[651] the central mesencephalic reticular formation, the long-lead burst neurons in the rostral pons and midbrain,[627] and the fastigial nucleus.[490] Omnipause cells send inhibitory projections, which are mainly crossed, to EBN in the pons, to IBN in the medulla, and to the riMLF.[481,500]

Omnipause neurons discharge continuously except immediately before and during saccades, when they pause. Omnipause cells cease discharging during saccades in any direction, hence their name. Omnipause cells also cease discharging during blinks,[289] and their discharge rate is modulated by static vergence angle.[95] When omnipause cells are experimentally stimulated in the monkey, the animal is unable to make saccades or quick phases in any direction, although other types of movements, such as vestibular slow phases, can still be elicited.[755] If omnipause cells are stimulated during a saccade, the eye decelerates abruptly in mid-flight (Fig. 3–11).[349,350] Based on these findings, it appears that omnipause cells tonically inhibit all burst cells, and when a saccade

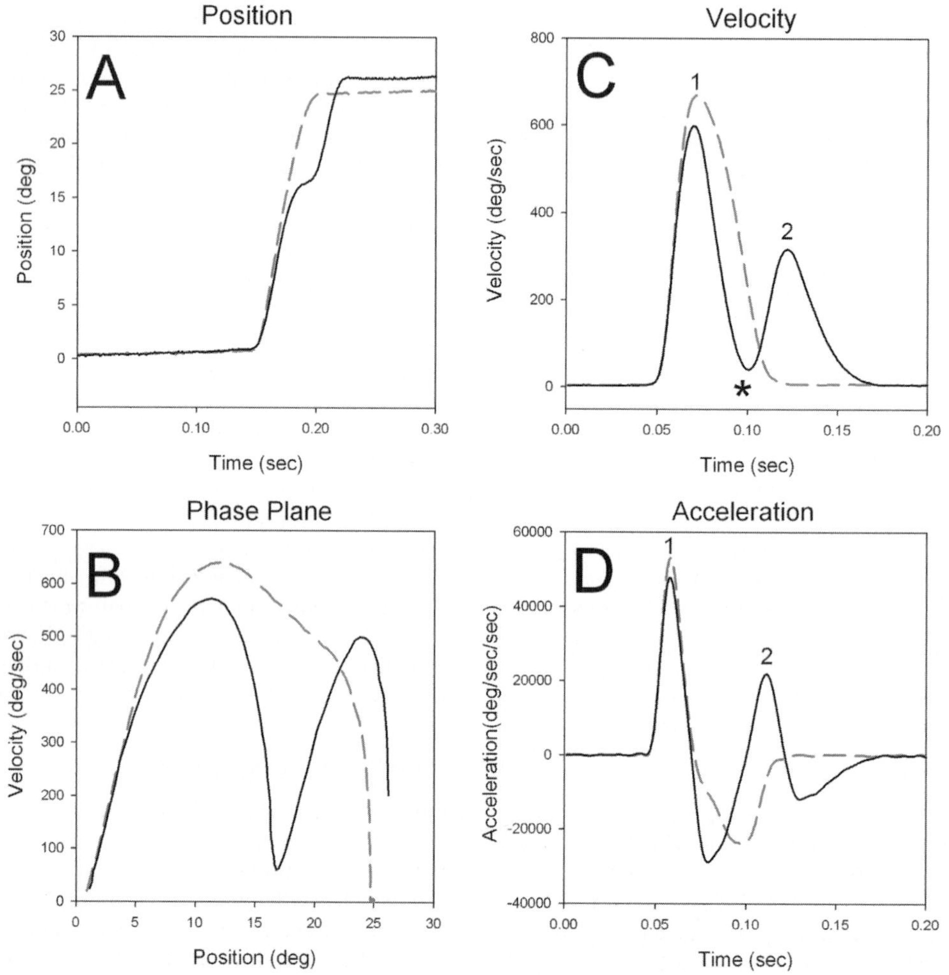

Figure 3–11. Experimental interruption of saccades in monkey. To interrupt saccades in mid-flight, omnipause neurons were stimulated at 400 Hz, with a 20-ms train of bipolar pulses, applied 4 ms–5 ms after saccade onset. Control saccades are shown in gray dashed lines and interrupted saccades in solid black line. (A) Comparison of position records of individual control and interrupted saccade trials. Note how the final position of interrupted saccade is greater than the control. (B) Phase plane plots of the same two saccades shown in A, demonstrating the abrupt fall in velocity with stimulation. (C) Average eye velocity traces are shown from 12 normal control trials and 16 trials in which saccades were interrupted by stimulation of omnipause neurons. During interrupted saccade trials, after the first velocity peak (1) eye velocity drops to 41.3 degrees per second (*) before increasing again to a second peak (2). (D) Acceleration responses corresponding to velocity records in C. (Data provided by courtesy of E. L. Keller.)

is called for, the omnipause cells themselves must be inhibited to permit the burst cells to discharge. By acting as an inhibitory switch, omnipause cells help maintain the necessary synchronization of the activity of premotor saccadic burst neurons to drive the eyes rapidly during the saccade and to keep the eyes still when the saccade is over. Recent studies in monkeys have shown that omnipause neurons may be inhibited by about 30% during smooth-pursuit movements,[444] suggesting that they have a more general function of gating visually mediated eye movements, as part of a visual fixation system.

Experimental lesions with excitotoxins or muscimol in the omnipause region cause slow horizontal and vertical saccades.[339,662] This effect is perhaps surprising, given the "high gain" properties of burst neurons, and one prediction of lesioning the "saccadic switch" would be uncontrollable saccadic oscillations, such as opsoclonus. An explanation for slow saccades may be that omnipause neurons exert a paradoxical influence on burst neurons. Since they are glycinergic, omnipause neurons normal inhibit burst neurons. However, it has been shown that glycine can actually facilitate N-methyl-D-aspartate (NMDA) receptor currents.[11] It has been postulated that when burst neurons synchronously receive a trigger signal from long-lead burst neurons (discussed next) and cessation of omnipause discharge, the result is a post-inhibitory rebound that produces the high acceleration typical of saccades.[447,448,448a] Thus, if omnipause neurons are lesioned, there will be no glycine to enhance the NMDA receptor currents (i.e., no post-inhibitory rebound), and saccades will be slower, depending solely on inputs from long-lead burst neurons.

What inhibits the omnipause neurons until the saccade is complete and the eye is on target? Intracellular electrophysiological studies indicate that omnipause neurons receive a powerful inhibitory input that completely turns them off just before a saccade is initiated;[770] this has been attributed to a "trigger signal," perhaps driven by inputs from the rostral pole of the superior colliculus. After this initial inhibition, the level of membrane hyperpolarization of omnipause neurons is temporally linked with current eye velocity, and this sustained hyperpolarization keeps omnipause neurons "off" for the remainder of the saccade. Since the discharge of excitatory burst neurons is also correlated with eye velocity during the saccade, they may be the source of sustained hyperpolarization of omnipause neurons via local inhibitory neurons called latch neurons (Fig. 3–9). Certain PPRF neurons have been identified that might serve as latch neurons.[444] Theoretically, should the latch circuit malfunction, then the eye would not get on target, but would prematurely decelerate; such behavior is encountered in certain disorders (see Prematurely Terminated Saccades).[332,591]

LONG-LEAD BURST NEURONS AND THE CENTRAL MESENCEPHALIC RETICULAR FORMATION

Neurons that start to discharge 40 ms or more before saccades are found throughout the brainstem. Some long-lead burst neurons (LLBN) lie in the pons and midbrain,[339a] and receive projections from the superior colliculus.[627] They project to pontine EBN, medullary IBN, and omnipause neurons; they also project to the nucleus reticularis tegmenti pontis (NRTP). These mesencephalic LLBN discharge before and during saccades to their "movement field." The portion of the mesencephalic reticular formation that lies just lateral to the CN III nucleus (central mesencephalic reticular formation, cMRF) [119] contains neurons that have reciprocal connections with the superior colliculus,[113,458] and it has been postulated that they may serve in a feedback loop.[742] These neurons also receive projections from the supplementary eye fields and fastigial nucleus; they project heavily to omnipause neurons and NRTP, and start to discharge more than 40 ms before saccades.[266] Within the population of cMRF neurons are some units with low background activity that could provide a "trigger signal" to the omnipause neurons; other units with high background activity could provide tonic inputs to omnipause neurons and specify saccade size via projections to NRTP.[288] Experimental lesions of the cMRF cause hypermetria of contralateral and upward saccades and hypometria of ipsilateral and downward saccades; fixation may be disrupted by large saccadic intrusions.[743] More rostral inactivation of the MRF impairs vertical saccades.[744]

Other LLBN lie in NRTP and project mainly to the cerebellum via the middle peduncle; some LLBN project to the PPRF.[627] Thus, it seems that LLBN may serve more than one function. Those LLBN that receive input from the superior colliculus may synchronize the onset and end of saccades, by virtue of their projections to omnipause and premotor burst neurons.[288,627]

Higher-Level Control of the Saccadic Pulse Generator

It is now clear that several distinct cortical areas are involved in the voluntary control of saccades. The anatomical connections of these areas and the way that they project to the brainstem saccadic pulse generator are summarized in the text and Boxes of Chapter 6, and in Figure 3–12. The two main brainstem targets of the cortical eye fields are the superior colliculus and the pontine nuclei, especially NRTP, which project, in turn, to the cerebellum. In comparison, direct projections from the cortical eye fields to the PPRF and riMLF are meager, although projections to omnipause neurons have been demonstrated.[678]

The superior colliculus, which receives inputs from all the cortical eye fields, may coordinate the discharge of burst and omnipause neurons. The importance of the superior colliculus is demonstrated by the finding that inactivation of collicular burst neurons blocks the effects of frontal eye field stimulation.[272] However, destructive lesions here do not

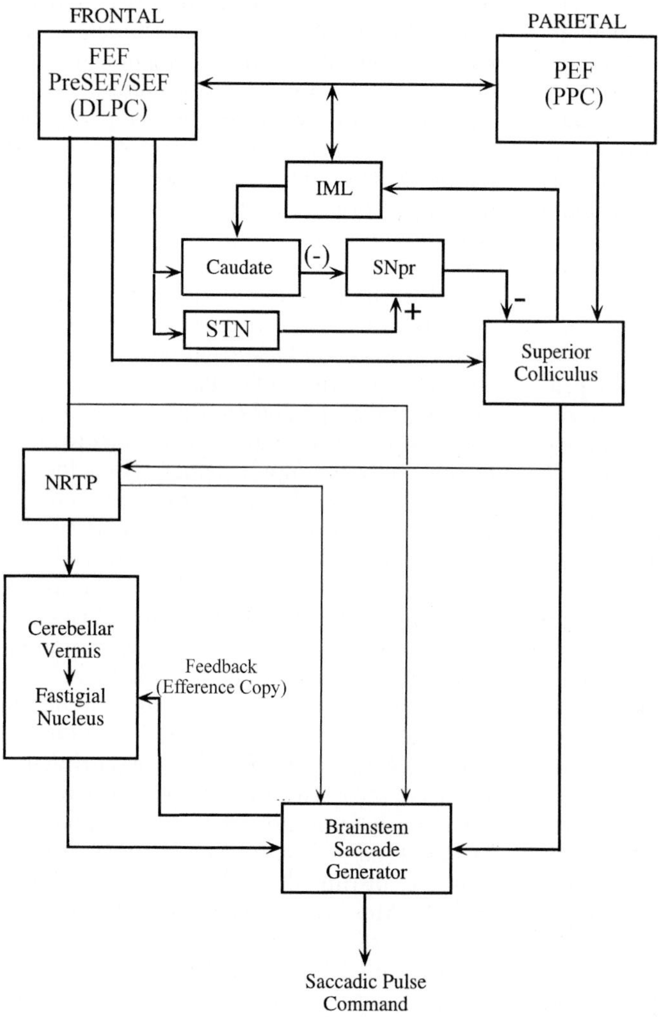

Figure 3–12. Block diagram of the major structures that project to the brainstem saccade generator (premotor burst neurons in PPRF and riMLF). Also shown are projections from cortical eye fields to superior colliculus. DLPC, dorsolateral prefrontal cortex; FEF, frontal eye fields; IML, intramedullary lamina of thalamus; NRTP, nucleus reticularis tegmenti pontis; PEF, parietal eye fields; PPC, posterior parietal cortex; SEF, supplementary eye fields; SNpr, substantia nigra, pars reticulata; STN, subthalamic nucleus. Not shown are the pulvinar, which has connections with the superior colliculus and both the frontal and parietal lobes, projections from the caudate nucleus to the subthalamic nucleus via globus pallidus, and the pathway that conveys efference copy from brainstem and cerebellum, via thalamus, to cerebral cortex. −, inhibition, +, excitation.

permanently abolish voluntary saccades,[17,271] and so the cortical projection to NRTP and the cerebellum also seems important. Conversely, saccades can still be made after destructive frontal eye field lesions. A crucial finding is that bilateral lesions of the frontal eye fields and the superior colliculus cause an enduring, severe deficit of voluntary saccades.[607] A similar defect occurs with combined bilateral lesions of the frontal and parietal eye fields.[409] Thus, parallel descending pathways are involved in generating voluntary saccades, and it appears that each is capable of performing spatial-to-temporal and retinotopic-to-craniotopic transformations of neural signals.

Superior Colliculus

VISUAL AND MOTOR LAYERS OF THE SUPERIOR COLLICULUS

The superior colliculus consists of seven layers.[669,761422,458,576] Early studies established that the dorsal layers of the superior colliculus are "visual" in terms of their properties and that the more ventral intermediate and deep layers are "motor."[10,24] The dorsal layers receive an orderly retinal projection, such that the visual field (which is compressed logarithmically relative to amplitude) is mapped onto its surface (Fig. 3–13A).[136] These layers receive visual inputs directly from the retina and from the striate cortex and send efferents to the pretectal nuclei, lateral geniculate body, and pulvinar.

The ventral layers contain a "motor map" (Fig. 3–13B) defined by the eye movements that are produced by electrical stimulation.[571,606] Although there are connections between the dorsal and the ventral layers,[456,457] in primates, cerebral cortical projections to the ventral superior colliculus are dominant. Furthermore, there is some independence between visually induced activity in the dorsal layers and movement activity in ventral layers, and there is a 40-ms delay between visual activity in the dorsal and ventral layers.[425,761] Thus, in primates, the superficial layers do not seem critical for generating eye movements, and the rest of this section will deal with only the connections and properties of the ventral layers of the superior colliculus.[410] To preview our discussion, the role of the superior colliculus depends on its retinotopic map, and the relative timing and level of neuronal activity across that map. The rostral pole is concerned with fixation and small saccades, and more caudal portions of the superior colliculus are important for target selection and initiation of eye and eye-head gaze shifts.

ANATOMICAL CONNECTIONS OF THE VENTRAL LAYERS OF THE SUPERIOR COLLICULUS

Afferents

Important projections to the ventral layers arise from striate, extrastriate and parietal cortex, and from the frontal lobes (Fig. 3–12).[576] Thus, the frontal eye field, supplementary eye field, and dorsolateral prefrontal cortex all project to the superior colliculus; some of these pathways are direct and some are via the basal ganglia, including the caudate nucleus and the pars reticulata of the substantia nigra (SNpr). In addition, the pedunculopontine tegmental nucleus (PPTN), which appears to promote saccade generation as part of a general effect on attention, sends nicotinic projections to the superior colliculus.[363–365]

The superior colliculus has reciprocal connections with the central mesencephalic reticular formation,[458] and receives inputs from the nucleus prepositus hypoglossi.[275] The rostral pole receives an input from the cerebellar fastigial nucleus.[423] Serotonin, acetylcholine, and gamma-amino butyric acid (GABA) have all been identified as transmitters in the ventral layers.

Efferents

The ventral layers project to critical structures in the brainstem that generate the premotor commands for saccades. These include the PPRF and riMLF, the nucleus prepositus hypoglossi, the nucleus reticularis tegmenti pontis (NRTP), the central mesencephalic reticular formation, and the vestibular nuclei. The ventral layers also send ascending projections to the FEF via the central and medial dorsal thalamus.[616,666] Descending outputs from the ventral layers of the superior colliculus are carried via an ipsilateral tectopontine pathway and a contralateral tectoreticular pathway. The latter crosses in the dorsal

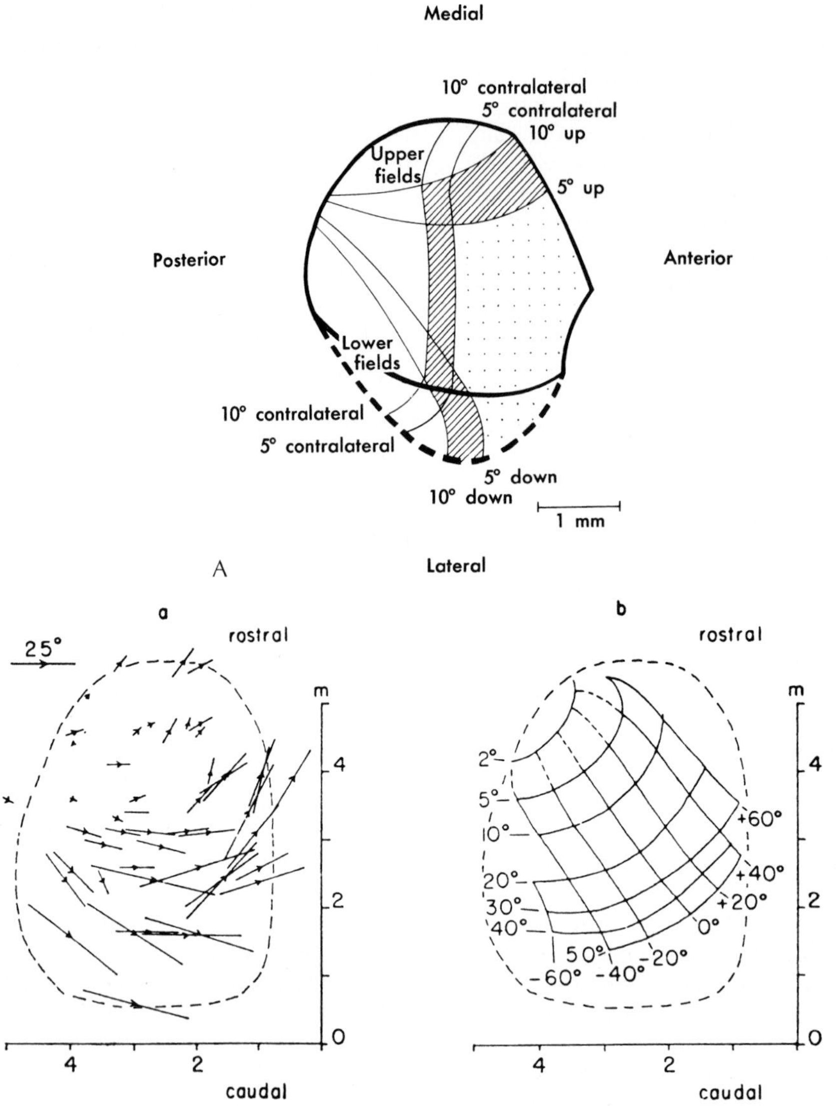

Figure 3–13. The topography of maps in the superior colliculus. (A) Representation of the visual field on the surface of the right colliculus. The stippled area represents the part of the contralateral visual field within 5 degrees of the fovea. Stippled and striped areas combined represent the part of the contralateral visual field within 10 degrees of the fovea. (Reproduced from Cynader M, Berman N. Receptive field organization of monkey superior colliculus. Neurophysiol 35, 187-201, 1972, with permission of the American Physiological Society.) (B) The motor map of the ventral layers of the left superior colliculus, based on stimulation studies. On the left, arrows indicate the direction and amplitude of saccades produced by stimulation. On the right are smoothed contours of the motor map. Isoamplitude lines (2 to 50 degrees) run from medial to lateral, and isodirection lines (–60 to +60 degrees) run from anterior to posterior. (Reprinted from Robinson DA. Eye movements evoked by collicular stimulation in the alert monkey. Vision Res 12, 1795-1808, 1972, with permission from Elsevier.)

tegmental decussation of Meynert and, as the predorsal bundle, lying ventral to the MLF, carries descending branches destined for the pontine and medullary reticular formation and ascending branches destined for the rostral midbrain.[252,457,458,458]

FUNCTIONAL ANATOMY OF THE SUPERIOR COLLICULUS REVEALED BY STIMULATION

Microstimulation of the ventral layers of the superior colliculus has provided many insights into the organization of this structure.[571,606] Stimulation of the rostral pole of the motor map suppresses saccades.[222] This "fixation zone" of the superior colliculus sends a monosynaptic excitatory projection to omnipause neurons,[101] which inhibit premotor burst neurons.

Stimulation more caudally induces saccades at latencies that imply disynaptic connections with premotor burst neurons;[351] it is suggested that long-lead burst neurons are interposed.[449] In general, the direction and size of the saccade are functions of the site of stimulation (above a certain threshold), rather than the strength of the stimulus. However, the current position of the eye also influences saccade size, with the amplitude of contralateral saccades increasing as the eye starts from progressively more ipsilateral positions. Furthermore, threshold required to stimulate a saccade is raised if the subjects actively fixates the target.[672] Nonetheless, once threshold has been reached, saccades occur in an 'all or none" fashion. The smallest saccades are elicited rostrally, the largest caudally. Saccades with upward components occur with more medial stimulation, those with downward components, with more lateral stimulation. Purely vertical saccades only occur with bilateral simultaneous stimulation of corresponding points.

This "motor map" is in polar coordinates (Fig. 3–13B), but lacks the 3-D (i.e., torsional) information required to implement Listing's law, which must be computed elsewhere.[729] Saccades of similar size (isoamplitude) correspond to lines running medial-to-lateral (largest with stimulation caudally), and saccades of similar direction (isodirection) correspond to lines running anterior to posterior (0 degree corresponding to a pure, horizontal, contralateral saccade). Stimulation in the caudal third of the ventral motor map produces combined eye-head gaze-shifts; both eye and head movements are directed contralateral to the side stimulated;[129] eye-head movements are discussed further in Chapter 7.

NEURAL ACTIVITY OF THE VENTRAL SUPERIOR COLLICULUS DURING SACCADES

The first studies of the activity of single neurons in the ventral layers of the superior colliculus in monkeys trained to make saccades to visual targets revealed a variety of cell types that showed responses related to either the visual stimulus, or to the saccadic movement, or to both.[171,671,760,762] Many subsequent studies have identified neurons with a range of properties. Thus, some neurons that respond to visual stimuli do so in anticipation of a saccade that will bring a target into their receptive field,[745] or show activity related to the likelihood that a target will be the goal of a saccade.[52,241] Quasivisual neurons hold in spatial register the amplitude and the direction of the upcoming required saccade (i.e., they encode the motor error signal necessary to acquire the target).[674] Neurons may even be active during covert shifts of visual attention, during which there is no eye movement.[321] Neurons also respond to auditory stimuli, either alone or in combination with visual stimuli, when the two are spatially aligned.[58] Such units may also have somatosensory receptive fields.[253,748] Thus, the superior colliculus neurons have multisensory properties, which are generally encoded in retinotopically coded movement fields.[253,335,748]

Two main populations of *saccade-related cells* have been defined in the ventral layers: build-up neurons, which have a prelude of activity before their saccade-related burst, and collicular-burst neurons, which are intermixed and slightly more dorsal.[410,471,761] Both build-up and saccadic-burst neurons project out of the superior colliculus, and may be extremes of a continuum rather than two separate types of cells.[471] The *rostral pole* of the motor map, corresponding to small saccades, projects to omnipause neurons, and may be important for sustaining fixation.[101,220,469,470]

Build-up neurons start to discharge when a visual stimulus becomes the target for a saccade.[472] Like collicular burst neurons, the location of build-up cell activity initially occurs at a site on the motor map related to the amplitude and direction of the upcoming saccade. However, unlike the location of discharging collicular burst cells, which remains constant throughout the eye movement, there appears to be a rostral spread of prelude activity of build-up neurons (a moving wave or hill) towards the rostral pole.[261,472] It had been postulated that this spread of activity amongst the build-up neurons population could achieve the spatial-temporal transformation of signals that is needed to provide the reticular burst neurons with the saccadic command. Thus, it was postulated that when the spreading wave of activity reached the fixation neurons at the rostral pole, the saccade would end.[472] However, electrophysiological studies have provided evidence against this hypothesis; the superior colliculus seems important in triggering, but not in steering or stopping, saccades.[13,624,661] The prelude of activity on build-up neurons is much smaller than the saccade-related burst, and its role in movement control is uncertain.

The site of maximum activity on the collicular motor map is related to the desired displacement, or change in eye orientation. During the course of a saccade, the site of maximum activity of the saccade-related burst neurons does not change, but their discharge rates decline as the eye approaches the target. Although it was found that the temporal discharge of collicular neurons decays in proportion to instantaneous motor error (the difference between current and desired eye position),[741] subsequent evidence found that their discharge is not calculating a dynamic motor error signal.[13,173,389,468]

Build-up and burst neurons located in the caudal part of the superior colliculus appear to encode the overall intended gaze displacement,[65] and their discharge properties are consistent with the notion that they indirectly drive premotor burst neurons in the brainstem reticular formation. Thus, when large target jumps elicit multiple small saccades to reach the goal, the locus of activity on the superior colliculus restarts after each small saccade at the locus corresponding to the remaining distance to the goal.[65] Thus, although the superior colliculus does not compute a dynamic motor error (e.g., to control saccade trajectory) during a saccade, it does represent the static motor error between saccades.

During more complex tasks, such as saccades to two sequentially flashed targets,[545] or visual search,[430,431] saccadic trajectories can become strongly curved if the brain starts going toward one target and then, in midflight, turns toward another target. Neurons in the ventral layers clearly encode the retinotopic location of each target, and the site with the highest activity switches during the saccade to indicate which target is the instantaneous goal. In these studies, it was found that the locus of activity on the superior colliculus corresponded to the locations of the target, but not to the direction and amplitude of subsequent saccades. These studies reveal that whenever the retinotopic location of the target does not match the ensuing saccade, the collicular activity always reflects the location of the target, and does not encode the saccade. In the context of early collicular studies that showed that monkeys can make saccades after superior colliculus lesions,[607] this dissociation leads to an important conclusion. The ventral superior colliculus does not encode saccadic eye movements, rather it encodes the current retinotopic goal; the movement needed to reach that goal is controlled from somewhere else, presumably the cerebellum.[508] The application of multi-electrode arrays,[544] and functional imaging,[455] may provide further insights into how ensembles of superior colliculus neurons contribute to a range of ocular motor behaviors.

EFFECTS OF PHARMACOLOGICAL INACTIVATION AND LESIONS OF THE SUPERIOR COLLICULUS

Insight into the role of the ventral layers of the superior colliculus in saccade generation has been gained by local injection of two agents: the GABA-A agonist muscimol, which increases normal GABA inhibition and thereby decreases neuronal activity, and the nonspecific GABA antagonist bicuculline, which increases neuron activity by decreasing normal GABA inhibition. Injection of muscimol into the rostral pole of the superior colliculus reduces latencies to those of express saccades; furthermore, steady fixation is disrupted by saccadic intrusions. Conversely, injection of bicuculline into the rostral pole increases saccadic latency, and sometimes no saccade is generated. Injection of muscimol or bicuculline into more caudal regions of the superior colliculus reverses their effects. Thus, inactivation with muscimol (or lidocaine) causes impaired initiation of saccades, which are hypometric and slow.[302,304,387] Caudal bicuculline injections cause fixation instability, with saccadic intrusions. Injection of nicotine into the superior colliculus produces express saccades for movements corresponding to the site of the injection.[12] These findings support the suggestion that the fixation neurons at the rostral pole of the superior colliculus suppress saccades both through excitation of omnipause neurons,[101] and by inhibiting collicular burst neurons.[760] However, inputs from structures other than the superior colliculus, such as cMRF, also influence omnipause neurons and the timing of saccadic onset.[188] If muscimol is injected locally into the superior colliculus at a point corresponding to small saccades (Fig. 3–13), and the monkey makes a large saccade, the saccade has a curved trajectory and the error depends on how far the goal is from the site of the lesion. This finding supports the hypothesis that the initial direction of a saccade is determined by a population average (such as the center of gravity of the distribution of activity),[387] which is displaced away from the area that has been pharmacologically inactivated.[548]

Conventional lesion studies have been less revealing than acute pharmacological inactivation, in part because of the effects of recovery and adaptation. Discrete electrolytic lesions of the superior colliculus cause an enduring increase in reaction time as well as some slowing of saccades,[271] but the accuracy of saccades recovers. Following larger surgical lesions, the frequency of spontaneous saccades is diminished during scanning of a visual scene, but not in complete darkness.[17] During fixation of a stationary target, the monkey without a superior colliculus is less easily distracted by peripheral stimuli and makes fewer saccades away from the fixation target. Saccadic accuracy is mildly impaired. Most important, short-latency express saccades are permanently abolished.[605] When lesions of the superior colliculus are combined with lesions of the caudal medial thalamus, [18] or with the frontal eye field (see Frontal Eye Field, in the following section), more long-lasting and severe ocular motor abnormalities are produced.[607]

Lesions restricted to the superior colliculi are rare in humans. One patient had undergone removal of an angioma from the right superior colliculus, and but also had evidence of dorsal midbrain syndrome.[291] Spontaneous horizontal saccades to the left occurred less frequently and were more commonly followed by corrective saccades; saccadic latency was normal. Another patient with a hematoma largely restricted to the right superior colliculus showed defects in latency and accuracy for contralateral saccades, and increased numbers of errors in the antisaccade task.[537] Recent functional imaging has demonstrated activation of the superior colliculus in humans engaged in visual search,[240,620] and showed increased inactivation for saccades made at decreased latency in response to testing with the gap paradigm.[483]

A SYNTHESIS OF THE INFLUENCE OF THE SUPERIOR COLLICULUS ON THE CONTROL OF SACCADES

In summary, based upon an intense research effort over the past 30 years, it appears that the superior colliculus plays an important role in target selection, and initiating saccades, and contributing to their speed. The superior colliculus may initiate saccades by providing a "trigger signal" to omnipause neurons, burst neurons, and possibly the cerebellum. However, another part of the brain, perhaps the frontal eye fields, must be able to adapt and provide a substitute for that trigger signal after superior colliculus lesions. Furthermore, cerebellar lesions lead to enduring saccadic dysmetria, implying that the superior colliculus alone cannot control saccades. Recent research has emphasized that whenever the target location and required eye movement differ, the superior colliculus always encodes the target location in retinal coordinates, but not the required eye movement.[508] Thus, it appears that the details of generating the saccade and getting it on target depend much more on the brainstem reticular formation and cerebellum, respectively. Clinicians seldom think about the superior colliculus when they interpret abnormal eye movements, partly because of the rarity of selective lesions in humans. It is also possible that the effects of superior colliculus lesions have been missed, since special testing for changes of saccade latency is usually needed. The new hypothesis that links collicular function to saccade latency and the initiation and speed of the saccade, but not to saccade accuracy, suggests future clinical tests that could more easily detect the consequences of superior colliculus lesions. Functional imaging studies are beginning to confirm a similar role for the superior colliculus in humans as in macaque.[240,483,620]

The Role of the Frontal Lobe

Since Ferrier stimulated the premotor cortical area 8 of monkeys and elicited contralateral eye movements,[195] several distinct areas of prefrontal cortex have been identified that contribute to the voluntary control of saccades. The best known is the *frontal eye field*, which was first identified in humans by electrical stimulation.[75,243,525] The location of the homologue of the frontal eye field in humans has been recently defined by functional imaging studies, and lies in the anterior wall of the precentral sulcus, close to the intersection with the superior frontal sulcus.[402] Three other areas, the *supplementary eye field*, *dorsolateral prefrontal cortex*, and *anterior cingulate cortex* have also been shown to influence voluntary saccades. In addition, other areas of cortex, such as in the dorsomedial frontal lobes, likely contribute to saccades made as a component of more complex behaviors.[455,499] As we discuss each cortical area, we will summarize studies in monkey that have defined its role, and supplement this with information from humans, based upon functional imaging, magnetic or intra-operative stimulation, and behavioral changes caused by lesions. The anatomical location and connections of these three areas are described in Chapter 6 and summarized in Figure 6–8, and Boxes 6–19, 6–20, and 6–21.

THE ROLE OF THE FRONTAL EYE FIELD

Effects of Microstimulation of Frontal Eye Field

In rhesus monkey, microstimulation studies have been crucial in defining the extent of the FEF (along the posterior portion of the arcuate sulcus—part of Brodmann area 8),[91] and have also provided insights into FEF function. Stimulation at any site on the FEF elicits a saccade of a specific direction and amplitude. A "motor map" is present with larger saccades evoked from stimulation of the dorsomedial portion of the FEF, and smaller saccades from stimulation of the ventrolateral part.[91] Usually, the movement is oblique, with a contralateral horizontal component; bilateral stimulation is required to elicit a purely vertical saccade. The latency from frontal eye field stimulation to the onset of a saccade is about 30 ms–45 ms, similar to that for stimulation in the superior colliculus. Stimulation in FEF at currents that are below the threshold needed to produce saccades may change properties of neurons in secondary visual areas; this finding presumably reflects a mechanism by which visual areas are normally advised of upcoming eye movements.[451,452] Intra-operative FEF stimulation in humans undergoing surgery for intractable epilepsy, at the posterior end of the middle frontal gyrus, produces eye movements that are directed contralaterally, often with an upward component; the direction sometimes depends on starting eye position.[75]

Microstimulation of the FEF can also *suppress* saccades under certain experimental conditions.[331] Thus, stimulation of a wide area of the FEF suppresses ipsiversive visually guided and memory-guided saccades at stimulus intensities lower than those for eliciting electrically evoked saccades. However, stimulation near the spur of the arcuate sulcus, which corresponds to the smooth-pursuit portion of FEF, suppresses both types of saccades in any direction. This part of the FEF projects to the "fixation region" at the rostral pole of the superior colliculus and also to omnipause neurons in the pons.[92,92,678] Stimulation is most effective in suppressing saccades when applied 40 ms–50 ms before saccade onset, probably having its effects at the level of the superior colliculus or PPRF. Stimulation of one FEF affects the activity of cells in the other FEF, in a manner conducive to coordination between the two eye fields.[608] In a patient with a frontal lobe tumor, per-operative stimulation over parts of the FEF arrested self-paced saccades.[441]

Physiological Properties of Frontal Eye Field Neurons

Only occasional FEF neurons discharge before spontaneous saccades made in complete darkness, though many neurons discharge after such movements. The most useful information about activity of single neurons in the FEF has been gained from experiments in which monkeys were trained to perform a variety of saccadic tasks for reward.[90,246] Different subpopulations of FEF neurons encode the visual stimulus,[69,70,596] the planned saccadic movement,[597] or both. Like the superior colliculus and parietal eye fields, some FEF cells show movement of their receptive fields that anticipate the visual consequences of planned saccades.[718] Although the discharge of FEF neurons is related to the amplitude and direction of voluntary saccades, their discharge during saccades does not dynamically encode signals such as motor error (the difference between current and desired eye position, which is required to guide the eyes to their target).[629]

Frontal eye field neurons also discharge for visual and motor aspects of *memory-guided saccades*.[208,719] FEF lesions in humans cause systematic errors of memory-guided saccades.[542] However, other cortical areas contribute,[43] notably dorsolateral prefrontal cortex (discussed below). When monkeys perform a double-step task, in which two target lights are flashed in succession before the eye has time to move, most units discharge not in relation to the retinal location of the second target but according to the saccade needed to acquire it.[246] Such cells behave similarly to quasivisual cells of the superior colliculus, since their activity encodes the desired change in eye position. Pharmacological inactivation of the mediodorsal thalamus, which relays corollary discharge from the superior colliculus to FEF, causes the second saccade in response to a double-step stimulus to become inaccurate,[667] implying that the FEF rely on efference copy information to correctly program the second saccade.

Neurons that appear to be concerned with *disengaging fixation* before a saccade increase their discharge when the fixation light is turned out, even before the new target becomes visible.[154] Some FEF neurons show properties indicating that they contribute to selection of the target to which a saccade will be made,[601] the decision whether to look at it or not,[270] and the process of visual scanning of a complex visual scene.[93,279]

The FEF appear to contribute to programming of the *antisaccade response* (Fig. 12–14). Thus, functional imaging studies indicate that FEF are activated bilaterally during both prosaccades and antisaccades, but more so for the latter. [126] Patients with FEF lesions show a normal percentage of errors on the antisaccade task, but their correct antisaccades are made at increased latency.[532,567] Thus, it has been suggested that, during the antisaccade task, triggering of the intentional, correct antisaccade depends upon FEF, whereas inhibition of reflexive misdirected saccades is due to dorsolateral prefrontal cortex, which is discussed below.[532]

The FEF are also activated during covert visual search, during which eye movements are suppressed.[161] Furthermore, magnetic stimulation over human FEF interferes with visual search tasks in which eye movements are not required.[463] Additional insights into the mechanism that suppresses saccade initiation can be gained from a *countermanding task*, in which monkeys are required to make visually guided saccades on most trials but, on a fraction of trials, to withhold a saccade on the basis of reappearance of the fixation cue.[600] Electrophysiological properties of FEF during this task have identified neurons that reflect behavioral responses, and indicate that these units are concerned with generation or suppression of saccades.

Effects of Frontal Eye Field Lesions on Saccade Generation

Acute pharmacological inactivation with muscimol causes a contralateral "ocular motor scotoma" with abolition of all reflex, visual, and voluntary saccades with sizes and directions corresponding to the injection site.[155] With unilateral muscimol inactivation of FEF, during attempted fixation there is a gaze shift towards the side of the lesion, and inappropriate saccades directed ipsilaterally may disrupt fixation. Thus, these results are similar to the effects of injecting these agents into the superior colliculus; inactivation of either structure causes substantial defects in reflex visual and voluntary saccades. Acute destructive lesions of the FEF in monkeys produce an increase of latency for contralateral saccades and a decrease of latency for ipsilateral movements; in other words, an increase of express saccades ipsilateral to the side of the lesion.[602]

More subtle changes in the generation of visually guided saccades are present with chronic experimental lesions of the FEF, including decreased frequency and size of movements,[607] and defects of saccades made to paired or multiple targets that are presented asynchronously.[602] In humans also, chronic lesions of the FEF cause relatively minor deficits. There is increased latency of visually guided saccades to contralateral targets, especially when tested using the overlap paradigm (fixation light remains on during testing, Fig. 3–2A).[85,414,567] Although abnormalities on the antisaccade task have been reported,[413] this may reflect additional involvement of dorsolateral prefrontal cortex, an issue discussed below.[532] Visual and memory-guided saccades are also inaccurate (see Box 12–21, Chapter 12).[233] In summary, the FEF in humans appears more concerned with voluntary than reflexive saccades, a view supported by functional imaging studies.[454]

ROLE OF THE SUPPLEMENTARY EYE FIELD

The supplementary eye field (SEF) lie just anterior to the supplementary motor cortex, in the dorsal medial portion of the frontal lobe;[612] in humans this corresponds to the upper part of the paracentral sulcus.[256] *Stimulation* in the SEF elicits saccades at low thresholds though at slightly longer latency than in the frontal eye fields.[612] Initial studies, using microstimulation, seemed to indicate that the eye was driven to a specific orbital position.[611] This was unlike the results of stimulation of the FEF, which produced an eye movement of specific size and direction, determined by the site stimulated. More recent evidence indicates that rostral SEF encodes saccades in an eye-centered frame whereas caudal SEF encodes saccades in a head-centered frame.[418,521,614]

Like the FEF, SEF contain neurons that discharge prior to voluntary saccades,[592] but also discharge during a range of more complex behaviors. Thus, SEF neurons also respond during *conditional learning*[114] and *antisaccades*.[614] Some SEF units fire before eye movements to the right or left end of a horizontal bar, irrespective of the location of the bar in the visual field; such neuronal activity is referred to as object-centered.[506] During a *countermanding task*, in which subjects make visually guided saccades on most trials but, on some, are required to withhold a saccade on the basis of reappearance of the fixation cue, SEF neurons are variously active after errors, after successful withholding, or in association with reinforcement.[688] Thus, SEF units show interesting differences from FEF neurons on the countermanding task,[600] and while some FEF neurons appear concerned with generation or suppression of saccades, neurons in the SEF (and the anterior cingulate cortex) respond on trials in which a saccade is erroneously not canceled and reward will not be given.[688] In comparison with other cortical eye fields, SEF appears most concerned with internally guided target selection based upon reward during prior trials.[19,106,117]

Neurons in SEF are active when monkeys are trained to make a *learned sequence of saccades*.[325,325,403] This finding is consistent with clinical studies that suggested that the SEF lesion, especially on the left side, disrupt the ability to carry out a learned sequence of saccades.[232,235] Inactivation of SEF in monkeys impairs the ability to respond to a double-step task,[665] and TMS over SEF in humans disrupts the order of responses to a double-step stimulus.[712] During testing of sequences of saccades (Fig. 3–2E), TMS studies have shown that the SEF could be crucial at two distinct times: during the learning phase (presentation of the visual targets), and just after the go signal, when the subject must initiate the sequence of saccades.[475] Further support for the notion that the SEF is concerned with eye movements that are programmed as part of learned, complex behaviors is supported by functional imaging studies in humans, which have demonstrated increased activation during a series of memory-guided saccades.[280,528] However, other cortical areas also contribute to longer-term memory of sequences of saccades, including the right medial temporo-occipital area, which was activated in the vicinity of the boundary between the parahippocampal and lingual gyri, as well as the parieto-occipital fissure.[255,538]

The role of the supplementary motor area (SMA) in general, and SEF in particular, has recently been linked to pre-supplementary motor cortex (pre-SMA), which is active during learning new sequences of movements,[292] including eye movements when they are contextually relevant to a task.[324,403] Microstimulation of pre-supplementary motor cortex in monkey reduces the reaction time of upcoming saccades.[324] One patient with a discrete lesion affecting one SEF had difficulty in changing the direction of his eye movements, especially when he had to reverse the direction of a previously established pattern of response.[319] Functional activation in parts of human pre-SMA in humans appear to corresponding to volition and conflict (Fig. 1–7, Chapter 1), whereas registration of success or failure activates the supplementary eye fields.[477] Therefore, SEF, SMA, and pre-SMA may work together to coordinate complex and sequential movements.[703] The cerebellum is also important for learning motor sequences, but cerebellar lesions do not impair visuomotor memory or spatial working memory.[488]

ROLE OF DORSOLATERAL PREFRONTAL CORTEX

Although not a conventional "eye field" (as defined by low threshold for stimulation of saccades), neurons in the dorsolateral prefrontal cortex (DLPC) of monkey, in the posterior third of the principal sulcus (see Fig. 6–8, Chapter 6), corresponding to Walker's area 46, contribute to the voluntary control of saccades (Box 6–21).[217,278] DLPC is reciprocally connected with posterior parietal cortex, and inactivation of either area similar reduces activity of the other's neurons during memory-guided saccades.[111] Networks of neurons in DLPC of monkey show an ability to hold specific visuospatial coordinates in a topographical memory map; thus, they are important for generating *saccades to remembered target locations*,[127,128,697] including visual search.[320] Some units in DLPC that respond to spatial signals show increased activity during a response for which reward is expected.[362] Both D1-dopamine and 5 hydroxytryptamine 2-A receptors appear to play an important facilitating role in this spatial working memory, and injection of antagonist for either transmitter impairs performance on memory-guided saccade takes.[598,599,758]

In humans, DLPC is activated when subjects make memory-guided saccades.[395,495,593,692] Patients with lesions affecting this area show defects of memory-guided saccades, with increased variability.[538,542] Functional imaging studies suggest that DLPC contributes to spatial memories for up to about 20 seconds;[593] thereafter other mechanisms assume importance for "medium-term" memory. Furthermore, single-pulse or repetitive transcranial magnetic stimulation over DLPC in normal subjects impairs the accuracy of memory-guided saccades, but only if delivered within a few seconds of target presentation.[84,473,493,494] Evidence for a substrate for medium-term spatial memory comes from studies of patients with lesions involving the parahippocampal cortex, who show inaccuracy of saccades made to target locations that were committed to memory up to 30 seconds previously.[541] Parahippocampal cortex may operate both serially with DLPC and in parallel through connections with posterior parietal cortex.[538] For spatial memory ranging up to minutes, the hippocampal formation may be important.[538] Patients with lesions affecting DLPC also show impaired ability to make "predictive saccades" that anticipate regularly occurring target jumps.[532]

Both the FEF and DLPC appear to contribute to programming of the *antisaccade response*, but in different ways. Thus, on the one hand, the right hemisphere DLPC is activated during antisaccades,[144,205] and patients with lesions affecting the DLPC have an increased percentage of errors in the antisaccade test.[532] On the other hand, patients with FEF lesions have a normal percentage of errors on the antisaccade task, but make their correct antisaccades at increased latency. Taken together, it appears that during the antisaccade task, inhibition of reflexive misdirected saccades is due to DLPC, whereas triggering of the correct antisaccade depends upon FEF.[538] Evidence from patients with subcortical lesions has indicated that increased errors on the antisaccade task can be ascribed to interruption of a pathway running from DLPC to the superior colliculus in the anterior limb, genu, or anterior part of posterior limb of the internal capsule.[125,230]

THE ROLE OF CINGULATE CORTEX

Cingulate cortex includes Brodmann areas 24 (anterior cingulate) and 23 (posterior cingulate). The anterior cingulate makes oligosynaptic connections with brainstem ocular motor structures.[455] Some, but not all, electrophysiological studies have suggested that the anterior cingulate cortex is important for monitoring the consequences of saccades, such as learning new motor sequences, particularly if they are rewarded.[328,480] Less is known about posterior cingulate cortex, where neurons discharge after saccades, in proportion to reward size, and expected saccade value.[427,505]

In humans, functional imaging demonstrates activation in the anterior cingulate cortex during self-paced saccades, memory-guided saccades, memorized triple saccades, and antisaccades.[23,162,205,280,529] Thus, it has been proposed that, in humans, there is a cingulate eye field, located in the posterior part of the anterior cingulate cortex, at the junction of Brodmann areas 23 and 24.[234]

Studies of two patients with small infarcts in the cingulate eye field on the right hemisphere caused increased saccadic reaction time and decreased gain for saccades made during the overlap task (Fig. 3–2A), and bilateral errors on the antisaccade task (Fig. 3–2D).[234] In a more recent study, surgical resections of tumors involving the anterior cingulate cortex also caused errors on the antisaccade task.[440] More electrophysiological and clinical studies are needed to clarify the role of cingulate cortex in the control of saccades.

The Role of the Parietal Lobe

The parietal lobe appears to influence the control of saccades in two principal ways. First, the posterior parietal cortex is important for shifts of visual attention, which may be accompanied by saccades. Second, the parietal eye fields (PEF) are directly involved in programming saccades to visual targets.

ROLE OF POSTERIOR PARIETAL CORTEX

Electrophysiological studies have shown that in monkey, area 7a of the inferior parietal lobule contains populations of neurons that respond to visual stimuli and discharge mainly after saccades have been made (Fig. 6–8).[46] It appears that the activity of some of these neurons is influenced not just by visual stimuli but also by eye and head position.[22,88,88] This finding has led to the hypothesis that a neural network of such cells could encode a visual target in spatial or craniotopic coordinates.[22,767] Furthermore, neurons in the posterior parietal lobe may be involved in representing visual locations during visual search, and maintaining a memory for the location of saccadic targets.[386]

Functional imaging studies in humans have demonstrated preferential activation in the right angular gyrus, during visually induced, but not internally generated, saccades,[454] and an analogous role has also been attributed to the supramarginal gyrus.[527]

In normal human subjects, a defect of memory-guided saccades is produced if transcranial magnetic stimulation is applied to the posterior parietal area early during the memory period.[476,515] If TMS is applied while subjects respond to double-step target jumps, and the stimulus is timed just after the first saccade, then the second saccade becomes inaccurate because of disruption of the craniotopic coding.[723] Antisaccades are also delayed by transcranial magnetic stimulation over parietal cortex; a similar effect is possible over frontal cortex if the stimulus is delivered later, suggesting flow of information from posterior to anterior during presaccadic processing.[704]

Acute human unilateral posterior parietal lesions, especially right-sided, cause contralateral *hemispatial neglect* and may confine saccades to the ipsilateral hemifield of gaze (Box 12–20, in Chapter 12).[453] Such patients show increased latency of visually guided saccades, and this is especially the case with right-sided lesions.[534] Because of hemineglect, patients have impaired ability to search contralateral space with saccades. In addition, such patients are unable to retain in working memory which targets they have seen before during visual search.[318] Thus, the defect of visual search in patients with parietal hemineglect combines a hemispatial attentive bias with an impaired memory for targets previously seen, which are reported as new.[676]

Bilateral posterior parietal lesions cause Balint's syndrome,[531] which includes difficulty initiating voluntary saccades to visual targets, and impaired visual scanning.[408] These deficits, which are described further in Chapter 12, may reflect disruption of the normal mechanisms by which posterior parietal cortex transforms visual signals into head or body-centered coordinates.

ROLE OF THE PARIETAL EYE FIELD

Animal Studies

In rhesus monkey, the PEF lies adjacent to area 7a, in the caudal third of the lateral bank of the intraparietal sulcus, an area called LIP (Fig. 6–8). *Electrical stimulation* on the lateral wall of the intraparietal sulcus produces saccades of similar direction irrespective of the starting position of the eye.[706] However, if the floor of the intraparietal sulcus and its underlying white matter are stimulated, the direction of the resulting eye movements appears to depend upon starting eye position. Thus, the summed output of the population of neurons in PEF may be concerned with saccades to targets coded in head-centered coordinates.[706]

Unlike area 7a, LIP neurons *discharge prior to* saccades;[46,47] some neurons also discharge during fixation (suppression of saccades).[60] Like cells in area 7a, the response of LIP neurons is influenced by eye position,[22] as well as other sensory modalities such as sounds.[400] These cells in LIP also show a shift of their visual response field that anticipates the consequence of the upcoming gaze-shift;[169,376] the phenomenon is also reported in other visual areas,[479] and corresponding changes have been seen in humans using functional imaging.[433,439] Thus, the ensemble activity of LIP neurons encodes the spatial and temporal dynamics of the monkey's attention across the visual field.[73]

Another important property of LIP neurons is their ability to remain active while the monkey is required to withhold eye movements and *remember the desired target location*.[47,518] Some neurons also encode a memory of motor error, similar to quasivisual cells found in the superior colliculus and frontal lobe.[83,120,426,540,575] During antisaccades, LIP neurons respond to the visual stimulus,[781] but show little saccade-related behavior.[250] Thus, LIP neurons appear to encode not so much the intended saccade, but rather the current locus of attention.[245,540]

Experimental *inactivation of LIP* causes increased latency for both visually and memory-guided saccades into contralateral hemispace.[399] Saccade dynamics are spared. Contralesional memory-guided saccades also become hypometric whereas ipsilesional saccades may be hypermetric. The accuracy of the second saccade in a contralateral double-step response is also impaired.[398] In addition, inactivation of LIP increases search time for a contralateral target during serial visual search, suggesting that one important contribution of LIP to oculomotor behavior is the selection of targets for saccades in the context of competing visual stimuli.[749] These results are consistent with the hypothesis of an attentional network contributing to fixation engagement and disengagement in a subregion of LIP.[61]

The PEF projects to the superior colliculus, and is important in the triggering of visually guided saccades.[194] Electrophysiological studies have revealed that, from parietal cortex to colliculus, there is a continuous evolution of signal processing, representing activity at nearly every stage of visuomotor transformation.[519,763] Moreover, the time course of the neural response suggests that monkey PEF accumulates sensory signals pertinent to the selection of targets for saccades.[635] Evidence from monkeys and humans indicates that the parietal-superior colliculus pathway runs in the most posterior region of the posterior limb of the internal capsule; lesions of this pathway impaired reflexive but not memory-guided saccades.[231]

Human Studies

In humans, functional imaging has located the PEF in the medial wall of the posterior half of the intraparietal sulcus, adjacent laterally to the anterior part of the angular gyrus and medially to the posterior part of the superior parietal lobule.[89,474] A similar area shows retinotopic activation during saccades to remembered targets.[634]

Lesions involving the PEF in humans cause prolonged latency of visually guided saccades during gap or overlap stimuli (Fig. 3–2).[476 534] Increased latency of visually guided saccades is more pronounced with right-sided parietal lesions, and is more prominent than with FEF or SEF lesions.[85,534] A similar effect results in normal subjects if transcranial magnetic stimulation is applied to the PEF region.[178,717a] It has been suggested that the greater latency that results when the fixation light is left on indicates that the PEF is important for disengagement of fixation before generating a saccade.[535]

Parietal lesions also impair the ability to make two saccades to two targets flashed in quick succession. In response to this double-step stimulus, the brain must take into account not only the retinal location of both targets, but also the effect of the eye movements.[170,281,281] Patients with right parietal lesions show errors when the first target appears in the left hemifield and the second in the right; the first saccade may be accurate, but the second is not. This deficit may be present even though there is no inattention or difficulty responding to the reverse order of presentation, or of making single saccades to left-sided targets. It appears that there has been disruption of the ability to monitor the size of the first saccade using efference copy.[170,281,281]

SUMMARY OF FRONTO-PARIETAL INFLUENCES ON THE CONTROL OF SACCADES

To summarize, the influence of frontal and parietal cortex on the control of saccades appears to be via two parallel descending pathways (Fig. 3–12). One pathway is via the frontal eye field to the superior colliculus (directly, and indirectly, via the basal ganglia).[285] The supplementary eye fields and dorsolateral prefrontal cortex also project to brainstem regions. Pathways from these prefrontal areas appear more concerned with preparation for self-generated changes in gaze as part of remembered, anticipated, or learned behavior.[297] The other pathway is directly from posterior parietal cortex to the superior colliculus. This pathway is more concerned with reorienting gaze to novel visual stimuli and in particular with shifting visual attention to the location of new targets appearing in extrapersonal space. However, the strong interconnections between parietal and frontal lobes and their common projection sites preclude a strict separation of function between the two pathways.[630] Thus, for example, lesions of both posterior parietal cortex and DLPC may impair memory-guided saccades.[533] Also important are connections between each cerebral hemisphere, since split-brain monkeys show impaired responses to double-step tasks when each stimulus is presented into a different visual hemifield.[66] Subsequent recovery implies that subcortical pathways, at least in monkey, are able to compensate for loss of interhemispheric connections. Finally, neurons in each of these cortical areas may modulate their activity when the correct behavior is to be rewarded.[117]

The Role of the Thalamus

Several different parts of the thalamus contribute to the programming of saccades, including the central nuclei of the internal medullary lamina, the mediodorsal nuclei, the ventrolateral nuclei, and the pulvinar. In humans, functional imaging has shown activation of the thalamus during voluntary saccades.[529]

THE ROLE OF THE INTERNAL MEDULLARY LAMINA

Neurons scattered throughout the internal medullary lamina (IML), which is the fiber pathway separating the medial from the lateral thalamic mass, show saccade-related properties.[610,610,615,702] IML neurons receive inputs from cortical and brainstem structures concerned with eye movements, including the superior colliculus, but project only to the cortex and basal ganglia. These connections suggest that IML might be important for relaying an efference copy of eye movement commands from the brainstem to the cortical eye fields.[616,666]

Electrical stimulation in the region of the IML elicits contralaterally directed saccades that may either be of fixed size and direction or directed to an orbital position. Neurons in IML discharge in relationship to spontaneous and visually guided, contralateral saccades.[615] During a visually guided delayed saccade task, neurons encode the visual stimulus, the delay, presaccadic and motor signals; some units appear to carry an efference copy of eye movements.[765] Consistent with the effects of stimulation, some units appear to encoded saccades in craniotopic rather than retinotopic coordinates. Other types of neurons in IML stop discharging during saccades but show a strong postsaccadic increase in activity, or discharge during steady fixation.[610,615]

Another important region is the mediodorsal nucleus, which serves as a thalamic gateway to prefrontal cortex,[701] and relays, amongst a range of other modalities, signals from the superior colliculus.[59,666] Thus, after inactivation of the mediodorsal thalamic nucleus with muscimol, on a double-step task, monkeys consistently show inaccuracy of the second saccade.[667] Consistent with this concept, tasks requiring a sequence of saccades (such as the double-step paradigm) are impaired when the central thalamus is affected by disease.[236] In Chapter 12, a patient with a thalamic metastasis is described, who made normal visually guided and memory-guided saccades, except when he made a smooth pursuit movement during the memory period. Thus, it appeared that he was unable to register a change of eye movement during the memory period, perhaps because of interruption of an efference copy of his pursuit movements.

A third region is the ventrolateral thalamus, which relays cerebellar signals to cerebral cortex concerned with self-triggered saccades.[700a] When disease affects the cerebellar thalamus, patients show impaired ability to adapt their saccades to novel visual demands as well as to responding correctly to double-step target displacements.[59,237]

THE ROLE OF THE PULVINAR

Two separate parts of the pulvinar, which has reciprocal connections with posterior parietal cortex,[390] are related to saccades. Each appears to make distinctive contributions to saccades. Neurons in the *inferior-lateral pulvinar* respond to retinal image motion when it is produced by a moving stimulus, but much less so if it is due to a saccade.[577] Thus, this region might contribute to the process of saccadic suppression, although this suggestion needs confirmation.

In the *dorsomedial pulvinar*, visually responsive neurons are not retinotopically organized and seem more important for shifts of attention towards salient features in the environment.[63,504,574] Injection of GABA antagonists and agonists into the dorsal medial portion of the lateral pulvinar facilitates or retards, respectively, the ability of an animal to shift its attention toward the contralateral visual field.[578] In humans, functional imaging supports that idea that the pulvinar is important for directing visual attention.[345,377]

Electrolytic lesions in the pulvinar of monkeys cause a paucity of saccades towards blank portions of the visual field, and gaze appears to be "captured" by visual stimuli.[720] Other studies, however, have revealed relatively normal patterns of visual search after pulvinar lesions.[62] As previously noted in the Behavior of the Saccadic System, normal subjects show a decrease in saccadic reaction time if the fixation point is turned off synchronously with the appearance of the visual target compared with leaving the fixation target on (overlap paradigm). However, patients with posterior thalamic lesions, but without hemineglect, show no such decrease in reaction time for visually triggered saccades.[551] This result confirmed older studies of the effects of pulvinar lesions in humans, which reported difficulties in disengaging visual fixation when a shift of attention is to be made.[498,785] Taken together, these experimental and clinical results suggest that the pulvinar in humans contributes to the mechanisms for shifting visual attention, but more research is needed.

The Role of the Basal Ganglia

Although the frontal and parietal eye fields project directly to the superior colliculus (Fig. 3–12), a second pathway running through the basal ganglia plays an important role, especially in selecting targets that will be rewarded.[297] In essence, the substantia nigra pars reticulata (SNpr) maintains a tonic inhibition of collicular-burst neurons. Thus, for a saccade to be initiated by this pathway, the caudate nucleus must disinhibit the SNpr. In turn, the caudate depends on cortical inputs to signal the need to suppress the tonic inhibition of the superior colliculus by SNpr. In considering what role this pathway could play in the control of saccades, we examine the properties of the caudate nucleus, SNpr, and the subthalamic nucleus. We then provide a synthesis of the possible overall function of the basal ganglia in the control of saccades, and consider the effects of human lesions.

THE ROLE OF THE CAUDATE NUCLEUS

The caudate (and parts of the putamen) receive inputs concerning the programming of saccades from the FEF, SEF, DLPC, and the intramedullary lamina (IML) region of the thalamus.[297] A second important input is a dopaminergic projection from the substantia nigra, pars compacta, which may convey reward-related signals. The caudate projects directly to the SNpr and, via the external segment of the globus pallidus, to the subthalamic nucleus.[482] Saccade-related neurons in the caudate lie at the junction of the head and body of this structure (the central longitudinal zone).

Projection neurons have a low rate of discharge that increases prior to saccades.[294,295,649] This presaccadic activity is related more to the behavioral context of the saccade than its size and direction.[296] Specifically, the activity of these caudate neurons shows a strong dependency on memory, expectation, attention, and reward.[296,329,348,750] Thus, some neurons change their discharge rate systematically, even before the appearance of the visual target, and usually fire more when the contralateral position is associated with reward.[383,384] Putative interneurons show less reward-related modulation of their activity.[649] Functional imaging studies in humans have demonstrated activation of the putamen and substantia nigra during memory-guided saccades.[496]

Experimental, unilateral dopamine depletion of the caudate and adjacent putamen causes impairment of contralaterally directed saccades.[346] The major deficit is for memory-guided saccades, which become hypometric, slow, and delayed.[368] In addition, there is contralateral hemineglect.[450] Dopamine also likely plays an important role in reward-contingent saccadic behavior, since studies of learning in patients with Parkinson's disease have shown that they become more sensitive to positive outcomes (carrot) than negative ones (stick) after they are administered dopamine medication.[207]

In a patient with bilateral lesions affecting the body of the caudate nucleus, memory-guided saccades were impaired whereas memory-guided finger-pointing was intact.[733] Patients with chronic lesions involving the putamen show deficits in saccades made to remembered locations and in anticipation of predictable target motion; visually guided saccades are intact.[734]

THE ROLE OF SUBSTANTIA NIGRA PARS RETICULATA

The saccade-related cells in SNpr lie in its lateral portion (near the cerebral peduncle) and project to the intermediate layers of the superior colliculus. Neurons in SNpr have high tonic discharge rates that decrease prior to voluntary saccades that are either visually guided or made to remembered target locations.[267,298,299–301] These neurons probably contribute to both target selection and saccade initiation.[53] Those SNpr neurons that decrease their discharge, and thereby disinhibit superior colliculus neurons, may show greater modulation of responses that are rewarded.[268,595]

The direct projections from the caudate nucleus to SNpr are mainly inhibitory. In addition, the SNpr receives excitatory projections from the subthalamic nucleus (Fig. 3–12). Stimulation of caudate neurons produces suppression or facilitation of SNpr neurons, the latter possibly due to a multisynaptic pathway.[293] However, neurons in the SNpr that seemed important for memory-guided saccades are usually inhibited by stimulation of the caudate.

The SNpr sends inhibitory projections to the superior colliculus, which are probably GABAergic. Injection of muscimol (a GABA agonist) into SNpr has a similar effect to injection of bicuculline (a GABA antagonist) into the superior colliculus: repetitive, irrepressible saccades occur, which are directed contralaterally to the side of the injection.[303] These saccadic intrusions appear to occur due to loss of the normal suppressive effect of SNpr on collicular-burst neurons rather than any effect on the fixation neurons at the rostral pole of the superior colliculus.[469]

THE ROLE OF THE SUBTHALAMIC NUCLEUS

Another basal ganglion, the subthalamic nucleus, contains neurons that discharge in relation to saccades.[421] The subthalamic nucleus appears to provide a second basal ganglionic pathway by which the cortical eye fields may influence the control of saccades via the basal ganglia (Fig. 3–12). The caudate nucleus projects, via the external segment of the globus pallidus, to the subthalamic nucleus.[482] This pathway appears to be double inhibitory, so that the overall effect of caudate inputs is excitation of the subthalamic nucleus. The subthalamic nucleus sends excitatory projections to the SNpr. Thus, it seems that the caudate has both a direct pathway to SNpr that is inhibitory, and an indirect pathway via the subthalamic nucleus that may be facilitatory. Consistent with this, stimulation of caudate neurons may produce either suppression or facilitation of SNpr neurons, the latter possibly due to the indirect pathway.[293]

In human patients undergoing placement of stimulating electrodes for treatment of Parkinson's disease, it has been possible to record single units in the ventral part of the subthalamic nucleus, where units discharge in relation to, but usually following, eye movements.[193] Discharge of some human subthalamic neurons is cued to self-paced saccades.

SYNTHESIS OF THE CONTRIBUTION OF BASAL GANGLIA TO THE CONTROL OF SACCADES IN THE CONTEXT OF CLINICAL DISORDERS

A simplified view of this basal ganglia pathway is that there are two serial, inhibitory links: a caudo-nigral inhibition that is only phasically active and a nigro-collicular inhibition that is tonically active. In addition, the subthalamic-nigral pathway is excitatory. Through these pathways, the basal ganglia appear to facilitate the initiation of more voluntary, self-generated types of saccades made in the context of learned behaviors, prediction, memory, and reward. Conversely, the basal ganglia could aid steady fixation by preventing unwanted reflexive saccades to stimuli that, at that particular moment, would be disruptive. As is discussed in Chapter 12, the means by which the frontal eye fields influence the superior colliculus is complex and might produce either difficulties in initiating or suppressing saccades. Both deficits have been described in patients with disorders affecting the basal ganglia, such as Huntington's disease.[382] However, the system is almost certainly more complex; for example, the direct and indirect caudate projections to SNpr may be serving different functions during complex behaviors.

Studies of the effects of human diseases affecting basal ganglia have focused on behavior such as memory-guided or predictive saccades. For example, memory-guided saccades are impaired after pallidotomy for Parkinson's disease,[76] but improved with subthalamic nucleus stimulation.[568] Pallidotomy increases saccadic intrusions on steady fixation— "square wave jerks."[33,497] In the future studies of patients with basal ganglionic disease, there is need for development of experimental strategies that involve reward for carrying out memory-guided and other saccade tasks.

The Cerebellar Contribution to Saccades

A major projection from the cortical eye fields is to the cerebellum, via the pontine nuclei (Fig. 3–12).[739] In addition, several important saccade-related structures in the brainstem project to the cerebellum. A role for the cerebellum in the control of saccades has been suspected since Hitzig[305] and Ferrier[195] elicited eye movements by electrical stimulation. Although more than one cerebellar area contributes to the programming of saccades, the dorsal vermis and caudal fastigial nucleus play key roles. The cerebellar hemispheres may also contribute to the control of saccades (Fig. 3–14),[279a,487] but their role has yet to be defined; the same is true of the basal interstitial nucleus.[699] Before reviewing these areas, we will first examine the role of a pontine nucleus that is a major relay for saccadic commands to the cerebellum.

NUCLEUS RETICULARIS TEGMENTI PONTIS

The nucleus reticularis tegmenti pontis (NRTP), which lies ventral to the rostral PPRF (see Fig. 6–3),[708] contains neurons that discharge in relation to a variety of eye movements, including saccades.[130] Its medial portion receives inputs from the frontal and supplementary eye fields.[652,677] The caudal part of NRTP receives inputs from the superior colliculus.[239] Portions of the NRTP project to the dorsal vermis and caudal fastigial nucleus.[490,768] The NRTP contains long-lead burst neurons, which project to the cerebellum and PPRF.[626]

Neurons in the caudal NRTP show similarities to collicular burst neurons, encoding the size and direction of saccades. However, unlike collicular neurons, they encode the 3-D eye displacement vectors.[730] Neurons in NRTP differ from those in riMLF by encoding both directions of torsional movement on each side of the brainstem. Microstimulation in NRTP elicits movements with an ipsilateral component that has a fixed torsional component. Inactivation of NRTP with muscimol caused torsional "errors" implying that NRTP normally ensures that saccadic eye movements obey Listing's law.[730] The influence of NRTP on the 3-D control of eye movements may depend upon its cerebellar projections.[655] The NRTP also contains neurons with activity related to pursuit and vergence, making it a possible site for coordination of these different classes of eye movements. The dorsolateral pontine nucleus (DLPN) also contains neurons that show saccade-related activity,[156] but generally seems more concerned with smooth pursuit. Pursuit and vergence aspects of the pontine nuclei are discussed in Chapters 4 and 8, respectively.

THE ROLE OF THE DORSAL VERMIS

The "ocular motor vermis" consists of lobules VI and VII (parts of the declive, folium, tuber, and pyramis); its anatomical connections are summarized in Box 6–12.[768] Purkinje cells in the dorsal vermis discharge about 15 ms before saccades in a preferred direction.[502] Stimulation of the vermis produces saccades with an ipsilateral component;[585] with currents near to threshold, a topographic organization is evident.[489] Stimulation of vermal lobule V evokes saccades that range from upward to horizontal, while stimulation of lobules VI and VII evokes saccades that range from horizontal to downward. The vertical component of the elicited saccade is larger when stimulation is more medial. Saccadic direction is largely dictated by the anatomic location of stimulation in the cerebellum just as it is in the frontal eye fields and in the superior colliculus. In contrast to the latter structures, though, saccades evoked by cerebellar stimulation are graded in amplitude and, to a minor extent, direction, as a function of stimulus intensity. Furthermore, the amplitude of the elicited saccade, and the amount of postsaccadic drift, depend upon the initial position of the eye in the orbit.

If the vermis is stimulated while the monkey is making a naturally occurring saccade, the saccade trajectory is modified more than if stimulation is applied during fixation.[352] This implies that the cerebellum may be directly involved in feedback control of the amplitude of individual saccades. Furthermore, if an animal's eyes are perturbed by cerebellar stimulation just prior to the generation of a voluntary saccade to a visual target, the ensuing saccade does not land on target.[242] This is unlike the accurate corrective movements that occur when the frontal eye field,[604] or the superior colliculus,[672] are stimulated just prior to a saccade.

Unilateral pharmacological decortication of the dorsal vermis causes marked ipsilateral hypometria and mild contralateral hypermetria, with a gaze deviation away from the side of the inactivation (see Box 12–4).[594] Ablative lesions of the dorsal vermis also cause saccadic dysmetria that is mainly hypometria.[696] The dysmetria concerns the saccadic pulse, and there is no post-saccadic drift as is seen after ablation of the cerebellar flocculus and paraflocculus,[779] or total cerebellectomy.[512] Symmetrical lesions cause bilateral hypometria of horizontal saccades, with a slight increase in saccadic latency. Asymmetrical lesions cause hypometria and increased latency of ipsilateral saccades, so that express and anticipatory saccades are abolished.[696] Centrifugal movements tend to be smaller and made at longer latency than centripetal movements. The dynamic characteristics of saccades are also affected, with abnormal waveforms, and decreased speed during both the acceleration and deceleration phases; these changes are not dependent of the starting position of the eye in the orbit. Finally, the ability to adapt saccades to visual demands is impaired by lesions of the dorsal vermis.[696]

How do the dorsal vermis (lobule VII) and the caudal part of the fastigial nucleus, to which it projects, play such key roles in governing the accuracy of saccades? Although Purkinje cells in the dorsal vermis show variability in the timing of their discharge with respect to each saccade, the populations of these neurons encode the time when a saccade must stop to land on target.[707] Consistent with

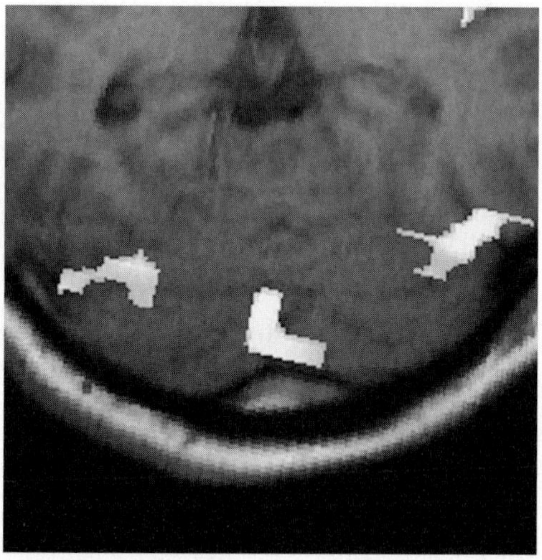

Figure 3–14. Activity of the cerebellum during a saccadic task as revealed by functional magnetic resonance imaging (fMRI). The subject was making voluntary, self-paced saccades between two visible targets. There is increased metabolic activity in the midline cerebellum (dorsal vermis and underlying fastigial nuclei) and also in the cerebellar hemispheres. Similar activation occurred if saccades were made in darkness between remembered target locations. (Courtesy Dr. Manabu Honda of Kyoto, Japan.) (From Honda M, Zee DS, Hallett M. Cerebellar control of voluntary saccadic eye movements in humans. Soc Neurosci Abstr 15, 1189, 1997.)

this scheme, after dorsal vermis lesions, the amplitude of saccades become more variable.[696]

THE ROLE OF THE FASTIGIAL NUCLEUS

Besides receiving inputs from Purkinje cells of the dorsal vermis, the caudal part of the fastigial nucleus, the fastigial oculomotor region (FOR), also receives a copy of the saccadic commands, which are relayed by NRTP from the frontal eye fields and superior colliculus.[490] The main projection from the fastigial nucleus crosses within the fellow fastigial nucleus, and enters the uncinate fasciculus, which runs in the dorsolateral border of the superior cerebellar peduncle, to reach the brainstem. Important projections of the caudal fastigial nucleus are to omnipause neurons, inhibitory burst neurons in the rostral medulla, excitatory burst neurons in the PPRF and riMLF, the mesencephalic reticular formation, thalamus, and the rostral pole of the superior colliculus.[423] Some of these connections are summarized in Box 6–13, and in Figure 3–12.

Neurons in the caudal fastigial nucleus discharge about 8 ms before onset of saccades with contralateral components, but generally towards the end of saccades with ipsilateral components.[213,283,501] These neurons also modulate their discharge according to saccade size and eye velocity, but not eye position.[360] Under normal circumstances, the fastigial nucleus might influence saccades by providing an early drive to premotor burst neurons during contralateral saccades and a late brake during ipsilateral ones.[213] These ideas are summarized in Figure 3–15.

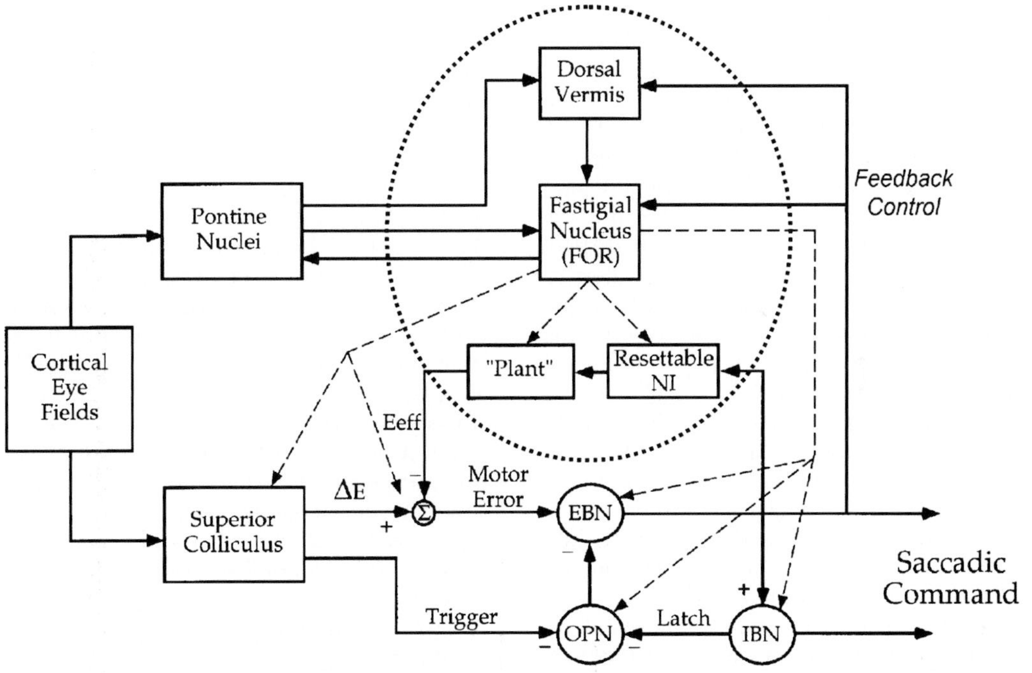

Figure 3–15. Hypothetical scheme for the role of the cerebellum in the generation of saccades. The superior colliculus, and probably the frontal eye field, provide a neural signal representing desired change in eye position (ΔE), which is compared with an efference copy of current eye position (Eeff), to give motor error, the signal that drives the premotor burst neurons (EBN). The superior colliculus rostral pole also provides the trigger signal to initiate the saccade, which inhibits omnipause neurons (OPN), which then stop inhibiting EBN, and (projection not shown) inhibitory burst neurons (IBN). The EBN project to IBN, which act as a latch circuit to stop OPN from discharging until the end of the saccade (when motor error is zero). The output of EBN and IBN constitute the saccadic command, which projects to ocular motoneurons. To generate Eeff, the output of EBN (and IBN, not shown) must be integrated (Resettable NI) and adjusted to account for non-linearities due to the orbital contents ("Plant"). This local feedback circuit may be partly located in the cerebellum. The dorsal vermis and fastigial ocular motor region (FOR) receive inputs from the pontine nuclei, such as NRTP, and climbing fiber inputs from the inferior olive (not shown). The dorsal vermis inhibits FOR, which projects to several elements of the brainstem saccade generator (broken lines), including EBN, IBN, and OPN. The dorsal vermis and FOR could lie within the internal saccadic feedback loop (dotted ellipsoid). −, inhibition, +, excitation.

Fastigial nucleus lesions produce marked hypermetria of saccades.[631,632] Destructive lesions are effectively bilateral because axons destined for the brainstem cross within the fastigial nucleus itself. A more effective way of demonstrating the contribution of the fastigial nucleus to saccade generation has been to use muscimol to pharmacologically inactivate the caudal fastigial nucleus on one side (see Box 12–4, Chapter 12).[581,584] A unilateral injection causes hypermetria of ipsilateral saccades (typical gain 1.3) and hypometria of contralateral saccades (typical gain of 0.7),[584] which affects saccades of all sizes.[330] The acceleration of ipsilateral saccades is increased and that of contralateral saccades is decreased. Hypermetria is slightly greater for centripetal (centering) saccades than centrifugal saccades. Vertical saccades show ipsipulsion (diagonal trajectory towards the side of inactivation) with unilateral fastigial nucleus lesions. With bilateral injections, all saccades, both horizontal and vertical, become hypermetric.[584] Microstimulation of the fastigial nucleus also inhibits its activity and has a similar effect to muscimol. Such stimulation only biases the trajectory of saccades if it is applied during the course of the movement.[244]

Complete cerebellectomy in trained monkeys creates an enduring saccadic pulse dysmetria.[512] In this case, all saccades overshoot, though the degree of overshoot is greatest for centripetally directed movements. The degree of saccadic hypermetria may be so great that the animal shows repetitive hypermetric saccades about the position of the target, a form of macrosaccadic oscillations (see Video Display: Disorders of Saccades). Monkeys with a complete removal of the cerebellum also show postsaccadic drift, implying pulse-step mismatch dysmetria. At the end of the rapid, pulse portion of the saccade, the eyes drift on, as a glissade, for a few hundred milliseconds, toward the final eye position. As noted above, saccadic pulse dysmetria can be attributed to involvement of the dorsal vermis and fastigial, whereas post-saccadic drift reflects involvement of the vestibulocerebellum (flocculus and paraflocculus).[779] Thus, the dorsal cerebellar vermis and underlying fastigial nuclei appear to function in controlling the size of the saccadic pulse, while the flocculus and paraflocculus seem to be responsible for appropriately matching the saccadic step to the pulse.

Scheme for the Control of Saccadic Metrics by the Dorsal Vermis and Fastigial Nucleus

Based on electrophysiology and the pharmacological inactivation studies summarized above, it is possible to offer a hypothetical scheme for way that the dorsal vermis and fastigial nucleus govern saccades to get the eye on target. Thus, early activity in one fastigial nucleus could be important for accelerating the eye at the beginning of a saccade, and the later activity in the other fastigial nucleus could be critical for stopping the eye on target. Thus, delay or abolition of the later, decelerating fastigial activity will cause hypermetria (Fig. 3–6) because the eye will not decelerate and stop on target. Central to this scheme is the concept that the brain monitors its own motor commands, referred to as corollary discharge or efference copy. Since saccades are brief, vision cannot be used to guide the eye to the target. However, the cerebellum could monitor a corollary discharge of the saccadic command and terminate the eye movement when it is calculated to be on target. How could this be achieved? Corollary discharge of all ocular motor signals are encoded on cell groups of the paramedian tracts (PMT), a group of neurons distributed throughout the brainstem to which all premotor ocular motor structures project.[100] The PMT cell groups project to the cerebellum and could, along with other mossy fiber projections from pontine nuclei, provide the cerebellum with the corollary discharge that it needs to stop the saccade on target. For vertical saccades, a different circuit including the posterior interpositus nucleus, which receives inputs from the ventral paraflocculus, could provide a similar role.[580] Such feedback of motor signals through the cerebellum requires that eye velocity signals be converted to a representation of current eye position by a resettable integrator.[508,511]

Thus, in patients with saccadic hypermetria (Fig. 3–6B) (see Video Display: Disorders of Saccades), feedback signals to the fastigial nucleus—which are required to stop the eye on target—could arrive late, or not at all.[691] Clinically, fastigial nucleus lesions are effectively bilateral, because the axons cross in the opposite nucleus; affected patients show bilateral hypermetria (Fig. 12–4). However, inter-

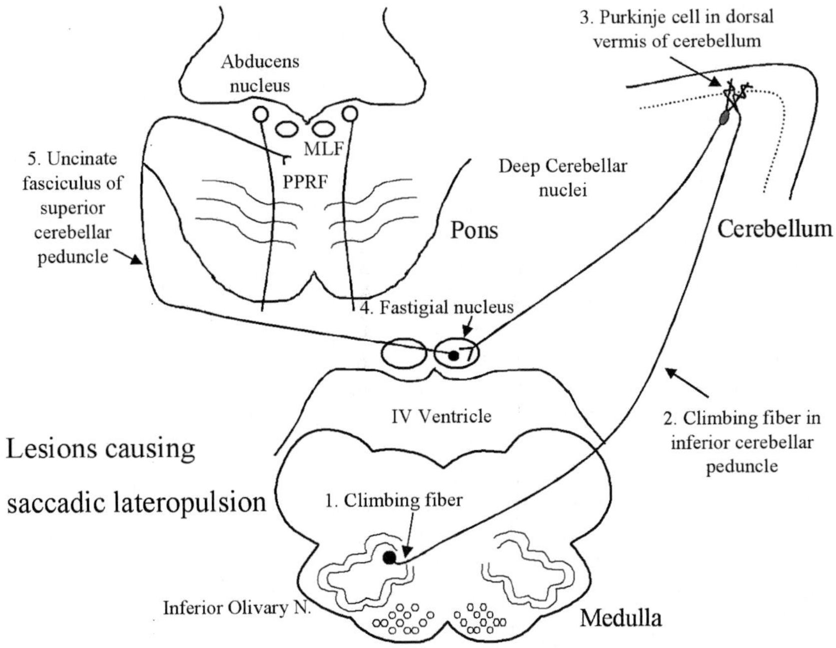

Figure 3–16. Hypothetical scheme to account for lateropulsion of saccades.[584,711,740] Interruption of climbing fibers originating from the inferior olivary nucleus may occur prior to their crossing in the medulla (1) or as they enter the inferior cerebellar peduncle (in Wallenberg's syndrome. (2). Loss of climbing fiber inputs to Purkinje cells in the dorsal vermis causes the latter to inhibit the fastigial nucleus (4), which causes ipsipulsion of saccades. Pharmacological inactivation of the dorsal vermis (3) causes contrapulsion (although clinical lesions produce bilateral hypometria). Interruption of crossed fastigial nucleus outputs in the superior cerebellar peduncle (uncinate fasciculus, 5) causes contrapulsion. Thus, contrapulsion arises at sites 1, 3 and 5, and ipsipulsion at sites 2–4.

ruption of inputs to the cerebellum in the inferior peduncle—as occurs in Wallenberg's syndrome—causes ipsipulsion (Fig. 3–16); it is postulated that increased activity of Purkinje cells causes a unilateral fastigial nucleus "lesion".[740] Interruption of the crossed output of the fastigial nucleus in the superior cerebellar peduncle causes contrapulsion of saccades (overshooting contralaterally, undershooting ipsilaterally).[683,740] Rarely, climbing fibers from the inferior olivary nucleus are lesioned before crossing the midline and passing into the inferior cerebellar peduncle;[711] this causes contrapulsion of saccades. Experimental studies indicate that lesions of the posterior interpositus nucleus may affect the accuracy of vertical saccades,[580] but this has not yet been documented clinically.

In sum, the cerebellum appears to be important for the control of saccadic accuracy, including both amplitude and direction, and possibly in correcting for position-dependent changes in the mechanical properties of the eye muscles and orbital tissues. This capability appears to function both in an "on-line" fashion, since cerebellar dysmetria is apparent immediately after inactivating the fastigial nuclei, as well as in the long term, as part of the process of adaptive control of saccade accuracy. This pivotal role of the cerebellum in the control of saccades is supported by finding that neither frontal eye field or superior colliculus lesions alone causes enduring changes in saccadic metrics; in each case, another area must be computing the size and dynamics of saccades, and the cerebellum seems the likely candidate. The role of the cerebellum is taken further in the next section, which attempts to identify its place in models for saccade generation.

MODELS FOR SACCADE GENERATION

With advances in knowledge of the saccadic system, quantitative hypotheses (models) to account for generation of these movements have grown in scale and complexity. Initial attempts used a classic control systems approach (see David A. Robinson's notes on the accompanying compact disc) whereas, more recently, neural-network models, which attempt to describe the contributions by distinct populations of neurons, are cast from a neuromimetic point of view. Here we briefly present a history of how saccadic models have developed, to provide the reader with a notion of the way that concepts about the generation of saccades have grown over the past half-century.[239a] Most of our account will be concerned with models of brainstem and cerebellar contributions to saccade generation, since the effects of cerebral cortex and basal ganglia on saccade dynamics are less well worked out. However, attempts have been made to model more complex aspects of saccadic behavior such as responses to remembered targets by neurons in LIP,[445,766] visual search by FEF,[446] and the role of the superior colliculus in a range of behaviors, including antisaccades.[713]

MODELS FOR HORIZONTAL SACCADES

Early notions of the generation of saccades proposed that the duration of the pulse of activity that creates saccades was predetermined or preprogrammed according to desired saccadic amplitude.[754] Studies of patients with slow saccades, however, led to an alternative hypothesis that suggested saccades are generated by a mechanism that drives the eyes to a particular orbital position rather than moves the eyes a specified distance.[777] By continuously comparing desired eye position and actual eye position (the latter is probably based on monitoring an internal, efference copy of the eye position command) the neurons that generate the saccadic pulse would be driven until the eye reaches the target, when they would automatically cease discharging. This is the original local-feedback model for saccades proposed by D.A. Robinson[572] (Fig. 3–17A). It has the advantage that it automatically generates the main sequence relationships between amplitude and peak velocity or duration for saccades (Fig. 3–2).[725] The model also accounts for slow but accurate saccades made both by some patients with neurological disease and by normal subjects taking various sedative or hypnotic medications.[336] It can also produce saccadic oscillations such as flutter if the omnipause neurons malfunction or are inhibited.[778] Although the notion of local feedback has sometimes been called into question,[339] the evidence to support it remains substantial. Thus, if a saccade is arrested in mid-flight by briefly stimulating the omnipause neurons, a new saccade is generated to get the eye on target within 70 ms (Fig. 3–11), which is shorter than could have been achieved by responding to the visual consequences of the arrested movement.[349,350] Furthermore, patients with slow saccades often get their eye on target,[411,777] and slow saccades induced by experimental inactivation of the rostral PPRF may be accurate.[49] Thus, it appears that a signal is used to ensure that the burst neurons discharge until the planned movement is achieved.

Subsequent physiological studies have called for modifications of the original Robinson model, while retaining the notion of local feedback control of saccade generation. One important revision is that the command signal is a desired change in eye position (Fig. 3–17B).[336] This signal would be compared continuously with an efference copy of the actual change in eye position, to determine when to terminate the saccade. Inherent in this modification of the local-feedback model is the idea of separate integrators, one common neural integrator for conversion of eye velocity to eye position commands (for all types of conjugate eye movements, discussed in Chapter 5) and a separate resettable neural integrator that operates specifically on saccadic velocity commands in the feedback loop that controls the duration of the saccadic pulse.[3,49,336,375,485,670,673]

At present, the anatomical basis for local feedback control of burst neurons and the resettable integrator for saccades is not understood.[249,609] One proposal is that the feedback involves long-lead burst neurons rather than premotor burst neurons.[622] In this model (Fig. 3–17C), long-lead burst neurons are also the proposed site for the second, saccade-specific integration. However, this model is not consistent with some anatomical projections of the superior colliculus,[101] cannot simulate the staircase of saccades that occurs with sustained stimulation of the superior colliculus, [86] and cannot account for saccadic oscillations such as flutter and opsoclonus.

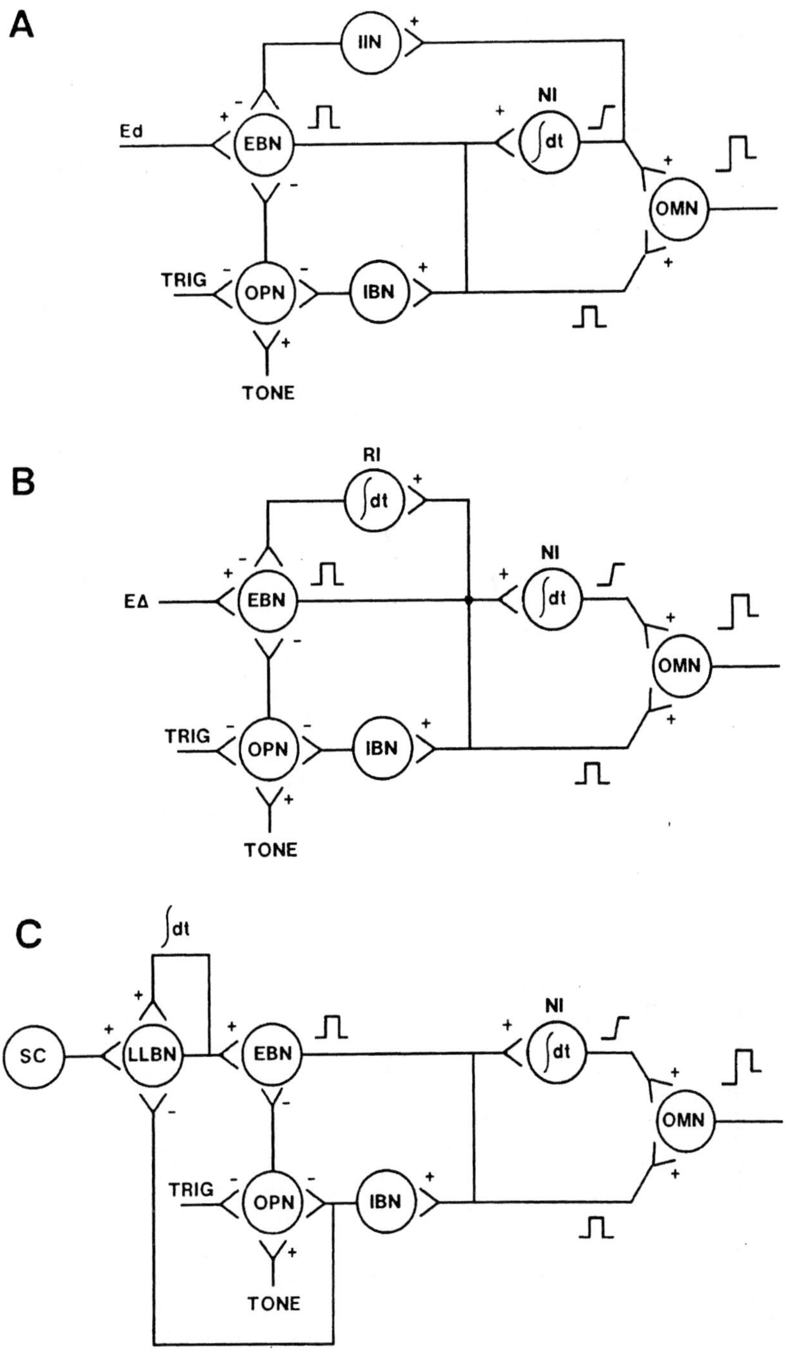

Figure 3–17. Models of the saccadic pulse generator. (A) Model after Robinson.[572] A desired eye position signal (Ed) excites burst neurons (EBN), which in turn project to the ocular motoneurons (OMN), to the neural integrator (NI) and to the inhibitory burst neurons (IBN). Omnipause neurons (OPN) have a tonic level of discharge (TONE) but are inhibited by a trigger signal (TRIG) when a saccade is desired. During the saccade, OPN are kept silent by IBN. The output of the NI is fed back as an efference copy of eye position to EBN via an inhibitory interneuron (IIN). When this signal becomes equal to Ed, the burst neurons cease discharging and the saccade is over. (B) Model after Jürgens and colleagues.[336] The input to the burst neurons is now a *desired change in eye position* (EΔ). This signal is compared with an efference copy of eye position, which is now derived from a separate, resettable neural integrator (RI) specific to the saccadic system. (C) Model modified from Scudder.[622] Long-lead burst neurons (LLBN) receive excitatory signals from the superior colliculus (SC) and are the site for the saccade-specific integration of velocity to position signals. The saccade is terminated by comparing the integral of an efference copy of saccade velocity (via IBN) and the integral of the input from the superior colliculus.

A second suggestion is that feedback control of saccades and the saccadic integrator involves the superior colliculus.[741] However, pharmacological inactivation of the superior colliculus does not produce effects consistent with predictions of this model,[13] as is discussed in the section on the superior colliculus.[508]

Third, it has been proposed that local feedback occurs via a cerebellar loop (Fig. 3–15).[389,511,549] This proposal is consistent with the anatomical connections between the premotor burst neurons, dorsal vermis and fastigial nucleus, and with experimental evidence that the cerebellum is important for getting saccades on target.[389,511,549] However, high-frequency oscillations, thought to be saccadic in origin,[555] occur in patients with lesions involving the fastigial nucleus that cause hypermetria (see Video Display: Disorders of Saccades). This and other observations have led to an alternative model to account for saccadic oscillations,[553] which depend on the synaptic connections between burst neurons (Fig. 3–10). Specifically, it has been shown that there are connections by which IBN inhibit IBN;[682] these form positive feedback loops that are potentially unstable. For example, during a saccade to the right, left-sided EBN will be inhibited by IBN. However, when the saccade is over, if EBN show post-inhibitory rebound,[447,448] they will start discharging again. It has been postulated that this is the mechanism underlying high-frequency saccadic oscillations, such as ocular flutter.[553]

MODELS FOR OBLIQUE SACCADES

The ocular motoneurons innervate extraocular muscles that rotate the eyes approximately in Cartesian coordinates (e.g., the medial and lateral rectus rotate the globe a specified distance horizontally). However, the saccade-related neurons in the superior colliculus and premotor burst neurons in the brainstem discharge for oblique movements, and so one aspect of modeling saccades is whether these structures encode the saccadic command in polar or Cartesian coordinates. In other words, do the two populations in the PPRF and riMLF become strongly coupled or do they remain independent? In one view of the way that oblique saccades are programmed, the "common source" saccade model, the command from the superior colliculus to burst neurons is specified in polar coordinates: an oblique (radial) velocity at angle θ.[727] Neural circuitry then converts this into a signal multiplied by cosine θ for the horizontal PPRF burst neurons and a signal multiplied by sine θ for the vertical riMLF burst neurons. This model predicts: (1) the horizontal and vertical components of oblique saccades may have different durations and peak velocities than when similar-sized movements are made as purely horizontal or vertical saccades; (2) the horizontal and vertical components will have synchronous onset and offset; (3) the peak velocities of the horizontal and vertical components of the saccade are scaled by cosine θ and sine θ, respectively; (4) the trajectory of the oblique saccade will be straight. An alternative hypothesis, the Cartesian coordinate model, proposes that the central command for the oblique saccade is broken down into horizontal and vertical eye displacement components before being sent to the horizontal and vertical burst neurons.[57,258] The critical predictions of this so-called independent model are: (1) the horizontal and vertical saccadic components of oblique saccades will have the same duration and peak velocity as when made as purely horizontal or vertical saccades; (2) although the horizontal and vertical components of oblique saccades will have a synchronous onset, they may end at different times; (3) the trajectory of oblique saccades could be curved.

Normal human saccades are so brief that it is often difficult to distinguish between the predictions of these two models. However, oblique saccades that have dissimilar horizontal and vertical components often appear curved,[39] and could have different times of offset of the two components.[258] Nonetheless, peak velocities of horizontal and vertical components are reported to be scaled as predicted by the common source model.[727]

Studies of patients with selective slowing of the vertical or horizontal components provide interesting results. Thus, patients with selective slowing of vertical saccades due to Niemann-Pick type C disease show markedly curved oblique saccades (Fig. 3–5B).[590] The initial movement is mainly horizontal and most of the vertical component occurs after the horizontal component has ended (i.e., the two components end at quite different times). After completion of the horizontal component of an oblique saccade, the eyes oscillate horizontally "in place" at 10 Hz–20 Hz until the vertical component ends (Fig. 3–5C). These horizontal oscillations probably occur because omnipause neurons are silent until the vertical component is complete, and after the horizontal component is over, the normal horizontal burst neurons lack a motor error signal to drive them and so oscillate until the whole saccade is completed. Similar oscillations are encountered during some oblique saccades made by normal subjects.[57] Curved oblique saccades are also encountered in patients with spinocerebellar ataxia who show selective slowing of horizontal saccades (see Video Display: Disorders of Saccades). Partial inactivation of the PPRF in monkey with lidocaine also produces oblique saccades with curved trajectories.[49]

Nonetheless, monkeys and some healthy humans make straight saccades during oblique movements. To account for straight trajectories of oblique saccades, a third model was suggested in which there was cross-coupling between the output of horizontal and vertical pulse generators.[258] However, other studies have shown that changes of peak velocity predicted by this model with coupled outputs do not occur, and suggested that it is more likely that it is the inputs that are coupled (common source).[49,57] A fourth model to account for the variable curving of oblique saccades encountered in humans and monkeys consists of a distributed network of neurons, which is able to simulate several characteristics of oblique saccades, with no cross-coupling between the two pulse generators.[550] Thus, the data are still somewhat conflicting and further studies of normal subjects and patients with selective slowing of horizontal or vertical saccades should provide the opportunity to test these several models.

NEUROMIMETIC MODELS FOR SACCADES IN TWO AND THREE DIMENSIONS

More recently, models have been developed that seek to account more realistically for the way that the brainstem and cerebellum control saccade generation. Thus, some models attempt to account for saccades interrupted by electrical stimulation of omnipause neurons,[25,219] as well as the curved trajectories encountered when more than one visual stimulus is presented in terms of activity of multiple populations of superior colliculus neurons.[26] Other efforts have modeled the resettable integrator for saccades as a population of neurons in the fastigial nucleus.[549]

The development of reliable methods to measure 3-D eye rotations has led to development of models to account for rotations of the eye in three planes during saccades. In fact, the position of saccadic eye rotations are essentially restricted to rotation about axes that lie in the frontal plane (Listing's plane—see Fig. 9–3 in Chapter 9), and so three degrees of freedom are reduced to two degrees. What remains to be settled is the mechanism that imposes Listing's law, and the relative contributions made by the mechanical and suspensory properties of the orbital tissues on the one hand,[142,510,558,619] and by neural factors on the other.[550,717] Specifically, rotations are noncommutative, which means that the brain must specify the order of rotations to get the eye to the correct tertiary position. The discovery of pulleys that guide the extraocular muscles (discussed in Chapter 9) may provide a means by which the brain can delegate at least some aspects of the complexities of 3-D rotations to a mechanical "analog computer" in the orbit.[141] This topic is discussed further in Chapter 9.

ADAPTIVE CONTROL OF SACCADIC ACCURACY

The first reports of adaptation in the saccadic system were in patients with partial abducens nerve palsies who preferred to view with their paretic eye, because it had better vision.[367] With the affected eye viewing, saccades made by the paretic eye were accurate even in the direction of the muscle weakness. The saccades of the nonparetic eye, on the other hand, were much larger and had post-saccadic drift. With the paretic eye covered and the "normal" eye viewing, the saccades of the nonparetic eye both overshot the target and showed post-saccadic drift. In other words, saccadic innervation had been readjusted (to both eyes, consistent with Hering's law of equal innervation) in an attempt to improve the performance of the habitually fixating but paretic eye. Both the pulse amplitude and the pulse-step match dysmetria created by the palsy had been repaired. Kommerell and colleagues[367] then patched the paretic eye of their patients continuously, requiring them to use their nonparetic eye. When examined after three days, the patients had readjusted the amplitude of the saccadic pulse and the pulse-step match so that saccades made by the nonparetic eye became accurate. In other words, the central nervous system changed saccadic innervation to meet best the visual needs of the habitually viewing eye.

It was subsequently shown that the change in saccadic amplitude was accomplished by prolonging the duration of the saccadic pulse alone, without an increase in its height.[5,323] If pulse height had increased, the peak velocity of saccades made by the normal eye would have increased; it did not. Moreover, the adaptive changes were specifically tailored to the mechanical needs dictated by the particular orbital positions from and to which the saccade was to be made.[513] Another clinical example of this adaptive capability concerns patients with internuclear ophthalmoplegia, who often show saccadic overshoot and backward postsaccadic drift in the abducting eye. This "abduction nystagmus" may be accounted for, in some patients, by the same mechanism that adjusts innervation conjugately in response to a peripheral muscle palsy.[167,775] Further discussion on saccadic changes in paralytic strabismus is provided in Chapter 9.

Experimentally Induced Saccadic Adaptation

In normal subjects, saccadic pulse dysmetria can be simulated by changing the position of the target just before the eye reaches it, forcing the subject to make a corrective saccade after every target jump.[310,429] After as few as 150 such trials, subjects automatically make saccades that are bigger or smaller, depending upon the particular nature of the induced dysmetria.[16,152,633,684] Saccadic adaptation also produces a recalibration of shifts of attention that accompany saccades.[428] The presence and timing of the post-saccadic visual error are important determinants of the amount (gain) of adaptation.[583,628,636]

A *pulse-step match dysmetria* can be simulated by making a large, projected visual stimulus drift briefly after every saccade. Both humans and monkeys soon learn to preprogram a postsaccadic drift of the eyes, by creating a pulse-step mismatch that nearly matches the artificial motion of the visual scene.[341,509]

Saccadic adaptation may be specific to the context of the stimulus conditions;[647] for example, adaptation for movements in one direction does not automatically lead to adaptation in another.[145] Adaptation may depend on orbital eye position and the vector of the movement; this is important for everyday life, when we make saccades from constantly changing starting positions in a range of directions.[15] Thus, adaptation with increased gain can be induced with the eyes in right gaze and with decreased gain in left gaze.[644] When adaptation is required for just one size of saccade, movements of other sizes or directions are less adapted.[491,687] When adaptation is required for two movements, averaging saccades (which fall between the two visual targets) also show some adaptation.[14] During adaptation in a context-based manner (such as a gain increase on right gaze and a gain decrease on left gaze), subjects adapt better if they are given rest period between each training state.[9] This is the phenomenon by which consolidation of motor learning is facilitated and has potential implications for rehabilitation of ocular motor and vestibular disorders by programs of eye movement training. Once induced, saccadic adaptation may last for days.[15a]

The visual features of the stimulus, such as color or visual background,[579] as well as otolithic signals,[645] have relatively small effects on the learning process compared with the nature of the saccadic response.[148] Thus, on the one hand, saccadic gain adaptation induced by step movements of a single target does not transfer to saccades made during scanning of an array of targets, or to remembered locations of single targets.[147] On the other hand, adaptation achieved during scanning an array of targets transfers to memory-guided saccades, but not to step movements of a single target.[147] Furthermore, adaptation of memory-guided saccades does not transfer to saccades during scanning or to single target jumps.[148]

Saccades induced by electrical stimulation of the superior colliculus in monkeys can be adapted if a visual stimulus is presented at a location different from where the eye movement ended.[437] This adaptation shows incomplete transfer to normal visually guided saccades, suggesting need for involvement of cortical areas in normal adaptation of saccades to single target jumps. However, adaptation of normal visually guided saccades does transfer to express saccades, suggesting the importance of cortical and cerebellar contributions.[309] Furthermore, adaptation to visually guided saccades transfers to express saccades. Briefly delaying the presentation of the post-saccadic target impedes adaptation, and has led to the suggestion that the brain compares the post-saccadic image with the one that would be predicted for the planned saccade.[36] All these findings emphasize the important role of context in motor learning, and suggest that multiple areas of the brain may be involved in facilitating motor learning, so that saccadic metrics are tailored to a specific environmental circumstance (see below).

Hypotheses to Account for Saccadic Adaptation

How can these diverse properties of saccadic adaptation be explained? Although results from adaptation experiments in monkeys may differ,[212,623] the transfer of adaptation from one type of saccade in human is specific and has suggested a hypothesis based on current notions of the control of saccades.[148] Thus, memory-guided saccade adaptation may depend on dorsolateral prefrontal cortex; scanning saccades adaptation on the frontal eye field; and adaptation of saccades to target jumps on the parietal eye field and superior colliculus. Such a hypothesis could be tested by studying saccadic adaptation in patients with discrete cortical lesions, and provides a tool to clinicians to investigate the cerebral control of saccades.[147] A model to account for the way that the superior colliculus could contribute to saccadic adaptation, by changes in the nature of the spreading of activation, has also been proposed.[257] Other aspects of saccadic adaptation such as occur following abducens nerve palsy are discussed under Adaptive Changes of Eye-Head Saccades in Chapter 7, Disconjugate Adaptation in Chapter 8, and Saccades in Paralytic Strabismus in Chapter 9.

Neural Substrate for Saccadic Adaptation: The Role of the Cerebellum

Which structures in the central nervous system participate in the adaptive control of saccadic accuracy? The most compelling evidence supports a role for the cerebellum. Thus, functional imaging of human subjects while they are carrying out a saccadic adaptation task shows selective activation in the cerebellar dorsal vermis, but not in the FEF or superior colliculus.[143] Furthermore, experimental cerebellectomy completely abolishes the adaptive capability—for both the pulse size and the pulse-step match.[512] Monkeys with lesions restricted to the *dorsal cerebellar vermis* cannot adapt the size of the saccadic pulse—they have pulse-size dysmetria.[48,696] *Fastigial nucleus* neurons show changes in their discharge properties after saccadic adapation,[625] and inactivation of the fastigial nucleus impairs saccadic adaptation.[322,582] Monkeys with *floccular lesions* show a different disturbance of saccadic adaptation: they cannot match the saccadic step to the pulse to eliminate pulse-step mismatch dysmetria.[513] Patients with cerebellar disease, especially cerebellar degeneration, show impaired saccadic adaptation.[685] Finally, neuronal activity in nucleus reticularis tegmenti pontis (NRTP), which projects to the cerebellum, shows changes during saccadic adaptation.[698]

Taken together, this evidence suggests that the repair of conjugate saccadic dysmetria is mediated by two different cerebellar structures. The dorsal cerebellar vermis and the fastigial nuclei control pulse size; the flocculus and paraflocculus control the pulse-step match. Does the cerebellar contribution to saccadic adaptation extend to all types of saccades? One patient with a midline cerebellar hemangioblastoma showed greater hypermetria for saccades made to single-target presentations than during saccadic scanning of a display of targets.[686] This finding implies that the cerebellum is also involved in context-specific motor learning. In fact, the cerebellum is ideally poised to implement context-specific motor learning as it has access to all the necessary afferent and corollary discharge signals to determine the context in which the next saccade is to occur.

The dorsal vermis and fastigial nucleus may also participate in the repair of disconjugate saccadic dysmetria, since patients with cerebellar disease show disconjugacy of saccades,[735] experimental vermal lesions cause saccadic disconjugacy,[695] and experimental inactivation by cooling of the fastigial nucleus causes disconjugate dysmetria.[737] Although visual signals are probably most important in providing the error signal that drives disconjugate saccadic adaptation, extraocular proprioception also contributes. Thus, monkeys deprived of proprioceptive information by section of the ophthalmic branch of the trigeminal nerve show abnormalities in disconjugate adaptation after surgically induced CN IV palsy, although it does not interfere with visually mediated adaptation.[396,397]

Other Areas Contributing to Saccadic Adaptation

Although the cerebellum projects to presaccadic circuits, there is evidence that it may not have the final word on saccadic behavior. For example, in normal monkeys that have undergone saccadic adaptation training, tasks requiring a sequence of saccades (such as the double-step paradigm) are performed appropriately, because even if the initial response is adapted (and inaccurate), the subsequent saccade gets the eye on target.[700] One possible explanation for this behavior relates to projections of cerebellar regions concerned with saccadic accuracy to cerebral cortex via the thalamus. Thus, inactivation or lesions of the dorsal vermis,[696] the fastigial nucleus,[582] or the ventrolateral thalamus to which the cerebellum projects,[237] all impair the ability to adapt saccades to new visual demands.

Inactivation of another pathway from the superior colliculus via the medial dorsal thalamus to the frontal eye field impairs the second saccade in the response to double-step stimuli in non-adapted monkeys, suggesting that this pathway is important so that the brain can keep a record of prior movements using corollary discharge signals to the cortex.[667] However, this pathway seems not to play a role in responses to saccadic adaptation since electrophysiological evidence indicates that the superior colliculus does not contribute to saccadic adaptation, although more rostral sites such as the frontal lobes and basal ganglia might.[172] In this regard, an interesting finding is that patients with Parkinson's disease have difficulties with adaptation of memory-guided, but not visually guided, saccades.[412]

SACCADES AND MOVEMENTS OF THE EYELIDS

Saccades are often accompanied by blinks, but only recently have their interactions been systematically studied.[189] At a cortical level, the FEF, SEF, and PEF are all activated during both saccades and blinks,[79] although there is perhaps more activation of the inferior precentral sulcus with blinks.[347] Here we focus on two aspects: the coordination of vertical saccades and eyelid movements, and the effects of blinks on saccades. The interaction of four separate forces determines the position of the eyelids. Upward forces are mainly due to the levator palpebrae superioris (LPS),[186] with Müller's smooth muscle, which bridges the LPS and its tendon, making a minor contribution. Downward forces are due to stretching of tendons and ligaments connected to LPS, and the orbicularis oculi muscle.[186]

The eyelids closely follow vertical gaze shifts, including saccades. Thus, eye and lid saccades show similar dynamic properties.[192,262] Upward lid saccades are due to a burst of activity in the LPS muscle and its motoneurons,[211] which lie in the unpaired, central caudal nucleus of the oculomotor nuclear complex (see Fig. 9–9 , Chapter 9). Downward lid saccades are due entirely to elastic forces, which close the eye when the LPS relaxes. The orbicularis oculi muscle is electrically silent except during blinks or voluntary lid closure. Thus, neural coordination of vertical gaze and lid position is due to a synkinesis between the vertically acting extraocular muscles and the LPS. How is this achieved?

The main elevator of the eye, the superior rectus, has a common embryology to LPS and these two muscles are connected by a common sheath of intermuscular fascia. However, the muscles are structurally different, and their motoneurons lie in distinct subnuclei of the oculomotor nucleus. It appears that a key structure in the coordination of vertical saccades is the M-group of neurons, which lie adjacent and medial to the caudal third of the riMLF, and project strongly to the LPS motoneurons, but also to subnuclei supplying the superior rectus and inferior oblique, and frontalis muscles.[312] The M-group appears to receive inputs from upward burst neurons in the riMLF, and may have connections with the nucleus of the posterior commissure. Thus, whereas lid retraction is a classic sign of posterior commissure lesions,[31] patients who have slow vertical saccades accompanied by lid lag but without lid retraction could have involvement of the M-group.[218,312]

Blinks typically occur 20 times per minute. During a blink, a burst of activity occurs in the normally quiescent orbicularis oculi muscle, while at the same time, tonic activity in the levator palpebrae ceases.[190] How do they affect eye movements? If blinks are made during fixation of a stationary target, the eyes transiently move down and toward the nose;[123] such movements are slower than saccades and are due to a co-contraction of all extraocular muscles except the superior oblique muscle.[191] Blinks are often made with saccades; the probability of a blink occurring increases with the size of the gaze shift.[191,192] Blinks caused substantial changes in the dynamic properties of horizontal saccades, decreasing peak velocity and increasing duration.[247,589] These changes are unlikely to be due to a summation of the down-and-inward movement produced by blinking and the saccade, since there is no direction preponderance in the slowing of saccades. Furthermore, saccades made with blinks show an increased incidence of dynamic overshoots (Fig. 3–18).[589]

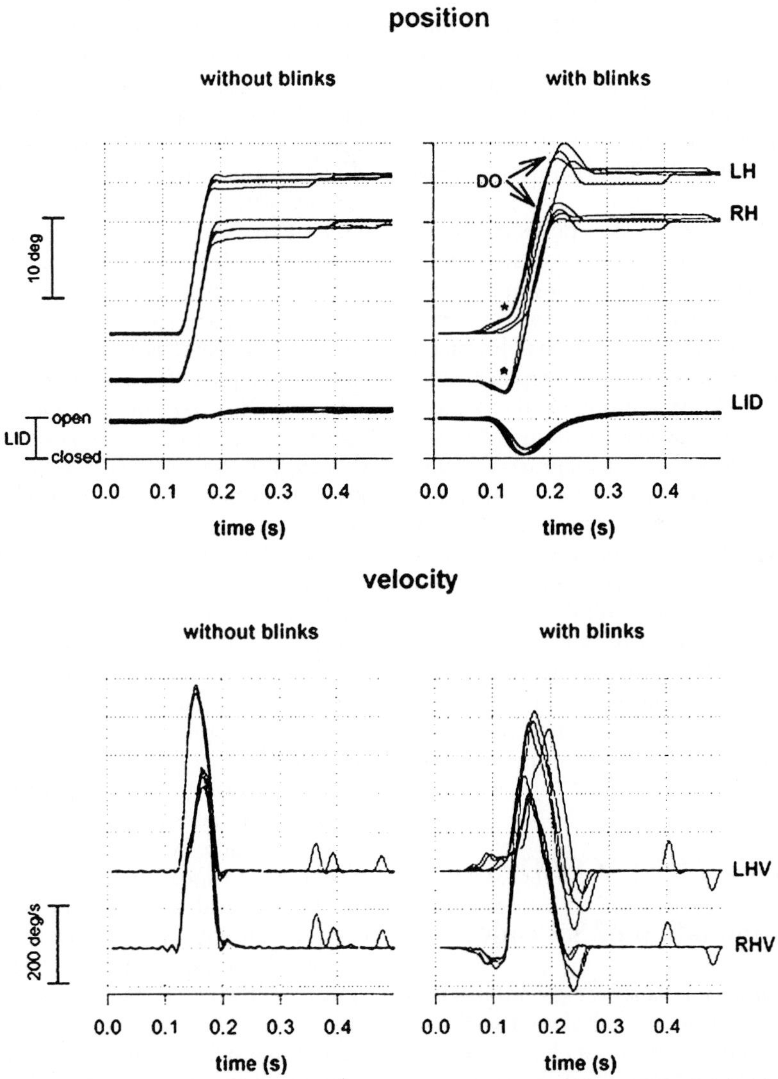

Figure 3–18. Effect of blinks on saccades from a normal subject. Position records are shown above and corresponding velocity traces below. Note that peak velocities are smaller, for similar-sized saccades, when the subject blinks with the saccade. Also note that dynamic overshoots (DO)—oppositely directed postsaccadic movements—occur more frequently with blinks. LH, left horizontal position; LHV, left horizontal velocity; RH, right horizontal position; RHV, right horizontal velocity. (Courtesy of Klaus G. Rottach.)

Electrophysiological studies have demonstrated suppression of discharge in superior colliculus burst neurons during blinks; after the blink, activity resumes and persists until the perturbed saccade is completed.[248] Since blink-perturbed saccades generally get on target, it seems likely that there is a mechanism, downstream from the superior colliculus, to compensate for the blink-induced saccade perturbation. It may even relate to the cerebellum, since vermal lesions lead not only to saccadic dysmetria but also a decrease in the blinks associated with saccades. It also seems likely that omnipause neurons are silent during both blinks and saccades and, if the blink outlasts the saccade, the eyes might briefly oscillate around the new eye position as a dynamic overshoot. Normal subjects and patients with opsoclonus or ocular flutter may show oscillations during blinks,[264, 290] or during eyelid closure.

Although blinks tend to slow down saccades, a paradoxical finding is that blinks may actually speed up abnormally slow saccades in patients with degenerative or other diseases.[773] In this case, the blink may cause a more synchronized and complete inhibition of the omnipause neurons, allowing the burst neurons a better chance to discharge. This may also be the mechanism that patients with ocular motor apraxia employ (along with a head movement) to initiate a saccade (see Video Display: Acquired Ocular Motor Apraxia). Whatever the mechanism, it is clear that studies of saccades must take into account the occurrence of blinks, which may substantially affect these eye movements. Furthermore, methods of eye movement recording that depend upon measuring a biological signal such as the corneal-retinal potential, may be confounded by lid movements (see Appendix B).

EXAMINATION OF SACCADES

Clinical Examination of Saccades

Saccadic eye movements are best examined at the bedside by instructing the patient to fixate alternately upon two targets—such as the tip of a pen and the examiner's nose. Saccades in each direction can be examined in each field of gaze in both the horizontal and vertical planes. The examiner should determine: Are saccades of normal velocity? Are they promptly initiated? Are they accurate? Do the eyes move together? (See Appendix A for a summary.)

Saccadic slowing, such as the lag of the adducting eye in internuclear ophthalmoplegia (INO), can be best appreciated when the patient is instructed to rapidly refixate between two widely spaced targets (see Video Display: Pontine Syndromes); identification of mild INO often requires measurement of eye movements.[210] Another useful technique to detect slow adduction is with a hand-held "optokinetic" drum or tape. Quick phases made by the affected eye are smaller and slower. If slowing of saccades occurs in only one plane of movement, it can be easily appreciated when the patient makes saccades between diagonally placed targets. The rapid, normal component is completed before the slower, orthogonally directed component, so that the saccade trajectory is strongly curved (see Fig. 3–5B and Video Display: Disorders of Saccades).

Saccade latencies can be appreciated by noting the time it takes the patient to initiate the saccade. Saccadic dysmetria can be inferred by the direction and size of corrective saccades made to acquire the fixation target (see Video Display: Disorders of Saccades). Since small saccades (as little as 1/2 degree) can be detected by careful observation, saccadic dysmetria can be easily observed clinically at the bedside. Normal individuals may undershoot the target by a few degrees when refixations are large, and saccadic overshoot may occur normally for centripetal and especially downward saccades. This tendency toward downward overshoot in normals may also appear when making horizontal refixations, when a slight downward component necessitates an upward corrective saccade. The dysmetria should disappear with repetitive refixations between the same targets.

If a saccade abnormality is detected, the strategy is to localize the disturbance within the hierarchical organization of the saccadic eye movement system (Table 3–1). First, establish whether or not the disease process affects reflexive types of saccades. Quick phases can be examined by spinning the patient in a swivel chair to elicit vestibular nystagmus or by using an optokinetic drum to elicit optokinetic nystagmus. Loss of quick phases usually points to a brainstem process affecting premotor burst neurons. Next, examine the ability of the patient to make a saccade to a suddenly appearing visual target. Determine if saccades can be made without a visual target or in response to auditory targets, or ask the patient to refixate under closed lids or behind Frenzel goggles. Loss of voluntary saccades with preservation of reflexive saccades and quick phases is characteristic of acquired ocular motor apraxia. One can also test the ability to make more volitional types of saccades by asking the patient to make saccades, rapidly, back and forth, between two stationary targets, first to command and then spontaneously. In Parkinson's disease, for example, the ability to make predictive saccades can be assessed by asking the patient to change fixation while the examiner holds up the index finger of each hand, positioned to elicit horizontal saccades across the patient's midline. Initially the patient is instructed to "look at the finger on your right, on your left," and so on until the patient falls into a predictable sequence set by the examiner's instructions. Then the examiner asks the patient to continue making such saccades on his or her own (i.e., without verbal cues). Certain patients, typically those with Parkinson's disease, make accurate saccades during verbal instructions but hypometric saccades when they are self-paced (see Video Display: Parkinsonian Disorders).

It is also possible to elicit antisaccades at the bedside. The examiner holds both hands up and asks the patient to look to the finger that does not move.[135] Errors on the antisaccade task, with saccades towards the visual stimulus are encountered with disease affecting the prefrontal cortex.

If saccade initiation seems impaired, observe gaze changes when the patient makes a combined eye-head movement to see if an accompanying head movement can facilitate the production of a saccade. Some patients with ocular motor apraxia employ this strategy (see Video Display: Acquired Ocular Motor Apraxia). The effect of blinks should also be noted since they may facilitate the ability to initiate saccades,[393] speed-up slow saccades,[773] or induce saccadic oscillations.[264] Finally, the effects of fatigue upon saccadic eye movements, for example in myasthenia gravis, may be tested by asking the patient to repetitively refixate between two targets.

During attempted steady fixation, extraneous saccadic eye movements (saccadic intrusions—which imply impaired ability to suppress saccades) should be noted. Subtle degrees of abnormal fixation behavior can be best appreciated during ophthalmoscopy. The motion of the optic nerve head of one eye is observed as the patient attempts to fixate a target with the other. In some patients, saccadic oscillations such as flutter and opsoclonus can be induced by blinks or by asking the patient to make a combined saccade-vergence movement.[68]

Measurement of Saccadic Eye Movements

While many abnormalities of saccadic velocity, initiation, and accuracy can be easily appreciated at the bedside, more subtle changes can be detected only by analysis of eye movement recordings. To obtain reliable recordings of saccade trajectories, one must have a measuring system with a high bandwidth (preferably greater than 150 Hz, which requires a digitization rate of at least 300 Hz), and which reproduces faithfully the saccade trajectory. These methodological issues are reviewed in Appendix B. The search coil and corneal reflection techniques usually meet these requirements as well as offering adequate sensitivity (<0.1 deg), and linear range (± 20 deg). Electrooculography (EOG), however, induces a number of artifacts in the eye movement trace due to movement of the lid, movement of the opposite eye, and a muscle action potential spike at the onset of the saccade.[158] With EOG, the speed of abducting saccades appears to be lower than that of adducting saccades though recordings with the search-coil and infrared reflection techniques indicate that the opposite is actually the case. EOG is unreliable for measurement of vertical saccades.

Saccadic gain (saccade amplitude/target amplitude) is the usual measure of saccadic accuracy. Saccadic amplitude is usually defined by the position of the eye at the start of the saccade and the position of the eye when the saccadic pulse is finished. (Conventionally, saccade onset is defined by the rise of eye velocity to some arbitrary value, such as 30 degrees per second, and saccade pulse offset is defined by the dropping of eye velocity below that value.) Saccadic gain can be tested using both stationary and moving targets; both target position and velocity are used in programming of moving targets,[259] and lesions in the posterior cerebral hemisphere may produce a specific deficit in saccade accuracy for moving targets.[77,484]

The most common measurements of saccadic dynamics are peak velocity and duration; both are conventionally plotted as a function of amplitude (Fig. 3–2). In addition, the shape of the velocity waveform and its skewness (the ratio of time-to-peak velocity to total saccadic duration, see Fig. 3–1) may be helpful. Postsaccadic drift, the unusual waveforms observed in myasthenia gravis, and some types of ocular oscillations are examples of saccadic abnormalities that are best detected with eye movement recordings. Recordings of eye movements are essential if one wants to analyze carefully quick phases of vestibular nystagmus induced in darkness, saccades made to auditory targets, and saccades made in combination with head movements. Comparison of latencies of saccades made in different behavioral contexts (e.g., gap-overlap tasks, antisaccades, predictive saccades, saccades on command) also requires quantitative measurements of eye movements. Measurement of saccades is also helpful to confirm the diagnosis of internuclear ophthalmoparesis. After measuring a range of horizontal saccades, the ratio of abducting/adducting peak velocity or peak acceleration is calculated for the patient and compared to a normative database.[209]

Even though certain properties of saccades—such as peak velocity—are relatively "machine-like," such measures are influenced by a number of factors, such as target luminance and attention, and possibly by the age of the patient. It is therefore essential to compare measurements in any patient with 95% confidence limits defined by an age-matched control group during similar testing in that laboratory.

PATHOPHYSIOLOGY OF SACCADIC ABNORMALITIES

The clinical disorders that cause saccadic abnormalities are described in Chapters 10 and 12, and some abnormalities are summarized in Table 3–3. Here our review aims to apply current knowledge about the normal generation of saccades to present a scheme for thinking about saccadic abnormalities (see also Video Display: Disorders of Saccades). From

Table 3–3. **Summary of Enduring Effects of Lesions on Saccades***

Site of Lesion	General Effects of Lesions
Motoneurons and ocular motor nerves	Slowed saccades; limited range of movement
Premotor burst neurons	Slow saccades
PPRF	Horizontally
RiMLF	Vertically and torsionally
Omnipause neurons	Saccadic oscillations (opsoclonus and flutter); Slow horizontal *and* vertical saccades
Cerebellar dorsal vermis (bilateral)	Saccadic hypometria
Cerebellar fastigial nucleus (bilateral)	Saccadic hypermetria
Superior colliculus	Loss of short-latency (express) saccades
Thalamus	Inaccurate responses to double-step stimuli
Parietal eye field	Increased latency of visually guided saccades Inaccurate responses to double-step stimuli Impaired visual search
Frontal eye field	Bilaterally increased latency to overlap stimuli, remembered targets, and in antisaccade task Contralateral hypometria to visual or remembered targets
Supplementary eye field (SEF) and pre-SEF	Impaired ability to make a remembered sequence of saccades, and to reverse the direction of a previously established pattern of response

Table 3–3. *(continued)*

Site of Lesion	General Effects of Lesions
Dorsolateral prefrontal cortex	Impaired ability to make saccades to remembered target locations and errors on the antisaccade task. Impaired visual search
Basal ganglia	Difficulties in initiating voluntary saccades in tasks that require learned or predictive behavior, and working memory (such as visual search)

*More than one behavioral disturbance has been attributed to certain lesions.

a pathophysiological point of view, abnormalities of saccades can be classified into disorders of the saccadic pulse, disorders of the saccadic step, or saccadic pulse-step mismatch (Fig. 3–19). For example, a change in the amplitude (size) (approximately width × height) of the saccadic pulse creates overshoot or undershoot (saccadic dysmetria). A decrease in the height of the saccadic pulse, which reflects discharge frequency, causes slow saccades. A mismatch between the saccadic pulse and step creates post-saccadic drift or glissades. If the saccadic step cannot be sustained, the eye drifts toward the central position after each eccentric saccade, creating gaze-evoked nystagmus. In addition, there may be disturbance of the voluntary initiation or suppression of saccades.

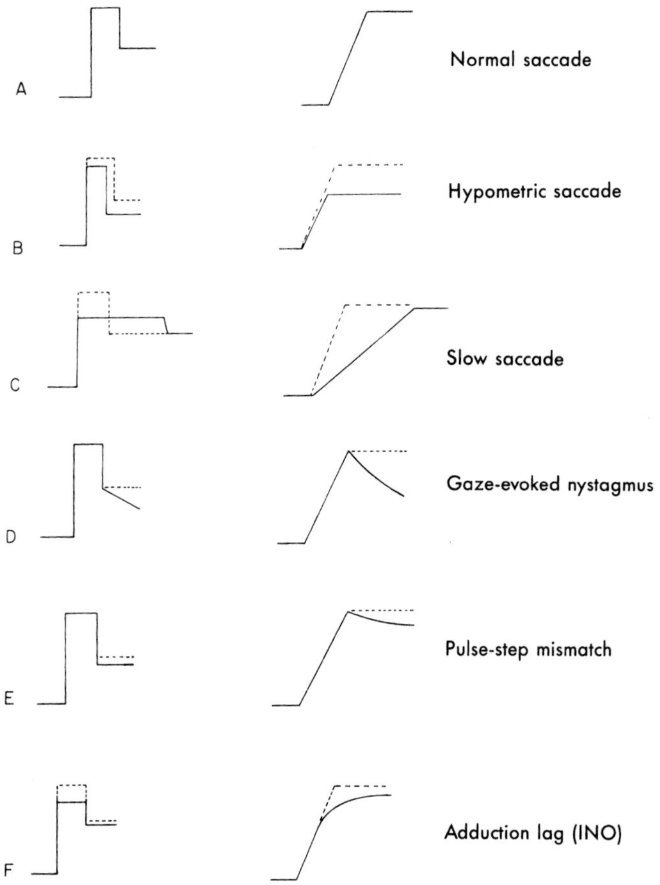

Figure 3–19. Disorders of the saccadic pulse and step. Innervation patterns are shown on the left, eye movements on the right. Dashed lines indicate the normal response. (A) Normal saccade. (B) Hypometric saccade: pulse amplitude (width × height) is too small but pulse and step are matched appropriately. (C) Slow saccade: decreased pulse height with normal pulse amplitude and normal pulse-step match. (D) Gaze-evoked nystagmus: normal pulse, poorly sustained step. (E) Pulse-step mismatch (glissade): step is relatively smaller than pulse. (F) Pulse-step mismatch due to internuclear ophthalmoplegia (INO): the step is larger than the pulse, and so the eye drifts onward after the initial rapid movement.

Disorders of Saccadic Velocity

Saccades are usually defined as being too slow or too fast if their peak velocities fall outside the normal peak velocity-amplitude relationship (main sequence, Fig. 3–3). Small-amplitude saccades that appear to be too fast usually occur when a saccade is interrupted in mid-flight, such that its final intended position is not reached. They are characteristic of myasthenia gravis (see Video Display: Diplopia and Strabismus).[51,507] Thus the saccade, rather than being too fast, is actually too small; this, in effect, increases its peak velocity-amplitude relationship. Abnormalities in the orbit, such as tumors, which restrict the motion of the globe in certain orbital positions can also lead to these seemingly fast saccades. Saccades that actually are faster than normal occur in some patients with saccadic oscillations such as flutter and opsoclonus (see Figs. 3–4 and 10–15)[64,778] (see Video Display: Disorders of Saccades), or macrosaccadic oscillations,[691] in patients with prematurely terminated saccades (Fig. 3–20),[591] and in some individuals who stutter.[166]

Slow saccades of restricted amplitude usually reflect abnormalities in the ocular motor periphery, such as an extraocular muscle or ocular motor nerve paresis, or in the medial longitudinal fasciculus (MLF), such as the slow adduction of internuclear ophthalmoplegia (see Video Display: Pontine Syndromes). Slow saccades occurring with a full ocular motor range are usually caused by central neurological disorders, summarized in Table 10–15 (see Video Display: Disorders of Saccades). Possibilities include direct disruption in the brainstem neural networks generating the saccadic pulse, either because of intrinsic disturbances of burst neurons, or because of failure to recruit a portion of burst cells. This latter problem could arise from a loss of higher-level excitatory inputs to burst cells or an abnormality in inhibition of omnipause cells. If the omnipause cells are at fault, slow saccades can be explained by desynchronization of the discharge of burst neurons or by failure to recruit a certain proportion of burst neurons during the saccade. Alternatively, slow saccade may occur because omnipause neurons no longer provide glycine, which can facilitate N-methyl-D-aspartate (NMDA) receptor currents;[11] thus, burst neurons may lack the post-inhibitory rebound that is postulated to produce the high acceleration typical of saccades.[447,448,448a]

Thus, while it was originally believed that slow saccades due to central disorders were pathognomonic of burst cell dysfunction, it has become apparent that disturbances of higher level structures including the cerebral hemispheres,[716] and superior colliculus,[302] can lead to saccade slowing. Nonetheless, selective

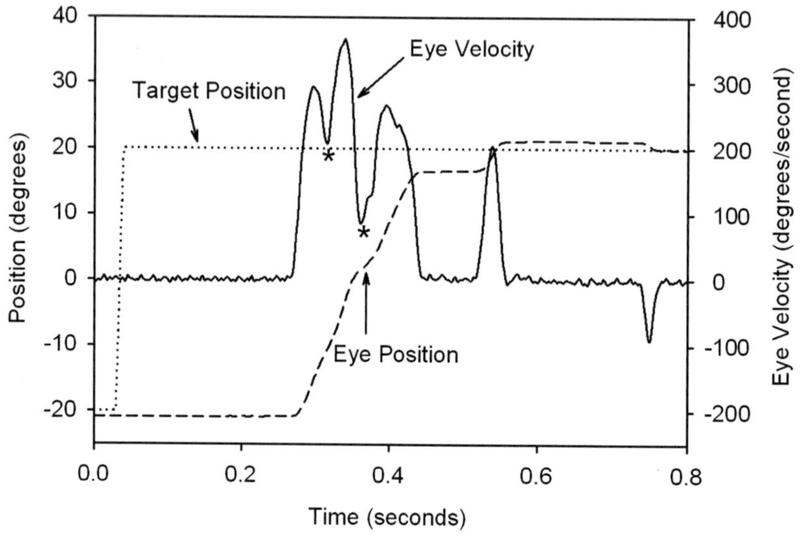

Figure 3–20. Representative records of horizontal saccades made by a patient with late-onset Tay-Sachs disease. The velocity record shows saccades with transient decelerations during which eye velocity declines, but not to zero, and then increases again (indicated by*). Thus these saccades appear to stall in mid-flight, a behavior similar to that induced by experimentally stimulating omnipause neurons during a saccade (Fig. 3–11).

slowing of horizontal saccades indicates pontine disease (PPRF), whereas selective slowing of vertical saccades suggests upper midbrain dysfunction (riMLF) (see Video Display: Midbrain Syndromes).[67] In patients with selective slowing of horizontal or vertical saccades, diagonal saccades often show a characteristically curved trajectory (Fig. 3–5B). Some patients with slow vertical saccades show curved trajectories even during vertical refixations; this might be an adaptive strategy that employs a normal horizontal component to completely inhibit omnipause neurons and so maximize the vertical component. In Gaucher's disease, a similar curved trajectory looping upwards is seen in association with slow horizontal saccades. Finally, saccadic velocities may be lower in drowsy, inattentive, or drug-intoxicated patients.[336,618,710]

Disorders of Saccadic Accuracy

Saccadic pulse dysmetria, especially hypermetria, is the hallmark of cerebellar disease. It is often asymmetric—*lateropulsion*, so that there is hypermetria of saccades in one direction and hypometria of saccades in the other. It is possible to offer a hypothesis that accounts for the direction of lateropulsion encountered in such patients (see Fig. 3–16 and Video Display: Disorders of Saccades). An important experimental finding, on which this hypothesis rests, is that pharmacological inactivation of the fastigial nucleus causes ipsipulsion (Fig. 3–16, site 4).[584] Thus, interruption of olivocerebellar climbing fibers within the medulla before they cross (Fig. 3–16, site 1), cause contrapulsion.[711] More commonly climbing fibers are interrupted within the inferior cerebellar peduncle (Fig. 3–16, site 2) in Wallenberg's syndrome, causing ipsipulsion. In both cases, interruption of climbing fibers may lead to increased simple-spike activity of Purkinje cells in the ipsilateral dorsal vermis, which, in turn, inhibits the underlying fastigial nucleus.[740] Conversely, removal of inhibition on fastigial nucleus neurons by pharmacological inactivation of the dorsal vermis (Fig. 3–16, site 3) causes contrapulsion,[594] although clinical lesions of the vermis are usually bilateral and so cause bilateral hypometria. Since the output of the fastigial nucleus is crossed, then lesions of the superior cerebellar peduncle (Fig. 3–16, site 5) cause contrapulsion—hypermetria of contralateral saccades and hypometria of ipsilateral saccades.

Patients with extreme degrees of saccadic hypermetria may show macrosaccadic oscillations: a series of hypermetric saccades made about the position of the target (see Video Display: Disorders of Saccades).[32,632] Occasionally, saccadic hypermetria reflects an adaptive response to a peripheral ocular motor deficit[367] or occurs after edrophonium is given to a myasthenic patient (see Video Display: Diplopia and Strabismus).[366]

Saccadic hypometria occurs with a variety of cerebellar and brain stem disorders. Postsaccadic drift, reflecting pulse-step match dysmetria, has been reported in patients with both central and peripheral ocular motor disorders. Visual defects may also lead to saccadic dysmetria. For example, patients with hemianopia may make hypermetric and hypometric saccades (depending on direction) to keep the target within the intact part of the visual field.[434,436,516] Patients with lesions in posterior parietal-temporal cortex may show saccadic dysmetria that is specific for moving, but not stationary, targets (Fig. 4–9).[391] Large unilateral lesions of the cerebral hemispheres may cause ipsilateral hypermetria and contralateral hypometria (see Video Display: Disorders of Smooth Pursuit), especially if there is neglect.[435] Unilateral hemispheric lesions may also lead to a biasing of vertical saccades toward the side of the lesion.[435,716]

Prematurely Terminated Saccades

In certain disorders saccades are very hypometric and the eye gets on target through a "staircase of small saccades." In Parkinson's disease, this occurs when patients make either memory-guided saccades,[355] or self-generated saccades (see Video Display: Parkinsonian Disorders). However, in such patients, the intersaccadic interval between each saccade in the series is no different from control subjects, about 200 ms.

Distinct from this phenomenon are transient decelerations, evident on the velocity records especially of larger saccades. Although normal subjects occasionally show this behavior for large saccades,[7] it is encountered during most gaze shifts in patients with some disorders affecting the brainstem and cerebellum, such as late-onset Tay-Sachs disease and

Wernicke's encephalopathy (Fig. 3–20).[332,591] Since the intersaccadic interval is shortened, and peak deceleration is increased for any saccadic pulse size (measured from peak velocity), it has been postulated that these disorders constitute a specific disorder of the "latch" circuit (Fig. 3–9) that normally inhibits omnipause neurons until the planned saccade is completed.[591] Support for this hypothesis is provided by similar findings when saccades are interrupted by experimental stimulation of the omnipause neurons (compare Fig. 3–11 and Fig. 3–20).[350] Note that transient decelerations also cause an abnormal velocity waveform with peak velocity/average velocity (Q) values that exceed 2.0 (see Saccadic Waveform).[374]

Disorders of Saccadic Initiation

Disorders of saccade initiation range from slight increases in saccadic reaction time, not perceptible at the bedside, to latencies greater than several seconds. The variability of reaction time may also be increased. Allowances must be made for the patient's age, state of consciousness, and level of attention. Saccadic latencies are increased in the presence of visual abnormalities such as amblyopia.[115] Patients with focal hemispheric lesions, especially those affecting the cortical "eye fields" may show increased latencies. Bilateral frontoparietal lesions produce a severe defect of saccade initiation called ocular motor apraxia (see Video Display: Acquired Ocular Motor Apraxia).[530] Such patients may be alert and cooperative but have impaired or delayed initiation of voluntary saccades, whereas random saccades and quick phases of nystagmus are normal.

Patients with disease of the basal ganglia such as Huntington's disease show a characteristic abnormality of saccadic initiation (see Box 12–17, in Chapter 12). Single saccades made in response to the sudden appearance of a visual target—reflexive saccades—are performed relatively normally with appropriate latencies and amplitudes. More volitional saccades, however, are impaired. Patients with Huntington's disease show a greater increase in latency for initiating saccades on command and during predictive tracking than for more reflexive saccades to novel visual stimuli.[381] Patients with Parkinson's disease show difficulties in making self-paced saccades between two visible targets (see Video Display: Parkinsonian Disorders).

Diffuse hemispheric disease may cause impaired ability to anticipate the location of a target moving in a predictable fashion.[354] Patients with Alzheimer's disease make express saccades in response to a gap stimulus, similar to normals, but also show greater variability of saccadic reaction times, probably due to difficulties with sustaining attention and suppressing reflexive movements.[8] Finally, in certain circumstances, saccadic latencies may actually be decreased, for example in some patients with progressive supranuclear palsy (PSP), in which the superior colliculus and its connections with the brainstem reticular formation may be involved.[536]

Inappropriate Saccades: Saccadic Intrusions and Oscillations

Saccades are inappropriate if they interfere with foveal fixation of an object of interest. Normally, subjects can suppress saccades during steady fixation. Saccadic intrusions are inappropriate movements that take the eye away from the target during attempted fixation (see Box 10–14 and Fig. 10–15, in Chapter 10). They occur spontaneously, without the appearance of a novel visual stimulus. They should be differentiated from excessive distractibility, wherein novel visual targets that are behaviorally irrelevant evoke inappropriate saccades. Excessive distractibility can be demonstrated in the antisaccade task (Fig. 3–2D).[776] When instructed to make a saccade in the direction opposite to that of a visual stimulus, patients with Huntington's disease, Alzheimer's disease, schizophrenia, and frontal lobe lesions make an inappropriate saccade to the visual target (see Fig. 12–14 in Chapter 12).[204,214,260,382,535,639] Patients with Parkinson's disease also make more errors on the antisaccade task.[112]

Several types of saccadic intrusions are recognized (Box 10–14, Chapter 10). At one end of the spectrum are *square-wave jerks*, which are small (typically 0.5 degrees), horizontal, involuntary saccades that take the eyes off the target and are followed, after an intersaccadic interval of about 250 ms, by a corrective saccade that brings the eyes back to the target (see Video Display: Parkinsonian Disorders). They may occur in normal individuals at frequencies of 20 per minute or greater;[1] they are reduced in frequency when subjects attempt to fix upon the remembered location of a target.[637] Normal subjects who have frequent square-wave jerks have no accompanying disorders of saccadic control.[251] Square-wave jerks are prominent in certain cerebellar disorders (especially Friedreich's ataxia) and PSP. These disorders may be due to dysfunction of saccade control by the superior colliculus or its inputs. Thus, microinjection of nicotine into the caudal superior colliculus in monkeys causes express saccades,[12] and nicotine is reported to increase square-wave jerk frequency in humans.[654] The superior colliculus has reciprocal connections with the central mesencephalic reticular formation, which is involved in PSP, and receives inhibitory projections from the substantia nigra, pars reticulata. Pallidotomy as therapy for Parkinson's disease is reported to increase the frequency of square-wave jerks,[33,497] perhaps by disrupting projections from the basal ganglia to the superior colliculus.

Another disorder that disrupts steady fixation is *macrosaccadic oscillations* (see Video Display: Disorders of Saccades). These may be an extreme form of saccadic hypermetria (Fig. 3–6), and are encountered in cerebellar disease that involves the fastigial nucleus or its output,[632] but are also reported with discrete pontine lesions that involved the region of the omnipause neurons.[32]

At the other end of the spectrum of saccadic abnormalities are back-to-back horizontal saccades without an intersaccadic interval. If such oscillations occur only in the horizontal plane, they are termed *ocular flutter*; if they occur in all directions, the oscillation is called *opsoclonus* (see Video Display: Disorders of Saccades). Some normal individuals can generate brief bursts of horizontal saccadic oscillations (voluntary flutter or "voluntary nystagmus") (see Video Display: Disorders of Saccades). Diseases associated with flutter and opsoclonus often also cause brainstem and cerebellar findings. Such oscillations probably reflect an inappropriate, repetitive, alternating discharge pattern of different groups of burst neurons. It was originally proposed that three factors contributed to saccadic oscillations without an intersaccadic interval: (1) the inherently high discharge rates (gain) of saccadic burst neurons, even for very small saccades; (2) the existence of central processing delays that make a system susceptible to oscillations; and (3) abnormalities of the brain stem omnipause cells (or their inputs), which normally inhibit burst neurons during fixation.[778] In support of this hypothesis, some patients manifest transient saccadic oscillations in association with blinks,[264] or vergence movements,[68] both of which inhibit omnipause neurons. Against the hypothesis that omnipause cell dysfunction is the primary cause of opsoclonus or flutter are two findings: (1) at autopsy some patients who had had opsoclonus showed no abnormalities in the region in which omnipause cells are located [566] and (2) pharmacological inactivation of the omnipause cell region in monkeys produces slow saccades,[339,662] not oscillations. Nonetheless, ocular flutter has been reported due to a pontine demyelinative lesion, with subsequent resolution of the oscillations as the patient recovered from the exacerbation of multiple sclerosis.[621]

An alternative hypothesis for flutter and opsoclonus is that saccadic oscillations arise because of the synaptic organization of premotor burst neurons (Fig. 3–10), in which positive feedback loops and post-inhibitory rebound properties of burst neurons predispose to saccadic oscillations.[447,448,553] Changes in the synaptic weighting of such circuits could produce oscillations whenever the omnipause neurons are inhibited.[556] In addition, cerebellar disease might, through projections of the fastigial nucleus to the premotor burst neurons, indirectly increase the likelihood of saccadic oscillations. Experimental lesions of the cerebellum in monkey have never led to flutter or opsoclonus, but this might be due to species differences. Patients with saccadic oscillations show activation of the fastigial nucleus on functional imaging,[282] but this might simply reflect increased frequency of saccades. New models for saccades that incorporate the membrane properties of burst neurons, or cerebellar neurons,[74] may provide suggestions for new treatments for opsoclonus. This is discussed further in Chapter 10.

SUMMARY

1. Saccades are rapid eye movements that change foveal fixation. They comprise both voluntary refixations and the quick phases of vestibular and optokinetic nystagmus. Saccades are characterized by a relatively invariant relationship between their amplitude and peak velocity (Fig.

3–3). The velocity of large saccades may exceed 500 degrees per second and their duration is generally less than 100 ms, which is less than the visual reaction time.
2. Saccades have many characteristics that suggest that they are under open loop or ballistic control. However, the saccadic system can acquire and use visual information continuously up to the initiation of the saccade to modify the amplitude and the direction of the impending saccade.
3. The main innervational change underlying saccadic eye movements is a pulse-step: the pulse is a saccadic eye velocity command that overcomes orbital viscous drag; the step is an eye position command that holds the eye in position against orbital elasticity (Fig. 1–3).
4. Excitatory burst neurons, within the pontine and mesencephalic reticular formation, generate the premotor commands for the horizontal and vertical components of saccades, respectively. Inhibitory burst neurons, located in the rostral medulla for horizontal saccades, assure reciprocal innervation by suppressing activity in motoneurons of antagonist muscles. Burst neurons are tonically inhibited by omnipause neurons except when a saccade is required. The duration of burst cell discharge appears to be under internal feedback control by neural pathways, since vision is too slow to guide saccades to their target.
5. The cerebral hemispheres can trigger saccades via parallel descending pathways (Fig. 3–12) to the superior colliculus and thence to the brainstem reticular formation. More volitional saccades (Table 3–1), made in the context of learned or remembered behavior, depend upon the frontal eye fields, which project both directly and indirectly (via the basal ganglia) to the superior colliculus. More reflexive saccades, to the locations of novel targets suddenly appearing in the external world, depend more upon direct projections from the parietal cortex to the superior colliculus. When the superior colliculus is damaged, recovery is probably mediated by direct projections from the frontal eye fields to the brain stem.
6. The basal ganglia, via serial, inhibitory projections, from the caudate nucleus to the substantia nigra pars reticulata and from the substantia nigra pars reticulata to the rostral pole of the superior colliculus, serve to inhibit extraneous reflexive saccades during attempted fixation and to facilitate volitional saccades in the context of remembered and learned behavior and reward.
7. The cerebellum (Fig. 3–15) calibrates saccadic amplitude (dorsal vermis and fastigial nucleus) and the saccadic pulse-step match (flocculus) for optimal visuo-ocular motor behavior. The cerebellum also influences the dynamics and the initiation (latency) of saccades.
8. Disorders of saccades consist of abnormalities of velocity, accuracy, initiation, prematurely terminated saccades, and the presence of saccadic intrusions and oscillations. Saccadic disorders can be classified according to whether the saccadic pulse, the saccadic step, or the pulse-step match is inappropriate (Fig. 3–19). Dysfunction of specific cell types within the brain stem reticular formation may account for various types of saccadic disorders.

REFERENCES

1. Abadi RV, Gowen E. Characteristics of saccadic intrusions. Vision Res 44, 2675–2690, 2004.
2. Abadi RV, Scallan CJ, Clement RA. The characteristics of dynamic overshoots in square-wave jerks, and in congenital and manifest latent nystagmus. Vision Res 40, 2813–2829, 2000.
3. Abel LA, Dell'Osso LF, Daroff RB. Analog model for gaze-evoked nystagmus. IEEE Trans Biomed Eng BME 25, 71–75, 1978.
4. Abel LA, Dell'Osso LF, Daroff RB, Parker L. Saccades in extremes of lateral gaze. Invest Ophthalmol Vis Sci 18, 324–327, 1979.
5. Abel LA, Schmidt D, Dell'Osso LF, Daroff RB. Saccadic system plasticity in humans. Ann Neurol 4, 313–318, 1978.
6. Abel LA, Troost BT, Dell'Osso LF. The effects of age on normal saccadic characteristics and their variability. Vision Res 23, 33–37, 1983.
7. Abel LA, Troost BT, Dell'Osso LF. Saccadic trajectories change with amplitude, not time. Neuro-ophthalmology 7, 309–314, 1987.
8. Abel LA, Unverzagt F, Yee RD. Effects of stimulus predictability and interstimulus gap on saccades in Alzheimer's disease. Dement Geriatr Cogn Disord 13, 235–243, 2002.
9. Aboukhalil A, Shelhamer M, Clendaniel R. Acquisition of context-specific adaptation is enhanced with rest intervals between changes in context state, suggesting a new form of motor consolidation. Neurosci Lett 369, 162–167, 2004.

10. Adamük E. Uber die Innervation der Augenbewegungen. Zentralbl Med Wissensch 8, 65–67, 1870.
11. Ahmadi S, Muth-Selbach U, Lauterbach A, et al. Facilitation of spinal NMDA receptor currents by spillover of synaptic released glycine. Science 300, 2094–2097, 2003.
12. Aizawa H, Kobayashi Y, Yamamoto M, Isa T. Injection of nicotine into the superior colliculus facilitates occurrence of express saccades in monkeys. J Neurophysiol 82, 1642–1646, 1999.
13. Aizawa H, Wurtz RH. Reversible inactivation of monkey superior colliculus. I. Curvature of saccadic trajectory. J Neurophysiol 79, 2082–2096, 1998.
14. Alahyane N, Koene A, Pelisson D. Transfer of adaptation from visually guided saccades to averaging saccades elicited by double visual targets. Eur J Neurosci 20, 827–836, 2004.
15. Alahyane N, Pelisson D. Eye position specificity of saccadic adaptation. Invest Ophthalmol Vis Sci 45, 123–130, 2004.
15a. Alahyane N, Pelisson D. Long-lasting modifications of saccadic eye movements following adaptation induced in the double-step target paradigm. Learn Mem 12, 433-443, 2005.
16. Albano JE, King WM. Rapid adaptation of saccadic amplitude in humans and monkeys. Invest Ophthalmol Vis Sci 30, 1883–1893, 1989.
17. Albano JE, Mishkin M, Westbrook LE, Wurtz RH. Visuomotor deficits following ablation of monkey superior colliculus. J Neurophysiol 48, 338–351, 1982.
18. Albano JE, Wurtz RH. Deficits in eye position following ablation of monkey superior colliculus, pretectum, and posterior-medial thalamus. J Neurophysiol 48, 318–337, 1982.
19. Amador N, Schlag-Rey M, Schlag J. Reward-predicting and reward-detecting neuronal activity in the primate supplementary eye field. J Neurophysiol 84, 2166–2170, 2000.
20. Amlot R, Walker R, Driver J, Spence C. Multimodal visual-somatosensory integration in saccade generation. Neuropsychologia 41, 1–15, 2003.
21. Anagnostou E, Kleiser R, Skrandies W. Electrophysiological correlates of human intrasaccadic processing. Exp Brain Res 130, 177–187, 2000.
22. Andersen RA, Bracewell RM, Barash S, Gnadt JW, Fogassi L. Eye position effects on visual, memory, and saccade-related activity in areas LIP and 7a of macaque. J Neurosci 10, 1176–1196, 1990.
23. Anderson TJ, Jenkins IH, Brooks DJ, et al. Cortical control of saccades and fixation in man. A PET study. Brain 117, 1073–1084, 1994.
24. Apter JT. Eye movements following strychninization of the superior colliculus of cats. J Neurophysiol 9, 73–86, 1946.
25. Arai K, Das S, Keller EL, Aiyoshi E. A distributed model of the saccade system: simulations of temporally perturbed saccades using position and velocity feedback. Neural Netw 12, 1359–1375, 1999.
26. Arai K, Keller EL. A model of the saccade-generating system that accounts for trajectory variations produced by competing visual stimuli. Biol Cybern 92, 21–37, 2005.
27. Arai K, McPeek RM, Keller EL. Properties of saccadic responses in monkey when multiple competing visual stimuli are present. J Neurophysiol 91, 890–900, 2004.
28. Araujo C, Kowler E, Pavel M. Eye movements during visual search: the costs of choosing the optimal path. Vision Res 41, 3613–3625, 2001.
29. Aslin RN, Shea SL. The amplitude and angle of saccades to double-step target displacements. Vision Res 27, 1925–1942, 1987.
30. Asrress KN, Carpenter RH. Saccadic countermanding: a comparison of central and peripheral stop signals. Vision Res 41, 2645–2651, 2001.
31. Averbuch-Heller L. Neurology of the eyelids. Curr Opin Ophthalmol 8, 27–34, 1997.
32. Averbuch-Heller L, Kori AA, Rottach K, et al. Dysfunction of pontine omnipause neurons causes impaired fixation: macrosaccadic oscillations with a unilateral pontine lesion. Neuro-ophthalmology 16, 99–106, 1996.
33. Averbuch-Heller L, Stahl JS, Hlavin ML, Leigh RJ. Square wave jerks induced by pallidotomy in parkinsonian patients. Neurology 52, 185–188, 1999.
34. Awater H, Burr D, Lappe M, Morrone MC, Goldberg ME. Effect of saccadic adaptation on localization of visual targets. J Neurophysiol 93, 3605–3614, 2005.
35. Bahcall DO, Kowler E. Illusory shifts in visual direction accompany adaptation of saccadic eye movements. Nature 400, 864–866, 1999.
36. Bahcall DO, Kowler E. The control of saccadic adaptation: implications for the scanning of natural visual scenes. Vision Res 40, 2779–2796, 2000.
37. Bahill AT, Clark MR, Stark L. Dynamic overshoot in saccadic eye movements is caused by neurological control signal reversals. Exp Neurol 48, 107–122, 1975.
38. Bahill AT, Clark MR, Stark L. The main sequence, a tool for studying human eye movements. Math Biosc 24, 191–204, 1975.
39. Bahill AT, Stark L. Neurological control of horizontal and vertical components of oblique saccadic eye movements. Math Biosci 27, 287–298, 1975.
40. Bahill AT, Stark L. Overlapping saccades and glissades are produced by fatigue in the saccadic eye movement system. Exp Neurol 48, 95–106, 1975.
41. Baizer JS, Bender DB. Comparison of saccadic eye movements in humans and macaques to single-step and double-step target movements. Vision Res 29, 485–495, 1989.
42. Baker JT, Harper TM, Snyder LH. Spatial memory following shifts of gaze. I. Saccades to memorized world-fixed and gaze-fixed targets. J Neurophysiol 89, 2564–2576, 2003.
43. Balan PF, Ferrera VP. Effects of gaze shifts on maintenance of spatial memory in macaque frontal eye field. J Neurosci 23, 5446–5454, 2003.
44. Ballard DH, Hayhoe MM, Pelz JB. Memory representations in natural tasks. J Cognitive Neuroscience 7, 66–80, 1995.
45. Baloh RW, Konrad HR, Sills AW, Honrubia V. The saccade velocity test. Neurology 25, 1071–1076, 1975.
46. Barash S, Bracewell RM, Fogassi L, Gnadt JW, Andersen RA. Saccade-related activity in the lateral intraparietal area. I. Temporal properties; comparison with area 7a. J Neurophysiol 66, 1095–1108, 1991.
47. Barash S, Bracewell RM, Fogassi L, Gnadt JW, Andersen RA. Saccade-related activity in the lateral intraparietal area. II. Spatial properties. J Neurophysiol 66, 1109–1124, 1991.
48. Barash S, Melikyan A, Sivakov A, et al. Saccadic dys-

metria and adaptation after lesions of the cerebellar cortex. J Neurosci 19, 10931–10939, 1999.
49. Barton EJ, Nelson JS, Gandhi NJ, Sparks DL. Effects of partial lidocaine inactivation of the paramedian pontine reticular formation on saccades of macaques. J Neurophysiol 90, 372–386, 2003.
50. Barton JJ, Cherkasova MV, Lindgren KA, Goff DC, Manoach DS. What is perseverated in schizophrenia? Evidence of abnormal response plasticity in the saccadic system. J Abnorm Psychol 114, 75–84, 2005.
51. Barton JJS, Jama A, Sharpe JA. Saccadic duration and intrasaccadic fatigue in myasthenic and nonmyasthenic ocular palsies. Neurology 45, 2065–2072, 1995.
52. Basso MA, Wurtz RH. Modulation of neuronal activity by target uncertainty. Nature 389, 66–69, 1997.
53. Basso MA, Wurtz RH. Neuronal activity in substantia nigra pars reticulata during target selection. J Neurosci 22, 1883–1894, 2002.
54. Beauvillain C, Dore K, Baudouin V. The 'center of gravity' of words: evidence for an effect of the word-initial letters. Vision Res 36, 589–603, 1996.
55. Becker W, Fuchs AF. Further properties of the human saccadic system: eye movements and correction saccades with and without visual fixation points. Vision Res 9, 1247–1258, 1969.
56. Becker W, Jürgens R. An analysis of the saccadic system by means of double step stimuli. Vision Res 19, 967–983, 1979.
57. Becker W, Jürgens R. Human oblique saccades: quantitative analysis of the relation between horizontal and vertical components. Vision Res 30, 893–920, 1990.
58. Bell AH, Meredith MA, van Opstal AJ, Munoz DP. Crossmodal integration in the primate superior colliculus underlying the preparation and initiation of saccadic eye movements. J Neurophysiol 93, 3659–3673, 2005.
59. Bellebaum C, Daum I, Koch B, Schwarz M, Hoffmann KP. The role of the human thalamus in processing corollary discharge. Brain 128, 1139–1154, 2005.
60. Ben HS, Duhamel JR. Ocular fixation and visual activity in the monkey lateral intraparietal area. Exp Brain Res 142, 512–528, 2002.
61. Ben HS, Duhamel JR, Bremmer F, Graf W. Visual receptive field modulation in the lateral intraparietal area during attentive fixation and free gaze. Cereb Cortex 12, 234–245, 2002.
62. Bender DB, Baizer JS. Saccadic eye movements following kainic acid lesions of the pulvinar in monkeys. Exp Brain Res 79, 467–478, 1990.
63. Benevento LA, Port JD. Single neurons with both form/color differential responses and saccade-related response in the non-retinotopic pulvinar of the behaving macque monkey. Vis Neurosci 12, 523–544, 1995.
64. Bergenius J. Saccade abnormalities in patients with ocular flutter. Acta Otolaryngol (Stockh) 102, 228–233, 1986.
65. Bergeron A, Matsuo S, Guitton D. Superior colliculus encodes distance to target, not saccade amplitude, in multi-step gaze shifts. Nat Neurosci 6, 404–413, 2003.
66. Berman RA, Heiser LM, Saunders RC, Colby CL. Dynamic circuitry for updating spatial representations: I. Behavioral evidence for interhemispheric transfer in the split-brain macaque. J Neurophysiol, 2005.
67. Bhidayasiri R, Riley DE, Somers JT, et al. Pathophysiology of slow vertical saccades in progressive supranuclear palsy. Neurology 57, 2070–2077, 2001.
68. Bhidayasiri R, Somers JT, Kim JI, et al. Ocular oscillations induced by shifts of the direction and depth of visual fixation. Ann Neurol 49, 24–28, 2001.
69. Bichot NP, Schall JD. Effects of similarity and history on neural mechanisms of visual selection. Nat Neurosci 2, 549–554, 1999.
70. Bichot NP, Thompson KG, Chenchal RS, Schall JD. Reliability of macaque frontal eye field neurons signaling saccade targets during visual search. J Neurosci 21, 713–725, 2001.
71. Biscaldi M, Fischer B, Aiple F. Saccadic eye movements of dyslexic and normal reading children. Perception 23, 45–64, 1994.
72. Biscaldi M, Fischer B, Hartnegg K. Voluntary saccadic control in dyslexia. Perception 29, 509–521, 2000.
73. Bisley JW, Goldberg ME. Neuronal activity in the lateral intraparietal area and spatial attention. Science 299, 81–86, 2003.
74. Blaes F, Fuhlhuber V, Korfei M, et al. Surface-binding autoantibodies to cerebellar neurons in opsoclonus syndrome. Ann Neurol 58, 313–317, 2005.
75. Blanke O, Seeck M. Direction of saccadic and smooth eye movements induced by electrical stimulation of the human frontal eye field: effect of orbital position. Exp Brain Res 150, 174–183, 2003.
76. Blekher T, Siemers E, Abel LA, Yee RD. Eye movements in Parkinson's disease: before and after pallidotomy. Invest Ophthalmol Vis Sci 41, 2177–2183, 2000.
77. Blohm G, Missal M, Lefevre P. Processing of retinal and extraretinal signals for memory guided saccades during smooth pursuit. J Neurophysiol, 2004.
78. Bloomberg JJ, Melvill Jones G, Segal B. Adaptive modification of vestibularly perceived rotation. Exp Brain Res 84, 47–56, 1991.
79. Bodis-Wollner I, Bucher SF, Seelos KC. Cortical activation patterns during voluntary blinks and voluntary saccades. Neurology 53, 1800–1805, 1999.
80. Boghen D, Troost BT, Daroff RB, Dell'Osso LF, Birkett JE. Velocity characteristics of normal human saccades. Invest Ophthalmol Vis Sci 13, 619–623, 1974.
81. Bollen E, Bax J, van Dijk JG, et al. Variability of the main sequence. Invest Ophthalmol Vis Sci 34, 3700–3704, 1993.
82. Bötzel K, Rottach K, Büttner U. Saccadic dynamic overshoot in normals and patients. Neuro-ophthalmology 13, 125–133, 1997.
83. Bracewell RM, Mazzoni P, Barash S, Andersen RA. Motor intention activity in the macaque's lateral intraparietal area. II. Changes of motor plan. J Neurophysiol 76, 1457–1464, 1996.
84. Brandt SA, Ploner CJ, Meyer BU, Leistner S, Villringer A. Effects of repetitive transcranial magnetic stimulation over dorsolateral prefrontal and posterior parietal cortex on memory-guided saccades. Exp Brain Res 188, 197–204, 1998.
85. Braun DI, Weber H, Mergner T, Schulte M. Saccadic reaction times in patients with frontal and parietal lesions. Brain 115, 1359–1386, 1992.
86. Breznen B, Gnadt JW. Analysis of the step response

of the saccadic feedback: computational models. Exp Brain Res 117, 181–191, 1997.
87. Bronstein AM, Kennard C. Predictive eye saccades are different from visually triggered saccades. Vision Res 27, 517–520, 1987.
88. Brotchie PR, Andersen RA, Snyder LH, Goodman SJ. Head position signals used by parietal neurons to encode locations of visual stimuli. Nature 375, 232–235, 1995.
89. Brotchie PR, Lee MB, Chen DY, et al. Head position modulates activity in the human parietal eye fields. Neuroimage. 18, 178–184, 2003.
90. Bruce CJ, Goldberg ME. Primate frontal eye fields. I. Single neurons discharging before saccades. J Neurophysiol 53, 603–635, 1985.
91. Bruce CJ, Goldberg ME, Bushnell MC, Stanton GB. Primate frontal eye fields. II. Physiological and anatomical correlates of electrically evoked eye movements. J Neurophysiol 54, 714–734, 1985.
91a. Bucci MP, Kapoula Z. Binocular coordination of saccades in 7 years old children in single word reading and target fixation. Vision Res, in press, 2005.
92. Burman DD, Bruce CJ. Suppression of task-related saccades by electrical stimulation in the primate's frontal eye field. J Neurophysiol 77, 2252–2267, 1997.
93. Burman DD, Segraves MA. Primate frontal eye field activity during natural scanning eye movements. J Neurophysiol 71, 1266–1271, 1994.
94. Burr DC, Morrone MC, Ross J. Selective suppression of the magnocellular visual pathway during saccadic eye movements. Nature 371, 511–513, 1997.
95. Busettini C, Mays LE. Pontine omnipause activity during conjugate and disconjugate eye movements in macaques. J Neurophysiol 90, 3838–3853, 2003.
96. Butler KM, Zacks RT, Henderson JM. Suppression of reflexive saccades in younger and older adults: age comparisons on an antisaccade task. Mem Cognit 27, 584–591, 1999.
97. Büttner U, Büttner-Ennever JA, Henn V. Vertical eye movement related unit activity in the rostral mesencephalic reticular formation of the alert monkey. Brain Res 130, 239–252, 1977.
98. Büttner-Ennever JA, Büttner U. The reticular formation. In Büttner-Enever JA (ed). Neuroanatomy of the Oculomotor System. New York, Elsevier, 1988, pp 119–176.
99. Büttner-Ennever JA, Cohen B, Pause M, Fries W. Raphe nucleus of pons containing omnipause neurons of the oculomotor system in the monkey, and its homologue in man. J Compar Neurol 267, 307–321, 1988.
100. Büttner-Ennever JA, Horn AK. Pathways from cell groups of the paramedian tracts to the floccular region. Ann N Y Acad Sci 781, 532–540, 1996.
101. Büttner-Ennever JA, Horn AK, Henn V, Cohen B. Projections from the superior colliculus motor map to omnipause neurons in monkey. J Comp Neurol 413, 55–67, 1999.
102. Cabel DW, Armstrong IT, Reingold E, Munoz DP. Control of saccade initiation in a countermanding task using visual and auditory stop signals. Exp Brain Res 133, 431–441, 2000.
103. Cai RH, Pouget A, Schlag-Rey M, Schlag J. Perceived geometrical relationships affected by eye-movement signals. Nature 386, 601–604, 1998.
104. Cairney S, Maruff P, Vance A, et al. Contextual abnormalities of saccadic inhibition in children with attention deficit hyperactivity disorder. Exp Brain Res 141, 507–518, 2001.
105. Campbell FW, Wurtz RH. Saccadic omission: why we do not see a grey out during a saccadic eye movement. Vision Res 18, 1297–1303, 1978.
106. Campos M, Breznen B, Bernheim K, Andersen RA. The supplementary motor area encodes reward expectancy in eye movement tasks. J Neurophysiol 94, 1325–1335, 2005.
107. Carpenter RH. Express saccades: is bimodality a result of the order of stimulus presentation? Vision Res 41, 1145–1151, 2001.
107a. Carpenter RH. Contrast, probability, and saccadic latency; evidence for independence of detection and decision. Curr Biol 14, 1576–1580, 2004.
108. Carpenter RHS. Movements of the Eyes. Pion, London, 1988.
109. Carter JE, Obler L, Woodward S, Albert M.L. The effect of increasing age on the latency for saccadic eye movements. J Gerontology 38, 318–320, 1983.
110. Castet E, Jeanjean S, Masson GS. Motion perception of saccade-induced retinal translation. Proc Natl Acad Sci U S A 99, 15159–15163, 2002.
111. Chafee MV, Goldman-Rakic PS. Inactivation of parietal and prefrontal cortex reveals interdependence of neural activity during memory-guided saccades. J Neurophysiol 83, 1550–1566, 2000.
112. Chan F, Armstrong IT, Pari G, Riopelle RJ, Munoz D.P. Deficits in saccadic eye-movement control in Parkinson's disease. Neuropsychologia 43, 784–796, 2005.
113. Chen B, May PJ. The feedback circuit connecting the superior colliculus and central mesencephalic reticular formation: a direct morphological demonstration. Exp Brain Res 131, 10–21, 2000.
114. Chen LT, Wise SP. Supplementary eye field contrasted with frontal eye field during acquisition of conditional oculomotor associations. J Neurophysiol 73, 1122–1134, 1995.
115. Ciuffreda KJ, Kenyon RV, Stark L. Increased saccadic latencies in amblyopic eyes. Invest Ophthalmol Vis Sci 17, 697–702, 1978.
116. Ciuffreda KJ, Kenyon RV, Stark L. Eye movements during reading: further case reports. Am J Optom Physiol Optics 62, 844–852, 1985.
117. Coe B, Tomihara K, Matsuzawa M, Hikosaka O. Visual and anticipatory bias in three cortical eye fields of the monkey during an adaptive decision-making task. J Neurosci 22, 5081–5090, 2002.
118. Cohen B, Komatsuzaki A. Eye movements induced by stimulation of the pontine reticular formation: evidence for integration in oculomotor pathways. Exp Neurol 36, 101–117, 1972.
119. Cohen B, Matsuo V, Fradin J, Raphan T. Horizontal saccades induced by stimulation of the central mesencephalic reticular formation. Exp Brain Res 57, 605–616, 1985.
120. Colby CL, Duhamel JR, Goldberg ME. Visual, presaccadic, and cognitive activation of single neurons in monkey lateral intraparietal area. J Neurophysiol 76, 2841–2852, 1996.
121. Collewijn H, Erkelens CJ, Steinman RM. Binocular co- ordination of human vertical saccadic eye movements. J Physiol (Lond) 404, 183–197, 1988.
122. Collewijn H, Erkelens CJ, Steinman RM. Binocular co-ordination of human horizontal saccadic eye movements. J Physiol (Lond) 404, 157–182, 1988.

123. Collewijn H, Van der Steen J, Steinman RM. Human eye movements associated with blinks and prolonged eyelid closure. J Neurophysiol 54, 11–27, 1985.
124. Colonius H, Ozyurt J, Arndt PA. Countermanding saccades with auditory stop signals: testing the race model. Vision Res 41, 1951–1968, 2001.
125. Condy C, Rivaud-Pechoux S, Ostendorf F, Ploner CJ, Gaymard B. Neural substrate of antisaccades. Role of subcortical structures. Neurology 63, 1571–1578, 2004.
126. Connolly JD, Goodale MA, Menon RS, Munoz DP. Human fMRI evidence for the neural correlates of preparatory set. Nat Neurosci 5, 1345–1352, 2002.
127. Constantinidis C, Franowicz MN, Goldman-Rakic PS. Coding specificity in cortical microcircuits: a multiple-electrode analysis of primate prefrontal cortex. J Neurosci 21, 3646–3655, 2001.
128. Constantinidis C, Franowicz MN, Goldman-Rakic PS. The sensory nature of mnemonic representation in the primate prefrontal cortex. Nat Neurosci 4, 311–316, 2001.
129. Cowie RJ, Robinson DL. Subcortical contributions to head movements in macaques. 1. Contrasting effects of electrical stimulation of a medial pontomedullary region and the superior colliculus. J Neurophysiol 72, 2648–2664, 1994.
130. Crandall WF, Keller EL. Visual and oculomotor signals in the nucleus reticularis tegmenti pontis in alert monkey. J Neurophysiol 54, 1326–1345, 1985.
131. Crawford JD, Cadera W, Vilis T. Generation of torsional and vertical eye position signals by the interstitial nucleus of Cajal. Science 252, 1551–1553, 1991.
132. Crawford JD, Guitton D. Visual-motor transformations required for accurate and kinematically correct saccades. J Neurophysiol 78, 1447–1467, 1997.
133. Crawford TJ, Higham S. Dyslexia and the centre-of-gravity effect. Exp Brain Res 137, 122–126, 2001.
133a. Crawford TJ, Hill S, Higham S. The inhibitory effect of a recent distracter. Vision Res 45, 3365–3378, 2005.
134. Currie JN, Goldberg ME, Matsuo V, Fitzgibbon EJ. Dyslexia with saccadic intrusions: a treatable reading disorder. Neurology 36 (Suppl), 134, 1986.
135. Currie JN, Ramsden B, McArthur C, Maruff P. Validation of a clinical antisaccade eye movement test in the assessment of dementia. Arch Neurol 48, 644–648, 1991.
136. Cynader M, Berman N. Receptive field organization of monkey superior colliculus. J Neurophysiol 35, 187–201, 1972.
137. Dassonville P, Schlag J, Schlag-Rey M. The use of egocentric and exocentric location cues in saccadic programming. Vision Res 35, 2191–2199, 1995.
138. de Brouwer S, Yuksel D, Blohm G, Missal M, Lefevre P. What triggers catch-up saccades during visual tracking? J Neurophysiol 87, 1646–1650, 2002.
139. De Luca M, Borrelli M, Judica A, Spinelli D, Zoccolotti P. Reading words and pseudowords: an eye movement study of developmental dyslexia. Brain Lang 80, 617–626, 2002.
140. De Luca M, Di Pace E, Judica A, Spinell D, Zoccolotti P. Eye movement patterns in linguistic and non-linguistic tasks in developmental surface dyslexia. Neuropsychologia 37, 1407–1420, 1999.
141. Demer JL. Pivotal role of orbital connective tissues in binocular alignment and strabismus. Invest Ophthalmol Vis Sci 45, 729–738, 2004.
142. Demer JL, Miller JM, Poukens V, Vinters HV, Glasgow BJ. Evidence for fibromuscular pulleys of the recti extraocular muscles. Invest Ophthalmol Vis Sci 36, 1125–1136, 1995.
143. Desmurget M, Pelisson D, Urquizai C, et al. Functional adaptation of reactive saccades in humans: a PET study. Exp Brain Res 132, 243–259, 2000.
144. Desouza JF, Menon RS, Everling S. Preparatory set associated with pro-saccades and anti-saccades in humans investigated with event-related FMRI. J Neurophysiol 89, 1016–1023, 2003.
145. Deubel H. Adaptivity of gain and direction in oblique saccades. In O'Regan JK, Levy-Schoen A (eds). Eye Movements: From Physiology to Cognition. New York, Elsevier, 1987, pp 181–190.
146. Deubel H. Sensory and motor aspects of saccade control. Eur Arch Psychiatr Neurol Sci 239, 17–22, 1989.
147. Deubel H. Separate adaptive mechanims for the control of reactive and volitional saccadic eye movements. Vision Res 35, 3529–3540, 1995.
148. Deubel H. In Gopher D, Koriat A (eds). Attention and Performance XVII. Cambridge, MIT Press, 1998.
149. Deubel H, Bridgeman B, Schneider WX. Immediate post-saccadic information mediates space constancy. Vision Res 38, 3147–3159, 1998.
150. Deubel H, Schneider WX, Bridgeman B. Post-saccadic target blanking prevents saccadic suppression of image displacement. Vision Res 36, 985–996, 1996.
151. Deubel H, Wolf W, Hauske G. Corrective saccades: effect of shifting the saccade goal. Vision Res 22, 353–364, 1982.
152. Deubel H, Wolf W, Hauske G. Adaptive gain control of saccadic eye movements. Human Neurobiol 5, 245–253, 1986.
153. Diamond MR, Ross J, Morrone MC. Extraretinal control of saccadic suppression. J Neurosci 20, 3449–3455, 2000.
154. Dias EC, Bruce CJ. Physiological correlate of fixation disengagement in the primate's frontal eye field. J Neurophysiol 72, 2532–2537, 1994.
155. Dias EC, Segraves MA. Muscimol-induced inactivation of monkey frontal eye field: effects on visually and memory-guided saccades. J Neurophysiol 81, 2191–2214, 1999.
156. Dicke PW, Barash S, Ilg UJ, Their P. Single-neuron evidence for a contribution of the dorsal pontine nuclei to both types of target-directed eye movements, saccades and smooth-pursuit. Eur J Neurosci 19, 609–624, 2004.
157. Dodge R. Five types of eye movement in the horizontal meridian plane of the field of regard. Am J Physiol 8, 307–329, 1919.
158. Doig HR, Boylan C. Presaccadic spike potentials with large horizontal eye movements. Electrocephal Clin Neurophysiol 73, 260–263, 1989.
159. Doma H, Hallett PE. Dependence of saccadic eye-movements on stimulus luminance and an effect of task. Vision Res 28, 915–924, 1988.
160. Doma H, Hallett PE. Rod-cone dependence of saccadic eye-movement latency in a foveating task. Vision Res 28, 899–913, 1988.
161. Donner T, Kettermann A, Diesch A, et al. Involvement of the human frontal eye field and mul-

tiple parietal areas in covert visual selection during conjunction search. Eur J Neurosci 12, 3407–3414, 2000.
162. Doricchi F, Pernai D, Inococcia C, et al. Neural control of fast-regular saccades and antisaccades: an investigation using positron emission tomography. Exp Brain Res 116, 50–62, 1997.
163. Dorris MC, Klein RM, Everling S, Munoz DP. Contribution of the primate superior colliculus to inhibition of return. J Cogn Neurosci 14, 1256–1263, 2002.
164. Dorris MC, Munoz DP. A neural correlate for the gap effect on saccadic reaction times in monkey. J Neurophysiol 73, 2558–2562, 1995.
165. Dorris MC, Munoz DP. Saccadic probability influences motor preparation signals and time to saccadic initiation. J Neurosci 18, 7015–7026, 1998.
166. Doslak MJ, Healey EC, Riese K. Eye movements of stutterers. Invest Ophthalmol Vis Sci 27, 1410–1414, 1986.
167. Doslak MJ, Kline LB, Dell'Osso LF, Daroff RB. Internuclear ophthalmoplegia: recovery and plasticity. Invest Ophthalmol Vis Sci 19, 1506–1511, 1980.
168. Doyle MC, Walker R. Multisensory interactions in saccade target selection: curved saccade trajectories. Exp Brain Res 142, 116–130, 2002.
169. Duhamel J-R, Colby CL, Goldberg ME. The updating of the representation of visual space in parietal cortex by intended eye movements. Science 255, 90–92, 1992.
170. Duhamel J-R, Goldberg ME, Fitzgibbon EJ, Sirigu A, Grafman J. Saccadic dysmetria in a patient with a right frontoparietal lesion: the importance of corollary disharge for accurate spatial-behavior. Brain 115, 1387–1402, 1992.
171. Edelman JA, Goldberg ME. Dependence of saccade-related activity in the primate superior colliculus on visual target presence. J Neurophysiol 86, 676–691, 2001.
172. Edelman JA, Goldberg ME. Effect of short-term saccadic adaptation on saccades evoked by electrical stimulation in the primate superior colliculus. J Neurophysiol 87, 1915–1923, 2002.
173. Edelman JA, Keller EL. Activity of visuomotor burst neurons in the superior colliculus accompanying express saccades. J Neurophysiol 76, 908–926, 1997.
173a. Edelman JA. Valenzuela N, Barton JJ. Antisaccade velocity, but not latency, results from a lack of saccade visual guidance. Vision Res, in press, 2005.
174. Eden GF, Stein JF, Wood HM, Wood FB. Differences in eye movements and reading problems in dyslexic and normal children. Vision Res 34, 1345–1358, 1997.
175. Eggert T, Ditterich J, Robinson FR, Straube A. Effects of intrasaccadic target steps on the latency of corrective saccades. Soc Neurosci Abstr 23, 757, 1997.
176. Eggert T, Guan Y, Bayer O, Büttner U. Saccades to moving targets. Ann N Y Acad Sci 1039, 149–159, 2005.
177. Eggert T, Sailer U, Ditterich J, Straube A. Differential effect of a distractor on primary saccades and perceptual localization. Vision Res 42, 2969–2984, 2002.
178. Elkington PT, Kerr GK, Stein JS. The effect of electromagnetic stimulation of the posterior parietal cortex on eye movements. Eye 6, 510–514, 1992.
179. Enright JT. Convergence during human vertical saccades: probable causes and perceptual consequences. J Physiol (Lond) 410, 45–65, 1989.
180. Epelboim J, Booth JR, Ashkenazy R, Taleghani A, Steinman RM. Fillers and spaces in text: the importance of word recognition during reading. Vision Res 37, 2899–2914, 1997.
181. Epelboim J, Booth JR, Steinman RM. Reading unspaced text: implications for theories of reading eye movements. Vision Res 34, 1735–1766, 1994.
182. Epelboim J, Booth JR, Steinman RM. Much ado about nothing: the place of space in text. Vision Res 36, 465–470, 1996.
183. Epelboim J, Steinman RM, Kowler E, et al. The function of visual search and memory in sequential looking tasks. Vision Res 35, 3401–3422, 1995.
184. Epelboim J, Steinman RM, Kowler E, et al. Gaze-shift dynamics in two kinds of sequential looking tasks. Vision Res 37, 2597–2607, 1997.
185. Erkelens CJ, Sloot OB. Initial directions and landing positions of binocular saccades. Vision Res 35, 3297–3303, 1995.
186. Ettl A, Pringlinger S, Kramer J, Koornneef L. Functional anatomy of the levator palpebrae superioris and its connective tissue system. Br J Ophthalmol 80, 702–707, 1996.
187. Evdokimidis I, Smyrnis N, Constantinidis TN, et al. The antisaccade task in a sample of 2,006 young men. I. Normal population characteristics. Exp Brain Res 147, 45–52, 2002.
188. Everling S, Paré M, Dorris MC, Munoz DP. Comparison of the discharge charactersitics of brain stem omipause neurons and superior colliculus fixation neurons in monkey: implications for control of fixation and saccade behavior. J Neurophysiol 79, 511–528, 1998.
189. Evinger LC. A brain stem reflex in the blink of an eye. News in Physiological Science 10, 147–153, 1995.
190. Evinger LC, Manning KA. Pattern of extraocular muscle activation during reflex blinking. Exp Brain Res 92, 502–506, 1993.
191. Evinger LC, Manning KA, Pellegrini JJ, et al. Not looking while leaping: the linkage of blinking and saccadic gaze shifts. Exp Brain Res 100, 337–344, 1994.
192. Evinger LC, Manning KA, Sibony PA. Eyelid movements. Mechanisms and normal data. Invest Ophthalmol Vis Sci 32, 387–400, 1991.
193. Fawcett AP, Dostrovsky JO, Lozano AM, Hutchison WD. Eye movement-related responses of neurons in human subthalamic nucleus. Exp Brain Res 162, 357–365, 2005.
194. Ferraina S, Pare M, Wurtz RH. Comparison of cortico-cortical and cortico-collicular signals for the generation of saccadic eye movements. J Neurophysiol 87, 845–858, 2002.
195. Ferrier D. The localization of function in the brain. Proc R Soc Lond (B Vol) 22, 229, 1874.
196. Findlay JM. Global visual processing for saccadic eye movements. Vision Res 22, 1033–1045, 1982.
196a. Findlay JM, Brown V. Eye scanning of multi-element displays: I. Scanpath planning. Vision Res, in press, 2005.
196b. Findlay JM, Brown V. Eye scanning of multi-element displays: II. Saccade planning. Vision Res, in press, 2005.
197. Fischer B, Weber H. Effects of stimulus conditions

on the performance of antisaccades in man. Exp Brain Res 116, 191–200, 1997.

198. Fischer B. The preparation of visually guided saccades. Rev Physiol Biochem Pharmacol 106, 2–35, 1987.
199. Fischer B, Gezeck S, Hartnegg K. On the production and correction of involuntary prosaccades in a gap antisaccade task. Vision Res 40, 2211–2217, 2000.
200. Fischer B, Hartnegg K, Mokler A. Dynamic visual perception of dyslexic children. Perception 29, 523–530, 2000.
201. Fischer B, Ramsperger E. Human express saccades: extremely short reaction times of goal directed eye movements. Exp Brain Res 57, 191–195, 1984.
202. Fischer B, Ramsperger E. Human express saccades: effects of randomization and daily practice. Exp Brain Res 64, 569–578, 1986.
203. Fischer B, Weber H. Express saccades and visual attention. Behavioral and Brain Sciences 16, 553–610, 1993.
204. Fletcher WA, Sharpe JA. Saccadic eye movement dysfunction in Alzheimer's disease. Ann Neurol 20, 464–471, 1986.
205. Ford KA, Goltz HC, Brown MR, Everling S. Neural processes associated with anti-saccade task performance investigated with event-related fMRI. J Neurophysiol, 94, 429–440, 2005.
206. Foville AL. Note sur une paralysie peu connue de certains muscles de l'oeil, et sa liaison avec quelques points dfe l'anatomie et la physiologie de la protubérance annulaire. Société de Anatomie (Paris) 33, 393–414, 1858.
207. Frank MJ, Seeberger LC, O'Reilly RC. By carrot or stick: cognitive reinforcement learning in Parkinsonism. Science 306, 1940–1943, 2004.
208. Friedman HR, Burman DD, Russo GS, et al. Neuronal activity in primate frontal eye field during memory guided saccades. Soc Neurosci Abstr 23, 844, 1997.
209. Frohman EM, Frohman TC, O'Suilleabhain P, et al. Quantitative oculographic characterisation of internuclear ophthalmoparesis in multiple sclerosis: the versional dysconjugacy index Z score. J Neurol Neurosurg Psychiatry 73, 51–55, 2002.
210. Frohman TC, Frohman EM, O'Suilleabhain P, et al. Accuracy of clinical detection of INO in MS: corroboration with quantitative infrared oculography. Neurology 61, 848–850, 2003.
211. Fuchs AF, Becker W, Ling L, Langer TP, Kaneko CRS. Discharge patterns of levator palpebrae superioris motoneurons during vertical lid and eye movements in the monkey. J Neurophysiol 68, 233–243, 1992.
212. Fuchs AF, Reiner D, Pong M. Transfer of gain changes from targeting to other types of saccades in the monkey: constraints on possible sites of gain adaptation. J Neurophysiol 76, 2522–2535, 1996.
213. Fuchs AF, Robinson FR, Straube A. Role of the caudal fastigial nucleus in saccade generation: I. Neuronal discharge patterns. J Neurophysiol 70, 1723–1740, 1993.
214. Fukushima J, Fukishima K, Chiba T, et al. Disturbances of voluntary control of saccadic eye movements in schizophrenic patients. Biol Psychiatry 23, 670–677, 1988.
215. Fukushima J, Hatta T, Fukushima K. Development of voluntary control of saccadic eye movements. I. Age-related changes in normal children. Brain Dev 22, 173–180, 2000.
216. Fuller JH. Eye position and target amplitude effects on human visual saccadic latencies. Exp Brain Res 109, 457–466, 1996.
217. Funahashi S, Bruce CJ, Goldman-Rakic PS. Neuronal activity related to saccadic eye movements in the monkey's dorsolateral prefrontal cortex. J Neurophysiol 65, 1464–1484, 1991.
218. Galetta SL, Raps EC, Liu GT, Saito NG, Kline LB. Eyelid lag without eyelid retraction in pretectal disease. J Neuro-ophthalmol 16, 96–98, 1996.
219. Gancarz G, Grossberg S. A neural model of the saccade generator in the reticular formation. Neural Netw. 11, 1159–1174, 1998.
220. Gandhi NJ, Keller EL. Spatial distribution and discharge characteristics of superior colliculus neurons antidromically activated from the omnipause region in monkey. J Neurophysiol 78, 2221–2225, 1997.
221. Gandhi NJ, Keller EL. Activity of the brain stem omnipause neurons during saccades perturbed by stimulation of the primate superior colliculus. J Neurophysiol 82, 3254–3267, 1999.
222. Gandhi NJ, Keller EL. Comparison of saccades perturbed by stimulation of the rostral superior colliculus, the caudal superior colliculus, and the omnipause neuron region. J Neurophysiol 82, 3236–3253, 1999.
223. Garbutt S, Han Y, Kumar AN, et al. Vertical optokinetic nystagmus and saccades in normal human subjects. Invest Ophthalmol Vis Sci 44, 3833–3841, 2003.
224. Garbutt S, Harwood MR, Harris CM. Comparison of the main sequence of reflexive saccades and the quick phases of optokinetic nystagmus. Br J Ophthalmol 85, 1477–1483, 2001.
225. Garbutt S, Harwood MR, Kumar AN, HanYH, Leigh RJ. Evaluating small eye movements in patients with saccadic palsies. Ann N Y Acad Sci 1004, 337–346, 2003.
226. Garbutt S, Riley DE, Kumar AN, et al. Abnormalities of optokinetic nystagmus in progressive supranuclear palsy. J Neurol Neurosurg Psychiatry 75, 1386–1394, 2004.
227. Garcia-Perez MA, Peli E. Intrasaccadic perception. J Neurosci 21, 7313–7322, 2001.
228. Gauthier GM, Nommay D, Vercher, J-L. The role of ocular muscle proprioception in visual localization of targets. Science 249, 58–61, 1990.
229. Gaveau V, Martin O, Prablanc C, et al. On-line modification of saccadic eye movements by retinal signals. Neuroreport 14, 875–878, 2003.
230. Gaymard B, Francois C, Ploner CJ, Condy C, Rivaud-Pechoux S. A direct prefrontotectal tract against distractibility in the human brain. Ann Neurol 53, 542–545, 2003.
231. Gaymard B, Lynch J, Ploner CJ, Condy C, Rivaud-Pechoux S. The parieto-collicular pathway: anatomical location and contribution to saccade generation. Eur J Neurosci 17, 1518–1526, 2003.
232. Gaymard B, Pierrot-Deseilligny C, Rivaud S. Impairment of sequences of memory-guided saccades after supplementary motor area lesions. Ann Neurol 28, 622–626, 1990.
233. Gaymard B, Ploner CJ, Rivaud-Pechoux S, Pierrot-Deseilligny C. The frontal eye field is involved in spatial short-term memory but not in reflexive saccade inhibition. Exp Brain Res 129, 288–301, 1999.

234. Gaymard B, Rivaud S, Cassarini JF, et al. Effects of anterior cingulate cortex lesions on ocular saccades in humans. Exp Brain Res 120, 173–183, 1998.
235. Gaymard B, Rivaud S, Pierrot-Deseilligny C. Role of the left and right supplementary motor areas in memory-guided saccade sequences. Ann Neurol 34, 404–406, 1993.
236. Gaymard B, Rivaud S, Pierrot-Deseilligny C. Impairment of extraretinal eye position signals after central thalamic lesions in humans. Exp Brain Res 102, 1–9, 1994.
237. Gaymard B, Rivaud-Pechoux S, Yelnik J, Pidoux B, Ploner CJ. Involvement of the cerebellar thalamus in human saccade adaptation. Eur J Neurosci 14, 554–560, 2001.
238. Gellman RS, Carl JR. Early responses to double-step targets are independent of step size. Exp Brain Res 87, 433–437, 1991.
239. Gerrits NM, Voogd J. The nucleus reticularis tegmenti pontis and the adjacent rostral paramedian pontine reticular formation: differential projections to the cerebellum and the caudal brainstem. Exp Brain Res 62, 29–45, 1986.
239a. Girard B, Berthoz A. From brainstem to cortex: Computational models of saccade generation circuitry. Prog Neurobiol 77, 215–251, 2005.
240. Gitelman DR, Parrish TB, Friston KJ, Mesulam,M.M. Functional anatomy of visual search: regional segregations within the frontal eye fields and effective connectivity of the superior colliculus. Neuroimage 15, 970–982, 2002.
241. Glimcher PW, Sparks DL. Movement selection in advance of action in the superior colliculus. Nature 355, 542–545, 1992.
242. Gochin PM, McElligott JG. Saccades to visual targets are uncompensated after cerebellar stimulation. Exp Neurol 97, 219–224, 1987.
243. Goday J, Luders H, Dinner DS, Morris HH, Wylie E. Versive eye movements elicited by cortical stimulation of the human brain. Neurology 40, 296–299, 1990.
244. Goffart L, Chen LL, Sparks DL. Saccade dysmetria during functional perturbation of the caudal fastigial nucleus in the monkey. Ann N Y Acad Sci 1004, 220–228, 2003.
245. Goldberg ME, Bisley J, Powell KD, Gottlieb J, Kusunoki M. The role of the lateral intraparietal area of the monkey in the generation of saccades and visuospatial attention. Ann N Y Acad Sci 956, 205–215, 2002.
246. Goldberg ME, Bruce CJ. Primate frontal eye fields. III. Maintenance of a spatially accurate saccade signal. J Neurophysiol 64, 489–508, 1990.
247. Goossens H.H, van Opstal AJ. Blink-perturbed saccades in monkey. I. Behavioral analysis. J. Neurophysiol. 83, 3411–3429, 2000.
248. Goossens HH, van Opstal AJ. Blink-perturbed saccades in monkey. II. Superior colliculus activity. J Neurophysiol 83, 3430–3452, 2000.
249. Goossens HHLM, van Opstal AJ. Local feedback signals are not distorted by prior eye movements: evidence from visually evoked double saccades. J Neurophysiol 78, 533–538, 1997.
250. Gottlieb J, Goldberg ME. Activity of neurons in the lateral intraparietal area of the monkey during an antisaccade task. Nat Neurosci 2, 906–912, 1999.
251. Gowen E, Abadi RV. Saccadic instabilities and voluntary saccadic behaviour. Exp Brain Res 164, 29–40, 2005.
252. Grantyn A, Brandi AM, Dubayle D, et al. Density gradients of trans-synaptically labeled collicular neurons after injections of rabies virus in the lateral rectus muscle of the rhesus monkey. J Comp Neurol 451, 346–361, 2002.
253. Groh JM, Sparks DL. Saccades to somatosensory targets. 2. Motor convergence in primate superior colliculus. J Neurophysiol 75, 428–438, 1996.
254. Groner R, Groner MT. Attention and eye movement control: an overview. Eur Arch Psychiatr Neurol Sci 239, 9–16, 1989.
255. Grosbras MH, Leonards U, Lobel E, et al. Human cortical networks for new and familiar sequences of saccades. Cereb Cortex 11, 936–945, 2001.
256. Grosbras MH, Lobel E, Van de Moortele PF, LeBihan D, Berthoz A. An anatomical landmark for the supplementary eye fields in human revealed with functional magnetic resonance imaging. Cereb Cortex 9, 705–711, 1999.
257. Grossberg SG, Roberts K, Aguilar M, Bullock D. A neural model of multimodal adaptive saccadic eye movement control by superior colliculus. J Neurosci 15, 9706–9725, 1997.
258. Grossman GE, Robinson DA. Ambivalence in modelling oblique saccades. Biol Cybern 58, 13–18, 1988.
259. Guan Y, Eggert T, Bayer O, Büttner U. Saccades to stationary and moving targets differ in the monkey. Exp Brain Res, 2004.
260. Guitton D, Buchtel HA, Douglas RM. Frontal lobe lesions in man cause difficulties in suppressing reflexive glances and in generating goal-directed saccades. Exp Brain Res 58, 455–472, 1985.
261. Guitton D, Munoz DP, Galiana HL. Gaze control in the cat: studies and modeling of the coupling between orienting eye and head movements in different behavioral tasks. J Neurophysiol 64, 509–531, 1990.
262. Guitton D, Simard R, Codère F. Upper eyelid movements measured with a search coil during blinks and vertical saccades. Invest Ophthalmol Vis Sci 32, 3298–3305, 1991.
263. Guthrie BL, Porter JD, Sparks DL. Corollary discharge provides accurate eye position information to the oculomotor system. Science 221, 1193–1195, 1983.
264. Hain TC, Zee DS, Mordes M. Blink-induced saccadic oscillations. Ann Neurol 19, 299–301, 1986.
265. Hallet PE. Primary and secondary saccades to goals defined by instructions. Vision Res 18, 1279–1296, 1997.
266. Handel A, Glimcher PW. Response properties of saccade-related burst neurons in the central mesencephalic reticular formation. J Neurophysiol 78, 2164–2175, 1997.
267. Handel A, Glimcher PW. Quantitative analysis of substantia nigra pars reticulata activity during a visually guided saccade task. J Neurophysiol 82, 3458–3475, 1999.
268. Handel A, Glimcher PW. Contextual modulation of substantia nigra pars reticulata neurons. J Neurophysiol. 83, 3042–3048, 2000.
269. Hanes DP, Carpenter RH. Countermanding saccades in humans. Vision Res 39, 2777–2791, 1999.
270. Hanes DP, Patterson WF, Schall JD. Role of frontal eye fields in countermanding saccades: visual, movement, and fixation activity. J Neurophysiol 79, 817–834, 1998.

271. Hanes DP, Smith MK, Optican LM, Wurtz R.H. Recovery of saccadic dysmetria following localized lesions in monkey superior colliculus. Exp Brain Res 160, 325, 2005.
272. Hanes DP, Wurtz RH. Interaction of the frontal eye field and superior colliculus for saccade generation. J Neurophysiol 85, 804–815, 2001.
273. Hanson MR, Hamid MA, Tomsak RL, Chou SS, Leigh RJ. Selective saccadic palsy caused by pontine lesions: clinical, physiological, and pathological correlations. Ann Neurol 20, 209–217, 1986.
274. Hartje W. Reading disturbances in the presence of oculomotor disorders. Eur Neurol 7, 249–264, 1972.
275. Hartwich-Young R, Nelson JS, Sparks DL. The perihypoglossal projections to the superior colliculus in the rhesus monkey. Vis Neurosci 4, 29–42, 1990.
276. Harwood MR, Harris CM. Time-optimality and the spectral overlap of saccadic eye movements. Ann N Y Acad Sci 956, 414–417, 2002.
277. Harwood MR, Mezey LE, Harris CM. The spectral main sequence of human saccades. J Neurosci 19, 9098–9106, 1999.
278. Hasegawa R, Sawaguchi T, Kubota K. Monkey prefrontal neuronal activity coding the forthcoming saccade in an oculomotor delayed matching-to-sample task. J Neurophysiol 79, 322–333, 1998.
279. Hasegawa RP, Matsumoto M, Mikami A. Search target selection in monkey prefrontal cortex. J Neurophysiol 84, 1692–1696, 2000.
279a. Hayakawa Y, Nakajima T, Takagi M, Fukuhara N, Abe H. Human cerebellar activation in relation to saccadic eye movements: A functional magnetic resonance imaging study. Ophthalmologica 216, 399–405, 2002.
280. Heide W, Binkofski F, Seitz RJ, et al. Activation of frontoparietal cortices during memorized triple-step sequences of saccadic eye movements: an fMRI study. Eur J Neurosci 13, 1177–1189, 2001.
281. Heide W, Blankenburg M, Zimmerman E. Cortical control of double-step saccades: implications for spatial orientation. Ann Neurol 38, 739–748, 1995.
282. Helmchen C, Rambold H, Erdmann C, et al. The role of the fastigial nucleus in saccadic eye oscillations. Ann N Y Acad Sci 1004, 229–240, 2003.
283. Helmchen C, Straube A, Büttner U. Saccade-related activity in the fastigial oculomotor region of the macaque monkey during spontaneous eye movements in light and darkness. Exp Brain Res 98, 474–482, 1994.
284. Helmholtz H. Treatise on Physiological Optics. Dover Press, New York, 1962.
285. Helminski JO, Segraves MA. Macaque frontal eye field input to saccade-related neurons in the superior colliculus. J Neurophysiol 90, 1046–1062, 2003.
286. Henn V, Hepp K, Vilis T. Rapid eye movement generation in the primate. Physiology, pathophysiology, and clinical implications. Rev Neurol (Paris) 145, 540–545, 1989.
287. Henn V, Lang W, Hepp K, Reisine H. Experimental gaze palsies in monkeys and their relation to human pathology. Brain 107, 619–636, 1984.
288. Hepp K, Henn V. Spatio-temporal recoding of rapid eye movement signals in the monkey paramedian pontine reticular formation (PPRF). Exp Brain Res 52, 105–120, 1983.
289. Hepp K, Henn V, Vilis T, Cohen B. In Wurtz RH, Goldberg ME (eds). The Neurobiology of Saccadic Eye Movements. Amsterdam, Elsevier, 1989, pp 105–212.
290. Herishanu Y, Abarbanel JM, Frisher S. Blink induced ocular flutter. Neuro-ophthalmology 7, 175–177, 1987.
291. Heywood S, Ratcliff G. Long-term oculomotor consequences of unilateral colliculectomy in man. In Lennerstrand G, Bach-y-Rita P (eds). Basic Mechanisms of Ocular Motility and their Clinical Implications. Pergamon Press, 1975, pp 561–564.
292. Hikosaka O, Nakamura K, Sakai K, Nakahara H. Central mechanisms of motor skill learning. Curr Opin Neurobiol 12, 217–222, 2002.
293. Hikosaka O, Sakamoto M, Miyashita N. Effects of caudate nucleus stimulation on substantia nigra cell activity in monkey. Exp Brain Res 95, 457–472, 1993.
294. Hikosaka O, Sakamoto M, Usui S. Functional properties of monkey caudate neurons. I. Activities related to saccadic eye movements. J Neurophysiol 61, 780–798, 1989.
295. Hikosaka O, Sakamoto M, Usui S. Functional properties of monkey caudate neurons. II. Visual and auditory responses. J Neurophysiol 61, 799–813, 1989.
296. Hikosaka O, Sakamoto M, Usui S. Functional properties of monkey caudate neurons. III. Activities related to expectation of target and reward. J Neurophysiol 61, 814–832, 1989.
297. Hikosaka O, TakikawaY, Kawagoe R. Role of the basal ganglia in the control of purposive saccadic eye movements. Physiol Rev 80, 953–978, 2000.
298. Hikosaka O, Wurtz RH. Visual and oculomotor functions of monkey substantia nigra pars reticulata. I. Relation of visual and auditory responses to saccades. J Neurophysiol 49, 1230–1253, 1983.
299. Hikosaka O, Wurtz RH. Visual and oculomotor functions of monkey substantia nigra pars reticulata. II. Visual responses related to fixation of gaze. J Neurophysiol 49, 1254–1267, 1983.
300. Hikosaka O, Wurtz RH. Visual and oculomotor functions of monkey substantia nigra pars reticulata. III. Memory-contingent visual and saccade responses. J Neurophysiol 49, 1268–1284, 1983.
301. Hikosaka O, Wurtz R.H. Visual and oculomotor functions of monkey substantia nigra pars reticulata. IV. Relation of substantia nigra to superior colliculus. J Neurophysiol 49, 1285–1301, 1983.
302. Hikosaka O, Wurtz RH. Modification of saccadic eye movements by GABA-related substances. I. Effect of muscimol and bicuculline in monkey superior colliculus. J Neurophysiol 53, 266–291, 1985.
303. Hikosaka O, Wurtz RH. Modification of saccadic eye movements by GABA-related substances. II. Effects of muscimol in monkey substantia nigra pars reticulata. J Neurophysiol 53, 292–308, 1985.
304. Hikosaka O, Wurtz RH. Saccadic eye movements following injection of lidocaine into the superior colliculus. Exp Brain Res 61, 531–539, 1986.
305. Hitzig E. Physiologische und klinische Untersuchungen uber das Gehirn. Gesammelte Abbandlungen. Part I. Hirschwald, Berlin, 1874.
306. Hodgson TL, Mort D, Chamberlain MM, et al. Orbitofrontal cortex mediates inhibition of return. Neuropsychologia 40, 1891–1901, 2002.
307. Honda H. The time courses of visual mislocalization and of extraretinal eye position signals at the time of vertical saccades. Vision Res 31, 1915–1921, 1991.
308. Honda H. Idiosyncratic left-right asymmetries of

saccadic latencies: examination in a gap paradigm. Vision Res 42, 1437–1445, 2002.
308a. Honda H. The remote distractor effect of saccade latencies in fixation-offset and overlap conditions. Vision Res 45, 2773-2779, 2005.
309. Hopp JJ, Fuchs AF. Investigating the site of human saccadic adaptation with express and targeting saccades. Exp Brain Res 144, 538–548, 2002.
310. Hopp JJ, Fuchs AF. The characteristics and neuronal substrate of saccadic eye movement plasticity. Progr Neurobiol 72, 27–53, 2004.
311. Horn AKE. The reticular formation. In Büttner-Ennever JA (ed). Neuroanatomy of the Oculomotor System. Prog Brain Res 151, 127–156, 2006.
312. Horn AKE, Büttner-Enever JA, Gayde M, Messoudi A. Neuroanatomical identification of mesencephalic premotor neurons coordinating eyelid with upgaze in the monkey and man. J Comp Neurol 420, 19–34, 2000.
313. Horn AKE, Büttner-Enever JA, Wahle P, Reichenberger I. Neurotransmitter profile of saccadic omnipause neurons in nucleus raphe interpositus. J Neuroscience 14, 2032–2046, 1994.
314. Horn AKE, Büttner-Ennever JA. Premotor neurons for vertical eye-movements in the rostral mesencephalon of monkey and man: the histological identification by parvalbumin immunostaining. J Comp Neurol 392, 413–427, 1998.
315. Horn AKE, Büttner-Ennever JA, Büttner U. Saccadic premotor neurons in the brainstem: functional neuroanatomy and clinical implications. Neuro-ophthalmology 16, 229–240, 1996.
316. Horn AKE, Büttner-Ennever JA, Suzuki Y, Henn V. Histological identification of premotor neurons for horizontal saccades in monkey and man by parvalbumin immunostaining. J Comp Neurol 359, 350–363, 1997.
317. Huaman AG, Sharpe JA. Vertical saccades in senescence. Invest Ophthalmol Vis Sci 34, 2588–2595, 1993.
318. Husain M, Mannan A, Hodgson T, et al. Impaired spatial working memory across saccades contributes to abnormal search in parietal neglect. Brain 124, 941–952, 2001.
319. Husain M, Parton A, Hodgson TL, Mort D, Rees G. Self-control during response conflict by human supplementary eye field. Nat Neurosci 6, 117–118, 2003.
320. Iba M, Sawaguchi T. Involvement of the dorsolateral prefrontal cortex of monkeys in visuospatial target selection. J Neurophysiol 89, 587–599, 2003.
321. Ignashchenkova A, Dicke PW, Haarmeier T, Their P. Neuron-specific contribution of the superior colliculus to overt and covert shifts of attention. Nat Neurosci 7, 56–64, 2004.
322. Inaba N, Iwamoto Y, Yoshida K. Changes in cerebellar fastigial burst activity related to saccadic gain adaptation in the monkey. Neurosci Res 46, 359–368, 2003.
323. Inchingolo P, Optican LM, Fitzgibbon EJ, Goldberg ME. In Schmid R, Zambarbieri D (eds). Oculomotor Control and Cognitive Processes. Amsterdam, Elsevier, 1991, pp 147–162.
324. Isoda M. Context-dependent stimulation effects on saccade initiation in the presupplementary motor area of the monkey. J Neurophysiol 92, 653–659, 2005.
325. Isoda M, Tanji J. Cellular activity in the supplementary eye field during sequential performance of multiple saccades. J Neurophysiol 88, 3541–3545, 2002.
326. Isotalo E, Zee DS, Lasker AG. Cognitive influences on predictive saccade tracking. Exp Brain Res 165, 461–469, 2005.
327. Israël I, Rivaud S, Gaymard B, Berthoz A, Pierrot-Deseilligny C. Cortical control of vestibular-guided saccades. Brain 118, 1169–1184, 1995.
328. Ito S, Stuphorn V, Brown JW, Schall JD. Performance monitoring by the anterior cingulate cortex during saccade countermanding. Science 302, 120–122, 2003.
329. Itoh H, Nakahara H, Hikosaka O, et al. Correlation of primate caudate neural activity and saccade parameters in reward-oriented behavior. J Neurophysiol 89, 1774–1783, 2003.
330. Iwamoto Y, Yoshida K. Saccadic dysmetria following inactivation of the primate fastigial oculomotor region. Neurosci Lett 325, 211–215, 2002.
331. Izawa Y, Suzuki H, Shinoda Y. Initiation and suppression of saccades by the frontal eye field in the monkey. Ann N Y Acad Sci 1039, 220–231, 2005.
332. Jack ARG, Currie JN, Harvey SK, et al. Perturbations of horizontal saccade velocity profiles in humans as a marker of brainstem dysfunction in Wernicke-Korsakoff syndrome. Soc Neurosci Abstr 23, 864.3, 1997.
333. Jacobs JB, Dell'Osso LF, Leigh RJ. Characteristics of braking saccades in congenital nystagmus. Doc Ophthalmol 107, 137–154, 2003.
334. Javal E. Essai sur la physiologie de la lecture. Annales d'Oculométrie 82, 242–253, 1879.
335. Jay MF, Sparks DL. Sensorimotor integration in the primate superior colliculus. II. Coordinates of auditory signals. J Neurophysiol 57, 35–55, 1987.
336. Jürgens R, Becker W, Kornhuber HH. Natural and drug-induced variations of velocity and duration of human saccadic eye movements: evidence for a control of the neural pulse generator by local feedback. Biol Cybern 39, 87–96, 1981.
337. Kajii N, Nazir TA, Osaka N. Eye movement control in reading unspaced text: the case of the Japanese script. Vision Res 41, 2503–2510, 2001.
338. Kalesnykas RP, Hallett PE. The differentiation of visually guided and anticipatory saccades in gap and overlap paradigms. Exp Brain Res 68, 115–121, 1987.
339. Kaneko CRS. Effect of ibotenic acid lesions of the omnipause neurons on saccadic eye movements in Rhesus macaques. J Neurophysiol 75, 2229–2242, 1996.
339a. Kaneko CR. Saccade-related, long-lead burst neurons in the monkey rostral pons. J Neurophysiol, in press, 2005.
340. Kapoula Z. Evidence for a range effect in the saccadic system. Vision Res 25, 1155–1157, 1985.
341. Kapoula Z, Optican LM, Robinson DA. Visually induced plasticity of postsaccadic ocular drift in normal humans. J Neurophysiol 61, 879–891, 1989.
342. Kapoula Z, Robinson DA. Saccadic undershoot is not inevitable: saccades can be accurate. Vision Res 26, 735–743, 1986.
343. Kapoula Z, Robinson DA, Hain TC. Motion of the eye immediately after a saccade. Exp Brain Res 61, 386–394, 1986.
344. Karn KS, Møller P, Hayhoe MM. Reference frames

in saccadic targeting. Exp Brain Res 115, 267–282, 1997.

345. Kastner S, O'Connor DH, Fukui MM, et al. Functional imaging of the human lateral geniculate nucleus and pulvinar. J Neurophysiol 91, 438–448, 2004.
346. Kato M, Miyashita N, Hikisaka O, et al. Eye movements in monkeys with local dopamine depletion in the caudate nucleus. 1. Deficits in spontaneous saccades. J Neurosci 15, 912–927, 1995.
347. Kato M, Miyauchi S. Human precentral cortical activation patterns during saccade tasks: an fMRI comparison with activation during intentional eyeblink tasks. Neuroimage 19, 1260–1272, 2003.
348. Kawagoe R, Takikawa Y, Hikosaka O. Expectation of reward modulates cognitive signals in the basal ganglia. Nat Neurosci 1, 411–416, 1998.
349. Keller EL, Edelman JA. Use of interrupted saccade paradigm to study spatial and temporal dynamics of saccadic burst cells in superior colliculus in monkey. J Neurophysiol 72, 2754–2770, 1994.
350. Keller EL, Gandhi NJ, Shieh JM. Endpoint accuracy in saccades interrupted by stimulation in the omnipause region in monkeys. Vis Neurosci 13, 1059–1067, 1996.
351. Keller EL, McPeek RM, Salz T. Evidence against direct connections to PPRF EBNs from SC in the monkey. J Neurophysiol 84, 1303–1313, 2000.
352. Keller EL, Slakey DP, Crandall WF. Microstimulation of the primate cerebellar vermis during saccadic eye movements. Brain Res 288, 131–143, 1983.
353. Kennard C. Scanpaths: the path to understanding abnormal cognitive processing in neurological disease. Ann N Y Acad Sci 956, 242–249, 2002.
354. Kennard C, Lueck CJ. Oculomotor abnormalities in diseases of the basal ganglia. Rev Neurol, Paris 145, 587–595, 1989.
355. Kimmig H, Haussmann K, Mergner T, Lucking CH. What is pathological with gaze shift fragmentation in Parkinson's disease? J Neurol 249, 683–692, 2002.
356. King WM, Fuchs AF. Reticular control of vertical saccadic eye movements by mesencephalic burst neurons. J Neurophysiol 42, 861–876, 1979.
357. Kinsler V, Carpenter RHS. Saccadic eye movements while reading music. Vision Res 35, 1447–1458, 1997.
358. Klein C, Foerster F. Development of prosaccade and antisaccade task performance in participants aged 6 to 26 years. Psychophysiology 38, 179–189, 2001.
359. Klein C, Jr, FB, Fischer B, Hartnegg K. Effects of methylphenidate on saccadic responses in patients with ADHD. Exp Brain Res 145, 121–125, 2002.
360. Kleine JF, Guan Y, Büttner U. Saccade-related neurons in the primate fastigial nucleus: what do they encode? J Neurophysiol 90, 3137–3154, 2003.
360a. Klier EM, Angelaki DE, Hess BJ. Roles of gravitational cues and efference copy signals in the rotational updating of memory saccades. J Neurophysiol 94, 468–478, 2005.
361. Knox PC, Weir CR, Murphy PJ. Modification of visually guided saccades by a nonvisual afferent feedback signal. Invest Ophthalmol Vis Sci 41, 2561–2565, 2000.
362. Kobayashi S, Lauwereyns J, Koizumi M, Sakagami M, Hikosaka O. Influence of reward expectation on visuospatial processing in macaque lateral prefrontal cortex. J Neurophysiol 87, 1488–1498, 2002.
363. Kobayashi Y, Inoue Y, Isa T. Pedunculo-pontine control of visually guided saccades. Prog Brain Res 143, 439–445, 2004.
364. Kobayashi Y, Inoue Y, Yamamoto M, Isa T, Aizawa H. Contribution of pedunculopontine tegmental nucleus neurons to performance of visually guided saccade tasks in monkeys. J Neurophysiol 88, 715–731, 2002.
365. Kobayashi Y, Saito Y, Isa T. Facilitation of saccade initiation by brainstem cholinergic system. Brain Dev 23 Suppl 1, S24–S27, 2001.
366. Komiyama A, Toda H, Johkura K. Edrophonium-induced macrosaccadic oscillations in myasthenia gravis. Ann Neurol 45, 522–525, 1999.
367. Kommerell G, Olivier D, Theopold H. Adaptive programming of phasic and tonic components in saccadic eye movements. Investigations in patients with abducens palsy. Invest Ophthalmol 15, 657–660, 1976.
368. Kori A, Miyashita N, Kato M, et al. Eye movements in monkeys with local dopamine depletion in the caudate nucleus. 2. Deficits in voluntary saccades. J Neurosci 15, 928–941, 1995.
369. Kori AA, Das VE, Zivotofsky AZ, Leigh RJ. Memory-guided saccadic eye movements: effects of cerebellar disease. Vision Res 38, 3181–3192, 1998.
370. Kowler E, Blaser E. The accuracy and precision of saccades to small and large targets. Vision Res 35, 1741–1754, 1995.
371. Krauzlis RJ, Miles FA. Decreases in the latency of smooth pursuit and saccadic eye movements produced by the "gap paradigm" in the monkey. Vision Res 36, 1973–1985, 1996.
372. Krauzlis RJ, Miles FA. Initiation of saccade during fixation or pursuit: Evidence in humans for a single mechanism. J Neurophysiol 76, 4175–4179, 1996.
373. Kristjansson A, Vandenbroucke MW, Driver J. When pros become cons for anti- versus prosaccades: factors with opposite or common effects on different saccade types. Exp Brain Res 155, 231–244, 2004.
374. Kumar AN, Han YH, Liao K, et al. Evaluating large saccades in patients with brain-stem or cerebellar disorders. Ann N Y Acad Sci 1039, 404–416, 2005.
375. Kustov AA, Robinson DL. Modified saccades evoked by stimulation of the macaque superior colliculus account for properties of the resettable inegrator. J Neurophysiol 73, 1724–1728, 1995.
376. Kusunoki M, Goldberg ME. The time course of perisaccadic receptive field shifts in the lateral intraparietal area of the monkey. J Neurophysiol 89, 1519–1527, 2003.
377. LaBèrge D, Buchsbaum MS. Positron emission tomographic measurements of pulvinar activity during an attention task. J Neurosci 10, 613–619, 1990.
378. Landolt E. Nouvelles recherches sur la physiologie des mouvements des yeux. Archives d'Ophtalmologie (Paris) 11, 385–395, 1891.
379. Langer TP, Kaneko CRS. Brainstem afferents to the oculomotor omnipause neurons in monkey. J Comp Neurol 295, 413–427, 1990.
380. Lappe M, Awater H, Krekelberg B. Postsaccadic visual references generate presaccadic compression of space. Nature 403, 892–895, 2000.
381. Lasker AG, Zee DS. Ocular motor abnormalities in Huntington's disease. Vision Res 37, 3639–3645, 1997.
382. Lasker AG, Zee DS, Hain TC, Folstein SE, Singer HS. Saccades in Huntington's disease: Initiation

defects and distractibility. Neurology 37, 364–370, 1987.
383. Lauwereyns J, Takikawa Y, Kawagoe R, et al. Feature-based anticipation of cues that predict reward in monkey caudate nucleus. Neuron 33, 463–473, 2002.
384. Lauwereyns J, Watanabe K, Coe B, Hikosaka O. A neural correlate of response bias in monkey caudate nucleus. Nature 418, 413–417, 2002.
385. Lebedev S, Van Gelder P, Tsui WH. Square-root relation between main saccade parameters. Invest Ophthalmol Vis Sci 37, 2750–2758, 1996.
386. Lee AC, Robbins TW, Owen AM. Episodic memory meets working memory in the frontal lobe: functional neuroimaging studies of encoding and retrieval. Crit Rev Neurobiol 14, 165–197, 2003.
387. Lee C, Rohrer WH, Sparks DL. Population coding of saccadic eye movements by neurons in the superior colliculus. Nature 332, 357–360, 1988.
388. Lee KM, Keller EL, Heinen SJ. Properties of saccades generated as a choice response. Exp Brain Res, 2005.
389. Lefèvre P, Quaia C, Optican LM. Distributed model of control of saccades by superior colliculus and cerebellum. Neural Network 11, 1175–1190, 1998.
390. Leichnetz GR. Connections of the medial posterior parietal cortex (area 7m) in the monkey. Anat Rec 263, 215–236, 2001.
391. Leigh RJ. The cortical control of ocular pursuit movements. Rev Neurol (Paris) 145, 605–612, 1989.
392. Leigh RJ, Kennard C. Using saccades as a research tool in the clinical neurosciences. Brain 127, 460–477, 2004.
393. Leigh RJ, Newman SA, Folstein SE, Lasker AG, Jensen BA. Abnormal ocular motor control in Huntington's chorea. Neurology 33, 1268–1275, 1983.
394. Lemij HG, Collewijn H. Differences in accuracy of human saccades between stationary and jumping targets. Vision Res 29, 1737–1748, 1989.
395. Leung HC, Gore JC, Goldman-Rakic PS. Sustained mnemonic response in the middle human frontal gyrus during on-line storage of spatial memoranda. Cogn Neurosci 14, 659–671, 2002.
396. Lewis RF, Zee DS, Gaymard B, Guthrie B. Extraocular muscle proprioception functions in the control of ocular alignment and eye movement conjugacy. J Neurophysiol 71, 1028–1031, 1994.
397. Lewis RF, Zee DS, Goldstein HP, Guthrie BL. Proprioceptive and retinal afference modify post-saccadic ocular drift. J Neurophysiol 82, 551–563, 1999.
398. Li CS, Andersen RA. Inactivation of macaque lateral intraparietal area delays initiation of the second saccade predominantly from contralesional eye positions in a double-saccade task. Exp Brain Res 137, 45–57, 2001.
399. Li CS, Mazzoni P, Andersen RA. Effect of reversible inactivation of macaque lateral intraparietal area on visual and memory saccades. J Neurophysiol 81, 1827–1838, 1999.
399a. Li N, Wei M, Angelaki DE. Primate memory saccade amplitude after intervened motion depends on target distance. J Neurophysiol 94, 722–733, 2005.
400. Linden JF, Grunewald A, Andersen RA. Responses to auditory stimuli in macaque lateral intraparietal area. II. Behavioral modulation. J Neurophysiol 82, 343–358, 1999.
401. Liversedge SP, Findlay JM. Saccadic eye movements and cognition. Trends Cogn Sci 4, 6–14, 2000.
402. Lobel E, Kehane P, Leonards U, et al. Localization of human frontal eye fields: anatomical and functional findings of functional magnetic resonance imaging and intracerebral electrical stimulation. J Neurosurg 95, 804–815, 2001.
403. Lu X, Matsuzawa M, Hikosaka O. A neural correlate of oculomotor sequences in supplementary eye field. Neuron 34, 317–325, 2002.
404. Ludwig CJ, Gilchrist ID. Target similarity affects saccade curvature away from irrelevant onsets. Exp Brain Res 152, 60–69, 2003.
405. Lueck CJ, Crawford TJ, Hansen HC, Kennard C. Increase in saccadic peak velocity with increased frequency of saccades in man. Vision Res 31, 1439–1443, 1991.
406. Lueck KL, Mendez MF, Perryman KM. Eye movement abnormalities during reading in patients with Alzheimer disease. Neuropsychiatry Neuropsychol Behav Neurol 13, 77 –82, 2000.
407. Luria AR, Karpov BA, Yarbuss AL. Disturbances of active visual perception with lesions of the frontal lobes. Cortex 2, 202–212, 1966.
408. Luria AR, Pravdine-Vinarskaya EN, Yarbuss AL. Disorders of ocular movement in a case of simultanagnosia. Brain 86, 219–228, 1963.
409. Lynch JC. Saccade initiation and latency deficits after combined lesions of the frontal and posterior eye fields in monkeys. J Neurophysiol 68, 1913–1916, 1992.
410. Ma TP, Graybiel AM, Wurtz RH. Location of saccade-related neurons in the macaque superior colliculus. Exp Brain Res 85, 21–35, 1991.
411. MacAskill MR, Anderson TJ, Jones RD. Suppression of displacement in severely slowed saccades. Vision Res 40, 3405–3413, 2000.
412. MacAskill MR, Anderson TJ, Jones RD. Adaptive modification of saccade amplitude in Parkinson's disease. Brain 125, 1570–1582, 2002.
413. Machado L, Rafal RD. Control of fixation and saccades during an anti-saccade task: an investigation in humans with chronic lesions of oculomotor cortex. Exp Brain Res 156, 55–63, 2004.
414. Machado L, Rafal RD. Control of fixation and saccades in humans with lesions of oculomotor cortex. Neuropsychology 18, 115–123, 2004.
415. MacKay DM. Visual stability. Invest Ophthalmol 11, 518–524, 1972.
416. Maioli C, Benaglio I, Siri S, Sosta K, Cappa S. The integration of parallel and serial processing mechanisms in visual search: evidence from eye movement recording. Eur J Neurosci 13, 364 –372, 2001.
417. Martinez-Conde S, Macknik SL, Hubel DH. The role of fixational eye movements in visual perception. Nat Rev Neurosci 5, 229–240, 2004.
418. Martinez-Trujillo JC, Wang H, Crawford JD. Electrical stimulation of the supplementary eye fields in the head-free macaque evokes kinematically normal gaze shifts. J Neurophysiol 89, 2961–2974, 2003.
419. Matin L. In Boff KR, Kaufman L, Thomas JP, (eds). Handbook of Human Perception and Performance. New York, Wiley, 1986, pp 20.2–20.45.
420. Matsumiya K, Uchikawa K. The role of presaccadic compression of visual space in spatial remapping across saccadic eye movements. Vision Res 43, 1969–1981, 2003.

421. Matsumura M, Kojima J, Gardiner TW, Hikosaka O. Visual and oculomotor functions of monkey subthalamic nucleus. J Neurophysiol 67, 1615–1632, 1992.
422. May PJ. The mammalian superior colliculus: laminar structure and connections. In Büttner-Ennever JA (ed). Neuroanatomy of the Oculomotor System. Prog Brain Res 151, 321–380, 2006.
423. May PJ, Hartwich-Young R, Nelson J, Sparks DL, Porter JD. Cerebellotectal pathways in the macaque: implications for collicular generation of saccades. Neuroscience 36, 305–324, 1990.
424. Mayfrank L, Mobashery M, Kimmig H, Fischer B. The role of fixation and visual attention in the occurrence of express saccades in man. Eur Arch Psychiatr Neurol Sci 235, 269–275, 1986.
425. Mays LE, Sparks DL. Dissociation of visual and saccade- related responses in superior colliculus neurons. J Neurophysiol 43, 207–232, 1980.
426. Mazzoni P, Bracewell RM, Barash S, Andersen RA. Motor intention activity in the macaque's lateral intraparietal area. I. Dissociation of motor plan from sensory memory. J Neurophysiol 76, 1439–1456, 1997.
427. McCoy AN, Crowley JC, Haghighian G, Dean HL, Platt ML. Saccade reward signals in posterior cingulate cortex. Neuron 40, 1031–1040, 2003.
427a. McDonald SA, Carpenter RH, Shillcock RC. An anatomically constrained, stochastic model of eye movement control in reading. Psychol Rev 112, 814–840, 2005.
428. McFadden SA, Khan A, Wallman J. Gain adaptation of exogenous shifts of visual attention. Vision Res 42, 2709–2726, 2002.
429. McLaughlin S. Parametric adjustment in saccadic eye movements. Percept Psychophys 2, 359–362, 1967.
430. McPeek RM, Han JH, Keller EL. Competition between saccade goals in the superior colliculus produces saccade curvature. J Neurophysiol 89, 2577–2590, 2003.
431. McPeek RM, Keller EL. Superior colliculus activity related to concurrent processing of saccade goals in a visual search task. J Neurophysiol 87, 1805–1815, 2002.
432. McPeek RM, Skavenski AA, Nakayama K. Concurrent processing of saccades in visual search. Vision Res 40, 2499–2516, 2000.
433. Medendorp WP, Goltz HC, Vilis T, Crawford JD. Gaze-centered updating of visual space in human parietal cortex. J Neurosci 23, 6209–6214, 2003.
434. Meienberg O. Clinical examination of saccadic eye movements in hemianopia. Neurology 33, 1311–1315, 1983.
435. Meienberg O, Harrer M, Wethren C. Oculographic diagnosis of hemineglect in patients with homonymous hemianopia. J Neurol 233, 97–101, 1986.
436. Meienberg O, Zangemeister WH, Rosenberg M, Hoyt WF, Stark L. Saccadic eye movement strategies in patients with homonymous hemianopia. Ann Neurol l 9, 537–544, 1981.
437. Melis BJ, van Gisbergen JAM. Short-term adaptation of electrically-induced saccades in monkey superior colliculus. J Neurophysiol 76, 1744 –1758, 1996.
438. Melvill Jones G. Predominance of anti-compensatory oculomotor response during rapid head rotation. Aerospace Med 35, 965–968, 1964.
439. Merriam EP, Genovese CR, Colby CL. Spatial updating in human parietal cortex. Neuron 39, 361–373, 2003.
440. Milea D, Lehericy S, Rivaud-Pechoux S, et al. Antisaccade deficit after anterior cingulate cortex resection. Neuroreport 14, 283–287, 2003.
441. Milea D, Lobel E, Lehericy S, et al. Intraoperative frontal eye field stimulation elicits ocular deviation and saccade suppression. Neuroreport 13, 1359–1364, 2002.
442. Miller JM. Egocentric localization of a perisaccadic flash by manual pointing. Vision Res 36, 837–851, 1996.
443. Miller JM, Robins D. Extraocular muscle forces in alert monkey. Vision Res 32, 1099–1113, 1992.
444. Missal M, Keller EL. Common inhibitory mechanism for saccades and smooth-pursuit eye movements. J Neurophysiol 88, 1880–1892, 2002.
445. Mitchell J, Zipser D. A model of visual-spatial memory across saccades. Vision Res 41, 1575–1592, 2001.
446. Mitchell JF, Zipser D. Sequential memory-guided saccades and target selection: a neural model of the frontal eye fields. Vision Res 43, 2669–2695, 2003.
447. Miura K, Optican LM. Membrane properties of medium-lead burst neurons may contribute to dynamical properties of saccades. Proceedings of the first international IEEE EMBS Conference on Neural Engineering, Capri Island, Italy, March 20–23, 2003 20–23.
448. Miura K, Optican LM. Membrane channel properties of premotor excitatory burst neurons may underlie saccade slowing after lesions of omnipause neurons. Neural Network, In Press, 2005.
448a. Miura K, Optican LM. Conductance-based model of excitatory burst neurons explains saccade slowing after lesions of omnipause neurons. Soc Neurosci Abstr 858.19, 2005.
449. Miyashita N, Hikosaka O. Minimal synaptic latency delay in the saccadic output pathway of the superior colliculus studied in awake monkey. Exp Brain Res 112, 187–196, 1996.
450. Miyashita N, Hikosaka O, Kato M. Visual hemineglect induced by unilateral striatal dopamine dificiency in monkeys. Neuroreport 6, 1257–1260, 1995.
450a. Montagnini A, Chelazzi L. The urgency to look: prompt saccades to the benefit of perception. Vision Res 45, 3391–3401, 2005.
451. Moore T, Armstrong KM. Selective gating of visual signals by microstimulation of frontal cortex. Nature 421, 370–373, 2003.
452. Moore T, Fallah M. Microstimulation of the frontal eye field and its effects on covert spatial attention. J Neurophysiol 91, 152–162, 2004.
452a. Morrone MC, Ross J, Burr D. Saccadic eye movements cause compression of time as well as space. Nat Neurosci 8, 950–954, 2005.
453. Morrow MJ. Craniotopic defects of smooth pursuit and saccadic eye movement. Neurology 46, 514–521, 1996.
454. Mort DJ, Perry RJ, Mannan SK, et al. Differential cortical activation during voluntary and reflexive saccades in man. Neuroimage 18, 231–246, 2003.
455. Moschovakis AK, Gregoriou GG, Ugolini G, et al. Oculomotor areas of the primate frontal lobes: a transneuronal transfer of rabies virus and [14C]-2-deoxyglucose functional imaging study. J Neurosci 24, 5726–5740, 2004.

456. Moschovakis AK, Highstein SM. The anatomy and physiology of primate neurons that control rapid eye movements. Ann Rev Neurosci 17, 465–488, 1994.
457. Moschovakis AK, Karabelas AB, Highstein SM. Structure-function relationships in the primate superior colliculus. I. Morphological classification of efferent neurons. J Neurophysiol 60, 232–262, 1988.
458. Moschovakis AK, Karabelas AB, Highstein SM. Structure-function relationships in the primate superior colliculus. II. Morphological identity of presaccadic neurons. J Neurophysiol 60, 263–302, 1988.
459. Moschovakis AK, ScudderCA, Highstein SM. Structure of the primate oculomotor burst generator. I. Medium-lead burst neurons with upward on-directions. J Neurophysiol 65, 203–217, 1991.
460. Moschovakis AK, Scudder CA, Highstein SM, Warren JD. Structure of the primate oculomotor burst generator. II. Medium-lead burst neurons with downward on-directions. J Neurophysiol 65, 218–229, 1991.
461. Mostofsky SH, Lasker AG, Cutting LE, Denckla MB, Zee DS. Oculomotor abnormalities in attention deficit hyperactivity disorder: a preliminary study. Neurology 57, 423–430, 2001.
462. Motter BC, Belky EJ. The guidance of eye movements during active visual search. Vision Res 38, 1805–1815, 1998.
463. Muggleton NG, Juan CH, Cowey A, Walsh V. Human frontal eye fields and visual search. J Neurophysiol 89, 3340–3343, 2003.
464. Munoz DP, Armstrong IT, Hampton KA, Moore KD. Altered control of visual fixation and saccadic eye movements in attention-deficit hyperactivity disorder. J Neurophysiol 90, 503–514, 2003.
465. Munoz DP, Broughton JR, Goldring JE, Armstrong IT. Age-related performance of human subjects on saccadic eye movement tasks. Exp Brain Res 12, 391–400, 1998.
466. Munoz DP, Corneil BD. Evidence for interactions between target selection and visual fixation for saccade generation in humans. Exp Brain Res 103, 168–173, 1995.
467. Munoz DP, Everling S. Look away: the anti-saccade task and the voluntary control of eye movement. Nat Rev Neurosci 5, 218–228, 2004.
468. Munoz DP, Waitzman DM, Wurtz RH. Activity of neurons in monkey superior colliculus during interrupted saccades. J Neurophysiol 75, 2562–2580, 1996.
469. Munoz DP, Wurtz RH. Fixation cells in monkey superior colliculus. I. Characteristics of cell discharge. J Neurophysiol 70, 559–575, 1993.
470. Munoz DP, Wurtz RH. Fixation cells in monkey superior colliculus. II. Reversible activation and deactivation. J Neurophysiol 70, 576–589, 1993.
471. Munoz DP, Wurtz RH. Saccade-related activity in monkey superior colliculus. I. Characteristics of burst and buildup cells. J Neurophysiol 73, 2313–2333, 1995.
472. Munoz DP, Wurtz RH. Saccade-related activity in monkey superior colliculus. II. Spread of activity during saccades. J Neurophysiol 73, 2334–2348, 1995.
473. Müri RM, Gaymard B, Rivard S, et al. Hemispheric asymmetry in cortical control of memory-guided saccades. A transcranial magnetic stimulation study. Neuropsychologia 38, 1105–1111, 2000.
474. Müri RM, Iba-Zizen MT, Derosier C, Cabanis EA, Pierrot-Deseilligny C. Location of the human posterior eye field with functional magnetic resonance imaging. J Neurol Neurosurg Psychiatry 60, 445–448, 1996.
475. Müri RM, Rosler KM, Hess CW. Influence of transcranial magnetic stimulation on the execution of memorised sequences of saccades in man. Exp Brain Res 101, 521–524, 1994.
476. Müri RM, Vermersch AI, Rivaud S, Gaymard B, Pierrot-Deseilligny C. Effects of single pulse transcranial magnetic stimulation over the prefrontal and posterior parietal cortices during memory-guided saccades in humans. J Neurophysiol 76, 2102–2106, 1997.
477. Nachev P, Rees G, Parton A, Kennard C, HusainM. Volition and conflict in human medial frontal cortex. Curr Biol 15, 122–128, 2005.
478. Nagel-Leiby S, Buchtel HA, Welch KMA. Cerebral control of directed visual attention and orienting saccades. Brain 113, 237–276, 1990.
479. Nakamura K, Colby CL. Updating of the visual representation in monkey striate and extrastriate cortex during saccades. Proc Natl Acad Sci U S A 99, 4026–4031, 2002.
480. Nakamura K, Roesch MR, Olson CR. Neuronal activity in macaque SEF and ACC during performance of tasks involving conflict. J Neurophysiol 93, 884–908, 2005.
481. Nakao S, Shiraishi Y, Oda H, Inagaki M. Direct inhibitory projection of pontine omnipause neurons to burst neurons in the Forel's field H controlling vertical eye movement-related motoneurons in the cat. Exp Brain Res 70, 632–636, 1988.
482. Nambu A, Tokuno H, Takada M. Functional significance of the cortico/subthalamo/pallidal 'hyperdirect' pathway. Neurosci Res 43, 111–117, 2002.
483. Neggers SF, Raemaekers MA, Lampmann EE, Postma A, Ramsey NF. Cortical and subcortical contributions to saccade latency in the human brain. Eur J Neurosci 21, 2853–2863, 2005.
484. Newsome WT, Wurtz RH, Dürsteler MR, Mikami A. Punctate chemical lesions of striate cortex in the macaque monkey: effect on visually guided saccades. Exp Brain Res 58, 392–399, 1985.
485. Nichols MJ, Sparks DL. Nonstationary properties of the saccadic system: new constraints on models of saccdic control. J Neurophysiol 73, 582–600, 1995.
486. Niemeier M, Crawford JD, Tweed DB. Optimal transsaccadic integration explains distorted spatial perception. Nature 422, 76–80, 2003.
487. Nitschke MF, Arp T, Stavrou G, Erdmann C, HeideW. The cerebellum in the cerebro-cerebellar network for the control of eye and hand movements—an fMRI study. Prog Brain Res 148, 151–164, 2004.
488. Nixon PD, Passingham RE. The cerebellum and cognition: cerebellar lesions impair sequence learning but not conditional visuomotor learning in monkeys. Neuropsychologia 38, 1054–1072, 2003.
489. Noda H, Fujikado T. Topography of the oculomotor area of the cerebellar vermis in macaques as determined by microstimulation. J Neurophysiol 58, 359–378, 1987.
490. Noda H, Sugita S, Ikeda Y. Afferent and efferent connections of the oculomotor region of the fastigial nucleus in the macaque monkey. J Comp Neurol 302, 330–348, 1990.
491. Noto CT, Watanabe S, Fuchs AF. Characteristics of

simian adaptation fields produced by behavioral changes in saccade size and direction. J Neurophysiol 81, 2798–2813, 1999.
492. Noton D, Stark L. Scanpaths in saccadic eye movements while viewing and recognizing patterns. Vision Res 11, 929–942, 1971.
493. Nyffeler T, Pierrot-Deseilligny C, Felblinger J, et al. Time-dependent hierarchical organization of spatial working memory: a transcranial magnetic stimulation study. Eur J Neurosci 16, 1823–1827, 2002.
494. Nyffeler T, Pierrot-Deseilligny C, Pflugshaupt T, et al. Information processing in long delay memory-guided saccades: further insights from TMS. Exp Brain Res 154, 109–112, 2004.
495. O'Driscoll GA, Alpert NM, Matthysse SW, et al. Functional neuroanatomy of antisaccade eye movements investigated with positron emission tomography. Proc Natl Acad Sci U S A 92, 925–929, 1995.
496. O'Sullivan EP, Jenkins IH, Henderson L, Kennard C, Brooks DJ. The functional anatomy of remembered saccades: a PET study. Neuroreport 6, 2141–2144, 1995.
497. O'Sullivan JD, Maruff P, Tyler P, et al. Unilateral pallidotomy for Parkinson's disease disrupts ocular fixation. J Clin Neurosci 10, 181–185, 2003.
498. Ogren MP, Mateer CA, Wyler AR. Alterations in visually related eye movements following left pulvinar damage in man. Neuropsychologia 22, 187–196, 1984.
499. Ohbayashi M, Ohki K, Miyashita Y. Conversion of working memory to motor sequence in the monkey premotor cortex. Science 301, 233–236, 2003.
500. Ohgaki T, Markham CH, Schneider JS, Curthoys IS. Anatomical evidence of the projection of pontine omnipause neurons to midbrain regions controlling vertical eye movements. J Comp Neurol 289, 610–625, 1989.
501. Ohtsuka K, Noda H. Saccadic burst neurons in the oculomotor region of the fastigial neurons in macaque monkeys. J Neurophysiol 65, 1422–1434, 1992.
502. Ohtsuka K, Noda H. Discharge properties of Purkinje cells in the oculomotor vermis during visually guided saccades in the macaque monkey. J Neurophysiol 74, 1828–1840, 1995.
503. Ohtsuka K, Sawa M, Takeda M. Accuracy of memory-guided saccades. Ophthalmologica 198, 53–56, 1989.
504. Olshausen BA, Anderson CH, Van Essen DC. A neurobiological model of visual attention and invariant pattern recognition based on dynamic routing of information. J Neurosci 13, 4700–4719, 1993.
505. Olson CR, Musil SY, Goldberg ME. Single neurons in posterior cingulate cortex of behaving macaque: eye movement signals. J Neurophysiol 76, 3285–3300, 1996.
506. Olson CR, Tremblay L. Macaque supplementary eye field neurons encode object-centered locations relative to both continuous and discontinuous objects. J Neurophysiol 83, 2392–2411, 2000.
507. Oohira A, Goto K, Ozawa T. Hypermetric saccades and adaptive response. Neuro-ophthalmology 3, 353–356, 1986.
508. Optican LM. Sensorimotor transformation for visually guided saccades. Ann N Y Acad Sci 1039, 132–148, 2005.
509. Optican LM, Miles FA. Visually induced adaptive changes in primate saccadic oculomotor control signals. J Neurophysiol 54, 940–958, 1985.
510. Optican LM, Quaia C. In Harris L, Jenkins M (eds). Vision and Action. New York, Cambridge University Press, 1998.
511. Optican LM, Quaia C. Distributed model of collicular and cerebellar function during saccades. Ann N Y Acad Sci 956, 164–177, 2002.
512. Optican LM, Robinson DA. Cerebellar-dependent adaptive control of primate saccadic system. J Neurophysiol 44, 1058–1076, 1980.
513. Optican LM, Zee DS, Miles FA. Floccular lesions abolish adaptive control of post-saccadic drift in primates. Exp Brain Res 64, 596–598, 1986.
514. Ottes FP, van Gisbergen JAM, Eggermont JJ. Metrics of saccade responses to visual double stimuli: two different modes. Vision Res 24, 1169–1179, 1984.
515. Oyachi H, Ohtsuka K. Transcranial magnetic stimulation of the posterior parietal cortex degrades accuracy of memory-guided saccades in humans. Invest Ophthalmol Vis Sci 36, 1441–1449, 1995.
516. Pambakian AL, Wooding DS, Patel N, et al. Scanning the visual world: a study of patients with homonymous hemianopia. J Neurol Neurosurg Psychiatry 69, 751–759, 2000.
517. Paré M, Munoz DP. Saccadic reaction time in the monkey: Advanced preparation of oculomotor programs is primarily responsible for express saccade occurrence. J Neurophysiol 76, 3666–3681, 1996.
518. Paré M, Wurtz RH. Monkey posterior parietal cortex neurons antidromically activated from superior colliculus. J Neurophysiol 78, 3493–3497, 1997.
519. Paré M, Wurtz RH. Progression in neuronal processing for saccadic eye movements from parietal cortex area lip to superior colliculus. J Neurophysiol 85, 2545–2562, 2001.
520. Park J, Schlag-Rey M, Schlag J. Spatial localization precedes temporal determination in visual perception. Vision Res 43, 1667–1674, 2003.
521. Park J, Schlag-Rey M, Schlag J. Frames of reference for saccadic command, tested by saccade collision in the supplementary eye field. J Neurophysiol, in press, 2005.
522. Paus T, Marrett S, Worsley KJ, Evans AC. Extraretinal modulation of cerebral blood flow in the human visual cortex: implications for saccadic suppression. J Neurophysiol 74, 2179–2183, 1995.
523. Pelisson D, Prablanc C. Kinematics of centrifugal and centripetal saccadic eye movements in man. Vision Res 28, 87–94, 1988.
524. Pelz JB, Hayhoe MM. The role of exocentric reference frames in the perception of visual direction. Vision Res 35, 2267–2275, 1995.
525. Penfield W, Jasper H. Epilepsy and the Functional Anatomy of the Human Brain. Little, Brown & Co., Boston, 1954.
526. Peng GC, Minor LB, Zee DS. Gaze position corrective eye movements in normal subjects and in patients with vestibular deficits. Ann N Y Acad Sci 1039, 337–348, 2005.
527. Perry RJ, Zeki S. The neurology of saccades and covert shifts in spatial attention: an event-related fMRI study. Brain 123, 2273–2288, 2000.
528. Petit L, Orssaud C, Tzourio N, et al. Functional anatomy of a prelearned sequence of horizontal saccades in humans. J Neurosci 16, 3714–3726, 1996.
529. Petit L, Orssaud C, Tzourio N, et al. PET study of voluntary saccadic eye movements in humans: basal ganglia-thalamocortical system and cingulate

cortex involvement. J Neurophysiol 69, 1009–1017, 1993.
530. Pierrot-Deseilligny C, Gautier JC, Loron P. Acquired ocular motor apraxia due to bilateral frontoparietal infarcts. Ann Neurol 23, 199–202, 1988.
531. Pierrot-Deseilligny C, Gray F, Brunet P. Infarcts of both inferior parietal lobules with impairment of visually guided eye movements, peripheral visual attention and optic ataxia. Brain 109, 81–97, 1986.
532. Pierrot-Deseilligny C, Muri RM, Ploner CJ, et al. Decisional role of the dorsolateral prefrontal cortex in ocular motor behaviour. Brain 126, 1460–1473, 2003.
533. Pierrot-Deseilligny C, Rivaud S, Gaymard B, Agid,Y. Cortical control of memory-guided saccades in man. Exp Brain Res 83, 607–617, 1991.
534. Pierrot-Deseilligny C, Rivaud S, Gaymard B, Agid Y. Cortical control of reflexive visually guided saccades in man. Brain 114, 1473–1485, 1991.
535. Pierrot-Deseilligny C, Rivaud S, Gaymard B, Müri RM, Vermersch AI. Cortical control of saccades. Ann Neurol 37, 557–567, 1995.
536. Pierrot-Deseilligny C, Rivaud S, Pillon B, FournierE, Agid,Y. Lateral visually-guided saccades in progressive supranuclear palsy. Brain 112, 471–487, 1989.
537. Pierrot-Deseilligny C, Rosa A, Masmoudi K, Rivaud S, Gaymard B. Saccade deficits after a unilateral lesion affecting the superior colliculus. J Neurol Neurosurg Psychiatry 54, 1106–1109, 1991.
538. Pierrot-Deseilligny C, Ploner CJ, Müri RM, Gaymard B, Rivaud-Pechoux S. Effects of cortical lesions on saccadic: eye movements in humans. Ann N Y Acad Sci 956, 216–229, 2002.
539. Pitt MC, Rawles JM. The effect of age on saccadic latency and velocity. Neuro-ophthalmology 8, 123–129, 1988.
540. Platt ML, Glimcher PW. Responses of intraparietal neurons to saccadic targets and visual distractors. J Neurophysiol 78, 1574–1589, 1997.
541. Ploner CJ, Gaymard BM, Rivaud-Pechoux S, et al. Lesions affecting the parahippocampal cortex yield spatial memory deficits in humans. Cereb Cortex 10, 1211–1216, 2000.
542. Ploner CJ, Rivaud-Pechoux S, Gaymard BM, Agid Y, Pierrot-Deseilligny C. Errors of memory-guided saccades in humans with lesions of the frontal eye field and the dorsolateral prefrontal cortex. J Neurophysiol 82, 1086–1090, 1999.
543. Pola J. Models of the mechanism underlying perceived location of a perisaccadic flash. Vision Res 44, 2799–2813, 2004.
544. Port NL, Sommer MA, Wurtz RH. Multielectrode evidence for spreading activity across the superior colliculus movement map. J Neurophysiol 84, 344–357, 2000.
545. Port NL, Wurtz RH. Sequential activity of simultaneously recorded neurons in the superior colliculus during curved saccades. J Neurophysiol 90, 1887–1903, 2003.
546. Prablanc C, Masse D, Echallier JF. Error-correcting mechanisms in large saccades. Vision Res 18, 557–560, 1978.
547. Pratt J. Visual fixation offsets affect both the initiation and the kinematic features of saccades. Exp Brain Res 118, 135–138, 1998.
548. Quaia C, Aizawa H, Optican LM, Wurtz RH. Reversible inactivation of monkey superior colliculus. I. Maps of saccadic deficits. J Neurophysiol 79, 2097–2110, 1998.
549. Quaia C, Lefevre P, Optican LM. Model of the control of saccades by superior colliculus and cerebellum. J Neurophysiol 82, 999–1018, 1999.
550. Quaia C, Optican LM. Model with distributed vectorial premotor bursters accounts for the component stretching of oblique saccades. J Neurophysiol 78, 1120–1134, 1997.
551. Rafal R, McGrath M, Machado L, Hindle J. Effects of lesions of the human posterior thalamus on ocular fixation during voluntary and visually triggered saccades. J Neurol Neurosurg Psychiatry 75, 1602–1606, 2004.
552. Rafal RD, Posner MI, Friedman JH, Inhoff AW, Bernstein E. Orienting of visual attention in progressive supranuclear palsy. Brain 111, 267–280, 1988.
553. Ramat S, Leigh RJ, Zee DS, Optican LM. Ocular oscillations generated by coupling of brainstem excitatory and inhibitory saccadic burst neurons. Exp Brain Res 160, 89–106, 2005.
554. Ramat S, Schmid R, Zambarbieri D. Eye-head coordination in darkness: formulation and testing of a mathematical model. J Vestib Res 13, 79–91, 2003.
555. Ramat S, Somers JT, Das VE, Leigh RJ. Conjugate ocular oscillations during shifts of the direction and depth of visual fixation. Invest Ophthalmol Vis Sci 40, 1681–1686, 1999.
556. Ramat S, Zee DS, Leigh RJ, Optican LM. Familial microsaccadic oscillations may be due to alterations in the inhibitory premotor circuit. Soc Neurosci Abstr 475.15, 2005.
557. Ramcharan EJ, Gnadt JW, Sherman SM. The effects of saccadic eye movements on the activity of geniculate relay neurons in the monkey. Vis Neurosci 18, 253–258, 2001.
557a. Ram-Tsur R, Caspi A, Gordon CR, Zivotofsky AZ. The saccadic system more readily co-processes orthogonal than co-linear saccades. Exp Brain Res 160, 398–403, 2005.
558. Raphan T. In Fetter M, Haslwanter T, Misslisch H, Tweed D (eds). Three-Dimensional Kinematics of Eye, Head, and Limb Movements. The Netherlands, Harwood Academic Publishing, 1997, pp 359–374.
559. Rayner K, Pollatsek A. Reading unspaced text is not easy: Comments on the implcations of Epelboim et al.'s (1994) study for models of eye movement control in reading. Vision Res 36, 461–470, 1996.
560. Rayner K, Juhasz B, Ashby J, Clifton C, Jr. Inhibition of saccade return in reading. Vision Res 43, 1027–1034, 2003.
561. Rayner K, Liversedge SP, White SJ, Vergilino-Perez D. Reading disappearing text: cognitive control of eye movements. Psychol Sci 14, 385–388, 2003.
562. Reddi BA, Asrress KN, Carpenter RH. Accuracy, information, and response time in a saccadic decision task. J Neurophysiol 90, 3538–3546, 2003.
563. Reppas JB, Usrey WM, Reid RC. Saccadic eye movements modulate visual responses in the lateral geniculate nucleus. Neuron 35, 961–974, 2002.
564. Reulen JPH. Latency of visually evoked saccadic eye movements. I. Saccadic latency and the facilitation model. Biol Cybern 50, 251–262, 1984.
565. Reulen JPH. Latency of visually evoked saccadic eye movements. II. Temporal properties of the facilitation mechanism. Biol Cybern 50, 263–271, 1984.
566. Ridley A, Kennard C, Scholtz CL, et al. Omnipause neurons in two cases of opsoclonus associated with

oat cell carcinoma of the lung. Brain 110, 1699–1709, 1987.
567. Rivaud S, Müri RM, Gaymard B, Vermersch AI, Pierrot-Deseilligny C. Eye movement disorders after frontal eye field lesions in humans. Exp Brain Res 102, 110–120, 1994.
568. Rivaud-Pechoux S, Vermersch AI, Gaymard B, et al. Improvement of memory guided saccades in parkinsonian patients by high frequency subthalamic nucleus stimulation. J Neurol Neurosurg Psychiatry 68, 381–384, 2000.
569. Rizzo M, Hurtig R, Damasio AR. The role of scanpaths in facial recognition and learning. Ann Neurol 22, 41–45, 1987.
570. Ro T, Pratt J, Rafal RD. Inhibition of return in saccadic eye movements. Exp Brain Res 130, 264–268, 2000.
571. Robinson DA. Eye movements evoked by collicular stimulation in the alert monkey. Vision Res 12, 1795–1808, 1972.
572. Robinson DA. In Lennerstrand F, Bach-y-Rita P (eds). Basic Mechanisms of Ocular Motility and their Clinical Implications. Oxford, Pergamon Press, 1975, pp 337–374.
573. Robinson DA, Kapoula Z, Goldstein HP. In Deecke L, Eccles JC, Mountcastle VB (eds). From Neuron to Action—An Appraisal of Fundamental and Clinical Research. New York, Springer, 1990, pp 89–96.
574. Robinson DL. Functional contributions of the primate pulvinar. Progress in Brain Res 95, 371–380, 1993.
575. Robinson DL, Bowman EM, Kertzman C. Covert orienting of attention in macaque. II. Contributions of parietal cortex. J Neurophysiol 74, 698–712, 1995.
576. Robinson DL, McClurkin JW. In Wurtz RH, Goldberg ME (eds). The Neurobiology of Saccadic Eye Movements. Amsterdam. Elsevier, 1989, pp 337–360.
577. Robinson DL, McClurkin JW, Kertzman C, Petersen SE. Visual responses of pulvinar and collicular neurons during eye movements of awake, trained macaques. J Neurophysiol 66, 485–496, 1991.
578. Robinson DL, Petersen SE. The pulvinar and visual salience. Trends Neurosci 15, 127–132, 1992.
579. Robinson F, Noto C, Watanabe S. Effect of visual background on saccade adaptation in monkeys. Vision Res 40, 2359–2367, 2000.
580. Robinson FR. Role of the cerebellar posterior interpositus nucleus in saccades I. Effect of temporary lesions. J Neurophysiol 84, 1289–1302, 2000.
581. Robinson FR, Fuchs AF. The role of the cerebellum in voluntary eye movements. Annu Rev Neurosci 24, 981–1004, 2001.
582. Robinson FR, Fuchs AF, Noto CT. Cerebellar influences on saccade plasticity. Ann N Y Acad Sci 956, 155–163, 2002.
583. Robinson FR, Noto CT, Bevans SE. Effect of visual error size on saccade adaptation in monkey. J Neurophysiol 90, 1235–1244, 2003.
584. Robinson FR, Straube A, Fuchs AF. Role of the caudal fastigial nucleus in saccade generation. II. Effects of muscimol inactivation. J Neurophysiol 70, 1741–1758, 1993.
585. Ron S, Robinson DA. Eye movements evoked by cerebellar stimulation in the alert monkey. J Neurophysiol 36, 1004–1022, 1973.
586. Ron S, Vieville T, Droulez J. Target velocity based prediction in saccadic vector programming. Vision Res 29, 1103–1114, 1989.
587. Ross J, Morrone MC, Goldberg ME, Burr DC. Changes in visual perception at the time of saccades. Trends Neurosci 24, 113–121, 2001.
588. Ross SM, Ross LE. Children's and adult's predictive saccades to square-wave targets. Vision Res 27, 2177–2180, 1987.
589. Rottach KG, Das VE, Wohlgemuth W, Zivotofsky AZ, Leigh RJ. Properties of horizontal saccades accompanied by blinks. J Neurophysiol 79, 2895–2902, 1998.
590. Rottach KG, von Maydell RD, Das VE, et al. Evidence for independent feedback control of horizontal and vertical saccades from Niemann-Pick type C disease. Vision Res 37, 3627–3638, 1997.
591. Rucker JC, Shapiro BE, Han YH, et al. Neuro-ophthalmology of late-onset Tay-Sachs disease (LOTS). Neurology 63, 1918–1926, 2004.
592. Russo GS, Bruce CJ. Supplementary eye field: representation of saccades and relationship between neural response fields and elicited eye movements. J Neurophysiol 84, 2605–2621, 2000.
593. Sakai K, Rowe JB, Passingham RE. Active maintenance in prefrontal area 46 creates distractor-resistant memory. Nat Neurosci 5, 479–483, 2002.
593a. Salman MS, Sharpe JA, Eizenman M, et al. Saccades in children. Vision Res, in press, 2005.
594. Sato H, Noda H. Saccadic dysmetria induced by transient functional decortication of the cerebellar vermis. Exp Brain Res 88, 455–458, 1992.
595. Sato M, Hikosaka O. Role of primate substantia nigra pars reticulata in reward-oriented saccadic eye movement. J Neurosci 22, 2363–2373, 2002.
596. Sato T, Murthy A, Thompson KG, Schall JD. Search efficiency but not response interference affects visual selection in frontal eye field. Neuron 30, 583–591, 2001.
597. Sato TR, Schall JD. Effects of stimulus-response compatibility on neural selection in frontal eye field. Neuron 38, 637–648, 2003.
598. Sawaguchi T. The effects of dopamine and its antagonists on directional delay-period activity of prefrontal neurons in monkeys during an oculomotor delayed-response task. Neurosci Res 41, 115–128, 2001.
599. Sawaguchi T, Goldman-Rakic PS. The role of D1-dopamine receptor in working memory: Local injections of dopamine antagonists into the prefrontal cortex of rhesus monkeys performing an oculomotor- delayed response task. J Neurophysiol 71, 515–528, 1994.
600. Schall JD. The neural selection and control of saccades by the frontal eye field. Philos. Trans R Soc Lond B Biol Sci 357, 1073–1082, 2002.
601. Schall JD, Hanes DP, Thompson KG, King DJ. Saccade target selection in frontal eye field of macaque. 1. Visual and premovement activation. J Neuroscience 15, 6905–6918, 1995.
602. Schiller PH, Chou IH. The effects of frontal eye field and dorsomedial frontal cortex lesions on visually guided eye movements. Nat Neurosci 1, 248–253, 1998.
603. Schiller PH, Haushofer J, Kendall G. An examination of the variables that affect express saccade generation. Vis Neurosci 21, 119–127, 2004.
603a. Schiller PH, Haushofer J. What is the coordinate frame utilized for the generation of express saccades in monkeys? Exp Brain Res 1–9, 2005.

604. Schiller PH, Sandell JH. Interactions between visually and electrically elicited saccades before and after superior colliculus and frontal eye field ablations in the Rhesus monkey. Exp Brain Res 49, 381–392, 1983.
605. Schiller PH, Sandell JH, Maunsell JHR. The effect of frontal eye field and superior colliculus lesions on saccadic latencies in the rhesus monkey. J Neurophysiol 57, 1033–1049, 1987.
606. Schiller PH, Stryker M. Single-unit recording and stimulation in superior colliculus of the alert rhesus monkey. J Neurophysiol 35, 915–924, 1972.
607. Schiller PH, True SD, Conway JL. Deficits in eye movements following frontal eye-field and superior colliculus ablations. J Neurophysiol 44, 1175–1189, 1980.
608. Schlag J, Dassonville P, Schlag-Rey M. Interaction of the two frontal eye fields before saccade onset. J Neurophysiol 79, 64–72, 1998.
609. Schlag J, Pouget A, Sadeghpour S, Schlag-Rey M. Interactions between natural and electrically evoked saccades. III. Is the nonstationarity the result of an integrator not instantaneously reset? J Neurophysiol 79, 903–910, 1998.
610. Schlag J, Schlag-Rey M. Visuomotor functions of central thalamus in monkey. II. Unit activity related to visual events, targeting, and fixation. J Neurophysiol 51, 1175–1195, 1984.
611. Schlag J, Schlag-Rey M. Does microstimulation evoke fixed-vector saccades by generating their vector or by specifying their goal? Exp Brain Res 68, 442–444, 1987.
612. Schlag J, Schlag-Rey M. Evidence for a supplementary eye field. J Neurophysiol 57, 179–200, 1987.
613. Schlag J, Schlag-Rey M, Dassonville P. Saccades can be aimed at the spatial location of targets flashed during pursuit. J Neurophysiol 64, 575–581, 1990.
614. Schlag-Rey M, Amador N, Sanchez H, Schlag J. Antisaccade performance predicted by neuronal activity in the supplementary eye field. Nature 390, 398–401, 1998.
615. Schlag-Rey M, Schlag J. Visuomotor functions of central thalamus in monkey. I. Unit activity related to spontaneous eye movements. J Neurophysiol 51, 1149–1174, 1984.
616. Schlag-Rey M, Schlag J. The central thalamus. In Wurtz RH, Goldberg ME (eds). The Neurobiology of Saccadic Eye Movements. Amsterdam, Elsevier, 1989, pp 361–390.
617. Schmid R, Ron S. A model of eye tracking of periodic square wave target motion. Biol Cybern 54, 179–187, 1986.
618. Schmidt D, Abel LA, Dell'Osso LF, Daroff RB. Saccadic velocity characteristics: Intrinsic variability and fatigue. Aviat Space Environ Med 50, 393–395, 1979.
619. Schnabolk C, Raphan T. Modeling three-dimensional velocity-to-position transformation in oculomotor control. J Neurophysiol 71, 623–637, 1994.
620. Schneider KA, Kastner S. Visual responses of the human superior colliculus: a high-resolution functional magnetic resonance imaging study. J Neurophysiol 94, 2491–2503, 2005.
621. Schon F, Hodgson TL, Mort D, Kennard C. Ocular flutter associated with a localized lesion in the paramedian pontine reticular formation. Ann Neurol 50, 413–416, 2001.
621a. Schreiber C, Missal M, Lefèvre P. Asynchrony between position and motion signals in the saccadic system. J Neurophysiol, in press, 2005.
622. Scudder CA. A new local feedback model of the saccadic burst generator. J Neurophysiol 59, 1455–1475, 1988.
623. Scudder CA, Batourina EY, Tunder GS. Comparison of two methods of producing adaptation of saccade size and implications for the site of plasticity. J Neurophysiol 79, 704–715, 1998.
624. Scudder CA, Kaneko CS, Fuchs AF. The brainstem burst generator for saccadic eye movements: a modern synthesis. Exp Brain Res 142, 439–462, 2002.
625. Scudder CA, McGee DM. Adaptive modification of saccade size produces correlated changes in the discharges of fastigial nucleus neurons. J Neurophysiol 90, 1011–1026, 2003.
626. Scudder CA, Moschovakis AK, Karabelas AB, Highstein SM. Anatomy and physiology of saccadic long-lead burst neurons recorded in the alert squirrel monkey. 2. Pontine neurons. J Neurophysiol 76, 353–370, 1996.
627. Scudder CA, Moschovakis AK, Karabelas AB, Highstein SM. Anatomy and physiology of saccadic long-lead burst neurons recorded in the alert squirrel monkey. 1. Descending projections from the mesencephalon. J Neurophysiol 76, 332–352, 1996.
628. Seeberger T, Noto C, Robinson F. Non-visual information does not drive saccade gain adaptation in monkeys. Brain Res 956, 374–379, 2002.
629. Segraves MA, Park K. The relationship of monkey frontal eye field activity to saccade dynamics. J Neurophysiol 69, 1880–1889, 1993.
630. Selemon LD, Goldman-Rakic PS. Common cortical and subcortical targets of the dorsolateral prefrontal and posterior parietal cortices in the rhesus monkey: evidence for a distributed neural network subserving spatially guided behavior. J Neurosci 8, 4049–4068, 1988.
631. Selhorst JB, Stark L, Ochs AL, Hoyt WF. Disorders in cerebellar ocular motor control. I. Saccadic overshoot dysmetria, an oculographic, control system and clinico- anatomic analysis. Brain 99, 497–508, 1976.
632. Selhorst JB, Stark L, Ochs AL, Hoyt WF. Disorders in cerebellar ocular motor control. II. Macrosaccadic oscillations, an oculographic, control system and clinico-anatomic analysis. Brain 99, 509–522, 1976.
633. Semmlow JL, Gauthier GM, Vercher J-L. Mechanisms of short-term saccadic adaptation. J Exper Psychol: Human Percept Perform 15, 249–258, 1989.
634. Sereno MI, Pitzalis S, Martinez A. Mapping of contralateral space in retinotopic coordinates by a parietal cortical area in humans. Science 294, 1350–1354, 2001.
635. Shadlen MN, Newsome WT. Neural basis of a perceptual decision in the parietal cortex (area LIP) of the rhesus monkey. J Neurophysiol 86, 1916–1936, 2001.
636. Shafer JL, Noto CT, Fuchs AF. Temporal characteristics of error signals driving saccadic gain adaptation in the macaque monkey. J Neurophysiol 84, 88–95, 2000.
637. Shaffer DM, Krisky CM, Sweeney JA. Frequency and metrics of square-wave jerks: influences of task-

demand characteristics. Invest Ophthalmol Vis Sci 44, 1082–1087, 2003.

638. Shafiq R, Stuart GW, Sandbach J, Maruff P, Currie J. The gap effect and express saccades in the auditory modality. Exp Brain Res 118, 221–229, 1998.
639. Shafiq-Antonacci R, Maruff P, Masters C, Currie J. Spectrum of saccade system function in Alzheimer disease. Arch Neurol 60, 1272–1278, 2003.
640. Shafiq-Antonacci R, Maruff P, Whyte S, et al. The effects of age and mood on saccadic function in older individuals. J Gerontol B Psychol Sci Soc Sci 54, 361–368, 1999.
641. Sharpe JA, Troost BT, Dell'Osso LF, Daroff RB. Comparative velocities of different types of fast eye movements in man. Invest Ophthalmol Vis Sci 14, 689–692, 1975.
642. Sharpe JA, Zackon DH. Senescent saccades. Effects of aging on their accuracy, latency and velocity. Acta Otolaryngol (Stockh) 104, 422–428, 1987.
643. Shelhamer M. Correlation dimension of optokinetic nystagmus as evidence of chaos in the oculomotor system. IEEC Trans Biomed Eng BME 39, 1319–1321, 1992.
644. Shelhamer M, Clendaniel RA. Context-specific adaptation of saccade gain. Exp Brain Res 146, 441–450, 2002.
645. Shelhamer M, Clendaniel RA, Roberts DC. Context-specific adaptation of saccade gain in parabolic flight. J Vestib Res 12, 211–221, 2002.
646. Shelhamer M, Joiner WM. Saccades exhibit abrupt transition between reactive and predictive; predictive saccade sequences have long-term correlations. J Neurophysiol 90, 2763–2769, 2003.
647. Shelhamer M, Zee DS. Context-specific adaptation and its significance for neurovestibular problems of space flight. J Vestib Res 13, 345–362, 2003.
648. Sheliga BM, Brown VJ, Miles FA. Voluntary saccadic eye movements in humans studied with a double-cue paradigm. Vision Res 42, 1897–1915, 2002.
649. Shimo Y, Hikosaka O. Role of tonically active neurons in primate caudate in reward-oriented saccadic eye movement. J Neurosci 21, 7804–7814, 2001.
650. Shimozaki SS, Hayhoe MM, Zelinksy GJ, et al. Effect of parietal lobe lesions on saccade targeting and spatial memory in a naturalistic visual search task. Neuropsychologia 41, 1365–1386, 2003.
651. Shook BL, Schlag-Rey M, Schlag J. Direct projection from the supplementary eye field to the nucleus raphe interpositus. Exp Brain Res 73, 215–218, 1988.
652. Shook BL, Schlag-Rey M, Schlag J. Primate supplementary eye field: I. Comparative aspects of mesencephalic and pontine connections. J Comp Neurol 301, 618–642, 1990.
653. Shupert C, Fuchs AF. Development of conjugate human eye movements. Vision Res 28, 585–596, 1988.
654. Sibony PA, Evinger C, Manning K, Pellegrini JJ. Nicotine and tobacco-induced nystagmus. Ann Neurol 28, 198, 1990.
655. Siebold C, Glonti L, Kleine J, Büttner U. Saccade-related activity in the fastigial nucleus of the monkey during 3-D eye movements. Soc Neurosci Abstr 23, 1298, 1997.
656. Sindermann F, Geiselmann B, Fischler M. Single motor unit activity in extraocular muscles in man during fixation and saccades. Electroencephalogr Clin Neurophysiol 45, 64–73, 1978.
657. Smit AE, van Gisbergen JAM. A short-latency transition in saccade dynamics during square-wave tracking and its significance for the differentiation of visually-guided and predictive saccades. Exp Brain Res 76, 64–74, 1989.
658. Smit AE, van Gisbergen JAM, Cools AR. A parametric analysis of human saccades in different experimental paradigms. Vision Res 27, 1745–1762, 1987.
659. Smyrnis N, Evdokimidis I, Stefanis NC, et al. Antisaccade performance of 1,273 men: effects of schizotypy, anxiety, and depression. J Abnorm Psychol 112, 403–414, 2003.
660. Smyrnis N, Evdokimidis I, Stefanis NC, et al. The antisaccade task in a sample of 2,006 young males. II. Effects of task parameters. Exp Brain Res 147, 53–63, 2002.
661. Soetedjo R, Kaneko CR, Fuchs AF. Evidence against a moving hill in the superior colliculus during saccadic eye movements in the monkey. J Neurophysiol 87, 2778–2789, 2002.
662. Soetedjo R, Kaneko CR, Fuchs AF. Evidence that the superior colliculus participates in the feedback control of saccadic eye movements. J Neurophysiol 87, 679–695, 2002.
663. Sogo H, Osaka N. Effects of inter-stimulus interval on perceived locations of successively flashed perisaccadic stimuli. Vision Res 42, 899–908, 2002.
664. Somers JT, Das VE, Dell'Osso LF, Leigh RJ. Saccades to sounds: effects of tracking illusory visual stimuli. J Neurophysiol 84, 96–101, 2000.
665. Sommer MA, Tehovnik EJ. Reversible inactivation of macaque dorsomedial frontal cortex: effects on saccades and fixations. Exp Brain Res 124, 429–446, 1999.
666. Sommer MA, Wurtz RH. What the brain stem tells the frontal cortex. I. Oculomotor signals sent from superior colliculus to frontal eye field via mediodorsal thalamus. J Neurophysiol 91, 1381–1402, 2004.
667. Sommer MA, Wurtz RH. What the brain stem tells the frontal cortex. II. Role of the SC-MD-FEF pathway in corollary discharge. J Neurophysiol 91, 1403–1423, 2004.
668. Sonderegger EN, Meienberg O, Ehrengruber H. Normative data of saccadic eye movements for routine diagnosis of ophthalmoneurological disorders. Neuro-ophthalmology 6, 257–269, 1986.
669. Sparks DL. The neural encoding of the location of targets for saccadic eye movements. J Exp Biol 146, 195–207, 1989.
670. Sparks DL. The brainstem control of saccadic eye movements. Nat Rev Neurosci 3, 952–964, 2002.
671. Sparks DL, Hartwich-Young R. The Neurobiology of Saccadic Eye Movements. Amsterdam, Elsevier, 1989, pp 213–255.
672. Sparks DL, Mays LE. Spatial localization of saccade targets. I. Compensation for stimulation-induced perturbations in eye position. J Neurophysiol 49, 45–63, 1983.
673. Sparks DL, Mays LE. Signal transformations required for the generation of saccadic eye movements. Ann Rev Neurosci 13, 309–336, 1990.
674. Sparks DL, Porter JD. Spatial localization of saccade targets. II. Activity of superior colliculus neurons preceding compensatory saccades. J Neurophysiol 49, 64–74, 1983.
675. Spiller WG. The importance in clinical diagnosis of paralysis of associated movements of the eyeballs (Blicklaehmung), especially of upward and downward associated movements. J Nerv Ment Dis 32, 417–448, 1919.

676. Sprenger A, Kompf D, Heide W. Visual search in patients with left visual hemineglect. Prog Brain Res 140, 395–416, 2002.
677. Stanton GB, Goldberg ME, Bruce CJ. Frontal eye field efferents in the macaque monkey: I. Subcortical pathways and topography of striatal and thalamic terminal fields. J Comp Neurol 271, 473–492, 1988.
678. Stanton GB, Goldberg ME, Bruce CJ. Frontal eye field efferents in the macaque monkey: II. Topography of terminal fields in midbrain and pons. J Comp Neurol 271, 493–506, 1988.
679. Starr MS, Rayner K. Eye movements during reading: some current controversies. Trends Cogn Sci 5, 156–163, 2001.
680. Stein J. The magnocellular theory of developmental dyslexia [abstract]. Dyslexia 7, 12–36, 2001.
681. Strassman A, Highstein SM, McCrea RA. Anatomy and physiology of saccadic burst neurons in the alert squirrel monkey. I. Excitatory burst neurons. J Comp Neurol 249, 337–357, 1986.
682. Strassman A, Highstein SM, McCrea RA. Anatomy and physiology of saccadic burst neurons in the alert squirrel monkey. II. Inhibitory burst neurons. J Comp Neurol 249, 358–380, 1986.
683. Straube A, Büttner U. Pathophysiology of saccadic contrapulsion in unilateral rostral cerebellar lesions. Neuro-ophthalmology 14, 3–7, 1994.
684. Straube A, Deubel H. Rapid gain adaptation affects the dynamics of saccadic eye movements in humans. Vision Res 35, 3451–3458, 1995.
685. Straube A, Deubel H, Ditterich J, Eggert,T. Cerebellar lesions impair rapid saccade amplitude adaptation. Neurology 57, 2105–2108, 2001.
686. Straube A, Deubel H, Spuler A, Büttner U. Differential effect of a bilateral deep cerebellar nuclei lesion on externally triggered saccades in humans. Neuro-ophthalmology 15, 67–74, 1995.
687. Straube A, Fuchs AF, Usher S, Robinson FR. Characteristics of saccadic gain adaptation in rhesus macaques. J Neurophysiol 77, 874–895, 1997.
688. Stuphorn V, Taylor TL, Schall JD. Performance monitoring by the supplementary eye field. Nature 408, 857–860, 2000.
689. Sugiuchi Y, Izawa Y, Takahashi M, Na J, Shinoda Y. Physiological characterization of synaptic inputs to inhibitory burst neurons from the rostral and caudal superior colliculus. J. Neurophysiol 93, 697–712, 2005.
690. Suzuki Y, Buttner-Ennever JA, Straumann D, et al. Deficits in torsional and vertical rapid eye movements and shift of Listing's plane after uni- and bilateral lesions of the rostral interstitial nucleus of the medial longitudinal fasciculus. Exp Brain Res 106, 215–232, 1995.
691. Swartz BE, Li S, Bespalova IN, et al. Pathogenesis of clinical signs in recessive cerebellar ataxia with saccadic intrusions and sensorimotor neuropathy (SCASI). Ann Neurol 54, 824–828, 2003.
692. Sweeney JA, Mintun MA, Kwee S, et al. Positron emission tomography study of voluntary saccadic eye movements and spatial working memory. J Neurophysiol 75, 454–468, 1996.
693. Sylvester R, Haynes JD, Rees G. Saccades differentially modulate human LGN and V1 responses in the presence and absence of visual stimulation. Curr Biol 15, 37–41, 2005.
694. Takagi M, Frohman EM, Zee DS. Gap-overlap effects on latencies of saccades, vergence and combined vergence-saccades in humans. Vision Res 35, 3373–3388, 1995.
695. Takagi M, Tamargo R, Zee DS. Effects of lesions of the cerebellar oculomotor vermis on eye movements in primate: binocular control. Prog Brain Res 142, 19–33, 2003.
696. Takagi M, Zee DS, Tamargo RJ. Effects of lesions of the oculomotor vermis on eye movements in primate: saccades. J Neurophysiol 80, 1911–1930, 1998.
697. Takeda K, Funahashi S. Prefrontal task-related activity representing visual cue location or saccade direction in spatial working memory tasks. J Neurophysiol 87, 567–588, 2002.
698. Takeichi N, Kaneko CR, Fuchs AF. Discharge of monkey nucleus reticularis tegmenti pontis (NRTP) neurons changes during saccade adaptation. J Neurophysiol 94, 1938–1951, 2005.
699. Takikawa Y, Kawagoe R, Miyashita N, Hikosaka O. Presaccadic omnidirectional burst activity in the basal interstitial nucleus in the monkey cerebellum. Exp Brain Res 121, 442–450, 1998.
700. Tanaka M. Contribution of signals downstream from adaptation to saccade programming. J Neurophysiol 90, 2080–2086, 2003.
700a. Tanaka M. Inactivation of the central thalamus delays self-timed saccades. Nat Neurosci, in press, 2005.
700b. Tanaka M. Effects of eye position on estimates of eye displacement for spatial updating. Neuroreport 16, 1261–1265, 2005.
701. Tanibuchi I, Goldman-Rakic PS. Dissociation of spatial-, object-, and sound-coding neurons in the mediodorsal nucleus of the primate thalamus. J Neurophysiol 89, 1067–1077, 2003.
702. Tanibuchi I, Goldman-Rakic PS. Comparison of oculomotor neuronal activity in paralaminar and mediodorsal thalamus in the rhesus monkey. J Neurophysiol 93, 614–619, 2005.
703. Tanji J. Sequential organization of multiple movements: involvement of cortical motor areas. Annu Rev Neurosci 24, 631–651, 2001.
704. Terao Y, Fukuda H, Ugawa Y, et al. Visualization of the information flow through human oculomotor cortical regions by transcranial magnetic stimulation. J Neurophysiol 80, 936–946, 1998.
705. Thiele A, Henning P, Kubischik M, Hoffmann KP. Neural mechanisms of saccadic suppression. Science 295, 2460–2462, 2002.
706. Their P, Andersen RA. Electrical microstimulation suggests two different forms of representation of head-centered space in the intraparietal sulcus of rhesus monkeys. Proc National Acad Sci U S A 93, 4962–4967, 1996.
707. Their P, Dicke PW, Haas R, Barash S. Encoding of movement time by populations of cerebellar Purkinje cells. Nature 405, 72–76, 2000.
708. Their P, Möck M. The oculomotor role of the pontine nuclei and the nucleus reticularis tegmenti pontis. In Büttner-Ennever JA (ed). Neuroanatomy of the Oculomotor System. Prog Brain Res 151, 293–320, 2006.
709. Thilo KV, Santoro L, Walsh V, Blakemore C. The site of saccadic suppression. Nat Neurosci 7, 13–14, 2004.
710. Thurston SE, Leigh RJ, Abel LA, Dell'Osso LF. Slow saccades and hypometria in anticonvulsant toxicity. Neurology 34, 1593–1596, 1984.
711. Tilikete C, Hermier M, Pelisson D, Vighetto A. Sac-

cadic lateropulsion and upbeat nystagmus: disorders of caudal medulla. Ann Neurol 52, 658–662, 2002.

712. Tobler PN, Müri RM. Role of human frontal and supplementary eye fields in double step saccades. Neuroreport 13, 253–255, 2002.

713. Trappenberg TP, Dorris MC, Munoz DP, Klein RM. A model of saccade initiation based on the competitive integration of exogenous and endogenous signals in the superior colliculus. J Cogn Neurosci 13, 256–271, 2001.

714. Trillenberg P, Zee DS, Shelhamer M. On the distribution of fast-phase intervals in optokinetic and vestibular nystagmus. Biol Cybern 87, 68–78, 2002.

715. Troost BT, Weber RB, Daroff RB. Hypometric saccades. Am J Ophthalmol 78, 1002–1005, 1974.

716. Tusa RJ, Zee DS, Herdman SJ. Effect of unilateral cerebral cortical lesions on ocular motor behavior in monkeys: saccades and quick phases. J Neurophysiol 56, 1590–1625, 1986.

717. Tweed D, Misslisch H, Fetter M. Testing models of the oculomotor velocity-to-position transformation. J Neurophysiol 72, 1425–1429, 1994.

717a. Tzelepi A, Yang Q, Kapoula Z. The effect of transcranial magnetic stimulation on the latencies of vertical saccades. Exp Brain Res 164, 67–77, 2005.

718. Umeno MM, Goldberg ME. Spatial properties in the monkey frontal eye field. 1. Predictive visual responses. J Neurophysiol 78, 1373–1383, 1997.

719. Umeno MM, Goldberg ME. Spatial processing in the monkey frontal eye field. II. Memory responses. J. Neurophysiol 86, 2344–2352, 2001.

720. Ungerleider LG, Christensen CA. Pulvinar lesions in monkeys produce abnormal scanning of a complex visual array. Neuropsychologia 17, 493–501, 1979.

721. Van Beuzekom AD, Van Gisbergen JA. Collicular microstimulation during passive rotation does not generate fixed gaze shifts. J Neurophysiol 87, 2946–2963, 2002.

722. Van Beuzekom AD, Van Gisbergen JA. Interaction between visual and vestibular signals for the control of rapid eye movements. J Neurophysiol 88, 306–322, 2002.

723. Van Donkelaar P, Müri RM. Craniotopic updating of visual space across saccades in the human posterior parietal cortex. Proc R Soc Lond B Biol Sci 269, 735–739, 2002.

724. Van Gelder P, Lebedev S, Tsui WH. Peak velocities of visually and nonvisually guided saccades in smooth-pursuit and saccadic tasks. Exp Brain Res 116, 201–215, 1997.

725. van Gisbergen JAM, Robinson DA, Gielen S. A quantitative analysis of generation of saccadic eye movements by burst neurons. J Neurophysiol 45, 417–442, 1981.

726. van Gisbergen JAM, van Opstal AJ, Roebroek JGH. Stimulus-induced modification of saccade trajectories. In O'Regan JK, Levy-Schoen A (eds). Eye Movements: From Physiology to Cognition. Elsevier, New York, 1987, pp 27–36.

727. van Gisbergen JAM, van Opstal AJ, Schoenmakers JJM. Experimental test of two models for the generation of oblique saccades. Exp Brain Res 57, 321–336, 1985.

728. van Leeuwen AF, Collewijn H, Erkelens CJ. Dynamics of horizontal vergence movements: interaction with horizontal and vertical saccades and relation with monocular preferences. Vision Res 38, 3943–3954, 1998.

729. van Opstal AJ, Hepp K, Hess BJ, Straumann D, Henn V. Two- rather than three-demensional representation of saccades in monkey superior colliculus. Science 252, 1313–1315, 1991.

730. van Opstal AJ, Hepp K, Suzuki Y, Henn V. Role of monkey nucleus reticularis tegmenti pontis in the stabilization of Listing's plane. J Neurosci 16, 7284–7296, 1996.

731. van Opstal AJ, van Gisbergen JAM. Skewness of saccadic velocity profiles: a unifying parameter for normal and slow saccades. Vision Res 27, 731–745, 1987.

732. van Opstal AJ, van Gisbergen JAM. Scatter in the metrics of saccades and properties of the collicular motor map. Vision Res 29, 1183–1196, 1989.

733. Vermersch AI, Gaymard BM, Rivaud-Pechaux S, et al. Memory guided saccade deficit after caudate nucleus lesion. J Neurol Neurosurg Psychiatry 66, 524–527, 1999.

734. Vermersch AI, Muri RM, Rivaud S, et al. Saccade disturbances after bilateral lentiform nucleus lesions in humans. J Neurol Neurosurg Psychiatry 60, 179–184, 1996.

735. Versino M, Hurko O, Zee DS. Disorders of binocular control of eye movements in patients with cerebellar dysfunction. Brain 119, 1933–1950, 1996.

736. Vilis T, Hepp K, Schwarz U, Henn V. On the generation of vertical and torsional rapid eye movements in the monkey. Exp Brain Res 77, 1–11, 1989.

737. Vilis T, Snow R, Hore J. Cerebellar saccadic dysmetria is not equal in the two eyes. Exp Brain Res 51, 343–350, 1983.

738. Vitu F, O'Regan JK, Inhoff AW, Topolski R. Mindless reading: eye-movement characteristics are similar in scanning letter strings and reading texts. Perception and Psychophysics 57, 352–364, 1997.

739. Voogd J, Barmack NH. Oculomotor cerebellum. In Büttner-Ennever JA (ed). Neuroanatomy of the Oculomotor System. Prog Brain Res 151, 231–268, 2006.

740. Waespe W, Wichmann W. Oculomotor disturbances during visual-vestibular interaction in Wallenberg's lateral medullary syndrome. Brain 113, 821–846, 1990.

741. Waitzman DM, Ma TP, Optican LM, Wurtz RH. Superior colliculus neurons provide the saccadic motor error signal. Exp Brain Res 72, 649–652, 1988.

742. Waitzman DM, Silakov VL, Cohen B. Central mesencephalic reticular formation (cMRF) neurons discharging before and during eye movements. J Neurophysiol 75, 1546–1572, 1996.

743. Waitzman DM, Silakov VL, Palma-Bowles S, Ayers AS. Effects of reversible inactivation of the primate mesencephalic reticular formation. I. Hypermetric goal-directed saccades. J Neurophysiol 83, 2260–2284, 2000.

744. Waitzman DM, Silakov VL, Palma-Bowles S, Ayers AS. Effects of reversible inactivation of the primate mesencephalic reticular formation. II. Hypometric vertical saccades. J Neurophysiol 83, 2285–2299, 2000.

745. Walker MF, Fitzgibbon EJ, Goldberg ME. Neurons in the monkey superior colliculus predict the visual result of impending saccadic eye movements. J Neurophysiol 73, 1988–2003, 1995.

746. Walker R, Deubel H, Schneider WX, Findlay JM.

Effect of remote distractors on saccade programming; evidence for an extended fixation zone. Vision Res 78, 1108–1119, 1997.
747. Walker R, Walker DG, Husain M, Kennard C. Control of voluntary and reflexive saccades. Exp Brain Res 130, 540–544, 2000.
748. Wallace MT, Wilkinson LK, Stein BE. Representation and integration of multiple sensory inputs in primate superior colliculus. J Neurophysiol 76, 1246–1266, 1996.
749. Wardak C, Olivier E, Duhamel JR. Saccadic target selection deficits after lateral intraparietal area inactivation in monkeys. J Neurosci 22, 9877–9884, 2002.
750. Watanabe K, Lauwereyns J, Hikosaka O. Neural correlates of rewarded and unrewarded eye movements in the primate caudate nucleus. J Neurosci 23, 10052–10057, 2003.
751. Weber H, Biscaldi M, Fischer B. Intertrial effects of randomization on saccadic reaction times in human observers. Vision Res 35, 2615–2642, 1995.
752. Weber H, Fischer B. Gap duration and location of attention focus modulate the occurrence of left right asymmetries in the saccadic reaction times of human subjects. Vision Res 35, 987–998, 1995.
753. Weber RB, Daroff RB. Corrective movements following refixation saccades: type and control system analysis. Vision Res 12, 467–475, 1972.
754. Westheimer G. Eye movement responses to a horizontally moving visual stimulus. Arch Ophthalmol 52, 932–941, 1954.
755. Westheimer G, Blair SM. Saccadic inhibition induced by brain-stem stimulation in the alert monkey. Invest Ophthalmol Vis Sci 12, 77–78, 1973.
756. Wexler M. Anticipating the three-dimensional consequences of eye movements. Proc Natl Acad Sci U S A 102, 1246–1251, 2005.
757. White JM, Sparks DL, Stanford TR. Saccades to remembered target locations: an analysis of systematic and variable errors. Vision Res 34, 79–92, 1994.
758. Williams GV, Rao SG, Goldman-Rakic PS. The physiological role of 5-HT2A receptors in working memory. J Neurosci 22, 2843–2854, 2002.
759. Wilmer JB, Richardson AJ, Chen Y, Stein JF. Two visual motion processing deficits in developmental dyslexia associated with different reading skills. J Cogn Neurosci 16, 528–540, 2004.
760. Wurtz RH. Vision for the control of eye movement. Invest Ophthalmol Vis Sci 37, 2131–2145, 1997.
761. Wurtz RH, Albano JE. Visual-motor function of the primate superior colliculus. Ann Rev Neurosci 3, 189–226, 1980.
762. Wurtz RH, Goldberg ME. Activity of superior colliculus in behaving monkey. III. Cells discharging before eye movements [abstract]. J Neurophysiol 35, 575–586, 1972.
763. Wurtz RH, Sommer MA, Pare M, Ferraina S. Signal transformations from cerebral cortex to superior colliculus for the generation of saccades. Vision Res 41, 3399–3412, 2001.
764. Wyatt HJ. Detecting saccades with jerk. Vision Res 38, 2147–2153, 1998.
765. Wyder MT, Massoglia DP, Stanford TR. Quantitative assessment of the timing and tuning of visual-related, saccade-related, and delay period activity in primate central thalamus. J Neurophysiol 90, 2029–2052, 2003.
766. Xing J, Andersen RA. Memory activity of LIP neurons for sequential eye movements simulated with neural networks. J Neurophysiol 84, 651–665, 2000.
767. Xing J, Andersen RA. Models of the posterior parietal cortex which perform multimodal integration and represent space in several coordinate frames. J Cogn Neurosci 12, 601–614, 2000.
768. Yamada J, Noda H. Afferent and efferent connections of the oculomotor cerebellar vermis in the macaque monkey. J Comp Neurol 265, 224–241, 1987.
769. Yarbus AL. Eye movements and vision. Plenum, New York, 1967.
770. Yoshida K, Iwamoto Y, Chimoto S, Shimazu H. Saccade-related inhibitory input to pontine omnipause neurons: an intracellular study in alert cats. J Neurophysiol 82, 1198–1208, 1999.
771. Young LR, Stark L. Variable feedback experiments testing a sampled data model for eye tracking movements. IEEE Trans Hum Factors Electron HFE-4, 38–51, 1963.
772. Zambarbieri D. The latency of saccades toward auditory targets in humans. Prog Brain Res 140, 51–59, 2002.
773. Zee DS, Chu FC, Leigh RJ, et al. Blink-saccade synkinesis. Neurology 33, 1233–1236, 1983.
774. Zee DS, Fitzgibbon EJ, Optican LM. Saccade-vergence interactions in humans. J Neurophysiol 68, 1624–1641, 1992.
775. Zee DS, Hain TC, Carl JR. Abduction nystagmus in internuclear ophthalmoplegia. Ann Neurol 21, 383–388, 1987.
776. Zee DS, Lasker AG. Antisaccades. Probing cognitive flexibility with eye movements. Neurology 63, 1554, 2004.
777. Zee DS, Optican LM, Cook JD, Robinson DA, Engel WK. Slow saccades in spinocerebellar degeneration. Arch Neurol 33, 243–251, 1976.
778. Zee DS, Robinson DA. A hypothetical explanation of saccadic oscillations. Ann Neurol 5, 405–414, 1979.
779. Zee DS, Yamazaki A, Butler PH, Gücer G. Effects of ablation of flocculus and paraflocculus on eye movements in primate. J Neurophysiol 46, 878–899, 1981.
780. Zee DS, Yee RD, Singer HS. Congenital ocular motor apraxia. Brain 100, 581–599, 1977.
781. Zhang M, Barash S. Persistent LIP activity in memory antisaccades: working memory for a sensorimotor transformation. J Neurophysiol 91, 1424–1441, 2004.
782. Zhou W, King WM. Binocular eye movements not coordinated during REM sleep. Exp Brain Res 117, 153–160, 1997.
783. Zhou W, King WM. Premotor commands encode monocular eye movements. Nature 393, 692–695, 1998.
784. Zihl J. Eye movement patterns in hemianopic dyslexia. Brain 118, 891–912, 1995.
785. Zihl J, Von Cramon D. The contribution of the "second" visual system to directed visual attention in man. Brain 102, 835–856, 1979.
786. Zingale CM, Kowler E. Planning sequences of saccades. Vision Res 27, 1327–1341, 1987.
787. Zivotofsky AZ, Rottach KG, Averbuch-Heller L, et al. Saccades to remembered targets: the effects of smooth pursuit and illusory stimulus-motion. J Neurophysiol 76, 3617–3632, 1996.

Chapter 4

Smooth Pursuit and Visual Fixation

THE PURPOSE OF SMOOTH PURSUIT

Smooth pursuit eye movements allow clear vision of objects moving within the visual environment—such as when we watch an eagle soaring in front of cliffs. Dodge [129] pointed out that this ability depends upon the generation of continuous eye movements that "keep the line of regard congruent with the line of interest." He demonstrated that the velocity of smooth pursuit eye movements matched the velocity of the target; that pursuit had "the character of habitual movements"; that it was continuous in nature with no "periods of rest"; and that vision remained clear throughout the movement. To achieve this last attribute, the image of a moving object must be attended to and kept on the fovea. Smeared images of the stationary background that move across the rest of the retina due to the eye movement are ignored, although they may be used to estimate the target's location in space.[64]

Although most research on smooth pursuit embodies Dodge's concept of eye movements that follow moving targets, F. A. Miles has suggested that the system actually evolved to keep the fovea pointed at a stationary target during self-motion.[318] As we walk through our environment, we induce an *optic flow* of images on the retina. The optic flow provides important information about the three-dimensional (3-D) layout of the environment and our direction of heading.[8a,19,180] However, excessive slip of images on the retina degrades vision. Smooth pursuit reduces image slip of an object of interest on the fovea, while optic flow still occurs on other parts of the retina. In other words, smooth-pursuit movements must be generated in response to local optic flow on the fovea, but not in response to optic flow on the rest of the retina. Furthermore, other visually mediated eye movements, such as the optokinetic responses to retinal image motion caused by head rotations and translations must be suppressed during smooth pursuit. The implication is that smooth pursuit depends on an ability to compensate for the effects of retinal image motion so that objects are correctly localized in space, and filter out visual motion inputs save for those at the focus of attention.[460] Once evolved, such a mechanism could also be used to pursue a small object moving across a complex background, or help to hold the image of a stationary object on the fovea when the observer was stationary—visual fixation. The illusion of motion of the stationary world during pursuit has been reported by a patient with posterior cortical lesions: the patient's symptom suggested that the mechanism to filter out image motion caused by eye movements had been disrupted.[181] Inadequate smooth pursuit is partially compensated by frequent saccades, which re-foveate the object of interest when the eye drifts off target. Nonetheless, patients with impaired smooth pursuit have impaired vision of moving targets.[181] Under natural circumstances, we often track moving targets with combined movements of eyes and head; this behavior is discussed in Chapter 7.

VISUAL FIXATION

Gaze Stability with and without Visual Fixation

To see a stationary object best, its image must be held steadily upon the fovea. As discussed in Chapter 1, visual acuity is influenced by either motion of the image, or displacement of it from the center of the fovea. For clear vision of higher spatial frequencies (e.g., a 20/20 Snellen optotype), motion of the image should be less than about 5 degrees per second and the image should lie within 0.5 degrees of the center of the fovea.[69,78,216] However, if images are perfectly stabilized on the retina, vision fades.[128,378,420,489] Visual fading occurs because, like other sensory systems, the visual system habituates its responses to persistent stimuli.[304]

During natural activities, the major threat to steady fixation comes from perturbations of the head.[175] However, even if the subject's head is stabilized using a bite-bar, gaze is still disrupted by involuntary eye movements.[140,249,304,419,420] An example is shown in Figure 4–1. The gaze instability during attempted fixation is more prominent in the torsional than the horizontal or vertical planes.[144,356] It has three main components: a high-frequency low-amplitude tremor, small saccades, and slow drifts. The frequency of the tremor ranges up to 150 Hz and its amplitude is less than 0.01 degree, which corresponds to less than the size of one photoreceptor.[249,286,412,420] It is uncertain whether ocular tremor aids vision.[304]

The small saccades, called microsaccades, are typically less than a third of a degree in amplitude, occur in all directions, and follow the main-sequence, like larger saccades.[505] Microsaccades can be suppressed during visual tasks that demand steady fixation, such as threading a needle, or sighting a gun.[122,420] They may also be influenced by attention shifts.[141,182] There has been doubt as to whether microsaccades serve any role for visual perception,[304] although some insights have been obtained from electrophysiological studies in primates. Microsaccades do cause bursts of spikes in the lateral geniculate

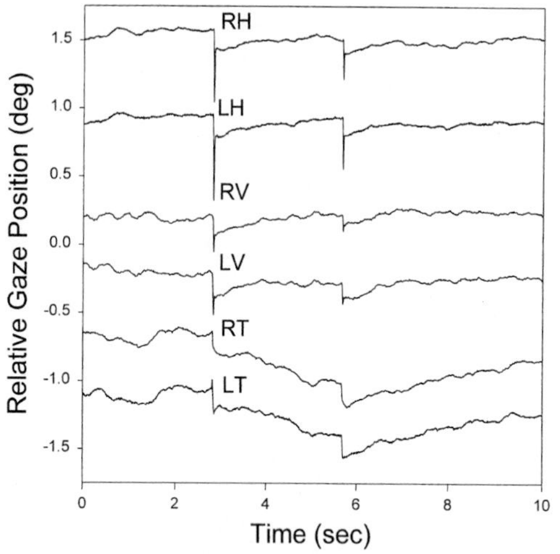

Figure 4–1. Gaze stability during fixation in a normal subject. The subject was viewing a small, stationary cross at a viewing distance of 1.2 meters in normal room illumination, with head stabilized. Three-dimensional rotations of both eyes were measured using the magnetic search coil technique. Gaze positions are relative, having been offset for clarity of display. RH: right horizontal; LH: left horizontal; RV: right vertical; LV: left vertical; RT: right torsional; LT: left torsional. Positive deflections indicate rightward, upward, and clockwise rotations, from the point of view of the subject. Note that small saccades and drifts occur; the drifts are greater in the torsional plane.

nucleus and primary visual cortex (V1) in monkeys, and the vigor of these bursts is influenced by the properties of the current visual stimulus.[302,303] Furthermore, psychophysical studies indicate that peripheral vision fades due to habituation when microsaccades are suppressed.[305] Thus, microsaccades may aid vision during fixation, and current research is seeking to clarify their role.

When a subject views a stationary target with the eyes close to center position, the slow drifts that occur during attempted fixation—and the image motion that they produce—are small (standard deviation of position is typically less than 0.1 degrees and of velocity is less than 0.25 degrees per second). When the eyes move away from the central to an eccentric position in the orbit, gaze-evoked nystagmus may develop because stability of gaze becomes susceptible to elastic restoring forces due to the passive properties of the orbital contents; this issue is discussed in Chapter 5. When a subject sits in darkness and attempts to look at the remembered location of a target, the velocity of slow drifts increases about fourfold above that when actually looking at the target (Fig. 4–2). This implies that during vision of the stationary target, any slip of images on the retina due to ocular drifts stimulates the brain to generate eye movements that will counter the drifts, and hold gaze steady. This response to drift of images upon the retina caused by instability of gaze during active fixation has been referred to as slow-control, or a field-holding reflex.[143,333] Eye drift is especially likely to occur in wake of saccade. Clear vision just after a saccade is critical since, during the saccade, the subject has been mainly blind to what has been happening in the visual world. There is evidence that the field-holding reflex is enhanced at that time. Thus, the ocular following response to motion of a large textured moving stimulus is increased if motion starts just after a saccade,[167,226] or during smooth pursuit.[427] These responses occur at ultra-short latencies (about 70 ms in humans)[167] and are not dependent on the subject attending to the visual stimulus. Furthermore, the shortest latency responses occur for images in the plane of fixation (i.e., for binocular images that lack disparity).[318] Thus, these pre-attentive ocular

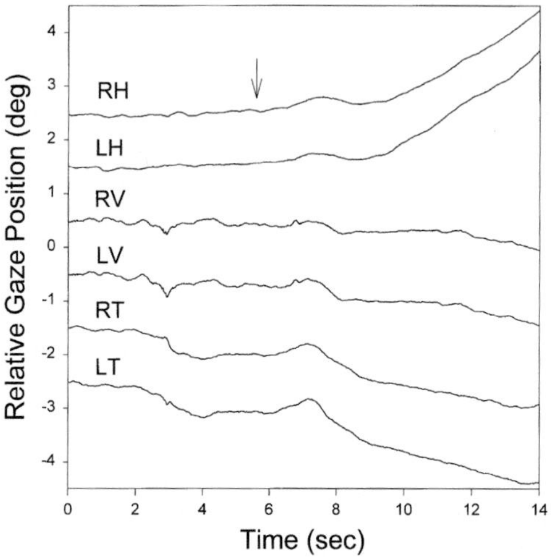

Figure 4–2. Comparison of gaze stability during fixation of a small red target light in a dark room and during attempted fixation of the remembered target location after it had been turned out (indicated by arrow). The subject had been instructed to suppress saccades. Note that increased drift occurs, especially horizontally, after the light is turned out. Conventions are similar to Figure 4–1.

following responses seem admirably suited to stabilize the eyes immediately after saccades and appear to be an important part of a visual fixation mechanism. The question then arises: Is there an independent visual fixation system distinct from smooth pursuit?

Evidence for and against an Independent Fixation System

One line of evidence that fixation differs from smooth pursuit comes from electrophysiological studies in monkeys. Thus, certain parietal lobe neurons discharge during steady fixation but not during smooth pursuit of a moving target.[296] Furthermore, some of these neurons respond to both the presence, or momentary disappearance, of the fixation stimulus.[45] Thus, the parietal lobe seems important in the engagement and disengagement of fixation. Microstimulation of neurons in the pursuit pathway—the medial superior temporal visual area,[245] the dorsolateral pontine nucleus,[310] or the posterior vermis[264] (see Fig. 6–6), produces changes in smooth eye velocity *only* if the monkey is already engaged in smooth pursuit; it does not produce pursuit if the object of regard is stationary. There is also electrophysiological evidence for a mechanism to suppress both saccades and pursuit during attempted fixation. Microstimulation of parts of the frontal eye fields,[68,213] and the rostral pole of the superior colliculus,[332] will suppress or delay the initiation of a visually triggered saccade. Stimulation of the rostral pole of the superior colliculus, which seems important for fixation, also suppresses ipsilateral smooth-pursuit movements; pharmacological inactivation increases ipsilateral pursuit. [35] Thus, the electrophysiological properties of both the saccadic and the pursuit systems are changed during active fixation of a stationary target, suggesting the influence of an independent, visual fixation system.

There is also evidence from behavioral studies that visual fixation differs from smooth pursuit. Most such studies have focused on differences between smooth pursuit of a moving target, and the eye movements that occur just after the target comes to a halt. In the latter case, retinal image slip is due to eye motion rather than target motion, and the function is therefore equivalent to visual fixation. During smooth pursuit of a moving target, and especially at the onset, small ocular oscillations may occur (Fig. 4–3).[382,384] These oscillations are usually absent or minor after the target for pursuit comes to a halt (Fig. 4–3),[202,260,263,273,295,384] suggesting that different mechanisms are involved in fixation than in pursuit. However, the presence of these oscillations might be due to other experimental factors. For example, oscillations do occur after the target stops if there is uncertainty about whether it will do so or speed up.[263] Thus, the oscillations that occur during smooth pursuit may be because the brain is placing greater reliance on visual inputs, and may not be related to whether retinal slip is due to target or eye motion.[263] Similarly, oscillations are present when patients who have lost vestibular function attempt to view a stationary target while they are rotated at constant speed in a chair;[273] in this situation, visual mechanisms must substitute for the vestibulo-ocular reflex.

Other attempts to identify an independent fixation system have involved comparisons of the dynamic properties of visually mediated eye movements when the eyes are either stationary or engaged in pursuit. First, the latency to onset of express saccades using the gap paradigm (Fig. 3–2B, Chapter 3), in which the fixation light is turned off before the new target is displayed, is approximately the same whether the target is stationary (fixation) or moving (smooth pursuit). Thus, the trigger for these saccades does not recognize the difference between fixation and pursuit.[55,262] Second, comparison of the ability to visually track a target that vibrates sinusoidally around a stationary target (corresponding to fixation) is no different from the response when similar vibrations that are superimposed upon ramp motion of the target (pursuit).[110] However, a single sine-wave cycle that increases the velocity of a ramp motion does produce a larger response than if the same sine wave is presented during fixation.[88] This latter finding has been interpreted as evidence for on-line control of pursuit gain rather than separate pursuit and fixation systems. A final line of evidence that does support an independent pursuit system is that patients are reported who show normal fixation of a stationary target, but whose eyes break into oscillations of the type seen in congenital nystagmus when they

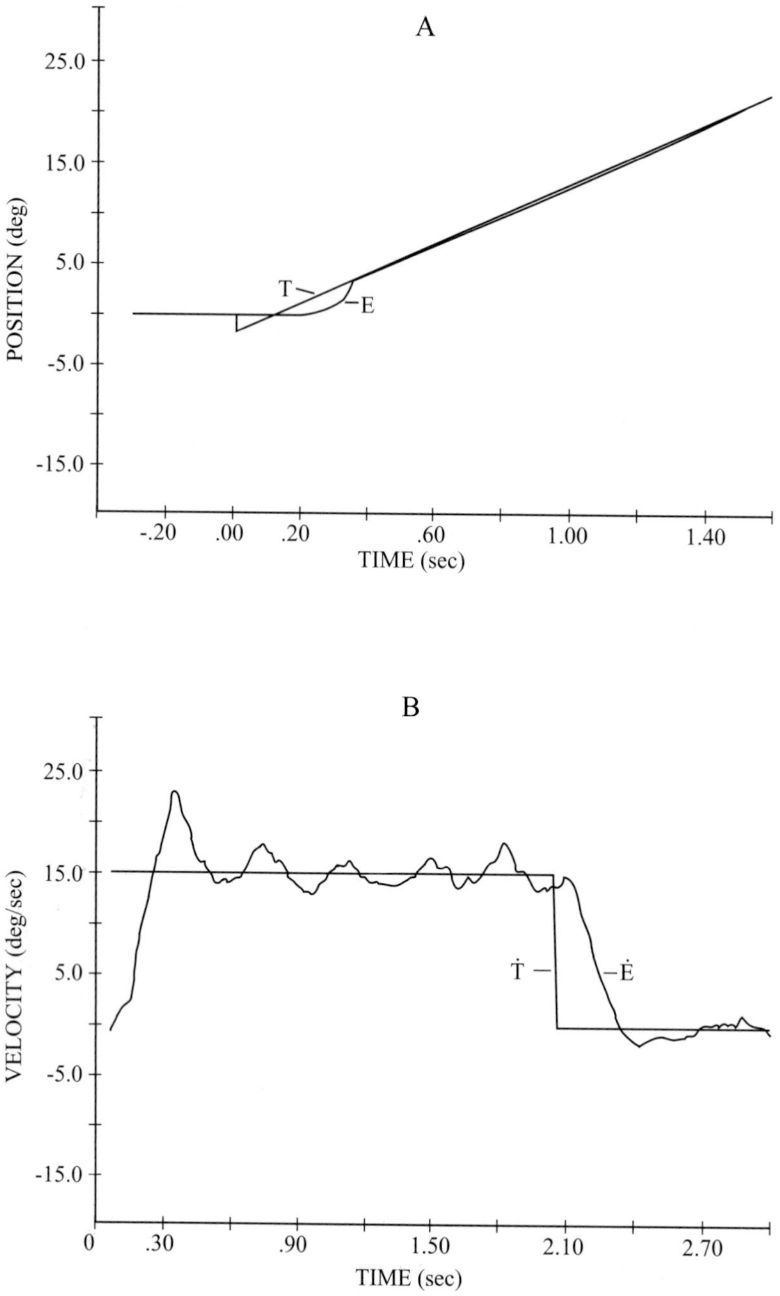

Figure 4–3. Initiation of smooth pursuit in response to a 15-degree per second step-ramp (Rashbass) stimulus, showing position (A) and velocity (B) plots of the response. In the velocity record, saccades have been removed. Positive values correspond to rightward movements. Note how, in A, the target (T) initially steps 1.8 degrees to the left (thereby creating a position error on the retina) and then immediately a smooth movement begins to the right at 15 degrees per second (creating a velocity error on the fovea). If the main response of the pursuit system were to the position stimulus, the initial movement would be in the direction of the initial target step (to the left). In fact, the eye (E) commences a smooth pursuit movement in response to the smooth movement of the target (to the right). In B target velocity (Ṫ) and eye velocity (Ė) records correspond to position records A. Target onset is at 0 seconds. After a latency of about 120 ms, the eye accelerates to a peak value (maximum slope) of 140 degrees per second/second. Eye velocity initially overshoots target velocity; thereafter, eye velocity oscillates ("rings") at a frequency of 2 Hz to 3 Hz. Note that when the target stops, the eye decelerates with a time course that approximates a negative exponential with a time constant of about 90 ms.

try to pursue a moving target (see Video Display: Disorders of Smooth Pursuit).[232]

To summarize the evidence: on the one hand, a fixation mechanism has been demonstrated for the suppression of saccades; this depends on known structures, such as the rostral pole of the superior colliculus, and is discussed further in Chapter 3. On the other hand, it is still debated as to whether retinal image motion is reduced by a separate fixation system when the target is stationary and by smooth pursuit when the target is moving. However, the ocular following responses to large textured moving stimuli, which occur at latencies as short as 70 ms, appear to constitute a field-holding visual fixation mechanism. These ocular following responses may also be part of the mechanism that stabilizes the fovea on a stationary target during locomotion. Thus, both ocular following and the translational vestibulo-ocular reflex (VOR) (but not the rotational VOR—see Chapter 2), obey Listing's law.[5,470]

STIMULUS FOR SMOOTH PURSUIT

In this section, we first examine attributes of stimuli that have been used to induce visual following eye movements, including smooth pursuit. We then discuss how smooth pursuit can be sustained either with stimuli that do not move or with non-visual stimuli. Finally, we review the role of stimulus predictability in generating the pursuit response.

Effects of Properties of the Visual Stimulus on Visual Following and Smooth Pursuit

GENERAL ASPECTS OF STIMULI THAT INDUCE OCULAR FOLLOWING

Although physics provides no special status for motion, which is simply displacement over time, several lines of evidence support the idea that the brain treats visual motion information separately from visual position information.[120,404] Perhaps best known is the waterfall illusion. It is induced by staring for some time at a moving object, such as a river or waterfall that occupies a substantial part of the visual field. Stationary objects viewed immediately afterwards in that same part of the visual field appear to move in the opposite direction. Thus, during the waterfall illusion, motion and position are dissociated, since the visual stimulus is seen as moving, and yet it remains in the same position on the retina. The waterfall illusion is not due to eye movements, such as optokinetic after-nystagmus;[396] rather it represents adaptation of the motion-vision system (recall that all sensory systems tend to habituate to persistent stimuli). The other line of evidence for an independent motion-vision system is based on electrophysiological studies that will be reviewed throughout this chapter. What sort of moving visual stimuli can drive smooth-tracking eye movements?

Ocular following responses can be driven by first-order or second-order motion stimuli.[79,206,287,404] First-order motion stimuli are defined by the spatial distribution of luminance. Examples of second-order motion stimuli, which depend on higher-level mechanisms, are contrast and flicker. Routinely, smooth pursuit is tested as subjects track a small spot of light, such as a laser spot projected onto a tangent screen in an otherwise dark room. However, this sort of visual stimulus is impoverished compared to what we see and track during natural activities. By studying ocular following responses to a range of first and second-order visual stimuli, and by pitting first-order against second-order motion,[82] insights have been gained into the mechanisms by which different areas of visual cortex process information on moving stimuli. Thus, the earliest visual following responses occur at latencies as short as 70 ms in response to large, textured moving stimuli; they are not influenced by factors such as attention to the stimulus.[167,404] As noted above, the ocular following responses are enhanced in the wake of a saccade, and seem well suited to serve as a field-holding visual fixation mechanism. Similar mechanisms probably aid alignment of the eyes;[405] these short-latency disparity vergence responses are described further in Chapter 8. Since primary visual cortex and some secondary visual areas do not respond to second-order visual stimuli,[347] it seems possible that testing patients with these two types of moving stimuli may prove useful diagnostically,[459] an issue that is discussed later in this chapter.

STIMULI FOR SMOOTH PURSUIT

When a small moving spot of light is used to stimulate smooth pursuit, the image of the target may not cover the fovea (it may be smaller); indeed, it may not lie on the fovea,[477,483] and such parafoveal tracking may be preferred if ambient light is poor, at which time rods are more efficient photoreceptors than cones. Pursuit tracking can also be triggered by objects moving in the far visual periphery and can begin before a saccade can be programmed. Nevertheless, foveal lesions do impair smooth pursuit of small targets.[381]

Experimentally, the responses to stimulation of various parts of the field of vision have been mapped by measuring the initial eye acceleration to targets that are projected onto specific portions of the retina in both humans[77] and monkeys.[455] Each trial starts during fixation of a stationary target so that the retinal location of the moving stimulus can be controlled. The fixation light is then turned out and a moving stimulus appears synchronously in the chosen part of the visual field. Since it takes about 100 ms for a pursuit eye movement to be initiated after the presentation of such stimuli (similar to Fig. 4–3), it follows that the first 100 ms of the pursuit movement will be due to stimulation of the selected portion of the retina. This technique is a sensitive way of measuring the open-loop response of pursuit that occurs before visual feedback is possible. The initial acceleration of the eye in response to horizontal, transient target motion is greater for target motions in the central than in the peripheral field, and is greater for targets moving towards the fovea than for targets moving away from the fovea. For vertical target motions, eye accelerations are greater for stimulus motion in the lower visual field, irrespective of whether the target is moving towards or away from the fovea. Bright targets elicit greater eye accelerations, at shorter latencies, than do dim targets. Attention to the target improves smooth-pursuit performance.[205]

Cues that signal the saliency of a target for smooth pursuit reduce latency to onset, provided they are located in a similar part of the visual field as the pursuit target.[185] Target saliency signaled, for example, by color, has greater effects on pursuit onset when target motion is directed towards the fovea.[322] Stationary distracters placed in the hemifield opposite to the moving target increase the latency to onset of pursuit.[240]

Another technique used to determine the relative influence of different parts of the retina (visual field) upon smooth pursuit is artificial stabilization of images upon the retina using electronic feedback.[131,480] For example, if a target is stabilized at the fovea, and optokinetic stimuli are presented to the peripheral visual field, the optokinetic response is partially suppressed.[369] However, the responses to such stimuli are affected not only by the visual stimulus but also by the subject's mental set.[13,100,106,131,462] Furthermore, because the moving stimuli are presented to one part of the eccentric retina, there is a displacement, or position-error component to the stimulus. Pursuit responses to target displacements are discussed in the next section.

When a subject pursues a larger stimulus, such as one that almost fills the visual field, the pursuit response is usually enhanced. This may be due, in part, to stimulation of a larger area of retina, but another factor that improves tracking is the freedom to select and attend to any feature of the visual stimulus.[461] When a full-field visual stimulus is used, the central 5–10 degrees of the visual field still dominates the response.[2a,463] As noted above, with sudden movement of full-field visual stimuli, humans generate ocular following responses at latencies as short as 70 ms.[167,404]

Under natural conditions, we pursue objects that move across a background provided by the stationary environment. As noted at the beginning of this chapter, under these conditions, slip of images of the stationary background occurs on the retina. Thus, a mechanism must exist to at least partly ignore the slip of images of the stationary background and focus attention on the relatively stable image of the moving target.[38] Another feature of natural stimuli for pursuit is that the moving object may be in a different depth plane than the background. When the moving target and the textured background lie in the same depth plane, there is a 10%–20% decrement in pursuit gain compared with tracking the same target in the absence of a background.[99,225,492] This effect is more pronounced for the onset of pursuit than during its maintenance,[231] and is influenced by the physical characteristics of the target and background.[192,479] The effect of the background is still present even if it is excluded from the path taken by the target, or seen only by one eye while the other sees only the moving target.[237] If, however, the target moves in a plane that is closer than the background (corresponding to natural conditions), pursuit is improved.[200,237] Taken together, these findings suggest that, under natural conditions, the smooth-pursuit response depends upon binocular visual inputs to generate a response appropriate to keep the eyes on a target moving through the environment.

If the background on which a small visual stimulus is projected moves—a rare event outside of the laboratory—there is a percept that a small target projected onto it moves in the opposite direction (the *Duncker illusion*).[136] Further, if a small target moves vertically over a horizontally moving background, subjects experience a strong illusion that the trajectory of the target is diagonal, but smooth pursuit follows the vertical target motion.[504] This finding illustrates how perception and pursuit can be dissociated, because of the low-level machine-like response of brainstem circuits.[503a,503b]

Subjects can be tested with more complex moving visual stimuli such as two-dimensional plaids, consisting of two sinusoidal gratings of different orientation. When two orthogonal moving gratings are presented, the ocular tracking response is best predicted by vector averaging of responses to each component grating. However, when plaids are constructed by summing one moving and one stationary grating with 45-degree orientation difference, ocular following shows two components: a shorter-latency response in the direction of grating motion, and, after a further 20 ms, a second component that brings the direction of the response to correspond with pattern motion.[306] Similarly, if subjects track line-figure diamonds, the initial eye movement is a vector average of the diamond's line segments, but the response eventually becomes tracking of the motion of the object.[307] The significance of these dissociated responses is that they have been generated by different functional components of the visual system, perhaps corresponding to the first-order and second-order motion. Such experimental paradigms can be used to better understand motion processing in visual areas of cerebral cortex.

Influence of Dynamic Properties of the Stimulus on Smooth Pursuit

What information about the movement of an image of a target does the pursuit system use? Is it target position (where) or target motion (at what speed)? In support of the importance of target motion, Rashbass,[376] and later Robinson,[382] showed that if a target abruptly jumps (steps) to one side of the fovea and then immediately begins a smooth movement in the opposite direction (a step-ramp stimulus; Figure 4–3), the subject will make a smooth eye movement in the direction of the ramp, but no saccade in the direction of the target step. In other words, the pursuit system responds to the ramp and the step appropriately, taking into account the motion of the ramp, which brings the target back to the fovea and so makes a saccade unnecessary.[386] In fact, cortical areas that abstract visual information about target motion project to both pursuit and saccade-generating mechanisms; this is discussed further in the section on Neural Substrate for Smooth Pursuit.

Although the rate of image motion on the retina is probably most important, particularly in initiating pursuit,[195] there is evidence that the smooth pursuit system may respond to both position and velocity errors.[52,77,263,366] The position error response is much more prominent when the eye is already tracking the target, and when the target jump is oppositely directed to the ongoing response.[441a] Furthermore, acceleration of the image of the target upon the retina also serves as a stimulus to pursuit.[288] Additional insights have been gained by studying responses to step-ramp stimuli that change direction; these show responses in which the saccadic component is mainly in response to position error while the pursuit component is principally influenced by target motion.[142] Furthermore, a sudden change in the direction of the stimulus being pursued may serve as a stimulus to pursuit independent from the mechanism determining eye speed.[411]

The interaction between pursuit and saccades has also been studied by simultaneously presenting two targets that move in different directions. Monkeys respond to such stimuli first with a pursuit movement that is the vector average of responses to the two individual target motions.[162] However, after the first saccade is made towards one of the targets, the pursuit movement is enhanced for movement of that target and suppressed for the other. Furthermore, if a saccade is evoked towards one of the moving targets by microstimulation of the monkey's frontal eye field or superior colliculus, that target is automatically chosen for subsequent pursuit.[163] These findings suggest that the saccadic command sets the agenda for the subsequent pursuit movement.

Pursuit Responses to Visual Stimuli that Do Not Move and Non-Visual Stimuli

Image motion on the retina is not the only stimulus capable of eliciting smooth pursuit movements. Some subjects can smoothly track their own outstretched finger while in darkness, probably using knowledge of the motor command to the limb (efference) and the consequent proprioceptive input (reafference).[164,308,417,418] Certain patients with acquired blindness can do the same.[277] By four years of age, children can pursue a partially occluded target or strobe-illuminated motion of their own finger.[435]

Few individuals can generate smooth eye movements without any perception, or short-term memory, of a moving stimulus.[195,221] However, most can do so in response to certain second-order visual stimuli, in which no image motion has actually occurred in the direction of the eye movement.[82] Examples of such stimuli are the apparent motion of sigma and phi phenomena,[39,40,73,98,145,462] and the motion of the imaginary center of a rolling wheel.[418] When subjects smoothly track such apparent motion, the perception of motion and the pursuit eye movements are highly correlated.[299] In normal subjects, the onset and maintenance of smooth pursuit deteriorates as a function of the spatial and temporal separation of flashed stimuli.[90]

A related finding is that patients with cortical lesions causing simultagnosia, defined as difficulty in seeing a single object in the presence of others, can still generate smooth pursuit at a time that they could not report seeing the target.[379] Thus, in addition to direct information about image motion from the retina, the brain can generate pursuit movements by using information about target motion from other sensory systems, by monitoring motor commands and by using higher-level perceptual representations of target motion.

Smooth Pursuit to Predictable Target Motion

THE RANGE OF PREDICTIVE PURSUIT BEHAVIOR

Another feature of the stimulus that greatly influences smooth-pursuit performance is the predictability of the target motion. In nature, both unpredictable movements (e.g., of a predator) and predictable motions (e.g., generated by the subject's hands) occur and must be pursued. One example of predictive behavior is that the eye will start to move in anticipation before the onset of target motion. These *anticipatory drifts* are small (less than 1.0 degrees per second) if the time of onset and the direction of target motion are unknown.[37,56,251-254] When the target light is kept on throughout the testing, real or apparent motion of the target is necessary to evoke anticipatory eye movements. However, if the target light is extinguished at the onset of a trial, following several prior, predictable, target motions, anticipatory drifts may increase to over 5 degrees per second.[37,56] They may be even faster and of short latency if subjects move the target with their own hands.[130,278] The movements are faster if the anticipatory movement starts from an eccentric eye position and moves centripetally.[434]

Once the target starts to move, a *predictive acceleration of the eye* occurs. For example, if on some trials of a predictable and repetitive nature the target light is extinguished just at the time that it would start to move, the eye may still accelerate.[37] If the target velocity is unexpectedly reduced, eye velocity may exceed it.[221] This behavior cannot depend upon actual motion of the target because that visual information has not yet reached the ocular motor neurons (due to the time taken for visual processing—over 70 ms). There is similar anticipation of the target stopping,[384,423] and of reversal of direction.[58,217a] In monkeys, extinguishing (blinking off) the moving target light is reported to cause a much greater decline of eye velocity than if an occluder is placed in front of the target,[89] a finding requiring confirmation in humans who have been given specific instructions.

Taken together, it appears that anticipatory drifts and early accelerations of the eye depend upon previous tracking experience, a form of memory that depends upon perceived motion.[30,56,57,473] This *memory for stimulus motion* is not simply limited to one direction or speed,[101a] but can extend to generate a series of anticipatory responses, suggesting that velocity information for each can be stored and released in the appropriate order.[29] Thus, if monkeys repeatedly track a target that initially moves horizontally but then changes direction after a predictable period, they will make the direction change even for probe trials, when the target continued to move horizontally.[313] This result suggests that the adapted behavior depends more on timing (duration of horizontal motion) rather than remembering a spatial location. Human subjects can voluntarily stop anticipatory pursuit movements to a cue,[217] and even countermand pursuit movements, similar to what has been described for saccades.[248] Furthermore, the timing of the response to auditory cues, the magnitude of the response itself, and selection of responses to one of two targets, can be independently controlled.[23,370] The store of memory for anticipatory smooth eye movements may exceed 14 seconds. [81] The same mechanisms appear to generate anticipatory responses during tracking of a visible or imagined head-fixed target during rotation in yaw.[27]

POSSIBLE MECHANISMS FOR PREDICTIVE PROPERTIES OF SMOOTH PURSUIT

After pursuit is initiated, subjects may be able to match almost perfectly the motion of a target moving in a regular waveform, such as a sine wave.[107,129,316] This predictive response is established rapidly—as soon as a quarter cycle after the onset of sinusoidal target motion. As discussed below in the section on Models of Smooth Pursuit, this behavior defies explanation by simple models of smooth pursuit that incorporate a delay due to visual processing. Certain unusual waveforms (such as a cubic function or sum of several different sine waves) also can be smoothly tracked, following a training period.[15,233,312] Other studies have shown that predictive features of smooth pursuit can be related to performance on the preceding trials.[21,22,25,221] This has led to the suggestions that prediction in smooth pursuit is due to storing of memories of eye movements and referring to them during tracking.[14,15,25,118] However, simply viewing repeated, predictable target motions can promote anticipatory smooth eye movements.[26]

A second possible mechanism, however, is an extrapolation of target behavior based upon the current stimulus to the pursuit system. This is evident if subjects track targets moving at constant speed and, at an unpredictable time, the target light is turned off.[37] Eye velocity falls about 200 ms after the target disappears, but not to zero; the eye continues to move at about 60% of target velocity for periods of up to four seconds. Because the amplitude of this "residual velocity" depended upon the previous target velocity, extrapolation seems likely.[37] Furthermore, the eye will start to speed up again before the target is turned back on, if this is done in a predictable fashion.[47,48] Although more than one predictive mechanism may aid smooth pursuit, there are differences between those subserving pursuit and predictive mechanisms underlying saccadic tracking. Thus, predictive mechanisms for pursuit are quickly established, whereas observation of several cycles of target jumps is generally required before predictive saccades can be generated.[503]

QUANTITATIVE ASPECTS OF SMOOTH PURSUIT

Having reviewed properties of the stimuli for smooth pursuit, here we summarize methods to quantify responses. Smooth-pursuit performance varies considerably among individuals and is affected by many factors such as the properties of the stimulus, attention, and age. Smooth-pursuit eye movements are sensitive to the effects of many medications (see Table 12–11, Chapter 12). Conventionally, pursuit is measured during tracking of predictable, sinusoidal target motion. There are advantages, however, to measuring the initiation of smooth pursuit and we will start by summarizing the properties of normal responses to such stimuli.

Onset of Pursuit

The initiation of smooth pursuit is most conveniently studied by measuring eye position and velocity in the first second following presentation of either a ramp or a step-ramp (Rashbass) stimulus (Fig. 4–3).[77,143a,384,455,481] The latency to onset of smooth pursuit in response to a ramp target motion is about 100 ms,[77] and is not substantially influenced by turning off a fixation target before a pursuit target appears, in the way that saccades are; thus, using the gap stimulus, there does not appear to be any express smooth pursuit.[236,261,325] If the ramp is proceeded by a step displacement in the opposite direction, the latency is greater, close to 150 ms, because the pursuit system is affected by the step stimulus.[77] Nevertheless, such step-ramp stimuli do have an advantage over pure ramp stimuli because they are less likely to stimulate saccades that often contaminate pursuit responses to ramp stimuli.

In humans or monkey, eye acceleration during the initial 40 ms of the pursuit response to a step-ramp stimulus is largely unrelated to the speed of the target, its brightness, or its position in the visual field.[260,455] Typical values for this initial eye acceleration are 40 degrees per second per second to 100 degrees per second per second, varying from subject to subject.[77,455] Thereafter, eye acceleration is a function of the velocity of image motion on the retina, and is decreased if the target is dimmer or if it stimulates more peripheral retina.[292,455] As target velocity is progressively increased, eye acceleration does not increase by the same amount; this has been called acceleration saturation.[288,384] Thus, the relationship between peak eye acceleration and target velocity is one measure of smooth pursuit initiation. Latency to onset, but not eye acceleration, may be influenced by the presence of a distracter.[241] In monkeys, the initial acceleration, but not latency, of pursuit onset is reduced if targets move across a textured background.[231,237]

Elderly human subjects show a decrease in initial acceleration, but no change in the latency to onset of pursuit.[328,424] Infants less than 12 weeks of age do show some pursuit responses; although they are relatively small and intermittent,[215,403] they may provide a means to estimate visual acuity.[283] By four months of age, smooth pursuit responses improve and are more related to target velocity.[364,467]

The initiation of smooth pursuit may show larger eye accelerations for vertical pursuit than for horizontal pursuit (the opposite of the case for predictable pursuit, as discussed in the next section); this difference may be evident during diagonal tracking (Fig. 4–4).[388] In the horizontal plane, pursuit accelerations are higher when the target moves towards the midline. In the vertical plane, responses are greater during stimulation of the inferior visual hemifield, irrespective of the direction of target movement.[455] Smooth-pursuit responses do not appear to correspond to the perceptions of target motion, which are stronger along the horizontal or vertical meridian than diagonally.[87] Initial acceleration is unaffected by whether the eye starts in a central or eccentric position.[300] If the target motion is towards the subject, and the trajectory is aligned with one eye, disjunctive smooth-pursuit movements are generated;[238] these are discussed further in Chapter 8.

The early phase of the response also shows damped pursuit oscillations—so-called "ringing"—at a frequency of 3 Hz–4 Hz and, often, an initial velocity overshoot of the target (Fig. 4–3); these findings are present in both the horizontal and vertical planes (Fig. 4–4).[388] Velocity overshoot and "ringing" during pursuit onset, however, are not present in every subject and are influenced by test conditions such as change in luminance of the target and background at stimulus onset. Moreover, the offset of smooth pursuit in response to cessation of target motion (Fig. 4–3) is usually different from the onset: after a latency slightly smaller than the onset, eye velocity declines exponentially to zero with a time constant of about 90 ms.[263,295,323] As discussed above, the lack of any sustained "ringing" during cessation of pursuit has been used as evidence that visual fixation is due to a different mechanism than smooth pursuit. However, in some reports such ringing at the time of pursuit onset might be caused by sudden change in luminance corresponding with presentation of the pursuit target. The onset of smooth pursuit is an open-loop, pre-programmed response; Learning is possible, similar to that of saccades; this is a form of pursuit adaptation, which is discussed in a following section.

Smooth Pursuit Responses during Sustained Tracking

Two types of stimuli are commonly used to test smooth pursuit: sine wave and constant velocity movements (ramps or saw-tooth wave-

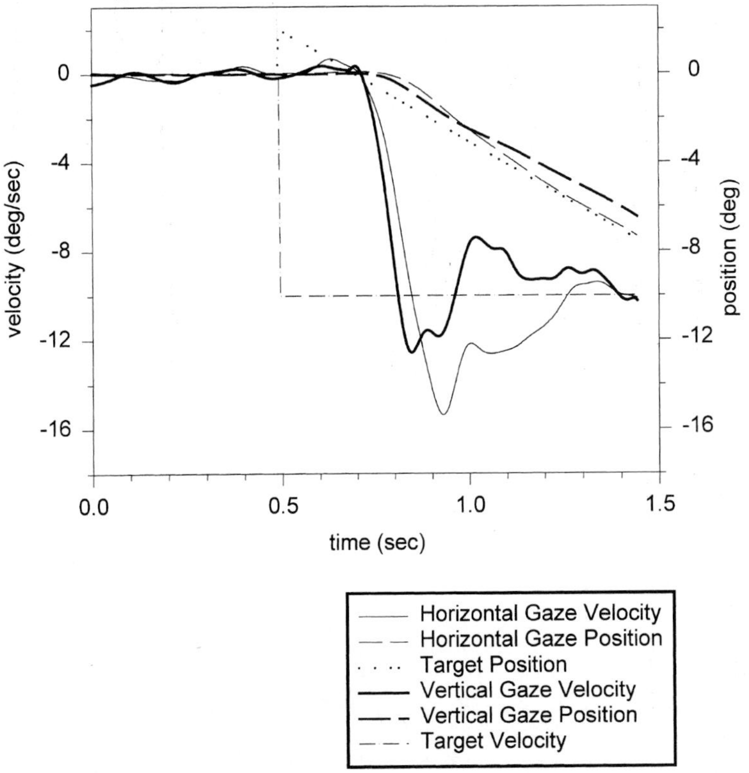

Figure 4–4. Comparison of horizontal and vertical components of the smooth-pursuit response to a diagonal (45-degree direction) step-ramp stimulus. Note that the velocity of the vertical eye component increases faster (higher acceleration of smooth pursuit initiation), although the horizontal component has a greater maximal velocity. Also note that both horizontal and vertical velocity components overshoot the target velocity and show transient oscillations. Positive values correspond to rightward and upward movements. (Rottach KG, Zivotofsky AZ, Das VE, Averbuch-Heller L, DiScenna AO, Poonyathalang A, Leigh RJ. Comparison of horizontal, vertical and diagonal smooth pursuit eye movements in normal human subjects. Vision Res 36, 2189–2195, 1996, with permission from Elsevier.)

forms). In addition, "pseudorandom" stimulus motion is sometimes used.

During smooth pursuit of a sinusoidal target motion, performance conventionally is evaluated by measuring gain (peak eye velocity/peak target velocity) and phase. Phase is a measure of the temporal synchrony between the target and the eye. During ideal pursuit tracking, the gain is close to 1.0 and the eye does not lag behind the target (i.e., phase shift is small). Breakdown in smooth pursuit of a sinusoidal stimulus is indicated by a decrease in gain and by the appearance of a phase lag of the eye with respect to the target at higher frequencies. Although gain and phase may be plotted as functions of frequency (as a Bode plot—see Fig. 2–6C), deterioration of smooth pursuit may also be related to increasing target acceleration.[288,384] Usually, target amplitude is kept constant so that an increase in target frequency is also accompanied by an increase in peak acceleration and in peak velocity. If, on the other hand, stimulus frequency is held constant, pursuit also declines if the amplitude of the target motion increases. A demonstration of this is shown in Figure 4–5A. The subject is able to pursue a target moving at a frequency of 1.0 Hz if its amplitude is small (5 degrees, peak-to-peak). If the frequency of the target movement is held at 1.0 Hz but its amplitude is increased, smooth pursuit deteriorates. Evidence to show that such deterioration is not due to target velocity is provided by the observation that, with constant-velocity targets (ramps), pursuit gain does not significantly deteriorate until target velocity exceeds about 100 degrees per second (Fig. 4–5B).[315] Up to this velocity saturation, gain is typically less

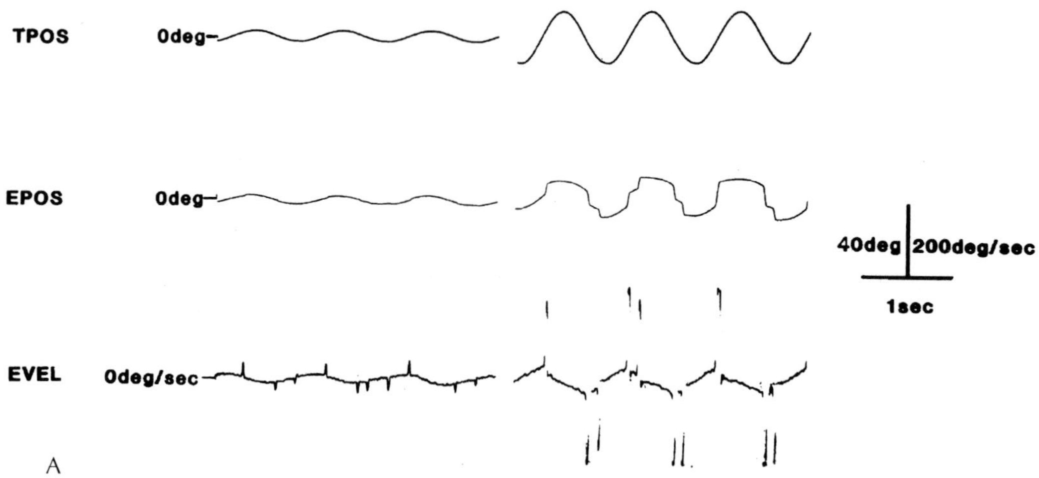

A

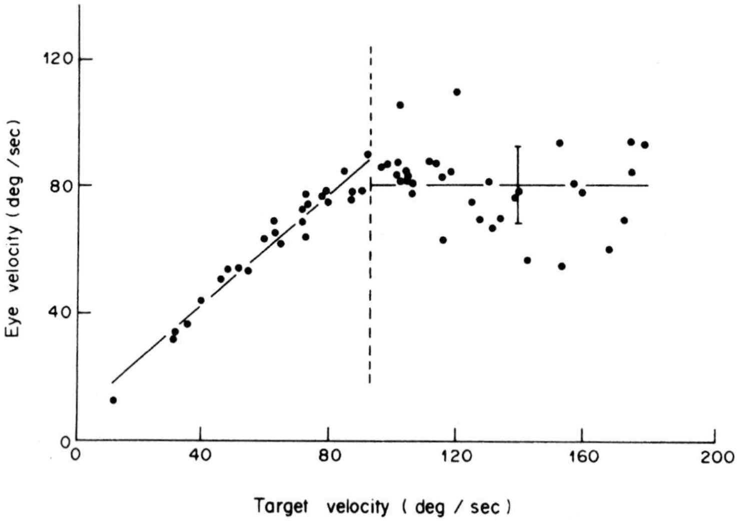

B

Figure 4–5. Quantitative aspects of smooth pursuit to predictable target motion. (A) Comparison of smooth pursuit at 1.0 Hz with target peak-to-peak amplitude of either 5 degrees (left) or 30 degrees (right). During tracking of the smaller amplitude movements, pursuit gain (peak eye velocity/peak target velocity) is greater than 0.8, but during tracking of the larger amplitude target, it falls to less than 0.5, and tracking is largely saccadic because of acceleration or velocity saturation. T POS: target position; E POS: eye position; E VEL: eye velocity. Upward deflections indicate rightward eye or target movements. (B) A demonstration in a normal subject of pursuit "velocity saturation," which becomes evident with target velocities above 93 degrees per second; below this, mean pursuit gain (eye velocity/target velocity) was 0.86 (From Meyer CH, Lasker AG, Robinson DA. The upper limit of smooth pursuit velocity. Vision Res 25, 561–563, 1985, with permission from Elsevier.)

than 1.0, but is fairly constant. Therefore, it is important to study pursuit responses with both constant velocity and with sinusoidal target motions. From the responses to constant-velocity stimuli, steady-state pursuit gain and the threshold of the velocity saturation of pursuit can be determined. From responses to sinusoidal stimuli, the acceleration saturation of smooth pursuit to predictable target motion can be determined. By analyzing the responses in this way, a number of characteristic pursuit deficits due to specific disorders have been defined. Examples are shown Figure 4–6 and are discussed in the final section of this chapter.

Generally, smooth pursuit of predictable target motions is superior to that of non-predictable motions such as step-ramps. For example, values of peak eye acceleration in response to predictable sinusoidal stimuli may

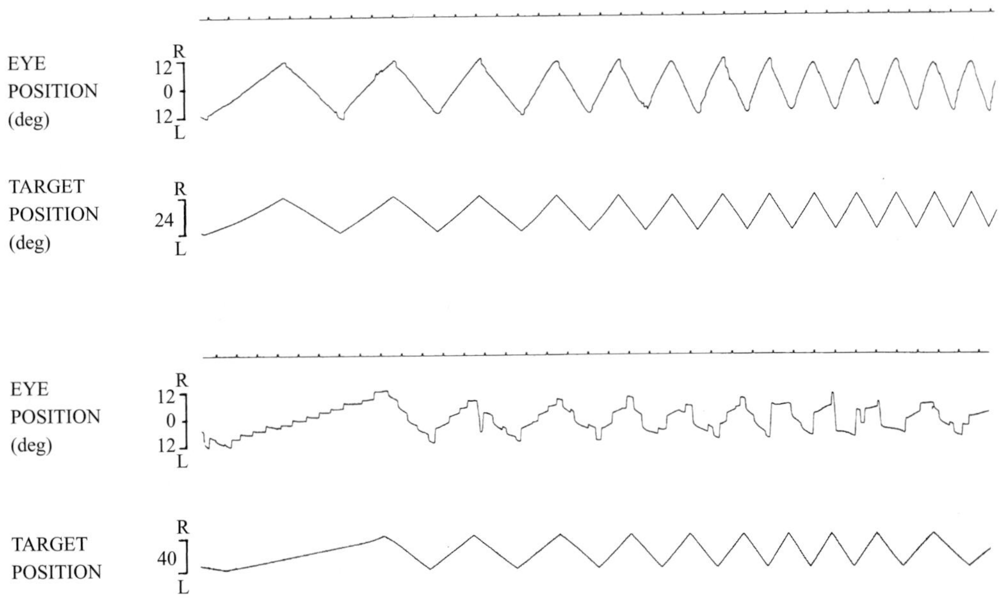

Figure 4–6. Comparison of smooth pursuit of a target moving in a triangular waveform by a normal subject (top panel) and a patient with cerebellar disease (bottom panel). In each panel, the calibration marks on the top line are seconds, the top trace shows horizontal eye position, and the bottom trace shows movement of the target (a small laser spot). The normal subject generates tracking eye movements that consist mainly of smooth pursuit movements with occasional small saccades. The patient with cerebellar disease can generate some smooth following movements, but their velocity (i.e., the slope of the position trace) is much less than that of the target. Consequently, the patient has to make "catch-up" saccades to place the image of the target on the fovea.

exceed 1000 degrees per second per second.[288] Horizontal smooth pursuit is usually superior to vertical smooth pursuit for sustained responses to predictable target motions;[18,388] in some subjects, this is the opposite to what is found during the onset of pursuit (Fig. 4–4), suggesting different mechanisms. Downward pursuit may be superior to upward pursuit.[222a] An important characteristic of the pursuit responses to predictable target motions is their variability. Even normal, young subjects show considerable inter-subject variability. For example, for target motion at a constant velocity of 30 degrees per second, gain ranges from below 0.8 to about 1.0.[268, 285,391] Some of the variability reflects differences in testing protocols and analysis procedures; thus it is important for each laboratory to determine its normal range of responses. Smooth pursuit gain is reduced if pursuit is performed with the eye in an eccentric position in the orbit; this cannot be ascribed to the effects of orbital mechanics, since pursuit initiation is not similarly affected.[300]

A number of studies have measured the deterioration of smooth pursuit that occurs with age.[361,402,413,495] The main change is a decrease of the steady-state gain for ramp target stimuli. With sinusoidal stimuli, there is a further decline in gain with high target accelerations (above about 400 degrees per second).[495] These changes should be kept in mind when evaluating elderly patients. Some technical points about how to make the different pursuit measurements are reviewed below, under Laboratory Evaluation of Fixation and Smooth Pursuit.

Smooth pursuit may also be tested with less predictable "pseudorandom" or "sum-of-sine waves" stimuli.[24,28,99,491] With such stimuli, pursuit tracking is optimized (minimal phase shift) at some frequency, at the expense of poorer tracking (larger phase shifts) at lower frequencies. Similar results have been reported for optokinetic responses.[482]

ADAPTIVE PROPERTIES OF SMOOTH PURSUIT

The brain uses vision to monitor the performance of smooth-pursuit eye movements. At one level, this amounts to a negative feedback control (an issue discussed further in the section on Models of Smooth Pursuit). Thus, with ability to adjust performance on a moment-by-moment basis, it may not seem necessary to have evolved an ability to plastically adapt the properties of the smooth-pursuit system. Adaptive properties are well developed for the vestibulo-ocular reflex, which is open loop; vestibular eye movements do not affect the motion-sensing organs in the ear.

Early suggestions of adaptive properties of smooth pursuit were reported from a patient with right abducens nerve palsy, who preferred to view with his paretic eye. It was noted that smooth pursuit by the normal left eye appeared to be too fast (see Fig. 4–7 and Video Display: Disorders of Smooth Pursuit).[355] One specific reason to be able to adapt the performance of pursuit movements to current visual demands arises from the long latency to onset of these movements (about 100 ms). There is a need to generate pursuit movements based on prior experience. Much work on adaptive properties of smooth pursuit has focused on initial responses to step-ramp stimuli.[156,220,348] Thus, if the target first steps away from center position and then ramps in the opposite direction, a sudden 90-degree change in the *direction* of target motion as it crosses midline can induce adaptive pursuit responses within 30 minutes of training.[186] If target *speed* is altered during the duration of catch-up saccades, adaptive changes occur in both pre- and post-saccadic eye speed; such changes are direction-specific, but generalize to target motions in different parts of the visual field than those used for training.[84] The contextual relevance of the cue is also important in governing pursuit adaptation; thus targets presented in specific fields of gaze are more likely to induce adaptive changes (since they may be called upon if there is an ocular motor paresis) than the color of the target.[436] There is also evidence that changes in motion perception occur during adaptation of smooth pursuit,[464] and that extraretinal signals are used in achieving adaptation.[298,472]

What is the neurobiological substrate for smooth-pursuit adaptation? Stimulation of neurons in the middle temporal (MT) visual area to coincide with pursuit responses can induce adaptive changes in the responses.[76] When subjects track asymmetric target motion (ramps upward with resetting steps downward), they develop downbeat nystagmus, a disorder often caused by disease affecting the flocculus.[301] The pathogenesis of downbeat nystagmus is discussed further in Chapter 10. Adaptation of the vestibulo-ocular reflex leads to changes in smooth pursuit, suggesting a shared mechanism underlying both systems, to which the cerebellar flocculus probably contributes.[75] In addition, the dorsal cerebellar vermis has been shown to be important for adaptive control of the initial 100 ms—the open-loop response—of pursuit tracking.[437]

NEURAL SUBSTRATE FOR SMOOTH PURSUIT

Here we present a hypothetical scheme for the generation of smooth-pursuit eye movements

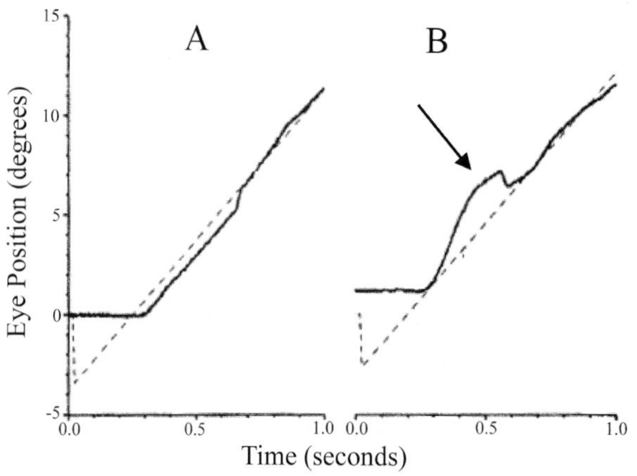

Figure 4–7. Comparison of pursuit responses to a 15-degrees/second step-ramp stimulus of the normal left eye in a patient with right sixth nerve palsy in unadapted and adapted states. (A) Unadapted state, in which the weak right eye had been patched for 9 days, allowing the left eye to view. The left eye lags a little behind the target (dashed line), requiring a catch-up saccade. (B) Adapted state, in which the weak right eye had been viewing for 9 days. Left eye velocity becomes much higher than the target velocity (arrow) before slowing down, and a back-up saccade is used to acquire the target. Oscillations are present during the latter part of the tracking response. (Reproduced from Optican LM, Zee DS, Chu FC. Adaptive response to ocular muscle weakness in human pursuit and saccadic eye movements. Neurophysiol 54, 110–122, 1985, with permission of the American Physiological Society.)

using information from both humans and monkeys. As we have stated elsewhere, caution is required in extrapolating results from different species, and in linking behavioral deficits to neuronal activity that is monitored by electrophysiological measures or functional imaging. Thus, the scheme summarized in Figure 4–8 and Figure 6–7 remains hypothetical.

There is general agreement that there are two functional divisions of the visual system, although there is some debate about how they should be defined.[82,120,222,294,459,465] Thus, one

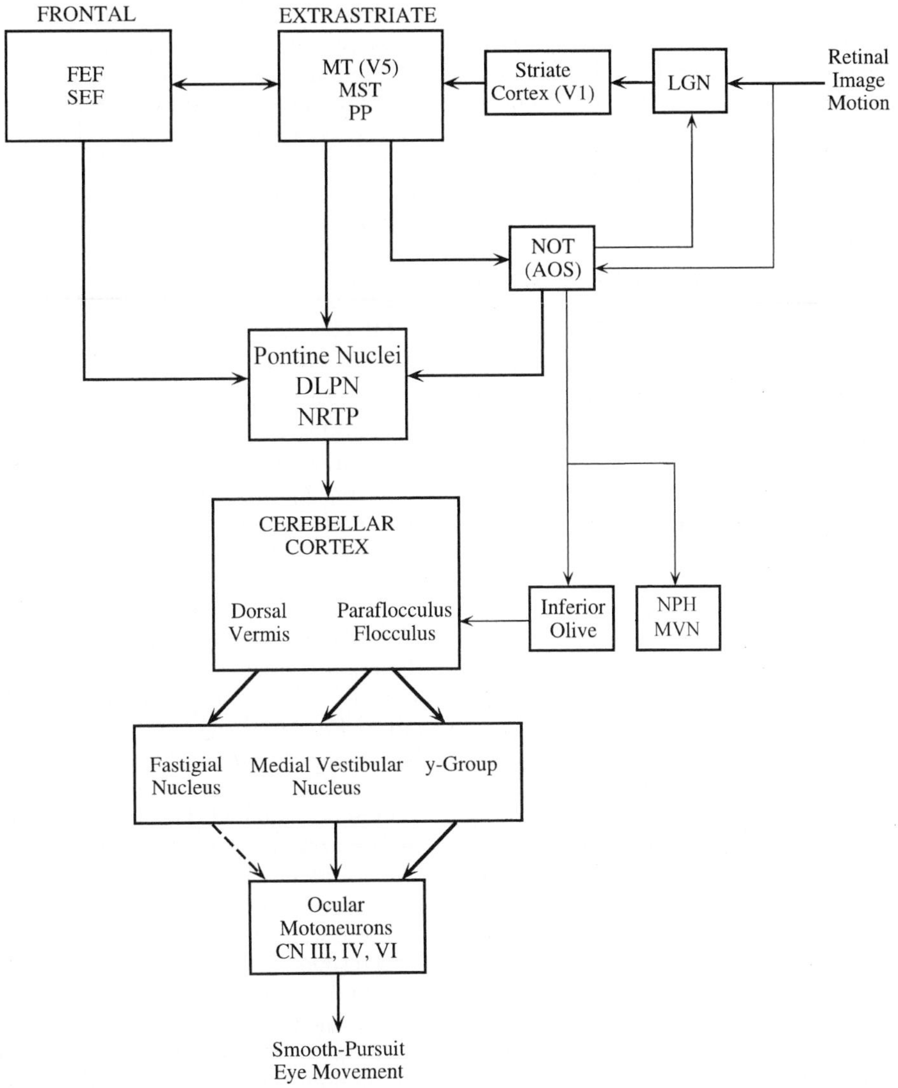

Figure 4–8. A hypothetical anatomic scheme for smooth-pursuit eye movements. Signals encoding retinal image motion pass via the lateral geniculate nucleus (LGN) to striate cortex (V1) and extrastriate areas. MT (V5): middle temporal visual area; MST: medial superior temporal visual area; PP: posterior parietal cortex; FEF: frontal eye fields; SEF: supplementary eye fields. The nucleus of the optic tract (NOT) and accessory optic system (AOS) receive visual motion signals from the retina but also from extrastriate cortical areas. Cortical areas concerned with smooth pursuit project to the cerebellum via pontine nuclei, including the dorsolateral pontine nuclei (DLPN) and nucleus reticularis tegmenti pontis (NRTP). The cerebellar areas concerned with smooth pursuit project to ocular motor neurons via fastigial, vestibular, and y-group nuclei; the pursuit pathway for fastigial nucleus efferents has not yet been defined. The NOT projects back to LGN. The NOT and AOS may influence smooth pursuit through their projections to the pontine nuclei, and indirectly, via the inferior olive and the nucleus prepositus (NPH)–medial vestibular nucleus (MVN) region.

scheme, which is primarily based in anatomy, equates vision of moving stimuli with retinal ganglion cells that project via the magnocellular layers of the lateral geniculate nucleus to layer 4Cα of primary visual (striate) cortex. A second anatomical scheme is primarily concerned with feature analysis (e.g., color) and projects via parvocellular layers of the lateral geniculate nucleus to layer 4Cβ of primary visual cortex. The latency of neurons in layer 4Cβ to flashing spots of light is about 20 ms longer than those in layer 4Cα.[345] Chemical lesions of the magnocellular pathway in the lateral geniculate nucleus impair but do not abolish smooth pursuit.[360] As mentioned above, a second division is based upon psychophysical and ocular following responses to first-order motion stimuli, which are luminance-defined versus second-order motion stimuli, which depend on higher-level mechanisms such as contrast and flicker.[79,82,120,206,287] At present, the contributions of different cortical areas to processing of first-order and second-order motion stimuli are still being elucidated.

Primary Visual Cortex and Smooth Pursuit

Primary visual cortex (V1, Brodmann area 17, striate cortex) contains neurons that respond to moving visual stimuli.[201] Such "complex" cells, however, have small visual fields and a narrow range of preferred target speeds. Neurons in V1 respond to first-order, but not second-order, motion stimuli.[347] Using step-ramp stimuli, it has been shown that unilateral lesions of striate cortex abolish smooth pursuit of targets moving in the defective hemifield, contralateral to the side of the lesion,[395] but pursuit remains intact for stimuli moving in any direction that are presented into the normal hemifield. During tracking of predictable target motion, smooth pursuit is usually normal due to the predictable properties of smooth pursuit and the sparing of the macular projection.[198]

Contributions of the Middle Temporal Visual Area

ANATOMICAL CONSIDERATIONS

Striate cortex projects to the middle temporal visual area (MT or V5) that, in rhesus monkey, lies in the superior temporal sulcus (see Fig. 6–8).[121,457,501] The projections from striate cortex to MT depend on arcuate, subcortical fiber bundles;[453] there is a direct pathway and an indirect pathway via peristriate cortex. The projections from striate cortex to MT are retinotopic and entirely ipsilateral. Most neurons in MT encode the speed, acceleration, and direction of moving visual stimuli; preferred stimulus velocity is typically 30 degrees per second.[291,309] Some neurons in MT have larger receptive fields than those in striate cortex. Neurons in MT show responses to second-order motion stimuli, such as stationary flashed targets,[92] but generally show stronger responses to first-order stimuli.[347]

PHYSIOLOGICAL PROPERTIES OF NEURONS IN MIDDLE TEMPORAL AREA

If complex visual stimuli such as two-dimensional plaids are presented, some neurons respond not to the direction of either component, but rather to the resultant global direction of the stimulus.[331] Similarly, in response to two small targets, which move in different directions, some MT neurons initially encode the vector average of the two motions; however, after about 450 ms, such neurons encode the direction of motion of the target that has been selected for smooth pursuit (winner-take-all).[377] Further insights have also been gained by presenting a set of moving dots that lie within a patch, which moves in a different direction than the component dots. Initially responses of MT neurons are to the local motion of the dots but eventually shift to respond to the global motion of the patch,[357,371] These neural responses are somewhat similar to the behavioral responses of humans who track line-figure diamonds; initially the eye movement is a vector average of the diamond's line segments, but the response eventually becomes tracking of the motion of the object. [307] Microstimulation in MT during tracking of a smoothly moving target increases smooth pursuit eye velocity, and may induce smooth eye movements even if the target is stationary.[174] Furthermore, MT stimulation that coincides with smooth tracking responses can induce pursuit adaptation.[76] Finally, there is evidence that neurons in MT contribute not only to behavioral responses, but also to speed perception.[293]

THE HUMAN HOMOLOGUE OF MIDDLE TEMPORAL AREA

Based on functional imaging studies, the probable homologue of MT in humans is located posterior to the superior temporal sulcus, at the junction of Brodmann areas 19, 37, and 39, close to the intersection of the ascending limb of the inferior temporal sulcus and the lateral occipital sulcus (see Fig. 6–7, Chapter 6).[9,135,471,502] Different regions of human MT may be activated during smooth pursuit, optic flow, or non-visual pursuit.[135]

EXPERIMENTAL AND HUMAN LESIONS OF MIDDLE TEMPORAL AREA

In monkeys, discrete chemical lesions of those portions of MT that encode visual inputs from the extrafoveal (peripheral) visual field cause a *scotoma for motion*, and these animals cannot estimate the speed of a moving target.[342] Normally, not only pursuit but also saccades are programmed to take into account the speed of target motion.[177] After MT lesions, the initiation of smooth pursuit is decreased, and the saccades to moving targets are dysmetric for stimuli presented in the affected portion of the visual field.[342] In contrast, saccades made to targets that are stationary within the affected field are normal. Thus, the deficit caused by a lesion of extrafoveal MT is one of visual processing of moving stimuli, rather than of pursuit per se. Moreover, this visual defect is accompanied by a selective loss of motion perception.[341]

Patients with selective lesions at the presumed human homologue of MT have defects of motion perception (akinetopsia) [409] and impairment of smooth pursuit,[272,448] similar to those described in monkeys with MT lesions (Fig. 4–9).

Contributions of the Medial Superior Temporal Visual Area

ANATOMICAL CONSIDERATIONS

Area MT in rhesus monkey projects to the medial superior temporal visual area (MST), which lies adjacent to MT in the superior temporal sulcus (see Fig. 6–8).[121,456] In addition, area MT projects via the major forceps and splenium of the corpus callosum to areas MT and MST of the contralateral hemisphere.[453] In rhesus monkey, area MST lies in the superior temporal sulcus (STS), and has two important divisions:[243,457] a ventrolateral portion (MSTl) and a dorsal region (MSTd).

PHYSIOLOGICAL PROPERTIES OF NEURONS IN VENTROLATERAL PORTION

The neurons in MSTl respond best to motion of small spots of light and seem concerned with *smooth pursuit*.[245] Their responses are also influenced by visual stimuli presented in the region surrounding their receptive field.[139] Neurons in MST differ from those in area MT by taking into account the effects of eye movements.[60,243,244,343,406,414] Such neurons also discharge during anticipatory pursuit movements or pursuit to imaginary target motion.[207,210] Thus, it seems likely that an *efference copy* of the eye movement command is sent to these neurons perhaps via thalamic nuclei.[438a] Human studies suggest that an efference copy of smooth pursuit movements is used in planning saccades, especially if visual cues are absent.[50,51,504] MST neurons also receive a vestibular signal; thus, during eye-head tracking, some MST neurons also encode target motion in world-centered coordinates.[209]

It seems that MST plays an important role during smooth pursuit of a small target across a textured background, or fixation of a stationary target during self-motion.[244] This summation of a visual signal and an efference copy of eye movement is similar to that proposed in certain models of smooth pursuit (Fig. 4–10B). Because these MST neurons combine visual and eye movement signals, they may encode the motion of the moving visual stimulus in a craniotopic (head-centered) rather than a retinotopic (eye-centered) frame of reference. Indeed, to understand the contributions of visual areas MT and MST to motion vision and smooth pursuit, it is necessary to consider how the population of neurons code responses to motion stimuli.[358,359,372,438]

PHYSIOLOGICAL PROPERTIES OF NEURONS IN DORSAL REGION

The neurons in MSTd seem particularly suited to *analysis of optic flow*,[134,166] and the direction of heading.[46] They have large receptive fields,

A

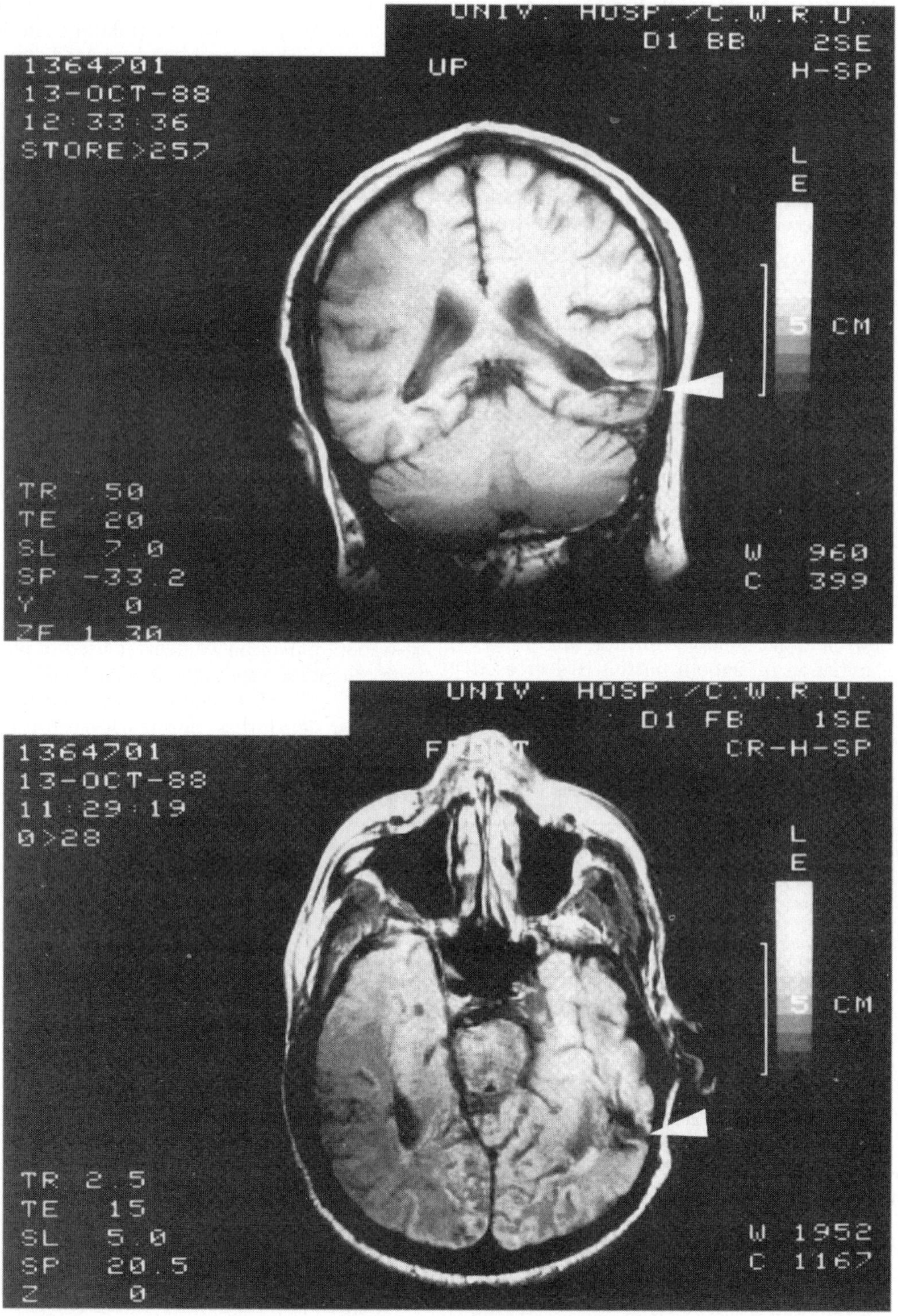
UNIV. HOSP./C.W.R.U.
D1 BB 2SE
1364701
13-OCT-88
12:33:36
STORE>257
UP
H-SP
LE
5 CM
TR 50
TE 20
SL 7.0
SP -33.2
Y 0
W 960
C 399
UNIV. HOSP./C.W.R.U.
D1 FB 1SE
1364701
13-OCT-88
11:29:19
0>28
CR-H-SP
LE
5 CM
TR 2.5
TE 15
SL 5.0
SP 20.5
Z 0
W 1952
C 1167

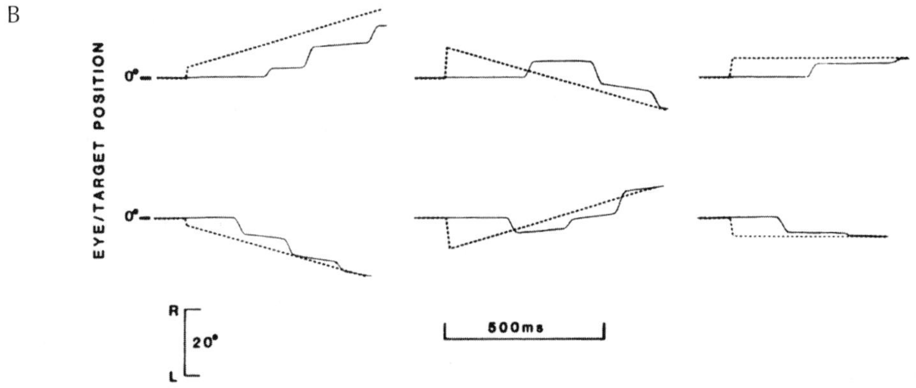

Figure 4–9. Effects of a lesion located at the temporo-occipital junction upon visual tracking.[448] (A) Magnetic resonance images demonstrating the location of the left-hemisphere infarct, the cortical involvement of which primarily affects Brodmann areas 37 and 19. (B) Typical responses of this patient to foveafugal step-ramps (left), foveapetal step-ramps (middle) and steps (right). Target motions are indicated by dotted lines and eye movement responses by solid lines. When step-ramps are presented in the right visual hemifield, pursuit initiation is impaired and saccades are inaccurate, compared with corresponding responses to targets presented in the left visual hemifield. By contrast, saccades made to steps are equally accurate in the right or the left visual hemifield. This tracking deficit is similar to that occurring after experimental lesions of the middle temporal visual area (MT) in monkey. R: right; L: left.

and respond at short latencies to rotations and expansions of visual stimuli, and to speed gradients across the visual field.[130,227] The response of individual neurons in MSTd to moving stimuli is influenced by the disparity between the locations of images of the same target on the two retinas;[390] such motion disparity information provides information about self-motion and the layout of the environ-ment. Vergence angle also influences their responses,[211] and some units respond to smooth vergence tracking.[6] Further, MSTd neurons receive vestibular inputs,[359] sense the direction of heading,[132] and seem able to contribute to spatial orientation, based on motion parallax information.[133] Like MT neurons, the activity of those in MST can be linked to perceptions of motion.[8,80,422]

Availability of an eye movement signal is important if the direction of heading is to be estimated while the eyes pursue a moving target.[60] In addition, a neural signal encoding head movement reaches some MST neurons.[446] Eye and head movement signals would seem to be important to enable smooth pursuit of a small target moving across a textured background while the subject is moving the head or walking. Certain neurons in MST respond to large-field stimuli moving in the opposite direction to that preferred by these same neurons during pursuit of small targets.[244]

THE HUMAN HOMOLOGUE OF MEDIAL SUPERIOR TEMPORAL VISUAL AREA

The human homologues of MT and MST probably lie adjacent, at the occipital-temporal-parietal junction. Thus, when subjects smoothly pursue a small target, there is activation of the lateral occipital-temporal cortex, an area close to the homologue of MT.[34] However, there is no activation in this area when subjects view a large moving stimulus with the eyes still; this finding implies that extraretinal signals—possibly related to eye movements—are reaching this area, which might be the human homologue of MST.[34] When targets are tracked attentively, additional activation occurs in the superior parietal lobule, intraparietal sulcus, precuneus, frontal eye field, and precentral sulcus.[61,105a] When human subjects view visual displays that simulate optic flow, functional imaging detects increased activity in the region of the right superior parietal lobe and dorsal cuneus (the probable homologue of V3 in monkey), and bilaterally on the ventral surface of the brain in the occipital-temporal (fusiform) gyrus.[67,111] Thus, multiple posterior cortical areas are active during the generation of smooth-pursuit eye movements during natural activities, such as locomotion.

EXPERIMENTAL AND HUMAN LESIONS OF MEDIAL SUPERIOR TEMPORAL VISUAL AREA

Experimental lesions of MSTl in monkey produce a unidirectional deficit of horizontal smooth pursuit for targets moving toward the side of the lesion, irrespective of the visual hemifield into which the stimulus falls.[137] In addition, a retinotopic deficit for motion detection, similar to that with MT lesions, occurs for targets presented in the contralateral visual field. Lesions of the adjacent foveal representation of MT produce a similar deficit.[138,245] Consistent with the effects of lesions, activation of MSTl (or foveal MT) by microstimulation during smooth pursuit increases eye velocity during tracking towards the side of stimulation and decreases eye velocity during tracking away from the side of stimulation.[245] During steady fixation, electrical stimulation produces lower eye velocity compared with stimulation during smooth pursuit.[245] Combined experimental lesions of MT and MST produce more permanent deficits.[487]

Unilateral, posterior cerebral lesions in humans that may involve the homologue of MST produce a tracking deficit similar to that in monkey, with impairment of ipsilateral pursuit and a defect of motion processing affecting the contralateral visual hemifield (Fig. 4–11).[33,272,327,448] Bilateral lesions involving MST are reported to cause inability to suppress image motion of the background during smooth-pursuit movements.[181]

Contribution of Posterior Parietal Cortex

In rhesus monkey, both MT and MST project via arcuate fiber bundles to posterior parietal cortex (area 7A), which lies ventral to the intraparietal sulcus (see Fig. 6–8).[453] In addition, posterior parietal cortex has reciprocal connections with MST. Neurons in posterior parietal cortex that modulate their activity during smooth-pursuit eye movements are influenced by the nature of the target being pursued (e.g., a scrap of food).[296] Neurons in the adjacent, multisensory ventral intraparietal area (VIP) also show velocity tuning during pursuit.[392] Microstimulation in the posterior parietal lobe may evoke smooth eye movements.[266]

The responses of visually sensitive neurons in posterior parietal cortex are influenced by current eye position, and so may encode the location of the visual stimulus in craniotopic coordinates.[7,63] This is consistent with the finding that unilateral posterior parietal lesions, especially right-sided, cause contralateral inattention and may contribute to ipsilateral gaze deviation or preference, and partially impair smooth pursuit and saccades in the contralateral hemifield of gaze.[54,324]

Although unidirectional pursuit deficits—poorer pursuit when the target moves towards the side of the lesion—have been ascribed to parietal lesions, these are probably due to involvement of other areas, such as MST, FEF, or their projections. It seems more likely that parietal lesions impair the ability to attend to the image of the moving target and "ignore" the smeared images of the stationary background consequent to the eye movement. Thus, patients with lesions affecting Brodmann area 40 show impaired smooth pursuit when the target moves across a structured background compared with pursuit across a dark background.[270] Impairment of the same mechanism may explain why patients with parietal lesions show relatively preserved responses to full-field visual stimuli, which demand less selective visual attention.[16]

Contributions of the Frontal Eye Field

Visual areas MT, MST, and posterior parietal cortex have reciprocal connections with the frontal eye field (FEF; Brodmann area 8) in monkeys (see Fig. 6–8).[271,415,416,453,456] Within a circumscribed part of the ventral (inferior) FEF, in the arcuate fundus and posterior bank, are a population of neurons that discharge for smooth pursuit, but not for saccades.[171] Microstimulation in this region produces smooth eye movements, usually with an ipsilateral component. Such evoked movements can be elicited even during attempted fixation,[171] but boost the responses of ongoing pursuit, suggesting that FEF controls pursuit gain.[439] Individual neurons increase their activity before and during pursuit in a preferred direction, and generally increase their discharge rate with eye velocity.[171,440,441] Typically, the onset of neuronal activity occurs 100 ms after target motion and 8ms–20 ms before the eye starts to move.[171,440] It has also been demonstrated that some caudal FEF neurons also discharge during pursuit of targets moving in both direction and depth (3-D motion).[158]

In humans, functional imaging indicates that the part of the FEF concerned with smooth pursuit also lies in the inferior lateral aspect of the FEF,[362,363] lying deep in the anterior wall of the central sulcus, reaching the fundus or deep posterior wall in some subjects.[387] Lesions of the FEF in monkeys and humans cause a predominantly ipsidirectional defect of the initiation, steady-state, and predictive aspects of the smooth response.[297,329] Although the pursuit may be impaired in both directions, optokinetic responses may be preserved.[228,229] Although the FEF seems important for predictive pursuit,[157] it does not appear to contribute to adaptive responses to step-ramp stimuli that change speed.[85]

Contributions of the Supplementary Eye Field

The supplementary eye field (SEF), which lies in the dorsomedial frontal lobe, also receives inputs from MST, the posterior parietal lobe, and the FEF.[203] The contributions of SEF appear to differ from those due to FEF.[442] The SEF contains neurons that discharge during smooth pursuit,[189] but such neurons may also carry a head velocity signal, and discharge during vergence pursuit.[154] Unlike FEF, pharmacological inactivation of the SEF does not impair smooth pursuit or VOR cancellation during eye-head tracking.[155] Electrical microstimulation in the SEF increases the velocity of anticipatory pursuit movements and decreases their latency.[320] This anticipatory pursuit facilitation is greater when stimulation is delivered near the end of the fixation period; no anticipatory smooth eye movements could be evoked during fixation unless there was an expectation of target motion.[320] Taken together, these reports indicate that the SEF is involved in the process of guiding anticipatory pursuit.[187,188,191,279,320,449]

Contributions of Other Cortical Areas

In humans, functional imaging indicates that other cortical areas may contribute to smooth pursuit, including the precuneus, anterior, and posterior cingulate cortices.[49,363] The anterior cingulate and pre-supplementary motor area (pre-SMA) may be important for pursuit responses to predictable target motions.[393] Further studies may clarify the role that each of these areas plays; indeed, the cerebral contributions to the initiation and maintenance of smooth pursuit are probably due to a distributed network of neurons in several cortical areas. Thus, for example, when subjects attend to a smooth-pursuit target that is intermittently blanked for a second, FEF, SEF, superior parietal lobe and intraparietal sulcus all maintain activation, and may be concerned in sustaining pursuit by using extraretinal signals and working memory.[282]

Thus, like the control of saccades, the posterior cortical areas seem more concerned with reflexive aspects of pursuit, whereas the frontal areas are important for internally generated and predictive aspects of smooth tracking.

Descending Pursuit Pathways to the Pons

Traditionally, the pursuit pathway has been viewed as a projection from posterior and anterior cortical areas to the cerebellum, via pontine nuclei; the cerebellum, in turn, projects to brainstem premotor areas, such as the vestibular nuclei (Fig. 6–7). Thus, in monkey, visual areas MT and MST project ipsilaterally through the *internal sagittal stratum*, the retrolenticular portion of the internal capsule, and the cerebral peduncle. The targets of this projection are the dorsolateral and lateral pontine nuclei.[59,169,453] The projections from MT and MST to the nucleus of the optic tract and accessory optic system are discussed in a separate section below.

In the human brain, the descending pathway is thought to originate in parieto-temporo-occipital cortex; it runs along the lateral surface of the lateral ventricle (internal sagittal stratum), turns medially above the temporal horn, and then toward the posterior limb of the internal capsule.[326,453] The FEF pursuit area projects to the caudate nucleus,[105] which has been shown to be important in monkeys who are rewarded for performing specific eye movement tasks.[196] A clinical lesion of the internal sagittal stratum that did not impair smooth pursuit was probably located posterior to the critical part of this pathway.[399,453] At a more caudal level in the pathway, an ipsilateral pursuit deficit has been reported with lesions affecting the posterior thalamus and adjacent retrolenticular portion of the internal capsule,[65] and with lesions of the dorsal midbrain.[494]

In monkeys, the terminations are scattered throughout several pontine nuclei including the *dorsolateral pontine nuclei* (DLPN) and the rostral portion of the *nucleus reticularis tegmenti pontis* (NRTP).[59,127,150,169,271] Pursuit-related neurons in these nuclei encode a variety of visual and ocular motor signals, including eye velocity.[124,334,351,353,430,433,447] Many neurons modulate their discharge during smooth pursuit of a small target in an otherwise dark room and show directional selectivity, with either ipsilateral or contralateral target motion. Some such neurons continue to discharge if the target light is briefly turned off while pursuit continues; this property implies that a non-visual signal (probably efference copy) encoding eye movement is reaching these neurons; this property is similar to that shown by some MST neurons.[343] Microstimulation in DLPN does not cause smooth eye movements during fixation, but accelerates the eye if the monkey is engaged in smooth pursuit;[230] this result is similar to stimulation in MST.[245] Microstimulation in rostral NRTP produces predominantly upward eye movements.[486]

Discrete chemical lesions of DLPN produce a deficit of smooth pursuit that is predominantly for ipsidirectional target motion.[311] An accompanying saccadic deficit to moving stimuli is directional, unlike the retinotopic defect that occurs following MT lesions.[311] Pharmacological inactivation of DLPN with muscimol impairs initiation of ipsilateral smooth pursuit and steady-state tracking.[352] Pharmacological inactivation of NRTP impairs smooth pursuit onset.[432] The major projections of the pontine nuclei are to the vestibulocerebellar paraflocculus and flocculus, and the dorsal vermis of the cerebellum but, based upon clinical studies the cerebellar hemispheres also contribute to pursuit.[425] One interpretation of these results is that projections from FEF concerned with the onset of smooth pursuit pass via NRTP to the dorsal vermis, whereas projections from MT and MST concerned with maintenance of smooth pursuit pass via DLPN to the flocculus and paraflocculus.[351,433]

It has been proposed that, similar to the saccadic system, cerebral areas concerned with smooth pursuit also project to ocular motoneurons via the *basal ganglia, superior colliculus, and brainstem reticular formation*.[256] Thus, the FEF pursuit area projects to the caudate nucleus,[105] which is activated during human smooth pursuit.[346] One target of the caudate nucleus is the substantial nigra, pars reticulata (SNpr), where some neurons cease discharge during pursuit; microstimulation of SNpr during pursuit onset may suppress ipsiversive, and enhance contraversive, pursuit responses.[36] The SNpr exerts important controls on the superior colliculus during programming of saccades (reviewed in Chapter 3); similar mechanisms might operate for smooth pursuit. Thus, in the rostral superior colliculus, neurons modulate their discharge during smooth pursuit in a way that suggests selectivity for stimuli that will be the targets for pursuit and saccades, including gap stimuli (fixation light turned off before target light is turned on).[35,257]

Although chemical lesions of the paramedian pontine reticular formation (PPRF) were reported to spare smooth pursuit,[193] some pontine neurons have been reported that carry both pursuit and saccadic signals, and may also contribute to the latch circuit for saccades (see Fig. 3–9, Chapter 3).[321] There is also anatomical evidence that pursuit signals from FEF are sent to the rostral interstitial nucleus of the medial longitudinal fasciculus (riMLF), which is important for generating vertical saccades.[488] Omnipause neurons, which are known to gate the onset and end of saccades, also decrease their discharge during smooth pursuit.[321]

A hypothetical scheme has been proposed that incorporates a mechanism that gates both smooth-pursuit and saccadic responses, and comprises the rostral pole of the superior colliculus (fixation zone), the omnipause neurons, and the latch neurons in the PPRF.[256] This suggestion will no doubt serve as the impetus to new experiments, but evidence strongly supports the pathway running from the pontine nuclei to the cerebellum as being critical for normal smooth tracking.

The Cerebellar Contribution

THE VESTIBULOCEREBELLUM AND SMOOTH PURSUIT

A major projection of the pontine nuclei is to the vestibulocerebellum (paraflocculus and ventral flocculus—see Figure 6–6, in Chapter 6).[169,339] These structures also receive mossy fiber inputs from the vestibular nucleus, nucleus prepositus hypoglossi, cell groups of the paramedian tracts,[72] and climbing fiber inputs from the contralateral inferior olive. The main efferent pathways of the paraflocculus and flocculus are to the ipsilateral superior and medial vestibular nuclei, and the y-group.[269] The paraflocculus may also project to the posterior interpositus and dentate nuclei.[340] The major anatomical connections are summarized in Box 6–10, in Chapter 6.

It currently appears that the ventral paraflocculus is more important for the control of smooth pursuit, and the flocculus for controlling the vestibulo-ocular reflex.[339,373] Purkinje cells in the paraflocculus and flocculus modulate their discharge according to gaze velocity and position during smooth pursuit or passive eye-head tracking (fixation of a head-fixed target during rotation in yaw).[235,284,289,290,319] If the monkey fixates a stationary target during passive head rotation, no significant modulation of these neurons occurs, consistent with gaze velocity remaining as zero. However, during active eye-head tracking, the flocculus may play a smaller role.[42-44] Some of these floccular neurons modulate their activity with ipsilateral, horizontal pursuit movements; others discharge preferentially for downward movements. Some neurons show transient bursts of activity that might help initiate pursuit.[255,260] Microstimulation of the ventral paraflocculus produces smooth eye movements within 10 ms, even during attempted fixation.[41] Typically the initial eye movement is upward and contralateral to the side of stimulation. After pursuit adaptation training, Purkinje cells show changes in both simple and complex-spike discharge rates, but it remains an open issue whether these changes reflect learning in the cerebellar cortex or elsewhere.[219]

Bilateral ablative lesions of the flocculus and paraflocculus greatly impair smooth pursuit.[373,499] Unilateral inactivation of the flocculus impairs ipsilateral smooth pursuit[43] (see Box 12–2). The deficit following lesions of the flocculus and paraflocculus is a low pursuit gain, differing from that following total cerebellectomy, which totally abolishes smooth pursuit.[474,475] This difference confirms that other areas of the cerebellum also contribute to smooth pursuit. Lesion studies suggest that the uvula may influence pursuit responses, although most of its neurons respond to large-field (optokinetic) rather than small moving visual stimuli.[190] Two other cerebellar regions also contain neurons that discharge for smooth pursuit: the dorsal vermis and the caudal fastigial nucleus.

THE DORSAL VERMIS AND SMOOTH PURSUIT

Lobules VI and VII of the dorsal vermis also receive inputs from the pontine nuclei, such as NRTP; other inputs are from the paramedian pontine reticular formation (PPRF), vestibular, and prepositus hypoglossi nuclei.[485] These anatomical connections are summarized in Box 6–12, in Chapter 6. Purkinje neurons in the dorsal vermis encode gaze velocity during smooth pursuit or combined eye-head tracking.[408,428,429] However, they differ from Purkinje cells in the vestibulocerebellum by also responding to retinal slip velocity during deficient pursuit or fixation. Thus, vermal Purkinje cells encode the sum of gaze velocity and retinal image velocity: target velocity in space.[223,431] Microstimulation evokes changes in smooth eye movement only during pursuit, not during fixation.[264] In humans, transcranial magnetic stimulation over the posterior cerebellum accelerates ipsilateral smooth pursuit.[349]

Experimental lesions of the dorsal vermis impair the onset of smooth pursuit, reducing initial acceleration by over 50%. In contrast, maintenance of pursuit of a target moving in a triangular waveform was preserved. The ability to adapt pursuit to novel visual demands was also impaired for the initial, open-loop period (see Box 12–4).[437] Cerebellar infarction that involves the posterior vermis impairs smooth pursuit, more so ipsilaterally with unilateral lesions.[458]

THE FASTIGIAL NUCLEUS AND SMOOTH PURSUIT

The caudal fastigial nucleus (the fastigial oculomotor region—FOR), which is important in the control of saccades, also contributes to smooth pursuit.[153] It receives inputs from the Purkinje cells of the dorsal vermis and also axon collaterals from pontine nuclei (see Box 6–13, in Chapter 6).[344] Neurons in the caudal fastigial nucleus discharge most vigorously during the acceleration phase of smooth pursuit at its onset; they sustain a lower firing rate during the subsequent, steady-state pursuit movement.[153] Although these neurons modulate their discharge during head movements, they do not encode gaze velocity. Their pattern of discharge at pursuit onset suggests that these neurons may help accelerate the eye during contralateral pursuit.[153] Thus, this pattern is similar to the activity of caudal fastigial nucleus neurons during saccades.[152]

Unilateral inactivation with muscimol decreases the acceleration of contralateral pursuit onset and increases the acceleration of ipsilateral pursuit onset; sustained pursuit is impaired in all directions, but most for horizontal, contralateral pursuit (see Box 12–4).[385] This pattern of pursuit asymmetry is similar to that reported in Wallenberg's syndrome (lateral medullary infarction), in which lateral medullary infarction interrupts olivary inputs to the cerebellar cortex, possibly leading to excessive inhibition of one fastigial nucleus.[469] Paradoxically, bilateral fastigial inactivation causes little net effect on eye acceleration during pursuit onset, but impairs sustained pursuit responses in all direction.[385] There is little effect on pursuit latency. Patients with bilateral lesions affecting the fastigial nucleus may appear to show preservation of pursuit,[70] if the onset of tracking is not tested.

Thus, it seems likely that while the dorsal vermis and caudal fastigial nucleus contribute to the onset of smooth pursuit, the vestibulocerebellum may be more important during steady-state tracking. Although the projections from the caudal fastigial nucleus to saccade-related structures are known, it is not clear how signals related to smooth pursuit reach ocular motoneurons.

The Accessory Optic System and Nucleus of the Optic Tract

In humans, the pathway that runs from extrastriate areas MT and MST, and the frontal eye fields, to the pontine nuclei and cerebellum appears to play the major role in generating smooth-pursuit eye movements. However, there is another pathway by which visual inputs can lead to smooth eye movements; this is via the accessory optic system (AOS) and the nucleus of the optic tract (NOT), and is summarized in Figure 4–8.[71,149,151,160,168,197,337,484]

The AOS comprises a group of midbrain nuclei that receive mainly contralateral retinal inputs via the accessory optic tract: the dorsal terminal nucleus (DTN), the lateral terminal nucleus (LTN), the medial terminal nucleus (MTN), and the interstitial terminal nucleus (ITN).[337] The retinal afferents to AOS encode retinal slip: neurons in DTN respond to horizontal stimulus motion, and neurons in LTN and MTN respond better to vertical motion. The AOS projects to the dorsal cap of the inferior olive, and the nucleus prepositus hypoglossi–medial vestibular nucleus (NPH-MVN) region. Although neurons in LTN do respond to moving visual fields, their responses saturate above 15 degrees per second.[336] Thus, the AOS may be more concerned with visual adaptation of the vestibulo-ocular reflex than with generation of smooth-pursuit or optokinetic eye movements per se.

The NOT is a pretectal nucleus that lies in the brachium of the superior colliculus, from which it receives its retinal inputs. It projects to the pontine nuclei, including DLPN and NRTP, and the inferior olive, but only weakly to the NPH-MVN region (Fig. 4–8).[71] The NOT also sends substantial projections to the magnocellular layers of the lateral geniculate nucleus, the pregeniculate nucleus, thalamic nuclei (including pulvinar), the mesencephalic reticular formation, and the superior colliculus. Neurons in NOT encode retinal error position, velocity, and acceleration;[108] this information is mainly provided to NOT by projections from MT, MST, and striate cortex.[125,126,197] An important aspect of the projections to NOT is that whereas neurons in MST variously show preferences for ipsilateral or contralateral stimulus motion, neurons in NOT respond only to ipsilateral stimuli.[151,335] This rectification of the output from cortical visual areas has been shown to depend on crossing, callosal projections of neurons.[197] A similar organization of other cortical areas—such as FEF—may explain why there appears to be no predominance of preferred direction based on neuronal activity, but lesions cause predominantly ipsilateral pursuit deficits. Thus, stimulation in NOT produces nystagmus with ipsilateral slow phases.[95] Most NOT units respond preferentially to movement of a large-field visual stimulus toward the side of recording; they respond to visual stimuli of up to 60 degrees per second.[208,335] Lesioning the NOT abolishes or impairs smooth pursuit and slow phases of optokinetic nystagmus directed towards the side of the lesion, although some recovery occurs.[224,484]

In sum, NOT appears to play an important role in the generation of eye movements to large, moving visual stimuli, such as the early and late components of optokinetic nystagmus.

Since NOT and DTN receive visual inputs from both retina and cortical visual areas, what are the relative contributions of each input to the optokinetic response? Bilateral occipital lobotomies in monkeys impair the optokinetic responses in three ways:[498] the initial high-acceleration, "pursuit" component of the response to a constant velocity stimulus is abolished;[94] the "velocity-storage" component is poor (low and variable gain) for high retinal-slip velocities; monocular optokinetic response is better when the stimulus moves temporal-nasally than nasal-temporally, a nasal-temporal asymmetry. These optokinetic properties are similar to those shown by the normal rabbit.[96] Unilateral hemisphere lesions, such as hemidecortication or localized destruction of area MST cause deficits 1 and 2 above, but not 3.[137]

How much does the accessory optic pathway contribute to the optokinetic responses in humans? In newborn babies, in whom pathways to the cerebral visual areas remain immature, optokinetic responses show certain similarities to those obtained in the rabbit;[96] for example, monocular optokinetic responses show temporal-nasal asymmetry.[11,394] Disappearance of this temporal-nasal asymmetry between 2 and 6 months of life implies that a pathway from retina to NOT and AOS is functioning in humans at birth but that, with the maturation of the cortical visual pathways, projections via extrastriate areas MT and MST to the brainstem supersede. However, when amblyopia or strabismus prevents normal development of binocular vision, nasal-temporal asymmetry of the optokinetic responses persists.[454] When binocular vision does not develop normally, the responses of NOT neurons are affected, and may contribute to the syndrome of latent nystagmus (see Smooth Pursuit, Visual Fixation, and Latent Nystagmus).[338]

Patients with bilateral occipital-lobe lesions that cause cortical blindness usually lack optokinetic responses; this is our experience and that reported by others.[66,466] One patient was reported to show a slow build-up of optokinetic nystagmus in one direction, with full-field stimulation, but there was some sparing of visual cortex when his brain was examined post-mortem.[443] Thus, although the NOT and AOS may contribute to visually induced eye movements, the transcortical pathway for optokinetic nystagmus is most important once binocular visual mechanisms are developed. One reason why the transcortical optokinetic mechanism has come to eclipse the brainstem optokinetic pathway in humans may be the evolution of frontal vision and the consequent changes in optic flow that occur during locomotion.[317] The normally developed cortical contribution to optokinetic nystagmus (OKN) in humans provides a directionally symmetrical monocular response, achieves stabilization of images in one depth plane during movement, and ensures that vergence mechanisms are provided with stable retinal images.[200,317]

Summary of Pursuit Pathway

Figure 4–8 summarizes important pathways for smooth pursuit. Retinal information on the speed and direction of a moving target is abstracted in visual cortex, especially area MT and MST. Such processing takes into account current eye movements, encodes the direction and speed of complex moving stimuli, and allows for the effects of relative motion of the background during pursuit (including the case of fixating a stationary target during self-motion). These signals are passed on to frontal areas, which may contribute to the initiation and predictive properties of the pursuit response. The extrastriate visual areas and frontal cortex concerned with pursuit project to pontine nuclei, especially the dorsolateral pontine nuclei (DLPN) and nucleus reticularis tegmenti pontis (NRTP), which contain cells encoding a mixture of eye movement signals and visual information. The NOT, which receives inputs from MT and MST, may also make an important contribution to pursuit by virtue of its projections to the pontine nuclei. The pontine nuclei project to the cerebellum, with DLPN mainly projecting to paraflocculus and flocculus, and NRTP to the dorsal vermis. The cerebellum plays a critical role in generating signals for pursuit from visual and ocular motor inputs. The dorsal vermis and fastigial nucleus may contribute mainly to the onset of pursuit, whereas the paraflocculus and flocculus mainly sustain the pursuit response. The output of the flocculus and paraflocculus is mainly through the vestibular nuclei and y-group (for vertical responses). Further details of the anatomical pathways involved in smooth pursuit may be found in Figure 6–7 of Chapter 6.

MODELS OF SMOOTH PURSUIT

Quantitative hypotheses—models—have played an important role in advancing our understanding of how the brain programs smooth-pursuit eye movements (See "Linear control systems in the oculomotor system" by David A. Robinson, on the accompanying DVD). Visually mediated eye movements, such as smooth pursuit, have traditionally been described as negative feedback control systems. What does this mean? Let us assume that, to start with, the eye is stationary, and a target of interest starts to move at velocity $\dot{T}$ (Fig. 4–10A). In this case, the stimulus to pursuit is the velocity of motion, or "slip," of the visual image of the target as it moves away from the fovea, across the retina. In this case, the "error signal," which is called retinal error velocity (REV in Fig. 4–10A) is equal to target velocity. Retinal error velocity is the signal used by the pursuit system to generate an eye velocity command, $\dot{E}$. Note that as soon as the eye starts to move, retinal error velocity is no longer equal to target velocity. Now, retinal error velocity is the difference between target velocity and eye velocity. This subtraction of eye velocity (via the visual feedback loop) from target velocity, to produce retinal-error velocity, is represented by the summing junction in Figure 4–10A. This subtraction reflects the physical fact that the retina is attached to the eye. The calculation of retinal error velocity is performed by the visual system based on the rate of image movement across the retina. The retinal error signal is "amplified" by the brain to generate an eye movement that will catch up with the target. This model, therefore, uses negative feedback with a central amplification; it is a simple velocity servo.

Ideally, we would want eye velocity ($\dot{E}$ in Fig. 4–10A) to increase until it matched target velocity ($\dot{T}$) so that the image of the moving target would be held steady on the fovea. However, the model shown in Figure 4–10A would not achieve this, because if the retinal error velocity were reduced to zero, then the stimulus for the eye movement would disappear, and the eye would slow down and fall behind the target. This model could achieve a steady state in which a constant, small retinal error velocity remains in order to sustain tracking. Intuitively, it is apparent that if the internal amplification factor (or *open-loop gain*, G_{OL}) is large, then small amounts of retinal slip will still drive an eye movement. A convenient measure of the overall tracking performance is the overall or *closed-loop* gain, G_{CL}, which is given by the ratio: eye velocity/target velocity. An equation relating G_{OL} and G_{CL} is given in Figure 4–10A. It can be seen that for eye speed to be close to target speed (G_{CL} close to 1.0), the value of G_{OL} must be large.

Negative feedback is widely used in physiologic control systems. It offers certain advantages: a prompt and accurate response to stimuli and a relative insensitivity to changes in internal parameters. Consider, for example, the effects of a decline of the value of the internal amplification factor or "open loop gain" G_{OL}. Such a decline might occur with disease. From the equation in Figure 4-10A, a decline of G_{OL} from 9.0 to 4.0 would cause G_{CL} to drop only from 0.9 to 0.8. So, a more than 50 percent reduction of G_{OL} would cause only a small effect on overall smooth pursuit gain. Negative feedback also carries a potential risk: oscillations caused by instability. Instability is more likely if the gain, G_{OL}, is high and if there are time delays in the system.

Although the model in Figure 4–10 is an over-simplified representation of smooth pursuit, it does make an interesting prediction. If normal closed-loop gain is close to 1.0 (near-perfect tracking), then G_{OL} must be large. This

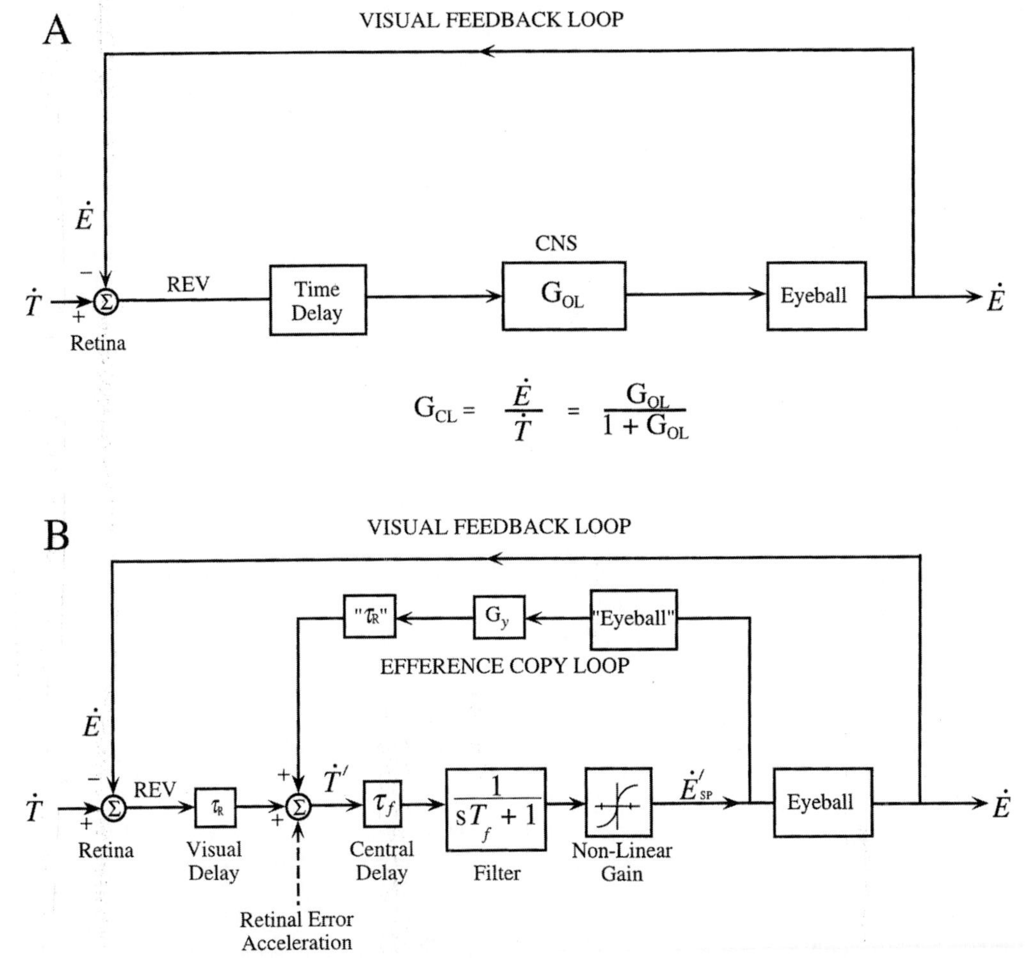

Figure 4–10. Models for smooth pursuit. (A) Negative feedback hypothesis. The target velocity ($\dot{T}$) and the eye velocity ($\dot{E}$) are compared at the retina indicated by the summing junction. The difference is the retinal image motion—the error velocity signal (REV)—which stimulates the pursuit system. G_{OL} is the open loop gain or amplification factor. It determines the velocity of the resulting pursuit eye movement (E). The time delay represents the time taken for neural processing. G_{CL} is the closed loop gain. CNS: central nervous system. (B) A pursuit model similar to that proposed by Yasui and Young.[490] In this scheme it is not the retinal error signal but an internal representation of the motion of the target in space, $\dot{T}'$, that drives the pursuit system. This internal representation of target velocity is constructed by combining retinal error velocity (REV), after the delay due to visual processing (τ_R), with an internal signal or efference copy of eye velocity smooth pursuit command ($\dot{E}'_{SP}$) at an internal summing junction. $\dot{T}'$ is subject to central processing delays (τf) and a low pass filter with time constant T_f (s is the Laplace operator) and drives the pursuit response according to a non-linear gain (the equivalent of G_{OL}—an "acceleration saturation"). G_y is the gain of the internal feedback loop that also takes into account the mechanical properties of the orbital tissues ("Eyeball"), and the delay due to visual processing ("τ_R"). An extension of the model would include the effects of retinal image acceleration.[258]

prediction can be tested experimentally by using a number of techniques to artificially open the visual feedback loop (i.e., dissociate retinal error velocity from the effects of eye movements that it stimulates). For example, the visual feedback loop is "opened" when one eye is immobilized and a moving stimulus is presented to it. In this case, eye movements can no longer affect the velocity at which images drift across the retina. The response to this open-loop stimulation can be studied by measuring the movements of the other eye, which is mobile but covered (to prevent visual feedback). Ter Braak was among the first to perform this experiment (an English translation of his paper can be found as an appendix to the monograph by Collewijn).[96] He used optokinetic stimulation in the rabbit and found that the open-loop gain, G_{OL}, was indeed high: the covered eye moved many times faster than the stimulus. Similar results have been reported in monkeys.[242] Patients with a complete unilateral ophthalmoplegia and with preservation of vision provide conditions suitable for measuring the open-loop gain.[172,176,274,426] Similar large values have been found for the open loop gain from these studies, particularly for low stimulus velocities. During chronic exposure to such an open loop situation, plastic adaptive changes, for example in the vestibulo-ocular reflex, are also stimulated.[426]

The feedback loop also can be opened in normal subjects by artificially stabilizing stimuli on the retina using electronic feedback systems.[131,480] Another method is to use photoflash after-images that are placed close to the fovea.[195] All these methods suffer from the drawback that, during this "open-loop" condition, the mental state of the subject may considerably influence the results.[13,274] Because there is a time delay in the pursuit response of approximately 100 ms, another method of studying the "open-loop" pursuit response is to measure the movement of the eye that occurs prior to the response of the visual system to that eye movement.[384] This technique measures the initial eye acceleration using step-ramp stimuli and was discussed in the section Onset of Pursuit. Since feedback tends to protect the closed-loop gain of the system, measuring the open-loop response directly is a more sensitive way of determining if there has been a change in the internal workings of the system.

The model of Figure 4–10A incorporates a time delay, which is about 100 ms, and is largely due to delays in the visual system. This delay has an important potential consequence: if the gain G_{OL} is large (high amplification), this negative feedback system would become unstable, with oscillations. Although damped oscillations ("ringing") occur during smooth pursuit, their magnitude is small and, overall, tracking is relatively stable, thus implying that a simple negative feedback model does not account for normal behavior. This discrepancy led Young and colleagues[490] to postulate that the stimulus to the pursuit system is not retinal error velocity per se, but an internal representation of the motion of the target in space (Fig. 4–10B). This internal representation of target velocity is obtained by combining retinal error velocity with an eye velocity signal, probably based on monitoring of motor commands (efference copy or corollary discharge). The effect of adding this positive, internal feedback loop is to cancel the outer, negative, visual feedback loop; the effective model is therefore "open-loop". However, if the efference copy loop did not exactly match the visual feedback loop (a plausible possibility, since the former depends on the performance of neurons, but the latter on physics), then certain features of pursuit onset—such as the oscillations at the beginning of the response (Fig. 4–3) could be explained.[263,367] This model has been extended further, to account for dynamic aspects of pursuit onset,[119,384] for the effects of pursuit adaptation such as occurs after extraocular muscle palsies,[355,384] and for the finding that acceleration of images on the retina also drives smooth pursuit onset.[91,259] It has been proposed that the pendular form of congenital nystagmus (discussed further in Chapter 10) could arise from the mechanism that causes oscillations at the onset of smooth pursuit.[214] Neuromimetic models have been proposed for smooth pursuit that attempts to incorporate neural networks that simulate the role of MST and account for predictive behavior.[407]

The model shown in Figure 4–10B has also been modified, in a number of ways, to account for the cessation of smooth pursuit, which may be equivalent to visual fixation.[12,202,368] One manifestation of an abnormal fixation mechanism is abnormal drifts, which lead to nystagmus (see A Pathophysiological Approach to the Diagnosis of Nystagmus in Chapter 10). In patients with nystagmus who also have disease affecting the visual pathways, such as demyelination in optic neuritis, prolongation of the delay due to visual feedback beyond 100 ms might be the cause of oscillations (see Video Display: Acquired Pendular Nystagmus and Figure 4–11A).[32] In normal subjects, it is possible to induce spontaneous ocular oscillations by experimentally increasing the latency of visual feedback during fixation (Fig. 4–11B).[478] However, the frequency of these induced oscillations is less than 2.5 Hz, which is lower than in most patients who have acquired pendular nystagmus in association with optic nerve demyelination.[173] Furthermore, when this experimental technique is applied to patients with acquired pendular nystagmus, it does not change the characteristics of the nystagmus but, instead, superimposes lower-frequency oscillations similar to those induced in normal subjects (Fig. 4–11C).[12] Thus, disturbance of visual fixation due to visual delays cannot solely account for the high-frequency oscillations that often characterize acquired pendular nystagmus.

During steady-state smooth pursuit of predictable target motion (such as a sine wave), many normal subjects can generate eye movements that match target movement with a gain of 1.0 and no phase shift.[107,503] Models such as those in Figure 4–10 cannot account for this behavior. The same problem occurs when such models are used to account for sustained visual fixation: the dynamic properties are better than could be accounted for the delays in the system, especially that due to visual processing.[202,263,478] The conclusion from this discrepancy between model predictions and observed behavior is that both sustained smooth pursuit of a moving target and fixation of a stationary one require a predictor mechanism. Several such models have been proposed,[25,234] with different topology and underlying assumptions. These models suggest experiments that are likely to produce new insights into how the brain generates visually mediated eye movements. Finally, for a more critical and detailed appraisal of models of smooth pursuit, the reader is referred to David A. Robinson's hand-written notes on the accompanying DVD.

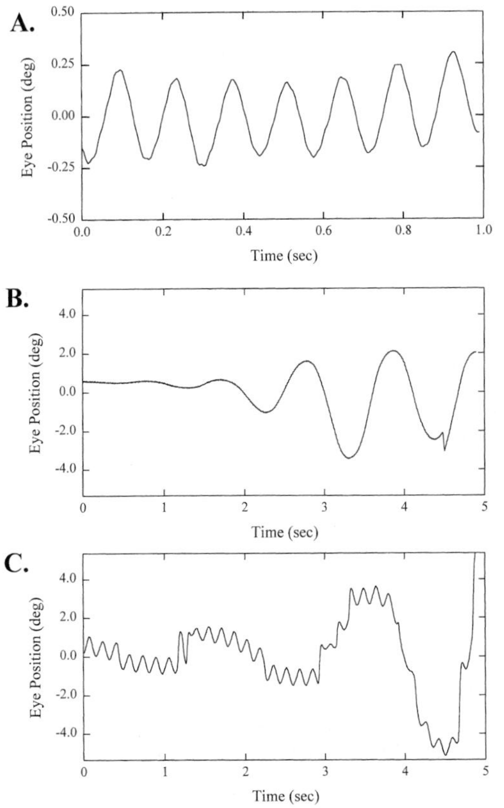

Figure 4–11. Effect of electronically delaying the visual consequences of eye movements during attempted fixation; details of the methodology are described elsewhere.[12] (A) Acquired pendular nystagmus during attempted fixation of a stationary target in a patient with multiple sclerosis. The frequency of these quasi-sinusoidal oscillations is over 6 Hz. (B) Effect of electronically delaying visual feedback by 480 ms in a normal subject, starting at time zero. The subject developed spontaneous ocular oscillations at about 1.0 Hz. (C) Effect of electronically delaying visual feedback by 480 ms in the patient whose nystagmus is shown in panel A. The oscillations of her nystagmus (essentially unchanged) were superimposed upon growing oscillations at about 0.67 Hz, which were induced by the electronic manipulation.

CLINICAL EXAMINATION OF FIXATION AND SMOOTH PURSUIT

Examining Fixation

First examine the patient's eyes while they are in primary position. This should be performed as the patient views an object located across the room, and which requires a visual discrimination, such as an optotype of a visual acuity chart. (Evaluation of the stability of fixation during eccentric gaze holding is discussed in Chapter 5.) Next, occlude one eye and observe the other eye to see if any abnormalities—particularly latent nystagmus—develop. Switch the cover and repeat this procedure for the other eye.

The most sensitive clinical method to evaluate fixation is with the ophthalmoscope: the patient fixates with one eye while the examiner views the optic disc of the other eye. Look for any drifts, nystagmus, or saccadic intrusions. If nystagmus is observed, examine one eye with the ophthalmoscope and transiently occlude the other, to determine if the nystagmus increases as fixation is prevented.

In evaluating visual fixation, remember that gaze is less steady in preschool children,[250] and may be disrupted by saccadic intrusions in some normal individuals, particularly the elderly.[2,194,400]

Examining Smooth Pursuit

Ask the patient to track a small target with the head still, such as a pencil tip held a meter or more before the eyes. Initially move the target at a low, uniform speed. Pursuit movements that do not match the target velocity necessitate corrective saccades. If these are catch-up saccades, then the pursuit gain is low. If pursuit gain is too high (for example, due to superimposed slow phases of nystagmus), then back-up saccades are seen (see Video Display: Disorders of Smooth Pursuit). During a series of regular to-and-fro movements of the test object, suddenly stop the target motion at a turnaround point and look for a brief continuation of pursuit; this tests the ability of the patient to use a predictive strategy. (See Appendix A for a summary.)

In evaluating smooth pursuit, recall that these movements depend upon the subject's ability to direct visual attention and are particularly susceptible to the influence of medications. Moreover, "normal" smooth pursuit depends upon the subject's age It is not well developed in young infants,[171a,265,364,389,410,467] and more variable in preschool children than in adults.[4,250] Smooth pursuit performance progressively deteriorates in old age.[241a,361,495] In evaluating smooth pursuit, recall that some normal subjects may show directional asymmetries, usually in the vertical plane and sometimes worse for downward tracking.[18] With these qualifications, it is usually possible, with experience, to determine clinically if pursuit is abnormal or, at least, if it warrants quantitative evaluation.

Certain special techniques are often useful for the clinical evaluation of pursuit. Uncooperative or inattentive patients, small children, or those thought to have hysterical blindness may be tested by slowly rotating a mirror held before their eyes; a mirror that is large and fills most of the visual field is a compelling stimulus for visual tracking. Hand-held optokinetic drums or tapes do not adequately test the optokinetic system but do stimulate pursuit. These are useful tools for demonstrating pursuit asymmetries (e.g., with cerebral hemispheric disease) and "reversed pursuit" seen in some patients with congenital nystagmus (see Video Display: Disorders of Smooth Pursuit). Although the corrective quick phases are most evident at the bedside, it is the direction and nature of the slow phases that should be analyzed. For example, a patient with a right posterior cerebral lesion may show fewer corrective quick phases when the drum is rotated to the right side. This is, in part, because the pursuit gain is lower to the right and, because the eyes deviate more slowly from the central position, fewer quick phases are needed.

In some patients, it will be difficult to test smooth pursuit because of spontaneous nystagmus. Sometimes this nystagmus is less prominent in the primary position or at some null point. In these patients, pursuit function can be inferred by testing cancellation or suppression of the vestibulo-ocular reflex with the eyes held in this orbital position (see Smooth Tracking with Eyes and Head in Chapter 7).[123,496] Patients often do this best by fixating their thumbnail with an arm outstretched, while they rotate their heads. Those who have muscle weakness can be rotated in a wheelchair while fixating the examiner's pointer, which rotates with the chair (see Video Display: Disorders of Smooth Pursuit). As with pursuit, the rotation should be gentle at first. With inadequate cancellation, the eyes will be continually taken off target by the slow phase of the vestibulo-ocular reflex and corrective saccades will be made. An asymmetrical deficit may imply a pursuit imbalance; for example, deficient cancellation of the VOR on rotation to the right corresponds to a low pursuit gain to the right. When there is a clear discrepancy between the performance of smooth pursuit and cancellation of the VOR (e.g., poor pursuit but good cancellation), then one should suspect an inadequate or asymmetrical VOR.

LABORATORY EVALUATION OF FIXATION AND SMOOTH PURSUIT

An essential prerequisite for smooth pursuit testing is to maintain the alertness and attention of the subject or patient; recording sessions should be kept as short as possible. The most commonly used stimulus for smooth pursuit is a small, bright spot of light, typically from a Helium-Neon laser, projected onto a dark or featureless screen. The position of the target light is usually controlled by mirror galvanometers that lie in the ray's path. A correction for the tangent error inherent in projecting the stimulus onto a flat screen is necessary for larger target movements; another solution is to project the target onto an arc at the center of which the subject sits. An alternative to a projected stimulus is a bright spot on a video screen. This method allows more precise control over the stimulus but the range of movement is usually less than the requisite plus and minus 20 degrees useful for clinical testing. Alternatively, a video image may be projected onto a large screen.

To investigate the onset of smooth pursuit, step-ramp or ramp stimuli of various velocities (typically 5 degrees per second to to 30 degrees per second) are used (Fig. 4–3). Several advantages are offered by non-predictable, step-ramp stimuli:

1. The initial response of smooth pursuit can be directly related to the stimulus, since there has not been time for any eye movement to influence the visual stimulus (the response is open-loop).
2. Because visual feedback tends to "compensate" for the system's inadequacies, it follows that the open-loop response to a step-ramp stimulus is a more sensitive index of dysfunction than the closed-loop response that occurs during maintenance of pursuit.
3. Using step-ramp stimuli, it is possible to stimulate selected portions of the extrafoveal visual field, a useful facility in studying, for example, patients with focal cerebral lesions who may have a retinotopic tracking deficit.

The response to step-ramp stimuli may be analyzed to determine: latency to onset of pursuit; average eye acceleration in first 100 ms ("open-loop" response); peak eye acceleration and the time taken to reach it and the velocity at that time; peak velocity of the first overshoot and the time to reach it; frequency of ringing; and steady-state gain.[384] The relationship between peak eye acceleration and target velocity is one measure of the initiation of smooth pursuit. In some studies, interactive computer programs have been used to identify valid trials, remove saccades, and average the responses to several trials. Averaging programs, however, may hide some of the dynamic features of the response owing to trial-to-trial variations. Blinks are reported to transiently slow smooth pursuit.[374]

Maintenance of smooth pursuit is usually tested with predictable waveforms such as constant velocity (ramp) and sinusoidal target motion. During smooth pursuit of a constant velocity target, the most useful measurement is gain (eye velocity/target velocity). Eye velocity may be estimated either from maximum smooth eye velocity for each trial,[391] or eye velocity as eye passes through primary position. For constant velocity waveforms, gain should be estimated for each of several trials at the same target velocity; then mean gain can be calculated. This should be done for several different target speeds (e.g., 5 degrees per second–50 degrees per second) and directions. These measurements are most easily accomplished by computer programs. Our experience is that interactive approaches, which allow the investigator to exclude saccades or blinks, are more reliable than automated methods.

For sinusoidal target motions, gain may be estimated from peak eye velocity/peak target velocity. The dependence of gain on peak target acceleration is a useful measure of the pursuit performance (see Models of Smooth Pursuit). Alternatively, using digitized data, it is possible to remove saccades and perform a Fourier transform of target and eye signals and thereby compute gain and phase.

A variety of indirect methods are commonly used to measure smooth pursuit performance. Attempts to quantify smooth pursuit by measuring frequency and number of saccades are prone to error, since saccadic abnormalities (e.g., square-wave jerks) may disrupt overall tracking but not necessarily imply impaired pursuit (i.e., pursuit gain may be normal). Similarly, power spectral measurements (e.g., natural logarithm of ratio of the power at target frequency to power at higher frequencies) or root-mean-square error are estimates of overall tracking, not just smooth pursuit. Finally, quantitative rating scales of pursuit as relatively "normal" or "deviant" are of little value in determining the nature of the deficit. (For quantitative aspects of smooth eye-head tracking, see the Evaluation of Eye-Head Movements, Chapter 7.)

ABNORMALITIES OF VISUAL FIXATION AND SMOOTH PURSUIT

Here we discuss the pathophysiology of abnormal visual fixation, abnormal pursuit initiation, abnormalities of pursuit to sustained target motion, and the relationship of visual fixation and smooth pursuit to latent nystagmus and infantile nystagmus syndrome (congenital nystagmus). In Chapters 10–12, these abnormalities are approached from the viewpoint of topological diagnosis.

Abnormalities of Visual Fixation

Steady fixation may be disrupted by slow drifts, nystagmus, or involuntary saccades. Since normal subjects show "miniature" movements of all three types (Fig. 4–1), determination of abnormal fixation behavior sometimes depends on statistical analysis of measured eye movements. One specific example of the problem of determining what is abnormal concerns *square-wave jerks* (see Fig. 10–15A and Video Display: Saccadic Oscillations and Intrusions). These are small, horizontal saccades (typically 0.5 deg–5.0 deg) that take the eye away from the fixation point and, after a period of about 200 ms, return it to the starting position. Many normal subjects show square-wave jerks when they attempt steady fixation.[2,194,398] During attempted fixation of the remembered location of a target, the frequency of square-wave jerks decreases, perhaps because of increased task demands, since there is also a decrease in their frequency during pursuit of faster targets, which requires greater attention.[397] The frequency of these saccadic intrusions increases with age and, in some elderly subjects, is as great as that occurring in certain neurological conditions, notably progressive supranuclear palsy, Friedreich's ataxia, and focal cerebral lesions.[2,400] Thus, disruption of fixation by square-wave jerks is only suggestive of an underlying neurological condition; they are discussed further in the section on Saccadic Intrusions in Chapter 10.

The presence of *nystagmus* during attempted visual fixation of a stationary target is abnormal. If the slow-phase velocity or intensity of such nystagmus is similar both during fixation and when fixation is prevented (e.g., by Frenzel goggles or in darkness), a disorder of the fixation system is inferred. If slow-phase velocity is reduced during attempted fixation, the fixation system is at least partially functioning and another ocular motor disorder (e.g., imbalance of vestibular drives) is present. A variety of conditions may lead to nystagmus during attempted fixation and are discussed in Chapter 10.

Disorders of the visual system lead to instability of gaze; an extreme example is blindness (see Fig. 10–8A of Chapter 10 and Video Display: Nystagmus and Visual Disorders).[277] This nystagmus characteristically changes direction over the course of seconds and minutes Fig. 10–8A),[275] a feature also encountered following experimental cerebellectomy.[383] Thus, the nystagmus that follows bilateral visual loss reflects a gaze-holding mechanism that has never been calibrated by visual inputs. Acquired lesions of the cerebellum without specific involvement of the visual pathways may disrupt fixation with saccadic intrusions and with slow drifts, especially in the vertical plane, that lead to nystagmus.[199,350] These abnormalities reflect the important role of the cerebellum in optimizing fixation to provide clearest vision.

Monocular loss of vision may lead to unstable gaze in the affected eye, predominantly due to slow, low-frequency vertical drifts.[275] These movements may reflect disturbance of a monocular fixation system or, perhaps, vertical vergence,[493] which, unlike horizontal vergence, only shows first-order responses to motion stimuli (see Chapter 8).[405,421]

As discussed in the section on Models of Smooth Pursuit, the pathogenesis of pendular oscillations in association with visual loss is undetermined. Experimental deprivation of information on retinal slip velocity during development causes a 4-Hz to 5-Hz pendular nystagmus,[102,314] a finding that may be pertinent to congenital forms of nystagmus, which are discussed below. When pendular nystagmus occurs in association with optic nerve demyelination due to multiple sclerosis, the size of the oscillations tends to be greatest in the eye with worse vision.[32] However, experimental studies (Fig. 4–11) indicate that visual delays cannot be the sole cause of their nystagmus.[12]

Abnormalities of Smooth Pursuit

ABNORMALITIES OF PURSUIT INITIATION

The advantages of studying the onset of pursuit are discussed above; in the case of cortical lesions, step-ramp stimuli are particularly valuable because they provide a method of controlling the location of the visual stimulus on the retina (i.e., in the visual field). Because of the latency of the pursuit system, the initial 100 ms of the response will reflect stimulation of the selected portion of the visual field and can be used to test the effects of *lesions affecting the cerebral hemispheres*. Thus, using step-ramp stimuli, it has been shown that experimental, unilateral lesions of *striate cortex* cause a loss of smooth pursuit for targets moving in the blind visual field;[395] this deficit is not evident during pursuit of a predictably moving target partly because of preserved macular vision.[198] In humans, bilateral occipital lobe lesions abolish or prevent the development of smooth pursuit.[380]

More important, it has been possible to identify distinct disturbances of ocular tracking due to lesions of *secondary visual areas*.[272,327] One such disturbance was exemplified by a patient who complained of difficulties in seeing moving, but not stationary, objects in his right visual hemifield, following a stroke (Fig. 4–9).[448] Routine perimetric testing of his visual fields was normal. Furthermore, testing of pursuit with predictable, sinusoidal stimuli showed little abnormality. Nevertheless, with step-ramp stimuli, his ocular motor deficits reflected a loss of the ability to estimate the speed of moving objects in the right visual hemifield. Specifically, the initiation of pursuit and planning of saccades to targets moving to right or left, within the right visual hemifield, were impaired. In contrast, saccades made to static target displacements were normal (Fig. 4–9). Thus, these deficits are similar to those described in monkeys after lesions of the *middle temporal visual area (MT or V5)*: a retinotopic defect for the perception of motion.[342] The lesion lay at the junction of temporo-occipital cortex (Fig. 4–9), consistent with subsequent functional imaging studies that localized the human homologue of MT to this region.[9,135,502]

A second, more common type of tracking deficit occurring with unilateral cerebral lesions consists of a directional pursuit deficit in which horizontal pursuit directed towards the side of the lesion is impaired compared with contralateral pursuit (Fig. 4–12B). Using step-ramp stimuli and measuring the onset of smooth pursuit, it has been demonstrated that this unidirectional deficit occurs irrespective of the visual hemifield into which the stimulus falls (Fig. 4–12C).[327,448] A retinotopic deficit such as that occurring with lesions of MT may or may not coexist. The unidirectional deficit may occur with lesions affecting posterior cortical areas and underlying white matter (Fig. 4–12A); this may be due to damage to the *medial superior temporal visual area (MST)* or its projections.[137] In addition, a unidirectional defect of smooth pursuit may occur following lesions of the frontal lobes that affect the frontal eye field,[329] or the supplementary eye field.[187,279]

In the future, better understanding of the disturbances of smooth ocular following due to lesions of the cerebral hemispheres may be made possible by presenting first-order and

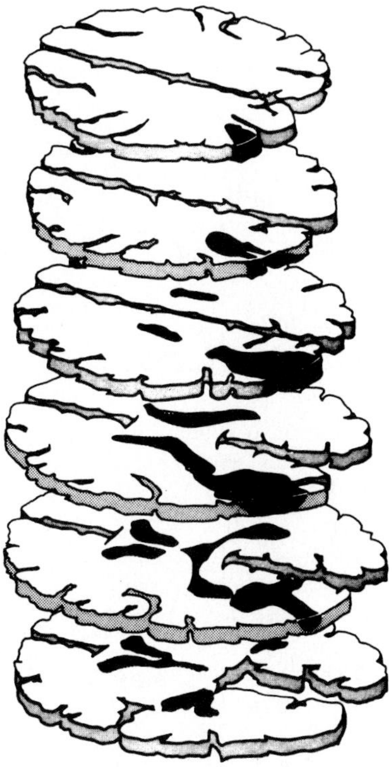

A

Figure 4–12. Asymmetric impairment of horizontal smooth pursuit due to unilateral lesions of the cerebral hemispheres. (A) Computer-generated three-dimensional reconstruction of the zones of lesion confluence associated with asymmetric reduction of pursuit gain in eight patients; ipsilateral pursuit velocities were consistently lower than contralateral velocities. The affected cortical areas included Brodmann 19 and the adjacent ventrocaudal aspect of area 39. (From Morrow MJ, Sharpe JA. Cerebral hemispheric localization of smooth pursuit asymmetry. Neurology 40, 284–292, 1990, with permission of Lippincott Williams and Wilkins.) *(continued)*

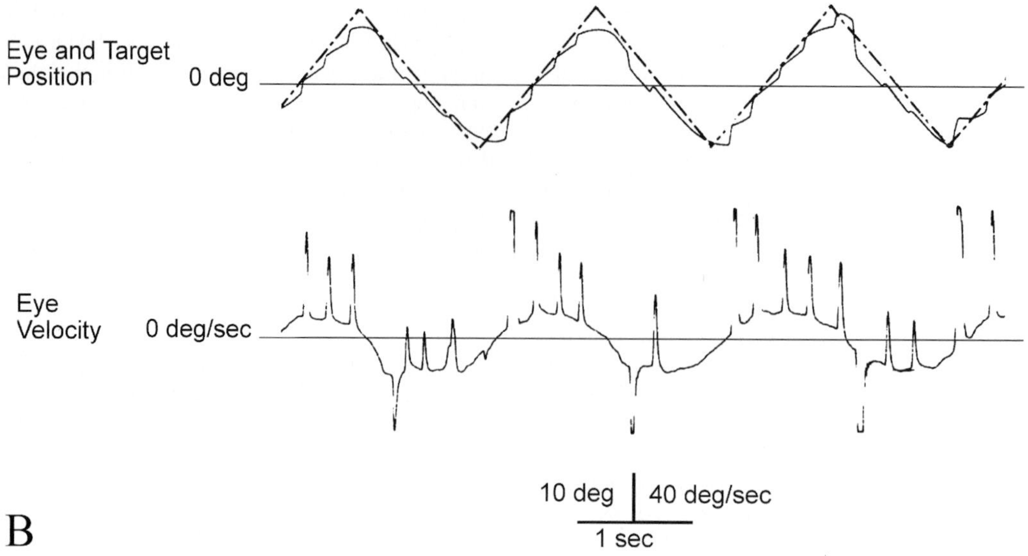

B

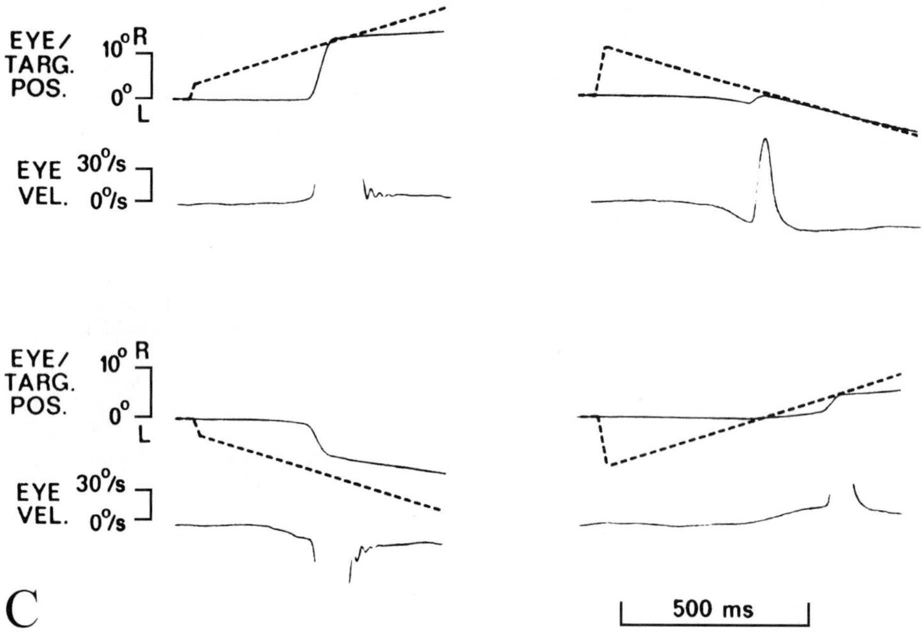

C

Figure 4–12. *(Continued)* (B) An example of asymmetric smooth pursuit in a patient with a porencephalic cyst of the right cerebral hemisphere. Note how smooth pursuit to the right (upward) is impaired, but corrective saccades are accurate. During tracking to the left, eye velocity exceeds target velocity, and "back-up" saccades are made. (C) Step-ramp responses to same patient as in (B). Pursuit initiation in response to rightward ramps is impaired compared to leftward ramps, regardless of the visual hemifield stimulated. In addition to this unidirectional pursuit deficit, saccades made to targets in the left visual hemifield are hypometric or delayed, suggesting a defect of motion processing in that hemifield. Thus this deficit is similar to that described after experimental lesions of the medial superior temporal visual area (MST) or the descending pursuit pathway in monkey.[448] R: right; L: left.

second-order motion stimuli, and combining measurement of the eye movements and psychophysical responses with functional imaging or the effects of lesions. Current evidence suggests that, in humans, visual areas V1 and V2 are mainly concerned with processing first-order motion, while areas V3 and the homologue of MST are more involved in processing second-order motion.[459]

The initiation of pursuit has also been investigated in patients with *latent nystagmus*.[454] By presenting step-ramp stimuli monocularly, it was possible to demonstrate a nasal-temporal asymmetry such that nasally directed target motion evoked a more vigorous onset of pursuit. This finding is evidence for maldevelopment of visual motion processing in patients with latent nystagmus and is discussed further below.

Another advantage offered by studying the initiation of smooth pursuit is that it measures the open-loop gain of the pursuit system; this is a sensitive index of smooth pursuit dysfunction. Three examples of how this strategy has proven effective are in studying adaptive changes occurring following extraocular muscle palsy, identifying pursuit abnormalities in some cases of congenital nystagmus, and in confirming a disorder of pursuit in schizophrenia. Each example is discussed further below or in Chapters 9–12. It seems likely that, in the future, the initiation of smooth pursuit will be tested in a variety of clinical conditions.

ABNORMALITIES OF PURSUIT TO SUSTAINED TARGET MOTION

Low gain pursuit is a common ocular motor abnormality. Attempts have been made to differentiate between a low steady-state pursuit gain in response to constant velocity target motions (i.e., reduced gain at both low and high target velocities—velocity saturation) and a reduction of pursuit gain with accelerating targets (e.g. sine waves)—so-called acceleration saturation. Low steady-state pursuit gain occurs with a variety of conditions, including old age,[361,413,495] Parkinson's disease,[476] progressive supranuclear palsy,[109] cerebellar disorders,[170,500] hepatic encephalopathy,[323a] and following large cerebral lesions (see Video Display: Disorders of Smooth Pursuit).[450] Impairment of smooth pursuit due to an abnormal acceleration saturation is seen with posterior cortical lesions,[276,326] Alzheimer's disease,[147] and schizophrenia.[285]

Studies of the effects of *predictive aspects of smooth pursuit* have shown impairment in schizophrenia.[74,285] Several mechanisms have been proposed, including impaired motion perception,[83] and extra-retinal factors, [444] but tracking may also be impaired because of saccadic mechanisms, which appear to constitute an independent problem.[204] In contrast, predictive aspects of pursuit are preserved in patients with Alzheimer's disease,[147] or Parkinson's disease,[281] who otherwise show poor tracking. Large lesions of the cerebral hemispheres causing predominantly ipsilateral tracking deficits have been reported to impair,[62] but not abolish,[280] predictive aspects of smooth pursuit. Frontal lesions may impair predictive smooth pursuit more than posterior lesions.[187] Smooth anticipatory eye drifts that precede predictable target stepping are absent in patients with cerebellar disease who have impaired smooth pursuit.[330]

Excessively high tracking gain may reflect *pursuit adaptation* in response to extraocular muscle palsy (see Video Display: Disorders of Smooth Pursuit, and Fig. 4–7). For example, a patient with right abducens palsy viewed from that eye for several days, his normal left eye being patched. Smooth pursuit responses of his normal left eye were then tested using step-ramp stimuli. Eye velocity to the right was greater than that of the target (Fig. 4–7B) and tracking was unstable with pendular oscillations.[355] These findings imply that pursuit adaptation, rather than simple negative feedback, is used to optimize smooth-tracking performance.[384]

An *asymmetry of sustained horizontal smooth pursuit* is seen with certain lesions affecting *cerebral cortex* (see Video Display: Disorders of Smooth Pursuit, and Fig. 4–12B). Thus, some patients with unilateral lesions of the cerebral hemispheres show impaired tracking of targets moving towards the side of the lesion. This has been most commonly reported with lesions restricted to posterior cortical areas and underlying white matter (Fig. 4–12A),[326,448] but also occurs with frontal lobes lesions,[279,329] and is invariable with large lesions such as hemidecortication.[401,450] Clinically, this pursuit deficit can often be brought out with hand-held "optokinetic" drums or tapes.[20,93,103,148,247] This impairment of smooth pursuit is independent of homonymous hemianopia or visual neglect, but this requires application of step-ramp stimuli, which control the position of the stimulus in the visual field (Fig. 4–12C).[272,327]

In occasional patients with unilateral lesions of the cerebral hemispheres, pursuit away from the side of the lesion may also have reduced gain, though not usually so much as ipsilaterally.[279,326] In other patients, particularly those with large lesions such as *hemidecortication* or involvement of the posterior internal capsule,[31] pursuit eye movements away from the side of the lesion may be *faster than the target* (i.e., smooth pursuit gain exceeds 1.0). An example is shown in Figure 4–12B. One consequence of such increased gain for contralateral pursuit is that the moving target is held in the visual hemifield ipsilateral to the side of the lesion, where the ability to estimate target speed is likely to be normal;[272] responses to moving stimuli presented into the visual hemifield contralateral to the side of the lesion may be impaired. After an acute large hemispheric lesion, there may be a *pursuit defect in craniotopic coordinates*, with difficulty moving the eyes in the contralateral orbital hemirange. Especially with right-sided lesions, there may also be contralateral neglect. However, within the remaining field of movement, responses to stimulus motion towards the intact hemisphere are greater.[324]

An ipsilateral pursuit deficit similar to that due to hemispheric disease may be encountered with unilateral lesions at lower points in the *descending pursuit pathway* (Fig. 4–8) such as in the thalamus,[65] midbrain tegmentum,[494] dorsolateral pontine nucleus,[165,445] and cerebellum.[475] However, because of the "double decussation" of the smooth-pursuit pathway (see Fig. 6–7), lesions involving the vestibular nucleus or pontine projections to the cerebellum may cause a greater impairment of either ipsilateral[468] or contralateral smooth pursuit.[17,159,218]

Disturbance of *vertical smooth pursuit* occurs with bilateral internuclear ophthalmoplegia (INO).[375] Lesions affecting the superior cerebellar peduncle, which conveys pursuit signals from the y-group nucleus to the oculomotor nucleus, may also impair smooth pursuit.[86,365] An unusual *directional disturbance of smooth pursuit* has been reported in three patients with cavernous angiomas involving the middle cerebellar peduncle. They all showed torsional nystagmus during vertical pursuit (see Video Display: Disorders of Smooth Pursuit). This finding suggests that pursuit signals might be encoded in the same planes as the labyrinthine semicircular canals, perhaps during cerebellar processing.[146] Lesions restricted to either the paramedian pontine or mesencephalic reticular formation impair saccades but tend to spare horizontal and vertical smooth pursuit.[184,193]

In some patients with asymmetry of pursuit, nystagmus is present during fixation with the eyes near to primary position. Thus, horizontal nystagmus is reported in some patients with unilateral cerebral lesions, particularly those with increased gain of contralateral pursuit.[401] This nystagmus is low-amplitude, with slow phases drifting away from the side of the lesion at a few degrees per second. Such nystagmus has been hypothesized to indicate an *imbalance of pursuit tone*. Another circumstance in which an imbalance of pursuit drives has been postulated as a cause of nystagmus concerns downbeat nystagmus.[497] As discussed in Chapter 10, several distinct hypotheses have been proposed to explain this form of nystagmus, but the "pursuit imbalance hypothesis" remains a possible mechanism, since it has been recently shown that normal subjects develop downbeat nystagmus after carrying out repetitive, asymmetric vertical smooth pursuit.[301]

Finally, smooth-pursuit performance is sometimes improved in patients with loss of vestibular function.[53] This is presumably an adaptation so that smooth-pursuit eye movements can be used to partially compensate for the vestibular loss. This issue is discussed further in Chapters 2 and 11.

Smooth Pursuit, Visual Fixation, and Latent Nystagmus

Individuals with latent nystagmus,[3,115] a congenital form of nystagmus (see Video Display: Congenital Forms of Nystagmus), show abnormalities of smooth pursuit during monocular viewing. Latent nystagmus is brought out or exaggerated by covering one eye (hence, "latent" nystagmus (see Video Display: Congenital Forms of Nystagmus and Fig. 10–12)). The quick phases of both eyes beat away from the covered eye. Latent nystagmus is almost always associated with strabismus and lack of development of normal binocular vision and stereopsis. The asymmetry of pursuit associated with latent nystagmus is more marked at the onset than during maintenance.[454] Furthermore, if moving stimuli are briefly presented after pursuit is underway, nasalward and temporalward image motion is equally effective in modulating eye velocity.[239] This suggests that defect is more related to pursuit initiation than maintenance. Vertical optokinetic stimulation induces nystagmus with an inappropriate horizontal component, which cannot be accounted for by ongoing latent nystagmus, and which probably reflects maldevelopment of motion processing mechanisms.[161]

Insights into the pathogenesis of latent nystagmus have been provided by studies of monkeys reared under a range of experimental conditions that preclude normal development of binocular vision. Thus, surgically creating strabismus in the first two months of life causes latent nystagmus.[239] Electrophysiological studies indicate that neurons in MT in such strabismic monkeys have normal responses but are rarely driven binocularly. Binocular lid suture for the first 25–40 days of life also causes strabismus, latent nystagmus, and asymmetric optokinetic responses that affect optokinetic after-nystagmus, which implies disturbance of the *velocity-storage mechanism* (which is discussed in Chapter 2).[451,452] How can these results be explained?

The activity of neurons in the nucleus of the optic tract (NOT) of adult monkeys raised with binocular eyelid sutures during the first days of life shows a large proportion of units that are dominated by the contralateral eye, in contrast to normal animals in which NOT units are sensitive to stimuli to either eye.[338] Furthermore, some NOT neurons respond preferentially to contraversive visual motion, which is rare in NOT of normal monkeys, where most neurons are sensitive to ipsiversive visual motion. Pharmacological inactivation of NOT with muscimol abolishes latent nystagmus in these monkeys. Thus, NOT appears to play an important role in the generation of latent nystagmus as well as asymmetric monocular optokinetic responses in monkeys raised with binocular lid sutures.

However, more than one mechanism seems likely. Thus, if bilateral lid sutures are extended to 55 days, pendular nystagmus also occurs. Moreover, if infant monkeys are reared with an opaque contact lens over one eye that is alternated daily, they develop strabismus, but no latent nystagmus or optokinetic abnormalities. In such monkeys, neurons in primary visual cortex (V1), but not in visual area MT, lack binocular responses.[452] Monkeys reared in a 3-Hz strobe environment, which prevents visual image motion, develop pendular nystagmus but no strabismus. Finally, for latent nystagmus to develop, some residual binocular vision is probably necessary (which is possible through thin eyelids if the tarsal plate is removed). Thus, it appears that disruption of sensory fusion during infancy causes strabismus and, if some form of vision from each eye is present, NOT responses become monocular, which causes optokinetic deficits and latent nystagmus. Pendular nystagmus develops in infant monkeys deprived of visual motion information.[452]

Despite this body of evidence, it remains possible that other factors such as abnormal extraocular proprioception,[212] or disturbance of either directed visual attention or egocentric localization play a role in the pathogenesis of LN.[114,246] Thus, some subjects can change direction of their nystagmus by "attempting" to view with one or the other eye, without change in visual inputs. Further discussion may be found in the section on latent nystagmus in Chapter 10.

Smooth Pursuit in Patients with Infantile Nystagmus Syndrome (Congenital Nystagmus)

Some individuals with congenital nystagmus (see Video Display: Congenital Forms of Nystagmus) maintain adequate "foveation periods" (periods when the image of the target is close to the fovea and eye velocity is similar to target velocity) during smooth pursuit.[116] Other individuals pursue poorly, probably because of associated visual defects rather than the congenital nystagmus per se. Finally, some affected individuals respond to a step-ramp pursuit stimulus with a reversal of their nystagmus slow phase that is in the direction opposite to the target ramp (see Video Display: Disorders of Smooth Pursuit).[232] Some individuals with congenital nystagmus seem to show an "inversion of smooth-pursuit or optokinetic responses."[183] For example, when they watch a hand-held optokinetic drum, the quick phases are directed to the same side as that to which the drum rotates. It has been shown, however, that the velocity of the moving optokinetic stimulus does not influence the slow-phase velocity of the nystagmus.[1] One interpretation of this last phenomenon is that smooth pursuit causes the nystagmus null point (i.e., orbital eye position at which eye velocity is zero) to shift to some other point.[112,267] An alternative explanation is that, in some individuals, velocity feedback signals due to proprioception or efference copy are processed incorrectly, with an inversion of sign, leading to a wrongly directed smooth pursuit command.[354] Recent surgical therapies for congenital nystagmus are based on the notion that disrupting proprioceptive feedback, by severing and then reattaching the extraocular tendons from the eye, will diminish the ocular oscillations.[113]

"Inversion of optokinetic responses" has also been found in albino rabbits when stimulation was limited to the anterior visual field (temporal retina).[101] Such animals showed a spontaneous nystagmus when their posterior visual fields were covered. A variety of albino species show anomalies of their visual pathways.[178,179] Evidence for abnormal decussation of temporal retinal fibers has been found in patients with ocular albinism.[104] Congenital nystagmus is a cardinal feature of human albinism.[97] Absence of crossing of nasal fibers in achiasmatic patients,[10] or mutant sheep dogs,[117] is associated with congenital seesaw nystagmus. The relationship between this misrouting of the visual pathways and congenital nystagmus has yet to be determined. However, it has been suggested that the pendular form of congenital nystagmus (discussed further in Chapter 10) may arise from oscillations within the pursuit system itself.[214]

SUMMARY

1. Smooth pursuit eye movements enable continuous clear vision of objects moving within the environment. Smooth pursuit may have evolved to provide continuous foveal vision of a stationary object during self-motion. There is some evidence for separate neural mechanisms that are more concerned with either visual fixation of a stationary target or smooth pursuit of a target that moves.
2. The principal stimulus for pursuit eye movements is the motion of the image of a target across the retina and especially the foveal and perifoveal region. Under certain circumstances, the perception of image motion may be sufficient, and even nonvisual stimuli such as proprioception can also generate smooth tracking movements. Smooth-pursuit responses are greatly influenced by the predictability of target motion.
3. Smooth pursuit can be quantified by measuring its onset and its maintenance. Step-ramp stimuli, presented in a nonpredictable sequence, can be used to measure the onset of smooth pursuit and especially the open-loop response, which is a sensitive index of pursuit malfunction. Step-ramp stimuli also permit one to assay the contribution of a specified portion of the retina (visual field) to the generation of the pursuit response. During maintenance of smooth pursuit, gain (eye velocity/target velocity) is the most useful measurement. If sinusoidal stimuli are used, the effects upon gain of increasing peak velocity and peak acceleration of the stimulus can be determined.
4. Like other classes of eye movements, smooth pursuit is under adaptive control, even though it uses visual feedback. Pursuit adaptation becomes evident following ocular nerve palsy. Experimental studies have shown that cortical areas concerned with motion vision play a key role in the adaptive response.
5. The pursuit pathway (Fig. 6–8) begins with a visual subsystem for analyzing movement; it starts at the retina and runs to the magnocellular portion of the lateral geniculate nucleus, the striate cortex, secondary visual areas (MT and MST), the dorsolateral pontine nucleus, cerebellum, vestibular nuclei, brainstem reticular formation, and the ocular motor nuclei. Study of discrete lesions along this pathway has provided insight into visual processing of moving targets. Unilateral lesions along this pathway pro-

duce a predominantly ipsilateral deficit of smooth pursuit. The frontal and supplementary eye fields also contribute to smooth pursuit, and may be important in generating responses to predictable target motions. An accessory optic system and the nucleus of the optic tract may play a role in activating the transcortical-pontine-cerebellar pursuit pathway Figure 4–8.

6. The pursuit response shows considerable inter-subject variability. Pursuit is influenced by alertness and by a variety of drugs, and declines in old age. Impaired pursuit (reduced gain) is a nonspecific finding of many diffuse neurologic disorders. Cortical lesions cause distinct deficits of smooth pursuit (Fig. 4–12). Abnormalities of smooth pursuit may be encountered in some individuals with congenital forms of nystagmus, and provide insights into the underlying mechanisms.

REFERENCES

1. Abadi RV, Dickinson CM. The influence of preexisting oscillations on the binocular optokinetic response. Ann Neurol 17, 578–586, 1985.
2. Abadi RV, Gowen E. Characteristics of saccadic intrusions. Vision Res 44, 2675–2690, 2004.
2a. Abadi RV, Howard IP, Ohmi M, Lee EE. The effect of central and peripheral field stimulation on the rise time and gain of human optokinetic nystagmus. Perception 34, 1015–1024, 2005.
3. Abadi RV, Scallan CJ. Waveform characteristics of manifest latent nystagmus. Invest Ophthalmol Vis Sci 41, 3805–3817, 2000.
4. Accardo AP, Pensiero S, Dapozzo S, Perissutti P. Characteristics of horizontal smooth pursuit eye movements to sinusoidal stimulation in children of primary school age. Vision Res 35, 539–548, 1995.
5. Adeyemo BO, Angelaki DE. Similar kinematic properties for ocular following and smooth pursuit eye movements. J Neurophysiol 93, 1710–1717, 2004.
6. Akao T, Mustari MJ, Fukushima J, Kurkin SA, Fukushima K. Discharge characteristics of pursuit neurons in the MST during vergence eye movements. J Neurophysiol 93, 2415–2434, 2004.
7. Andersen RA, Essick GK, Siegel RM. Encoding of spatial location by posterior parietal neurons. Science 230, 456–458, 1985.
8. Andersen RA, Shenoy KV, Crowell JA, Bradley DC. Neural mechanisms for self-motion perception in area MST. Int Rev Neurobiol 44, 219–233, 2000.
8a. Angelaki DE, Hess BJ. Self-motion-induced eye movements: effects on visual acuity and navigation. Nat Rev Neurosci 6, 966–976, 2005.
9. Annese J, Gazzaniga MS, Toga AW. Localization of the human cortical visual area MT based on computer aided histological analysis. Cereb Cortex 15, 1044–1053, 2005.
10. Apkarian P, Bour LJ, Barth PG, Wennigerprick L, Verbeeten B. Non-decussating retinal-fugal fibre syndrome—An inborn achiasmatic malformation associated with visuotopic misrouting, visual evoked potential ipsilateral asymmetry and nystagmus. Brain 118, 1195–1216, 1995.
11. Atkinson J. Human visual development over the first 6 months of life. A review and hypothesis. Human Neurobiol 3, 61–74, 1984.
12. Averbuch-Heller L, Zivotofsky AZ, Das VE, DiScenna AO, Leigh RJ. Investigations of the pathogenesis of acquired pendular nystagmus. Brain 188, 369–378, 1995.
13. Bahill AT, Harvey DR. Open-loop experiments for modeling the human eye movement system. IEEE Trans SMC 16, 240-250, 1986.
14. Bahill AT, McDonald JD. Model emulates human smooth pursuit system producing zero-latency target tracking. Biol Cybern 48, 213–222, 1983.
15. Bahill AT, McDonald JD. Smooth pursuit eye movements in response to predictable target motions. Vision Res 23, 1573–1583, 1983.
16. Baloh RW, Yee RD, Honrubia V. Optokinetic nystagmus and parietal lobe lesions. Ann Neurol 7, 269–276, 1980.
17. Baloh RW, Yee RD, Honrubia,V. Eye movements in patients with Wallenberg's syndrome. Ann N Y Acad Sci 374, 600-613, 1981.
18. Baloh RW, Yee RD, Honrubia V, Jacobson K. A comparison of the dynamics of horizontal and vertical smooth pursuit in normal human subjects. Aviat Space Environ Med 59, 121–124, 1988.
19. Banks MS, Ehrlich SM, Backus BT, Crowell JA. Estimates of heading during real and simulated eye movements. Vision Res 36, 431–443, 1996.
20. Barany R. Zur Klinik und Theorie des Eisenbahnnystagmus. Acta Otolaryngol 3, 260–265, 1921.
21. Barnes GR, Asselman PT. The mechanism of prediction in human smooth pursuit eye movements. J Physiol (Lond) 439, 439–461, 1991.
22. Barnes GR, Asselman PT. Pursuit of intermittently illuminated moving targets in the human. J Physiol (Lond) 445, 617–637, 1992.
23. Barnes GR, Donelan SF. The remembered pursuit task: evidence for segregation of timing and velocity storage in predictive oculomotor control. Exp Brain Res 129, 57–67, 1999.
24. Barnes GR, Donnelly SF, Eason RD. Predictive velocity estimation in the pursuit reflex response to pseudo-random and step displacement stimuli in man. J Physiol (Lond) 389, 111–136, 1987.
25. Barnes GR, Goodbody S, Collins S. Volitional control of anticipatory ocular pursuit responses under stabilized image conditions in humans. Exp Brain Res 106, 301–317, 1995.
26. Barnes GR, Grealy M, Collins S. Volitional control of anticipatory ocular smooth pursuit after viewing, but not pursuing, a moving target: evidence for a re-afferent velocity store. Exp Brain Res 116, 445–455, 1997.
27. Barnes GR, Paige GD. Anticipatory VOR suppression induced by visual and nonvisual stimuli in humans. J Neurophysiol 92, 1501–1511, 1004.

28. Barnes GR, Ruddock CJS. Factors affecting the predictability of pseudo-random motion stimuli in the pursuit reflex of man. J Physiol (Lond) 408, 137–165, 1989.
29. Barnes GR, Schmid AM. Sequence learning in human ocular smooth pursuit. Exp Brain Res 144, 322–335, 2002.
30. Barnes GR, Schmid AM, Jarrett CB. The role of expectancy and volition in smooth pursuit eye movements. Prog Brain Res 140, 239–254, 2002.
31. Barton JJ, Sharpe JA. Ocular tracking of step-ramp targets by patients with unilateral cerebral lesions. Brain 121, 1165–1183, 1998.
32. Barton JJS, Cox TA. Acquired pendular nystagmus in multiple sclerosis—Clinical observations and the role of optic neuropathy. J Neurol Neurosurg Psychiatry 56, 262–267, 1993.
33. Barton JJS, Sharpe JA, Raymond JE. Retinoptic and directional defects in motion discrimination in humans with cerebral lesions. Ann Neurol 37, 665–675, 1995.
34. Barton JJS, Simpson T, Kiriakopoulos E, et al. Functional MRI of lateral occipitotemporal cortex during pursuit and motion perception. Ann Neurol 40, 387–398, 1996.
35. Basso MA, Krauzlis RJ, Wurtz RH. Activation and inactivation of rostral superior colliculus neurons during smooth-pursuit eye movements in monkeys. J Neurophysiol 84, 892–908, 2000.
36. Basso MA, Pokorny JJ, Liu P. Activity of monkey substantia nigra pars reticulata neurons during smooth pursuit eye movements. Eur J Neurosci 22, 448–464, 2005.
37. Becker W, Fuchs AF. Prediction in the oculomotor system: smooth pursuit during transient disappearance of a visual target. Exp Brain Res 57, 562–575, 1985.
38. Bedell HE, Chung ST, Patel SS. Attenuation of perceived motion smear during vergence and pursuit tracking. Vision Res 44, 895–902, 2004.
39. Behrens F, Collewijn H, Grusser O-J. Velocity step responses of the human gaze pursuit system. Experiments with sigma-movement. Vision Res 25, 893–905, 1985.
40. Behrens F, Grusser O-J. On the additivity of sigma- and phi- movement in visual perception and oculomotor control. Human Neurobiol 1, 121–127, 1982.
41. Belknap DB, Noda H. Eye movements evoked by microstimulation in the flocculus of the alert macaque. Exp Brain Res 67, 352–362, 1987.
42. Belton T, McCrea RA. Contribution of the cerebellar flocculus to gaze control during active head movements. J. Neurophysiol 81, 3105–3109, 1999.
43. Belton T, McCrea RA. Role of the cerebellar flocculus region in cancellation of the VOR during passive whole body rotation. J Neurophysiol 84, 1599–1613, 2000.
44. Belton T, McCrea RA. Role of the cerebellar flocculus region in the coordination of eye and head movements during gaze pursuit. J Neurophysiol 84, 1614–1626, 2000.
45. Ben HS, Duhamel JR. Ocular fixation and visual activity in the monkey lateral intraparietal area. Exp Brain Res 142, 512–528, 2002.
46. Ben HS, Page W, Duffy C, Pouget A. MSTd neuronal basis functions for the population encoding of heading direction. J Neurophysiol 90, 549–558, 2003.
47. Bennett SJ, Barnes GR. Human ocular pursuit during the transient disappearance of a visual target. J Neurophysiol 90, 2504–2520, 2003.
48. Bennett SJ, Barnes GR. Predictive smooth ocular pursuit during the transient disappearance of a visual target. J Neurophysiol 92, 578–590, 2004.
49. Berman RA, Colby CL, Genovese CR, et al. Cortical networks subserving pursuit and saccadic eye movements in humans: an FMRI study. Hum Brain Mapp 8, 209–225, 1999.
50. Blohm G, Missal M, Lefevre P. Interaction between smooth anticipation and saccades during ocular orientation in darkness. J Neurophysiol 89, 1423–1433, 2003.
51. Blohm G, Missal M, Lefevre P. Processing of retinal and extraretinal signals for memory guided saccades during smooth pursuit. J Neurophysiol 93, 1510–1522, 2004.
52. Blohm G, Missal M, Lefevre P. Direct evidence for a position input to the smooth pursuit system. J Neurophysiol 94, 712–721, 2005.
53. Bockisch CJ, Straumann D, Hess K, Haslwanter T. Enhanced smooth pursuit eye movements in patients with bilateral vestibular deficits. Neuroreport 15, 2617–2620, 2004.
54. Bogousslavsky J, Regli F. Pursuit gaze defects in acute and chronic unilateral parieto-occipital lesions. Eur Neurol 25, 10–18, 1986.
55. Boman DK, Braun DI, Hotson J. Stationary and pursuit visual fixation share similar behavior. Vision Res 36, 751–763, 1996.
56. Boman DK, Hotson JR. Stimulus conditions that enhance anticipatory slow eye movements. Vision Res 28, 1157–1165, 1988.
57. Boman DK, Hotson JR. Motion perception prominence alters anticipatory slow eye movements. Exp Brain Res 74, 555–562, 1989.
58. Boman DK, Hotson JR. Predictive smooth pursuit eye movements near abrupt changes in motion direction. Vision Res 32, 675–689, 1992.
59. Boussaoud D, Desimone R, Ungerleider L. Subcortical connections of visual areas MST and FST in macques. Vis Neurosci 9, 291–302, 1992.
60. Bradley DC, Maxwell M, Andersen RA, Banks MS, Shenoy KV. Mechanisms of heading perception in primate visual cortex. Science 273, 1544–1547, 1996.
61. Brandt SA, Dale AM, Wenzel R, et al. Sensory, motor and attentional components of eye movement induced cortex activation. Soc Neurosci Abstr 23, 2223, 1997.
62. Braun DI, Boman DK, Hotson JR. Anticipatory smooth eye movements and predictive pursuit after unilateral lesions in human brain. Exp Brain Res 110, 111–116, 1996.
63. Bremmer F, Distler C, Hoffmann K.-P. Eye position effects in monkey cortex. II. Pursuit- and fixation-related activity in posterior parietal areas LIP and 7A. J Neurophysiol 77, 962–977, 1997.
64. Brenner E, Smeets JB, van den Berg AV. Smooth eye movements and spatial localisation. Vision Res 41, 2253–2259, 2001.
65. Brigell M, Goodwin JA. Hypometric saccades and low-gain pursuit resulting from a thalamic hemorrhage. Ann Neurol 15, 374–378, 1984.

66. Brindley GS, Gautier-Smith PC, Lewin W. Cortical blindness and the functions of the non-geniculate fibers of the optic tracts. J Neurol Neurosurg Psychiatry 32, 259–264, 1969.
67. Bucher SF, Dieterich M, Seelos KC, Brandt T. Sensorimotor cerebral activation during optokinetic nystagmus. A functional MRI study. Neurology 49, 1370–1377, 1997.
68. Burman DD, Bruce CJ. Suppression of task-related saccades by electrical stimulation in the primate's frontal eye field. J Neurophysiol 77, 2252–2267, 1997.
69. Burr DC, Ross J. Contrast sensitivity at high velocities. Vision Res 22, 479–484, 1982.
70. Büttner U, Straube A, Spuler A. Saccadic dysmetria and "intact" smooth pursuit eye movements after bilateral deep cerebellar nuclei. J Neurol Neurosurg Psychiatry 57, 832–834, 1994.
71. Büttner-Ennever JA, Cohen B, Horn AKE, Reisine H. Efferent pathways of the nucleus of the optic tract in monkey and their role in eye movements. J Comp Neurol 373, 90–107, 1996.
72. Büttner-Ennever JA, Horn AK. Pathways from cell groups of the paramedian tracts to the floccular region. Ann N Y Acad Sci 781, 532–540, 1996.
73. Butzer F, Ilg UJ, Zanker JM. Smooth-pursuit eye movements elicited by first-order and second-order motion. Exp Brain Res 115, 61–70, 1997.
74. Calkins ME, Iacono WG, Curtis CE. Smooth pursuit and antisaccade performance evidence trait stability in schizophrenia patients and their relatives. Int J Psychophysiol 49, 139–146, 2003.
75. Carey MR, Lisberger SG. Signals that modulate gain control for smooth pursuit eye movements in monkeys. J Neurophysiol 91, 623–631, 2004.
76. Carey MR, Medina JF, Lisberger SG. Instructive signals for motor learning from visual cortical area MT. Nat Neurosci 6, 813–819, 2005.
77. Carl JR, Gellman RS. Human smooth pursuit: stimulus-dependent responses. J Neurophysiol 57, 1446–1463, 1987.
78. Carpenter RHS. The visual origins of ocular motility. In Carpenter RHS (ed). Eye Movements. Vol 8. MacMillan Press, London, 1991, pp 1–10.
79. Cavanagh P, Mather G. Motion: the long and short of it. Spat Vis 4, 103–129, 1989.
80. Celebrini S, Newsome WT. Neuronal and psychophysical sensitivity to motion signals in extrastriate cortex area MST of the macaque monkey. J Neurosci 14, 4109–4124, 1994.
81. Chakraborti SR, Barnes GR, Collins CJ. Factors affecting the longevity of a short-term velocity store for predictive oculomotor tracking. Exp Brain Res 144, 152–158, 2002.
82. Chen KJ, Sheliga BM, FitzGibbon EJ, Miles FA. Initial ocular following in humans depends critically on the Fourier components of the motion stimulus. Ann N Y Acad Sci 1039, 260–271, 2005.
83. Chen Y, Nakayama K, Levy D, Matthysse S, Holzman P. Processing of global, but not local, motion direction is deficient in schizophrenia. Schizophr Res 61, 215–227, 2003.
84. Chou IH, Lisberger SG. Spatial generalization of learning in smooth pursuit eye movements: implications for the coordinate frame and sites of learning. J Neurosci 22, 4728–4739, 2002.
85. Chou IH, Lisberger SG. The role of the frontal pursuit area in learning in smooth pursuit eye movements. J Neurosci 24, 4124–4133, 2004.
86. Chubb MC, Fuchs AF. Contribution of y group of vestibular nuclei and dentate nucleus of cerebellum to generation of vertical smooth eye movements. J Neurophysiol 48, 75–99, 1982.
87. Churchland AK, Gardner JL, Chou I, Priebe NJ, Lisberger SG. Directional anisotropies reveal a functional segregation of visual motion processing for perception and action. Neuron 37, 1001–1011, 2003.
88. Churchland AK, Lisberger SG. Gain control in human smooth-pursuit eye movements. J Neurophysiol 87, 2936–2945, 2002.
89. Churchland MM, Chou IH, Lisberger SG. Evidence for object permanence in the smooth-pursuit eye movements of monkeys. J Neurophysiol 90, 2205–2218, 2003.
90. Churchland MM, Lisberger SG. Apparent motion produces multiple deficits in visually guided smooth pursuit eye movements of monkeys. J Neurophysiol 84, 216–235, 2000.
91. Churchland MM, Lisberger SG. Experimental and computational analysis of monkey smooth pursuit eye movements. J Neurophysiol 86, 741–759, 2001.
92. Churchland MM, Lisberger SG. Shifts in the population response in the middle temporal visual area parallel perceptual and motor illusions produced by apparent motion. J. Neurosci. 21, 9387–9402, 2001.
93. Cogan DG, Loeb DR. Optokinetic response and intracranial lesions. Arch Neurol Psychiatry 61, 183–187, 1949.
94. Cohen B, Matsuo V, Raphan T. Quantitative analysis of the velocity characteristics of optokinetic nystagmus and optokinetic after-nystagmus. J Physiol (Lond) 270, 321–344, 1977.
95. Cohen B, Reisine H, Yokota JI, Raphan T. The nucleus of the optic tract. Ann NY Acad Sci 656, 277–296, 1992.
96. Collewijn H. The Oculomotor System of the Rabbit and its Plasticity. Springer, New York, 1981.
97. Collewijn H, Apkarian P, Spekreijse H. The oculomotor behavior of human albinos. Brain 108, 1–28, 1985.
98. Collewijn H, Curio G, Grusser O-J. Spatially selective visual attention and generation of eye pursuit movements. Human Neurobiol 1, 129–139, 1982.
99. Collewijn H, Tamminga EP. Human smooth and saccadic eye movements during voluntary pursuit of different target motions on different backgrounds. J Physiol (Lond) 351, 217–250, 1984.
100. Collewijn H, Tamminga EP. Human fixation and pursuit in normal and open-loop conditions: effects of central and peripheral retinal targets. J Physiol (Lond) 379, 109–129, 1986.
101. Collewijn H, Winterson BJ, Dubois MFW. Optokinetic eye movements in albino rabbits: Inversion in the anterior visual field. Science 199, 1351–1353, 1978.
101a. Collins CJ, Barnes GR. Scaling of smooth anticipatory eye velocity in response to sequences of discrete target movements in humans. Exp Brain Res 1–10, 2005.
102. Conway JL, Timberlake GT, Skavenski AA. Oculomotor changes in cats reared without experiencing continuous retinal image motion. Exp Brain Res 43, 229–232, 1981.

103. Cords R. Optisch-motorisches Feld und optisch-motorische Bahn. Ein Beitrag zur Physiologie und Pathologie der Rindeninnervation der Augenmuskeln. Albrecht von Graefe's Arch Ophthalmol 117, 58–113, 1926.
104. Creel D, O'Donnell FE Jr., Witkop CJ. Visual system anomalies in human ocular albinos. Science 201, 931–933, 1978.
105. Cui DM, YanYJ, Lynch JC. Pursuit subregion of the frontal eye field projects to the caudate nucleus in monkeys. J Neurophysiol 89, 2678–2684, 2003.
105a. Culham JC, Brandt SA, Cavanagh P, Kanwisher NG, Dale AM, Tootell RB. Cortical fMRI activation produced by attentive tracking of moving targets. J Neurophysiol 80, 2657–2670, 1998.
106. Cushman WB, Tangney JF, Steinman RM, Ferguson JL. Characteristics of smooth eye movements with stabilized targets. Vision Res 24, 1003–1009, 1984.
107. Dallos PJ, Jones RW. Learning behavior of the eye fixation control system. IEEE Trans Automat Control AC-8, 218–227, 1963.
108. Das VE, Economides JR, Ono S, Mustari MJ. Information processing by parafoveal cells in the primate nucleus of the optic tract. Exp Brain Res 140, 301–310, 2001.
109. Das VE, Leigh RJ. Visual-vestibular interaction in progressive supranuclear palsy. Vision Res 40, 2077–2081, 2000.
110. Das VE, Leigh RJ, Thomas CW, et al. Modulation of high–frequency vestibulo-ocular reflex during visual tracking in humans. J Neurophysiol 74, 624–632, 1995.
111. de Jong BM, Shipp S, Skidmore B, Frackowiak RS, Zeki S. The cerebral activity related to the visual perception of forward motion in depth. Brain 117, 1039–1054, 1994.
112. Dell'Osso LF. Evaluation of smooth pursuit in the presence of congenital nystagmus. Neuro-ophthalmology 6, 383–406, 1986.
113. Dell'Osso LF. Development of new treatments for congenital nystagmus. Ann N Y Acad Sci 956, 361–379, 2002.
114. Dell'Osso LF, Abel LA, Daroff RB. Latent/manifest latent nystagmus reversal using an ocular prosthesis. Implications for vision and ocular dominance. Invest Ophthalmol Vis Sci 28, 1873–1876, 1987.
115. Dell'Osso LF, Schmidt D, Daroff RB. Latent, manifest latent, and congenital nystagmus. Arch Ophthalmol 97, 1877–1885, 1979.
116. Dell'Osso LF, Van der Steen J, Steinman RM, Collewijn H. Foveation dynamics in congenital nystagmus. II: Smooth pursuit. Documenta Ophthlamologica 79, 25–49, 1992.
117. Dell'Osso LF, Williams RW. Ocular motor abnormalities in achiasmatic mutant Belgian sheepdogs: Unyoked eye movements in a mammal. Vision Res 35, 109–116, 1994.
118. Deno DC, Crandall WF, Sherman K, Keller EL. Characterization of prediction in the primate visual smooth pursuit system. BioSystems 34, 107–128, 1995.
119. Deno DC, Keller EL, Crandall WF. Dynamical neural network organization of the visual pursuit system. IEEE Trans Biomed Eng 36, 85–92, 1989.
120. Derrington AM, Allen HA, Delicato LS. Visual mechanisms of motion analysis and motion perception. Annu Rev Psychol 55, 181–205, 2004.
121. Desimone R, Ungerleider L. Multiple visual areas in the caudal superior temporal sulcus of the macaque. J Comp Neurol 248, 164–189, 1986.
122. Di RF, Pitzalis S, Spinelli D. Fixation stability and saccadic latency in elite shooters. Vision Res 43, 1837–1845, 2003.
123. Dichgans J, von Reutern GM, Rommelt U. Impaired suppression of vestibular nystagmus by fixation in cerebellar and noncerebellar patients. Archiv Psychiat Nervenkr 226, 183–199, 1978.
124. Dicke PW, Barash S, Ilg UJ, Their P. Single-neuron evidence for a contribution of the dorsal pontine nuclei to both types of target-directed eye movements, saccades and smooth-pursuit. Eur J Neurosci 19, 609–624, 2004.
125. Distler C, Hoffmann KP. Cortical input to the nucleus of the optic tract and dorsal terminal nucleus (NOT-DTN) in macaques: a retrograde tracing study. Cereb Cortex 11, 572–580, 2001.
126. Distler C, Mustari MJ, Hoffmann KP. Cortical projections to the nucleus of the optic tract and dorsal terminal nucleus and to the dorsolateral pontine nucleus in macaques: a dual retrograde tracing study. J Comp Neurol 444, 144–158, 2002.
127. Distler C, Mustari MJ, Hoffmann KP. Cortical projections to the nucleus of the optic tract and dorsal terminal nucleus and to the dorsolateral pontine nucleus in macaques: a dual retrograde tracing study. J Comp Neurol 444, 144–158, 2002.
128. Ditchburn RW, Ginsborg BL. Vision with a stabilized retinal image. Nature 170, 36–37, 1952.
129. Dodge R. Five types of eye movement in the horizontal meridian plane of the field of regard. Am J Physiol 8, 307–329, 1919.
130. Domann R, Bock O, Eckmiller R. Interaction of visual and non-visual signals in the initiation of smooth pursuit eye movements in primates. Behavioural Brain Res 32, 95–99, 1989.
131. Dubois MFW, Collewijn H. Optokinetic reactions in man elicited by localized retinal motion stimuli. Vision Res 19, 1105–1115, 1979.
132. Duffy CJ, Wurtz RH. Response of monkey MST neurons to optic flow stimuli with shifted centers of motion. J Neurosci 15, 5192–5208, 1995.
133. Duffy CJ, Wurtz RH. Medial superior temporal area neurons respond to speed patterns in optic flow. J Neurosci 17, 2839–2851, 1997.
134. Duffy CJ, Wurtz RH. Planar directional contributions to optic flow responses in MST neurons. J Neurophysiol 77, 782–796, 1997.
135. Dukelow SP, De Souza JF, Culham JC, et al. Distinguishing subregions of the human MT+ complex using visual fields and pursuit eye movements. J Neurophysiol 86, 1991–2000, 2001.
136. Duncker K. Uber induzierte bewegung (Induced motion). In Ellis WD (ed). A Source Book on Gestalt Psychology. Humanities Press, New York, 1929, pp 180–259.
137. Dürsteler MR, Wurtz RH. Pursuit and optokinetic deficits following chemical lesions of cortical areas MT and MST. J Neurophysiol 60, 940–965, 1988.
138. Dürsteler MR, Wurtz RH, Newsome WT. Directional pursuit deficits following lesions of the

foveal representation within the superior temporal sulcus of the macaque monkey. J Neurophysiol 57, 1262–1287, 1987.
139. Eifuku S, Wurtz RH. Responses to motion in extrastriate area MSTl: center-surround interactions. J Neurophysiol 80, 282–296, 1998.
140. Eizenman M, Hallett PE, Frecker RC. Power spectra for ocular drift and tremor. Vision Res 25, 1635–1640, 1985.
141. Engbert R, Kliegel R. Microsaccades keep the eye's balance during fixation. Psychol Sci 15, 431–436, 2004.
142. Engel KC, Anderson JH, Soechting JF. Oculomotor tracking in two dimensions. J Neurophysiol 81, 1597–1602, 1999.
143. Epelboim J, Kowler E. Slow control with eccentric targets: Evidence against a position-corrective model. Vision Res 33, 361–380, 1993.
143a. Erkelens CJ. Coordination of smooth pursuit and saccades. Vision Res, in press, 2005.
144. Ferman L, Collewijn H, Jansen TC, van den Berg AV. Human gaze stability in the horizontal, vertical and torsional direction during horizontal head movements, evaluated with a three-dimensional scleral induction coil technique. Vision Res 27, 811–828, 1987.
145. Fetter M, Buettner UW. Stimulus characteristics influence the gain of smooth pursuit eye movements in normal subjects. Exp Brain Res 79, 388–392, 1990.
146. FitzGibbon EJ, Calvert PC, Dieterich MD, Brandt T, Zee DS. Torsional nystagmus during vertical pursuit. J Neuro-ophthalmology 16, 79–90, 1996.
147. Fletcher WA, Sharpe JA. Smooth pursuit dysfunction in Alzheimer's disease. Neurology 38, 272–277, 1988.
148. Fox JC, Holmes G. Optic nystagmus and its value in the localization of cerebral lesions. Brain 49, 333–371, 1926.
149. Fredericks CA, Giolli RA, Blanks RHI, Sadun AA. The human accessory optic system. Brain Res 454, 116–122, 1988.
150. Fries W. Pontine projection from striate and prestriate visual cortex in the macaque monkey: An anterograde study. Vis Neurosci 4, 205–216, 1990.
151. Fuchs AF, Mustari MJ. The optokinetic response in primates and its possible neuronal substrate. In Miles FA, Wallman J (eds). Visual Motion and its Role in the Stabilization of Gaze. Elsevier, New York, 1993, pp 343–369.
152. Fuchs AF, Robinson FR, Straube A. Role of the caudal fastigial nucleus in saccade generation: I. Neuronal discharge patterns. J Neurophysiol 70, 1723–1740, 1993.
153. Fuchs AF, Robinson FR, Straube A. Participation of the caudal fastigial nucleus in smooth-pursuit eye movements. 1. Neuronal activity. J Neurophysiol 72, 2714–2728, 1994.
154. Fukushima J, Akeo T, Akeichi N, et al. Pursuit-related neurons in the supplementary eye fields: discharge during pursuit and passive whole body rotation. J Neurophysiol 91, 2809–2825, 2004.
155. Fukushima K, Fukushima J, Sato T. Vestibular-pursuit interactions: gaze-velocity and target-velocity signals in the monkey frontal eye fields. Ann N Y Acad Sci 871, 248–259, 1999.
156. Fukushima K, Tanaka M, Suzuki Y, Fukushima J, Yoshida T. Adaptive changes in human smooth pursuit eye movement. Neurosci Res 25, 391–398, 1996.
157. Fukushima K, Yamanobe T, Shinmei Y, Fukushima J. Predictive responses of periarcuate pursuit neurons to visual target motion. Exp Brain Res 145, 104–120, 2002.
158. Fukushima K, Yamanobe T, Shinmei Y, et al. Coding of smooth eye movements in three-dimensional space by frontal cortex. Nature 419, 157–162, 2002.
159. Furman JM, Hurtt MR, Hirsch WL. Asymmetrical ocular pursuit with posterior fossa tumors. Ann Neurol 30, 208–211, 1991.
160. Gamlin PD. The pretectum: connections and oculomotor-related roles. In Büttner-Ennever JA (ed). Neuroanatomy of the Oculomotor System. Prog Brain Res 151, 381–408, 2006.
161. Garbutt S, Han Y, Kumar AN, et al. Disorders of vertical optokinetic nystagmus in patients with ocular misalignment. Vision Res 43, 347–357, 2003.
162. Gardner JL, Lisberger SG. Linked target selection for saccadic and smooth pursuit eye movements. J Neurosci 21, 2075–2084, 2001.
163. Gardner JL, Lisberger SG. Serial linkage of target selection for orienting and tracking eye movements. Nat Neurosci 5, 892–899, 2002.
164. Gauthier GM, Hofferer J-M. Eye tracking of self-moved targets in the absence of vision. Exp Brain Res 26, 121–139, 1976.
165. Gaymard B, Pierrot-Deseilligny C, Rivaud S, Velut S. Smooth pursuit eye movement deficits after pontine nuclei lesions in humans. J Neurol Neurosurg Psychiatry 56, 799–807, 1993.
166. Geesaman BJ, Andersen RA. The analysis of complex motion patterns by form/cue invariant MSTd neurons. J Neurosci 16, 4716–4732, 1996.
167. Gellman RS, Carl JR, Miles FA. Short latency ocular-following responses in man. Vis Neurosci 5, 107–122, 1990.
168. Giolli RA, Blanks RH, Lui F. The accessory optic system: basic organization with an update on connectivity, neurochemistry and function. In Büttner-Ennever JA (ed). Neuroanatomy of the Oculomotor System. Prog Brain Res 151, 409–444, 2006.
169. Glickstein M, Gerritts N, Kralj-Hans I, et al. Visual pontocerebellar projections in the macaque. J Comp Neurol 349, 51–72, 1994.
170. Gomez CM, Thompson RM, Gammack JT, et al. SCA6: Gaze-evoked and vertical nystagmus, Purkinje cell degeneration, and variable age of onset despite stable CAG repeat size. Ann Neurol 42, 933–950, 1997.
171. Gottlieb JP, MacAvoy M, Bruce CJ. Neural responses related to smooth-pursuit eye movements and their correspondence with electrically elicited smooth eye movements in the primate frontal eye field. J Neurophysiol 72, 1634–1653, 1994.
171a. Gredeback G, von Hofsten C, Karlsson J, Aus K. The development of two-dimensional tracking: a longitudinal study of circular pursuit. Exp Brain Res 163, 204–213, 2005.
172. Gresty M, Halmagyi M. Following eye movements

in the absence of central vision. Acta Otolaryngol (Stockh) 87, 477–483, 1979.
173. Gresty MA, Ell JJ, Findley LJ. Acquired pendular nystagmus: its characteristics, localising value and pathophysiology. J Neurol Neurosurg Psychiatry 45, 431–439, 1982.
174. Groh JM, Born RT, Newsome WT. How is a sensory map read out? Effects of microstimulation in visual area MT on saccades and smooth pursuit eye movements. J Neurosci 17, 4312–4330, 1997.
175. Grossman GE, Leigh RJ, Abel LA, Lanska DJ, Thurston SE. Frequency and velocity of rotational head perturbations during locomotion. Exp Brain Res 70, 470–476, 1988.
176. Grüsser O-J, Kulikowski J, Pause M, Wollensak J. Optokinetic nystagmus, sigma-optokinetic nystagmus and eye pursuit movements elicited by stimulation of an immobilized human eye. J Physiol (Lond) 320, 21–22P, 1981.
177. GuanY, Eggert T, Bayer O, ButtnerU. Saccades to stationary and moving targets differ in the monkey. Exp Brain Res, 2004.
178. Guillery RW, Hickey TL, Kaas JH, et al. Abnormal central visual pathways in the brain of an albino green monkey (Cercopithecus aethiops). J Comp Neurol 226, 165–183, 1984.
179. Guillery RW, Okoro AN, Witkop CJ Jr. Abnormal visual pathways in the brain of a human albino. Brain Res 96, 373–377, 1975.
180. Haarmeier T, Bunjes F, Lindner A, Berret E, Their P. Optimizing visual motion perception during eye movements. Neuron 32, 527–535, 2001.
181. Haarmeier T, Their P, Repnow M, Petersen D. False perception of motion in a patient who cannot compensate for eye movements. Nature 389, 849–852, 1997.
182. Hafed ZM, Clark JJ. Microsaccades as an overt measure of covert attention shifts. Vision Res 42, 2533–2545, 2002.
183. Halmagyi GM, Gresty MA, Leech J. Reversed optokinetic nystagmus (OKN): mechanism and clinical significance. Ann Neurol 7, 429–435, 1980.
184. Hanson MR, Hamid MA, Tomsak RL, Chou SS, Leigh RJ. Selective saccadic palsy caused by pontine lesions: clinical, physiological, and pathological correlations. Ann Neurol 20, 209–217, 1986.
185. Hashimoto K, Suehiro K, Kawano K. Temporospatial properties of the effects of bottom-up attention on smooth pursuit initiation in humans. Exp Brain Res 156, 88–93, 2004.
186. Hayakawa Y, Tagaki M, Abe H, et al. Cross-axis adaptation of pursuit initiation in humans. Invest Ophthalmol Vis Sci 42, 668–674, 2001.
187. Heide W, Kurzidim K, Kömpf D. Deficits of smooth pursuit eye movements after frontal and parietal lesions. Brain 119, 1951–1969, 1996.
188. Heinen SJ. In Fuchs AF, Brandt T, Büttner U, Zee DS (eds). Contemporary Ocular Motor and Vestibular Research: A Tribute to David A. Robinson. Thieme Medical, Stuttgart, 1994, pp 408–410.
189. Heinen SJ. Single neuron activity in the dorsomedial frontal cortex during smooth pursuit eye movements. Exp Brain Res 104, 357–361, 1995.
190. Heinen SJ, Keller EL. The function of the cerebellar uvula in monkey during optokinetic and pursuit eye movements: single-unit responses and lesion effects. Exp Brain Res 110, 1–14, 1996.
191. Heinen SJ, Liu M. Single-neurons activity in the dorsomedial frontal cortex during smooth-pursuit eye movements to predictable target motion. Vision Res 14, 853–865, 1997.
192. Heinen SJ, Watamaniuk SN. Spatial integration in human smooth pursuit. Vision Res 38, 3785–3794, 1998.
193. Henn V, Lang W, Hepp K, Reisine H. Experimental gaze palsies in monkeys and their relation to human pathology. Brain 107, 619–636, 1984.
194. Herishanu YO, Sharpe JA. Normal square wave jerks. Invest Ophthalmol Vis Sci 20, 268–272, 1981.
195. Heywood S, Churcher J. Eye movements and the after-image. I. Tracking the after-image. Vision Res 11, 1163–1168, 1971.
196. Hikosaka O, TakikawaY, Kawagoe R. Role of the basal ganglia in the control of purposive saccadic eye movements. Physiol Rev 80, 953–978, 2000.
197. Hoffmann K-P, Distler C, Ilg U. Callosal and superior temporal sulcus contributions to receptive field properties in the macaque monkey's nucleus of the optic tract and dorsal terminal nucleus of the accessory optic tract. J Comp Neurol 321, 150–162, 1992.
198. Horton JC, Hoyt WF. The representation of the visual field in human striate cortex. A revision of the classic Holmes map. Arch Ophthalmol 109, 816–824, 1991.
199. Hotson JR. Cerebellar control of fixation eye movements. Neurology 32, 31–36, 1982.
200. Howard IP, Marton C. Visual pursuit over textured backgrounds in different depth planes. Exp Brain Res 90, 625–629, 1997.
201. Hubel DH, Wiesel TN. Brain and Visual Perception. Oxford University Press, New York, 2005.
202. Huebner WP, Leigh RJ, Seidman, SH, et al. Experimental tests of a superposition hypothesis to explain the relationship between the vestibuloocular reflex and smooth pursuit during horizontal combined eye-head tracking in humans. J Neurophysiol 68, 1775–1792, 1992.
203. Huerta MF, Kaas JH. Supplementary eye fields as defined by intracortical microstimulation: connections in macaques. J Comp Neurol 293, 299–330, 1990.
204. Hutton SB, Huddy V, Barnes TR, et al. The relationship between antisaccades, smooth pursuit, and executive dysfunction in first-episode schizophrenia. Biol Psychiatry 56, 553–559, 2004.
205. Hutton SB, Tegally D. The effects of dividing attention on smooth pursuit eye tracking. Exp Brain Res 2005.
206. Ilg UJ. Commentary: smooth pursuit eye movements: from low-level to high-level vision. Prog Brain Res 140, 279–298, 2002.
207. Ilg UJ. Visual-tracking neurons in area MST are activated during anticipatory pursuit eye movements. Neuroreport 14, 2219–2223, 2003.
208. Ilg UJ, Hoffmann K-P. Responses of neurons of the nucleus of the optic tract and dorsal terminal nucleus of the accessory optic tract in the awake monkey. Eur J Neurosci 8, 92–105, 1996.
209. Ilg UJ, Schumann S, Their P. Posterior parietal cortex neurons encode target motion in world-centered coordinates. Neuron 43, 145–151, 2004.
210. Ilg UJ, Their P. Visual tracking neurons in primate area MST are activated by smooth-pursuit eye movements of an "imaginary" target. J Neurophysiol 90, 1489–1502, 2003.
211. InoueY, Takemura A, Kawano K, Kitama K, Miles FA. Dependence of short-latency ocular following

and associated activity in the medial superior temporal area (MST) on ocular vergence. Exp Brain Res 121, 135–144, 1998.
212. Ishikawa S. In Reinecke RD (ed). Third Meeting of the International Strasbismological Association, Kyoto, Japan. Grune and Stratton, New York, 1979, pp 203–214.
213. IzawaY, Suzuki H, ShinodaY. Initiation and suppression of saccades by the frontal eye field in the monkey. Ann N Y Acad Sci 1039, 220–231, 2005.
214. Jacobs JB, Dell'Osso LF. Congenital nystagmus: hypotheses for its genesis and complex waveforms within a behavioral ocular motor system model. J Vis 4, 604–625, 2004.
215. Jacobs M, Harris CM, Shawkat F, Taylor D. Smooth pursuit development in infants. Aust N Z J Ophthalmol 25, 199–206, 1997.
216. Jacobs RJ. Visual resolution and contour interaction in the fovea and periphery. Vision Res 19, 1187–1195, 1979.
217. Jarrett CB, Barnes GR. The volitional inhibition of anticipatory ocular pursuit using a stop signal. Brain Res Cogn Brain Res 17, 759–769, 2003.
217a. Jarrett C, Barnes G. The use of non-motion-based cues to pre-programme the timing of predictive velocity reversal in human smooth pursuit. Exp Brain Res 164, 423–430, 2005.
218. Johnston JL, Sharpe JA, Morrow MJ. Paresis of contralateral smooth pursuit and normal vestibular smooth eye movements after unilateral brainstem lesions. Ann Neurol 31, 495–502, 1992.
219. Kahlon M, Lisberger SG. Changes in the responses of Purkinje cells in the floccular complex of monkeys after motor learning in smooth pursuit eye movements. J Neurophysiol 84, 2945–2960, 2000.
220. Kahlon M, Lisberger SJ. Coordinate system for learning in the smooth pursuit eye movements of monkeys. J Neurosci 16, 7270–7283, 1996.
221. Kao GW, Morrow MJ. The relationship of anticipatory smooth eye movement to smooth pursuit initiation. Vision Res 34, 3027–3036, 1994.
222. Kaplan E. In Chapula LM, Werner JS (eds). The Visual Neurosciences. MIT Press, Cambridge, MA, 2003, pp 481–493.
222a. Kasahara S, Akao T, Fukushima J, Kurkin S, Fukushima K. Further evidence for selective difficulty of upward eye pursuit in juvenile monkeys: effects of optokinetic stimulation, static roll tilt, and active head movements. Exp Brain Res 1–16, 2005.
223. Kase M, Noda H, Suzuki DA, Miller DC. Target velocity signals of visual tracking in vermal Purkinje cells of the monkey. Science 205, 717–720, 1979.
224. Kato I, Harada K, Hasegawa T, Ikarashi T. Role of the nucleus of the optic tract of monkeys in optokinetic nystagmus and optokinetic after-nystagmus. Brain Res 474, 16–26, 1988.
225. Kaufman SR, Abel LA. The effects of distraction on smooth pursuit in normal subjects. Acta Otolaryngol (Stockh) 102, 57–64, 1986.
226. Kawano K, Miles FA. Short-latency ocular following responses of monkey. II. Dependence on a prior saccadic eye movement. J Neurophysiol 56, 1355–1380, 1986.
227. Kawano K, Shidara M, Watanabe Y, Yamane S. Neural activity in cortical area MST of alert monkey during ocular following responses. J Neurophysiol 71, 2305–2324, 1994.
228. Keating EG. Frontal eye field lesions impair predictive and visually-guided pursuit eye movements. Exp Brain Res 86, 311–323, 1991.
229. Keating EG, Pierre A, Chopra S. Ablation of the pursuit area in the frontal cortex of the primate degrades foveal but not optokinetic smooth eye movements. J Neurophysiol 76, 637–641, 1996.
230. Keller EL, Heinen SJ. Generation of smooth-pursuit eye movements: neuronal mechanisms and pathways. Neurosci Res 11, 79–107, 1991.
231. Keller EL, Khan NS. Smooth-pursuit initiation in the presence of a textured background in monkey. Vision Res 26, 943–955, 1986.
232. Kelly BJ, Rosenberg ML, Zee DS, Optican LM. Unilateral pursuit-induced congenital nystagmus. Neurology 39, 414–416, 1989.
233. Kettner RE, Leung HC, Peterson BW. Predictive smooth pursuit of complex two-dimensional trajectories in monkey: component interactions. Exp Brain Res 108, 221–235, 1996.
234. Kettner RE, Mahamud S, Leung HC, et al. Prediction of complex two-dimensional trajectories by a cerebellar model of smooth pursuit eye movement. J Neurophysiol 77, 2115–2130, 1997.
235. Kettner RE, Suh M, Davis D, Leung HC. Complex predictive eye pursuit in monkey: a model system for cerebellar studies of skilled movement. Arch Ital Biol 140, 331–340, 2002.
236. Kimmig H, Biscaldi M, Mutter J, Doerr JP, Fischer B. The initiation of smooth pursuit eye movements and saccades in normal subjects and in "express saccade makers". Exp Brain Res 144, 373–384, 2002.
237. Kimmig HG, Miles FA, Schwarz U. Effects of stationary textured backgrounds on the initiation of pursuit eye movements in monkeys. J Neurophysiol 68, 2147–2164, 1992.
238. King WM, Zhou W. Initiation of disjunctive smooth pursuit in monkeys—evidence that Hering's law of equal innervation is not obeyed by the smooth pursuit system. Vision Res 35, 3389–3400, 1995.
239. Kiorpes L, Walton PJ, O'Keefe LP, Movshon JA, Lisberger SG. Effects of early-onset artificial strabismus on pursuit eye movements and on neuronal responses in area MT of macaque monkeys. J Neurosci 16, 6537–6553, 1996.
240. Knox PC, Bekkour T. Non-target influences on the initiation of smooth pursuit. Prog Brain Res 140, 211–224, 2002.
241. Knox PC, Bekkour T. Spatial mapping of the remote distractor effect on smooth pursuit initiation. Exp Brain Res 154, 494–503, 2004.
241a. Knox PC, Davidson JH, Anderson D. Age-related changes in smooth pursuit initiation. Exp Brain Res 165, 1–7, 2005.
242. Koerner F, Schiller PH. The optokinetic response under open and closed loop conditions in the monkey. Exp Brain Res 14, 318–330, 1972.
243. Komatsu H, Wurtz RH. Relation of cortical areas MT and MST to pursuit eye movements. I. Localization and visual properties of neurons. J Neurophysiol 60, 580–603, 1988.
244. Komatsu H, Wurtz RH. Relation of cortical areas MT and MST to pursuit eye movements. III. Interaction with full-field visual stimulation. J Neurophysiol 60, 621–644, 1988.
245. Komatsu H, Wurtz RH. Modulation of pursuit eye

movements by stimulation of cortical areas MT and MST. J Neurophysiol 62, 31–47, 1989.
246. Kommerell G, Zee DS. Latent nystagmus. Release and suppression at will. Invest Ophthalmol Vis Sci 34, 1785–1792, 1993.
247. Kömpf D. The significance of optokinetic nystagmus asymmetry in hemispheric lesions. Neuro-ophthalmology 6, 61–64, 1986.
248. Kornylo K, Dill N, Saenz M, Krauzlis RJ. Cancelling of pursuit and saccadic eye movements in humans and monkeys. J Neurophysiol 89, 2984–2999, 2003.
249. Kowler E. The stability of gaze and its implications for vision. In Carpenter RHS (ed). Eye Movements. Vol 8. MacMillan Press, London,1991 pp 71–92.
250. Kowler E, Martins AJ. Eye movements of preschool children. Science 215, 997–999, 1982.
251. Kowler E, Martins AJ, Pavel M. The effect of expectations on slow oculomotor control—IV. Anticipatory smooth eye movements depend on prior target motions. Vision Res 24, 197–210, 1984.
252. Kowler E, Steinman RM. The effect of expectations on slow oculomotor control—I. Periodic target steps. Vision Res 19, 619–632, 1979.
253. Kowler E, Steinman RM. The effect of expectations on slow oculomotor control—II. Single target displacements. Vision Res 19, 633–646, 1979.
254. Kowler E, Steinman RM. The effect of expectations on slow oculomotor control—III. Guessing unpredictable target displacements. Vision Res 21, 191–203, 1981.
255. Krauzlis RJ. Population coding of movement dynamics by cerebellar Purkinje cells. Neuroreport 11, 1045–1050, 2000.
256. Krauzlis RJ. Recasting the smooth pursuit eye movement system. J Neurophysiol 91, 591–603, 2004.
257. Krauzlis RJ, Dill N, Kornylo K. Activity in the primate rostral superior colliculus during the "gap effect" for pursuit and saccades. Ann N Y Acad Sci 956, 409–413, 2002.
258. Krauzlis RJ, Lisberger SG. A control systems model of smooth pursuit eye movements with realistic emergent properties. Neural Computation 1, 116–122, 1989.
259. Krauzlis RJ, Lisberger SJ. A model of visually-guided smooth pursuit eye movements based on behavioral observations. J Comp Neurosci 1, 265–283, 1994.
260. Krauzlis RJ, Lisberger SJ. Temporal properties of visual motion signals for the initiation of smooth pursuit eye movements in monkeys. J Neurophysiol 72, 150–162, 1994.
261. Krauzlis RJ, Miles FA. Decreases in the latency of smooth pursuit and saccadic eye movements produced by the "gap paradigm" in the monkey. Vision Res 36, 1973–1985, 1996.
262. Krauzlis RJ, Miles FA. Initiation of saccade during fixation or pursuit: evidence in humans for a single mechanism. J Neurophysiol 76, 4175–4179, 1996.
263. Krauzlis RJ, Miles FA. Transitions between pursuit eye movements and fixation in the monkey: dependence on context. J Neurophysiol 76, 1622–1638, 1996.
264. Krauzlis RJ, Miles FA. Role of the oculomotor ver-mis in generating pursuit and saccades: effects of microstimulation. J Neurophysiol 80, 2046–2062, 1998.
265. Kremenitzer JP, Vaughan HG Jr, Kurtzberg D, Dowling K. Smooth-pursuit eye movements in the newborn infant. Child Development 50, 442–448, 1979.
266. Kurylo DD, Skavenski AA. Eye movements elicited by electrical stimulation of area PG in the monkey. J Neurophysiol 65, 1243–1253, 1991.
267. Kurzan R, Büttner U. Smooth pursuit mechanisms in congenital nystagmus. Neuro-ophthalmology 9, 313–325, 1989.
268. Langenegger T, Meienberg O. Slow conjugate eye movements. Normative data for routine diagnosis of ophthalmo-neurological disorders. Neuro-ophthalmology 8, 53–76, 1988.
269. Langer T, Fuchs AF, Chubb MC, Scudder CA, Lisberger SG. Floccular efferents in the rhesus macaque as revealed by autoradiography and horseradish peroxidase. J Comp Neurol 235, 26–37, 1985.
270. Lawden MC, Bagelmann H, Crawford TJ, Matthews TD, Kennard C. An effect of structured backgrounds on smooth pursuit eye movements in patients with cerebral lesions. Brain 118, 37–48, 1995.
271. Leichnetz GR. Inferior frontal eye field projections to the pursuit-related dorsolateral pontine nucleus, and middle temporal area (MT) in the monkey. Vis Neurosci 3, 171–180, 1989.
272. Leigh RJ. The cortical control of ocular pursuit movements. Rev Neurol (Paris) 145, 605–612, 1989.
273. Leigh RJ, Huebner WP, Gordon JL. Supplementation of the human vestibulo-ocular reflex by visual fixation and smooth pursuit. J Vestib Res 4, 347–353, 1994.
274. Leigh RJ, Newman SA, Zee DS, Miller NR. Visual following during stimulation of an immobile eye (the open loop condition). Vision Res 22, 1193–1197, 1982.
275. Leigh RJ, Thurston SE, Tomsak RL, Grossman GE, Lanska DJ. Effect of monocular visual loss upon stability of gaze. Invest Ophthalmol Vis Sci 30, 288–292, 1989.
276. Leigh RJ, Tusa RJ. Disturbance of smooth pursuit caused by infarction of occipitoparietal cortex. Ann Neurol 17, 185–187, 1985.
277. Leigh RJ, Zee DS. Eye movements of the blind. Invest Ophthalmol Vis Sci 19, 328–331, 1980.
278. Leist A, Freund H-J, Cohen B. Comparative characteristics of predictive eye-hand tracking. Human Neurobiol 6, 19–26, 1987.
279. Lekwuwa GU, Barnes GR. Cerebral control of eye movements. I. The relationship between cerebral lesion sites and smooth pursuit deficits. Brain 119, 473–490, 1996.
280. Lekwuwa GU, Barnes GR. Cerebral control of eye movements. II. Timing of anticipatory eye movements, predictive pursuit and phase errors in focal cerebral lesions. Brain 119, 491–505, 1996.
281. Lekwuwa GU, Barnes GR, Collins CJ, Limousin P. Progressive bradykinesia and hypokinesia of ocular pursuit in Parkinson's disease. J Neurol Neurosurg Psychiatry 66, 746–753, 1999.
282. Lencer R, Nagel M, Sprenger A, et al. Cortical mechanisms of smooth pursuit eye movements with target blanking. An fMRI study. Eur J Neurosci 19, 1430–1436, 2004.
283. Lengyel D, Gottlob I. Comparison between grating acuity measured by visual tracking and preferential looking in infants. Strabismus 11, 85–93, 2003.
284. Leung HC, Suh M, Kettner RE. Cerebellar flocculus and paraflocculus Purkinje cell activity during circular pursuit in monkey. J Neurophysiol 83, 13–30, 2000.
285. Levin S, Luebke A, Zee DS, Hain TC, Robinson DA. Smooth pursuit eye movements in schizophrenics.

Quantitative measurements with the search-coil technique. J Psych Res 22, 195–206, 1988.
286. Lewis RF, Zee DS, Hayman MR, Tamargo RJ. Oculomotor function in the rhesus monkey after deafferentation of the extraocular muscles. Exp Brain Res 141, 349–358, 2001.
287. Lindner A, Ilg UJ. Initiation of smooth-pursuit eye movements to first-order and second-order motion stimuli. Exp Brain Res 133, 450–456, 2000.
288. Lisberger SG, Evinger C, Johanson GW, Fuchs AF. Relationship between eye acceleration and retinal image velocity during foveal smooth pursuit in man and monkey. J Neurophysiol 46, 229–249, 1981.
289. Lisberger SG, Fuchs AF. Role of primate flocculus during rapid behavioral modification of vestibuloocular reflex. I. Purkinje cell activity during visually guided horizontal smooth-pursuit eye movements and passive head rotation. J Neurophysiol 41, 733–763, 1978.
290. Lisberger SG, Fuchs AF. Role of primate flocculus during rapid behavioral modification of vestibuloocular reflex. II. Mossy fiber firing patterns during horizontal head rotation and eye movement. J Neurophysiol 41, 764–777, 1978.
291. Lisberger SG, Movshon JA. Visual motion analysis for pursuit eye movements in area MT of macaque monkeys. J Neurosci 19, 2224–2246, 1999.
292. Lisberger SG, Pavelko TA. Topographic and directional organization of visual motion inputs for the initiation of horizontal and vertical smooth-pursuit eye movements in monkeys. J Neurophysiol 61, 173–185, 1989.
293. Liu J, Newsome WT. Correlation between speed perception and neural activity in the middle temporal visual area. J Neurosci 25, 711–722, 2005.
294. Livingstone M, Hubel D. Segregation of form, color, movement, and depth: anatomy, physiology, and perception. Science 240, 740–749, 1988.
295. Luebke AE, Robinson DA. Transition dynamics between pursuit and fixation suggest different systems. Vision Res 28, 941–946, 1988.
296. Lynch JC, MountcastleVB, Talbot WH, Yin TCT. Parietal lobe mechanisms for directed visual attention. J Neurophysiol 40, 362–389, 1977.
297. Macavoy MG, Gottlieb JP, Bruce CJ. Smooth-pursuit eye movement representation in the primate frontal eye field. Cereb Cortex 1, 95–102, 1991.
298. Madelain L, Krauzlis RJ. Effects of learning on smooth pursuit during transient disappearance of a visual target. J. Neurophysiol 90, 972–982, 2003.
299. Madelain L, Krauzlis RJ. Pursuit of the ineffable: perceptual and motor reversals during the tracking of apparent motion. J Vis 3, 642–653, 2003.
300. Mann CA, Morrow MJ. Effects of eye and head position on horizontal and vertical smooth pursuit. Invest Ophthalmol Vis Sci 38, 773–779, 1997.
301. Marti S, Bockisch CJ, Straumann D. Prolonged asymmetric smooth-pursuit stimulation leads to downbeat nystagmus in healthy human subjects. Invest Ophthalmol Vis Sci 46, 143–149, 2005.
302. Martinez-Conde S, Macknik SL, Hubel DH. The function of bursts of spikes during visual fixation in the awake primate lateral geniculate nucleus and primary visual cortex. Proc Natl Acad Sci U S A 99, 13920–13925, 2002.
303. Martinez-Conde S, Macknik SL, Hubel DH. Microsaccadic eye movements and firing of single cells in the striate cortex of macaque monkeys. Nat Neurosci 3, 251–258, 2000.
304. Martinez-Conde S, Macknik SL, Hubel DH. The role of fixational eye movements in visual perception. Nat Rev Neurosci 5, 229–240, 2004.
305. Martinez-Conde S, Macknik SL, Troncosa XG, Dyar TA. Microsaccades counteract visual fading during fixation. Neuron, in press, 2006.
306. Masson GS, Castet E. Parallel motion processing for the initiation of short-latency ocular following in humans. J Neurosci 22, 5149–5163, 2002.
307. Masson GS, Stone LS. From following edges to pursuing objects. J Neurophysiol 88, 2869–2873, 2002.
308. Mather JA, Lackner JR. The influence of efferent, proprioceptive, and timing factors on the accuracy of eye-hand tracking. Exp Brain Res 43, 406–412, 1981.
309. Maunsell JHR, Van Essen DC. Functional properties of neurons in middle temporal visual area of the macaque monkey. I. Selectivity for stimulus direction, speed, and orientation. J Neurophysiol 49, 1127–1147, 1983.
310. May JG, Keller EL, Crandall J. Changes in eye velocity during smooth pursuit tracking induced by microstimulation in the dorsolateral pontine nucleus of the macaque. Soc Neurosci Abstr 11, 79, 1985.
311. May JG, Keller EL, Suzuki DA. Smooth-pursuit eye movement deficits with chemical lesions in the dorsolateral pontine nucleus of the monkey. J Neurophysiol 59, 952–977, 1988.
312. McHugh DE, Bahill AT. Learning to track predictable target waveforms without a time delay. Invest Ophthalmol Vis Sci 26, 932–937, 1985.
313. Medina JF, Carey MR, Lisberger SG. The representation of time for motor learning. Neuron 45, 157–167, 2005.
314. Melvill Jones G, Mandl G, Cynader M, Outerbridge JS. Eye oscillations in strobe reared cats. Brain Res 209, 47–60, 1981.
315. Meyer CH, Lasker AG, Robinson DA. The upper limit of human smooth pursuit velocity. Vision Res 25, 561–563, 1985.
316. Michael JA, Melvill Jones G. Dependence of visual tracking capability upon stimulus predictability. Vision Res 6, 707–716, 1966.
317. Miles FA. In Miles FA, Wallman J (eds). Visual Motion and Its Role in the Stablization of Gaze. Elsevier, New York, 1993, pp 393–403.
318. Miles FA. The neural processing of 3-D visual information: evidence from eye movements. Eur J Neurosci 10, 811–822, 1998.
319. Miles FA, Fuller JH. Visual tracking and the primate flocculus. Science 189, 1000–1002, 1975.
320. Missal M, Heinen SJ. Supplementary eye fields stimulation facilitates anticipatory pursuit. J. Neurophysiol 92, 1257–1262, 2004.
321. Missal M, Keller EL. Common inhibitory mechanism for saccades and smooth-pursuit eye movements. J Neurophysiol 88, 1880–1892, 2002.
322. Miura K, Suehiro K, Yamamoto M, Kodaka Y, Kawano K. Initiation of smooth pursuit in humans. Dependence on target saliency. Exp Brain Res 141, 242–249, 2001.
323. Mohrmann H, Their P. The influence of structured visual background on smooth-pursuit initiation, steady-state pursuit and smooth pursuit termination. Biol Cybern 73, 83–93, 1995.

323a. Montagnese S, Gordon HM, Jackson C, et al. Disruption of smooth pursuit eye movements in cirrhosis: relationship to hepatic encephalopathy and its treatment. Hepatology 42, 772–781, 2005.
324. Morrow MJ. Craniotopic defects of smooth pursuit and saccadic eye movement. Neurology 46, 514–521, 1996.
325. Morrow MJ, Lamb NL. Effects of fixation target timing on smooth-pursuit initiation. Exp Brain Res 111, 262–270, 1996.
326. Morrow MJ, Sharpe JA. Cerebral hemispheric localization of smooth pursuit asymmetry. Neurology 40, 284–292, 1990.
327. Morrow MJ, Sharpe JA. Retinoptic and directional deficits of smooth pursuit initiation after posterior cerebral hemispheric lesions. Neurology 43, 595–603, 1993.
328. Morrow MJ, Sharpe JA. Smooth pursuit initiation in young and elderly subjects. Vision Res 33, 203–210, 1993.
329. Morrow MJ, Sharpe JA. Deficits of smooth-pursuit eye movement after unilateral frontal lobe lesions. Ann Neurol 37, 443–451, 1995.
330. Moschner C, Crawford TJ, Heide W, et al. Deficits of smooth pursuit initiation in patients with degenerative cerebellar lesions. Brain 122 (Pt 11), 2147–2158, 1999.
331. Movshon JA, Adelson EH, Gizzi MS, Newsome WT. In Chagas C, Gattass R, Gross C (eds). Pattern Recognition Mechanisms. Vatican Press, Rome, 1985, pp 117–151.
332. Munoz DP, Wurtz RH. Fixation cells in monkey superior colliculus. II. Reversible activation and deactivation. J Neurophysiol 70, 576–589, 1993.
333. Murphy BJ, Kowler E, Steinman RM. Slow oculomotor control in the presence of moving backgrounds. Vision Res 15, 1263–1268, 1975.
334. Mustari M, Fuchs A, Wallman J. Response properties of dorsolateral pontine units during smooth pursuit in the rhesus macaque. J Neurophysiol 60, 664–686, 1988.
335. Mustari MJ, Fuchs AF. Discharge patterns of neurons in the pretectal nucleus of the optic tract (NOT) in the behaving primate. J Neurophysiol 64, 77–90, 1989.
336. Mustari MJ, Fuchs AF. Response properties of single units in the lateral terminal nucleus of the accessory optic system in the behaving primate. J Neurophysiol 61, 1207–1220, 1989.
337. Mustari MJ, Fuchs AF, Kaneko CR, Robinson FR. Anatomical connections of the primate pretectal nucleus of the optic tract. J Comp Neurol 349, 111–128, 1994.
338. Mustari MJ, Tusa RJ, Burrows AF, Fuchs AF, Livingston CA. Gaze-stabilizing deficits and latent nystagmus in monkeys with early-onset visual deprivation: role of the pretectal not. J Neurophysiol 86, 662–675, 2001.
339. Nagao S, Kitamura T, Nakamura N, Hiramatsu T, Yamada J. Differences of the primate flocculus and ventral paraflocculus in the mossy and climbing fiber input organization. J Comp Neurol 382, 480–498, 1997.
340. Nagao S, Kitamura T, Nakamura N, Hiramatsu T, Yamada J. Location of efferent terminals of the primate flocculus and ventral paraflocculus revealed by anterograde axonal transport methods. Neurosci Res 27, 257–269, 1997.
341. Newsome WT, Paré EB. A selective impairment of motion perception following lesions of the middle temporal visual area (MT). J Neurosci 8, 2201–2211, 1988.
342. Newsome WT, Wurtz RH, Dürsteler MR, Mikami A. Deficits in visual motion processing following ibotenic acid lesions of the middle temporal visual area of the macaque monkey. J Neurosci 5, 825–840, 1985.
343. Newsome WT, Wurtz RH, Komatsu H. Relation of cortical areas MT and MST to pursuit eye movements. II. Differentiation of retinal from extraretinal inputs. J Neurophysiol 60, 604–620, 1988.
344. Noda H, Sugita S, Ikeda Y. Afferent and efferent connections of the oculomotor region of the fastigial nucleus in the macaque monkey. J Comp Neurol 302, 330–348, 1990.
345. Nowak LG, Munk MHJ, Girard P, Bullier J. Visual latencies in areas V1 and V2 on the macaque monkey. Vis Neurosci 12, 371–384, 1995.
346. O'Driscoll GA, Wolff AL, Benkelfat C, et al. Functional neuroanatomy of smooth pursuit and predictive saccades. Neuroreport 11, 1335–1340, 2000.
347. O'Keefe LP, Movshon JA. Processing of first- and second-order motion signals by neurons in area MT of the macaque monkey. Vis Neurosci 15, 305–317, 1998.
348. Ogawa T, Fujita M. Adaptive modifications of human postsaccadic pursuit eye movements induced by a step-ramp-ramp paradigm. Exp Brain Res 116, 83–96, 1997.
349. Ohtsuka K, Enoki T. Transcranial magnetic stimulation over the posterior cerebellum during smooth pursuit eye movements in man. Brain 121, 429–435, 1998.
350. Ohtsuka K, Mukuno K, Sakai H, Ishikawa S. Instability of eye position in the dark in cerebellar degeneration. Ophthalmologica (Basel) 196, 35–39, 1988.
351. Ono S, Das VE, Economides JR, Mustari MJ. Modeling of smooth pursuit-related neuronal responses in the DLPN and NRTP of the rhesus macaque. J Neurophysiol 93, 108–116, 2005.
352. Ono S, Das VE, Mustari MJ. Role of the dorsolateral pontine nucleus in short-term adaptation of the horizontal vestibuloocular reflex. J Neurophysiol 89, 2879–2885, 2003.
353. Ono S, Das VE, Mustari MJ. Gaze-related response properties of DLPN and NRTP neurons in the rhesus macaque. J Neurophysiol 91, 2484–2500, 2004.
354. Optican LM, Zee DS. A hypothetical explanation of congenital nystagmus. Biol Cybern 50, 119–134, 1984.
355. Optican LM, Zee DS, Chu FC. Adaptive response to ocular muscle weakness in human pursuit and saccadic eye movements. J Neurophysiol 54, 110–122, 1985.
356. Ott D, Seidman SH, Leigh RJ. The stability of human eye orientation during visual fixation. Neurosci Lett 142, 183–186, 1992.
357. Pack C, Born RT. Temporal dynamics of a neural solution to the aperture problem in visual area MT of macaque brain. Nature 409, 1040–1042, 2001.
358. Pack C, Grossberg S, Mingolla E. A neural model of

smooth pursuit control and motion perception by cortical area MST. J Cogn Neurosci 13, 102–120, 2001.
359. Page WK, Duffy CJ. Heading representation in MST: sensory interactions and population encoding. J Neurophysiol 89, 1994–2013, 2003.
360. Page WK, King WM, Merigan W, MaunsellJ. Magnocellular or parvocellular lesions in the lateral geniculate nucleus of monkeys cause minor deficits of smooth pursuit eye movements. Vision Res 34, 223–239, 1997.
361. Paige GD. Senescence of human visual-vestibular interactions: smooth pursuit, optokinetic, and vestibular control of eye movements with aging. Exp Brain Res 98, 355–372, 1994.
362. Petit L, Clarke VP, Ingeholm J, Haxby JV. Dissociation of saccade-related and pursuit-related activation in human frontal eye fields as revealed by fMRI. J Neurophysiol 77, 3386–3390, 1997.
363. Petit L, Haxby JV. Functional anatomy of pursuit eye movements in humans as revealed by fMRI. J Neurophysiol 82, 463–471, 1999.
364. Phillips JO, Finocchio DV, Ong L, Fuchs AF. Smooth pursuit in 1- to 4-month-old human infants. Vision Res 37, 3009–3020, 1997.
365. Pierrot-Deseilligny C, Rivaud S, Samson Y, Cambon H. Some instructive cases concerning the circuitry of smooth ocular pursuit in the brainstem. Neuro-ophthalmology 9, 31–42, 1989.
366. Pola J, Wyatt HJ. Target position and velocity: The stimuli for smooth pursuit eye movements. Vision Res 20, 523–534, 1980.
367. Pola J, Wyatt HJ. Offset dynamics of human smooth pursuit eye movements: effects of target presence and subject attention. Vision Res 37, 2579–2595, 1997.
368. Pola J, Wyatt HJ. The role of target position in smooth pursuit deceleration and termination. Vision Res 41, 655–669, 2001.
369. Pola J, Wyatt HJ, Lustgarten M. Visual fixation of a target and suppression of optokinetic nystagmus: effects of varying target feedback. Vision Res 35, 1079–1087, 1995.
370. Poliakoff E, Collins CJ, Barnes GR. Target selection for predictive smooth pursuit eye movements. Exp Brain Res 155, 129–133, 2004.
371. Priebe NJ, Churchland MM, Lisberger SG. Reconstruction of target speed for the guidance of pursuit eye movements. J Neurosci 21, 3196–3206, 2001.
372. Priebe NJ, Lisberger SG. Estimating target speed from the population response in visual area MT. J Neurosci 24, 1907–1916, 2004.
373. Rambold H, Churchland A, Selig Y, Jasmin L, Lisberger SG. Partial ablations of the flocculus and ventral paraflocculus in monkeys cause linked deficits in smooth pursuit eye movements and adaptive modification of the VOR. J Neurophysiol 87, 912–924, 2002.
374. Rambold H, El Baz I, Helmchen C. Blink effects on ongoing smooth pursuit eye movements in humans. Exp Brain Res, 2004.
375. Ranalli PJ, Sharpe JA. Vertical vestibulo-ocular reflex, smooth pursuit and eye-head tracking dysfunction in internuclear ophthalomoplegia. Brain 111, 1299–1317, 1988.
376. Rashbass C. The relationship between saccadic and smooth tracking eye movements. J Physiol (Lond) 159, 326–338, 1961.
377. Recanzone GH, Wurtz RH, Schwarz U. Responses of MT and MST neurons to one and two moving objects in the receptive field. J Neurophysiol 78, 2904–2915, 1997.
378. Riggs LA, Ratliff F. The effects of counteracting the normal movements of the eye. J Opt Soc of America 42, 872–873, 1952.
379. Rizzo M, Hurtig R. Looking but not seeing: Attention, perception, and eye movements in simultanagnosia. Neurology 37, 1642–1648, 1987.
380. Rizzo M, Hurtig R. The effects of bilateral visual cortex lesions on the development of eye movements and perception. Neurology 39, 406–413, 1989.
381. Roberts DK, Noda H. Effect of a parafoveal microlesion made with an argon laser on smooth-pursuit eye movements of monkeys. Exp Neurol 93, 631–641, 1986.
382. Robinson DA. The mechanics of human smooth pursuit eye movement. J Physiol (Lond) 180, 569–591, 1965.
383. Robinson DA. The effect of cerebellectomy on the cat's vestibulo-ocular integrator. Brain Res 71, 195–207, 1974.
384. Robinson DA, Gordon JL, Gordon SE. A model of the smooth pursuit eye movement system. Biol Cybern 55, 43–57, 1986.
385. Robinson FR, Straube A, Fuchs AF. Participation of the caudal fastigial nucleus in smooth-pursuit eye movements. 2. Effects of muscimol inactivation. J Neurophysiol 78, 848–859, 1997.
386. Ron S, Vieville T, Droulez J. Target velocity based prediction in saccadic vector programming. Vision Res 29, 1103–1114, 1989.
387. Rosano C, Kristy CM, Welling JS, et al. Pursuit and saccadic eye movement subregions in human frontal eye field: a high-resolution fMRI investigation. Cereb Cortex 12, 107–115, 2002.
388. Rottach KG, Zivotofsky A, Das VE, et al. Comparison of horizontal, vertical and diagonal smooth pursuit eye movements in normal human subjects. Vision Res 36, 2189–2195, 1996.
389. Roucoux A, Culee C, Roucoux M. Development of fixation and pursuit eye movements in human infants. Behav Brain Res 10, 133–139, 1983.
390. Roy J-P, Wurtz RH. The role of disparity-sensitive cortical neurons in signalling the direction of self-motion. Nature 348, 160–162, 1990.
391. Schalén L. Quantification of tracking eye movements in normal subjects. Acta Otolaryngol (Stockh) 90, 404–413, 1980.
392. Schlack A, Hoffmann KP, Bremmer F. Selectivity of macaque ventral intraparietal area (area VIP) for smooth pursuit eye movements. J Physiol 551, 551–561, 2003.
393. Schmid A, Rees G, Frith C, Barnes G. An fMRI study of anticipation and learning of smooth pursuit eye movements in humans. Neuroreport 12, 1409–1414, 2001.
394. Schor CM. Subcortical binocular suppression affects the development of latent and optokinetic nystagmus. Am J Optom Physiol Opt 60, 481–502, 1983.
395. Segraves MA, Goldberg ME, Deng SY, et al. The role of striate cortex in the guidance of eye movements in the monkey. J Neurosci 7, 3040–3058, 1987.

396. Seidman SH, Leigh RJ, Thomas CW. Eye movements during the motion after-effect. Vision Res 32, 167–171, 1992.
397. Shaffer DM, Krisky CM, Sweeney JA. Frequency and metrics of square-wave jerks: influences of task-demand characteristics. Invest Ophthalmol Vis Sci 44, 1082–1087 2003.
398. Shallo-Hoffmann J, Petersen J, Mühlendyck H. How normal are "normal" square wave jerks. Invest Ophthalmol Vis Sci 30, 1009–1011, 1989.
399. Sharpe JA, Deck JHN. Destruction of the internal sagittal stratum and normal smooth pursuit. Ann Neurol 4, 473–476, 1978.
400. Sharpe JA, Herishanu YO, White OB. Cerebral square wave jerks. Neurology 32, 57–62, 1982.
401. Sharpe JA, Lo AW, Rabinovitch HE. Control of the saccadic and smooth pursuit systems after cerebral hemidecortication. Brain 102, 387–403, 1979.
402. Sharpe JA, Sylvester TO. Effect of aging on horizontal smooth pursuit. Invest Ophthalmol Vis Sci 17, 465–468, 1978.
403. Shea SL, Aslin RN. Oculomotor responses to step-ramp targets by young human infants. Vision Res 30, 1077–1092, 1990.
404. Sheliga BM, Chen KJ, FitzGibbon EJ, Miles FA. Initial ocular following in humans: a response to first-order motion energy. Vision Res 45, 3307–3321, 2005.
405. Sheliga BM, Chen KJ, FitzGibbon EJ, Miles FA. Short-latency disparity vergence in humans: evidence for early spatial filtering. Ann N Y Acad Sci 1039, 252–259, 2005.
406. Shenoy KV, Crowell JA, Andersen RA. Pursuit speed compensation in cortical area MSTd. J Neurophysiol 88, 2630–2647, 2002.
407. Shibata T, Tabata H, Schaal S, Kawato M. A model of smooth pursuit in primates based on learning the target dynamics. Neural Networks 18, 213–224, 2005.
408. Shinmei Y, Yamanobe T, Fukushima J, Fukushima K. Purkinje cells of the cerebellar dorsal vermis: simple-spike activity during pursuit and passive whole-body rotation. J Neurophysiol 87, 1836–1849, 2002.
409. Shipp S, de Jong BM, Zihl J, Frackowiak RSJ, Zeki S. The brain activity related to residual motion vision in a patient with bilateral lesions of V5. Brain 117, 1023–1038, 1994.
410. Shupert C, Fuchs AF. Development of conjugate human eye movements. Vision Res 28, 585–596, 1988.
411. Soechting JF, Mrotek LA, Flanders M. Smooth pursuit tracking of an abrupt change in target direction: vector superposition of discrete responses. Exp Brain Res 160, 245–258, 2005.
412. Spauschus A, Marsden J, Halliday DM, Rosenberg JR, Brown P. The origin of ocular microtremor in man. Exp Brain Res 126, 556–562, 1999.
413. Spooner JW, Sakala SM, Baloh RW. Effect of aging on eye tracking. Arch Neurol 37, 575–576, 1980.
414. Squatrito S, Maioli MG. Encoding of smooth pursuit direction and eye position by neurons of area MSTd of macaque monkey. J Neurosci 17, 3847–3860, 1997.
415. Stanton GB, Bruce CJ, Goldberg ME. Topography of projections to posterior cortical areas from the macaque frontal eye fields. J Comp Neurol 353, 291–305, 1995.
416. Stanton GB, Friedman HR, Dias EC, Bruce CJ. Cortical afferents to the smooth-pursuit region of the macaque monkey's frontal eye field. Exp Brain Res 165, 179–192, 2005.
417. Steinbach MJ. Pursuing the perceptual rather than the retinal stimulus. Vision Res 16, 1371–1376, 1976.
418. Steinbach MJ, Held R. Eye tracking of observer-generated target movements. Science 161, 187–188, 1968.
419. Steinman RM, Cushman WB, Martins AJ. The precision of gaze. Human Neurobiol 1, 97–109, 1982.
420. Steinman RM, Haddad GM, Skavenski AA. Miniature eye movement. Science 181, 810–819, 1973.
421. Stevenson SB. Visual processing in vertical disparity control. Ann N Y Acad Sci 456, 492–494, 2002.
422. Stone LS, Krauzlis RJ. Shared motion signals for human perceptual decisions and oculomotor actions. J Vis 3, 725–736, 2003.
423. Stork S, Neggers SF, Musseler J. Intentionally-evoked modulations of smooth pursuit eye movements. Hum Mov Sci 21, 335–348, 2002.
424. Straube A, Scheuerer W, Eggert T. Target velocity and age influence the initial smooth pursuit response in humans. Neuro-ophthalmology 18, 191–198, 1997.
425. Straube A, Scheuerer W, Eggert T. Unilateral cerebellar lesions affect initiation of ipsilateral smooth pursuit eye movements in humans. Ann Neurol 42, 891–898, 1997.
426. Straumann D, Henn V. Open-loop syndrome: one plegic and one amaurotic eye. Clin Vision Sci 7, 129–132, 1992.
427. Suehiro K, Miura K, Kodaka Y, et al. Effects of smooth pursuit eye movement on ocular responses to sudden background motion in humans. Neurosci Res 35, 329–338, 1999.
428. Suzuki DA, Keller EL. The role of the posterior vermis of monkey cerebellum in smooth-pursuit eye movement control. I. Eye and head movement-related activity. J Neurophysiol 59, 1–18, 1988.
429. Suzuki DA, Keller EL. The role of the posterior vermis of monkey cerebellum in smooth-pursuit eye movement control. II. Target velocity-related Purkinje cell activity. J Neurophysiol 59, 19–40, 1988.
430. Suzuki DA, May JG, Keller EL, Yee RD. Visual motion response properties of neurons in dorsolateral pontine nucleus of alert monkey. J Neurophysiol 63, 37–59, 1990.
431. Suzuki DA, Noda H, Kase M. Visual and pursuit eye movement-related activity in posterior vermis of monkey cerebellum. J Neurophysiol 46, 1120–1139, 1981.
432. Suzuki DA, Yamada T, Hoedema R, Yee RD. Smooth-pursuit eye-movement deficits with chemical lesions in macaque nucleus reticularis tegmenti pontis. J Neurophysiol 82, 1178–1186, 1999.
433. Suzuki DA, Yamada T, Yee RD. Smooth-pursuit eye-movement-related neuronal activity in macaque nucleus reticularis tegmenti pontis. J Neurophysiol 89, 2146–2158, 2003.
434. Tabata H, Hashimoto K, Inaba N, Kawano K. Centripetal bias on preparation for smooth pursuit eye movements based on the anticipation. Exp Brain Res 156, 392–395, 2004.
435. Tajik-Parvinchi DJ, Lillakas L, Irving E, Steinbach M.J. Children's pursuit eye movements: a developmental study. Vision Res 43, 77–84, 2003.
436. Takagi M, Abe H, Hasegawa S, et al. Context-specific

adaptation of pursuit initiation in humans. Invest Ophthalmol Vis Sci 41, 3763–3769, 2000.
437. Takagi M, Zee DS, Tamargo RJ. Effects of lesions of the oculomotor cerebellar vermis on eye movements in primate: smooth pursuit. J Neurophysiol 83, 2047–2062, 2000.
438. Takemura A, Kawano K, Quaia C, Miles FA. Population coding in cortical area MST. Ann N Y Acad Sci 956, 284–296, 2002.
438a. Tanaka M. Involvement of the central thalamus in the control of smooth pursuit eye movements. J Neurosci 25, 5866–5876, 2005.
439. Tanaka M, Lisberger SG. Regulation of the gain of visually guided smooth-pursuit eye movements by frontal cortex. Nature 409, 191–194, 2001.
440. Tanaka M, Lisberger SG. Role of arcuate frontal cortex of monkeys in smooth pursuit eye movements. I. Basic response properties to retinal image motion and position. J Neurophysiol 87, 2684–2699, 2002.
441. Tanaka M, Lisberger SG. Role of arcuate frontal cortex of monkeys in smooth pursuit eye movements. II. Relation to vector averaging pursuit. J Neurophysiol 87, 2700–2714, 2002.
441a. Tarnutzer AA, Zee DS, Ramat S, Straumann D. Pursuit responses to target steps during ongoing tracking. Soc Neurosci Abstr 475.13, 2005.
442. Tehovnik EJ, Sommer MA, Chou IH, Slocum WM, Schiller PH. Eye fields in the frontal lobes of primates. Brain Res Brain Res Rev 32, 413–448, 2000.
443. Ter Braak JWG, Schenk VWD, Van Vliet AGM. Visual reactions in a case of long-standing cortical blindness. J Neurol Neurosurg Psychiatry 34, 140–147, 1971.
444. Thaker GK, Ross DE, Buchanan RW, Adami HM, Medoff DR. Smooth pursuit eye movements to extra-retinal motion signals: deficits in patients with schizophrenia. Psychiatry Res 88, 209–219, 1999.
445. Their P, Bachor A, Faiss J, Dichgans J, Koenig E. Selective impairment of smooth-pursuit eye movements due to an ischemic lesion of the basal pons. Ann Neurol 29, 443–448, 1991.
446. Their P, Erickson RG. Vestibular inputs to visual-tracking neurons in area MST of awake rhesus monkeys. Ann N Y Acad Sci 656, 960–963, 1992.
447. Their P, Koehler W, Buettner UW. Neuronal activity in the dorsolateral pontine nucleus of the alert monkey modulated by visual stimuli and eye movements. Exp Brain Res 70, 496–512, 1988.
448. Thurston SE, Leigh RJ, Crawford T, Thompson A, Kennard C. Two distinct deficits of visual tracking caused by unilateral lesions of cerebral cortex in humans. Ann Neurol 23, 266–273, 1988.
449. Tian J-R, Lynch JC. Slow and saccadic eye movements evoked by microstimulation in the supplementary eye field of the Cebus monkey. J Neurophysiol 74, 2204–2210, 1995.
450. Troost BT, Daroff RB, Weber RB, Dell'Osso LF. Hemispheric control of eye movements. II. Quantitative analysis of smooth pursuit in an hemispherectomy patient. Arch Neurol 27, 449–452, 1972.
451. Tusa RJ, Mustari MJ, Burrows AF, Fuchs AF. Gaze-stabilizing deficits and latent nystagmus in monkeys with brief, early-onset visual deprivation: eye movement recordings. J Neurophysiol 86, 651–661, 2001.
452. Tusa RJ, Mustari MJ, Das VE, Boothe RG. Animal models for visual deprivation-induced strabismus and nystagmus. Ann N Y Acad Sci 956, 346–360, 2002.
453. Tusa RJ, Ungerleider L. Fiber pathways of cortical areas mediating smooth pursuit eye movements in monkeys. Ann Neurol 23, 174–183, 1988.
454. Tychsen L, Lisberger SG. Maldevelopment of visual motion processing in humans who had strabismus with onset in infancy. J Neurosci 6, 2495–2508, 1986.
455. Tychsen L, Lisberger SG. Visual motion processing for the initiation of smooth-pursuit eye movements in humans. J Neurophysiol 56, 953–968, 1986.
456. Ungerleider LG, Desimone R. Cortical connections of visual area MT in the macaque. J Comp Neurol 248, 190–222, 1986.
457. Ungerleider LG, Desimone R. Projections to the superior temporal sulcus from the central and peripheral field representations of V1 and V2. J Comp Neurol 248, 147–163, 1986.
458. Vahedi K, Rivaud S, Amarenco P, Pierrot-Deseilligny C. Horizontal eye movement disorders after posterior vermis infarctions. J Neurol Neurosurg Psychiatry 58, 91–94, 1995.
459. Vaina LM, Soloviev S. First-order and second-order motion: neurological evidence for neuroanatomically distinct systems. Prog Brain Res 144, 197–212, 2004.
460. van Beers RJ, Wolpert DM, Haggard P. Sensorimotor integration compensates for visual localization errors during smooth pursuit eye movements. J Neurophysiol 85, 1914–1922, 2001.
461. van den Berg AV, Collewijn H. Human smooth pursuit: effects of stimulus extent and of spatial and temporal constraints of the pursuit trajectory. Vision Res 26, 1209–1222, 1986.
462. Van der Steen J, Tamminga EP, Collewijn H. A comparison of oculomotor pursuit of a target in circular real, beta or sigma motion. Vision Res 23, 1655–1661, 1983.
463. Van Die GC, Collewijn H. Control of human optokinetic nystagmus by the central and peripheral retina: effects of partial visual field masking, scotopic vision and central retinal scotomata. Brain Res 383, 185–194, 1986.
464. van Donkelaar P, Miall RC, Stein JF. Changes in motion perception following oculomotor smooth pursuit adaptation. Percept Psychophysiol 62, 378–385, 2000.
465. Van Essen D, Gallant JL. Neural mechanisms of form and motion processing in the primate visual system. Neuron 13, 1–10, 1994.
466. Verhagen WIM, Huygens PLM, Mulleners WM. Lack of opkinetic nystagmus and visual motion perception in acquired cortical blindness. Neuro-ophthalmology 17, 211–216, 1997.
467. Von Hofsten C, Rosander K. Development of smooth pursuit tracking in young infants. Vision Res 37, 1799–1810, 1997.
468. Waespe W, Martin P. Pursuit eye movements in a patient with a lesion involving the vestibular nuclear complex. Neuro-ophthalmology 7, 195–202, 1987.
469. Waespe W, Wichmann W. Oculomotor disturbances during visual-vestibular interaction in Wallenberg's lateral medullary syndrome. Brain 113, 821–846, 1990.

470. Walker MF, Shelhamer M, Zee DS. Eye-position dependence of torsional velocity during interaural translation, horizontal pursuit, and yaw-axis rotation in humans. Vision Res 44, 613–620, 2004.
471. Watson JD, Myers R, Frackowiak RS, et al. Area V5 of the human brain: evidence from a combined study using positron emission tomography and magnetic resonance imaging. Cereb Cortex 3, 79–94, 1993.
472. Weir CR, Knox PC. Modification of smooth pursuit initiation by a nonvisual, afferent feedback signal. Invest Ophthalmol Vis Sci 42, 2297–2302, 2001.
473. Wells SG, Barnes GR. Predictive smooth pursuit eye movements during identification of moving acuity targets. Vision Res 39, 2767–2775, 1999.
474. Westheimer G, Blair SM. Oculomotor defects in cerebellectomized monkeys. Invest Ophthalmol 12, 618–621, 1973.
475. Westheimer G, Blair SM. Functional organization of primate oculomotor system revealed by cerebellectomy. Exp Brain Res 21, 463–472, 1974.
476. White OB, Saint-Cyr JA, Tomlinson RD, Sharpe J. Ocular motor deficits in Parkinson's disease. II: control of saccadic and smooth pursuit systems. Brain 106, 571–587, 1983.
477. Winterson BJ, Steinman RM. The effect of luminance on human smooth pursuit of perifoveal and foveal targets. Vision Res 18, 1165–1172, 1978.
478. Wolpert DM, Miall RC, Kerr GK, Stein JF. Ocular limit cycles induced by delayed retinal feedback. Exp Brain Res 96, 173–180, 1993.
479. Worfolk R, Barnes GR. Interaction of active and passive slow eye movement systems. Exp Brain Res 90, 589–598, 1992.
480. Wyatt HJ, Pola J. Smooth pursuit eye movements under open-loop and closed-loop conditions. Vision Res 23, 1121–1131, 1983.
481. Wyatt HJ, Pola J. Smooth eye movements with step-ramp stimuli: the influence of attention and stimulus extent. Vision Res 27, 1565–1580, 1987.
482. Wyatt HJ, Pola J. Predictive behavior of optokinetic eye movements. Exp Brain Res 73, 615–626, 1988.
483. Wyatt HJ, Pola J, Fortune B, Posner M. Smooth pursuit eye movements with imaginary targets defined by extrafoveal cues. Vision Res 34, 803–820, 1994.
484. Yakushin SB, Gizzi M, Reisine H, et al. Functions of the nucleus of the optic tract (NOT). II. Control of ocular pursuit. Exp Brain Res 131, 433–447, 2000.
485. Yamada J, Noda H. Afferent and efferent connections of the oculomotor cerebellar vermis in the macaque monkey. J Comp Neurol 265, 224–241, 1987.
486. Yamada T, Suzuki DA, Yee RD. Smooth pursuit like eye movements evoked by microstimulation in macaque nucleus reticularis tegmenti pontis. J Neurophysiol 76, 3313–3324, 1996.
487. Yamasaki DS, Wurtz RH. Recovery of function after lesions in the superior temporal sulcus in the monkey. J Neurophysiol 66, 651–673, 1991.
488. Yan YJ, Cui DM, Lynch JC. Overlap of saccadic and pursuit eye movement systems in the brain stem reticular formation. J Neurophysiol 86, 3056–3060, 2001.
489. Yarbus AL. Eye Movements and Vision. Plenum, New York, 1967.
490. Yasui S, Young LR. Perceived visual motion as effective stimulus to pursuit eye movement system. Science 190, 906–908, 1975.
491. Yasui S, Young LR. On the predictive control of foveal eye tracking and slow phases of optokinetic and vestibular nystagmus. J Physiol (Lond) 347, 17–33, 1984.
492. Yee RD, Daniels SA, Jones OW, Baloh RW, Honrubia V. Effects of an optokinetic background on pursuit eye movements. Invest Ophthalmol Vis Sci 24, 1115–1122, 1983.
493. Yee RD, Jelks GW, Baloh RW, Honrubia V. Uniocular nystagmus in monocular visual loss. Ophthalmology 86, 511–518, 1979.
494. Zackon DH, Sharpe JA. Midbrain paresis of horizontal gaze. Ann Neurol 16, 495–504, 1984.
495. Zackon DH, Sharpe JA. Smooth pursuit in senescence. Acta Otolaryngol (Stockh) 104, 290–297, 1987.
496. Zee DS. Suppression of vestibular nystagmus. Ann Neurol 1, 207, 1977.
497. Zee DS, Friendlich AR, Robinson DA. The mechanism of downbeat nystagmus. Arch Neurol 30, 227–237, 1974.
498. Zee DS, Tusa RJ, Herdman SJ, Butler PH, Gücer G. Effects of occipital lobectomy upon eye movements in primate. J Neurophysiol 58, 883–907, 1987.
499. Zee DS, Yamazaki A, Butler PH, Gücer G. Effects of ablation of flocculus and paraflocculus on eye movements in primate. J Neurophysiol 46, 878–899, 1981.
500. Zee DS, Yee RD, Cogan DG, Robinson DA, Engel WK. Ocular motor abnormalities in hereditary cerebellar ataxia. Brain 99, 207–234, 1976.
501. Zeki S. A Vision of the Brain. Blackwell Scientific, London, 1993.
502. Zeki S, Watson JD, Lueck CJ, et al. A direct demonstration of functional specialization in human visual cortex. J Neurosci 11, 641–649, 1997.
503. Zhao DL, Lasker AG, Robinson DA. In Fuchs AF, Brandt T, Büttner U, Zee DS (eds). Contemporary Ocular Motor and Vestibular Research: A Tribute to David A. Robinson. Thieme Medical, Stuttgart, 1994, pp 171–180.
503a. Zivotofsky AZ. A dissociation between perception and action in open-loop smooth-pursuit ocular tracking of the Duncker Illusion. Neurosci Lett 376, 81–86, 2005.
503b. Zivotofsky AZ, Goldberg ME, Powell KD. Rhesus monkeys behave as if they perceive the Duncker Illusion. J Cogn Neurosci 17, 1011–1017, 2005.
504. Zivotofsky AZ, Rottach KG, Averbach-Huller L, et al. Saccades to remembered targets: the effects of smooth pursuit and illusory stimulus-motion. J Neurophysiol 76, 3617–3632, 1996.
505. Zuber BL, Stark L. Microsaccades and the velocity-amplitude relationship for saccadic eye movements. Science 150, 1459–1460, 1965.

Chapter 5

Gaze Holding and the Neural Integrator

This chapter deals with the neural mechanism that holds gaze steady when the eyes are turned away from the central position. This function depends on the ability of networks of neurons to integrate velocity signals into position commands (mathematical integration in the Newtonian sense). This remarkable ability of the central nervous system is not just a matter of local interest to ocular motor scientists. Indeed, it has attracted the attention of the neuroscience community because it provides an accessible system to investigate the way that the brain stores a form of memory.[7] Testing the ability to hold the eye steadily at an eccentric position is also a routine component of the neurological examination.

The ability to holding the eyes steady in lateral gaze depends on more than visual fixation (discussed in Chapter 4), since eccentric gaze remains relatively steady in darkness.[13,108] In Chapter 1, we pointed out that the orbital contents impose elastic restoring forces that tend to pull the eyes back to central position. To counteract these forces, and hold the eyes steady in an eccentric position in the orbit, the extraocular muscles must contract tonically. Such a tonic contraction is achieved by a sustained rate of discharge of the ocular motoneurons.

The mechanical forces that act on the eye are illustrated in the experiment shown in Figure 5–1.[110] The subject viewed a stationary visual target with one eye while vision from the other eye was occluded with a sheet of opaque paper at a distance of about 5 cm. After applying topical anesthetic to the non-fixating eye, it was mechanically displaced, using ophthalmic forceps, into eccentric positions of (A) intorsion, (B) extorsion, or (C) horizontal abduction. After the eye was suddenly released from each of these eccentric positions, it sprang back to a "central" position of rest (see Video

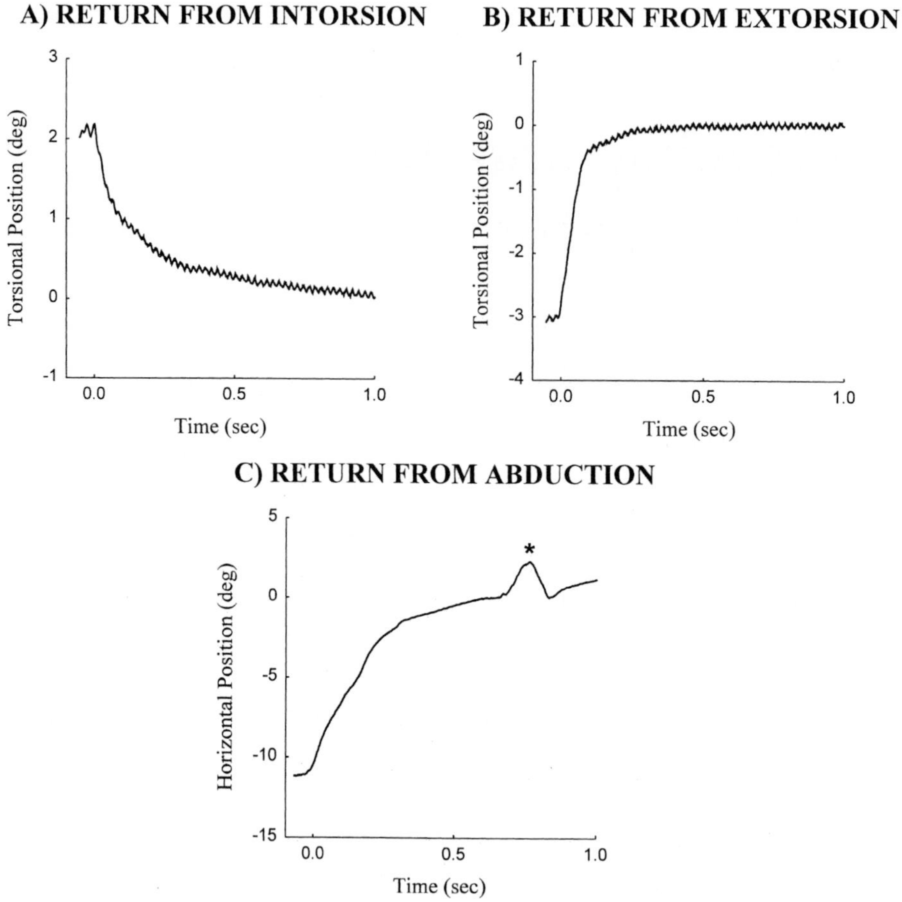

Figure 5–1. Experimental data from a normal human subject to show the time course of the return to resting position after the eye was mechanically displaced into an eccentric position in the orbit and then suddenly released. The time course of return was fit by a single exponential function, and the time constants were: (A) 323 ms after release from intorsion; (B) 58 ms after release from extorsion; and (C) 183 ms after release from abduction. The asterisk in (C) indicates a blink. (Reprinted from Seidman SH, Leigh RJ, Tomsak RL, Grant MP, Dell'Osso LF. Dynamic properties of the human vestibulo-ocular reflex during head rotations in roll. Vision Res 35, 679–689, 1995, with permission from Elsevier.)

Display: Disorders of Gaze Holding). The time course of this return reflected the mechanical forces acting on the eye, which depend on the direction of eye displacement. The brain must take into account these mechanical forces in programming all types of eye movements.

Our approach in this chapter will be, first, to explore what neural signals the ocular motoneurons must generate to hold the eye in an eccentric position; second, to outline quantitative aspects of this gaze-holding function; third, to identify the neurobiological substrate for normal gaze holding; fourth, to apply these principles to the clinical examination; and finally, to review clinical disorders that impair the ability to hold steady, eccentric gaze.

NEURAL CODING OF THE OCULAR MOTOR SIGNAL

The Need for a Neural Integrator of Ocular Motor Signals

To understand the neural basis for the gaze-holding mechanism, it is helpful to consider the way that brainstem neurons encode eye movement signals. The activity of any single neuron is represented by its frequency of spike discharges. Although differences exist between the physiological properties of each member of the pool of ocular motoneurons (including the way that individual units encode the move-

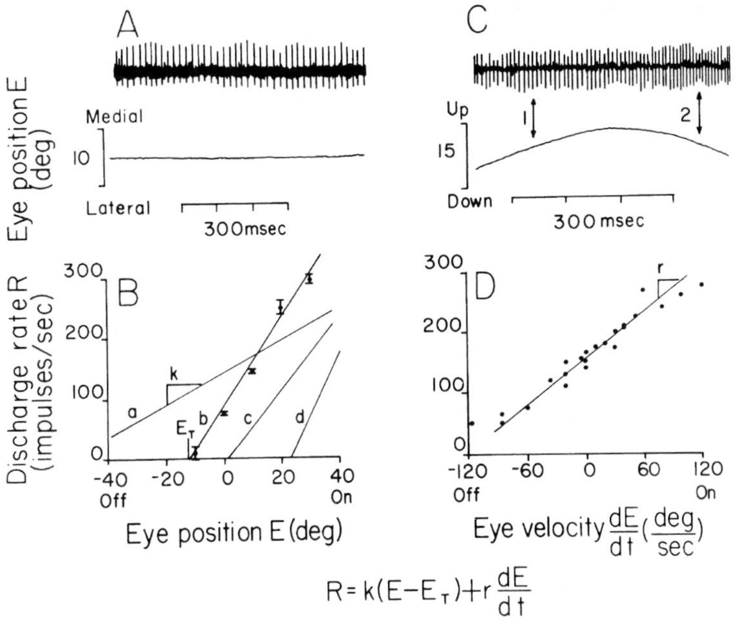

Figure 5–2. Discharge properties of ocular motor neurons during fixation and smooth pursuit. (A) The neuron discharges at a steady rate during fixation. (B) The discharge rate (R) of four ocular motor neurons is compared with eye position (E) during fixation. For each neuron, this relationship is approximately linear, although the slope (k) varies from unit to unit, as does the threshold (given by the intercept E_T). Typical means and standard deviations (bars) of R are shown for cell b. (C) During smooth pursuit, the eye passes through the same position at times 1 and 2, but the discharge rate of the neuron is different because the velocity of the eye is different at the two times. (D) The relationship between eye velocity (dE/dt) and neuron discharge rate is shown. Its slope is r. These relationships are expressed by the equation at the bottom, which describes how ocular motor neurons discharge according to both eye position and velocity. (From Robinson DA. The functional behavior of the peripheral oculomotor apparatus: a review. In Kommerell G (ed). Disorders of Ocular Motility. Neurophysiology and Clinical Aspects. JF Bergman, Munich, 1978, pp 46, with permission.)

ment of one or both eyes),[18,30,34,43,47,117,120] it is possible to make some general statements. The discharge frequency of neurons within the ocular motor nuclei varies linearly with eye position during fixation (Fig. 5–2A and 2B).[55] In addition, during conjugate movements, these ocular motoneurons modulate their discharge in proportion to eye velocity (Fig. 5–2C and 2D). This combination of velocity and position information is necessary to compensate for the restrictions imposed upon eye movements and fixation by the mechanical properties of the orbital contents. The viscous drag of the orbital contents slows down eye movements; the elastic restoring forces tend to pull the eye back towards its central position in the orbit. Thus, a combined velocity-position signal on the ocular motoneurons takes care of the forces applied on the eyeball by its suspensory tissues. The next question is: How do velocity and position signals arrive on the ocular motoneurons? To preview our discussion, this depends on the ability of neurons to integrate (in the mathematical sense) velocity signals into position signals.

Consider the neural signal required to program a saccade (Fig. 5–3A). A pulse of innervation, generated by burst neurons (B), projects to ocular motoneurons (OM). The pulse is a velocity command that causes a phasic contraction of the extraocular muscles, which overcomes the viscous drag of the orbit and rotates the eye rapidly through angle E to its destination. This same pulse signal is sent to cells within the neural integrator (NI), which generate a step of innervation. The step is a position command that causes a tonic contraction of the extraocular muscles, which resists the elastic restoring forces of the orbit and holds the eye steady at its new eccentric position. Hence, ocular motoneurons carry information about both eye position and velocity—a combined pulse and step. Although we have presented a simplified scheme for saccades as our example, ocular motoneurons encode velocity and position commands for all types of eye movements.

An important fact is that while ocular motoneurons encode combined velocity-position commands, the raw sensory or premotor inputs, from which the final ocular motor command is assembled, primarily encode velocity signals. For example, vestibular afferents[41] and secondary vestibular neurons[127] carry information on head velocity. Saccadic burst cells discharge at rates that reflect saccadic eye velocity.[125] For the pursuit system, cells within cortical visual areas,[74] brainstem nuclei,[95] and cerebellum,[45,89] all encode combinations of retinal error velocity and eye velocity signals. Moreover, during combined movements of the head and eyes, it is gaze velocity (i.e., eye velocity in space) that is encoded, for example, by Purkinje cells of the cerebellum.[89] Yet, because of the forces imposed on the eyeball by its supporting tissues (Fig. 5–1), a position signal clearly is required in order to hold the eye away from center position. Therefore, a *mathematical integration* is necessary to convert velocity-coded information to position-coded signals. Theoretical and experimental evidence suggest a common neural network that integrates all conjugate eye movement commands;[10,51,107] this is referred to as the *neural integrator*. Such a concept also provides

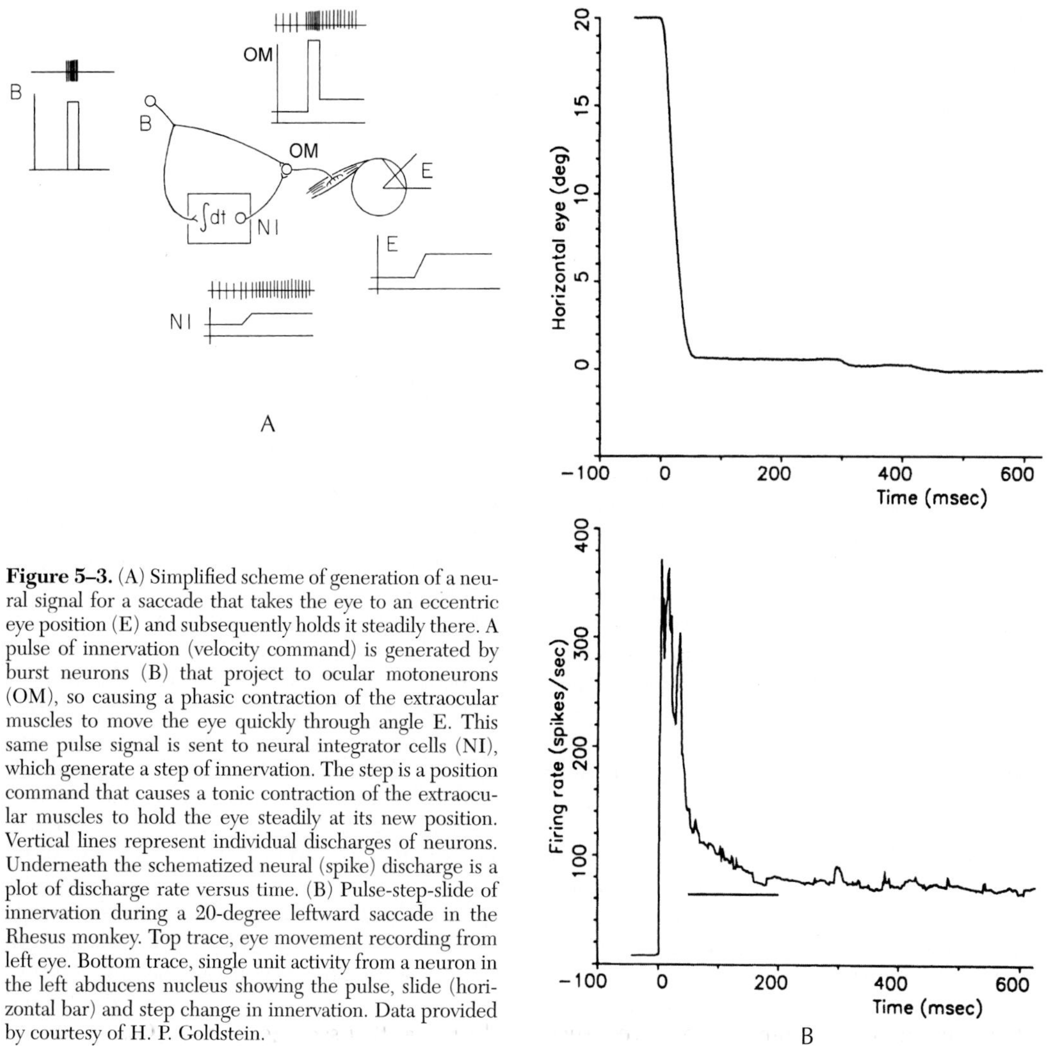

Figure 5–3. (A) Simplified scheme of generation of a neural signal for a saccade that takes the eye to an eccentric eye position (E) and subsequently holds it steadily there. A pulse of innervation (velocity command) is generated by burst neurons (B) that project to ocular motoneurons (OM), so causing a phasic contraction of the extraocular muscles to move the eye quickly through angle E. This same pulse signal is sent to neural integrator cells (NI), which generate a step of innervation. The step is a position command that causes a tonic contraction of the extraocular muscles to hold the eye steadily at its new position. Vertical lines represent individual discharges of neurons. Underneath the schematized neural (spike) discharge is a plot of discharge rate versus time. (B) Pulse-step-slide of innervation during a 20-degree leftward saccade in the Rhesus monkey. Top trace, eye movement recording from left eye. Bottom trace, single unit activity from a neuron in the left abducens nucleus showing the pulse, slide (horizontal bar) and step change in innervation. Data provided by courtesy of H. P. Goldstein.

an explanation for how one type of eye movement (such as a saccade or smooth pursuit) may influence another type of movement (such as the vestibulo-ocular reflex), since their signals are fed to a common neural network.[32] Integration of vergence signals also occurs, and is discussed in Chapter 8.

Special Demands on the Neural Integrator

The concept of a velocity-position neural signal (such as the saccadic pulse-step shown in Fig. 5–3) that moves the eye against the viscous and elastic forces of the orbit helps in interpreting gaze-holding abnormalities at the bedside. However, the orbital mechanics are more complicated than this description. This is evident, for example, in the different centripetal drifts that occur after the eye is pulled to different eccentric positions and suddenly released (compare the curves in Fig. 5–1). The mechanical properties of the orbit are nonlinear, especially as the eye moves out toward the extremes of gaze. Furthermore, the brain must actually program a *pulse-slide-step* in order to avoid drift at the end of the saccade (Fig. 5–3B).[98,119] For gaze to be held steady and vision to remain clear, the neural integrator must take these factors into account.

Certain neural signals need more integration than others. For example, more than one integration occurs between vestibular afferents and the ocular motoneurons that generate the horizontal angular vestibulo-ocular reflex.[115] The further integration of the vestibular signal is called the *velocity-storage mechanism*,[105] and represents a perseveration or prolongation of the signal from the semicircular canals, which is important during sustained rotations of the head and body. Most evidence suggests that the neural integrator and the velocity-storage mechanism depend upon separate anatomical connections; the neural substrate for velocity storage is reviewed in Chapter 2.

When we view and follow the movements of a near target, it becomes necessary to move the eyes by different amounts. Theoretical considerations[35] and electrophysiological studies suggest that some neurons contributing to the neural integrator network may encode the position of a single eye.[82,119,138] This aspect of interaction between conjugate and vergence eye movements is discussed under Saccade-Vergence Interactions, in Chapter 8.

QUANTITATIVE ASPECTS OF NEURAL INTEGRATION

Consider, once more, the neural command for a saccade (Fig. 5–3). The step of innervation is essential to hold the eye steady at the end of the movement. The step is generated by the neural integrator from a pulse of innervation (Fig. 5–4A). The step holds the eye steady in its new, eccentric position in the orbit, opposing the elastic forces that would rotate the eye back to center position. If the performance of the neural integrator is perfect, then the saccadic pulse (an eye velocity command) is converted into a step (a position command; Fig. 5–4A). If the integrator does not function perfectly (Fig. 5–4B), the eye position signal decays with time and the integrator is said to be "leaky" (just as water might leak from a hole at the bottom of a bucket). The elastic restoring forces of the orbit rotate the eye back toward the central position with a time course that approximates a negative (decaying) exponential (Fig. 5–4C). The rate of this centripetal drift of the eyes indicates the time constant of the neural integrator. Specifically, 63% of the drift back to the midline occurs during an interval equal to one time constant; so, for example, if it takes 2 seconds to drift back 63%, the time constant would be 2 seconds. The time constant, therefore, is a quantitative measure of the fidelity of integration: the longer the time constant, the better the integration. Another useful approach is to plot eye velocity versus eye position.[92] Nystagmus slow phases that have a negative exponential waveform appear as a linear slope, the gradient of which provides a measure of the time constant. Nystagmus with linear (constant-velocity) slow phases produces a horizontal line on such velocity-position plots.

When a leaky integrator causes centripetal drift of the eye, corrective saccades are required to carry the eye back to the desired eccentric position in the orbit. A convenient, approximate method to measure the time constant of the neural integrator is to measure the ratio of eye displacement from the midline immediately after an eccentrically directed saccade to the initial velocity of the centripetal drift after that saccade (Fig. 5–3C).

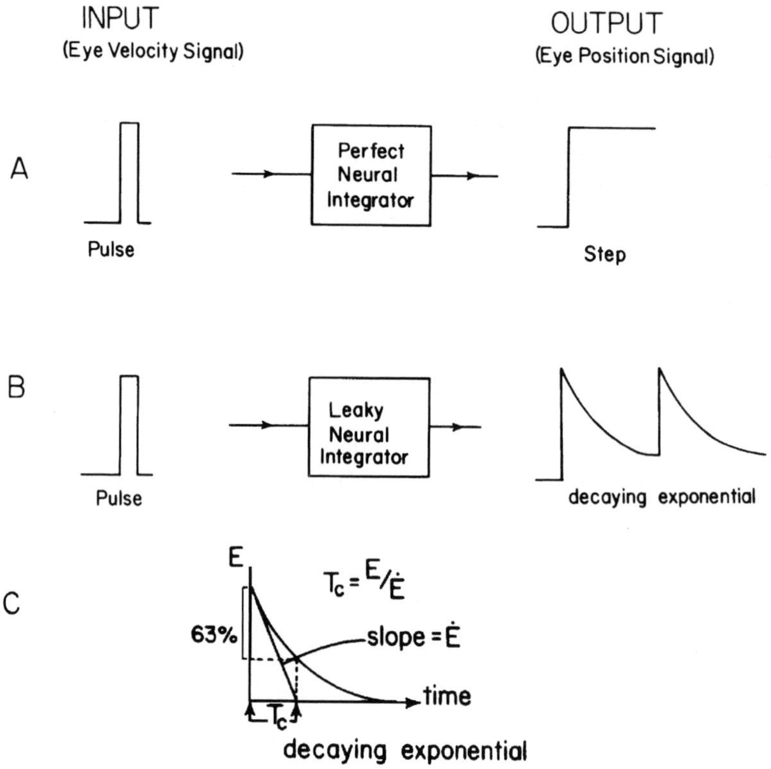

Figure 5–4. Quantitative aspects of the neural integrator. (A) For saccades, the input to the neural integrator is a pulse, which may be thought of as an eye velocity signal. If neural integration is perfect, then the output will be a step, which may be thought of as an eye position signal. (B) If the integration of eye velocity signals is imperfect (i.e., if the neural integrator is "leaky"), then the eye position signal will be a decaying exponential. Thus, the eye will drift back toward the midline until a corrective quick-phase puts the eye back on target. This causes gaze-evoked nystagmus. (C) The centripetal drift of the eyes that occurs with a leaky integrator can be described by its time constant (T_c), given by the time at which the eye has drifted 63% of the way back to the midline. Thus, the "leakier" the integrator, the shorter the time constant. A convenient way of calculating the time constant is from the ratio of the initial displacement of the eye from midline (E) to the initial velocity of eye drift (Ė).

Normal subjects do not have "perfect" neural integrators. Thus, in darkness, when vision cannot be used for ocular stabilization, healthy individuals show a drift of the eyes back from eccentric gaze to central position with a time constant of between 20 and 70 seconds; [13] the rate of this drift is influenced by the mental percept of the subject and sensory context.[26,108] If disease or drugs impair the process of neural integration, the time constant may become much smaller. In darkness, centripetal drifts due to deficient integration are corrected by quick phases of nystagmus;[63] in the light, visual fixation can also help to suppress any spontaneous drift (see Chapter 4).

The way in which the brain is able to hold the eyes still—the neural integrator function—has been conceptualized in many ways.[2,68,107,112,113,123,133] Recent attempts to model the neural integrator have simulated the behavior of networks of neurons.[10,54] We will review these studies after discussing the anatomical pathways involved in gaze holding.

NEURAL SUBSTRATE FOR GAZE HOLDING

The neural integrator depends upon a distributed network of neurons lying in the brainstem and cerebellum. Collectively, these circuits perform mathematical integration of vestibular, optokinetic, saccadic, and pursuit eye velocity commands. For horizontal, conjugate eye movements, the nucleus prepositus hypoglossi and the adjacent medial vestibular nucleus are most important. For vertical and torsional conjugate movements, the interstitial nucleus of

Cajal plays an important role. The cerebellum also contributes to normal gaze holding, and for this purpose, it may receive important inputs from the cell groups of the paramedian tracts (PMT) (see Box 6–4, Chapter 6). Inactivation of components of the PMT cell groups impairs the activity of the neural integrator.[96] The paramedian pontine reticular formation (PPRF) is no longer thought to contribute to neural integration because lesions there spare the ability to hold eccentric gaze.[61]

The Contribution of the Nucleus Prepositus Hypoglossi and Medial Vestibular Nucleus to Gaze Holding

ANATOMY, PHYSIOLOGY, AND PHARMACOLOGY

The nucleus prepositus hypoglossi (NPH) is one member of the *perihypoglossal complex of nuclei* and lies just medial to the vestibular nuclei and caudal to the abducens nucleus (see Fig. 6–1). Other perihypoglossal nuclei are the nucleus intercalatus and the nucleus of Roller, which may also contribute to the control of eye movements. The main afferent and efferent connections of the NPH are summarized in Table 5–1.[77,83] The NPH receives projections from every structure that projects to the abducens nucleus.[14] Both the NPH and the parvocellular portion of the adjacent medial vestibular nucleus (MVN) contain neurons that encode the position of each eye as well as eye velocity signals.[82,85,119] These regions project mainly to motoneurons supplying the non-twitch extraocular muscle fibers,[129] a finding that is discussed further in Chapter 9.

Acetylcholine is a neurotransmitter in NPH,[97] including the projections of NPH to the abducens nucleus.[84] Vestibular inputs to NPH may utilize nitric oxide and gaba-aminobutyric

Table 5–1. **Principal Connections of the Nucleus Prepositus Hypoglossi (NPH)[14,59,83]**

Structure	Characteristics
	INPUTS
Vestibular nuclei	Bilateral projections, especially from the medial and ventral lateral nuclei
Contralateral NPH	
Brain stem reticular formation	
Medullary reticular formation	Mainly contralateral
PPRF	Mainly ipsilateral
RiMLF	Mainly ipsilateral
Interstitial nucleus of Cajal	Bilateral
Mesencephalic reticular formation	Bilateral
Ocular motor nuclei	Bilateral, including oculomotor internuclear neurons
Cerebellar fastigial nuclei	Bilateral
Others	Raphe nuclei, nucleus of the optic tract
	OUTPUTS
Ocular motor nuclei	Abducens and trochlear nuclei, bilaterally; oculomotor nucleus, mainly ipsilaterally
Vestibular nuclei	Bilaterally, heavy to medial nucleus, but also to other nuclei, including y-group
Cerebellum	Bilateral, to cortex of vestibulocerebellum and posterior vermis
Interstitial nucleus of Cajal	Bilateral
Brainstem reticular formation	Medullary and pontine reticular formation
Superior colliculus	Contralateral
Others	Dorsal cap of inferior olive; raphe nuclei

NPH, nucleus prepositus hypoglossi; PPRF, paramedian pontine reticular formation; riMLF, rostral interstitial nucleus of the medial longitudinal fasciculus.

acid (GABA).[91] N-methyl-D-aspartate (NMDA) and AMPA-kainate glutamate receptors are both present in NPH.[11,97,102] The NPH sends a strong projection to the abducens nucleus via its rostro-lateral "marginal" zone,[77] where it abuts the medial vestibular nucleus.[47]

EFFECTS OF CHEMICAL AND PHARMACOLOGICAL INACTIVATION OF NUCLEUS PREPOSITUS HYPOGLOSSI-MEDIAL VESTIBULAR NUCLEUS

Studies in monkeys and cat of the effects of chemical lesions or pharmacological inactivation have defined the crucial role of the NPH-MVN region in neural integration of ocular motor signals.[23,27,52,69,70,88] Figure 5–5 summarizes effects of injecting the excitotoxin ibotenate into the NPH-MVN region in a monkey.[23] At the beginning of the experimental session (Fig. 5–5A) the monkey held steady horizontal gaze between saccades in the light or in darkness. Unilateral injection of an excitotoxin produced an acute, partial failure of both ipsilateral and contralateral gaze holding (Figs. 5–5B and 5C), and a shift of the null or neutral point (the eye position where eye velocity is zero) towards the side of the lesion. Bilateral excitotoxin lesions of NPH and MVN abolished neural integration for all horizontal, conjugate eye movements. Horizontal saccades were still possible, and were of normal velocity, but the eye could not be held at its new position, and drifted rapidly back to central position with a time constant of about 200 ms, a value close to that determined by the mechanical properties of the orbital tissues (Fig. 5–5D). Saccades did not over shoot the target, however, implying that their local feedback mechanism, which requires a special resettable integrator, was spared. This aspect of the feedback control of saccades is discussed further in Chapter 3. Besides saccades, the other conjugate horizontal eye movement systems—vestibular, optokinetic, and smooth-pursuit—were also

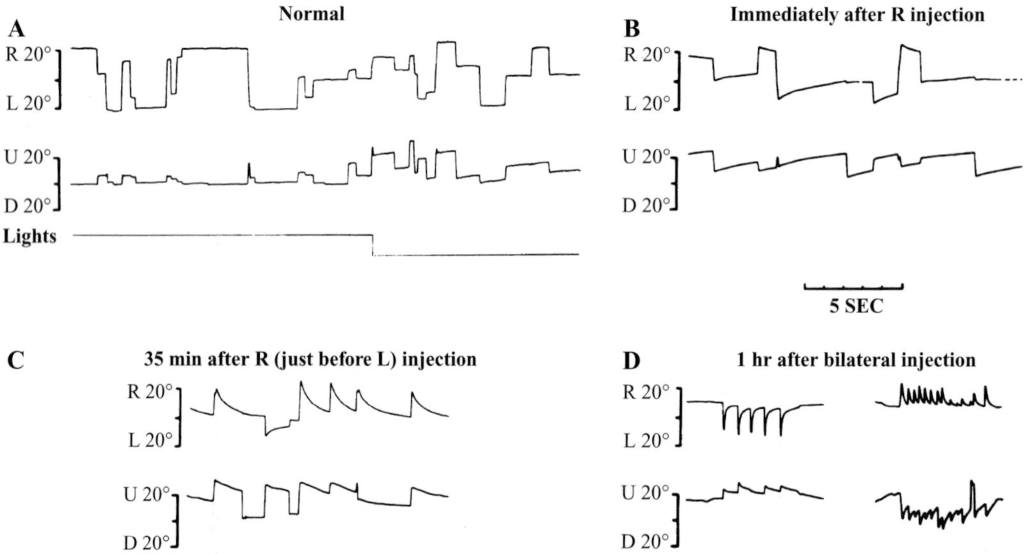

Figure 5–5. Saccadic eye movements before and after injection of an excitotoxin (ibotenate) into the medial vestibular nucleus and adjacent nucleus prepositus hypoglossi, first on the right and then the left side. (A) Target-directed and spontaneous saccades recorded from a normal monkey. In the first half of the record, the fixation light was alternated between right and left 20 degrees. For the second half, spontaneous eye movements were recorded in total darkness. Notice that even in total darkness, horizontal gaze holding is steady. The upward drift in darkness is a form of downbeat nystagmus found in many normal rhesus monkeys. (B–D) Each panel shows spontaneous saccades recorded in total darkness from the same monkey as in (A), at various times after the injection of 30 μg of ibotenate, as indicated. The records in (D) (following bilateral lesions) are two excerpts from a continuous record to demonstrate that eye position drifts centripetally after both leftward and rightward saccades. The time constant of the horizontal drift decreases progressively from 2 to 0.6 to 0.2 in (B–D). (A–D) were recorded at the same time scale as indicated. R: right; L: left; U: up; D: down. (Reproduced from Cannon SC, Robinson DA. Loss of the neural integrator of the oculomotor system from brain stem lesions in monkey. Neurophysiol 57, 1383–1409, 1987, used with permission of the American Physiological Society.)

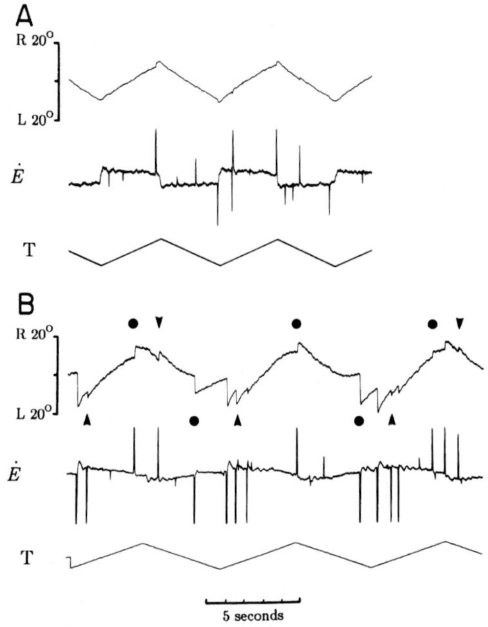

Figure 5–6. Pursuit eye movements before and after bilateral injection of excitotoxin (kainic acid) into MVN/NPH. (A) Eye position (E), eye velocity (Edot), and target position (T) recorded in a normal monkey during smooth pursuit of a small target moving in a triangular waveform. (B) Eye movements recorded during smooth pursuit in the same task 22 hours after injection of kainic acid. Null point is close to zero. When the eyes move centrifugally, catch-up saccades are needed (filled circles); when centripetal, back-up saccades occur (arrows). (Reproduced from Cannon SC, Robinson DA. Loss of the neural integrator of the oculomotor system from brain stem lesions in monkey. Neurophysiol 57, 1383–1409, 1987, used with permission of the American Physiological Society.)

affected (Fig. 5–6). Neurotoxic lesions confined to NPH and sparing MVN cause milder defects of neural integration.[69,70]

Electrolytic lesions in the midline of the pons, just caudal to the abducens nuclei, disable the horizontal neural integrator;[9] this effect may be due to interruption of commissural connections between the right and left NPH-MVN regions.[8,10]

Pharmacological inactivation has confirmed the important role for NPH-MVN and has also provided information of the neurotransmitters that contribute to neural integration of horizontal ocular motor signals. Thus, microinjection of the GABA-A agonist muscimol or the non-specific GABA antagonist bicuculline inactivate the neural integrator, causing it to become leaky (Fig. 5–7, K too small).[11,88,118] Paradoxically, injections of either bicuculline,[118] or muscimol,[11] into the more lateral parts of the medial vestibular nucleus sometimes cause instability of gaze holding, in which the eye drifts away from the central position with increasing velocity. The latter finding implies that the neural integrator has become unstable (Fig. 5–7, K too large).

Injection of NMDA agonists and antagonists into NPH-MVN also cause partial integrator

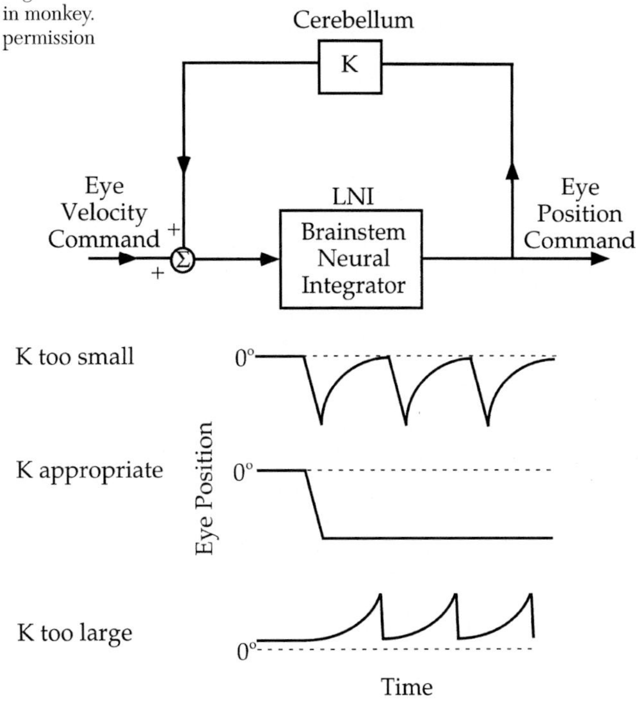

Figure 5–7. An hypothesis of the cerebellar influence on the brain stem neural integrator. A positive feedback loop with a gain of K improves the time constant of an inherently leaky brain stem neural integrator (NI). The effects of varying the value of K are shown on the right. If K is appropriate, neural integration would be perfect and the eyes would be held steady in their new position in the orbit after an eye movement. If K is too small, the integration becomes imperfect (leaky) and the eyes drift back, with a negative exponential time course, toward the central position; gaze-evoked nystagmus results. If K is too large, the neural integrator becomes unstable and the eyes drift away from the central position with a positive exponential time course (increasing velocity) also causing nystagmus.[133]

failure.[11,28,87] Evidence from brain-slice preparations indicates that glutamatergic projections from the paramedian pontine reticular formation (PPRF) to NPH act on AMPA-kainate receptors.[97] Cholinergic antagonists also impair gaze holding.[97] Glycine and strychnine apparently have no role in NPH-MVN.[11]

Vertical gaze holding is also impaired following bilateral NPH-MVN lesions; following vertical saccades, centripetal drift has a time constant of about 2.5 seconds.[23] This result implies that other structures and pathways are important for vertical gaze holding, such as the interstitial nucleus of Cajal. Clinical lesion involving the nucleus intercalatus and the nucleus of Roller have been reported to cause upbeat nystagmus, suggesting that either of these structures may relay vertical eye position signals to the cerebellum.[64,67,71,92,101]

The Interstitial Nucleus of Cajal and Vertical Gaze Holding

ANATOMY AND PHYSIOLOGY

The anatomical connections of the interstitial nucleus of Cajal (INC) are summarized in Figure 6–5 and Box 6–6. The INC receives vertical and torsional saccadic inputs from the rostral interstitial nucleus of the medial longitudinal fasciculus (riMLF) and vestibular inputs via the medial longitudinal fasciculus (MLF) and other ascending pathways. It contains neurons that encode burst-tonic (velocity-position) signals.[30,44,46,47] Projections of the INC to ocular motoneurons may be exclusively via the posterior commissure.[73]

EFFECTS OF PHARMACOLOGICAL INACTIVATION

Pharmacological inactivation of the INC with muscimol causes deficits of gaze-holding deficit for torsional and vertical eye positions (neural integrator failure), with time constants of about 350 ms.[60] This integrator failure is most evident after saccades that take the eye to a tertiary eye position (combined horizontal and vertical displacement from primary position).[30]. With unilateral lesions, a vestibular imbalance is also present, manifest as spontaneous torsional nystagmus (fast phases towards the side of the lesion) with a vertical component; additionally, there is a shift of Listing's plane to the contralesional side.[60] Experimental inactivation or lesions of the *posterior commissure*, which contains INC projections, also disables the vertical neural integrator.[99]

Although the INC appears to play a crucial role for holding vertical and torsional gaze steady after saccades, the *torsional vestibular responses* appear to show different properties. For example, when normal subjects rotate their head in roll to a new position, the eyes counterroll, but then drift back towards a new torsional position with a time constant of 2 to 3 seconds.[110] At the end of the drift, the new torsional position (static counterroll) compensates for only about 10% of the head roll that induced it. Some studies have questioned whether or how the otolithic signals need integration.[94] Experimental inactivation of INC has produced conflicting results. On the one hand it has been reported to have no effect on static eye position after counterrolling.[60] On the other hand, 3-D measurement of the shift of the end-position suggests that there may be some integration of otolithic signals.[31,49] Another view is that otolithic signals undergo two integrations,[58] an issue dealt with in Chapter 2. Thus, the contribution of INC to the torsional vestibular movements is less clear than for saccades, when it plays an important role in sustaining torsional eye position at the end of the movement, in accordance with Listing's law. [30]

The Contribution of the Cerebellum to Gaze Holding

Lesions of the cerebellum,[25,53,106,130] especially the flocculus and paraflocculus,[121,126,136] make the neural integrator deficient. The centripetal drift following a saccade to an eccentric horizontal position typically has a time constant of 1.5 seconds. It has been suggested that a function of the cerebellum is to improve the performance of an inherently leaky neural integrator in the brain stem.[68,106,133] Thus, NPH projects both eye velocity and eye positions to the flocculus.[40] One way in which the cerebellum could perform this function is shown in Figure 5–7. Although hypothetical, this scheme may help clinicians interpret nystagmus with velocity-increasing or velocity-decreasing slow-phase waveforms. The effects of the cerebellum on neural integration are represented, in this scheme, by a gain, K, in a positive feedback loop between the cerebellum and brain stem. Anatomical evidence for such a pathway exists; the NPH-MVN region has reciprocal connections with the vestibulocerebellum, and the flocculus receives inputs from the cell groups of the paramedian tracts (PMT),[20,21] which relay ocular motor signals from a variety of brain stem structures (see Fig. 6–3 and Box 6–4 of Chapter 6). Such a feedback loop implies that neurons excite themselves and so perseverate their own activity—an action that is, in effect, integration. Genetic disorders of the P/Q calcium channels, which are abundant in cerebellum, are associated with reduced time constants of gaze holding in affected mice, thus providing an animal model to study the contributions of the cerebellum to the neural integrator.[116]

Experimental inactivation of constituents of the PMT cell groups causes neural integration to become deficient.[96] If the value of K is appropriate, integration is nearly perfect. If the value of K falls, the integrator becomes leaky, with exponentially decaying drifts of the eyes back to the neutral position. This is the waveform of gaze-evoked nystagmus. If K rises above the appropriate value, then the integrator becomes unstable, with exponentially increasing velocity drifts of the eyes away from the midline. This last waveform has been reported in patients with downbeating nystagmus (see Video Display: Disorders of Gaze Holding),[133] upbeating nystagmus (see Fig. 10–3, Chapter 10), and in monkeys with floccular lesions.[136] A further possibility is that the integrator could become unstable and then oscillate; this has been postulated as a mechanism to account for acquired pendular nystagmus, and this is considered further under Abnormalities of the Neural Integrator.

The time constant of the neural integrator has been shown to be under adaptive control, and can even be made to have a time constant of integration that is different for saccades and vestibular eye movements.[76,122] The cerebellar flocculus appear to play a key role in this adaptation.[16] Thus, patients with cerebellar disease are often unable to use visual information to correct abnormalities of the neural integrator and consequently have persistent gaze-evoked nystagmus.

How a Network of Neurons Could Function as the Neural Integrator

The simple scheme shown in Figure 5–7 does not account for some of the actual properties of the gaze-holding network.[10,22,24] For example, relatively small changes in the feedback loop gain, K, would cause the network to become leaky or unstable, but in reality, the gaze-holding network is quite stable. A second factor is that neurons that carry an eye-velocity signal to the neural integrator have a background discharge rate; it is modulation about this background discharge that encodes eye velocity. The properties of gaze holding indicate that although the modulated signal is integrated, the background activity is not. Third, cells in the NPH-MVN region encode not just eye position but also, to varying extents, eye velocity, which the scheme in Figure 5–7 would not predict. Fourth, the integrator must be relatively robust to the effects of lesions; some integration must still be possible after loss of a proportion of its constituent neurons.[23] Fifth, the properties of the neural integrator can be changed, such as during adaptation to novel visual-vestibular demands.[52,75] A neural network approach has been able to address some of these problems and also to represent the anatomical way that the neural integrator is anatomically distributed (Fig. 5–8).

A network of neurons, in which cells excite themselves through connections with other cells, can sustain its activity after initial stimulation without further input. This integrating network is conceptually similar to Lorente de Nó's *system of reverberating collaterals*.[81] In practice, if each neuron inhibits its neighbors and is, in turn, inhibited by them, the overall effect is a positive feedback loop.[22,24] Such a model, unlike the model shown in Figure 5–7, integrates velocity-modulated signals, but not the background activity.[24] Because the inhibition is distributed over many cells and synapses, the network is robust to the effect of lesions and also accounts for some of the subtle differences in waveforms of gaze-evoked nystagmus in patients with various neurologic diseases. For example, an initial rapid centripetal drift (smaller time constant) followed by a slower drift (larger time constant),[2,24] might be explained by the tendency of neural

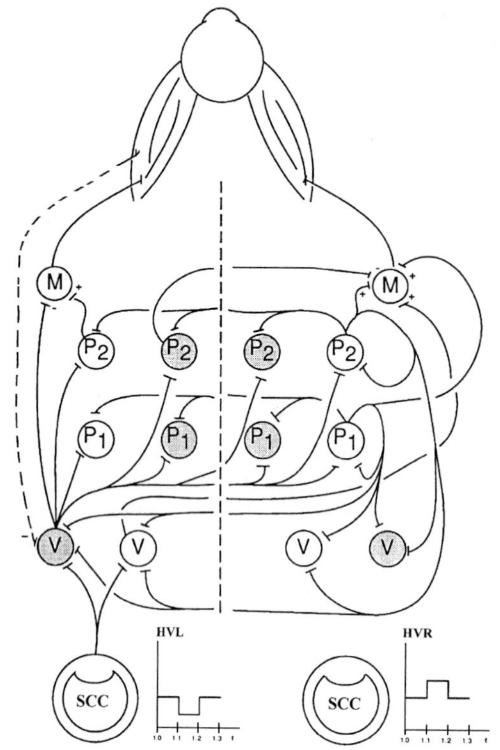

Figure 5–8. Neural network model of the ocular motor integrator, redrawn from Arnold and Robinson.[10] Light units are excitatory, dark units are inhibitory. Afferents from each semicircular canal (SCC) project to both excitatory and inhibitory vestibular (V) units. Each V unit projects to every unit of the nucleus prepositus hypoglossi (P1 and P2 units), and to the contralateral motoneuron (M) unit if it is excitatory and the ipsilateral M unit if it is inhibitory. Each P unit projects to every P unit of the same type (P1 or P2) but not to P units of the other type, as well as to all V units and to the ipsilateral M unit if it is excitatory and the contralateral M unit if it is inhibitory. The output of the M units goes through a first-order lag with a 200-ms time constant (not shown) that represents the transfer function of the eye and its muscles. The pathway conveying proprioceptive feedback of eye position from the extraocular muscles to all V units is indicated by the broken line at left. Note that not all connections are shown. The insets at bottom show head velocity input signals from the left (HV_L) and right (HV_R) semicircular canals, reflecting a rapid head rotation to the right.

networks to form "clusters" of neurons with strong connection; similar properties have been observed electrophysiologically in NPH neurons.[38] It has proved possible to "train" a network of neurons to simulate normal gaze-holding behavior using a Hebbian learning rule, in which correlated activity between pre- and post-synaptic neurons strengthens the synapse between them, whereas uncorrelated activity weakens the synapse.[10] When such a network has been trained, each unit carries a weighted combination of eye position and velocity. The trained network is capable of simulating adaptation to new visual-vestibular demands. Furthermore, if the model is arranged into left and right sides, the synaptic development that occurs during training leads to the formation of an inhibitory commissure. "Lesioning" this commissure in the model disables the neural integrator in much the same way that a midline lesion in the pons, just caudal to the abducens nucleus, does.[9,10]

Thus, the neural network shown in Figure 5–8 can be applied to understand better *clinical disorders of gaze holding*. For example, if the network became unstable, it could account for nystagmus with increasing velocity waveforms.[12,133] Furthermore, if the neural integrator network were governed by a feedback control, such as the PMT cell groups that project to the cerebellum, then it would have the potential to oscillate. One prediction of this hypothesis is that saccades would influence such oscillations. This is because saccadic pulses transiently silence the neural network and would therefore be expected to "reset" the oscillations, causing a phase shift between oscillations just before and just after the rapid eye movement. This theoretical prediction was tested experimentally in patients with acquired pendular nystagmus due to multiple sclerosis, and it was confirmed that these oscillations were indeed "reset" —larger effects occurring with larger saccades (see Fig. 10–9, Chapter 10 and Video Display: Acquired Pendular Nystagmus).[33]

Experimental validation for some of these concepts has been provided from studies of the goldfish, in which a relatively small number of cells contribute to the neural integrator for eye movements. In these studies, electrophysiological evidence supports the notion of integration by the network of neurons rather than by cell membrane properties or pacemaker currents.[6] This reductionist model has also proven useful in investigating the dependence of neural integration on feedback circuits between neurons,[4,100] as well as studying how visual conditions can be used to adapt the properties of the integrator, making it leaky or unstable.[5,86]

One unresolved aspect of neural integration of ocular motor signals concerns *3-D eye rotations*. When a sphere rotates first in one direction and then in another, the final eye position is not the same if the rotations were performed in the reverse order. This non-commutative property of the rotation of spheres also means that, in a vectorial sense, eye position is not the exact integral of eye velocity. This geometric property has led to the hypothesis that the brain uses a non-commutative operator to convert eye velocity to eye position.[124] However, given the demonstration of pulleys (see Fig. 9–1, in Chapter 9) that constrain movement of the tendons of extraocular muscle,[36] it has been proposed that, for most eye movements (less than 40 degrees amplitude), three simple integrators, one for each direction, will account for observed behavior.[104,109] Theoretical considerations suggest that the fibromuscular pulleys simplify the computations that the brain must make in order to take into account the non-commutative nature of rotations,[103] and electrophysiological studies support this viewpoint.[48,72] Nonetheless, a number of experimental studies, reviewed in Chapter 9, have provided evidence for a neural contribution to the programming of some 3-D eye movements.[131] Networks of neurons could provide such 3-D innervation by transforming an eye-velocity command to a command for a change in eye position that depended on eye position itself.[10]

CLINICAL EVALUATION OF GAZE HOLDING

The fidelity of the neural integrator is tested at the bedside by noting the patient's ability to hold the eyes in an eccentric position in the orbit (see Appendix A for a summary). When the integrator is leaky (i.e., has a low time constant) the eyes will drift back toward the central position; this necessitates corrective saccades, and gaze-evoked nystagmus will result (see Video Display: Disorders of Gaze Holding). The term gaze-paretic nystagmus, although in common use, is probably best avoided because it implies a paresis of gaze, which may or may not accompany nystagmus with centripetal drifts. For example, gaze-evoked nystagmus was reported when looking to the left in a patient with a right-sided abducens nucleus lesion that caused complete right gaze palsy.[93]

Before testing gaze stability in eccentric positions, examine the eyes during fixation in the central position and note any nystagmus. An ophthalmoscopic examination will often help to determine the presence and nature of any drift of the eyes, both with and without fixation (if the fixating eye is covered for a short period). Next, examine the eye movements as the patient fixates to the right, left, up, and down. Repeat this examination behind Frenzel goggles to exclude the effects of visual fixation. If gaze-evoked nystagmus occurs, is it only present at extremes of gaze and is it symmetrical on looking right, left, up, and down? With sustained efforts at eccentric gaze, does the nystagmus diminish? On returning the eyes to central position, does transient nystagmus occur with slow phases towards the direction of prior gaze? (This phenomenon, rebound nystagmus, is discussed below, under the section on Pathogenesis of Centripetal and Rebound Nystagmus). The presence of gaze-evoked nystagmus in the light often implies more than just a leaky integrator: the visual fixation and stabilization reflexes are probably impaired, and hence smooth pursuit and cancellation of the vestibulo-ocular reflex may be abnormal.

Recording of eye movements will help establish the nature of the slow-phase component during attempted eccentric fixation in both light and darkness. The time constant of drift (see Fig. 5–4C), when measured in normal subjects in darkness, varies considerably but is typically 20 to 70 seconds.[13,39] Some normal subjects show a low-velocity unidirectional drift.[63] Centripetal drift caused by an inadequate (leaky) integrator due to disease may have a time constant of a few seconds. Rarely, disease of the gaze-holding mechanism causes nystagmus with an increasing-velocity slow-phase waveform that is evident clinically (see Video Display: Disorders of Gaze Holding).

The centripetal drifts of gaze-evoked nystagmus may appear to have a linear rather than a decaying exponential waveform (compare Fig. 10–1A and 1B, in Chapter 10). This nystagmus may still be due to a deficient neural integrator; exponential decay may not be obvious if the integrator is only slightly leaky, if there are corrective saccades, or if visual-following reflexes reduce the drift. In addition, lesions affecting the vestibular nuclei that impair gaze holding may also cause a vestibular imbalance leading to nystagmus with more linear slow phases (see Alexander's law, below). In practice, the best way to show that slow phases of nystagmus have a negative exponential waveform is to record eye movements in darkness.

ABNORMALITIES OF THE NEURAL INTEGRATOR: GAZE-EVOKED NYSTAGMUS

Disease affecting the neural integrator causes an inadequately sustained eye position signal. This is manifest by drift of the eyes back from an eccentric position to the central position and corrective quick phases that produce gaze-evoked nystagmus (see Video Display: Disorders of Gaze Holding). As noted previously, even normal subjects do not have a "perfect" neural integrator; most individuals will show some centripetal drift when in darkness. Some normal subjects show deficient gaze holding even when fixating a visual target. This "physiological" or "end-point" nystagmus usually occurs when such individuals are in extreme lateral gaze or upgaze.[3,37,39,114] In some normal subjects, a small amount of mixed vertical (downbeat) torsional nystagmus may appear on extreme lateral gaze. Certain normal subjects, however, develop gaze-evoked nystagmus even with modest eye deviations, such as at 20 degrees eccentricity.[3] End-point nystagmus usually comes on soon after turning the eyes to an eccentric position,[114] and may dampen after several seconds. It may be asymmetric (e.g., present on looking to the right but not to the left), and be of greater amplitude in the abducting eye.[114] The slow-phase drift may be a decaying exponential (Fig. 5–4C) or have a more constant-velocity (linear) waveform. Some individuals show small-amplitude, pendular oscillations, increasing-velocity waveforms, or small saccadic intrusions on far eccentric fixation;[1] usually measurement of eye movements is necessary to appreciate these details. Important points in differentiating "physiological nystagmus" from the effects of disease are low amplitude (slower drift) and the absence of other ocular motor abnormalities (see Box 10–8, in Chapter 10).[19] Quick phases of end-point nystagmus may increase or decrease when the subject imagines a target location in darkness, rather than viewing it;[1,39] slow-phase drift persists. Prolonged attempts to maintain extreme lateral gaze lead to "fatigue nystagmus" in some normal subjects,[3,39] but this probably represents a different mechanism than the more common finding of nystagmus that develops soon after the eye reaches its eccentric position.

Although a leaky neural integrator produces gaze-evoked nystagmus, this does not produce great functional disability, since the eyes are used mostly near the central position. When the eyes are held in an eccentric position in the orbit, each quick phase (saccade) resets the level of activity of the neural integrator so that the eye position is corrected before the eye drifts far off target. Only if the velocity of centripetal drifts is high will vision be noticeably degraded.

Pathogenesis of Deficient Neural Integration

In the clinic, the most common cause of gaze-evoked nystagmus is *drugs*, usually sedatives, tranquilizers, anticonvulsants, or alcohol (see Table 12–11, in Chapter 12). Such nystagmus may occur in the horizontal or vertical plane. Although the exact site of action of such agents is not always unknown, it seems likely that either the cerebellum or the vestibular nuclei may be affected.[84]

A variety of *cerebellar disorders* cause gaze-evoked nystagmus, and usually reflect involvement of the vestibulocerebellum (flocculo-nodular lobe) or its connections (see Box 12–2, in Chapter 12).[56,137] Other abnormalities of eye movements, especially impairment of smooth pursuit and impaired cancellation of the VOR when fixing upon a target moving with the head, usually co-exist.[19] Brain stem lesions affecting the NPH and MVN, which are essential for neural integration, impair gaze holding, but also often cause vestibular imbalance.[111] Loss of neurons from the medial vestibular and prepositus hypoglossi nuclei has been reported in a patient who suffered lithium intoxication.[29] Prior to her death from respiratory failure, she lost voluntary and reflexive eye movements, except for what may have been saccades followed by a rapid centripetal drift.

When a *vestibular imbalance* occurs, due either to a peripheral or central lesion, gaze-evoked nystagmus is often superimposed. Such interaction of vestibular nystagmus and gaze-evoked nystagmus is the basis for *Alexander's law*: nystagmus due to a vestibular lesion is more intense when the patient looks in the direction of the quick phases.[63,108] In other words, slow-phase velocity is greatest when the eye is turned away from the direction of drift. The effect of deficient gaze holding is small during natural behavior of the VOR, but is evident during sustained stimulation (rotational or caloric) and especially with imbalance due to lesions.[37,108] It has been postulated that, faced with a persisting vestibular imbalance (i.e., a false signal), the nervous system disables the neural integrator and the time constant of centripetal drift falls.[62,108] In this way, centripetal drift due to a leaky neural integrator can be used to counteract the vestibular nystagmus in one field of gaze. The negative-exponential waveforms that characterize a leaky neural integrator are difficult to discern in patients when a vestibular imbalance is also present.[108] However, if the slow-phase velocity of a unidirectional nystagmus varies with orbital position, impaired integration can be inferred. Such waveforms have been identified following experimental lesions of the peripheral vestibular organ or nerve in monkeys.[42] Bilateral experimental vestibular neurectomy causes gaze-evoked nystagmus, probably because of the effects on resting discharge rate of neurons in vestibular nuclei.[128]

Vertical gaze-evoked nystagmus can be caused by drugs, and by brain stem and cerebellar lesions that also disrupt horizontal gaze holding. Other causes of vertical gaze-evoked nystagmus include bilateral internuclear ophthalmoplegia, and lesions affecting the posterior commissure.[15] Both the medial longitudinal fasciculus and the posterior commissure convey signals that encode vertical eye position. Downbeat nystagmus present with the eye close to center position is often accompanied by horizontal and vertical gaze-evoked nystagmus. Systematic, 3-D measurements of downbeat nystagmus have indicated that, in some patients with downbeat nystagmus, the underlying defect is one of the neural integrator.[50] Similarly, in patients with upbeat nystagmus, in whom there was involvement of the nucleus intercalatus and nucleus of Roller (parts of the perihypoglossal group), disruption of the vertical neural integrator has been postulated.[64,67,92]

Sometimes, disease causes an *unstable neural integrator* manifest by nystagmus with exponentially increasing slow phases. This finding is indicative of an unstable rather than a leaky neural integrator. Nystagmus with increasing-velocity waveforms is most commonly encountered in the horizontal plane as a feature of congenital nystagmus. It also occurs in some patients with cerebellar disease, who show horizontal or vertical nystagmus that is made worse by looking in the direction of the slow phases (see Video Display: Disorders of Gaze Holding).[12,133] We have attempted to interpret this finding by the simple integrator model in Figure 5–7. Nystagmus with slow phases that variably increase or decrease in velocity and have a variable neutral point has been reported in blind individuals (see Video Display: Nystagmus and Visual Disorders),[79,80] and following experimental occipital lobectomy.[134] In such cases, it seems that deprivation of visual or vestibular inputs can cause the neural integrator to become "uncalibrated," with a variable, inappropriate performance. Similar drifts of the eyes are reported following experimental cerebellectomy.[106]

Pathogenesis of Centripetal Nystagmus and Rebound Nystagmus

Persistent effort at maintaining eccentric gaze usually reduces the intensity of gaze-evoked nystagmus and may actually cause a reversal of direction—so-called centripetal nystagmus (Box 10–7, Chapter 10).[78] If the patient then returns the eyes to the central position, a transient nystagmus may be observed with slow phases occurring in the direction of former gaze; this is called rebound nystagmus (see Video Display: Disorders of Gaze Holding).[17,65,66] Rebound nystagmus occurs in normal subjects after prolonged, eccentric gaze.[114]

In one study of five normal subjects, rebound nystagmus was elicited after varying degrees and durations of eccentric fixation of a continuously illuminated light emitting diode (LED).[57] After holding eccentric gaze, subjects returned their eyes to an LED flashing on for 10 ms every second. This stimulus enabled the subjects to keep their eyes near a specific orbital position but provided little retinal slip information for fixation-pursuit mechanisms to suppress rebound nystagmus. Thresholds and amplitudes of rebound nystagmus were determined with the flashing LED located at 0 degrees. Eccentric gaze for a constant duration of 16 seconds elicited rebound nystagmus with an initial slow-phase velocity of 0.3 degrees per second after fixation at 30 degrees. Initial slow-phase eye velocity of rebound nystagmus increased to 6.8 degrees per second after far eccentric fixation at 60 degrees. With a constant eccentricity of 55 degrees, slow-phase velocity of rebound nystagmus increased from 0.3 degrees per second after 4 seconds of gaze holding to 5.8 degrees per second after 16 seconds and then remained about 6 degrees per second for longer durations. Rebound nystagmus also depended on orbital position, implying that a velocity bias alone could not account for rebound nystagmus. When the flashing LED alternated between ± 20 degrees subjects showed a centripetal drift superimposed on the bias. The centripetal drift presumably reflected a decrease in the time constant of the central gaze-holding network, the neural integrator. By measuring the velocity of rebound nystagmus at ± 20 degrees, the time constant, the velocity bias, and the consequent shift in the null (no drift) position were calculated. The development of the bias (up to 8 degrees per second), the decrease in time constant (to 4–5 s), and the calculated shift in the null (as far as 75 degrees) varied with the degree and duration of prior eccentric gaze. As rebound nystagmus decayed, the velocity bias disappeared well before the time constant returned to normal.

These results suggest that rebound nystagmus reflects a shift of the null in the direction of prior eccentric gaze; it may reflect the actions of a physiological mechanism to optimize ocular stability in eccentric positions of gaze. The shift in the null reflects two processes: development of a velocity bias, and a decrease in the time constant of the neural integrator, which, together determine the exact location of the null. Since, after eccentric gaze, the time course of the decay of the bias and of the recovery of the time constant were different, the two components of rebound nystagmus may reflect separate neural mechanisms.[57]

Clinicians most frequently encounter rebound nystagmus in patients with cerebellar disease (Fig. 10–7),[17,66,90] and rebound nystagmus also occurs in monkeys with lesions in the flocculus and paraflocculus.[135] Rebound nystagmus also has been reported in monkeys with bilateral lesions restricted to the NPH and MVN.[23] On the other hand, rebound nystagmus in one patient, who had a choroid plexus papilloma involving the flocculus and nodulus, disappeared when the vestibular nucleus was invaded by tumor.[132]

Since rebound nystagmus can occur following eccentric gaze holding in the dark, it cannot simply be a response to retinal slip.[57] Moreover, rebound nystagmus occurs in both normals and patients who have impaired pursuit,[17] so abnormalities of the pursuit system are unlikely to be primarily responsible for it. We examined one patient with an absent horizontal vestibulo-ocular reflex who still developed rebound nystagmus. Bilateral vestibular hypofunction resulted in loss of optokinetic afternystagmus implying that the velocity-storage mechanism is disabled (see Chapter 2). Thus, it is unlikely that rebound nystagmus arose from the velocity-storage mechanism. More likely, the generation of rebound nystagmus is related to the function of the gaze-holding networks within NPH-MVN and depends upon the ability to internally monitor eye movement signals (i.e., efference copy or proprioception) and activate compensatory eye drifts. Rebound nystagmus only occurred during the recovery phase following lesions of the NPH and MVN, indicating that some neural integrator function may be necessary for its generation.[23]

Centripetal nystagmus in eccentric gaze, which consists of centrifugally directed slow phases and centripetally directed quick phases,[78] likely reflects instability in the gaze-holding networks, similar to the velocity-increasing waveforms of downbeat nystagmus seen in some patients with cerebellar disease.

SUMMARY

1. For normal conjugate eye movements, the ocular motor neurons carry a neural signal that contains velocity and position components. Such a signal is necessary to hold the eyes steady at an eccentric position in the orbit (see Fig. 1–3, Chapter 1). The position-coded ocular motor signal is obtained from the velocity-coded signal by a process of mathematical integration. Electrophysiological evidence indicates that a common neural network integrates all conjugate eye movement commands; this network is called the neural integrator.
2. For horizontal, conjugate eye movements, the nucleus prepositus hypoglossi and medial vestibular nuclei are of prime importance for holding steady, eccentric gaze. Unilateral lesions of this NPH-MVN region cause partial, bilateral loss of gaze holding; bilateral lesions abolish

the horizontal neural integrator. For vertical eye movements, midbrain structures, especially the interstitial nucleus of Cajal, contribute to neural integration. The vestibulocerebellum also contributes to the integration of ocular motor signals, and this role may depend on feedback of eye movement signals by the cell groups of the paramedian tracts. Thus, a network of interconnected neurons may achieve mathematical integration of ocular motor signals. Knowledge about the neurotransmitters used in these circuits has guided treatment of abnormal eye movements such as nystagmus (Chapter 10).

3. Inadequate neural integration causes a progressive decay in the eye-position signal and consequent negative exponential drift of the eyes back from an eccentric to a neutral position (Fig. 5–4B). Clinically, this is manifest as gaze-evoked nystagmus. Such impaired integration is a common side effect of medications and is caused by disease affecting the vestibulocerebellum and brain stem. Deficient neural integration also impairs vestibular, optokinetic, and pursuit eye movements. Vestibular lesions lead to a deficient neural integrator, in addition to causing a tonic vestibular imbalance. This combination of deficits follows Alexander's law—nystagmus with a slow-phase velocity that increases when the eyes are brought to a position in the orbit in the direction of the quick phases.
4. The nervous system can partially compensate for deficient integrator function by programming oppositely directed, adaptive drifts of the eyes that are apparent as rebound nystagmus. If the nervous system is deprived of vision (blindness), the neural integrator loses its calibration and is unable to hold gaze steady.

REFERENCES

1. Abadi RV, Scallan CJ. Ocular oscillations on eccentric gaze. Vision Res 41, 2895–2907 2001.
2. Abel LA, Dell'Osso LF, Daroff RB. Analog model for gaze-evoked nystagmus. IEEE Trans Biomed. Eng 25, 71–75, 1978.
3. Abel LA, Parker L, Daroff RB, Dell'Osso LF. End-point nystagmus. Invest Ophthalmol Vis Sci 17, 539–544, 1977.
4. Aksay E, Baker R, Seung HS, Tank DW. Correlated discharge among cell pairs within the oculomotor horizontal velocity-to-position integrator. J Neurosci 23, 10852–10858, 2003.
5. Aksay E, Baker R, Seung HS, Tank DW. Visual adaptation of the the oculomotor horizontal velocity-to-position integrator (Check). Proc Natl Acad Sci U S A 23, 10852–10858, 2005.
6. Aksay E, Gamkrelidze G, Seung HS, Baker R, Tank DW. In vivo intracellular recording and perturbation of persistent activity in a neural integrator. Nat Neurosci 4, 184–193, 2001.
7. Aksay E, Major G, Goldman MS, et al. History dependence of rate covariation between neurons during persistent activity in an oculomotor integrator. Cereb Cortex 13, 1173–1184, 2003.
8. Anastasio TJ. Neural network models of velocity storage in the horizontal vestibulo-ocular reflex. Biol Cybern 64, 187–196, 1991.
9. Anastasio TJ, Robinson DA. Failure of the oculomotor neural integrator from a discrete midline lesion between the abducens nuclei in the monkey. Neurosci Lett 127, 82–86, 1991.
10. Arnold DB, Robinson DA. The oculomotor integrator: testing of a neural network model. Exp Brain Res 113, 57–74, 1997.
11. Arnold DB, Robinson DA, Leigh RJ. Nystagmus induced by pharmacological inactivation of the brainstem ocular motor integrator in monkey. Vision Res 39, 4286–4295, 1999.
12. Barton JJS, Sharpe JA. Oscillopsia and horizontal nystagmus with accelerating slow phases following lumbar puncture in the Arnold-Chiari malformation. Ann Neurol 33, 418–421, 1993.
13. Becker W, Klein H-M. Accuracy of saccadic eye movements and maintenance of eccentric eye positions in the dark. Vision Res 13, 1021–1034, 1973.
14. Belknap DB, McCrea RA. Anatomical connections of the prepositus and abducens nuclei in the squirrel monkey. J Comp Neurol 268, 13–28, 1988.
15. Bhidayasiri R, Plant GT, Leigh RJ. A hypothetical scheme for the brainstem control of vertical gaze. Neurology 54, 1985–1993, 2000.
16. Blazquez PM, Hirata Y, Heiney SA, Green AM, Highstein SM. Cerebellar signatures of vestibulo-ocular reflex motor learning. J Neurosci 23, 9742–9751, 2003.
17. Bondar RL, Sharpe JA, Lewis AJ. Rebound nystagmus in olivocerebellar atrophy: a clinicopathological correlation. Ann Neurol 15, 474–477, 1984.
18. Broussard DM, De Charms RC, Lisberger SG. Inputs from the ipsilateral and contralateral vestibular apparatus to behaviorally characterized abducens neurons in rhesus monkeys. J Neurophysiol 74, 2445–2459, 1995.
19. Büttner U, Grundei T. Gaze-evoked nystagmus and smooth pursuit deficits: their relationship studied in 52 patients. J Neurol 242, 384–389, 1995.
20. Büttner-Ennever JA, Horn AK. Pathways from cell groups of the paramedian tracts to the floccular region. Ann N Y Acad Sci 781, 532–540, 1996.
21. Büttner-Ennever JA, Horn AK, Schmidtke K. Cell groups of the medial longitudinal fasciculus and paramedian tracts. Rev Neurol (Paris) 145, 533–539, 1989.
22. Cannon SC, Robinson DA. An improved neural-network model for the neural integrator of the oculomotor system: more realistic neuron behavior. Biol Cybern 53, 93–108, 1985.

23. Cannon SC, Robinson DA. Loss of the neural integrator of the oculomotor system from brain stem lesions in monkey. J Neurophysiol 57, 1383–1409, 1987.
24. Cannon SC, Robinson DA, Shamma S. A proposed neural network for the integrator of the oculomotor system. Biol Cybern 49, 127–136, 1983.
25. Carpenter RHS. Cerebellectomy and the transfer function of the vestibulo-ocular reflex in the decerebrate cat. Proc Royal Soc (Lond) B 181, 353–374, 1972.
26. Chan WW, Galiana HL. Integrator function in the oculomotor system is dependent on sensory context. J Neurophysiol 93, 3709–3717, 2005.
27. Cheron G, Godaux E. Disabling of the oculomotor neural integrator by kainic acid injections in the prepositus-vestibular complex of the cat. J Physiol 394, 267–290, 1987.
28. Cheron G, Mettens P, Godaux E. Gaze holding defect induced by injections of ketamine in the cat brainstem. Neuroreport 3, 97–100, 1992.
29. Corbett JJ, Jacobson DM, Thompson HS, Hart MN, Albert DW. Downbeating nystagmus and other ocular motor defects caused by lithium toxicity. Neurology 39, 481–487, 1989.
30. Crawford JD, Cadera W, Vilis T. Generation of torsional and vertical eye position signals by the interstitial nucleus of Cajal. Science 252, 1551–1553, 1991.
31. Crawford JD, Tweed DB, Vilis T. Static ocular counterroll is implemented through the 3-D neural integrator. J Neurophysiol 90, 2777–2784, 2003.
32. Das VE, Dell'Osso LF, Leigh RJ. Enhancement of the vestibulo-ocular reflex by prior eye movements. J Neurophysiol 81, 2884–2892, 1999.
33. Das VE, Oruganti P, Kramer PD, Leigh RJ. Experimental tests of a neural-network model for ocular oscillations caused by disease of central myelin. Exp Brain Res 133, 189–197, 2000.
34. Dean P. Simulated recruitment of medial rectus motoneurons by abducens internuclear neurons: synaptic specificity vs. intrinsic motoneuron properties. J Neurophysiol 78, 1531–1549, 1997.
35. Dell'Osso LF. Evidence suggesting individual ocular motor control of each eye (muscle). J Vestib Res 4, 335–345, 1994.
36. Demer JL. Pivotal role of orbital connective tissues in binocular alignment and strabismus. Invest Ophthalmol Vis Sci 45, 729–738, 2004.
37. Doslak MS, Dell'Osso LF, Daroff RB. Alexander's law: a model and resulting study. Ann Otol Rhino Laryngol 91, 316–322, 1982.
38. Draye JP, Cheron G, Libert G, Godaux E. Emergence of clusters in the hidden layer of a dynamic recurrent neural network. Biol Cybern 76, 365–374, 1997.
39. Eizenman M, Cheng P, Sharpe JA, Frecker RC. Endpoint nystagmus and ocular drift: an experimental and theoretical study. Vision Res 30, 863–877, 1990.
40. Escudero M, Cheron G, Godaux E. Discharge properties of brain stem neurons projecting to the flocculus in the alert cat. II. Prepositus hypoglossal nucleus. J Neurophysiol 76, 1775–1785, 1996.
41. Fernandez C, Goldberg JM. Physiology of peripheral neurons innervating semicircular canals of the squirrel monkey. II. Response to sinusoidal stimulation and dynamics of peripheral vestibular system. J Neurophysiol 34, 661–675, 1971.
42. Fetter M, Zee DS. Recovery from unilateral labyrinthectomy in rhesus monkey. J Neurophysiol 59, 370–393, 1988.
43. Fuchs AF, Scudder CA, Kaneko CRS. Discharge patterns and recruitment order of identified motoneurons and internuclear neurons in the monkey abducens nucleus. J Neurophysiol 60, 1874–1895, 1988.
44. Fukushima K. The interstitial nucleus of Cajal and its role in the control of movements of head and eyes. Progr Neurobiol 29, 107–192, 1987.
45. Fukushima K. Roles of the cerebellum in pursuit-vestibular interactions. Cerebellum 2, 223–232, 2003.
46. Fukushima K, Kaneko CR. Vestibular integrators in the oculomotor system. Neurosci Res 22, 249–258, 1995.
47. Fukushima K, Kaneko CR, Fuchs AF. The neuronal substrate of integration in the oculomotor system. Progr Neurobiol 39, 609–639, 1992.
48. Ghasia FF, Angelaki DE. Do motoneurons encode the noncommutativity of ocular rotations? Neuron 47, 1–13, 2005.
49. Glasauer S, Dieterich M, Brandt T. Central positional nystagmus simulated by a mathematical ocular motor model of otolith-dependent modification of Listing's plane. J Neurophysiol 86, 1546–1554, 2001.
50. Glasauer S, Hoshi M, Kempermann U, Eggert T, Buttner U. Three-dimensional eye position and slow phase velocity in humans with downbeat nystagmus. J Neurophysiol 89, 338–354, 2003.
51. Godaux E, Cheron G. The hypothesis of the uniqueness of the oculomotor neural integrator: direct experimental evidence in the cat. J Physiol 492, 517–527, 1996.
52. Godaux E, Mettens P, Cheron G. Differential effect of injections of kainic acid into the prepositus and the vestibular nuclei of the cat. J Physiol 472, 459–482, 1993.
53. Godaux E, Vanderkelen B. Vestibulo-ocular reflex, optokinetic response and their interactions in the cerebellectomized cat. J Physiol (Lond) 346, 155–170, 1984.
54. Goldman MS, Levine JH, Major G, Tank DW, Seung HS. Robust persistent neural activity in a model integrator with multiple hysteretic dendrites per neuron. Cereb Cortex 13, 1185–1195, 2003.
55. Goldstein HP, Robinson DA. Hysteresis and slow drift in abducens unit activity. J Neurophysiol 55, 1044–1056, 1986.
56. Gomez CM, Thompson RM, Gammack JT, et al. SCA6: Gaze-evoked and vertical nystagmus, Purkinje cell degeneration, and variable age of onset despite stable CAG repeat size. Ann Neurol 42, 933–950, 1997.
57. Gordon SE, Hain TC, Zee DS, Fetter M. Rebound nystagmus. Soc Neurosci Abstr 12, 1091, 1986.
58. Green AM, Angelaki DE. Resolution of sensory ambiguities for gaze stabilization requires a second neural integrator. J Neurosci 23, 9265–9275, 2003.
59. Hartwich-Young R, Nelson JS, Sparks DL. The perihypoglossal projection to the superior colliculus in the rhesus monkey. Vis Neurosci 4, 29–42, 1990.
60. Helmchen C, Rambold H, Fuhry L, Büttner U. Deficits in vertical and torsional eye movements after uni- and bilateral muscimol inactivation of the interstitial nucleus of Cajal of the alert monkey. Exp Brain Res 119, 436–452, 1998.
61. Henn V, Lang W, Hepp K, Reisine H. Experimental gaze palsies in monkeys and their relation to human pathology. Brain 107, 619–636, 1984.
62. Hess K. Do peripheral-vestibular lesions in man

affect the position integrator of the eyes? Neurosci Lett (Suppl 10), S242–S243, 1982.
63. Hess K, Reisine H, Dürsteler MR. Normal eye drift and saccadic drift correction in darkness. Neuro-ophthalmology 5, 247–252, 1985.
64. Hirose G, Ogasarwa T, Shirakawa T, et al. Primary position upbeat nystagmus due to unilateral medial medullary infarction. Ann Neurol 43, 403–405, 1998.
65. Hood JD. Further observations on the phenomenon of rebound nystagmus. Ann N Y Acad Sci 374, 532–539, 1981.
66. Hood JD, Kayan A, Leech J. Rebound nystagmus. Brain 96, 507–526, 1973.
67. Janssen JC, Larner AJ, Morris H, Bronstein AM, Farmer SF. Upbeat nystagmus: clinicoanatomical correlation. J Neurol Neurosurg Psychiatry 65, 380–381, 1998.
68. Kamath BY, Keller EL. A neurological integrator for the oculomotor control system. Mathematical Biosciences 30, 341–352, 1976.
69. Kaneko CR. Eye movement deficits after ibotenic acid lesions of the nucleus prepositus hypoglossi in monkeys. I. Saccades and fixation. J Neurophysiol 78, 1753–1768, 1997.
70. Kaneko CR. Eye movement deficits following ibotenic acid lesions of the nucleus prepositus hypoglossi in monkeys II. Pursuit, vestibular, and optokinetic responses. J. Neurophysiol 81, 668–681, 1999.
71. Keane JR, Itabashi HH. Upbeat nystagmus: clinicopathologic study of two patients. Neurology 37, 491–494, 1987.
72. Klier EM, Meng H, Angelaki DE. Abducens nerve/nucleus stimulation produces knematically correct three-dimensional eye movement [abstract]. Soc Neurosci Abstr. 2005.
73. Kokkoroyannis T, Scudder CA, Balaban CD, Highstein SM, Moschovakis AK. Anatomy and physiology of the primate interstitial nucleus of Cajal .1. Efferent projections. J Neurophysiol 75, 725–739, 1996.
74. Komatsu H, Wurtz R. Relation of cortical areas MT and MST to pursuit eye movements. III. Interaction with full-field visual stimulation. J Neurophysiol 60, 621–644, 1988.
75. Kramer P, Shelhamer M, Zee DS. Short-term vestibulo-ocular adaptation: influence of context. Otolaryngol Head Neck Surg 119, 60–64, 1998.
76. Kramer PD, Shelhamer MJ, Zee DS. Short-term adaptation of the phase of the vestibulo-ocular reflex (VOR) in normal human subjects. Exp Brain Res 106, 318–326, 1995.
77. Langer T, Kaneko CRS, Scudder CA, Fuchs AF. Afferents to the abducens nucleus in the monkey and cat. J Comp Neurol 245, 379–400, 1986.
78. Leech J, Gresty M, Hess K, Rudge P. Gaze failure, drifting eye movements, and centripetal nystagmus in cerebellar disease. Br J Ophthalmol 61, 774–781, 1977.
79. Leigh RJ, Thurston SE, Tomsak RL, Grossman GE, Lanska DJ. Effect of monocular visual loss upon stability of gaze. Invest Ophthalmol Vis Sci 30, 288–292, 1989.
80. Leigh RJ, Zee DS. Eye movements of the blind. Invest Ophthalmol Vis Sci 19, 328–331, 1980.
81. Lorente de Nó F. Vestibulo-ocular reflex arc. Arch Neurol Psychiatr 30, 625–633, 1933.
82. McConville K, Tomlinson RD, King WM, Paige G, Na EQ. Eye position signals in the vestibular nuclei: consequences for models of integrator function. J Vestib Res 4, 391–400, 1994.
83. McCrea RA, Horn AKE. Nucleus prepositus. In Büttner-Ennever JA (ed). Neuroanatomy of the Oculomotor System. Prog Brain Res 151, 205–230, 2006.
84. McElligott JG, Spencer RF. Neuropharmacological aspects of the vestibulo-ocular reflex. In Anderson JH, Beitz AJ (eds). Neurochemistry of the Vestibular System. CRC Press, Boca Raton, 2000, pp 199–222.
85. McFarland JL, Fuchs AF. Discharge patterns in nucleus prepositus hypoglossi and adjacent medial vestibular nucleus during horizontal eye movement in behaving macaques. J Neurophysiol 68, 319–332, 1992.
86. Mensh BD, Aksay E, Lee DD, Seung HS, Tank DW. Spontaneous eye movements in goldfish: oculomotor integrator performance, plasticity, and dependence on visual feedback. Vision Res 44, 711–726, 2004.
87. Mettens P, Cheron G, Godaux E. NMDA receptors are involved in temporal integration in the oculomotor system of the cat. Neuroreport 5, 1333–1336, 1994.
88. Mettens P, Godaux E, Cheron G, Galiana HL. Effect of muscimol microinjections into the prepositus hypoglossi and the medial vestibular nuclei on cat eye movements. J Neurophysiol 72, 785–802, 1994.
89. Miles FA, Fuller J. Visual tracking and the primate flocculus. Science 189, 1000–1002, 1975.
90. Morales-Garcia C, Cardenas JL, Arriagada C, Otte J. Clinical significance of rebound nystagmus in neuro-otological diagnosis. Ann Otol Rhinol Laryngol 87, 238–242, 1978.
91. Moreno-López B, Escudero M, Delgado-Garcia JM, Estrada C. Nitric oxide production by brain stem neurons is required for normal performance of eye movements in alert animals. Neuron 17, 739–745, 1996.
92. Munro NA. The role of the nucleus intercalatus in vertical gaze holding. J Neurol Neurosurg Psychiatry 66, 552–553, 1999.
93. Müri RM, Chermann JF, Cohen L, Rivaud S, Pierrot-Deseilligny C. Ocular motor consequences of damage to the abducens nucleus area in humans. J Neuroophthalmol 16, 191–195, 1996.
94. Musallam WS, Tomlinson RD. Model for the translational vestibuloocular reflex (VOR). J Neurophysiol 82, 2010–2014, 1999.
95. Mustari MJ, Fuchs AF, Wallman J. Response properties of dorsolateral pontine units during smooth pursuit of the rhesus macaque. J Neurophysiol 60, 664–686, 1988.
96. Nakamagoe K, Iwamoto Y, Yoshida K. Evidence for brainstem structures participating in oculomotor integration. Science 288, 857–859, 2000.
97. Navarro-Lopez JD, Alvarado JC, Marquez-Ruiz J, et al. A cholinergic synaptically triggered event participates in the generation of persistent activity necessary for eye fixation. J Neurosci 24, 5109–5118, 2004.
98. Optican LM, Miles FA. Visually induced adaptive changes in primate saccadic oculomotor control signals. J Neurophysiol 54, 940–958, 1985.
99. Partsalis AM, Highstein SM, Moschovakis AK. Lesions of the posterior commissure disable the vertical neural integrator of the primate oculomotor system. J Neurophysiol 71, 2582–2585, 1994.

100. Pastor AM, De la Cruz RR, Baker R. Eye position and eye velocity integrators reside in separate brainstem nuclei. Proc Natl Acad Sci U S A 91, 807–811, 1994.
101. Pierrot-Deseilligny C, Milea D. Vertical nystagmus: clinical facts and hypotheses. Brain 128, 1237–1246, 2005.
102. Priesol AJ, Jones GE, Tomlinson RD, Broussard DM. Frequency-dependent effects of glutamate antagonists on the vestibulo-ocular reflex of the cat. Brain Res 857, 252–264, 2000.
103. Quaia C, Optican LM. Commutative saccadic generator is sufficient to control a 3-D ocular plant with pulleys. J Neurophysiol 79, 3197–3215, 1998.
104. Raphan T. Modeling control of eye orientation in three dimensions. I. Role of muscle pulleys in determining saccadic trajectory. J Neurophysiol 79, 2653–2667, 1998.
105. Raphan T, Matsuo V, Cohen B. Velocity storage in the vestibulo-ocular reflex arc (VOR). Exp Brain Res 35, 229–248, 1979.
106. Robinson DA. The effect of cerebellectomy on the cat's vestibulo-ocular integrator. Brain Res 71, 195–207, 1974.
107. Robinson DA. Oculomotor control signals. In Lennerstrand G, Bach-y-Rita P (eds). Basic Mechanisms of Ocular Motility and their Clinical Implications. Pergamon Press, Oxford, 1975, pp 337–374.
108. Robinson DA, Zee DS, Hain TC, Holmes A, Rosenberg LF. Alexander's law: its behavior and origin in the human vestibulo-ocular reflex. Ann Neurol 16, 714–722, 1984.
109. Schnabolk C, Raphan T. Modeling three-dimensional velocity-to-position transformation in oculomotor control. J Neurophysiol 71, 623–638, 1994.
110. Seidman SH, Leigh RJ, Tomsak RL, Grant MP, Dell'Osso LF. Dynamic properties of the human vestibulo-ocular reflex during head rotations in roll. Vision Res 35, 679–689, 1995.
111. Seo SW, Shin HY, Kim SH, et al. Vestibular imbalance associated with a lesion in the nucleus prepositus hypoglossi area. Arch Neurol 61, 1440–1443, 2004.
112. Seung HS. How the brain keeps the eyes still. Proc Natl Acad Sci U S A 93, 13339–13344, 1996.
113. Seung HS, Lee DD, Reis BY, Tank DW. Stability of the memory of eye position in a recurrent network of conductance-based model neurons. Neuron 26, 259–271, 2000.
114. Shallo-Hoffmann J, Schwarze H, Simonsz HJ, Muhlendyck H. A reexamination of end-point and rebound nystagmus in normals. Invest Ophthalmol Vis Sci 31, 388–392, 1990.
115. Skavenski AA, Robinson DA. Role of abducens neurons in vestibuloocular reflex. J Neurophysiol 36, 724–738, 1973.
116. Stahl JS, James RA. Neural Integrator Function in Murine CACNA1A Mutants. Ann N Y Acad Sci 1039, 580–582, 2005.
117. Stahl JS, Simpson JI. Dynamics of abducens nucleus neurons in the awake rabbit. J Neurophysiol 73, 1383–1395, 1995.
118. Straube A, Kurzan R, Büttner U. Differential effects of bicuculline and muscimol microinjections into the vestibular nuclei on simian eye movements. Exp Brain Res 86, 347–358, 1991.
119. Sylvestre PA, Choi JT, Cullen KE. Discharge dynamics of oculomotor neural integrator neurons during conjugate and disjunctive saccades and fixation. J Neurophysiol 90, 739–754, 2003.
120. Sylvestre PA, Cullen KE. Dynamics of abducens nucleus neuron discharges during disjunctive saccades. J Neurophysiol 88, 3452–3468, 2002.
121. Takemori S, Cohen B. Loss of visual suppression of vestibular nystagmus after flocculus lesions. Brain Res 72, 213–224, 1974.
122. Tiliket C, Shelhamer M, Roberts D, Zee DS. Short-term vestibulo-ocular reflex adaptation in humans. I. Effect on the ocular motor velocity-to-position neural integrator. Exp Brain Res 100, 316–327, 1994.
123. Tweed D, Misslisch H, Fetter M. Testing models of the oculomotor velocity-to-position transformation. J Neurophysiol 72, 1425–1429, 1994.
124. Tweed D, Vilis T. Implications of rotational kinematics for the oculomotor system in three dimensions. J Neurophysiol 58, 832–849, 1987.
125. Van Gisbergen JAM, Robinson DA, Gielen S. A quantitative analysis of the generation of saccadic eye movements by burst neurons. J Neurophysiol 45, 417–442, 1981.
126. Waespe W, Cohen B, Raphan T. Role of the flocculus and paraflocculus in optokinetic nystagmus and visual-vestibular interactions: effects of lesions. Exp Brain Res 50, 9–33, 1983.
127. Waespe W, Henn V. Neuronal activity in the vestibular nuclei of the alert monkey during vestibular and optokinetic stimulation. Exp Brain Res 27, 523–538, 1977.
128. Waespe W, Wolfensberger M. Optokinetic nystagmus (OKN) and optokinetic after-responses after bilateral vestibular neurectomy in the monkey. Exp Brain Res 60, 263–269, 1985.
129. Wasicky R, Horn AK, Buttner-Ennever JA. Twitch and nontwitch motoneuron subgroups in the oculomotor nucleus of monkeys receive different afferent projections. J Comp Neurol 479, 117–129, 2004.
130. Westheimer G, Blair SM. Oculomotor defects in cerebellectomized monkeys. Invest Ophthalmol 12, 618–621, 1973.
131. Wong AM. Listing's law: clinical significance and implications for neural control. Surv. Ophthalmol 49, 563–575, 2004.
132. Yamazaki A, Zee DS. Rebound nystagmus: EOG analysis of a case with a floccular tumour. Br J Ophthalmol 63, 782–786, 1979.
133. Zee DS, Leigh RJ, Mathieu-Millaire F. Cerebellar control of ocular gaze stability. Ann Neurol 7, 37–40, 1980.
134. Zee DS, Tusa RJ, Herdman SJ, Butler PH, Gucer G. Effects of occipital lobectomy upon eye movements in primate. J Neurophysiol 58, 883–907, 1987.
135. Zee DS, Yamazaki A, Butler PH, Gücer G. Effects of ablation of flocculus and paraflocculus on eye movements in primate. J Neurophysiol 46, 878–899, 1981.
136. Zee DS, Yamazaki A, Butler PH, Gücer G. Effects of ablation of flocculus and paraflocculus on eye movements in primate. J Neurophysiol 46, 878–899, 1981.
137. Zee DS, Yee RD, Cogan DG, Robinson DA, Engel WK. Ocular motor abnormalities in hereditary cerebellar ataxia. Brain 99, 207–234, 1976.
138. Zhou W, King WM. Premotor commands encode monocular eye movements. Nature 393, 692–695, 1998.

Chapter 6

Synthesis of the Command for Conjugate Eye Movements

HYPOTHETICAL PATHWAYS FOR GAZE CONTROL

This chapter provides an anatomic scheme for the synthesis of neural commands for conjugate eye movements. We present a hypothesis to account for the way in which neural signals for vestibular, optokinetic, saccadic, and pursuit eye movements, and the gaze-holding mechanism (neural integrator), project to ocular motoneurons. At the outset, the reader should realize that we draw on findings from studies of both humans and monkeys to forge this hypothesis. Although such an approach carries the risk of making inaccurate suppositions, it also enhances the opportunities for experimental tests in both patients and monkeys.

Our approach is from the bottom up. First we discuss the brainstem machinery responsible for all conjugate eye movements—reflex or voluntary. Second, we summarize the role of the cerebellum. Finally, we review the pathways responsible for voluntary eye movements. Although most of our account concerns anatomy, we will recapitulate important neurophysiologic points, and summarize what is currently known about the neurotransmitters for these pathways. We will also outline the effects of certain well-defined lesions and so lay out an anatomic basis for the topological diagnosis of clinical conditions that are discussed in Chapter 12.

BRAINSTEM CONNECTIONS FOR HORIZONTAL CONJUGATE MOVEMENTS

The tegmentum of the pons contains the neural machinery that ultimately controls horizontal conjugate eye movements (Fig. 6–1).[186] The most important structure is the *abducens nucleus*,[53] which controls conjugate movements of both the ipsilateral lateral rectus and the contralateral medial rectus muscles (Box 6–1), and so may be regarded as the "horizontal gaze center." The abducens nucleus houses four distinct subpopulations of neurons (see Fig. 1B on compact disk).[114] *Abducens motoneurons*, which innervate the lateral rectus muscle, comprise twitch and non-twitch motoneurons, named for the different types of extraocular muscle fibers that they supply.[60] Non-twitch motoneurons lie around the medial perimeter of the nucleus, the nerve exit zone, but also centrally in the nucleus. Twitch motoneurons lie throughout the abducens nucleus except rostromedially. The possible roles of twitch and non-twitch motoneurons (in abducens, trochlear, and oculomotor nuclei) are discussed in Chapter 9. Abducens internuclear neurons are grouped lateral to the nerve exit zone in the rostral nucleus, and in a central strip in the caudal nucleus. A fourth group is the cell groups of the paramedian tracts (PMT), which are discussed below.

Abducens internuclear neurons project up the contralateral *medial longitudinal fasciculus (MLF)* (Box 6–2) to contact medial rectus motoneurons of the oculomotor nucleus (Fig. 6–1).[66,175] Thus, the axons of the abducens nerve, together with those of the abducens internuclear neurons that course in the MLF, encode conjugate horizontal eye movements.[214,355] Abducens motoneurons and internuclear neurons are partially intermingled but show some morphologic differences.[265] Abducens motoneurons have no axon collaterals, but the internuclear neurons send collaterals to the cell groups of the paramedian tracts (PMT cell groups), which lie in the midline of the brainstem and, in turn, project to the cerebellum.[62,265] Abducens motoneurons and internuclear neurons are pharmacologically distinct: the motoneurons use acetylcholine, and the internuclear neurons use glutamate and aspartate.[69,267,309,410] Although both populations of neurons show qualitatively similar electrophysiological properties, internuclear neurons show a lower sensitivity for eye position and a higher sensitivity for eye velocity.[128]

How do signals for each functional class of eye movement reach the abducens nucleus? Figure 6–1 summarizes monosynaptic excitatory and inhibitory projections to the abducens nucleus, and indicates neurotransmitters that have been postulated for these projections.[267] Vestibular and optokinetic inputs reach the abducens nucleus from the vestibular nuclei; some of these axons pass through the ipsilateral abducens nucleus en route to the contralateral abducens nucleus.[264] Excitatory saccadic commands originate from burst neurons that lie in the ipsilateral paramedian pontine reticular formation (PPRF) (Fig. 6–2 and Box 6–3), rostral to the abducens nucleus.[191,418] Inhibitory saccadic commands originate from

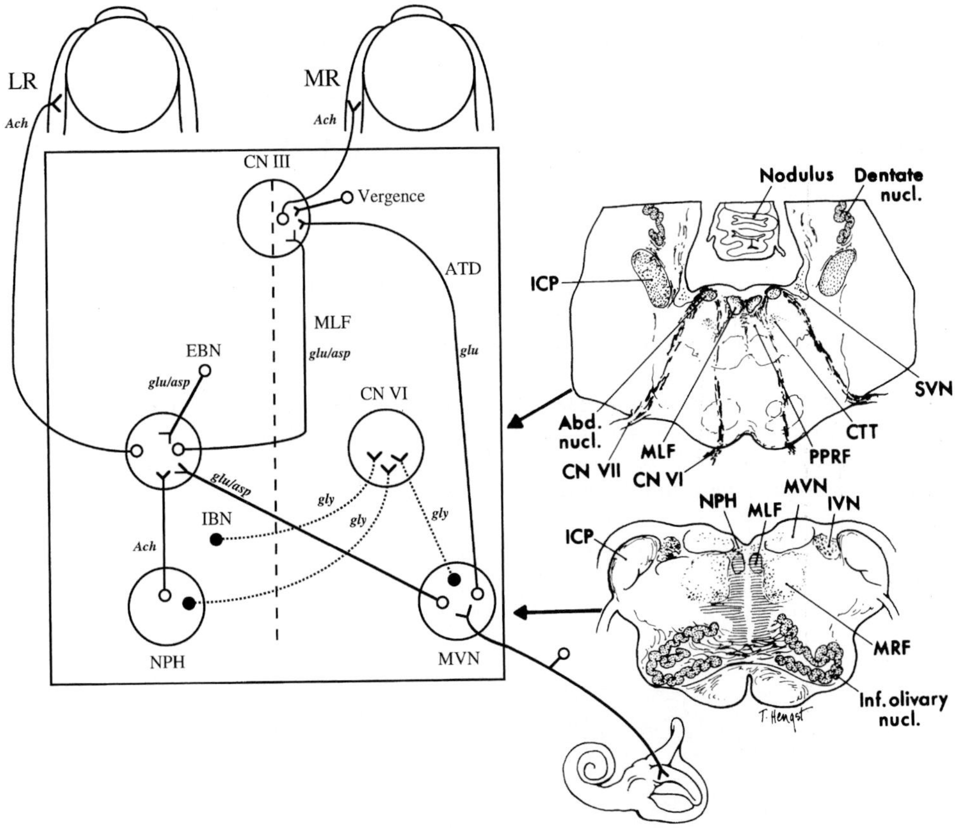

Figure 6–1. Anatomic scheme for the synthesis of signals for horizontal eye movements. The abducens nucleus (CN VI) contains abducens motoneurons that innervate the ipsilateral lateral rectus muscle (LR), and abducens internuclear neurons that send an ascending projection in the contralateral medial longitudinal fasciculus (MLF) to contact medial rectus (MR) motoneurons in the contralateral third nerve nucleus (CN III). From the horizontal semicircular canal, primary afferents on the vestibular nerve project mainly to the medial vestibular nucleus (MVN), where they synapse and then send an excitatory connection to the contralateral abducens nucleus and an inhibitory projection to the ipsilateral abducens nucleus. Saccadic inputs reach the abducens nucleus from ipsilateral excitatory burst neurons (EBN) and contralateral inhibitory burst neurons (IBN). Eye position information (the output of the neural integrator) reaches the abducens nucleus from neurons within the nucleus prepositus hypoglossi (NPH) and adjacent MVN. The medial rectus motoneurons in CN III also receive a command for vergence eye movements. Putative neurotransmitters for each pathway are shown: Ach: acetylcholine; asp: aspartate; glu: glutamate; gly: glycine. The anatomic sections on the right correspond to the level of the arrow heads on the schematic on the left. Abd. nucl.: abducens nucleus; CN VI: abducens nerve; CN VII: facial nerve; CTT: central tegmental tract; ICP: inferior cerebellar peduncle; IVN: inferior vestibular nucleus; Inf. olivary nucl.: inferior olivary nucleus; MVN: medial vestibular nucleus; MRF: medullary reticular formation; SVN: superior vestibular nucleus. (Transverse sections redrawn from Carpenter MB: Human Neuroanatomy, ed. 7. Williams & Wilkins, Baltimore, 1976.)

Box 6–1. Abducens Nucleus

- The conjugate, horizontal gaze center that houses abducens motoneurons, abducens internuclear neurons, and PMT neurons*
- Axons of abducens twitch and non-twitch motoneurons project in the sixth cranial nerve to innervate the ipsilateral lateral rectus muscle
- Axons of abducens internuclear neurons cross the midline to ascend in the medial longitudinal fasciculus to contact contralateral medial rectus motoneurons in the oculomotor nucleus

(For related clinical disorders, see Box 12–5, Chapter 12; *PMT neurons are defined in Box 6–4.)

Box 6–2. Medial Longitudinal Fasciculus (MLF)

- Conveys axons from neurons concerned with horizontal, vertical, and torsional conjugate gaze
- For horizontal gaze: Axons from abducens internuclear neurons, which carry the conjugate eye movement command, project to medial rectus motoneurons in the contralateral oculomotor nucleus
- For vertical and torsional gaze: Axons from vestibular nuclei, which carry signals contributing to smooth pursuit, the rotational vestibulo-ocular reflex and otolith-ocular reflexes and gaze holding project to the oculomotor and trochlear nuclei, and the interstitial nucleus of Cajal

(For related clinical disorders, see Box 12–7, in Chapter 12.)

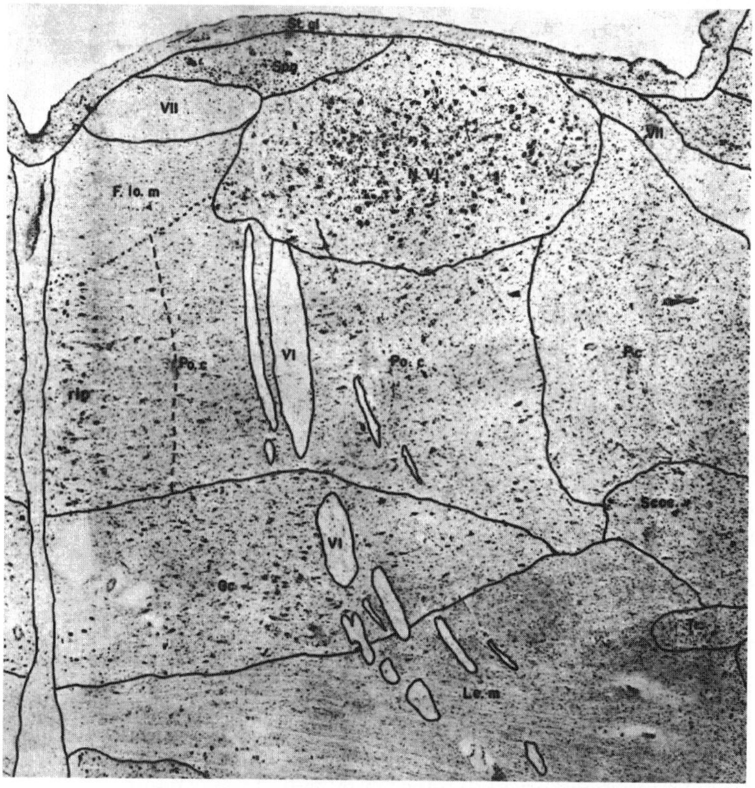

Figure 6–2. Human brainstem section showing pontine tegmentum at the level of the abducens nucleus (N.VI). The close relationship between the medial longitudinal fasciculus (F.lo.m), nucleus reticularis pontis caudalis (Po.c), which houses excitatory saccadic burst neurons, and nucleus raphe interpositus (rip), which is the location of omnipause neurons, is evident. VI: abducens nerve; VII: facial nerve; Gc: nucleus gigantocellularis; Le.m: medial lemniscus; Pc: nucleus parvocellularis; Scoe.v: nucleus subcoeruleus, subnucleus ventralis; Spg: Nucleus suprageniculatus; St.gl: Stratum gliosum subependymale; Tr: nucleus trapezoidalis. (Reproduced from Olszewski and Baxter,[322] with permission of S. Karger AG, Basel.)

Box 6–3. Paramedian Pontine Reticular Formation (PPRF)

- A physiologically defined entity that houses the vital machinery for horizontal saccades, including excitatory and inhibitory burst neurons (which lie in the rostral medulla) and omnipause neurons
- Excitatory burst neurons lie in the dorsomedial nucleus reticularis pontis caudalis (nrpc), rostral to the level of the abducens nucleus, receive inhibitory inputs from omnipause neurons and inhibitory burst neurons, and project monosynaptically to the ipsilateral abducens nucleus
- Inhibitory burst neurons lie in the medial portion of the nucleus paragigantocellularis dorsalis (pgd), caudal to the abducens nucleus (rostral medulla), receive inhibitory inputs from omnipause neurons, other inhibitory burst neurons, and ipsilateral excitatory burst neurons; project monosynaptically to the contralateral abducens nucleus
- Omnipause neurons lie in the nucleus raphe interpositus (rip), close to the midline, at the level of the abducens nucleus, receive inputs from long-lead burst neurons, the rostral pole (fixation zone) of the superior colliculus, and fastigial nucleus, and project to excitatory and inhibitory burst neurons for horizontal and vertical saccades

(For related clinical disorders, see Box 12–6, in Chapter 12.)

burst neurons located contralaterally, in the paramedian reticular formation caudal to the abducens nucleus, at the pontomedullary junction.[191,419] Inhibitory burst neurons are driven by monosynaptic projections from ipsilateral excitatory burst neurons (see Chapter 3). Pursuit signals are relayed from the cerebellum, in part via the vestibular nuclei.[127,228] The output of the gaze-holding network (neural integrator) reaches the abducens nucleus from the nucleus prepositus hypoglossi (NPH) and adjacent medial vestibular nucleus (MVN).[21,228] The abducens nucleus also receives a projection from the contralateral medial rectus subdivision of the oculomotor complex (oculomotor internuclear neurons), which contributes to the control of conjugate gaze.[81,228]

In addition to inputs via the MLF, medial rectus motoneurons receive direct projections from neurons in the ipsilateral vestibular nucleus via the *ascending tract of Deiters* (see Fig. 2–3, Chapter 2),[266,309,365] which runs lateral to the MLF and may play a role in adjusting the vestibular responses during near-viewing.[77,78] Medial rectus motoneurons also receive inputs for vergence eye movements from neurons in the mesencephalic reticular formation, which lie dorsolateral to the oculomotor nucleus.[56,263]

All the neurons that project to the abducens nucleus also send axon collaterals to a continuum of cell clusters that lie close to the MLF and other paramedian tracts in the caudal pons and medulla; these have been called the *cell groups of the paramedian tracts* (PMT) (see Box 6–4 and Fig. 6–3).[61,62] One of these cell groups lies in the rostral-medial part of the abducens nucleus.[114] The PMT cell groups, in turn, project to the cerebellar flocculus, paraflocculus, and vermis of the cerebellum.[52,62] In this way, the cerebellum may receive feedback about all motor signals flowing to the abducens nucleus. The possible role of the PMT pathway is discussed further under the section on the Cerebellar Influences on Gaze.

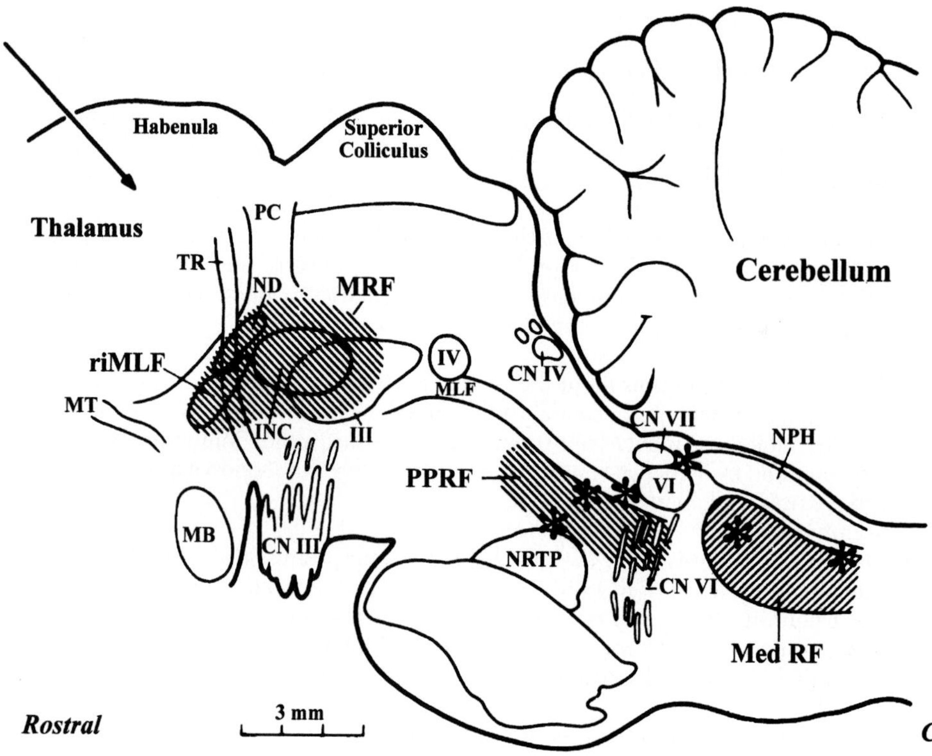

Figure 6–3. A sagittal section of the monkey brain stem showing the location of the rostral interstitial nucleus of the medial longitudinal fasciculus (riMLF) and other structures important in the control of vertical and horizontal gaze. The shaded areas indicate the mesencephalic reticular formation (MRF), paramedian pontine reticular formation (PPRF), and medullary reticular formation (Med RF). The asterisks indicate the location of cell groups of the paramedian tracts, which project to the flocculus. III: oculomotor nucleus; IV: trochlear nucleus; VI: abducens nucleus; CN III: rootlets of the oculomotor nerve; CN IV: trochlear nerve; CN VI: rootlets of the abducens nerve; INC: interstitial nucleus of Cajal; MB: mammillary body; MT: mammillothalamic tract; ND: nucleus of Darkschewitsch; NRTP: nucleus reticularis tegmenti pontis; PC: posterior commissure; NPH: nucleus prepositus hypoglossi; TR: tractus retroflexus. The arrow refers to the Horsley-Clarke plane of section. (Adapted from Büttner-Ennever JA, Horn AKE. Pathways from cell groups of the paramedian tracts of the floccular region. Ann NY Acad Sci 781, 532–540, 1996, with permission of the New York Academy of Sciences.)

Box 6–4. Cell Groups of the Paramedian Tracts (PMT)

- Clusters of neurons scattered along the midline fiber tracts in the pons and medulla
- Receive inputs from essentially all structures that project to ocular motoneurons
- Project to the flocculus, paraflocculus and vermis of the cerebellum
- May provide the flocculus with an "efference copy" of eye movement commands for gaze holding or more long-term adaptation

(For possible clinical significance, see Pathogenesis of Central Vestibular Nystagmus, and Pathogenesis of Nystagmus Occurring with Visual System Disorders in Chapter 10.)

Interpretation of the Effects of Discrete Lesions on Pathways for Horizontal Gaze

A test of the validity of the anatomic scheme shown in Figure 6–1 is its ability to account for the effects of discrete lesions on horizontal eye movements (see Video Display: Pontine Syndromes). *Lesions of the abducens nucleus* produce paralysis of both the ipsilateral lateral rectus and contralateral medial rectus for all conjugate eye movements (see Box 12–5).[30,68,268,273,291] Vergence is spared, since these movements mainly depend on projections that pass directly to medial rectus motoneurons. Saccadic, pursuit, optokinetic, and vestibular movements are still present in the contralateral hemifield, but are impaired when directed towards the side of the lesion. Contraversive saccades are preserved because they depend on the intact abducens nucleus, which receives projections from excitatory burst neurons in the ipsilateral PPRF. Saccades directed towards the side of the lesion are also present in the contralateral hemifield of movement, but they are slow. This is because they must now depend solely on projections to the intact abducens nucleus from the inhibitory burst neurons of the contralateral medullary reticular formation, so that saccadic peak velocity becomes a function of antagonist muscle relaxation rather than agonist contraction. Another finding with abducens nerve palsies is horizontal gaze-evoked nystagmus on looking contralaterally. This nystagmus is probably due to involvement of fibers of passage from the medial vestibular nucleus, which provide an eye position signal to the contralateral abducens nucleus.[291] This explanation is supported by the report that a discrete experimental lesion made between the abducens nuclei caused profound, bilateral gaze-holding failure.[4] Alternatively, it might be due to involvement of the PMT cell group that lies at the rostral pole of the abducens nucleus, and probably contributes to horizontal gaze holding via its projections to the cerebellum.[62,291]

Lesions of the medial longitudinal fasciculus produce *internuclear ophthalmoplegia* (INO) (see Box 12–7), which is characterized by paresis of adduction for conjugate movements on the side of the lesion (see Video Display: Pontine Syndromes).[70,116,137] Adduction is still possible with convergence, because of direct vergence inputs to medial rectus motoneurons (see Figure 6–1) (see Video Display: Pontine Syndromes). Thus, when INO is produced experimentally by lidocaine blockade of the MLF between the levels of the trochlear and abducens nuclei, the vergence response is preserved or even increased.[137] More rostral lesions of the MLF may impair vergence if the medial rectus motoneurons, or their vergence inputs, are involved. With complete lesions of the MLF, the eye does not adduct across the midline with any conjugate movements, implying that extra-MLF pathways, such as the ascending tract of Deiters, can only play a minor role in the horizontal vestibulo-ocular reflex. A combined lesion of one MLF and the abducens nucleus on the same side produces paralysis of all conjugate movements save for abduction of the eye contralateral to the side of the lesion— "one-and-a-half" syndrome (see Box 12–8).[122,342] This syndrome could has also been attributed to an infarction that bilaterally affects the MLF and the abducens nucleus on one side.[123]

Discrete *lesions of the paramedian pontine reticular formation (PPRF)* cause loss of saccades and quick phases of nystagmus to the side of the lesion (see Box 12–6).[149,173] Experimental lesions in the PPRF, using excitotoxins that spare fibers of passage, leave smooth pursuit, the vestibulo-ocular reflex, and gaze-holding ability intact;[173] similar sparing is sometimes encountered with clinical lesions.[163,218] Often, however, lesions of the pons that affect the PPRF also involve axons conveying vestibular and pursuit inputs to the abducens nucleus.[344] Furthermore, lesions that affect the excitatory burst neurons may also affect omnipause neurons, which lie in the adjacent nucleus raphe interpositus, close to the midline at the level of the abducens nerve (Fig. 6–2),[57,189,322] and which inhibit all burst neurons except during saccades. Involvement of omnipause neurons might account for the slowing of vertical, as well as horizontal, saccades that is sometimes reported after bilateral pontine lesions.[163,173]

Unilateral lesions affecting the vestibular nuclei—such as in Wallenberg's syndrome (lateral medullary infarction) (see Fig. 12–2)—may produce an ocular motor imbalance manifest by spontaneous nystagmus, skew deviation, and the ocular tilt reaction. An additional finding—lateropulsion of saccades (see

Video Display: Medullary Syndromes)—may reflect interruption of axons running in the inferior cerebellar peduncle from the inferior olivary nucleus to the cerebellum (Fig. 3–16).[457] Bilateral, experimental lesions of the nucleus prepositus hypoglossi -medial vestibular complex—the NPH-MVN region—abolish the gaze-holding mechanism (neural integrator) for eye movements in the horizontal plane (Chapter 5).[12,64]

BRAINSTEM CONNECTIONS FOR VERTICAL AND TORSIONAL MOVEMENTS

The ocular motoneurons concerned with vertical and torsional eye movements lie in the oculomotor nucleus and trochlear nucleus. How do these motoneurons receive signals for each functional class of eye movement? A partial dichotomy is evident, with vertical saccadic commands and gaze-holding (neural integrator) innervation being generated in the midbrain, and vestibular and pursuit signals arising from the lower brainstem.[186]

The Substrate for Vertical Saccades

Vertical and torsional saccades are generated in the *rostral interstitial nucleus of the medial longitudinal fasciculus (riMLF)*, a region of the rostral mesencephalon in the prerubral fields, rostral to the tractus retroflexus and caudal to the mammillothalamic tract (Box 6–5) (see Fig. 6–3 and Fig. 6–4).[52,54,187] In the past, this structure has also been called the nucleus of the prerubral fields and the nucleus of the fields of Forel. Although the riMLF lies adjacent to other mesencephalic reticular nuclei, particularly the interstitial nucleus of Cajal, its physiologic properties and anatomic connections make it a distinct functional entity. It contains several morphological types of neurons that include medium-sized excitatory burst neurons for vertical and torsional saccades and quick phases.[50,96,286–288] Corresponding inhibitory

Box 6–5. Rostral Interstitial Nucleus of the Medial Longitudinal Fasciculus (riMLF)

- A wing-shaped structure that lies dorsomedial to red nucleus, rostral to INC, and caudal to the posterior branch of the thalamo-subthalamic paramedian artery
- Houses most burst neurons for vertical and torsional saccades; burst neurons for clockwise movements (right eye extorts, left eye intorts) lie in the right riMLF; those for counterclockwise movements lie in the left riMLF
- Receives inputs from omnipause neurons in the pontine nucleus raphe interpositus, superior colliculus, nucleus of the posterior commissure, long-lead burst neurons of midbrain and rostral PPRF, cerebellar fastigial nucleus, and contralateral riMLF via the ventral commissure
- Projects predominantly to the ipsilateral oculomotor and trochlear nuclei, each burst neuron sending axon collaterals to motoneurons supplying yoke muscle pairs (Hering's law for vertical movements); projections to motoneurons innervating the superior rectus and inferior oblique are bilateral, crossing within the oculomotor nucleus complex
- Also projects to the ipsilateral interstitial nucleus of Cajal, to cell groups of the paramedian tracts, and to the spinal cord (for head movements)

(For related clinical disorders, see Box 12–10, in Chapter 12.)

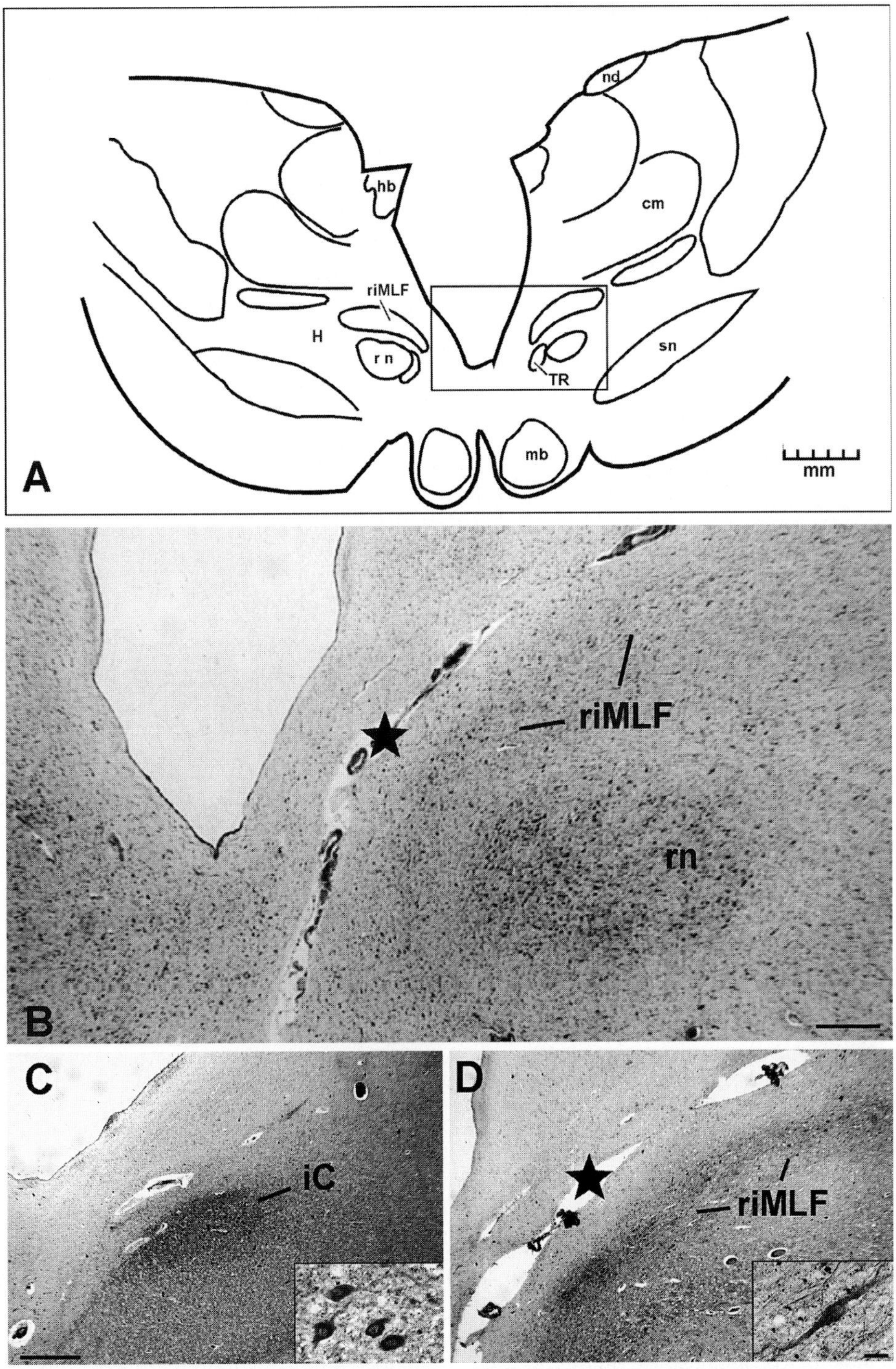

Figure 6–4. Transverse section of rostral mesencephalon of human brainstem showing structures important for vertical gaze. (A) Schematic showing location of riMLF with respect to the rostral pole of the red nucleus (rn), substantia nigra (sn), H-fields of Forell (H) , habenular (hb), centromedian nucleus of the thalamus (cm), nucleus of Darkschweitz (nd), mammillary body (mb), and the tractus retroflexus (TR), which separates the riMLF from the more caudal interstitial nucleus of Cajal (iC). (B) Nissl stained section showing riMLF, which is dorsally bordered by the posterior thalamo-subthalamic paramedian artery (star). (C) and (D) are microphotographs immunocytochemically labeled with PAV-antibodies.[190] The iC is highlighted by its PAV content and forms a compact nucleus; the inset shows that iC neurons are round and densely packed. The riMLF contains elongated neurons (presumed burst neurons) that are oriented parallel to the mediolateral axis of the riMLF. Scale bar: 500 μm (B,C,D); 30 μm (insets of C,D). (Courtesy of A.K.E. Horn, Munich, Germany.)

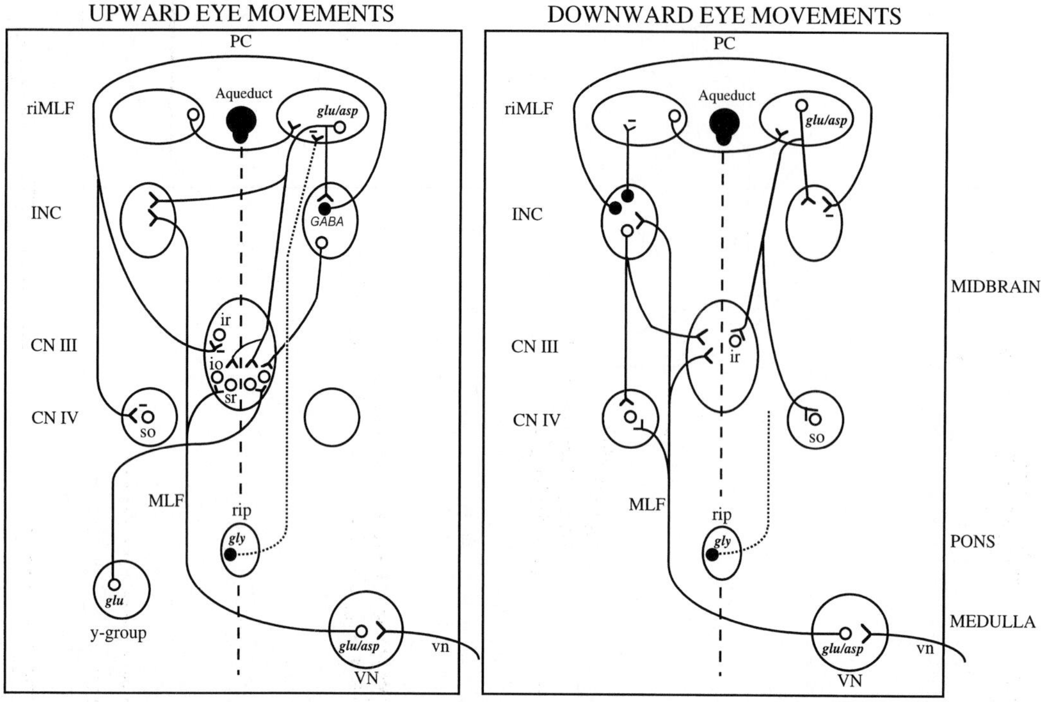

Figure 6–5. Anatomic hypothetical scheme for the synthesis of upward, downward, and torsional eye movements. From the vertical semicircular canals, primary afferents on the vestibular nerve (vn) synapse in the vestibular nuclei (VN) and ascend in the medial longitudinal fasciculus (MLF), as well as the crossing ventral tegmental tract and brachium conjunctivum (not shown) to contact neurons in the trochlear nucleus (CN IV), oculomotor nucleus (CN III), and the interstitial nucleus of Cajal (INC). (For clarity, only excitatory vestibular projections are shown; more details about vestibular projections may be found in Figure 2–3 and Table 2–2 of Chapter 2.) The rostral interstitial nucleus of the medial longitudinal fasciculus (riMLF), which lies in the prerubral fields, contains excitatory saccadic burst neurons. It receives an inhibitory input from omnipause neurons of the nucleus raphe interpositus (rip), which lie in the pons (for clarity, this projection is only shown for upward movements). Excitatory burst neurons in riMLF project to the motoneurons of CN III and CN IV, and also send an axon collateral to INC. Each riMLF neuron sends axon collaterals to yoke-pair muscles (Hering's law). Projections to the elevator subnuclei, which innervate the superior rectus (sr) and inferior oblique (io) motoneurons may be bilateral due to axon collaterals crossing at the level of the CN III nucleus.[286-288] Inhibitory burst neurons for upward saccades lie in the INC and project, via the posterior commissure (PC), to inferior rectus (ir) and superior oblique (so) motoneurons; corresponding projections for downward saccades are less well understood, and are not shown.[186,192] The INC provides a gaze-holding signal, and projects to vertical motoneurons. The INC also probably sends inhibitory projections to riMLF and the contralateral INC (shown only in Downward Eye Movement panel, for clarity). Signals contributing to vertical smooth pursuit and eye-head tracking reach CN III from the y-group via the brachium conjunctivum and crossing ventral tegmental tract. Neurotransmitters: asp=aspartate; glu=glutamate; gly=glycine. Inhibitory projections are indicated by black cell bodies and a negative sign at the synapse.

burst neurons may reside in the adjacent interstitial nucleus of Cajal,[192] which is described below. Each riMLF contains neurons that burst for upward and downward eye movements, but for torsional quick phases in only one direction. Thus, the right riMLF discharges for quick phases that are directed clockwise with respect to the subject;[286,288] that is, the top poles of both eyes rotate toward the side that is activated. In the cat, neurons projecting to muscles that depress the eye (inferior rectus and superior oblique) may be located more rostrally, whereas projections to muscles that elevate the eye (superior rectus and inferior oblique) lie more caudally;[464] it is unclear whether this is also the case in primates. The postulated projections of the riMLF and the associated neurotransmitters are summarized in Figure 6–5. Each riMLF projects predominantly to the ipsilateral oculomotor and trochlear nuclei; however, projections to motoneurons innervating the elevator muscles appear to be bilateral, with axon collaterals probably crossing to the opposite side at the level of the motoneurons, and not in the posterior commissure.[286–288] Furthermore, each burst neuron in the riMLF appears to send axon collaterals to motoneurons supplying yoke muscle pairs; this appears to be part of the neural substrate for Hering's law of equal innervation in the vertical plane.[281,285] Axons from the riMLF neurons also send collaterals to the interstitial nucleus of Cajal (bilaterally for upward burst neurons), and to the PMT cell groups,[62] which project to the cerebellum. The riMLF receives an ascending projection from omnipause neurons in the pons.[52,303]

Interpretation of Effects of Discrete Lesions on Substrate for Vertical Saccades

The anatomic scheme shown in Figure 6–5 has been tested by studying the effects of discrete lesions on vertical saccades (see Video Display: Midbrain Syndromes). Unilateral, *experimental lesions of the riMLF* using excitotoxins that spare fibers of passage, cause a mild defect in vertical movements, consisting of slowing of downward saccades (see Box 12–10).[425] This slowing probably occurs because each nucleus contains burst neurons for both upward and downward movements, but projections to motoneurons innervating depression are ipsilateral, whereas those innervating the elevators may be bilateral.[286–288] On the other hand, a severe, specific defect of torsional quick phases is produced.[425] For example, with a lesion of the right riMLF, torsional quick phases, clockwise from the point of view of the subject (extorsion of the right eye and intorsion of the left eye—with top poles rotating towards the side of the lesion) are lost; in addition, there is a static, contralesional torsional deviation, with torsional nystagmus beating contralesionally. Similarly, a lesion of the left riMLF impairs counterclockwise quick phases. Unilateral riMLF lesions in humans are reported to produce similar but generally more severe defects, probably partly due to involvement of adjacent structures.[171,239]

Bilateral experimental lesions of the riMLF in monkeys abolish vertical and torsional saccades,[425] but vertical gaze holding, vestibular eye movements, and pursuit are preserved, as are horizontal saccades. Patients with discrete, bilateral infarction in the region of the riMLF usually show deficits of either downward saccades (see Video Display: Midbrain Syndromes) or both upward and downward saccades.[55,352]

Box 6–6. Interstitial Nucleus of Cajal (INC)

- Contains several populations of neurons: One set makes major contribution to the neural integrator (gaze-holding mechanism) for vertical and torsional gaze; another contributes to eye-head coordination in roll; inhibitory vertical burst neurons may also reside in INC
- Receives inputs from burst neurons in the riMLF, the vestibular nuclei, and the y-group
- Commissural projections are contralateral (via the posterior commissure) to ocular motoneurons of CN III and CN IV and to the opposite INC
- Ascending projections are to mesencephalic reticular formation, zona incerta, riMLF, and nuclei of the central thalamus
- Descending projections are to nucleus gigantocellularis of pontine reticular formation (for head movements), vestibular nuclei, PMT cell groups in medulla, and cervical cord

(For related clinical disorders, see Box 12–11, in Chapter 12.)

Box 6–7. Posterior Commissure

- Contains axons from INC projecting to contralateral CN III, CN IV, and INC
- Also contains axons from the nucleus of the posterior commissure projecting to contralateral riMLF and INC, which may be important for upgaze; and to the "M" group of neurons, which may be important for coordination of vertical eye and lid movements

(For related clinical disorders, see Box 12–12, in Chapter 12.)

The Substrate for Vertical Gaze Holding

A critical structure for *vertical gaze holding* (the neural integrator) is the *interstitial nucleus of Cajal (INC)* (Box 6–6). This nucleus contains several distinct populations of neurons.[479] In the monkey, some neurons in the INC encode the complete, vertical, burst-tonic, ocular motor signal.[213] The INC receives inputs from the vestibular nuclei, y-group, and axon collaterals from burst neurons in the riMLF.[215, 217] In addition, the INC may house inhibitory burst neurons for vertical and torsional saccades.[192] The INC projects to vertical motoneurons in the oculomotor and trochlear subnuclei on the contralateral side of the brainstem via the *posterior commissure* (Box 6–7).[217]

The INC also contains neurons that project to motoneurons of the neck and trunk muscles, and appears to coordinate combined eye-head movements in torsional and vertical planes. Stimulation near the INC in the monkey produces an *ocular tilt reaction* (see Fig. 11–5) that consists of an *ipsilateral* head tilt and a synkinetic ocular reaction: depression and extorsion of the eye ipsilateral to the stimulation and elevation and intorsion of the contralateral eye;[467] similar findings have been reported in a human patient.[248]

Interpretation of Effects of Discrete Lesions on Substrate for Vertical Gaze Holding

Pharmacological *inactivation of the INC* with muscimol causes impaired vertical and torsional gaze holding after a saccade carries the eye to a tertiary (oblique) position.[92,93] The vertical range of saccades is impaired, but these movements are not slowed.[170] The gaze-holding signal following a vestibular eye movement may also depend on ascending signals from the nucleus prepositus hypoglossi. Experimental *inactivation of the posterior commissure* with lidocaine causes failure of vertical gaze-holding function, with centripetal drifts of the eyes following vertical saccades.[330] Larger destructive lesions severely limit vertical eye movements, especially upward;[333,334] it is possible that such lesions also affect other structures, such as the nucleus of the posterior commissure,[287] which normally contribute to upward gaze.

Experimental, unilateral lesions of the INC also cause an *ocular tilt reaction* with *contralateral* head tilt, skew deviation with hypertropia of the ipsilateral eye, extorsion of the contralateral eye, and intorsion of the ipsilateral eye (see Video Display: Disorders of the Vestibular System). This pattern of ocular tilt reaction is similar to that produced by stimulation of the contralateral utricular nerve,[424] and is encountered clinically with a variety of brainstem lesions that involve central otolithic pathways.[39] Bilateral inactivation or lesions of INC restrict the vertical ocular motor range, and cause upbeat nystagmus and neck retroflexion.[170]

The Neural Substrate for Vertical Vestibular and Smooth Pursuit

The neural signals necessary for vertical vestibular and pursuit eye movements as well as contributions to the vertical gaze-holding command ascend from the medulla and pons to the midbrain. The MLF is an important route for these projections, but the brachium conjunctivum (superior cerebellar peduncle) and other pathways, including the ventral tegmental tract, which crosses at the rostral pole of the nucleus reticularis tegmenti pontis,[445] are also involved. Details of ascending vestibular projections are summarized in Figure 2–3 and Table 2–2 of Chapter 2. The ascending axons concerned with vertical eye movements arise from vestibular nucleus neurons that have been called position-vestibular-pause cells.[440] They carry an eye position signal and a head velocity signal and cease discharging during vertical saccades. These fibers also convey an eye velocity signal during vertical smooth pursuit, but during combined eye-head tracking (see Chapter 7), when the eyes may be nearly stationary in the orbits, a head velocity signal is still present on these axons. This vestibular signal must be canceled by another equal and opposite signal, which also projects to the oculomotor and trochlear nuclei. One mechanism that might make possible such *cancellation of the* vestibulo-ocular reflex during vertical eye-head tracking is a gaze velocity signal that ascends from the dorsal portion of the *y-group* (Box 6–8), a small collection of cells that cap the inferior cerebellar peduncle.[67,80,331,332,384,413] The y-group receives afferents from flocculus Purkinje cells, and projects to the oculomotor and trochlear nuclei via the brachium conjunctivum and the crossing ventral tegmental tract.

Interpretation of Effects of Discrete Lesions on Substrate for Vertical Pursuit and Vestibular Eye Movements

Consistent with these projections, *bilateral lesions of the medial longitudinal fasciculus* cause bilateral INO, and impair vertical vestibular and smooth-pursuit movements, but spare vertical saccades (see Box 12–7).[116,364] In addition, partial loss of the vertical eye position signal causes vertical gaze-evoked nystagmus. Unilateral INO also impairs the vertical vestibulo-ocular responses when the contralateral posterior canal is stimulated, but the defect is smaller during stimulation of the contralateral anterior canal,[95] since its central connections partially ascend in pathways other than the MLF, such as the crossing ventral tegmental tract (Fig. 2–3).[363,445]

Other Midbrain Neurons that Contribute to Control of Vertical Gaze

The *nucleus of the posterior commissure* (nPC) contains neurons that burst for upward saccades,[286,287] and project through the posterior

Box 6–8. y-Group

- A small collection of cells that cap the inferior cerebellar peduncle. Receives afferents from flocculus Purkinje cells, and projects to the oculomotor and trochlear nuclei via the brachium conjunctivum and a crossing ventral tegmental tract
- Dorsal y-group cells increase their discharge during upward smooth pursuit, optokinetic following, and combined eye-head tracking (vestibulo-ocular reflex suppression), but show no consistent modulation during vestibulo-ocular reflex in darkness
- Along with flocculus, may contribute to adaptation of the vertical vestibulo-ocular reflex

(For functional significance, see Neural Substrate for Eye-Head Pursuit, in Chapter 7 and Electrophysiological Aspects of Vestibulocerebellum control of the vestibulo-ocular reflex in Chapter 2.)

commissure to contact the riMLF, INC, and the intralaminar thalamic nuclei.[52]

The *central mesencephalic reticular formation* (cMRF) (Box 6–9), which contains the nucleus subcuneiformis, plays an important role in the control of horizontal and vertical saccades.[84,459] It receives inputs from the PPRF, nucleus of the posterior commissure, fastigial nucleus, and cortical eye fields, and has reciprocal connections with the superior colliculus, which is discussed in Chapter 3. The cMRF also projects to the omnipause neurons and nucleus reticularis tegmenti pontis (NRTP),[83, 159,459] so that it may play an important role in gating saccades. Experimental lesions of the cMRF cause hypermetria of contralateral and upward saccades and hypometria of ipsilateral and downward saccades.[458,460,461] In addition, fixation is disrupted by saccadic intrusions directed away from the side of inactivation (see Box 12–13). Human lesions affecting the mesencephalic reticular formation cause contralateral saccadic palsy,[473] possibly interrupting descending pathways to the contralateral PPRF.

Additional midbrain regions that may contribute to saccades include the *zona incerta*,[255] and the *periaqueductal gray matter*, which contain neurons, some of which discharge in relation to vertical saccades and vertical eye position, and other that cease discharging during vertical saccades. The function of these neurons is presently unknown.[208]

An important structure in the coordination of vertical saccades and eyelid movements is the *M-group of neurons*, which lies rostral to the interstitial nucleus of Cajal and medial to riMLF. The M-group appears to receive inputs from upward burst neurons in the riMLF, and may have connections with the nucleus of the posterior commissure. It projects to both the elevator subnuclei of the eye (superior rectus and inferior oblique) and the motoneurons of the levator palpebrae superioris in the central caudal subdivision of the oculomotor nucleus.[188] It is postulated that M-group lesions would disrupt lid-eye coordination during vertical saccades.[63] The nucleus of Darkschewitsch doe not seem to be involved in the control of eye movements.[52]

CEREBELLAR INFLUENCES ON GAZE

The cerebellum (Fig. 6–6) optimizes eye movements so that they are calibrated to ensure clearest vision. Two main subdivisions of the cerebellum play an important role in the control of eye movements: (1) the vestibulocerebellum (flocculus, paraflocculus, nodulus, and ventral uvula) and (2) the dorsal vermis of

Box 6–9. Central Mesencephalic Reticular Formation (cMRF)

- Extending rostral and caudal to the posterior commissure; in coronal section, a line extending laterally from the aqueduct divides into dorsal (nucleus cuneiformis) and ventral segment (nucleus subcuneiformis)
- Reciprocal, topographically arranged connections with motor superior colliculus; receives projections from PPRF, nucleus of posterior commissure, fastigial nucleus, cortical eye fields
- Projects to nucleus reticularis tegmenti pontis (NRTP) and omnipause neurons in nucleus raphe interpositus in the pons
- May contribute to programming of both horizontal and vertical saccades through reciprocal connections with superior colliculus and brainstem nuclei

(For related clinical disorders, see Box 12–13, in Chapter 12.)

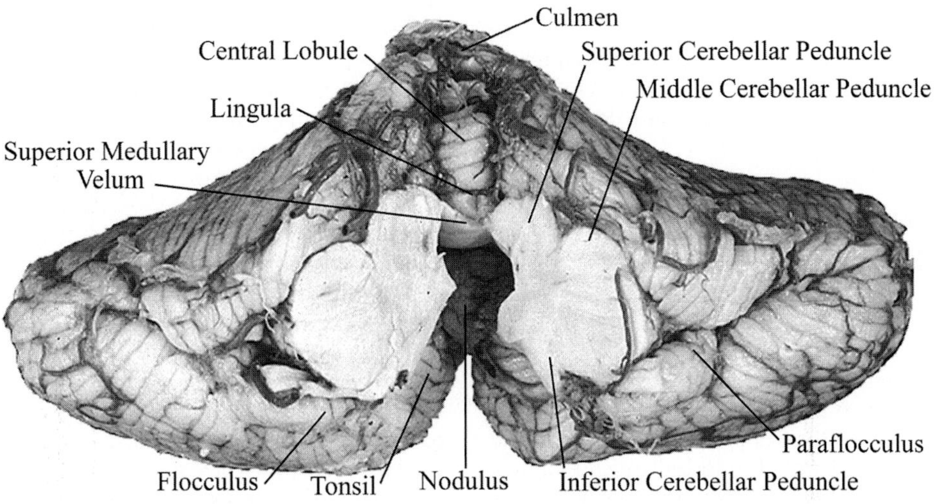

A

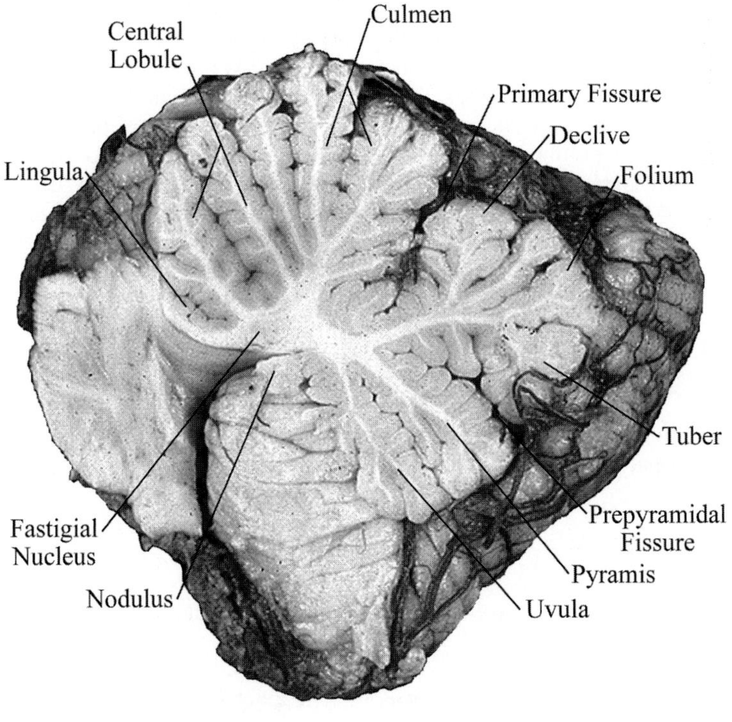

B

Figure 6–6. Gross anatomy of the human cerebellum. (A) Inferior surface, after removal from brain stem by transection of cerebellar peduncles. (B) View of sagittally sectioned cerebellum showing lobules of the cerebellar vermis.

the posterior lobe, and the underlying posterior portion of the fastigial nucleus.[452] Here we focus on contributions of the cerebellum to conjugate eye movements; influences on vergence and ocular alignment are discussed in Chapter 8.

Contributions of the Flocculus and Paraflocculus

The flocculi are paired structures which, in the human brain, lie adjacent to the tonsils (paraflocculi), ventral to the inferior cerebellar peduncle, and next to the eighth cranial nerve (Fig. 6–6 and Box 6–10).[453,454] In primates, the caudal five folia of the flocculi receive mossy fiber inputs mainly from the vestibular nucleus and nerve, the nucleus prepositus hypoglossi (NPH), the nucleus reticularis tegmenti pontis, and the mesencephalic reticular formation. The adjacent ventral paraflocculi receive inputs mainly from the contralateral pontine nuclei.[299] Both the flocculi and paraflocculi receive climbing fiber inputs from the contralateral inferior olivary nucleus (Figs. 6–1 and 3–16), which may provide information important for adaptive ocular motor control.[21,147,227,299] On the basis of this pattern of inputs, it is suggested that the flocculus is more important for controlling the vestibulo-ocular reflex, whereas the paraflocculus mainly contributes to smooth pursuit.[299,452,454]

One further important input to the flocculus is from the cell groups of the paramedian tracts (PMT), which receive inputs from essentially all premotor structures that project to ocular motoneurons (Box 6–4).[61,62] The PMT cell groups provide a larger projection to the flocculus than does the vestibular nuclei. One PMT cell group in the medulla—nucleus pararaphales—receives inputs from the INC and projects via the ventrolateral surface of the medulla and inferior cerebellar peduncle to the flocculus and ventral paraflocculus.[62] Neurons in another probable PMT cell group— the nucleus incertus—have been shown to contain "burst-tonic" neurons,[79] and so it seems possible that the PMT cell groups send an efference copy of eye movement commands to the flocculus.[61] Such a signal could be important for normal function of the gaze-holding (neural integrator) network, or for the adaptive control of eye movements. Inactivation of components of the PMT cell groups causes failure of the neural integrator.[301]

The main efferent pathways of the flocculus and paraflocculus are to the ipsilateral superior and medial vestibular nuclei, and the y-group.[226,300] The Purkinje cells in the flocculus

Box 6–10. Vestibulocerebellum: Flocculus and Paraflocculus

- Main floccular inputs are from the vestibular nuclei, nucleus prepositus hypoglossi, inferior olivary nucleus, and cells group of the paramedian tracts (PMT)
- Dorsal and ventral paraflocculus receive main inputs from pontine nuclei
- Main outputs are to ipsilateral superior and medial vestibular nuclei, and y-group
- Important for stabilizing the eyes with respect to a visual scene or object. Contribute to vestibulo-visual interactions, gaze holding, smooth-pursuit or combined eye-head tracking, and to plasticity of the vestibulo-ocular reflex—by providing the brainstem with signals necessary for adaptive changes

(For related clinical disorders, see Box 12–2, in Chapter 12.)

that project to vestibular nucleus neurons may influence the generation of compensatory eye movements during self-rotation,[78,456] regulate the phase of the vestibulo-ocular reflex,[99,412] and contribute to the transformation of vestibular and visual signals into a common frame of reference.[97,221] In addition, the floccular Purkinje cells play an important role in the adaptive control of both the vestibulo-ocular reflex and smooth pursuit.[65,244,361] Although some Purkinje cells in both the flocculus and ventral paraflocculus encode gaze velocity discharge during smooth pursuit and combined eye-head tracking,[243,272] as noted above, the ventral paraflocculus seems more concerned with control of smooth pursuit, while the flocculus is more concerned with governance of the vestibulo-ocular reflex.[299,362]

Interpretation of Effects of Discrete Lesions on the Flocculus and Paraflocculus

Surgical lesions of the flocculus and paraflocculus in monkeys produce a characteristic syndrome that is similar to that encountered clinically in patients with the Arnold-Chiari malformation (see Table 12–1 and Video Display: Cerebellar Syndromes).[475] This includes downbeat nystagmus, impaired smooth pursuit and eye-head tracking, as well as impaired gaze holding (deficient neural integrator). The gaze-holding deficit probably reflects loss of the contribution of the cerebellum to the fidelity of the brainstem neural integrator, which lies in the medial vestibular nuclei and the nucleus prepositus hypoglossi.[12,64] Pharmacological inactivation of the flocculus impairs ipsilateral smooth pursuit and cancellation of the vestibulo-ocular reflex during passive rotation,[23] but not during active eye-head tracking.[24] Another important deficit caused by floccular-parafloccular lesions is loss of ability to adapt the properties of the vestibulo-ocular reflex in response to visual demands.[360]

Contributions of the Nodulus and Ventral Uvula

The nodulus, which is the midline portion of the flocculo-nodular lobe, lying immediately caudal to the inferior medullary velum, and the adjacent ventral uvula receive afferents from the vestibular nuclei, nucleus prepositus hypoglossi, inferior olivary nucleus, and vestibular nerve (Fig. 6–6 and Box 6–11).[379,383,452,462] The nodulus and ventral uvula project to the vestibular nuclei and control the velocity-storage mechanism of the vestibulo-ocular reflex, by which the response of this reflex to low-frequency stimuli is enhanced.[406,455] The effects of velocity storage are best illustrated by considering the duration of nystagmus that ensues following the onset of a sustained, constant-velocity rotation: such nystagmus lasts two or three times longer than could be accounted for by the mechanical properties of the cupula and endolymph.

Box 6–11. Vestibulocerebellum: Nodulus and Ventral Uvula

- Main afferents are medial and inferior vestibular nuclei, nucleus prepositus hypoglossi, inferior olivary nucleus, and vestibular nerve
- Main projections are to the vestibular nuclei
- Controls velocity-storage mechanism of the vestibulo-ocular reflex, by which responses of secondary vestibular neurons are prolonged beyond those in primary vestibular neurons

(For related clinical disorders, see Box 12–3, in Chapter 12.)

Interpretation of Effects of Discrete Lesions on the Nodulus and Ventral Uvula

Some examples of lesions of this part of the vestibulocerebellum are shown on the Video Displays: Cerebellar Syndromes and Periodic Alternating Nystagmus. In monkeys, lesions of the nodulus and uvula maximize the velocity-storage effect; maneuvers that will usually reduce it, such as pitching the head forward during post-rotational nystagmus, are ineffective.[455] Similar effects are seen in patients with midline cerebellar tumors that involve the nodulus.[158] In addition, when monkeys that have nodular lesions are placed in darkness, they develop periodic alternating nystagmus.[455] Thus, to clinicians, the most important result produced by lesions affecting the nodulus and ventral uvula is periodic alternating nystagmus,[138] which may be present during attempted visual fixation if adjacent flocculus and paraflocculus are also involved (Chapter 10).

Contributions of the Dorsal Vermis

Lobules VI and VII of the *dorsal vermis* (parts of the declive, folium, tuber, and pyramis) (Fig. 6–6 and Box 6–12) receive mossy fiber inputs from the paramedian pontine reticular formation (PPRF), nucleus reticularis tegmenti pontis (NRTP), dorsolateral and dorsomedial pontine nuclei, vestibular nuclei, and nucleus prepositus hypoglossi, as well as climbing fiber inputs from the inferior olivary nucleus.[41,435,452,472] The projection from the NRTP may relay information necessary for the planning of saccades from the frontal eye field and superior colliculus to the cerebellum,[91,435,472] whereas those from the dorsolateral pontine nuclei seem more concerned with smooth pursuit.[296,323,435,438]

Purkinje cells in the dorsal vermis discharge before saccades,[169,319] and the population of neurons may send a "stop" signal to the fastigial nuclei to end a saccade on target.[437] Dorsal vermis Purkinje cells also encode target velocity during smooth pursuit and combined eye-head tracking.[422] Stimulation of the vermis produces saccades.[377] With currents near to threshold, a topographic organization is evident: upward saccades are evoked from the anterior part, downward saccades from the posterior part, and ipsilateral, horizontal saccades from the lateral part.[310]

Interpretation of Effects of Discrete Lesions on the Dorsal Vermis

Lesions of the dorsal vermis produce saccadic dysmetria, typically hypometria (see Video Display: Cerebellar Syndromes). Unilateral pharmacological decortication causes marked ipsilateral hypometria and mild contralateral hypermetria, with a gaze deviation away from the side of the inactivation.[381] Surgical lesions of the dorsal vermis in monkey cause saccadic hypometria, impaired onset of smooth pursuit,

Box 6–12. Cerebellar Dorsal Vermis (Lobules VI AND VII)

- Receives mossy fiber inputs from nucleus reticularis tegmenti pontis (NRTP), PPRF, dorsolateral and dorsomedial pontine nuclei, vestibular nuclei, nucleus prepositus hypoglossi, and climbing fiber inputs from the inferior olivary nucleus
- Main projection is to underlying caudal fastigial nucleus
- Purkinje cells in the dorsal vermis discharge before saccades and encode gaze velocity during smooth-pursuit and combined eye-head tracking. Microstimulation produces contralaterally directed saccades.

(For related clinical disorders, see Box 12–4, in Chapter 12.)

and impaired ability to adapt saccades or pursuit to novel visual demands.[427,429] Patients with lesions involving the posterior vermis also show impaired smooth pursuit, predominantly towards the side of the lesion.[448] Dorsal vermis lesions also cause disturbances of binocular alignment of the eyes, which is discussed further in Chapter 8.[428] Interpretation of these findings is aided by considering the structure to which the dorsal vermis sends its inhibitory projections: the fastigial nucleus.

Contributions of the Fastigial Nucleus

The main projection of the Purkinje cells of the dorsal vermis is to the caudal part of the fastigial nucleus—the most medial of the deep cerebellar nuclei (Fig. 6–6 and Box 6–13).[472] This fastigial oculomotor region (FOR) also receives climbing fiber inputs from the inferior olivary nucleus, and axon collaterals from mossy fibers projecting to the dorsal vermis from pontine nuclei, especially NRTP.[152,311,472] Thus, the fastigial nucleus receives a "copy" of the saccadic commands, which are relayed by NRTP from the frontal eye fields and superior colliculus.[311] The main projection from the fastigial nucleus crosses through the other fastigial nucleus, and enters the uncinate fasciculus, which runs in the dorsolateral border of the superior cerebellar peduncle, to reach the brainstem. The main targets of the caudal fastigial nucleus are the omnipause neurons, and the premotor burst neurons in the medulla, pons, and midbrain. In addition, the nucleus of the posterior commissure, the mesencephalic reticular formation, and the rostral pole of the superior colliculus receive inputs from the fastigial nucleus.[262,311] There are also smaller projections to other structures, including NRTP, the dorsolateral pontine nuclei, vestibular nuclei, the caudal superior colliculus, and the nucleus prepositus hypoglossi.[19,21,152]

Neurons in the caudal fastigial nucleus discharge in relation both to saccades,[126,172,318] and the onset of smooth pursuit,[127] in a manner which suggests that the eye is accelerated towards the opposite side. As discussed in Chapter 3, it is possible that the fastigial nucleus on one side fires early to help start a saccade, whereas inputs to the fastigial nucleus on the other side cause it to fire later, perhaps sending a signal to stop the eye on target.[324,437]

Interpretation of Effects of Discrete Lesions on the Fastigial Nucleus

Clinical lesions that involve the fastigial nuclei lesions produce marked hypermetria of saccades (see Video Display: Cerebellar Syndromes).[399] Such destructive lesions are effectively bilateral because of the crossing of axons destined for the brainstem within the fastigial nucleus itself (Fig. 3–16, Chapter 3). The nature of the defect has been clarified using muscimol to induce pharmacological inactivation of one side of the caudal fastigial nucleus.[373] The main

Box 6–13. Fastigial Nucleus

- Receives inputs from the dorsal vermis, inferior olivary nucleus, and axon collaterals from mossy fibers projecting to the dorsal vermis from pontine nuclei
- Main projection from the fastigial nucleus crosses and runs in uncinate fasciculus of the brachium conjunctivum to reach PPRF, riMLF, nucleus of the posterior commissure, the mesencephalic reticular formation, superior colliculus, omnipause neurons
- Neurons in the caudal fastigial nucleus (FOR) discharge prior to and during saccades and smooth pursuit; earlier discharge occurs for movements contralaterally, and late discharge occurs for movements ipsilaterally

(For related clinical disorders, see Box 12–4, in Chapter 12.)

effect is markedly hypermetric ipsilateral saccades and hypometric contralateral saccades (ipsipulsion). Additionally, there is a tonic gaze deviation towards the side of inactivation, and onset of smooth pursuit is impaired for targets moving contralaterally.[374] The posterior interpositus nucleus appears to have similar effects on vertical saccades; inactivation causes hypermetria of upward saccades and hypometria of downward saccades.[372] Based on electrophysiological studies, it seems possible that hypermetria with fastigial nucleus lesions occurs because of interruption of the normal feedback required to stop the eye on target.[324]

These findings are similar to the lateropulsion (ipsipulsion) encountered in Wallenberg's syndrome (lateral medullary infarction) (see Fig. 3–16 and Video Display: Medullary Syndromes). In that disorder, interruption of olivocerebellar climbing fibers within the restiform body are postulated to cause increased activity of Purkinje cells in the ipsilateral dorsal vermis, which, in turn, inhibits the underlying fastigial nucleus.[457] Patients with fastigial nucleus lesions have prominent saccadic hypermetria, but smooth pursuit may appear normal,[51] unless its onset (beginning) is specifically tested.

THE CEREBRAL HEMISPHERES AND VOLUNTARY CONTROL OF EYE MOVEMENTS

Approaches to Studying the Cerebral Control of Eye Movements in Humans

In developing a hypothetical scheme for the voluntary control of eye movements in humans, we have drawn on several different lines of evidence, each of which has inherent strengths and weaknesses. What are the methodological limitations?

First, the anatomy of cerebral cortex shows substantial differences between the various species of monkeys studied and humans (Fig. 6–8).[254] Second, caution is required in extrapolating results of electrophysiological studies in monkeys to account for behavior in humans, since mental set is inferred from the animals' responses that, unlike in most human experiments, are influenced by reward.[82,230,442] Third, functional imaging, including proton emission tomography (PET) and functional magnetic resonance imaging (fMRI), has held the promise of identifying cortical areas homologous to those that have been well defined in monkeys, but such studies have often yielded discrepant results, partly reflecting use of different test paradigms.[290,449] Another pitfall of functional imaging is that inferred local changes in cerebral metabolism may represent excitation or inhibition. Furthermore, there is evidence that just thinking about eye movements—without actually making them—may cause metabolic changes in areas such as the frontal eye field.[35,225] Application of functional imaging to monkeys may help define homology with cortical areas in humans.[200] Fourth, direct electrical stimulation of cerebral cortex during operations has limited availability;[271] however, implanted subdural arrays of electrodes in patients requiring surgical treatment of epilepsy have provided new insights about the frontal eye field.[32,148] Fifth, the non-invasive technique of transcranial magnetic stimulation (TMS), which transiently perturbs local cortical activity, will not induce eye movements, only delay or inhibit them. This technique has provided information on the sequence of programming that takes place in different cortical areas, but TMS over cortical eye fields also affects shifts of visuospatial attention and visual selection made without eye movements.[156,289] Finally, studies of the behavioral effects of discrete lesions, using paradigms that test specific aspects of the voluntary control of eye movements are of abiding importance and are the key to many of our interpretations. However, the most useful data for interpreting everyday function are behavioral changes that occur with acute lesions or pharmacological inactivation, since the effects of adaptation and recovery modify or abolish acute behavioral deficits quite rapidly.

Even when these and other techniques are optimally applied,[200a] selection of which behaviors to test is crucial. First, it is usually advantageous to test a range of behaviors between pure reflex and most voluntary, since hemispheric lesions may affect all but the most reflex responses (see Video Display: Acquired Ocular Motor Apraxia). Recall that, for example, rapid eye movements include reflex quick phases of nystagmus, saccades that respond to the changing highlights of the environment, and premeditated saccadic refixations (see

Table 3–1, Chapter 3). Second, the effects of attentional factors may profoundly influence voluntary eye movements, and electrophysiological evidence has linked increased attention with enhanced neural performance.[88,411] Thus, on the one hand, ocular following responses of a large textured pattern occurs at very short latencies and are relatively independent of how much attention the subject pays to it.[75] On the other hand, tracking a small target moving across a textured background occurs with a greater latency, and requires focused visual attention and the ability to suppress consequent motion of the image of the background on the retina.[157] A number of ingenious paradigms have been developed to probe other aspects of voluntary control and target selection.[298] Third, association areas of cortex that receive sensory signals that are disparate both in timing and modality (e.g., visual or vestibular) must transform them so that they are synchronized and in similar coordinates, and also take into account the current position of eye, head, and body in space.[238,471] Finally, although our scheme is presented as a series of operations by different cortical and subcortical centers, parallel distributed processing of signals conveying visual, ocular motor, efference copy or proprioception, and cognitive factors seems required to achieve the extensive repertoire of voluntary eye movements.

Our approach will be (1) to summarize the contributions of posterior, largely sensory cortical areas; (2) to review the role played by parietal cortex and the pulvinar; (3) to examine the properties of neurons in several frontal areas and the thalamic nuclei to which they are connected; and (4) to discuss the parallel, descending pathways by which volition controls eye movements. The reader should realize that what we present is a working hypothesis, which will be modified as new information becomes available, and present data are reinterpreted.

Contributions of Posterior Cortical Areas to Gaze Control

PRIMARY VISUAL CORTEX AND GAZE CONTROL

Striate cortex (visual area V1, Brodmann area 17) (Figs. 6–7 and 6–8) is of fundamental importance in the control of visually guided eye movements (Box 6–14).[193] A separate visual pathway for the perception of motion starts in retinal ganglion cells that project via the magnocellular layers of the lateral geniculate nucleus to layer 4Cα of striate cortex.[207,246] Although some neurons in striate cortex respond to moving visual stimuli, such cells have small receptive fields. Moreover, V1 neurons respond only to motion in the frontal plane of first-order stimuli, which are defined by the spatial distribution of luminance, and not by second-order motion stimuli such as contrast or flicker, which are thought to depend on higher-level mechanisms.[315]

In monkeys, experimental, unilateral *lesions of striate cortex* impair eye movements because of the lack of visual input; saccadic and pursuit eye movements can still be made if the visual stimulus falls in the intact visual hemifield.[397] If moving targets are presented in the visual hemifield contralateral to the lesion, however, saccades are inaccurate and no smooth pursuit is generated. Although monkeys tend to show partial recovery from bilateral occipital lobe lesions, so that they eventually regain some smooth-pursuit function,[474] human beings with occipital lobe lesions show limited recovery.[17] The deficit is greater with larger lesions, and smooth pursuit is impaired more than saccades.[368] Complete, bilateral lesions of the occipital lobes that produce cortical blindness probably abolish optokinetic nystagmus in humans,[450] although some visual discriminative capacity may remain.[465]

CONTRIBUTIONS OF SECONDARY VISUAL AREAS

Since primary visual cortex is limited in its ability to extract information about moving stimuli, further processing is necessary before a pursuit or saccadic eye movement can be programmed; this is largely performed in the middle temporal visual area (MT or V5) and the adjacent medial superior temporal visual area (MST) (Box 6–14 and Fig. 6–8). Striate cortex projects both directly and indirectly to MT;[443] in addition, MT receives inputs that bypass striate cortex,[120] perhaps via the superior colliculus and pulvinar.[375]

Middle Temporal Visual Area (MT, V5)

As reviewed in Chapter 4, neurons in *area MT* have larger receptive fields than those in striate

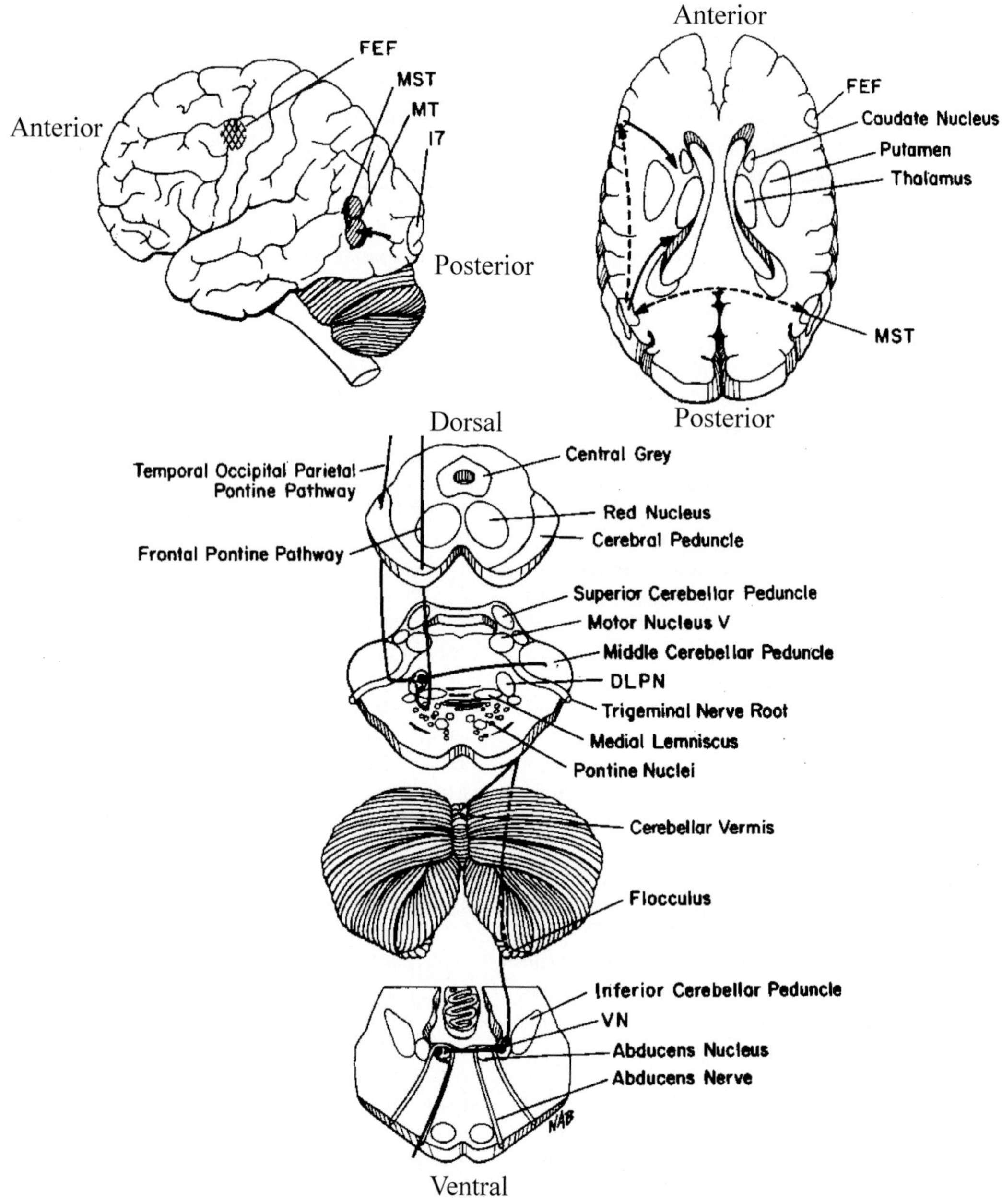

Figure 6–7. A hypothetical scheme for horizontal smooth pursuit. Primary visual cortex (V1) projects to the homologue of the middle temporal visual area (MT) that, in humans, lies at the temporal-occipital-parietal junction. MT projects to the homologue of the medial superior temporal visual area (MST) and also to the frontal eye field (FEF). MST also receives inputs from its contralateral counterpart. MST projects through the retrolenticular portion of the internal capsule and the posterior portion of the cerebral peduncle to the dorsolateral pontine nucleus (DLPN). The DLPN also receives inputs important for pursuit from the frontal eye field; these inputs descend in the medial portion of the cerebral peduncle. In addition, nucleus reticularis tegmenti pontis (NRTP), which is not shown, relays FEF projections to the dorsal vermis. The DLPN projects, mainly contralaterally, to the flocculus, paraflocculus and ventral uvula of the cerebellum; projections also pass to the dorsal vermis. The flocculus projects to the ipsilateral vestibular nuclei (VN), which in turn project to the contralateral abducens nucleus. Note that the sections of brainstem are in different planes from those of the cerebral hemispheres.

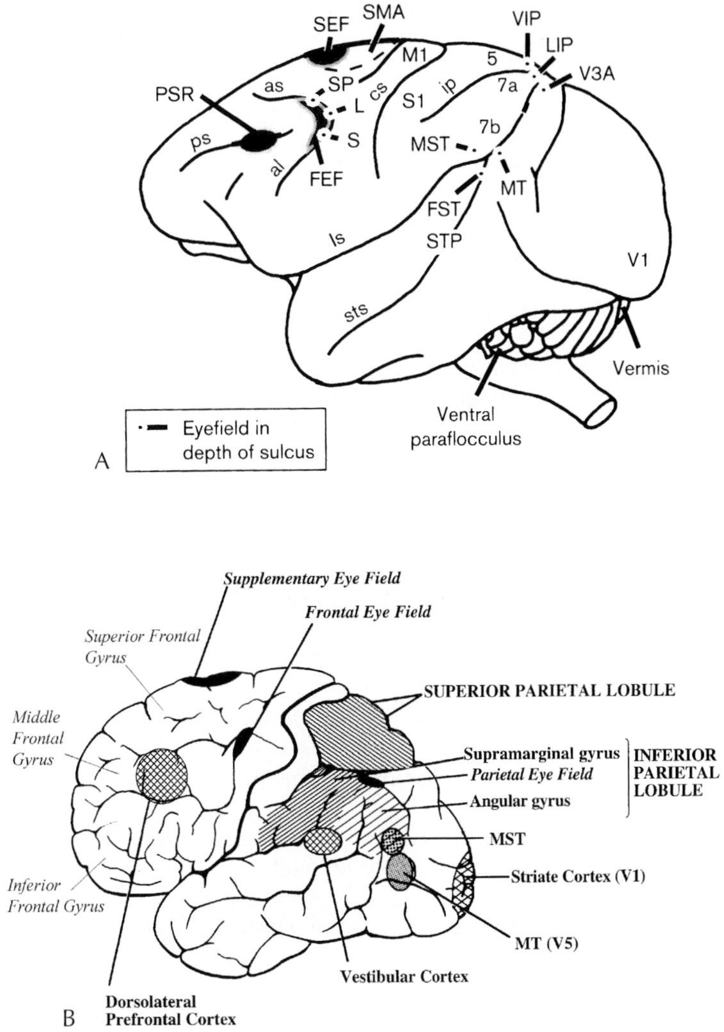

Figure 6–8. Probable location of cortical areas important for eye movements in rhesus monkey (A) and human brain (B). al: lateral arcuate sulcus; as: superior arcuate sulcus; cs: central sulcus; FEF: frontal eye field; FST: fundus of the superior temporal area; ip: intraparietal sulcus; L: large saccade region of FEF; LIP: lateral intraparietal area; M1: primary motor cortex; MST: medial superior temporal visual area; MT: middle temporal visual area; ps: principal sulcus; PSR: principal sulcus region; S: small saccade region of FEF; S1: primary sensory cortex; SEF: supplementary eye field; SMA: supplementary motor area; SP: smooth pursuit region of FEF; STP: superior temporal polysensory area; sts: superior temporal sulcus; V1: primary visual cortex; V3A: parietal visual area V3a; VIP: ventral intraparietal area; 5: area 5; 7: area 7; numbers refer to Brodmann's areas. In humans, MT and MST may form a contiguous cortical area. (Panel A reproduced from Büttner-Ennever JA, Horn AK. Anatomical substrates of oculomotor control. Curr Opin Neurobiol 7, 872–879, 1997, with permission of Elsevier.)

cortex and encode the speed and direction of target movements in three dimensions,[259] contributing to the generation of smooth pursuit movements.[356] Area MT also seems important for perception of speed [245]and stereopsis.[101] Functional imaging studies have demonstrated the *human homologue of MT* to be located at the temporo-parieto-occipital junction, posterior to the superior temporal sulcus, at the junction of Brodmann areas 19, 37, and 39, close to the intersection of the ascending limb of the inferior temporal sulcus and the lateral occipital sulcus.[112,441,476] The anterior part of the superior temporal sulcus shows activation during second–order motion stimuli.[312] Histological analysis of human brains has identified a region with a characteristic tangential band of myelination that occupies cortical layers III and IV, and corresponds to an area bordered dorsally by the lateral occipital sulcus, and ventrally by the inferior occipital sulcus;[10] this may correspond to MT localized by function imaging.

Experimental *lesions of MT* corresponding to extrafoveal retina cause a scotoma for motion in the contralateral visual field: stationary objects are perceived appropriately but motion perception is disrupted.[306] The consequences of lesions of extrafoveal MT for eye movements are that saccades can still be made accurately to stationary targets in the affected visual field, but moving stimuli cannot be tracked accurately by saccades or smooth pursuit.[154,308] Patients with cortical lesions have

Box 6–14. Posterior Cortical Areas

Primary Visual Cortex (Striate Cortex, V1)

- Fundamentally important for control of visually guided eye movements, but receptive fields are small, and unable to analyze complex visual stimuli

Middle Temporal Visual Area (MT, V5)

- Human homologue lies at occipito-temporo-parietal junction, at junction of Brodmann areas 19, 37, and 39
- Receives inputs from primary visual cortex (V1)
- Projects to FEF, MST, other cortical areas concerned with visual motion, and to dorsolateral pontine nuclei
- Encodes speed and direction of visual stimuli in three dimensions

Medial Superior Temporal Visual Area (MST)

- Human homologue lies close to MT at occipito-temporo-parietal junction
- Receives visual inputs from area MT, and vestibular and ocular motor signals
- Projects to FEF and other cortical areas concerned with visual motion, and to dorsolateral pontine nuclei
- Encodes moving visual stimuli and may also carry eye movement and vestibular signals

(For related clinical disorders, see Box 12–19, in Chapter 12.)

been described who have defects of smooth pursuit and saccades to targets presented within part of the contralateral visual field (Fig. 4–9);[278,439] these defects are similar to those reported with MT lesions in monkeys.[113,306] In humans, cortical lesions presumed to affect area MT also impair the perception of motion (akinetopsia).[15,16,402,478]

Medial Superior Temporal Visual Area (MST)

Visual area MT, in turn, projects to MST,[103,117] which, in monkey, consists of two parts: ventrolateral (MSTl) and dorsal (MSTd). Neurons in MSTl have properties that make them well suited for contributing to smooth pursuit across textured backgrounds. Thus, these neurons not only encode moving visual stimuli but also appear to carry an eye movement signal.[199,307] Neurons in MSTd seem concerned with analyzing the optic flow that occurs during locomotion, since they encode visual, ocular motor, and vestibular signals.[26,325,326] The *human homologues of MT and MST* probably lie adjacent, at the occipital-temporal-parietal junction, and while two visual areas may not be distinguishable in humans (MT+), there is some evidence of differential activation, according to the nature and location of the visual stimulus.[112] with the anterior part of the superior temporal sulcus responding to second-order motion stimuli.[312] Interestingly, responses to peripheral moving stimuli in MT and MST are greater in congenitally deaf individuals than in normals.[20]

Experimental lesions of area MST, or in the foveal representation of MT, cause a deficit primarily of horizontal smooth pursuit for targets moving toward the side of the lesion. In addition, a retinotopic deficit for motion detection, similar to that with extrafoveal lesions of MT, is present for targets presented in the contralateral visual hemifield.[113] In humans, posterior cerebral lesions involving the homologue of MST produce a deficit in tracking similar to that in monkey, with impairment of ipsilateral pursuit (Fig. 4–12), and a defect of motion processing affecting the contralateral visual hemifield.[15,278,439]

Contributions of the Middle Temporal Visual Area and Medial Superior Temporal Visual Area to Descending Pathways for Smooth Pursuit

The projections of areas MT and MST are important components of a neural pathway contributing to smooth pursuit (Fig. 6–7),[443] which runs ipsilaterally through the retrolenticular portion of the internal capsule,[277] and the posterior portion of the cerebral peduncle to reach the dorsolateral pontine nuclei (DLPN) and the nucleus reticularis tegmenti pontis (NRTP).[146,260,296323,423] These pontine nuclei also receive inputs related to smooth pursuit from the frontal eye field. The dorsolateral pontine nuclei project to the paraflocculus,[147] and the dorsal vermis of the cerebellum.[41] These cerebellar areas project, in turn, to the brainstem, via the vestibular and fastigial nuclei.[127,226] The effects of lesions at various points along this "pursuit pathway" are discussed in Chapter 4.

It has also been shown that MT and MST are important for mediating *optokinetic nystagmus*.[113] A subcortical visual pathway, which is discussed in Chapter 4 and includes the nucleus of the optic tract and dorsal terminal nucleus, receives a separate projection from MT and MST.[108] An accessory optic pathway also exists in human brain,[125] and it also receives inputs from MT and MST.[443] Its role in humans had been in doubt, but recent studies indicate that in disorders of binocular visual development, the accessory optic pathway does not mature normally and may play an important role in the pathogenesis of latent nystagmus (discussed in Chapter 10).[297]

Contributions of the Temporal Lobe to Gaze Control

Many areas of cerebral cortex receive vestibular inputs,[37,237] including area MST,[326] and the frontal eye fields.[130] However, a cortical area that may be important for the perception of vestibular sensation has been localized in the posterior aspect of the superior temporal gyrus, the parieto-insular-vestibular cortex (PIVC) (Fig. 6–8) using functional imaging during vestibular and optokinetic stimulation,[37,47,107] and by studying the effects of cortical lesions (see Box 6–15 and also Chapter 2).[39,40] This localization confirms the

Box 6–15. Posterior Temporal Lobe ("Vestibular Cortex")

- In humans, one component of vestibular cortex corresponds to the posterior aspect of the superior temporal gyrus—parieto-insular-vestibular cortex (PIVC)
- Clinical lesions cause contralateral tilts of subjective visual vertical, abolish circularvection, and cause memory-guided saccades to become inaccurate if the subject is turned during the memory period

(For related clinical disorders, see Box 12–19, in Chapter 12; for vestibular sensation see Chapter 2.)

stimulation studies of Penfield.[335] Clinical lesions affecting this area of temporal cortex cause contraversive tilts of the subjective visual vertical,[40] abolish the sense of self-rotation (circularvection) that normally occurs with optokinetic stimulation,[420] and impair memory-guided saccades if patients are rotated to a new position during the memory period.[202]

Other areas of the medial temporal lobes, such as the hippocampus, make important contributions to programming of memory-guided saccades,[348] and will be discussed further in relation to control of saccades by the frontal lobes.

Contributions of the Parietal Lobe to Gaze Control

The parietal lobe has important influences upon all classes of eye movements by virtue of its role in directing visual attention to objects in extrapersonal space. In addition, the "parietal eye field" (PEF) has a direct role in programming saccades. Substantial progress has been achieved in understanding parietal lobe contributions to the control of eye movements in the rhesus monkey, but particular caution is necessary in extrapolating these results to humans, because of differences in anatomy and hemispheric specialization between the two species.

CONTRIBUTIONS OF THE POSTERIOR PARIETAL CORTEX

The inferior parietal lobule of the monkey, specifically the caudomedial portion that has been called area 7a or PG, contains populations of neurons that respond to visual stimuli and discharge during a range of eye movements (see Fig. 6–8A and Box 6–16).[5,253] In monkeys, these neurons receive inputs from secondary visual areas, such as MST, and from the pulvinar, superior colliculus, cingulate cortex, and the intralaminar thalamic nuclei.[6,72,305] Parietal area 7a projects to the dorsolateral prefrontal cortex and to the cingulate gyrus, but only weakly to the frontal eye field.[6] A medial parietal eye field might be present in adjacent area 7m.[235,436]

Area 7a contains a variety of neurons that discharge during active visual fixation, in relation to saccades, or during smooth pursuit. Their visual receptive fields are large, often crossing the midline. Neurons that discharge in relationship to saccades usually do so *after* the eye movement is made.[14] Furthermore, neurons that are active during smooth pursuit seem more concerned with directing attention to the stimulus than with encoding its dynamic properties.[253] An important property of area 7 neurons is that their activity is influenced not just by visual stimuli, but also by eye and head position.[8,42] Thus, it has been postulated that a neural network of such neurons could play an

Box 6–16. Posterior Parietal Cortex

- The human homologue of area 7a in the rhesus monkey may lie in the inferior parietal lobule, corresponding to portions of Brodmann areas 39 and 40
- In monkey, area 7a receives inputs from secondary visual areas, such as MST, the pulvinar, superior colliculus, cingulate cortex, and the intralaminar thalamic nuclei
- Area 7a projects to dorsolateral prefrontal cortex and to the cingulate gyrus, but only weakly to the frontal eye field
- Important for directing visual attention in extrapersonal space; to this end, visually responsive neurons modulate their discharge according to eye position

(For related clinical disorders, see Box 12–20, in Chapter 12.)

important role in transforming visual signals from retinal into spatial or craniotopic coordinates.[471]

Neurons with similar properties have been demonstrated in another subdivision of the parietal lobe, the ventral intraparietal area (VIP), which lies in the fundus of the intraparietal sulcus in monkeys (Fig. 6–8A).[110] Area VIP may be important for building an internal, multisensory representation of extrapersonal space,[110] and contains neurons that respond during smooth pursuit.[389]

A region homologous to area 7a in the human brain probably corresponds to portions of the Brodmann areas 39 and 40, including parts of the supramarginal gyri and angular gyri (see Fig. 6–8B).[280,336] Clinically, unilateral posterior parietal lesions, especially right-sided, cause contralateral neglect and may produce ipsilateral gaze deviation or preference, and impair the ability to make saccades and smooth pursuit in the contralateral hemifield of gaze.[36,276] After the acute phase, the latency of visually guided saccades remains bilaterally increased and memory-guided saccades are inaccurate.[349] During visual search, parietal lobe patients may show a double-deficit consisting of hemispatial neglect, and impaired memory of where their search has previously led them.[197]

Unilateral parietal lesions have also been thought to cause greater impairment of pursuit when the target moves towards the side of the lesion, but such deficits may be partly due to involvement of adjacent MT and MST or their projections. A defect that may be more specific for parietal lobe lesions, especially when Brodmann's area 40 is involved, is impaired smooth pursuit when the target moves across a structured background, compared with pursuit across a dark background.[232] This defect may be due to an impaired ability to attend to the image of the moving target and "ignore" the smeared images of the stationary background consequent to the eye movement.

Bilateral posterior parietal lesions cause Balint's syndrome,[345] features of which are disturbance of visual attention (simultanagnosia), inaccurate arm pointing (optic ataxia), and difficulty initiating voluntary saccades to visual targets (ocular motor apraxia). These deficits, which are discussed further in Chapter 12 and in the Video Display: Acquired Ocular Motor Apraxia, could be due to disruption of the neural mechanisms by which posterior parietal cortex internally represents the locations of objects in extrapersonal space.

CONTRIBUTION OF THE PARIETAL EYE FIELD (PEF)

In rhesus monkeys, the parietal eye field (PEF) corresponds to an area called the lateral intraparietal area (LIP), which lies adjacent to area 7a, in the caudal third of the lateral bank of the intraparietal sulcus (Box 6–17). Functional imaging studies indicate that, in humans, the PEF lies within the medial wall of

Box 6–17. Parietal Eye Field (PEF)

- The human PEF lies around the horizontal portion of the intraparietal sulcus, in adjacent parts of the superior part of the angular gyrus and the supramarginal gyrus, corresponding to Brodmann areas 39 and 40
- Receives inputs from secondary visual areas
- Projects to the frontal eye field and the superior colliculus
- Important for triggering visually guided saccades to reflexively explore the visual environment

(For related clinical disorders, see Box 12–20, in Chapter 12.)

the posterior half of the intraparietal sulcus, adjacent to the anterior part of the angular gyrus and posterior part of the superior parietal lobule (Fig. 6–8).[43,293] LIP receives inputs from secondary visual areas and projects strongly to the frontal eye field and the superior colliculus.[6,34,250]

Saccade-related neurons in LIP discharge *before* saccades.[14] Other neurons discharge during fixation.[25] As in area 7a, the response of LIP neurons is influenced by eye position,[7] and neurons show a shift of their visual fields to anticipate the consequences of upcoming gaze shifts.[223] LIP neurons can also hold in memory the location of a desired target location,[14,327] thereby contributing to the ability to make a series of shifts of gaze,[470] and a corresponding series of shifts of attention.[150]

Experimental inactivation of LIP causes increased latency for both visually and memory-guided saccades into contralateral hemispace.[241] Perhaps more revealing is the impaired ability to make two saccades to two targets flashed in quick succession. In response to this "double-step" stimulus, the brain must take into account not only the retinal location of the two targets, but also the effect of the eye movements, since planning the second eye movement requires knowledge of the first in order to be accurate. After LIP inactivation in monkeys, when the first saccade stepped into the contralesional field, the second saccade became more inaccurate.[240] Patients with right parietal lesions show similar deficits if the first target appears in the left hemifield and the second in the right; the first saccade may be accurate, but the second is not.[111,166] Such a deficit may be present even though there is no inattention or difficulty responding to the reverse order of presentation, or of making single saccades to left-sided targets. Taken together, these results suggest a disruption of the ability to monitor the size of the first saccade using efference copy,[111,166] and as further evidence for transformation by the population of LIP from retinotopic eye-centered into head-centered coordinates.[240]

Contributions of the Pulvinar to Gaze Control

The pulvinar is the posterior and largest portion of the thalamus (Box 6–18).[71] It has reciprocal connections with striate, peristriate, parietal, and frontal cortex.[74,98,195,337,370,371,376,447] The pulvinar receives inputs from retina and superior colliculus, but inputs from the cortex seem most important.[27,90,203] Indeed, the evolution of the pulvinar appears to have paralleled that of association cortex.

Three regions of the pulvinar contain neurons that show visual responses: inferior, lateral, and dorsomedial. Neurons in the first two regions are retinotopically organized. They send a projection to visual area MT.[375] Neuro-

Box 6–18. Pulvinar

- Posterior, largest part of thalamus
- Receives inputs from striate, peristriate, parietal and frontal cortex; smaller inputs from retina and superior colliculus
- Projects to striate, peristriate, parietal, and frontal cortex
- Inferior and lateral pulvinar project to visual area MT and may be important in dealing with the visual consequences of eye movements
- Dorsomedial pulvinar projects to parietal lobe and seems concerned with shifts of attention

(For related clinical disorders, see Box 12–15, in Chapter 12.)

physiologic evidence suggests that these two regions may be important in dealing with the visual effects of eye movements (for example, the visual blur produced by a saccade), because neurons here do respond to moving visual stimuli, but they respond much less if the motion of images on the retina is caused by an eye movement.[370]

Visually responsive cells in the dorsomedial pulvinar are not retinotopically organized, and have large receptive fields; some show sensitivity to visual features such as color.[29,256] They respond vigorously if the visual stimulus is a cue for active behavior, such as a saccade. Like neurons in the inferior parietal lobe, to which they project, these pulvinar neurons seem more concerned with shifts of attention than with eye movements per se. Other neurons in the dorsomedial pulvinar discharge for saccades and quick phases, even in the dark, but these neurons do not encode the amplitude and direction of such movements and so are probably signaling that an eye movement has occurred that might be efference copy. Pharmacological manipulation of cells in dorsomedial pulvinar, using microinjection of GABA-related drugs, has confirmed that this region is involved in shifts in spatial attention towards salient features.[320,369,371] Functional imaging studies in humans support the notion that the pulvinar is important for directing visual attention.[209,224]

Normal human subjects show a decrease in the reaction time of visually triggered saccades if the fixation point is turned off synchronously with the appearance of the visual target, rather than leaving the fixation light on. Patients with posterior thalamic lesions involving the pulvinar show no such reduction in reaction time for visually triggered saccades; however, voluntary saccades are similar to normals.[357] This result is consistent with prior studies that had reported difficulties in disengaging visual fixation when a shift of attention was to be made.[317,447,477] Thus, current experimental and clinical data indicate that the pulvinar contributes to the mechanisms for shifting visual attention.

The pulvinar has proven to be a challenging area for electrophysiologists to link neuronal discharge to behavior.[71] Nonetheless, it is undoubtedly important in controlling shifts of attention and gaze, and more basic and clinical studies are needed.

Contributions of the Frontal Lobe to Gaze Control

The frontal lobes contain several areas important in the voluntary control of saccades, smooth pursuit and vergence. These areas include the frontal eye field (FEF), the supplementary eye field (SEF), and the dorsolateral prefrontal cortex (DLPC). In addition, cingulate cortex and the intralaminar thalamic nuclei, with which the frontal and supplementary eye fields have reciprocal connections, may contribute to the control of gaze.

CONTRIBUTIONS OF THE FRONTAL EYE FIELD

Anatomical Location and Connections

Although the FEF is long-known to contribute to the voluntary control of gaze,[185] a clear definition of its role has required the application of modern electrophysiological and anatomic studies, and novel test paradigms to demonstrate defects in patients (Box 6–19). Definition of the boundaries of FEF depends on the technique used. Thus, in rhesus monkeys, FEF, defined by microstimulation that evokes eye movements, lies in a circumscribed zone along the posterior portion of the arcuate sulcus (part of Brodmann area 8).[45] Combined functional imaging and anatomical studies have suggested that FEF in monkeys also includes the caudal part of the pre-arcuate convexity and part of premotor cortex.[282] In humans, stimulation studies using subdural electrode arrays implanted in patients prior to surgery for intractable epilepsy, suggest that the FEF is located at the posterior end of the middle frontal gyrus, immediately anterior to the precentral sulcus.[33] High-resolution fMRI during saccadic tasks indicates that the human FEF lies in the anterior wall of the precentral sulcus, close to the intersection with the superior frontal sulcus;[247,378] specific chemoarchitecture may identify the location.[378a]

The FEF receives inputs from posterior visual cortical areas, inferior parietal cortex, the parietal eye fields (PEF),[119] contralateral FEF, supplementary eye field, prefrontal cortex, central thalamic nuclei, substantia nigra pars reticulata, superior colliculus, and cerebellar dentate nucleus.[196,251,414,416,417] The FEF also receives afferents from regions concerned

Box 6–19. The Frontal Eye Field (FEF)

- In humans, the FEF is located around the lateral part of the precentral sulcus, involving adjacent areas of the precentral gyrus, the middle frontal gyrus, and the superior frontal gyrus, and corresponding to confluent portions of Brodmann areas 6 and 4, but not 8
- Receives inputs from posterior visual cortical areas, inferior parietal cortex, contralateral FEF, SEF, DLPC, intralaminar thalamic nuclei, substantia nigra pars reticulata, superior colliculus, and cerebellar dentate nucleus
- Projects to contralateral FEF, SEF, and posterior visual cortical areas; superior colliculus (both directly and via caudate and substantia nigra pars reticulata); nucleus reticularis tegmenti pontis; and nucleus raphe interpositus (pontine omnipause neurons)
- FEF probably contributes to all voluntary and visually guided saccades, to smooth pursuit and vergence

(For related clinical disorders, see Box 12–21, in Chapter 12.)

with smooth pursuit, including visual areas MT and MST.[415] The projections of the FEF are discussed further in the section of this chapter on Descending Parallel Pathways that Control Saccades. Important targets include the caudate and putamen, subthalamic nucleus, superior colliculus, nucleus reticularis tegmenti pontis (NRTP), and the omnipause neurons of the pontine raphe.[195,236,417]

Frontal Eye Field Contributions to Saccades

In monkeys, neurons in the FEF do not become active before every saccade, only those made purposively.[44] A topographic "motor map" is present, with larger saccades evoked from stimulation of the dorsomedial portion of the FEF, and smaller saccades from stimulation of the ventrolateral part.[45] Different subpopulations of FEF neurons encode the visual stimulus, the planned saccadic movement, or both.[151] Cells with visual responsiveness anticipate the visual consequences of planned saccades.[446]

In humans, subdural electrode arrays indicate that human FEF shows visual responses that correspond to the direction of movement induced by electrical stimulation.[31] Functional imaging studies have demonstrated increased FEF activation during all visually guided saccades, reflex or voluntary;[9,109,426] repetitive saccades made in darkness;[340,341] and memory-guided saccades.[316,426] In addition, activation of the right FEF is reported during antisaccades.[86,314,426] Antisaccades are delayed by TMS over frontal cortex; the same effect can be achieved if the stimulus is delivered earlier over parietal cortex, suggesting flow of information from posterior to anterior during presaccadic processing.[434]

The influence of the FEF on eye movements has been demonstrated using the technique of pharmacological inactivation.[106] Muscimol injection causes a contralateral ocular motor scotoma with abolition of all reflex visual and voluntary saccades with sizes and directions corresponding to the injection site on the FEF map. In addition, during fixation, there is a gaze shift towards the side of the lesion and inappropriate ipsilateral saccades may disrupt steady fixation. Acute destructive lesions of the FEF in monkeys produce an increase of latency for contralateral saccades and a decrease of latency for ipsilateral movements (that is, an increase of express saccades ipsilateral to the side of the lesion).[386] Recovery from acute FEF lesions is rapid but incomplete, and patients show enduring effects on the latency and accuracy of visual and memory-guided saccades,[366] especially when directed contralaterally.[354]

Frontal Eye Field Contributions to Smooth Pursuit

In rhesus monkey, neurons active during smooth pursuit lie in the ventral (inferior) part of FEF, in the arcuate fundus and posterior bank.[153] Such FEF neurons also modulate their discharge during smooth eye-head tracking, implying that they receive vestibular signals.[129] Neurons that discharge during pursuit project to the ipsilateral dorsolateral pontine nuclei (see Fig. 6–7). In humans, functional imaging indicates that the part of FEF concerned with smooth pursuit lies in the lower anterior wall and adjacent fundus of the precentral sulcus, occasionally extending to the deeper part of the posterior wall of the sulcus.[339,378] Inactivation of FEF with muscimol severely impairs smooth pursuit.[400] Lesions of the FEF in monkeys and humans cause a predominantly ipsidirectional defect of smooth pursuit that especially involves predictive aspects of the tracking response.[167,257,279]

Frontal Eye Field Contributions to Fixation

Some FEF neurons also appear to be concerned with disengaging fixation prior to a saccade; their discharge increases when the fixation light is turned out, even before the new target becomes visible.[105] Other neurons appear to promote fixation; if microstimulation of these neurons is timed to coincide with the visual stimulus for a saccade, the eye movement may be suppressed.[45,48] Microstimulation near the spur of the arcuate sulcus, which corresponds to the smooth-pursuit portion of FEF, suppresses visual and memory-guided saccades in any direction.[206] This part of the FEF projects to the "fixation region" at the rostral pole of the superior colliculus and also to omnipause neurons in the pons.[48,417] In humans, functional imaging demonstrates activation of the FEF area during active fixation of a stationary target,[338] or during the increased fixation demands made by the antisaccade task.[89]

Frontal Eye Field Contributions to Vergence and Complex Behaviors

The FEF plays a role in vergence eye movements, whether these are made alone or in combination with saccades or smooth pursuit.[132,136] Some FEF neurons discharge for smooth tracking in three dimensions.[222] Thus, FEF neurons show a range of responses to disparity of visual stimuli and the ocular motor responses to them.[118]

Neurons in FEF are also active during complex behaviors such as memory-guided saccades,[446] countermanding saccades,[160] predictive tracking,[131] and visual search.[49] In a patient with a frontal lobe tumor, per-operative stimulation over the FEF arrested self-paced saccades.[271]

CONTRIBUTIONS OF THE SUPPLEMENTARY EYE FIELD (SEF)

Anatomical Location and Connections

The dorsomedial frontal lobe of monkeys contains neurons that discharge before contralateral saccades; this region has been designated the supplementary eye field (SEF) (Box 6–20).[391] Based on functional imaging studies during saccade tasks, the SEF in humans lies on the dorsomedial surface of the hemisphere, in the upper part of the paracentral sulcus, 7 mm anterior to the area of supplementary cortex activated by hand movements, and corresponding to the medial portion of Brodmann area 6.[155,340]

The SEF has reciprocal connections with the FEF, dorsolateral prefrontal cortex, cortex surrounding the cingulate, intraparietal and superior temporal sulci, the thalamus, and the claustrum.[18,403,405] Like the FEF, the SEF projects to the caudate and putamen, superior colliculus, nucleus reticularis tegmenti pontis, and other pontine nuclei, including the pontine omnipause neurons in the nucleus raphe interpositus.[194,282,404,405] Projections from the FEF and SEF convergence in the caudate nucleus.[329] On the other hand, the SEF has more extensive connections with prefrontal and skeletomotor areas and fewer connections with vision-related structures than does the FEF.[194]

Supplementary Eye Field Contribution to Saccades

Saccade-related neurons in monkey SEF show some properties similar to those in FEF,[380] but also respond during a variety of more complex behaviors,[76] such as antisaccades (Fig 3–2).[3] There is evidence that rostral SEF encodes

Box 6–20. The Supplementary Eye Field (SEF)

- In humans, the SEF lies on the dorsomedial surface of the hemisphere, in the posteriomedial portion of the superior frontal gyrus
- Receives inputs from FEF, prefrontal, cingulate, parietal, and temporal cortex; thalamus; and claustrum
- Projects to FEF; prefrontal, cingulate, parietal, and temporal cortex; thalamus; claustrum; caudate nucleus; superior colliculus; nucleus reticularis tegmenti pontis; and pontine omnipause neurons
- SEF seems important for programming saccades as part of learned or complex behaviors

(For related clinical disorders, see Box 12–21, in Chapter 12.)

saccades in an eye-centered frame whereas caudal SEF encodes saccades in a head-centered frame.[328] Neurons in SEF are also active when monkeys are trained to make a learned sequence of saccades.[201]

During a *countermanding task*, in which subjects make visually guided saccades on most trials but are required on some to withhold a saccade (on the basis of reappearance of the fixation cue), some SEF neurons respond on trials in which saccades are erroneously not cancelled, and reward will not be given.[421] Thus, in comparison with the other cortical eye fields, SEF appears most concerned with internally guided target selection based on prior trials that were rewarded.[3,82]

Functional imaging studies in humans have demonstrated increased SEF activation during single memory-guided saccades,[9,316,426] or a series of them,[165,340] and during antisaccades.[314,426] Activation during visually guided saccades may occur if the task involves predictable behavior.[124]

Inactivation of SEF in monkeys impairs the ability to respond to a double-step task.[407] Studies of patients with lesions involving the SEF show impaired ability to make a sequence of saccades to an array of visible targets in the order that they were turned on.[140,142] This defect in the ability to make a memorized series of saccades seems more pronounced with left-sided lesions. Functional imaging studies in humans have demonstrated increased SEF activation during a series of memory-guided saccades.[165] Taken together, this evidence suggests an important role for the SEF in the planning of series of saccades as part of complex or learned behaviors. However, as discussed below, other cortical areas also contribute to the ability to make saccades in a remembered sequence.

Supplementary Eye Field Contribution to Smooth Tracking

The SEF contains neurons that discharge during smooth pursuit,[168] and they may also carry a head velocity signal, and discharge during tracking of a target moving in both direction and depth.[129] Electrical microstimulation in the SEF increases the velocity of anticipatory pursuit movements and decreases their latency.[274] This anticipatory pursuit facilitation is greater when stimulation is delivered near the end of the fixation period. In patients, predictive aspects of smooth pursuit may also be impaired when lesions involve the SEF.[167] In sum, the SEF pursuit area seems to be involved in the process of guiding anticipatory smooth tracking.[94]

SUPPLEMENTARY EYE FIELD AND THE PRE-SUPPLEMENTARY MOTOR AREA (PRE-SMA)

The cortical area anterior to SEF, referred to as the *pre-supplementary motor area (pre-SMA)*, seems important for switching responses during more challenging tasks. For example, during a task that combines repetitive saccadic responses with sudden changes in the rule in which stimuli are presented, pre-SMA neurons are active. Together with SEF and cingulate cortex, pre-SMA may play a critical role in switching behavioral set.[82] Thus, anterior pre-SMA is activated during conflicts between choosing one of two possible behavioral responses, whereas posterior pre-SMA seems more concerned with the decisional process.[298] Support for such a proposal comes from a report of a patient with a discrete lesion affecting one SEF, who showed difficulty in changing the direction of his eye movements, especially when he had to reverse the direction of a previously established pattern of response.[198] Other areas rostral to FEF, SEF, and PEF may also be activated during more challenging cognitive tasks.[269]

CONTRIBUTIONS OF THE DORSOLATERAL PREFRONTAL CORTEX

Anatomical Location, Connections, and Physiology

Goldman-Rakic and colleagues demonstrated that DLPC is an important component of the working memory that makes it possible to make saccades to previously presented target locations (Box 6–21).[13,87,133,430] In monkeys, DLPC lies in the posterior third of the principal sulcus on the dorsolateral convexity of the frontal lobe (Fig. 6–8), corresponding to Walker's area 46. In humans, the homologue of the DLPC lies on the dorsolateral surface of the frontal lobe, anterior to the FEF, occupying approximately the middle third of the middle frontal gyrus and adjacent cortex, corresponding to Brodmann's areas 46 and 9.[134,358,359] It is suggested that the ability of neurons in DLPC to hold in memory the spatial location of targets depends on its reciprocal connections with a number of other areas, including posterior parietal cortex,[73] FEF, SEF and limbic cortex (including parahippocampal and cingulate cortex). It also receives inputs from the thalamus and medial pulvinar, and projects to the caudate, putamen, claustrum, thalamic nuclei, superior colliculus, and PPRF.[72,282,398]

In human subjects, the DLPC are activated when subjects make memory-guided saccades or antisaccades,[242,292,316,426] these results are consistent with properties of neurons in monkey DLPC.

Effects of Dorsolateral Prefrontal Cortex Lesions and Inactivation on Memory-Guided Saccades

Experimental lesions of DLPC in monkeys disrupt the performance of saccades to remem-

Box 6–21. Dorsolateral Prefrontal Cortex (DLPC)

- In humans, lies on the dorsolateral surface of the frontal lobe, occupying the middle frontal gyrus and adjacent cortex, corresponding to Brodmann areas 46 and 9
- Receives inputs from FEF, SEF, posterior parietal cortex and limbic cortex (including parahippocampal and cingulate cortex), thalamus, and medial pulvinar
- Projects to the FEF, SEF, posterior parietal and limbic cortex, caudate and putamen, superior colliculus, and PPRF
- DLPC is important for programming saccades to remembered locations and antisaccades (For related clinical disorders, see Box 12–21, in Chapter 12.)

bered target locations.[135] Pharmacological inactivation of DLPC with D1-dopamine antagonists impairs the accuracy of contralateral memory-guided saccades. Both D1-dopamine and 5 hydroxytryptamine 2-A receptors are involved in this spatial working memory, and injection of antagonist for either transmitter impairs memory guided saccade tasks.[385,468] Patients with chronic lesions involving the DLPC show increased variability of the gain of memory-guided saccades.[354]

Several insights have been gained into how DLPC controls saccades by the technique of transcranial magnetic stimulation (TMS), which briefly inactivates underlying cortex. First, TMS over DLPC increases the number of express saccades during a gap task, *i.e.*, it decreases saccadic reaction time (Fig. 3–2).[294] This result suggests that DLPC normally inhibits the superior colliculus. Second, when subjects attempt to look to the location of a target shown a few seconds before ("short-term spatial memory"), TMS applied over the DLPC during the memory period causes saccades to become inaccurate.[38,295] Third, when TMS is applied over DLPC after longer memory periods (28 s), there is less impairment of memory-guided saccades, indicating that other regions are contributing to this "intermediate spatial memory."[313] Thus, patients with lesions involving the parahippocampal cortex show inaccuracy of saccades made to target locations that were memorized up to 30 seconds previously.[353] For "long-term spatial memory" ranging up to minutes, the hippocampal formation may be important.[346,348]

The DLPC, along with the FEF, makes important contributions to programming of antisaccades (Fig. 3–2). Thus, functional imaging shows that the DLPC in the right hemisphere is activated during antisaccades,[104] and patients with lesions affecting the DLPC have an increased percentage of errors in the antisaccade test.[347] At present, one view is that, during the antisaccade task, inhibition of reflexive misdirected saccades appears to be due to DLPC, whereas triggering of the correct antisaccade depends upon FEF.[347] Patients with lesions affecting the anterior limb, the genu, or the anterior part of the posterior limb of the internal capsule show increased errors on the antisaccade task, and this may be because of disrupted projections of DLPC to the superior colliculus.[85]

Role of Cingulate Cortex

The evidence for a cingulate eye field is mainly based on human studies, and the demonstration that anterior cingulate cortex has oligosynaptic connections with brainstem ocular motor structures, implying that it makes important contributions to the voluntary control of eye movements.[282]

On the one hand, functional imaging has demonstrated activation of the anterior cingulate cortex during self-paced saccades in darkness,[341] memory-guided saccades,[9] memorized triple saccades,[165] and antisaccades.[109] On the other hand, activation of the posterior cingulate gyrus is reported during reflexive, but not intentional, saccades.[280]

Studies of patients with focal lesions has led to the proposal that there is a cingulate eye field, located in the posterior part of the anterior cingulate cortex, at the junction of Brodmann areas 23 and 24.[141] Thus, in two patients with small infarcts in this area on the right hemisphere, saccadic reaction time was increased and gain decreased for saccades made during the overlap task, and for memory-guided saccades.[141] Both patients also made bidirectional errors on the antisaccade task and during sequences of saccades to remembered target locations. Patients with tumor resections involving the anterior cingulate cortex also showed deficits on the antisaccade task.[270]

Electrophysiological evidence from monkey suggests that anterior cingulate neurons are active when monkeys carry out a saccade-countermanding task, signaling when errors occurred or when reinforcement was withheld,[204] but not in relationship to conflict posed on tasks that require a choice between two responses.[302] Neurons located in the posterior cingulate cortex are reported to discharge during or after eye movements,[321] and neuronal activity may be related to directing visual attention.[100] Thus, much work is needed to clarify the contributions made by the anterior and posterior cingulate in the control of gaze but, as for other cortical areas, studies of the effects of clinical lesions may have provided the first clues.

Contributions of the Intralaminar Thalamic Nuclei

The FEF, SEF, and PEF all have reciprocal connections with thalamic neurons that lie near the upper wing of the internal medullary lamina (IML—the fiber pathway that separates the medial from the lateral thalamic mass) (Box 6–22).[390,392,433,469] These saccade-related neurons are scattered throughout adjacent portions of the central lateral, superior central lateral, and dorsomedial nuclei. In addition to frontal cortical areas, the intralaminar thalamic nuclei also receive inputs from the pontine reticular formation, cerebellum, tectum, and pretectum. On the other hand, the intralaminar nuclei do not project to brainstem structures concerned with eye movements.[393]

Neurons in these central thalamic nuclei encode a range of signals that include the location of goals for memory-guided saccades, suggesting a role in context-dependent linkage of sensory signals with saccadic commands.[432,469] Neurons in the ventrolateral thalamus encode pursuit-related signals, and may serve as a relay from cerebellum to cortex rather than a direct pursuit pathway, since inactivation has only modest effects on pursuit behavior.[432] Taking together the broad range of properties of thalamic neurons during saccades and pursuit, it was suggested that these thalamic neurons are an important source of efference copy to the cortical eye fields,[393] and recent studies have supported this hypothesis. Thus, inactivation of the medial dorsal thalamus in monkey, an important relay between the superior colliculus and FEF, causes errors on double-step tasks.[408] The latter deficit implies lost ability to hold in register the first saccade while planning the second.

In humans, functional imaging has shown thalamic activation when subjects make voluntary saccades.[341] Patients with lesions affecting the central thalamic nuclei show similar functional deficits to the effects of medial dorsal nucleus inactivation in monkeys. Thus, there is an inaccuracy of memory-guided saccades only if gaze is perturbed during the memory period.[22,143] An illustrative case is presented in Chapter 12. Another defect reported with lesions of the ventrolateral thalamus, which relays cerebellar inputs to the FEF, is an impaired ability to adapt saccades to novel visual demands.[144] In sum, the thalamic nuclei seem important for monitoring the consequences of both saccades and smooth pursuit, but much remains unknown about how this is achieved and whether the thalamus make more direct contributions to eye movements.

DESCENDING, PARALLEL PATHWAYS THAT CONTROL VOLUNTARY GAZE

We first describe the descending pathways from the several eye fields of cerebral cortex

Box 6–22. Intralaminar Thalamic Nuclei

- Portion of thalamus lying near the upper wing of the internal medullary lamina (IML), the fiber pathway that separates the medial and lateral thalamic masses
- Receives inputs from FEF, SEF, PEF, PPRF, cerebellum, superior colliculus, and pretectum
- Project to the striatum, FEF SEF, PEF, and cingulate gyri, but not to brainstem structures concerned with eye movements
- Might be a source of efference copy information for cortical areas

(For related clinical disorders, see Box 12–15, in Chapter 12.)

and then discuss the influence that each may have on the generation of saccades. No direct projection exists from cortical neurons to ocular motoneurons;[205] instead, several intermediate structures play important roles, including the caudate, putamen, subthalamic nucleus, substantia nigra pars reticulata, superior colliculus, and brainstem reticular formation. The descending pathway for smooth pursuit is summarized in Figure 6–7.

Reports of the projections of the *FEF* are based on how this eye field is defined, and although microstimulation has been the standard method, [416,417] novel techniques such as using rabies virus as a tracer, are providing a new view.[282] Each FEF projects to its counterpart and also to other cortical areas concerned with visual processing, such as inferior parietal cortex.[196] The descending projections of the FEF initially run in the anterior limb of the internal capsule; clinical lesions here and in the adjacent deep frontal region increase saccadic latency.[350]

Below the level of the internal capsule, several separate pathways can be discerned (Figure 6–9 and Figure 3–12 of Chapter 3).[236] One projection, via the anterior limb of the internal capsule, goes to the caudate and adjacent putamen, which in turn project, via the pars reticulata of the substantia nigra (SNpr),

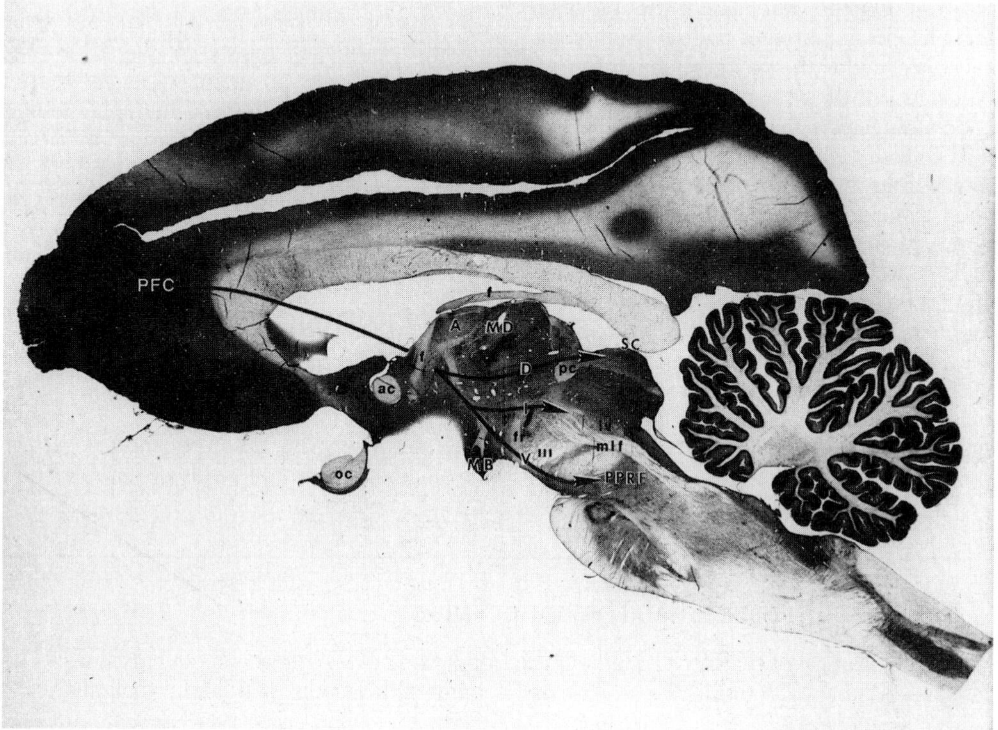

Figure 6–9. Projections from prefrontal cortex to ocular motor structures in the monkey. From prefrontal cortex (PFC—frontal eye field and caudal sulcus principalis), a unified projection runs in the anterior limb of the internal capsule and then divides into a dorsal prefrontofugal system (D—"transthalamic" pathway) and a ventral prefrontofugal system (V—classic "pedunculo-tegmental" pathway). The transthalamic pathway traverses and projects to the dorsomedial (MD) and intralaminar thalamic nuclei and the superior colliculus (SC). The pedunculo-tegmental pathway descends in the most medial portion of the cerebral peduncle, decussating partially in the upper pons, and contacting neurons in the nucleus reticularis tegmenti pontis and in the nucleus raphe interpositus of the paramedian pontine reticular formation (PPRF). An intermediate prefrontofugal system (I—"prefrontal oculomotor bundle") becomes evident at the border of the diencephalon and mesencephalon and contacts cell groups adjacent to the oculomotor nuclear complex, which may include the nucleus of the posterior commissure and the rostral interstitial nucleus of the medial longitudinal fasciculus. A = anterior thalamic nucleus; ac = anterior commissure; f = fornix; III = oculomotor nerve, iv = trochlear nerve; MB = mammillary body; mlf = medial longitudinal fasciculus; pc = posterior commissure. (Modified from Leichnetz GR. The prefrontal cortico-oculomotor trajectories in the monkey. A possible explanation for the effects of stimulation/lesion experiments on eye movement. J Neurol Sci 49, 387–396, 1981, with permission of Elsevier.)

to the superior colliculus. A transthalamic pathway starts in the anterior limb of the internal capsule and projects to the dorsomedial and intralaminar thalamic nuclei, to the ipsilateral superior colliculus and, perhaps, to certain midbrain reticular nuclei such as the riMLF.[236] A pedunculopontine pathway runs from the internal capsule in the most medial aspect of the cerebral peduncle.[236] Its main projections are to the superior colliculus and to the nucleus reticularis tegmenti pontis (NRTP) (Fig. 6–3) that, in turn, projects to the cerebellum.

The PPRF and especially the midline pontine raphe nuclei that house saccadic omnipause cells also receive projections from the FEF.[236,395] A direction projection from FEF to saccadic premotor burst neurons seems unlikely to be important since inactivation of the superior colliculus blocks saccade generation during FEF stimulation.[162] A partial ocular motor decussation, first defined on the basis of stimulation studies,[28,46] may occur between the levels of the trochlear and abducens nuclei.[234]

The *SEF* also projects to the caudate, putamen, superior colliculus, nucleus reticularis tegmenti pontis, and pontine omnipause neurons.[194,404] The *DLPC* projects to parts of the caudate and putamen nucleus, the superior colliculus, and PPRF.[11,398] It is proposed that interruption of DLPC projections to the superior colliculus, either in the anterior limb, genu, or anterior part of the posterior limb of the internal capsule,[85] or in the pedunculopontine pathway,[139] cause increased errors on the antisaccade task.

The *PEF* projects to the superior colliculus.[6,250] How do these multiple projections from frontal and parietal cortex to the caudate nucleus, superior colliculus, and pontine nuclei (see Fig. 3–12, in Chapter 3) differ in the influence they exert on the voluntary control of saccades?

Contributions of the Striatal-Nigral-Collicular Pathway

A pathway through the caudate and adjacent putamen seems important for generation of saccades as part of more complex behaviors that involve memory, expectations, and reward.[164] The caudate and putamen receive inputs from the FEF,[417] SEF,[194] and DLPC.[11] Some eye-movement related neurons in the caudate nucleus discharge for memory-guided saccades,[177] and the general properties of these cells suggest that they are concerned with complex aspects of ocular motor behavior that are necessary, for example, in predicting environmental changes,[178,219] and whether the behavior will be rewarded.[230,231,431] Dopaminergic neurons in substantial nigra pars compacta that project to the caudate nucleus respond to reward contingency but not to the spatial localization of the stimulus.[211] Cholinergic interneurons in the caudate nucleus respond by pausing their discharge to visual cues that indicate saccade goals that will be rewarded.[401] Dopaminergic projections to the caudate appear to modulate spatially selective signals in caudate neurons which, in turn, influence saccade behavior.[211,431]

Functional imaging studies in humans have demonstrated activation of the putamen and substantia nigra during memory-guided saccades.[316] Experimental lesions of the caudate and putamen in monkeys produced ipsilateral gaze deviation, heminegelect, and impairment of contralateral spontaneous, visually mediated, and memory-guided saccades.[210,219,275] Patients with chronic lesions affecting the putamen (and globus pallidus) show deficits in saccades made to remembered locations and in anticipation of predictable target motion; visually guided saccades are unaffected.[451]

The caudate and putamen send projections to the non-dopaminergic substantia nigra pars reticulata (SNpr); these projections are probably GABAergic. Neurons in the SNpr have high tonic discharge rates that decrease before voluntary saccades that are either visually guided or made to remembered target locations.[179–182] They also show reward-related decreases in discharge during saccades.[382] The SNpr, in turn, sends inhibitory projections to the superior colliculus; these projections are also GABAergic. In addition, the SNpr receives excitatory projections from the subthalamic nucleus, which contains neurons that discharge in relation to saccades.[258] The subthalamic nucleus appears to provide a second basal ganglionic pathway by which the cortical eye fields could influence saccades. In addition, the caudate nucleus sends projections to the subthalamic nucleus via the external segment of the globus pallidus.[304] In patients with Parkinson's disease, subthalamic nucleus stimulation causes improved accuracy of memory-guided saccades.[367]

A simplified view of this basal ganglia pathway is that it is composed of two serial, inhibitory links: a caudo-nigral inhibition, which is only phasically active, and a nigro-collicular inhibition, which is tonically active. If frontal cortex causes caudate neurons to fire, then the nigro-collicular inhibition is removed and the superior colliculus is able to activate a saccade. Studies of the effects of pharmacologically inactivating,[183,184] or chemically lesioning,[210,219] the nuclei in this pathway have supported this hypothesis. However, stimulation of caudate neurons can produce either suppression or facilitation of SNpr neurons, and this suggests that the facilitation may be due to a multisynaptic pathway,[176] perhaps via the subthalamic nucleus, whereas inhibition is due to the direct pathway from caudate to SNpr. Furthermore, the pedunculopontine tegmental nucleus (PPTN), which promotes saccade generation as part of a general effect on attention, sends nicotinic projections to the superior colliculus.[216] Thus, the means by which the frontal eye field influences the superior colliculus is complex and might produce difficulties in either initiating or suppressing saccades. Both deficits have been described in patients with disorders affecting the basal ganglia, such as Huntington's disease.[229]

Descending Pathways to the Superior Colliculus for Gaze Control

The FEF, SEF, PEF, and DLPC all project directly to the superior colliculus.[194,250,397,417] FEF projections to ventral layers of the superior colliculus play an important role in programming a range of voluntary eye movements,[115] and pharmacological inactivation of collicular target neurons blocks the effect of stimulating the FEF.[162] In addition, the frontal lobe areas also project indirectly to the superior colliculus via the basal ganglia.

As summarized in Chapter 3, the superior colliculus is a multi-layered structure;[261] while the dorsal layers of the superior colliculus are "visual" in terms of their properties the more ventral are motor.[283,284,409] In primates, the ventral layers are most pertinent for the control of eye movements, and contain a motor map (Fig. 3–13), that predicts the size and direction of saccades that will be induced by microstimulation. Neurons at the rostral pole of this motor map seem important for maintaining steady fixation, and project to omnipause neurons;[59] more caudally located neurons project to burst neurons in the PPRF. Although long thought to be exclusively concerned with saccades, there is now evidence that the superior colliculus may also contribute to smooth-pursuit and vergence eye movements.[220,463] Discrete experimental lesions of the superior colliculus cause an enduring deficit of saccades; their latency is increased and they are slightly slow.[161] Current views emphasize the role of the superior colliculus in target selection and saccade initiation, but not in steering the eye to accurately to the target.[324]

Corticopontine Projections for Gaze Control

A direct pathway has been defined from the FEF to the PPRF, probably to long-lead burst neurons and to the omnipause neurons that lie in the nucleus raphe interpositus (see Fig. 6–2).[395,396] However, acute inactivation of the superior colliculus prevents electrical stimulation of the FEF from inducing saccades, indicating that any direct pathway from FEF to PPRF normally has only a minor influence on saccade generation. Furthermore, this projection is small compared to that going from FEF via the nucleus reticularis tegmenti pontis (NRTP) to the cerebellum. This latter pathway may explain why monkeys are still able to initiate saccades after ablation of the superior colliculus. Although, the cerebellum may be important in optimizing saccadic metrics (discussed in Chapter 3), it is not essential for the initiation of saccades, as they persist even after total cerebellectomy.[466]

Relative Importance of Descending Pathways for Gaze Control

Studies of the effects of restricted, experimental lesions have provided insights into the relative roles of the descending pathways for saccades. In monkeys, acute pharmacological inactivation of the superior colliculus substantially impairs the ability to make saccades.[233]

The enduring effects of discrete lesions of the superior colliculus are increased latency and slowing of saccades.[161] Thus, collicular lesions abolish short-latency or "express" saccades that occur if the fixation light is turned out prior to the appearance of a peripheral visual target (gap task, see Fig. 3–2).[387] Larger lesions cause reduced frequency of spontaneous saccades, and less distractibility on a fixation task.[1] Under normal circumstances, disappearance of the fixation light presumably releases the superior colliculus from inhibitory inputs, so the appearance of the visual target can then elicit a short-latency, "express" saccade.[121] If damage extends to the pretectum and adjacent posterior thalamus (possibly also affecting descending pathways for saccades), the deficit consists of an enduring hypometria without corrective saccades, suggesting that the correct motor error signal required to initiate a corrective saccade no longer reaches the superior colliculus.[2]

Similarly, acute pharmacological inactivation of the FEF substantially impairs saccades, but chronic lesions cause minor deficits that affect visual search and saccades to remembered targets.[102] In contrast, combined bilateral lesions of FEF and superior colliculi produce a severe and enduring deficit of eye movements, with a greatly restricted range of movement.[387,388] Acute, reversible lesions of the FEF and superior colliculus also cause marked hypometria of saccades and a restricted range of movement.[212] Severe deficits of saccadic and pursuit eye movements also follow combined, bilateral lesions of parietal-occipital and frontal cortex in monkeys.[249] With unilateral, combined parieto-frontal lesions, saccades to visual targets in contralateral hemispace are impaired;[252] with hemidecortication, the deficit is more enduring.[444]

In humans, the relative importance of the descending ocular motor pathways is less well defined. Functional imaging has recently shown increased blood flow in the superior colliculi during visual search,[145,394] and this may clarify their role. Isolated lesions of the superior colliculus are reported to cause increased latency and inaccuracy of visually guided saccades,[351] and a paucity of spontaneous saccades contralateral to the side of the lesion.[174] As previously summarized, frontal lobe lesions in humans cause hypometria of visually guided and memory-guided saccades directed contralateral to the lesion and impairment of smooth pursuit of targets moving towards the side of the lesion. No reports exist of combined lesions of the frontal eye fields and superior colliculi in humans. However, combined lesions of frontal and parietal cortex cause loss of ability to make voluntary saccades—ocular motor apraxia (see Video Display: Acquired Ocular Motor Apraxia).[343] Overall, it seems likely that during normal, ocular motor behavior, the frontal and parietal lobes of humans complement each other. The FEFs direct the eyes towards an object or a location of behavioral interest, while the parietal lobes are more concerned with reflexly induced saccades. Finally, although the contributions of the FEF, parietal lobes, and superior colliculus have been defined best for saccades, it seems likely that each of these areas also influence pursuit and vergence, and so allow for changes in gaze in three-dimensional space using all types of eye movements.

SUMMARY

1. The abducens nucleus is the center for conjugate, horizontal eye movements and receives inputs for each functional class of eye movement (Fig. 6–1). The abducens nucleus contains two main groups of neurons: motoneurons that send axons to the ipsilateral lateral rectus muscle, and internuclear neurons that project, via the contralateral medial longitudinal fasciculus, to synapse in the oculomotor nucleus on medial rectus motoneurons. The abducens motoneurons and internuclear neurons receive inputs for horizontal saccades from the PPRF, vestibular, and pursuit inputs from the vestibular nuclei, and the gaze-holding signal from the prepositus–medial vestibular nuclear complex.
2. The oculomotor and trochlear nuclei receive inputs for vertical saccades from the rostral interstitial nucleus of the medial longitudinal fasciculus (riMLF), which lies in the prerubral fields (Fig. 6–5). The interstitial nucleus of Cajal (INC) is important for vertical gaze holding. Vertical vestibular and pursuit signals ascend to the oculomotor and trochlear nuclei from the lower brainstem.

3. The cerebellum (Fig. 6–6) ensures that all classes of eye movements and gaze holding are calibrated to provide clearest vision. The vestibulocerebellum, which consists of the flocculus, paraflocculus, and nodulus, is important for steady gaze holding, smooth ocular tracking, and optimal performance of the vestibulo-ocular reflex. The dorsal vermis and underlying fastigial nucleus have an important role in programming accurate saccades and the initiation of smooth pursuit.
4. Primary visual cortex is essential for accurate saccades and for generating smooth pursuit and optokinetic eye movements. The parietal-occipital-temporal lobe junction contains secondary visual areas important for detecting the speed and direction of moving targets in three dimensions and generating an eye-tracking response. This area of posterior cortex gives rise to an ipsilateral pathway to brainstem and cerebellum, which is important for smooth-pursuit eye movements (Fig. 6–7).
5. Parietal cortical areas contribute to shifting visual attention and also to initiating saccades (Fig. 6–8). The visual responses of some neurons in parietal cortex are influenced by the current direction of gaze. The dorsomedial pulvinar projects to parietal cortex and contributes to shifts of attention.
6. Frontal cortex contains three areas that contribute to programming of saccades (Fig. 6–8). The frontal eye field (FEF) contains neurons that discharge before visually guided and memory-guided saccades. The dorsomedial, supplementary motor area seems important for control of sequences of memory-guided saccades and complex ocular motor behaviors. Dorsolateral prefrontal cortex (DLPC) probably contributes to programming of saccades to remembered target locations and plays an important role during antisaccades. The latter is a special case of saccades made to a location where there is no visual information immediately available.
7. The eye fields of the frontal lobes project, in parallel descending pathways, to the superior colliculus, the brainstem reticular formation, and, via pontine nuclei, to the cerebellum (Fig. 6–9). Indirect pathways involve the caudate nuclei and the pars reticulata of the substantia nigra (SNpr). Combined lesions of the frontal eye fields and the parietal eye fields, or of the frontal eye fields and the superior colliculi, cause profound and enduring ocular motor deficits.

REFERENCES

1. Albano JE, Mishkin M, Westbrook LE, Wurtz RH. Visuomotor deficits following ablation of monkey superior colliculus. J Neurophysiol 48, 338–351, 1982.
2. Albano JE, Wurtz RH. Deficits in eye position following ablation of monkey superior colliculus, pretectum, and posterior-medial thalamus. J Neurophysiol 48, 318–337, 1982.
3. Amador N, Schlag-Rey M, Schlag J. Primate antisaccade. II. Supplementary eye field neuronal activity predicts correct performance. J Neurophysiol 91, 1672–1689, 2004.
4. Anastasio TJ, Robinson DA. Failure of the oculomotor neural integrator from a discrete midline lesion between the abducens nuclei in the monkey. Neurosci Lett 127, 82–86, 1991.
5. Andersen RA. Multimodal integration for the representation of space in the posterior parietal cortex. Philos Trans R Soc Lond B Biol Sci 352, 1421–1428, 1997.
6. Andersen RA, Asanuma C, Essick GK, Siegel RM. Cortico-cortical connections of anatomically and physiologically defined subdivisions within the inferior parietal lobe. J Comp Neurol 296, 65–113, 1990.
7. Andersen RA, Bracewell RM, Barash S, Gnadt JW, Fogassi L. Eye position effects on visual, memory, and saccade-related activity in areas LIP and 7a of macaque. J Neurosci 10, 1176–1196, 1990.
8. Andersen RA, Mountcastle VB. The influence of the angle of gaze upon the excitability of the light-sensitive neurons of the posterior parietal cortex. J Neurosci 3, 532–548, 1983.
9. Anderson TJ, Jenkins IH, Brooks DJ, et al. Cortical control of saccades and fixation in man. A PET study. Brain 117, 1073–1084, 1994.
10. Annese J, Gazzaniga MS, Toga AW. Localization of the human cortical visual area MT based on computer aided histological analysis. Cereb Cortex 15, 1044–1053, 2005.
11. Arikuni T, Kubota K. The organization of prefrontocaudate projections and their laminar origin in the macaque monkey: a retrograde study using HRP-gel. J Comp Neurol 244, 492–510, 1986.
12. Arnold DB, Robinson DA. The oculomotor integrator: testing of a neural network model. Exp Brain Res 113, 57–74, 1997.
13. Balan PF, Ferrera VP. Effects of spontaneous eye movements on spatial memory in macaque periarcuate cortex. J Neurosci 23, 11392–11401, 2003.
14. Barash S, Bracewell RM, Fogassi L, Gnadt JW, Andersen RA. Saccade-related activity in the lateral

intraparietal area. I. Temporal properties; comparison with area 7a. J Neurophysiol 66, 1095–1108, 1991.
15. Barton JJS, Sharpe JA, Raymond JE. Retinoptic and directional defects in motion discrimination in humans with cerebral lesions. Ann Neurol 37, 665–675, 1995.
16. Barton JJS, Sharpe JA, Raymond JE. Directional defects in pursuit and motion perception in humans with unilateral cerebral lesions. Brain 119, 1535–1550, 1996.
17. Barton JJS, Sharpe JA. Motion direction discrimination in blind hemifields. Ann Neurol 41, 255–264, 1997.
18. Bates JF, Goldman-Rakic PS. Prefrontal connections of the medial motor area in the rhesus monkey. J Comp Neurol 336, 211–228, 1993.
19. Batton RR, Jayaraman A, Ruggiero D, Carpenter MB. Fastigial efferent projections in the monkey: an autoradiographic study. J Comp Neurol 174, 281–306, 1977.
20. Bavelier D, Tomann A, Hutton C, et al. Visual attention to the periphery is enhanced in congenitally deaf individuals. J Neurosci 20, RC93, 2000.
21. Belknap DB, McCrea RA. Anatomical connections of the prepositus and abducens nuclei in the squirrel monkey. J Comp Neurol 268, 13–28, 1988.
22. Bellebaum C, Daum I, Koch B, Schwarz M, Hoffmann KP. The role of the human thalamus in processing corollary discharge. Brain 128, 1139–1154, 2005.
23. Belton T, McCrea RA. Role of the cerebellar flocculus region in cancellation of the VOR during passive whole body rotation. J Neurophysiol 84, 1599–1613, 2000.
24. Belton T, McCrea RA. Role of the cerebellar flocculus region in the coordination of eye and head movements during gaze pursuit. J Neurophysiol 84, 1614–1626, 2000.
25. Ben HS, Duhamel JR, Bremmer F, Graf W. Visual receptive field modulation in the lateral intraparietal area during attentive fixation and free gaze. Cereb Cortex 12, 234–245, 2002.
26. Ben HS, Page W, Duffy C, Pouget A. MSTd neuronal basis functions for the population encoding of heading direction. J Neurophysiol 90, 549–558, 2003.
27. Bender DB. Visual activation of neurons in the primate pulvinar depends on cortex but not colliculus. Brain Res 279, 258–261, 1983.
28. Bender MB, Shanzer S. In Bender MB (ed). The Oculomotor System. Harper and Row, New York, 1964, pp 81–140.
29. Benevento LA, Port JD. Single neurons with both form/color differential responses and saccade-related responses in the nonretinotopic pulvinar of the behaving macaque monkey. Vis Neurosci 12, 523–544, 1995.
30. Bennett AH, Savill T. A case of permanent conjugate deviation of the eyes and head, the result of a lesion limited to the sixth nucleus; with remarks on associated lateral movements of the eyeballs, and rotation of the head and neck. Brain 12, 102–116, 1889.
31. Blanke O, Marand S, Thut G, et al. Visual activity in the human frontal eye field. Neuroreport 10, 925–930, 1999.
32. Blanke O, Seeck M. Direction of saccadic and smooth eye movements induced by electrical stimulation of the human frontal eye field: effect of orbital position. Exp Brain Res 150, 174–183, 2003.
33. Blanke O, Spinelli L, Thut G, et al. Location of the human frontal eye field as defined by electrical cortical stimulation: anatomical, functional and electrophysiological characteristics. Neuroreport 11, 1907–1913, 2000.
34. Blatt GJ, Andersen RA, Stoner GR. Visual receptive field organization and cortico-cortical connections of the lateral intraparietal area (LIP) in the macaque. J Comp Neurol 299, 421–445, 1990.
35. Bodis-Wollner I, Bucher SF, Seelos KC, et al. Functional MRI mapping of occipital and frontal cortical activity during voluntary and imagined saccades. Neurology 49, 416–420, 1997.
36. Bogousslavsky J, Regli F. Pursuit gaze defects in acute and chronic unilateral parieto-occipital lesions. Eur Neurol 25, 10–18, 1986.
37. Bottini G, Sterzi R, Paulesu E, et al. Identification of the central vestibular projections in man: a positron emission tomography activation study. Exp Brain Res 99, 164–169, 1994.
38. Brandt SA, Ploner CJ, Meyer BU, Leistner S, Villringer A. Effects of repetitive transcranial magnetic stimulation over dorsolateral prefrontal and posterior parietal cortex on memory-guided saccades. Exp Brain Res 118, 197–204, 1998.
39. Brandt T, Dieterich M. Vestibular syndromes in the roll plane: topographic diagnosis from brain stem to cortex. Ann Neurol 36, 337–347, 1994.
40. Brandt T, Dieterich M, Danek A. Vestibular cortex lesions affect the perception of verticality. Ann Neurol 35, 403–412, 1994.
41. Brodal P. Further observations on the cerebellar projections from the pontine nuclei and the nucleus reticularis tegmenti pontis in the rhesus monkey. J Comp Neurol 204, 44–55, 1982.
42. Brotchie PR, Andersen RA, Snyder LH, Goodman SJ. Head position signals used by parietal neurons to encode locations of visual stimuli. Nature 375, 232–235, 1995.
43. Brotchie PR, Lee MB, Chen DY, et al. Head position modulates activity in the human parietal eye fields. Neuroimage 18, 178–184, 2003.
44. Bruce CJ, Goldberg ME. Primate frontal eye fields. I. Single neurons discharging before saccades. J Neurophysiol 53, 603–635, 1985.
45. Bruce CJ, Goldberg ME, Bushnell MC, Stanton GB. Primate Frontal Eye Fields. II. Physiological and anatomical correlates of electrically evoked eye movements. J Neurophysiol 54, 714–734, 1985.
46. Brucher JM. L'aire oculogyre frontale du singe. Ses fonctions et ses voies efférentes. Arscia, Brussels, 1964.
47. Bucher SF, Dieterich M, Wiesmann M, et al. Cerebral functional magnetic resonance imaging of vestibular, auditory, and nociceptive areas during galvanic stimulation. Ann Neurol 44, 120–125, 1998.
48. Burman DD, Bruce CJ. Suppression of task-related saccades by electrical stimulation in the primate's frontal eye field. J Neurophysiol 77, 2252–2267, 1997.
49. Burman DD, Segraves MA. Primate frontal eye field activity during natural scanning eye movements. J Neurophysiol 71, 1266–1271, 1994.
50. Büttner U, Büttner-Ennever JA, Henn V. Vertical eye movement related unit activity in the rostral mesen-

cephalic reticular formation of the alert monkey. Brain Res 130, 239–252, 1977.

51. Büttner U, Straube A, Spuler A. Saccadic dysmetria and "intact" smooth pursuit eye movements after bilateral deep cerebellar nuclei lesions. J Neurol Neurosurg Psychiatry 57, 832–834, 1995.
52. Büttner-Ennever J, Büttner U. The reticular formation. In Büttner-Enever JA (ed). Neuroanatomy of the Oculomotor System. Elsevier, New York,1988, pp 119–176.
53. Büttner-Ennever JA. The extraocular motor nuclei. In Büttner-Ennever JA (ed). Neuroanatomy of the Oculomotor System. Prog Brain Res 151, 95–126, 2006.
54. Büttner-Ennever JA, Büttner U. A cell group associated with vertical eye movements in the rostral mesencephalic reticular formation of the monkey. Brain Res 151, 31–47, 1978.
55. Büttner-Ennever JA, Büttner U, Cohen B, Baumgartner G. Vertical gaze paralysis and the rostral interstitial nucleus of the medial longitudinal fasciculus. Brain 105, 125–149, 1982.
56. Büttner-Ennever JA, Cohen B, Horn AK, Reisine H. Pretectal projections to the oculomotor complex of the monkey and their role in eye movements. J Comp Neurol 366, 348–359, 1996.
57. Büttner-Ennever JA, Cohen B, Pause M, Fries W. Raphe nucleus of the pons containing omnipause neurons of the oculomotor system in the monkey, and its homologue in man. J Comp Neurol 267, 307–321, 1988.
58. Büttner-Ennever JA, Horn AK. Anatomical substrates of oculomotor control. Curr Opin Neurobiol 7, 872–879, 1997.
59. Büttner-Ennever JA, Horn AK, Henn V, Cohen B. Projections from the superior colliculus motor map to omnipause neurons in monkey. J Comp Neurol 413, 55–67, 1999.
60. Büttner-Ennever JA, Horn AK, Scherberger H, D'Ascanio P. Motoneurons of twitch and nontwitch extraocular muscle fibers in the abducens, trochlear, and oculomotor nuclei of monkeys. J Comp Neurol 438, 318–335, 2001.
61. Büttner-Ennever JA, Horn AK, Schmidtke K. Cell groups of the medial longitudinal fasciculus and paramedian tracts. Rev Neurol (Paris) 145, 533–539, 1989.
62. Büttner-Ennever JA, Horn AKE. Pathways from cell groups of the paramedian tracts to the floccular region. Ann N Y Acad Sci 781, 532–540, 1996.
63. Büttner-Ennever JA, Jenkins C, Armin-Parsa H, Horn AKE, Elston JS. A neuroanatomical analysis of lid-eye coordination in cases of ptosis and downgaze paralysis. Clin Neuropathol 15, 313–318, 1996.
64. Cannon SC, Robinson DA. Loss of the neural integrator of the oculomotor system from brain stem lesions in monkey. J Neurophysiol 57, 1383–1409, 1987.
65. Carey MR, Lisberger SG. Signals that modulate gain control for smooth pursuit eye movements in monkeys. J Neurophysiol 91, 623–631, 2004.
66. Carpenter MB, Batton RR, III. Abducens internuclear neurons and their role in conjugate horizontal gaze. J Comp Neurol 189, 191–209, 1980.
67. Carpenter MB, Cowie RJ. Connections and oculomotor projections of the superior vestibular nucleus and cell group 'y'. Brain Res 336, 265–287, 1985.
68. Carpenter MB, McMasters RE, Hanna GR. Disturbances of conjugate horizontal eye movements in the monkey. I. Physiological effects and anatomical degeneration resulting from lesions of the abducens nucleus and nerve. Arch Neurol 8, 231–247, 1963.
69. Carpenter MB, Periera AB, Guha N. Immunocytochemistry of oculomotor afferents in the squirrel monkey (Saimiri sciureus). J Hirnforschung 33, 151–167, 1992.
70. Carpenter MB, Strominger NL. The medial longitudinal fasciculus and disturbances of conjugate horizontal eye movements in the monkey. J Comp Neurol. 125, 41–65, 1965.
71. Casanova C. The visual functions of the pulvinar. In Chapula LM, Werner JS (eds). The Visual Neurosciences. MIT Press, Cambridge, Massachusetts, 2003 pp 592–608.
72. Cavada C, Goldman-Rakic PS. Posterior parietal cortex in rhesus monkeys: I. Parcellation of areas based on distinctive limbic and sensory corticocortical connections. J Comp Neurol 287, 393–421, 1989.
73. Chafee MV, Goldman-Rakic PS. Matching patterns of activity in primate prefrontal area 8a and parietal area 7ip neurons during a spatial working memory task. J Neurophysiol 79, 2919–2940, 1998.
74. Chalupa LM. A review of cat and monkey studies implicating the pulvinar in visual function. Behav Biol 20, 149–167, 1977.
75. Chen KJ, Sheliga BM, FitzGibbon EJ, Miles FA. Initial ocular following in humans depends critically on the Fourier components of the motion stimulus. Ann N Y Acad Sci 1039, 260–271, 2005.
76. Chen LL, Wise SP. Supplementary eye field contrasted with the frontal eye field during acquisition of conditional oculomotor associations. J Neurophysiol 73, 1122–1134, 1995.
77. Chen-Huang C, McCrea RA. Viewing distance related sensory processing in the ascending tract of Deiters vestibulo-ocular reflex pathway. J Vestib Res 8, 175–184, 1998.
78. Chen-Huang C, McCrea RA. Effects of viewing distance on the responses of horizontal canal-related secondary vestibular neurons during angular head rotation. J Neurophysiol 81, 2517–2537, 1999.
79. Cheron G, Dufief M-P, Gerrits N, Godaux E. Properties of nucleus incertus neurons of the cat projecting to the cerebellar flocculus. Ann N Y Acad Sci 781, 589–593, 1996.
80. Chubb MC, Fuchs AF. Contribution of y group of vestibular nuclei and dentate nucleus of cerebellum to generation of vertical smooth eye movements. J Neurophysiol 48, 75–99, 1982.
81. Clendaniel RA, Mays LE. Characteristics of antidromically identified oculomotor internuclear neurons during vergence and versional eye movements. J Neurophysiol 71, 1111–1127, 1994.
82. Coe B, Tomihara K, Matsuzawa M, Hikosaka O. Visual and anticipatory bias in three cortical eye fields of the monkey during an adaptive decision-making task. J Neurosci 22, 5081–5090, 2002.
83. Cohen B, Büttner-Ennever JA. Projections from the superior colliculus to a region of the central mesencephalic reticular formation (cMRF) associated with horizontal saccadic eye movements. Exp Brain Res 57, 167–176, 1984.

84. Cohen B, Waitzman DM, Büttner-Ennever JA, Matsuo V. Horizontal saccades and the central mesencephalic reticular formation. Progr Brain Res 64, 243–256, 1986.
85. Condy C, Rivaud-Pechoux S, Ostendorf F, Ploner CJ, Gaymard B. Neural substrate of antisaccades: role of subcortical structures. Neurology 63, 1571–1578, 2004.
86. Connolly JD, Goodale MA, Menon RS, Munoz DP. Human fMRI evidence for the neural correlates of preparatory set. Nat Neurosci 5, 1345–1352, 2002.
87. Constantinidis C, Franowicz MN, Goldman-Rakic PS. The sensory nature of mnemonic representation in the primate prefrontal cortex. Nat Neurosci 4, 311–316, 2001.
88. Corbetta M. Frontoparietal cortical networks for directing attention and the eye to visual locations - identical, independent, or overlapping neural systems? Proc Natl Acad Sci U S A 95, 831–838, 1998.
89. Cornelissen FW, Kimmig H, Schira M, et al. Event-related fMRI responses in the human frontal eye fields in a randomized pro- and antisaccade task. Exp Brain Res 145, 270–274, 2002.
90. Cowey A, Stoerig P, Bannister M. Retinal ganglion cells labelled from the pulvinar nucleus in macaque monkeys. Neuroscience 61, 691–705, 1994.
91. Crandall WF, Keller EL. Visual and oculomotor signals in nucleus reticularis tegmenti pontis in alert monkey. J Neurophysiol 54, 1326–1345, 1985.
92. Crawford JD. The oculomotor neural integrator uses a behavior-related coordinate system. J Neurosci 14, 6911–6923, 1994.
93. Crawford JD, Cadera W, Vilis T. Generation of torsional and vertical eye position signals by the interstitial nucleus of Cajal. Science 252, 1551–1553, 1991.
94. Crawford TJ, Bennett D, Lekwuwa G, Shaunak S. Deakin JF. Cognition and the inhibitory control of saccades in schizophrenia and Parkinson's disease. Prog Brain Res 140, 449–466, 2002.
95. Cremer PD, Migliaccio AA, Halmagyi GM, Curthoys IS. Vestibulo-ocular reflex pathways in internuclear ophthalmoplegia. Ann Neurol 45, 529–533, 1999.
96. Crossland WJ, Hu XJ, Rafols JA. Morphological study of the rostral interstitial nucleus of the medial longitudinal fasciculus in the monkey, Macaca mulatta, by Nissl, Golgi, and computer reconstruction and rotation methods. J Comp Neurol 347, 47–63, 1994.
97. Cullen KE, Roy JE. Signal processing in the vestibular system during active versus passive head movements. J Neurophysiol 91, 1919–1933, 2004.
98. Cusick CG, Scripter JL, Darensbourg JG, Weber JT. Chemoarchitectonic subdivisions of the visual pulvinar in monkey and their connectional relations with the middle temporal and rostral dosrolateral visual areas, MT and DLr. J Comp Neurol 336, 1–30, 1993.
99. De Zeeuw CI, Wylie DR, Stahl JS, Simpson JI. Phase relations of Purkinje cells in the rabbit flocculus during compensatory eye movements. J Neurophysiol 74, 2051–2064, 1995.
100. Dean HL, Crowley JC, Platt ML. Visual and saccade-related activity in macaque posterior cingulate cortex. J Neurophysiol 92, 3056–3068, 2004.
101. DeAngelis GC, Cumming BG, Newsome WT. Cortical area MT and the perception of stereoscopic depth. Nature 394, 677–680, 1998.
102. Deng SY, Goldberg ME, Segraves MA, Ungerleider L, Mishkin M. The effects of unilateral ablation of the frontal eye fields on saccadic performance in the monkey. In Keller EL, Zee DS (eds). Adaptive Processes in Visual and Oculomotor Systems. Pergamon, Oxford,1986, pp 201–208.
103. Desimone R, Ungerleider LG. Multiple visual areas in the caudal superior temporal sulcus of the macaque. J Comp Neurol 248, 164–189, 1986.
104. DeSouza JF, Menon RS, Everling S. Preparatory set associated with pro-saccades and anti-saccades in humans investigated with event-related FMRI. J Neurophysiol 89, 1016–1023, 2003.
105. Dias EC, Bruce CJ. Physiological correlate of fixation disengagement in the primate's frontal eye field. J Neurophysiol 72, 2532–2537, 1994.
106. Dias EC, Segraves MA. Muscimol-induced inactivation of monkey frontal eye field: effects on visually and memory-guided saccades. J Neurophysiol 81, 2191–2214, 1999.
107. Dieterich M, Bense S, Stephan T, Yousry TA, Brandt T. fMRI signal increases and decreases in cortical areas during small-field optokinetic stimulation and central fixation. Exp Brain Res 148, 117–127, 2003.
108. Distler C, Mustari MJ, Hoffmann KP. Cortical projections to the nucleus of the optic tract and dorsal terminal nucleus and to the dorsolateral pontine nucleus in macaques: a dual retrograde tracing study. J Comp Neurol 444, 144–158, 2002.
109. Doricchi F, Perani D, Incoccia C, et al. Neural control of fast-regular saccades and antisaccades: an investigation using positron emission tomography. Exp Brain Res 116, 50–62, 1997.
110. Duhamel J-R, Colby CL, Goldberg ME. Ventral intraparietal area of the macaque: congruent visual and somatic response properties. J Neurophysiol 79, 126–136, 1998.
111. Duhamel J-R, Goldberg ME, FitzGibbon EJ, Sirigu A, Grafman J. Saccadic dysmetria in a patient with a right frontoparietal lesion: the importance of corollary discharge for accurate spatial-behavior. Brain 115, 1387–1402, 1992.
112. Dukelow SP, De Souza JF, Culham JC, et al. Distinguishing subregions of the human MT+ complex using visual fields and pursuit eye movements. J Neurophysiol 86, 1991–2000, 2001.
113. Dürsteler MR, Wurtz RH. Pursuit and optokinetic deficits following chemical lesions of cortical areas MT and MST. J Neurophysiol 60, 940–965, 1988.
114. Eberhorn AC, Horng A, Hartig W, et al. Distribution of functional cell groups in the abducens nucleus of monkey and man. Soc Neurosci Abstr 881.6, 2004.
115. Everling S, Munoz DP. Neuronal correlates for preparatory set associated with pro-saccades and anti-saccades in the primate frontal eye field. J Neurosci 20, 387–400, 2000.
116. Evinger LC, Fuchs AF, Baker R. Bilateral lesions of the medial longitudinal fasciculus in monkeys: Effects on the horizontal and vertical components of voluntary and vestibular induced eye movements. Exp Brain Res 28, 1–20, 1977.
117. Felleman DJ, Van Essen DC. Distributed hierarchical processing in the primate cerebral cortex. Cerebr Cortex 1, 1–47, 1991.
118. Ferraina S, Pare M, Wurtz RH. Disparity sensitivity

of frontal eye field neurons. J. Neurophysiol. 83, 625–629, 2000.
119. Ferraina S, Pare M, Wurtz RH. Comparison of cortico-cortical and cortico-collicular signals for the generation of saccadic eye movements. J Neurophysiol 87, 845–858, 2002.
120. Ffytche DH, Guy CN, Zeki S. The parallel visual motion inputs into areas V1 and V5 of human cerebral cortex. Brain 118, 1375–1394, 1995.
121. Fischer B, Ramsperger E. Human express saccades: extremely short reaction times of goal directed eye movements. Exp Brain Res 57, 191–195, 1984.
122. Fisher CM. Some neuro-ophthalmological observations. J Neurol Neurosurg Psychiatry 30, 383–392, 1967.
123. Fisher CM. Neuroanatomic evidence to explain why bilateral internuclear ophthalmoplegia may result from occlusion of a unilateral pontine branch artery. J Neuroophthalmol 24, 39–41, 2004.
124. Fox PT, Fox JM, Raichle ME, Burde RM. The role of cerebral cortex in the generation of voluntary saccades: a positron emission tomographic study. J Neurophysiol 54, 348–369, 1985.
125. Fredericks CA, Giolli RA, Blanks RHI, Sadun AA. The human accessory optic system. Brain Res 454, 116–122, 1988.
126. Fuchs AF, Robinson FR, Straube A. Role of the caudal fastigial nucleus in saccade generation: I. Neuronal discharge patterns. J Neurophysiol 70, 1723–1740, 1993.
127. Fuchs AF, Robinson FR, Straube A. Participation of the caudal fastigial nucleus in smooth-pursuit eye movements .1. Neuronal activity. J Neurophysiol 72, 2714–2728, 1994.
128. Fuchs AF, Scudder CA, Kaneko CRS. Discharge patterns and recruitment order of identified motoneurons and internuclear neurons in the monkey abducens nucleus. J Neurophysiol 60, 1874–1895, 1988.
129. Fukushima J, Akao T, Takeichi N, et al. Pursuit-related neurons in the supplementary eye fields: discharge during pursuit and passive whole body rotation. J Neurophysiol 91, 2809–2825, 2004.
130. Fukushima K, Fukushima J, Sato T. Vestibular-pursuit interactions: gaze-velocity and target-velocity signals in the monkey frontal eye fields. Ann N Y Acad Sci 871, 248–259, 1999.
131. Fukushima K, Yamanobe T, Shinmei Y, Fukushima J. Predictive responses of periarcuate pursuit neurons to visual target motion. Exp Brain Res 145, 104–120, 2002.
132. Fukushima K, Yamanobe T, Shinmei Y, et al. Coding of smooth eye movements in three-dimensional space by frontal cortex. Nature 419, 157–162, 2002.
133. Funahashi S, Bruce CJ, Goldman-Rakic PS. Mnemonic coding of visual space in the monkey's dorsolateral prefrontal cortex. J Neurophysiol 61, 331–349, 1989.
134. Funahashi S, Bruce CJ, Goldman-Rakic PS. Neuronal activity related to saccadic eye movements in the monkey's dorsolateral prefrontal cortex. J Neurophysiol 65, 1464–1483, 1991.
135. Funahashi S, Bruce CJ, Goldman-Rakic PS. Dorsolateral prefrontal lesions and oculomotor delayed-response performance: evidence for mnemonic "scotomas". J Neurosci 13, 1479–1497, 1993.
136. Gamlin PD, Yoon K. An area for vergence eye movement in primate frontal cortex. Nature 407, 1003–1007, 2000.
137. Gamlin PDR, Gnadt JW, Mays LE. Lidocaine-induced unilateral internuclear ophthalmoplegia: effects on convergence and conjugate eye movements. J Neurophysiol 62, 82–95, 1989.
138. Garbutt S, Thakore N, Rucker JC, et al. Effects of visual fixation and convergence in periodic alternating nystagmus due to MS. Neuro-ophthalmology 28, 221–229, 2004.
139. Gaymard B, Francois C, Ploner CJ, Condy C, Rivaud-Pechoux S. A direct prefrontotectal tract against distractibility in the human brain. Ann Neurol 53, 542–545, 2003.
140. Gaymard B, Pierrot-Deseilligny C, Rivaud S. Impairment of sequences of memory-guided saccades after supplementary motor area lesions. Ann Neurol 28, 622–626, 1990.
141. Gaymard B, Rivaud S, Cassarini JF, et al. Effects of anterior cingulate cortex lesions on ocular saccades in humans. Exp Brain Res 120, 173–183, 1998.
142. Gaymard B, Rivaud S, Pierrot-Deseilligny C. Role of the left and right supplementary motor areas in memory-guided saccade sequences. Ann Neurol 34, 404–406, 1993.
143. Gaymard B, Rivaud S, Pierrot-Deseilligny C. Impairment of extraretinal eye position signals after central thalamic lesions in humans. Exp Brain Res 102, 1–9, 1994.
144. Gaymard B, Rivaud-Pechoux S, Yelnik J, Pidoux B, Ploner CJ. Involvement of the cerebellar thalamus in human saccade adaptation. Eur J Neurosci 14, 554–560, 2001.
145. Gitelman DR, Parrish TB, Friston KJ, Mesulam MM. Functional anatomy of visual search: regional segregations within the frontal eye fields and effective connectivity of the superior colliculus. Neuroimage 15, 970–982, 2002.
146. Glickstein M, Cohen JL, Dixon B, et al. Corticopontine visual projections in macaque monkeys. J Comp Neurol 190, 209–229, 1980.
147. Glickstein M, Gerritts N, Kralj-Hans I, et al. Visual pontocerebellar projections in the macaque. J Comp Neurol 349, 51–72, 1994.
148. Godoy J, Luders H, Dinner DS, Morris HH, Wyllie E. Versive eye movements elicited by cortical stimulation of the human brain. Neurology 40, 296–299, 1990.
149. Goebel HH, Komatsuzaki A, Bender MB, Cohen B. Lesions of the pontine tegmentum and conjugate gaze paralysis. Arch Neurol 24, 431–440, 1971.
150. Goldberg ME, Bisley J, Powell KD, Gottlieb J, Kusunoki M. The role of the lateral intraparietal area of the monkey in the generation of saccades and visuospatial attention. Ann N Y Acad Sci 956, 205–215, 2002.
151. Goldberg ME, Bruce CJ. Primate frontal eye fields. III. Maintenance of a spatially accurate saccade signal. J Neurophysiol 64, 489–508, 1990.
152. Gonzalo-Ruiz A, Leichnetz GR, Smith DJ. Origin of cerebellar projections to the region of the oculomotor complex, medial pontine reticular formation, and superior colliculus in new world monkeys: A retrograde horseradish peroxidase study. J Comp Neurol 268, 508–526, 1988.
153. Gottlieb JP, MacAvoy MG, Bruce CJ. Neural

responses related to smooth-pursuit eye movements and their correspondence with electrically elicited smooth eye movements in the primate frontal eye field. J Neurophysiol 72, 1634–1653, 1994.
154. Groh JM, Born RT, Newsome WT. How is a sensory map read out? Effects of microstimulation in visual area MT on saccades and smooth pursuit eye movements. J Neurosci 17, 4312–4330, 1997.
155. Grosbras MH, Lobel E, Van de Moortele PF, LeBihan D, Berthoz A. An anatomical landmark for the supplementary eye fields in human revealed with functional magnetic resonance imaging. Cerebr Cortex 9, 705–711, 1999.
156. Grosbras MH, Paus T. Transcranial magnetic stimulation of the human frontal eye field: effects on visual perception and attention. J Cogn Neurosci 14, 1109–1120, 2002.
157. Haarmeier T, Their P, Repnow M, Petersen D. False perception of motion in a patient who cannot compensate for eye movements. Nature 389, 849–852, 1997.
158. Hain TC, Zee DS, Maria BL. Tilt suppression of vestibulo-ocular reflex in patients with cerebellar lesions. Acta Otolaryngol (Stockh) 105, 13–20, 1988.
159. Handel A, Glimcher PW. Response properties of saccade-related burst neurons in the central mesencephalic reticular formation. J Neurophysiol 78, 2164–2175, 1997.
160. Hanes DP, Patterson WF, Schall JD. Role of frontal eye fields in countermanding saccades: visual, movement, and fixation activity. J Neurophysiol. 79, 817–834, 1998.
161. Hanes DP, Smith MK, Optican LM, Wurtz RH. Recovery of saccadic dysmetria following localized lesions in monkey superior colliculus. Exp Brain Res 160, 325, 2005.
162. Hanes DP, Wurtz RH. Interaction of the frontal eye field and superior colliculus for saccade generation. J Neurophysiol 85, 804–815, 2001.
163. Hanson MR, Hamid MA, Tomsak RL, Chou SS, Leigh RJ. Selective saccadic palsy caused by pontine lesions: clinical, physiological, and pathological correlations. Ann Neurol 20, 209–217, 1986.
164. Harting JK, Updyke BV. Oculomotor-related pathways of the basal ganglia. In Büttner-Ennever JA (ed). Neuroanatomy of the Oculomotor System. Prog Brain Res 151, 466, 2006.
165. Heide W, Binkofski F, Seitz RJ, et al. Activation of frontoparietal cortices during memorized triple-step sequences of saccadic eye movements: an fMRI study. Eur J Neurosci 13, 1177–1189, 2001.
166. Heide W, Blankenburg M, Zimmerman E. Cortical control of double-step saccades: implications for spatial orientation. Ann Neurol 38, 739–748, 1995.
167. Heide W, Kurzidim K, Kompf D. Deficits of smooth pursuit eye movements after frontal and parietal lesions. Brain 119 (Pt 6), 1951–1969, 1996.
168. Heinen SJ. Single neuron activity in the dorsomedial frontal cortex during smooth pursuit eye movements. Exp Brain Res 104, 357–361, 1995.
169. Helmchen C, Büttner U. Saccade-related Purkinje cell activity in the oculomotor vermis during spontaneous eye movements in the light and darkness. Exp Brain Res 103, 198–208, 1995.
170. Helmchen C, Rambold H, Fuhry L, Büttner U. Deficits in vertical and torsional eye movements after uni- and bilateral muscimol inactivation of the interstitial nucleus of Cajal of the alert monkey. Exp Brain Res 119, 436–452, 1998.
171. Helmchen C, Rambold H, Kempermann U, Büttner-Ennever JA, Büttner U. Localizing value of torsional nystagmus in small midbrain lesions. Neurology 59, 1956–1964, 2002.
172. Helmchen C, Straube A, Büttner U. Saccade-related activity in the fastigial oculomotor region of the macaque monkey during spontaneous eye movements in light and darkness. Exp Brain Res 98, 474–482, 1994.
173. Henn V, Lang W, Hepp K, Reisine H. Experimental gaze palsies in monkeys and their relation to human pathology. Brain 107, 619–636, 1984.
174. Heywood S, Ratcliff G. Long-term oculomotor consequences of unilateral colliculectomy in man. In Lennerstand G, Bach-y-Rita P (eds). Basic Mechanisms of Ocular Motility and their Clinical Implications. Pergamon, Oxford, 1986, pp 561–564.
175. Highstein SM, Baker R. Excitatory termination of abducens internuclear neurons on medial rectus motoneurons: relationship to syndrome of internuclear ophthalmoplegia. J Neurophysiol 41, 1647–1661, 1978.
176. Hikosaka O, Sakamoto M, Miyashita N. Effects of caudate nucleus stimulation on substantia nigra cell activity in monkey. Exp Brain Res 95, 457–472, 1993.
177. Hikosaka O, Sakamoto M, Usui S. Functional properties of monkey caudate neurons. I. Activities related to saccadic eye movements. J Neurophysiol 61, 780–798, 1989.
178. Hikosaka O, Sakamoto M, Usui S. Functional properties of monkey caudate neurons. III. Activities related to expectation of target and reward. J Neurophysiol 61, 814–832, 1989.
179. Hikosaka O, Wurtz RH. Visual and oculomotor functions of monkey substantia nigra pars reticulata. I. Relation of visual and auditory responses to saccades. J Neurophysiol 49, 1230–1253, 1983.
180. Hikosaka O, Wurtz RH. Visual and oculomotor functions of monkey substantia nigra pars reticulata. II. Visual responses related to fixation of gaze. J Neurophysiol 49, 1254–1267, 1983.
181. Hikosaka O, Wurtz RH. Visual and oculomotor functions of monkey substantia nigra pars reticulata. III. Memory-contingent visual and saccade responses. J Neurophysiol 49, 1268–1284, 1983.
182. Hikosaka O, Wurtz RH. Visual and oculomotor functions of monkey substantia nigra pars reticulata. IV. Relation of substantia nigra to superior colliculus. J Neurophysiol 49, 1285–1301, 1983.
183. Hikosaka O, Wurtz RH. Modification of saccadic eye movements by GABA-related substances. I. Effect of muscimol and bicuculline in monkey superior colliculus. J Neurophysiol 53, 266–291, 1985.
184. Hikosaka O, Wurtz RH. Modification of saccadic eye movements by GABA-related substances. II. Effects of muscimol in monkey substantia nigra pars reticulata. J Neurophysiol 53, 292–308, 1985.
185. Holmes G. The cerebral integration of the ocular movements. Br Med J 2, 107–112, 1938.
186. Horn AK. The reticular formation. In Büttner-Ennever JA (ed). Neuroanatomy of the Oculomotor System. Prog Brain Res 151, 33–79, 2006.
187. Horn AK, Büttner-Ennever JA. Premotor neurons for vertical eye movements in the rostral mesen

cephalon of monkey and human: histologic identification by parvalbumin immunostaining. J Comp Neurol 392, 413–427, 1998.
188. Horn AK, Büttner-Ennever JA, Gayde M, Messoudi A. Neuroanatomical identification of mesencephalic premotor neurons coordinating eyelid with upgaze in the monkey and man. J Comp Neurol 420, 19–34, 2000.
189. Horn AK, Büttner-Ennever JA, Wahle P, Reichenberger I. Neurotransmitter profile of saccadic omnipause neurons in nucleus raphe interpositus. J Neurosci 14, 2032–2046, 1994.
190. Horn AKE, Büttner-Ennever JA, Büttner U. Saccadic premotor neurons in the brainstem: functional neuroanatomy and clinical implications. Neuro-ophthalmology 16, 229–240, 1996.
191. Horn AKE, Büttner-Ennever JA, Suzuki Y, Henn,V. Histological identification of premotor neurons for horizontal saccades in monkey and man by parvalbumin immunostaining. J Comp Neurol 359, 350–363, 1997.
192. Horn AKE, Helmchen C, Wahle P. GABAergic neurons in the rostral mesencephalon of the macaque monkey that control vertical eye movements. Ann N Y Acad Sci 1004, 19–28, 2003.
193. Hubel DH, Wiesel TN. Brain and Visual Perception. Oxford University Press, New York, 2005.
194. Huerta MF, Kaas JH. Supplementary eye fields as defined by intracortical microstimulation: connections in macaques. J Comp Neurol 293, 299–330, 1990.
195. Huerta MF, Krubitzer LA, Kaas JH. Frontal eye field as defined by intracortical microstimulation in squirrel monkeys, owl monkeys, and macaque monkeys: I. Subcortical connections. J Comp Neurol 253, 415–439, 1986.
196. Huerta MF, Krubitzer LA, Kaas JH. Frontal eye field as defined by intracortical microstimulation in squirrel monkeys, owl monkeys, and macaque monkeys. II. Cortical connections. J Comp Neurol 265, 332–361, 1987.
197. Husain M, Mannan S, Hodgson T, et al. Impaired spatial working memory across saccades contributes to abnormal search in parietal neglect. Brain 124, 941–952, 2001.
198. Husain M, Parton A, Hodgson TL, Mort D, Rees G. Self-control during response conflict by human supplementary eye field. Nat Neurosci 6, 117–118, 2003.
199. Ilg UJ, Their P. Visual tracking neurons in primate area MST are activated by smooth-pursuit eye movements of an “imaginary” target. J Neurophysiol 90, 1489–1502, 2003.
200. Inoue M, Mikami A, Ando I, Tsukada H. Functional brain mapping of the macaque related to spatial working memory as revealed by PET. Cerebr Cortex 14, 106–119, 2004.
200a. Ioannides AA, Fenwick PBC, Liu L. Widely distributed magnetoencephalography spike related to planning and execution of human saccades. J Neurosci 25, 7950–7967, 2005.
201. Isoda M, Tanji J. Cellular activity in the supplementary eye field during sequential performance of multiple saccades. J Neurophysiol 88, 3541–3545, 2002.
202. Israël I, Rivaud S, Gaymard B, Berthoz A, Pierrot-Deseilligny C. Cortical control of vestibular-guided saccades. Brain 118, 1169–1184, 1995.
203. Itaya S, van Hoesen G. Retinal projections to the inferior and medial pulvinar nuclei in the old-world monkey. Brain Res 269, 223–230, 1983.
204. Ito S, Stuphorn V, Brown JW, Schall JD. Performance monitoring by the anterior cingulate cortex during saccade countermanding. Science 302, 120–122, 2003.
205. Iwatsubo T, Kuzuhara S, Kanemitsu A, Shimada H, Toyokura Y. Corticofugal projections to the motor nuclei of the brainstem and spinal cord in humans. Neurology 40, 309–312, 1990.
206. Izawa Y, Suzuki H, Shinoda Y. Initiation and suppression of saccades by the frontal eye field in the monkey. Ann. N Y Acad Sci 1039, 220–231, 2005.
207. Kaplan E. The M, P, and K pathway of the primate visual system. In Chapula LM, Werner JS (eds). The Visual Neurosciences. MIT Press, Cambridge, MA, 2003 pp 481–493.
208. Kase M, Nagata R, Kato M. Saccade-related activity of periaqueductal gray matter of the monkey. Invest Ophthalmol Vis Sci 27, 1165–1169, 1986.
209. Kastner S, O'Connor DH, Fukui MM, et al. Functional imaging of the human lateral geniculate nucleus and pulvinar. J Neurophysiol 91, 438–448, 2004.
210. Kato M, Miyashita N, Hikosaka O, et al. Eye movements in monkeys with local dopamine depletion in the caudate nucleus. I. Deficits in spontaneous saccades. J Neurosci 15, 912–927, 1995.
211. Kawagoe R, Takikawa Y, Hikosaka O. Reward-predicting activity of dopamine and caudate neurons—a possible mechanism of motivational control of saccadic eye movement. J Neurophysiol 91, 1013–1024, 2004.
212. Keating EG, Gooley SG. Saccadic disorders caused by cooling the superior colliculus or the frontal eye field, or from combined lesions of both structures. Brain Res 438, 247–255, 1988.
213. King WM, Fuchs AF, Magnin M. Vertical eye movement-related responses of neurons in midbrain near interstitial nucleus of Cajal. J Neurophysiol 46, 549–562, 1981.
214. King WM, Lisberger SG, Fuchs AF. Responses of fibers in medial longitudinal fasciculus (MLF) of alert monkeys during horizontal and vertical conjugate eye movements evoked by vestibular or visual stimuli. J Neurophysiol 39, 1135–1149, 1976.
215. King WM, Precht W, Dieringer N. Synaptic organization of frontal eye field and vestibular afferents to the interstitial nucleus of Cajal in cat. J Neurophysiol 43, 912–928, 1980.
216. Kobayashi Y, Inoue Y, Isa T. Pedunculo-pontine control of visually guided saccades. Prog Brain Res 143, 439–445, 2004.
217. Kokkoroyannis T,Scudder CA, Balaban CD, Highstein SM, Moschovakis AK. Anatomy and physiology of the primate interstitial nucleus of Cajal. 1. Efferent projections. J Neurophysiol 75, 725–739, 1996.
218. Kommerell G, Henn V, Bach M, Lücking CH. Unilateral lesion of the paramedian pontine reticular formation. Loss of rapid eye movements with preservation of vestibulo-ocular reflex and pursuit. Neuro-ophthalmology 7, 93–98, 1987.

219. Kori A, Miyashita N, Kato M, et al. Eye movements in monkeys with local dopamine depletion in the caudate nucleus. II. Deficits in voluntary saccades. J Neurosci 15, 928–941, 1995.
220. Krauzlis RJ. Recasting the smooth pursuit eye movement system. J Neurophysiol 91, 591–603, 2004.
221. Krauzlis RJ, Lisberger SG. Directional organization of eye movement and visual signals in the floccular lobe of the monkey cerebellum. Exp Brain Res 109, 289–302, 1996.
222. Kurkin S, Takeicho N, Akao T, et al. Neurons in the caudal frontal eye fields of monkeys signal three-dimensional tracking. Ann N Y Acad Sci 1004, 262–270, 2003.
223. Kusunoki M, Goldberg ME. The time course of perisaccadic receptive field shifts in the lateral intraparietal area of the monkey. J Neurophysiol 89, 1519–1527, 2003.
224. LaBerge D, Buchsbaum MS. Positron emission tomographic measurements of pulvinar activity during an attention task. J Neurosci 10, 613–619, 1990.
225. Lang W, Petit L, Hollinger P, et al. A positron emission tomography study of oculomotor imagery. Neuroreport 5, 921–924, 1994.
226. Langer T, Fuchs AF, Chubb MC, Scudder CA, Lisberger SG. Floccular efferents in the rhesus macaque as revealed by autoradiography and horseradish peroxidase. J Comp Neurol 235, 26–37, 1985.
227. Langer T, Fuchs AF, Scudder CA, Chubb MC. Afferents to the flocculus of the cerebellum in the rhesus macaque as revealed by retrograde transport of horseradish peroxidase. J Comp Neurol 235, 1–25, 1985.
228. Langer T, Kaneko CR, Scudder CA, Fuchs AF. Afferents to the abducens nucleus in the monkey and cat. J Comp Neurol 245, 379–400, 1986.
229. Lasker AG, Zee DS, Hain TC, Folstein SE, Singer HS. Saccades in Huntington's disease: initiation defects and distractability. Neurology 37, 364–370, 1987.
230. Lauwereyns J, Takikawa Y, Kawagoe R, et al. Feature-based anticipation of cues that predict reward in monkey caudate nucleus. Neuron 33, 463–473, 2002.
231. Lauwereyns J, Watanabe K, Coe B, Hikosaka O. A neural correlate of response bias in monkey caudate nucleus. Nature 418, 413–417, 2002.
232. Lawden MC, Bagelmann H, Crawford TJ, Matthews TD, Kennard C. An effect of structured backgrounds on smooth pursuit eye movements in patients with cerebral lesions. Brain 118, 37–48, 1995.
233. Lee C, Rohrer W, Sparks DL. Population coding of saccadic eye movements by neurons in the superior colliculus. Nature 332, 357–360, 1988.
234. Leichnetz GR. The prefrontal cortico-oculomotor trajectories in the monkey. A possible explanation for the effects of stimulation/lesion experiments on eye movement. J Neurol Sci 49, 387–396, 1981.
235. Leichnetz GR. Connections of the medial posterior parietal cortex (area 7m) in the monkey. Anat Rec 263, 215–236, 2001.
236. Leichnetz GR, Smith DJ, Spencer RF. Cortical projections to the paramedian tegmental and basilar pons in the monkey. J Comp Neurol 228, 388–408, 1984.
237. Leigh RJ. Human vestibular cortex. Ann Neurol 35, 383–384, 1994.
238. Leigh RJ, Rottach KG, Das VE. Transforming sensory perceptions into motor commands: evidence from programming of eye movements. Ann N Y Acad Sci 835, 353–362, 1997.
239. Leigh RJ, Seidman SH, Grant MP, Hanna JP. Loss of ipsidirectional quick phases of torsional nystagmus with a unilateral midbrain lesion. J Vestib Res 3, 115–122, 1993.
240. Li CS, Andersen RA. Inactivation of macaque lateral intraparietal area delays initiation of the second saccade predominantly from contralesional eye positions in a double-saccade task. Exp. Brain Res. 137, 45–57, 2001.
241. Li CS, Mazzoni P, Andersen RA. Effect of reversible inactivation of macaque lateral intraparietal area on visual and memory saccades. J Neurophysiol 81, 1827–1838, 1999.
242. Linden DE, Bittner JA, Muckli L, et al. Cortical capacity constraints for visual working memory: dissociation of fMRI load effects in a fronto-parietal network. Neuroimage 20, 1518–1530, 2003.
243. Lisberger SG, Fuchs AF. Role of primate flocculus during rapid behavioral modification of vestibulo-ocular reflex. I. Purkinje cell activity during visually guided horizontal smooth-pursuit eye movements and passive head rotation. J Neurophysiol 41, 733–763, 1978.
244. Lisberger SG, Miles FA, Zee DS. Signals used to compute errors in monkey vestibuloocular reflex: possible role of flocculus. J Neurophysiol 52, 1140–1153, 1984.
245. Liu J, Newsome WT. Correlation between speed perception and neural activity in the middle temporal visual area. J Neurosci 25, 711–722, 2005.
246. Livingstone M, Hubel D. Segregation of form, color, movement, and depth: anatomy, physiology, and perception. Science 240, 740–749, 1988.
247. Lobel E, Kahane P, Leonards U, et al. Localization of human frontal eye fields: anatomical and functional findings of functional magnetic resonance imaging and intracerebral electrical stimulation. J Neurosurg 95, 804–815, 2001.
248. Lueck CJ, Hamlyn P, Crawford TJ, et al. A case of ocular tilt reaction and torsional nystagmus due to direct stimulation of the midbrain in man. Brain 114, 2069–2079, 1991.
249. Lynch JC. Saccade initiation and latency deficits after combined lesions of the frontal and posterior eye fields in monkeys. J Neurophysiol 68, 1913–1916, 1992.
250. Lynch JC, Graybiel AM, Lobeck L. The differential projection of two cytoarchitectonic subregions of the inferior parietal lobule of macaque upon the deep layers of the superior colliculus. J Comp Neurol 235, 241–254, 1985.
251. Lynch JC, Hoover JE, Strick PL. Input to the primate frontal eye field from the substantia nigra, superior colliculus, and dentate nucleus demonstrated by transneuronal transport. Exp Brain Res 100, 181–186, 1994.
252. Lynch JC, McLaren J. Deficits of visual attention and saccadic eye movements after lesions of parietooccipital cortex in monkeys. J Neurophysiol 61, 74–90, 1989.

253. Lynch JC, Mountcastle VB, Talbot WH, Yin TCT. Parietal lobe mechanisms for directed visual attention. J Neurophysiol 40, 362–389, 1977.
254. Lynch JC, Tian J-R. Cortico-cortical networks and cortico-subcortical loops for the higher control of eye movements. In Büttner-Ennever JA (ed). Neuroanatomy of the Oculomotor System. Prog Brain Res 151, 467–508, 2006.
255. Ma TP, Hu XJ, Anavi Y, Rafols JA. Organization of the zona incerta in the macaque: a Nissl and Golgi study. J Comp Neurol 320, 273–290, 1992.
256. Ma TP, Lynch JC, Donahoe DK, Attallah H, Rafols JA. Organization of the medial pulvinar nucleus in the macaque. Anat Rec 250, 220–237, 1998.
257. MacAvoy MG, Gottlieb JP, Bruce CJ. Smooth-pursuit eye movement representation in the primate frontal eye field. Cerebr Cortex 1, 95–102, 1991.
258. Matsumura M, Kojima J, Gardiner TW, Hikosaka O. Visual and oculomotor functions of monkey subthalamic nucleus. J Neurophysiol 67, 1615–1632, 1992.
259. Maunsell JHR, Van Essen DC. Functional properties of neurons in middle temporal visual area of the macaque monkey. I. Selectivity for stimulus direction, speed, and orientation. J Neurophysiol 49, 1127–1147, 1983.
260. May JG, Keller EL, Suzuki DA. Smooth-pursuit eye movement deficits with chemical lesions in the dorsolateral pontine nucleus of the monkey. J Neurophysiol 59, 952–977, 1988.
261. May PJ. The mammalian superior colliculus: Laminar structure and connections. In Büttner-Ennever JA (ed). Neuroanatomy of the Oculomotor System. Prog Brain Res 151, 321–380, 2006.
262. May PJ, Hartwich-Young R, Nelson J, Sparks DL, Porter JD. Cerebellotectal pathways in the macaque: implications for collicular generation of saccades. Neuroscience 36, 305–324, 1990.
263. Mays LE. Neural control of vergence eye movements: convergence and divergence neurons in the midbrain. J Neurophysiol 51, 1091–1108, 1984.
264. McCrea R, Strassman A, May E, Highstein S. Anatomical and physiological characteristics of vestibular neurons mediating the horizontal vestibulo-ocular reflex of the squirrel monkey. J Comp Neurol 264, 547–570, 1987.
265. McCrea RA, Strassman A, Highstein SM. Morphology and physiology of abducens motoneurons and internuclear neurons intracellularly injected with horseradish peroxidase in alert squirrel monkeys. J Comp Neurol 243, 291–308, 1986.
266. McCrea RA, Strassman A, Highstein SM. Anatomical and physiological characteristics of vestibular neurons mediating the vertical vestibulo-ocular reflexes of the squirrel monkey. J Comp Neurol 264, 571–594, 1987.
267. McElligot JG, Spencer RF. Neuropharmacological aspects of the vestibulo-ocular reflex. In Beitz AJ, Anderson JH (eds). Neurochemistry of the Vestibular System. CRC Press, Boca Raton, 2000, pp 199–222.
268. Meienberg O, Büttner-Ennever JA, Kraus-Ruppert R. Unilateral paralysis of conjugate gaze due to lesion of the abducens nucleus. Clinico-pathological case report. Neuro-ophthalmology 2, 47–52, 1981.
269. Merriam EP, Colby CL, Thulborn KR, et al. Stimulus-response incompatibility activates cortex proximate to three eye fields. Neuroimage 13, 794–800, 2001.
270. Milea D, Lehericy S, Rivaud-Pechoux S, et al. Antisaccade deficit after anterior cingulate cortex resection. Neuroreport 14, 283–287, 2003.
271. Milea D, Lobel E, Lehericy S, et al. Intraoperative frontal eye field stimulation elicits ocular deviation and saccade suppression. Neuroreport 13, 1359–1364, 2002.
272. Miles FA, Fuller JH. Visual tracking and the primate flocculus. Science 189, 1000–1002, 1975.
273. Miller NR, Biousse V, Hwang T, et al. Isolated acquired unilateral horizontal gaze paresis from a putative lesion of the abducens nucleus. J Neuroophthalmol 22, 204–207, 2002.
274. Missal M, Heinen SJ. Supplementary eye fields stimulation facilitates anticipatory pursuit. J Neurophysiol 92, 1257–1262, 2004.
275. Miyashita N, Hikosaka O, Kato M. Visual hemineglect induced by unilateral striatal dopamine deficiency in monkeys. Neuroreport 6, 1257–1260, 1995.
276. Morrow MJ. Craniotopic defects of smooth pursuit and saccadic eye movement. Neurology 46, 514–521, 1996.
277. Morrow MJ, Sharpe JA. Cerebral hemispheric localization of smooth pursuit asymmetry. Neurology 40, 284–292, 1990.
278. Morrow MJ, Sharpe JA. Retinotopic and directional deficits of smooth pursuit initiation after posterior cerebral hemispheric lesions. Neurology 43, 595–603, 1993.
279. Morrow MJ, Sharpe JA. Deficits of smooth-pursuit eye movement after unilateral frontal lobe lesions. Ann Neurol 37, 443–451, 1995.
280. Mort DJ, Perry J, Mannan SK, et al. Differential cortical activation during voluntary and reflexive saccades in man. Neuroimage 18, 231–246, 2003.
281. Moschovakis AK. Are laws that govern behavior embedded in the structure of the CNS? The case of Hering's law. Vision Res 35, 3207–3216, 1995.
282. Moschovakis AK, Gregoriou GG, Ugolini G, et al. Oculomotor areas of the primate frontal lobes: a transneuronal transfer of rabies virus and [14C]-2-deoxyglucose functional imaging study. J Neurosci 24, 5726–5740, 2004.
283. Moschovakis AK, Karabelas AB, Highstein SM. Structure-function relationships in the primate superior colliculus. I. Morphological classification of efferent neurons. J Neurophysiol 60, 232–262, 1988.
284. Moschovakis AK, Karabelas AB, Highstein SM. Structure-function relationships in the primate superior colliculus. II. Morphological identity of presaccadic neurons. J Neurophysiol 60, 263–301, 1988.
285. Moschovakis AK, Scudder CA, Highstein SM. A structural basis for Hering's law: projections to extraocular motoneurons. Science 248, 1118–1119, 1990.
286. Moschovakis AK, Scudder CA, Highstein SM. Structure of the primate oculomotor burst generator. I. Medium-lead burst neurons with upward on-directions. J Neurophysiol 65, 203–217, 1991.
287. Moschovakis AK, Scudder CA, Highstein SM. The microscopic anatomy and physiology of the mammalian saccadic system. Progr Neurobiol 50, 133–254, 1996.
288. Moschovakis AK, Scudder CA, Highstein SM,

Warren JD. Structure of the primate oculomotor burst generator. II. Medium-lead burst neurons with downward on-directions. J Neurophysiol 65, 218–229, 1991.
289. Muggleton NG, Juan CH, Cowey A, Walsh,V. Human frontal eye fields and visual search. J Neurophysiol 89, 3340–3343, 2003.
290. Müri RM. MRI and fMRI analysis of oculomotor function. In Büttner-Ennever JA (ed). Neuroanatomy of the Oculomotor System. Prog Brain Res 151, 509–532, 2006.
291. Müri RM, Chermann JF, Cohen L, Rivaud S, Pierrot-Deseilligny C. Ocular motor consequences of damage to the abducens nucleus area in humans. J Neuro-ophthalmol 16, 191–195, 1996.
292. Müri RM, Heid O, Nirkko AC, et al. Functional organisation of saccades and antisaccades in the frontal lobe in humans: a study with echo planar functional magnetic resonance imaging. J Neurol Neurosurg Psychiatry 65, 374–377, 1998.
293. Müri RM, Iba-Zizen MT, Derosier C, Cabanis EA, Pierrot-Deseilligny C. Location of the human posterior eye field with functional magnetic resonance imaging. J Neurol Neurosurg Psychiatry 60, 445–448, 1996.
294. Müri RM, Rivaud S, Gaymard B, et al. Role of the prefrontal cortex in the control of express saccades. A transcranial magnetic stimulation study. Neuropsychologia 37, 199–206, 1999.
295. Müri RM, Vermersch AI, Rivaud S, Gaymard B, Pierrot-Deseilligny C. Effects of single-pulse transcranial magnetic stimulation over the prefrontal and posterior parietal cortices during memory-guided saccades in humans. J Neurophysiol 76, 2102–2106, 1996.
296. Mustari MJ, Fuchs AF, Wallman J. Response properties of dorsolateral pontine units during smooth pursuit in the rhesus macaque. J Neurophysiol 60, 664–686, 1988.
297. Mustari MJ, Tusa RJ, Burrows AF, Fuchs AF, Livingston CA. Gaze-stabilizing deficits and latent nystagmus in monkeys with early-onset visual deprivation: role of the pretectal not. J Neurophysiol. 86, 662–675, 2001.
298. Nachev P, Rees G, Parton A, Kennard C, Husain M. Volition and conflict in human medial frontal cortex. Curr Biol 15, 122–128, 2005.
299. Nagao S, Kitamura T, Nakamura N, Hiramatsu T, Yamada J. Differences of the primate flocculus and ventral paraflocculus in the mossy and climbing fiber input organization. J Comp Neurol 382, 480–498, 1997.
300. Nagao S, Kitamura T, Nakamura N, Hiramatsu T, Yamada J. Location of efferent terminals of the primate flocculus and ventral paraflocculus revealed by anterograde axonal transport methods. Neurosci Res 27, 257–269, 1997.
301. Nakamagoe K, Iwamoto Y, Yoshida K. Evidence for brainstem structures participating in oculomotor integration. Science 288, 857–859, 2000.
302. Nakamura K, Roesch MR, Olson CR. Neuronal activity in macaque SEF and ACC during performance of tasks involving conflict. J Neurophysiol 93, 884–908, 2005.
303. Nakao S, Shiraishi Y, Oda H, Inagaki M. Direct inhibitory projection of pontine omnipause neurons to burst neurons in the Forel's field H controlling vertical eye movement-related motoneurons in the cat. Exp Brain Res 70, 632–636, 1988.
304. Nambu A, Tokuno H, Takada,M. Functional significance of the cortico/subthalamo/pallidal 'hyperdirect' pathway. Neurosci Res 43, 111–117, 2002.
305. Neal JW, Pearson RCA, Powell TPS. The connections of area PG, 7a, with cortex in the parietal, occipital and temporal lobes of the monkey. Brain Res 532, 249–264, 1997.
306. Newsome WT, Pare EB. A selective impairment of motion perception following lesions of the middle temporal visual area (MT). J Neurosci 8, 2201–2211, 1988.
307. Newsome WT, Wurtz RH, Komatsu H. Relation of cortical areas MT and MST to pursuit eye movements. II. Differentiation of retinal from extraretinal inputs. J Neurophysiol 60, 604–620, 1988.
308. Newsome WT, Wurtz RH, Dursteler MR, Mikami A. Deficits in visual motion processing following ibotenic acid lesions of the middle temporal visual area of the macaque monkey. J Neurosci 5, 825–840, 1985.
309. Nguyen LT, Spencer RF. Abducens internuclear and ascending tract of Deiters inputs to medial rectus motoneurons in the cat oculomotor nucleus: neurotransmitters. J Comp Neurol 411, 73–86, 1999.
310. Noda H, Fujikado T. Topography of the oculomotor area of the cerebellar vermis in macaques as determined by microstimulation. J Neurophysiol 58, 359–378, 1987.
311. Noda H, Sugita S, Ikeda Y. Afferent and efferent connections of the oculomotor region of the fastigial nucleus in the macaque monkey. J Comp Neurol 302, 330–348, 1990.
312. Noguchi Y, Kaneoke Y, Kakigi R, Tanabe HC, Sadato N. Role of the superior temporal region in human motion perception. Cerebr Cortex 15, 1592–1601, 2005.
313. Nyffeler T, Pierrot-Deseilligny C, Plugshaupt T, et al. Information processing in long delay memory-guided saccades: further insights from TMS. Exp Brain Res 154, 109–112, 2004.
314. O'Driscoll GA, Alpert NM, Matthysse SW, et al. Functional neuroanatomy of antisaccade eye movements investigated with positron emission tomography. Proc Natl Acad Sci U S A 92, 925–929, 1995.
315. O'Keefe LP, Movshon JA. Processing of first- and second-order motion signals by neurons in area MT of the macaque monkey. Vis Neurosci 15, 305–317, 1998.
316. O'Sullivan EP, Jenkins IH, Henderson L, Kennard C, Brooks DJ. The functional anatomy of remembered saccades: a PET study. Neuroreport 6, 2141–2144, 1995.
317. Ogren MP, Mateer CA, Wyler AR. Alterations in visually related eye movements following left pulvinar damage in man. Neuropsychologia 22, 187–196, 1984.
318. Ohtsuka K, Noda H. Saccadic burst neurons in the oculomotor region of the fastigial neurons in macaque monkeys. J Neurophysiol 65, 1422–1434, 1992.
319. Ohtsuka K, Noda H. Discharge properties of Purkinje cells in the oculomotor vermis during visu-

ally guided saccades in the macaque monkey. J Neurophysiol 74, 1828–1840, 1995.
320. Olshausen BA, Anderson CH, Van Essen DC. A neurobiological model of visual attention and invariant pattern recognition based on dynamic routing of information. J Neurosci 13, 4700–4719, 1993.
321. Olson CR, Musil SY, Goldberg ME. Single neurons in posterior cingulate cortex of behaving macaque: eye movement signals. J Neurophysiol 76, 3285–3300, 1996.
322. Olszewski J, Baxter D. Cytoarchitecture of the Human Brain Stem. Karger, Basel, 1954.
323. Ono S, Das VE, Mustari MJ. Gaze-related response properties of DLPN and NRTP neurons in the rhesus macaque. J Neurophysiol 91, 2484–2500, 2004.
324. Optican LM. Sensorimotor transformation for visually guided saccades. Ann N Y Acad Sci 1039, 132–148, 2005.
325. Page WK, Duffy CJ. MST neuronal responses to heading direction during pursuit eye movements. J Neurophysiol 81, 596–610, 1999.
326. Page WK, Duffy CJ. Heading representation in MST: sensory interactions and population encoding. J Neurophysiol 89, 1994–2013, 2003.
327. Paré M, Wurtz RH. Monkey posterior parietal cortex neurons antidromically activated from superior colliculus. J Neurophysiol 78, 3493–3497, 1997.
328. Park J, Schlag-Rey M, Schlag J. Frames of reference for saccadic command, tested by saccade collision in the supplementary eye field. J Neurophysiol, in press, 2005.
329. Parthasarathy HB, Schall JD, Graybiel AM. Distributed but convergent ordering of corticostriatal projections: analysis of the frontal eye field and the supplementary eye field in the macaque monkey. J Neurosci 12, 4468–4488, 1992.
330. Partsalis AM, Highstein SM, Moschovakis AK. Lesions of the posterior commissure disable the vertical neural integrator of the primate oculomotor system. J Neurophysiol 71, 2582–2585, 1994.
331. Partsalis AM, Zhang Y, Highstein SM. Dorsal y group in the squirrel monkey. I. Neuronal responses during rapid and long-term modifications of the vertica VOR. J Neurophysiol 73, 615–631, 1995.
332. Partsalis AM, Zhang Y, Highstein SM. Dorsal y group in the squirrel monkey. II. Contribution of the cerebellar flocculus to neuronal responses in normal and adapted animals. J Neurophysiol 73, 632–650, 1997.
333. Pasik P, Pasik T, Bender MB. The pretectal syndrome in monkeys. I. Disturbances of gaze and body posture. Brain 92, 521–534, 1969.
334. Pasik T, Pasik P, Bender MB. The pretectal syndrome in monkeys. II. Spontaneous and induced nystagmus and "lightning" eye movements. Brain 92, 871–884, 1969.
335. Penfield W. Vestibular sensation and the cerebral cortex. Ann Otol Rhinol Laryngol 66, 691–698, 1957.
336. Perry RJ, Zeki S. The neurology of saccades and covert shifts in spatial attention: an event-related fMRI study. Brain 123, 2273–2288, 2000.
337. Petersen SL, Robinson DL, Morris JD. Contributions of the pulvinar to visual spatial attention. Neuropsychologia 25, 97–105, 1987.
338. Petit L, Dubois S, Tzourio N, et al. PET study of the human foveal fixation system. Hum Brain Mapp 8, 28–43, 1999.
339. Petit L, Haxby JV. Functional anatomy of pursuit eye movements in humans as revealed by fMRI. J Neurophysiol 82, 463–471, 1999.
340. Petit L, Orssaud C, Tzourio N, et al. Functional anatomy of a prelearned sequence of horizontal saccades in humans. J Neurosci 16, 3714–3726, 1996.
341. Petit L, Orssaud C, Tzourio N, et al. PET study of voluntary saccadic eye movements in humans: basal ganglia-thalamocortical system and cingulate cortex involvement. J Neurophysiol 69, 1009–1017, 1993.
342. Pierrot-Deseilligny C, Chain F, Serdaru M, Gray F, Lhermitte F. The "one-and-a-half" syndrome. Electro-oculographic analyses of five cases with deductions about the physiological mechanisms of lateral gaze. Brain 104, 665–699, 1981.
343. Pierrot-Deseilligny C, Gautier J-C, Loron P. Acquired ocular motor apraxia due to bilateral fronto-parietal infarcts. Ann Neurol 23, 199–202, 1988.
344. Pierrot-Deseilligny C, Goasguen J, Chain F, Lapresle J. Pontine metastasis with dissociated bilateral horizontal gaze paralysis. J Neurol Neurosurg Psychiatry 47, 159–164, 1984.
345. Pierrot-Deseilligny C, Gray F, Brunet P. Infarcts of both inferior parietal lobules with impairment of visually guided eye movements, peripheral visual attention and optic ataxia. Brain 109, 81–97, 1986.
346. Pierrot-Deseilligny C, Milea D, Müri RM. Eye movement control by the cerebral cortex. Curr Opin Neurol 17, 17–25, 2004.
347. Pierrot-Deseilligny C, Müri RM, Ploner CJ, et al. Decisional role of the dorsolateral prefrontal cortex in ocular motor behaviour. Brain 126, 1460–1473, 2003.
348. Pierrot-Deseilligny C, Müri RM, Rivaud-Pechoux S, Gaymard B, Ploner CJ. Cortical control of spatial memory in humans: the visuooculomotor model. Ann Neurol 52, 10–19, 2002.
349. Pierrot-Deseilligny C, Rivaud S, Gaymard B, Agid Y. Cortical control of memory-guided saccades in man. Exp Brain Res 83, 607–617, 1991.
350. Pierrot-Deseilligny C, Rivaud S, Penet C, Rigolet MH. Latencies of visually guided saccades in unilateral hemispheric cerebral lesions. Ann Neurol. 21, 138–148, 1987.
351. Pierrot-Deseilligny C, Rosa A, Masmoudi K, Rivaud S, Gaymard B. Saccade deficits after a unilateral lesion affecting the superior colliculus. J Neurol Neurosurg Psychiatry 54, 1106–1109, 1991.
352. Pierrot-Deseilligny CH, Chain F, Gray F, et al. Parinaud's syndrome: electro-oculographic and anatomical analyses of six vascular cases with deductions about vertical gaze organization in the premotor structures. Brain 105, 667–696, 1982.
353. Ploner CJ, Gaymard BM, Rivaud-Pechoux S, et al. Lesions affecting the parahippocampal cortex yield spatial memory deficits in humans. Cereb Cortex 10, 1211–1216, 2000.
354. Ploner CJ, Rivaud-Pechoux S, Gaymard,BM, Agid Y, Pierrot-Deseilligny C. Errors of memory-guided saccades in humans with lesions of the frontal eye field and the dorsolateral prefrontal cortex. J Neurophysiol 82, 1086–1090, 1999.
355. Pola J, Robinson DA. Oculomotor signals in medial longitudinal fasciculus of the monkey. J Neurophysiol 41, 245–259, 1978.

356. Priebe NJ, Lisberger SG. Estimating target speed from the population response in visual area MT. J Neurosci 24, 1907–1916, 2004.
357. Rafal R, McGrath M, Machado L, Hindle J. Effects of lesions of the human posterior thalamus on ocular fixation during voluntary and visually triggered saccades. J Neurol Neurosurg Psychiatry 75, 1602–1606, 2004.
358. Rajkowska G, Goldman-Rakic PS. Cytoarchitectonic definition of prefrontal areas in the normal human cortex. I. Remapping of areas 9 and 46 using quantitative criteria. Cereb Cortex 5, 307–322, 1995.
359. Rajkowska G, Goldman-Rakic PS. Cytoarchitectonic definition of prefrontal areas in the normal human cortex. II. Variability in locations of areas 9 and 46 and relationship to Talairach coordinate system. Cereb Cortex 5, 323–337, 1995.
360. Rambold H, Churchland A, Selig Y, Jasmin L, Lisberger SG. Partial ablations of the flocculus and ventral paraflocculus in monkeys cause linked deficits in smooth pursuit eye movements and adaptive modification of the VOR. J Neurophysiol 87, 912–924, 2002.
361. Rambold H, Churchland A, Selig Y, Jasmin L, Lisberger SG. Partial ablations of the flocculus and ventral paraflocculus in monkeys cause linked deficits in smooth pursuit eye movements and adaptive modification of the VOR. J Neurophysiol 87, 912–924, 2002.
362. Rambold H, Churchland A, Selig Y, Jasmin L, Lisberger SG. Partial ablations of the flocculus and ventral paraflocculus in monkeys cause linked deficits in smooth pursuit eye movements and adaptive modification of the VOR. J Neurophysiol 87, 912–924, 2002.
363. Ranalli PJ, Sharpe JA. Upbeat nystagmus and the ventral tegmental pathway of the upward vestibulo-ocular reflex. Neurology 38, 1329–1330, 1988.
364. Ranalli PJ, Sharpe JA. Vertical vestibulo-ocular reflex, smooth pursuit and eye-head tracking dysfunction in internuclear ophthalmoplegia. Brain 111, 1299–1317, 1988.
365. Reisine H, Highstein SM. The ascending tract of Deiters' conveys a head velocity signal to medial rectus motoneurons. Brain Res 170, 172–176, 1979.
366. Rivaud S, Muri RM, Gaymard B, Vermersch AI, Pierrot-Deseilligny C. Eye movement disorders after frontal eye field lesions in humans. Exp Brain Res 102, 110–120, 1994.
367. Rivaud-Pechoux S, Vermersch AI, Gaymard B, et al. Improvement of memory guided saccades in parkinsonian patients by high frequency subthalamic nucleus stimulation. J Neurol Neurosurg Psychiatry 68, 381–384, 2000.
368. Rizzo M, Robin DA. Bilateral effects of unilateral visual cortex lesions in human. Brain 119, 951–963, 1996.
369. Robinson DL. Functional contributions of the primate pulvinar. Prog. Brain Res 95, 371–380, 1993.
370. Robinson DL, McClurkin JW, Kertzman C, Petersen SE. Visual responses of pulvinar and collicular neurons during eye movements of awake, trained macaques. J Neurophysiol 66, 485–496, 1991.
371. Robinson DL, Petersen SE. The pulvinar and visual salience. Trends Neurosci 15, 127–132, 1992.
372. Robinson FR. Role of the cerebellar posterior interpositus nucleus in saccades I. Effect of temporary lesions. J Neurophysiol 84, 1289–1302, 2000.
373. Robinson FR, Straube A, Fuchs AF. Role of the caudal fastigial nucleus in saccade generation. II. Effects of muscimol inactivation. J Neurophysiol 70, 1741–1758, 1993.
374. Robinson FR, Straube A, Fuchs AF. Participation of caudal fastigial nucleus in smooth pursuit eye movements. II. Effects of muscimol inactivation. J Neurophysiology 78, 1997.
375. Rodman HR, Gross CG, Albright TD. Afferent basis of visual response properties in area MT of the macaque. I. Effect of striate cortex removal. J Neurosci 9, 2033–2050, 1989.
376. Romanski LM, Giguere M, Bates JF, Goldman-Rakic PS. Topographic organization of medial pulvinar connections with prefrontal cortex in the rhesus monkey. J Comp Neurol 379, 313–332, 1997.
377. Ron S, Robinson DA. Eye movements evoked by cerebellar stimulation in the alert monkey. J Neurophysiol 36, 1004–1022, 1973.
378. Rosano C, Krisky CM, Welling JS, et al. Pursuit and saccadic eye movement subregions in human frontal eye field: a high-resolution fMRI investigation. Cereb Cortex 12, 107–115, 2002.
378a. Rosano C, Sweeney JA, Melchitzky DS, Lewis DA. The human precentral sulcus: chemoarchitecture of a region corresponding to the frontal eye fields. Brain Res 972, 16–30, 2003.
379. Rubertone JA, Haines DE. Secondary vestibulocerebellar projections to flocculonodular lobe in a prosimian primate, Galago senegalensis. J Comp Neurol 200, 255–272, 1981.
380. Russo GS, Bruce CJ. Supplementary eye field: representation of saccades and relationship between neural response fields and elicited eye movements. J Neurophysiol 84, 2605–2621, 2000.
381. Sato H, Noda H. Saccadic dysmetria induced by transient functional decortication of the cerebellar vermis. Exp Brain Res 88, 455–458, 1992.
382. Sato M, Hikosaka O. Role of primate substantia nigra pars reticulata in reward-oriented saccadic eye movement. J Neurosci 22, 2363–2373, 2002.
383. Sato Y, Kanda K-I, Ikarashi K, Kawasaki T. Differential mossy fiber projections to the dorsal and ventral uvula in the cat. J Comp Neurol 279, 149–164, 1989.
384. Sato Y, Kawasaki T. Target Neurons of floccular caudal zone inhibition in y-group nucleus of vestibular nuclear complex. J Neurophysiol 57, 460–480, 1987.
385. Sawaguchi T, Goldman-Rakic PS. The role of D1-dopamine receptor in working memory: Local injections of dopamine antagonists into the prefrontal cortex of rhesus monkeys performing an oculomotor- delayed response task. J Neurophysiol 71, 515–528, 1994.
386. Schiller PH, Chou IH. The effects of frontal eye field and dorsomedial frontal cortex lesions on visually guided eye movements. Nat Neurosci 1, 248–253, 1998.
387. Schiller PH, Sandell JH, Maunsell JHR. The effect of frontal eye field and superior colliculus lesions on saccadic latencies in the rhesus monkey. J Neurophysiol 57, 1033–1049, 1987.
388. Schiller PH, True SD, Conway JL. Deficits in eye

movements following frontal eye-field and superior colliculus ablations. J Neurophysiol 44, 1175–1189, 1980.
389. Schlack A, Hoffmann KP, Bremmer F. Selectivity of macaque ventral intraparietal area (area VIP) for smooth pursuit eye movements. J Physiol 551, 551–561, 2003.
390. Schlag J, Schlag-Rey M. Visuomotor functions of central thalamus in monkey. II. Unit activity related to visual events, targeting, and fixation. J Neurophysiol 51, 1175–1195, 1984.
391. Schlag J, Schlag-Rey M. Evidence for a supplementary eye field. J Neurophysiol 57, 179–200, 1987.
392. Schlag-Rey M, Schlag J. Visuomotor functions of central thalamus in monkey. I. Unit activity related to spontaneous eye movements. J Neurophysiol 51, 1149–1174, 1984.
393. Schlag-Rey M, Schlag J. The central thalamus. Rev Oculomot Res 3, 361–390, 1989.
394. Schneider KA, Kastner S. Visual responses of the human superior colliculus: a high-resolution functional magnetic resonance imaging study. J Neurophysiol 94, 2491–2503, 2005.
395. Schnyder H, Reisine H, Hepp K, Henn V. Frontal eye field projection to the paramedian pontine reticular formation traced with wheat germ agglutinin in the monkey. Brain Res 329, 151–160, 1985.
396. Segraves MA. Activity of monkey frontal eye field neurons projecting to oculomotor regions of the pons. J Neurophysiol 68, 1967–1985, 1992.
397. Segraves MA, Goldberg ME, Deng SY, et al. The role of striate cortex in the guidance of eye movements in the monkey. J Neurosci 7, 3040–3058, 1987.
398. Selemon LD, Goldman-Rakic PS. Common cortical and subcortical targets of the dorsolateral prefrontal and posterior parietal cortices in the rhesus monkey: evidence for a distributed neural network subserving spatially guided behavior. J Neurosci 8, 4049–4068, 1988.
399. Selhorst JB, Stark L, Ochs AL, Hoyt WF. Disorders in cerebellar ocular motor control. II. Macrosaccadic oscillations: an oculographic, control system, and clinico-anatomical analysis. Brain 99, 509–522, 1976.
400. Shi D, Friedman HR, Bruce CJ. Deficits in smooth-pursuit eye movements after muscimol inactivation within the primate's frontal eye field. J Neurophysiol 80, 458–464, 1998.
401. Shimo Y, Hikosaka O. Role of tonically active neurons in primate caudate in reward-oriented saccadic eye movement. J Neurosci 21, 7804–7814, 2001.
402. Shipp S, de Jong BM, Zihl J, Frackowiak RSJ, Zeki S. The brain activity related to residual motion vision in a patient with bilateral lesions of V5. Brain 117, 1023–1038, 1994.
403. Shook BL, Schlag-Rey M, Schlag J. Direct projection from the supplementary eye field to the nucleus raphe interpositus. Exp Brain Res 73, 215–218, 1988.
404. Shook BL, Schlag-Rey M, Schlag J. Primate supplementary eye field: I. Comparative aspects of mesencephalic and pontine connections. J Comp Neurol 301, 618–642, 1990.
405. Shook BL, Schlag-Rey M, Schlag J. Primate supplementary eye field. II. Comparative aspects of connections with thalamus, corpus striatum, and related forebrain nuclei. J Comp Neurol 307, 562–583, 1991.
406. Solomon D, Cohen B. Stimulation of the nodulus and uvula discharges velocity storage in the vestibulo-ocular reflex. Exp Brain Res 102, 57–68, 1994.
407. Sommer MA, Tehovnik EJ. Reversible inactivation of macaque dorsomedial frontal cortex: effects on saccades and fixations. Exp Brain Res 124, 429–446, 1999.
408. Sommer MA, Wurtz RH. What the brain stem tells the frontal cortex. II. Role of the SC-MD-FEF pathway in corollary discharge. J Neurophysiol 91, 1403–1423, 2004.
409. Sparks DL, Hartwich-Young R. The Neurobiology of Saccadic Eye Movements. Elsevier, Amsterdam,1989, pp 213–255.
410. Spencer RF, Baker R. Histochemical localization of acetycholinesterase in relation to motor neurons and internuclear neurons of the cat abducens nucleus. J Neurocytology 15, 137–154, 1986.
411. Spitzer H, Desimone R, Moran J. Increased attention enhances both behavioral and neuronal performance. Science 240, 338–340, 1988.
412. Stahl JS, Simpson JI. Dynamics of rabbit vestibular nucleus neurons and the influence of the flocculus. J Neurophysiol 73, 1396–1413, 1995.
413. Stanton GB. Afferents to oculomotor nuclei from area "y" in Macaca mulatta: An anterograde degeneration study. J Comp Neurol 192, 377–385, 1980.
414. Stanton GB, Bruce CJ, Goldberg ME. Topography of projections to the frontal lobe from the macaque frontal eye fields. J Comp Neurol 330, 286–301, 1993.
415. Stanton GB, Friedman HR, Dias EC, Bruce CJ. Cortical afferents to the smooth-pursuit region of the macaque monkey's frontal eye field. Exp Brain Res 165, 179–192, 2005.
416. Stanton GB, Goldberg ME, Bruce CJ. Frontal eye field efferents in the macaque monkey: I. Subcortical pathways and topography of striatal and thalamic terminal fields. J Comp Neurol 271, 473–492, 1988.
417. Stanton GB, Goldberg ME, Bruce CJ. Frontal eye field efferents in the macaque monkey: II. Topography of terminal fields in midbrain and pons. J Comp Neurol 271, 493–506, 1988.
418. Strassman A, Highstein SM, McCrea RA. Anatomy and physiology of saccadic burst neurons in the alert squirrel monkey. I. Excitatory burst neurons. J Comp Neurol 249, 337–357, 1986.
419. Strassman A, Highstein SM, McCrea RA. Anatomy and physiology of saccadic burst neurons in the alert squirrel monkey. II. Inhibitory burst neurons. J Comp Neurol 249, 358–380, 1986.
420. Straube A, Brandt T. Importance of the visual and vestibular cortex for self-motion perception in man (circularvection). Human Neurobiol 6, 211–218, 1987.
421. Stuphorn V, Taylor TL, Schall JD. Performance monitoring by the supplementary eye field. Nature 408, 857–860, 2000.
422. Suzuki DA, Keller EL. The role of the posterior vermis of monkey cerebellum in smooth-pursuit eye movement control. I. Eye and head movement-related activity. J Neurophysiol 59, 1–18, 1988.
423. Suzuki DA, Yamada T, Yee RD. Smooth-pursuit eye-movement-related neuronal activity in macaque nucleus reticularis tegmenti pontis. J Neurophysiol 89, 2146–2158, 2003.
424. Suzuki JI, Tokumasu K, Goto K. Eye movements

from single utricular nerve stimulation in the cat. Acta Otolaryngol (Stockh) 68, 350–362, 1969.
425. Suzuki Y, Büttner-Ennever JA, Straumann D, et al. Deficits in torsional and vertical rapid eye movements and shift of Listing's plane after uni- and bilateral lesions of the rostral interstitial nucleus of the medial longitudinal fasciculus. Exp Brain Res 106, 215–232, 1995.
426. Sweeney JA, Mintun MA, Kwee S, et al. Positron emission tomography study of voluntary saccadic eye movements and spatial working memory. J Neurophysiol 75, 454–468, 1996.
427. Takagi M, Zee DS, Tamargo R. Effects of lesions of the oculomotor vermis on eye movements in primate: saccades. J Neurophysiol 80, 1911–1930, 1998.
428. Takagi M, Tamargo R, Zee DS. Effects of lesions of the cerebellar oculomotor vermis on eye movements in primate: binocular control. Prog Brain Res 142, 19–33, 2003.
429. Takagi M, Zee DS, Tamargo RJ. Effects of lesions of the oculomotor cerebellar vermis on eye movements in primate: smooth pursuit. J Neurophysiol 83, 2047–2062, 2000.
430. Takeda K, Funahashi S. Prefrontal task-related activity representing visual cue location or saccade direction in spatial working memory tasks. J Neurophysiol 87, 567–588, 2002.
431. Takikawa Y, Kawagoe R, Hikosaka O. Reward-dependent spatial selectivity of anticipatory activity in monkey caudate neurons. J Neurophysiol 87, 508–515, 2002.
432. Tanaka M. Involvement of the central thalamus in the control of smooth pursuit eye movements. J Neurosci 25, 5866–5876, 2005.
433. Tanibuchi I, Goldman-Rakic PS. Comparison of oculomotor neuronal activity in paralaminar and mediodorsal thalamus in the rhesus monkey. J Neurophysiol 93, 614–619, 2005.
434. Terao Y, Fukuda H, Ugawa Y, et al. Visualization of the information flow through human oculomotor cortical regions by transcranial magnetic stimulation. J Neurophysiol 80, 936–946, 1998.
435. Thielert CD, Their P. Patterns of projections from the pontine nuclei and the nucleus reticularis tegmenti pontis to the posterior vermis in the rhesus monkey: a study using retrograde tracers. J Comp Neurol 337, 113–126, 1993.
436. Their P, Andersen RA. Electrical microstimulation distinguishes distinct saccade-related areas in the posterior parietal cortex. J Neurophysiol 80, 1713–1735, 1998.
437. Their P, Dicke PW, Haas R, Barash S. Encoding of movement time by populations of cerebellar Purkinje cells. Nature 405, 72–76, 2000.
438. Their P, Möck,M. The oculomotor role of the pontine nuclei and the nucleus reticularis tegmenti pontis. In Büttner-Ennever JA (ed). Neuroanatomy of the Oculomotor System. Prog Brain Res 151, 293–320, 2006.
439. Thurston SE, Leigh RJ, Crawford T, Thompson A, Kennard C. Two distinct deficits of visual tracking caused by unilateral lesions of cerebral cortex in man. Ann Neurol 23, 266–273, 1988.
440. Tomlinson RD, Robinson DA. Signals in vestibular nucleus mediating vertical eye movements in the monkey. J Neurophysiol 51, 1121–1136, 1984.
441. Tootell RB, Taylor JB. Anatomical evidence for MT and additional cortical visual areas in humans. Cerebr Cortex 5, 39–55, 1995.
442. Tsujimoto S, Sawaguchi T. Neuronal activity representing temporal prediction of reward in the primate prefrontal cortex. J Neurophysiol 93, 3687–3692, 2005.
443. Tusa RJ, Ungerleider L. Fiber pathways of cortical areas mediating smooth pursuit eye movements in monkeys. Ann Neurol 23, 174–183, 1988.
444. Tusa RJ, Zee DS, Herdman SJ. Effect of unilateral cerebral cortical lesions on ocular motor behavior in monkeys: Saccades and quick phases. J Neurophysiol 56, 1590–1625, 1986.
445. Uchino Y, Sasaki M, Isu N, et al. Second-order vestibular neuron morphology of the extra-MLF anterior canal pathway in the cat. Exp Brain Res 97, 387–396, 1994.
446. Umeno MM, Goldberg ME. Spatial properties in the monkey frontal eye field. 1. Predictive visual responses. J Neurophysiol 78, 1373–1383, 1997.
447. Ungerleider LG, Christensen CA. Pulvinar lesions in monkeys produce abnormal eye movements during visual discrimination training. Brain Res 136, 189–196, 1977.
448. Vahedi K, Rivaud S, Amarenco P, Pierrot-Deseilligny C. Horizontal eye movement disorders after posterior vermis infarctions. J Neurol Neurosurg Psychiatry 58, 91–94, 1995.
449. Van Essen DC, Drury HA. Structural and functional analysis of human cerebral cortex using a surface-based atlas. J Neurosci 17, 7079–7102, 1997.
450. Verhagen WIM, Huygens PLM, Mulleners WM. Lack of optokinetic nystagmus and visual motion perception in acquired cortical blindness. Neuro-ophthalmology 17, 211–216, 1997.
451. Vermersch AI, Muri RM, Rivaud RS, et al. Saccade disturbances after bilateral lentiform nucleus lesions in humans. J Neurol Neurosurg Psychiatry 60, 179–184, 1996.
452. Voogd J. The human cerebellum. J Chemical Anatomy 26, 243–252, 2003.
453. Voogd J, Barmack NH. Oculomotor cerebellum. In Büttner-Ennever JA (ed). Neuroanatomy of the Oculomotor System. Prog Brain Res 151, 231–268, 2006.
454. Voogd J, Wylie DR. Functional and anatomical organization of floccular zones: A preserved feature in vertebrates. J Comp Neurol 470, 107–112, 2004.
455. Waespe W, Cohen B, Raphan T. Dynamic modification of the vestibulo-ocular reflex by the nodulus and uvula. Science 228, 199–202, 1985.
456. Waespe W, Henn V. Visual-vestibular interaction in the flocculus of the alert monkey. II. Purkinje cell activity. Exp Brain Res 43, 349–360, 1981.
457. Waespe W, Wichmann W. Oculomotor disturbances during visual-vestibular interaction in Wallenberg's lateral medullary syndrome. Brain 113, 821–846, 1990.
458. Waitzman DM, Silakov VL. Effects of reversible lesions of the central mesencephalic reticular formation (cMRF) on primate saccadic eye movements. Soc Neurosci Abstr 20, 1399, 1994.
459. Waitzman DM, Silakov VL, Cohen B. Central mesencephalic reticular formation (cMRF) neurons dis-

charging before and during eye movements. J Neurophysiol 75, 1546–1572, 1996.
460. Waitzman DM, Silakov VL, Palma-Bowles S, Ayers AS. Effects of reversible inactivation of the primate mesencephalic reticular formation. I. Hypermetric goal-directed saccades. J Neurophysiol 83, 2260–2284, 2000.
461. Waitzman DM, Silakov VL, Palma-Bowles S, Ayers AS. Effects of reversible inactivation of the primate mesencephalic reticular formation. II. Hypometric vertical saccades. J Neurophysiol 83, 2285–2299, 2000.
462. Walberg F, Dietrichs E. The interconnection between the vestibular nuclei and the nodulus: a study of reciprocity. Brain Res 449, 47–53, 1988.
463. Walton MM, Mays LE. Discharge of saccade-related superior colliculus neurons during saccades accompanied by vergence. J Neurophysiol 90, 1124–1139, 2003.
464. Wang SF, Spencer RF. Spatial organization of premotor neurons related to vertical upward and downward saccadic eye movements in the rostral interstitial nucleus of the medial longitudinal fasciculus (riMLF) in the cat. J Comp Neurol 366, 163–180, 1996.
465. Weiskrantz L. Blindsight. In Chapula LM, Werner JS (eds). The Visual Neurosciences. MIT Press, Cambridge, Massachusetts, 2003, pp 657–669.
466. Westheimer G, Blair SM. Oculomotor defects in cerebellectomized monkeys. Invest Ophthalmol 12, 618–621, 1973.
467. Westheimer G, Blair SM. The ocular tilt reaction—a brainstem oculomotor routine. Invest Ophthalmol 14, 833–839, 1975.
468. Williams GV, Rao SG, Goldman-Rakic PS. The physiological role of 5-HT2A receptors in working memory. J Neurosci 22, 2843–2854, 2002.
469. Wyder MT, Massoglia DP, Stanford TR. Contextual modulation of central thalamic delay-period activity: representation of visual and saccadic goals. J Neurophysiol 91, 2628–2648, 2004.
470. Xing J, Andersen RA. Memory activity of LIP neurons for sequential eye movements simulated with neural networks. J Neurophysiol 84, 651–665, 2000.
471. Xing J, Andersen RA. Models of the posterior parietal cortex which perform multimodal integration and represent space in several coordinate frames. J Cogn Neurosci 12, 601–614, 2000.
472. Yamada J, Noda H. Afferent and efferent connections of the oculomotor cerebellar vermis in the macaque monkey. J Comp Neurol 265, 224–241, 1987.
473. Zackon DH, Sharpe JA. Midbrain paresis of horizontal gaze. Ann Neurol 16, 495–504, 1984.
474. Zee DS, Tusa RJ, Herdman SJ, Butler PH, Gucer G. Effects of occipital lobectomy upon eye movements in primate. J Neurophysiol 58, 883–907, 1987.
475. Zee DS, Yamazaki A, Butler PH, Gucer G. Effects of ablation of flocculus and paraflocculus on eye movements in primate. J Neurophysiol 46, 878–899, 1981.
476. Zeki S, Watson JD, Leucke CJ, et al. A direct demonstration of functional specialization in human visual cortex. J Neurosci 11, 641–649, 1997.
477. Zihl J, Von Crammon D. The contribution of the "second" visual system to directed visual attention in man. Brain 102, 835–856, 1979.
478. Zihl J, Von Crammon D, Mai N. Selective disturbance of movement vision after bilateral brain damage. Brain 106, 313–340, 1983.
479. Zuk A, Gwyn DG, Rutherford JG. Cytoarchitecture, neuronal morphology, and some efferent connections of the interstitial nucleus of Cajal. J Comp Neurol 212, 278–292, 1982.

Chapter 7

Eye-Head Movements

OCULAR MOTOR AND CEPHALOMOTOR SYSTEMS

When most animals visually track or acquire targets, they use a combination of eye and head movements. Likewise, in response to perturbations of the body that occurs during locomotion, both eye and head movements are used to reflexively stabilize the line of sight. This behavioral cooperation is reflected in the anatomic and physiologic similarities between the head (cephalomotor) and the eye (ocular motor) control systems. With the evolution of a fovea and a large ocular motor range, however, it became advantageous to be able to move the eyes with the head still. Therefore, primates in general and humans in particular have evolved a high degree of independent control of the head and eyes. Even so, we frequently move our eyes and head together, and an analysis of the effects of disease on eye movements must consider the interactions between the ocular motor and cephalomotor control systems. Rotations of the head are usually described as having components in one or more of three planes: horizontal (yaw, rotation about the Z or vertical axis), sagittal (pitch, rotation about the Y or inter-aural axis), and torsional or frontal (roll, rotation about the X or nasal-occipital axis). Likewise, displacements or translations of the head are described as having components along one or more of three axes: bob (vertical), surge (anterior-posterior), and heave (lateral).

STABILIZATION OF THE HEAD

Head perturbations that occur during locomotion are a major threat to clear vision. Although the vestibulo-ocular reflex (VOR) can compensate for head rotations by producing compensatory eye rotations, its ability to do so is limited; for example, when head velocities exceed approximately 350 degrees per second, saturation is reached and the reflex no longer works adequately.[170] Stabilization of the head in space reduces demands made of the VOR. How well is the head stabilized during locomotion?

Measurement of the rotational perturbations of the head during walking or running in place indicates that angular head velocity usually does not exceed 100 degrees per second, even during running (Fig. 7–1A).[55,91,92,99,113,168] The predominant frequencies of head perturbations principally lie in the range 0.5 Hz–5.0 Hz (Fig. 7–1B), although some harmonic frequencies may be as high as 20 Hz. The predominant frequency of vertical head perturbations (i.e., pitch rotations) is usually twice that of horizontal perturbations (i.e., yaw rotations).[91] The reason for this is that the head is perturbed vertically (up and down) with each heel strike, which typically occurs at about 2 Hz,[128] but rotates horizontally (right and left) with each successive pair of steps.

During locomotion, the angle of head orientation in the sagittal plane with respect to gravity is held quite constant (standard deviation of 3 degrees).[168] This head orientation may optimize the sensitivity of the otolith organs to linear accelerations. During fast walking or running, the head may bob up and down by as

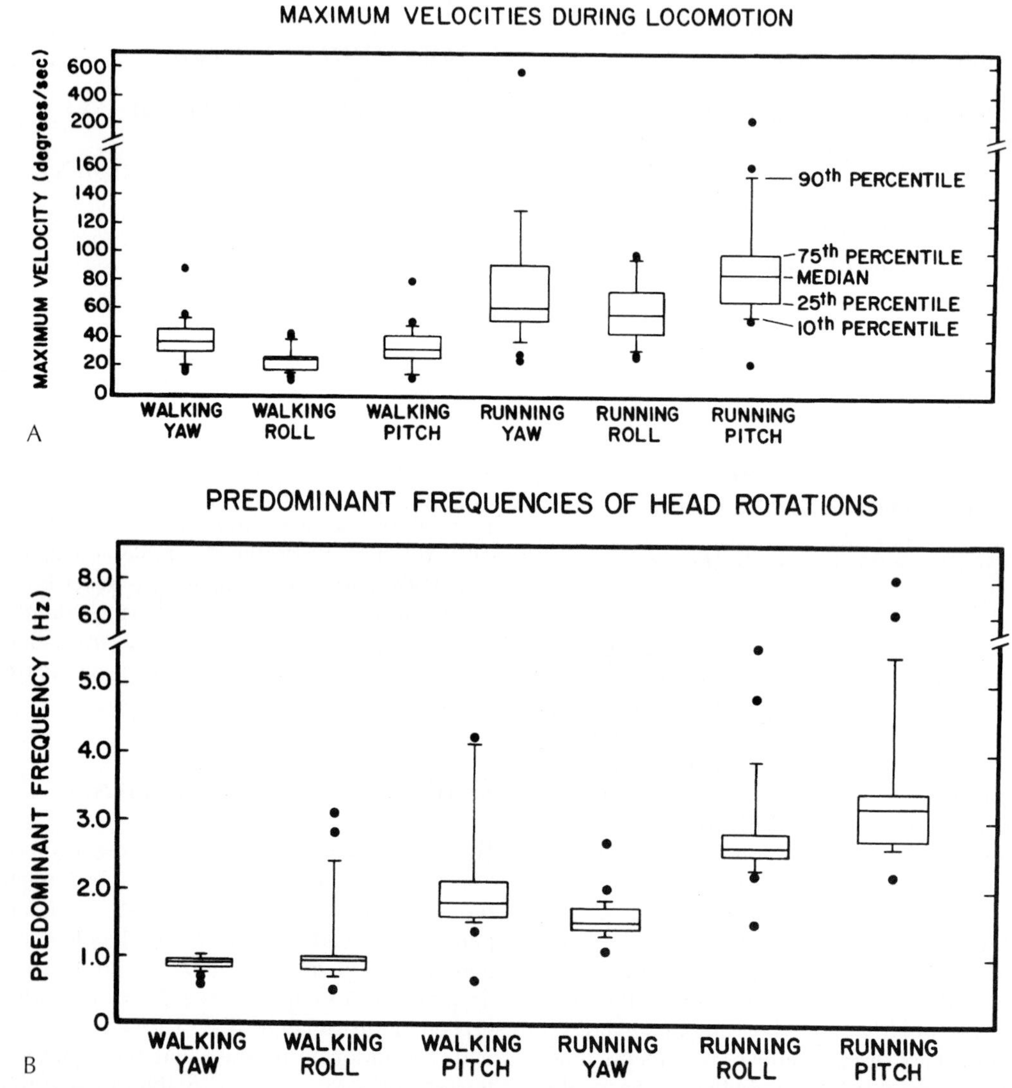

Figure 7–1. Summary of the ranges of (A) maximum velocity and (B) frequency of rotational head perturbations occurring during walking or running in place. Distribution of data from 20 normal subjects is displayed as Tukey box graphs, which show selected percentiles of the data. All values beyond the 10th and 90th percentiles are graphed individually as points. (Adapted from King et al.[113])

much as 6 cm, and this becomes especially important if subjects view near targets.[40,92] In normal subjects, head translations and rotations are synchronized so that when the head bobs up, it pitches down, and as it heaves laterally, it rotates medially.[40,99,168] In this way, the direction orientation of the naso-occipital axis of the head is held fairly steady.[145]

What mechanisms stabilize the orientation of the head during locomotion? Four main factors have been identified in humans: (1) Passive mechanical forces due to the inertial mass of the head and the muscles and tissues that support it.[87,93] Although the mass of the head tends to make it resistant to perturbations, its eccentric carriage on the series of joints that form the neck predisposes it to oscillations, especially in pitch.[88] Head inertia contributes to head stability for head perturbations with frequencies exceeding 3.0 Hz.[110] (2) The vestibulo-collic reflex (VCR),[153] by which the vestibular system activates neck muscles to stabilize the head with respect to space. Head pitch rotations that compensate for bob translations during walking are absent in patients with deficient vestibular function,[169] and this has been taken as evidence that the vestibulo-collic reflex generates this compensatory response.[99,145] (3) The cervico-collic reflex (CCR), the stretch reflex of the neck muscles, which acts to stabilize the position with respect to the trunk. The way in which the VCR and CCR work together is complex. Thus, during perturbations of the head, the VCR and CCR work together to stabilize the head in space. However, during perturbations of the body, the CCR could detract from the ability of the VCR to hold the head steady in space. These two reflexes appear to work together, with the VCR being more prominent, to prevent oscillations of the head.[158,159] (4) Voluntary control of tone in the neck muscles, which may assume importance in developing compensatory strategies if vestibular function is lost.[87,163] The relative importance of each of these mechanisms is discussed further in the section Disorders of Head and Gaze Stabilization.

VOLUNTARY CONTROL OF EYE-HEAD MOVEMENTS

During natural activities, we commonly use a combined eye-head saccade to shift gaze towards a novel visual target, to scan the environment,[119] and during eye-hand activities.[43] However, head movements also occur during a variety of behaviors besides gaze-shifts, such as during communication and eating. Thus, independent control of eye and head movements is to be expected. Just how independent eye and head movements are during voluntary gaze shifts is unclear. In cats, they seem to be closely coupled,[94] but care is required in extrapolating such findings to primates, who have a larger ocular motor range and may use eye-head movements independently for more complex behaviors.[166]

In discussing gaze shifts achieved by combined movements of eye and head, it is necessary to distinguish between eye position in the head ("eye position") and eye position in space ("the angle of gaze" or, simply, "gaze"). During viewing of distant targets, gaze is the sum of eye position and head position. During viewing of a near target, a correction is necessary to account for the eyes not being at the center of rotation of the head (see Laboratory Evaluation of Eye-Head Movements). As is discussed below, current evidence suggests that the brain is able to plan eye-head movements to visual or auditory targets by encoding a continuum of reference frames, from eye-, to head-, to body- or world-center scheme.[83,118,131,213,227]

Rapid Gaze Shifts Achieved by Combined Eye-Head Movements

Rapid gaze shifts that are achieved by combined, rapid eye-head movements (eye-head saccades or gaze saccades) serve two related, but separate functions: (1) they bring the image of an object, detected in the retinal periphery, to the fovea, where it can be seen best; and (2) they reorient the head and eyes in space so that a new part of the visual scene can be viewed using ocular saccades.[122] The second type of rapid gaze change is the predominant one made by afoveate animals,[32] and it assumes particular importance in animals with a limited ocular motor range. Note also that quick phases of nystagmus, which occur during vestibular stimulation, do not bring a specific object to the fovea. The purpose of quick phases is to keep the eyes within the working ocular motor range (i.e., prevent the eyes reaching the mechanical limits of the orbits and to reorient the eyes towards the oncoming visual scene (Fig. 1–6, Chapter 1).[139]

DYNAMIC PROPERTIES OF HEAD SACCADES

Examples of eye-head saccades are shown in Figure 7–2, with a comparison of a similar sized eye saccade and eye-head saccade shown in panel A. Although the head component shows more variability than the gaze component,[122,166] certain properties are similar to ocular saccades. Thus, during eye-head saccades, the velocity of the head increases with the amplitude of the head movement (Fig. 7–3A and 3B). This main sequence of head movements differs from the main sequence of eye saccades in that the former shows no saturation for larger movements and is more variable (compare with Fig. 3–3 in Chapter 3).[6,126,195,201,202,228] Unlike the saccade main sequence, the speed of head movements are under some voluntary control. Like ocular saccades, eye-head shifts of gaze obey Listing's law,[115,206,208] which is discussed further in Chapter 9.

Other properties of eye-head saccades emphasize *differences* between the eye and head components. Thus, the waveforms of

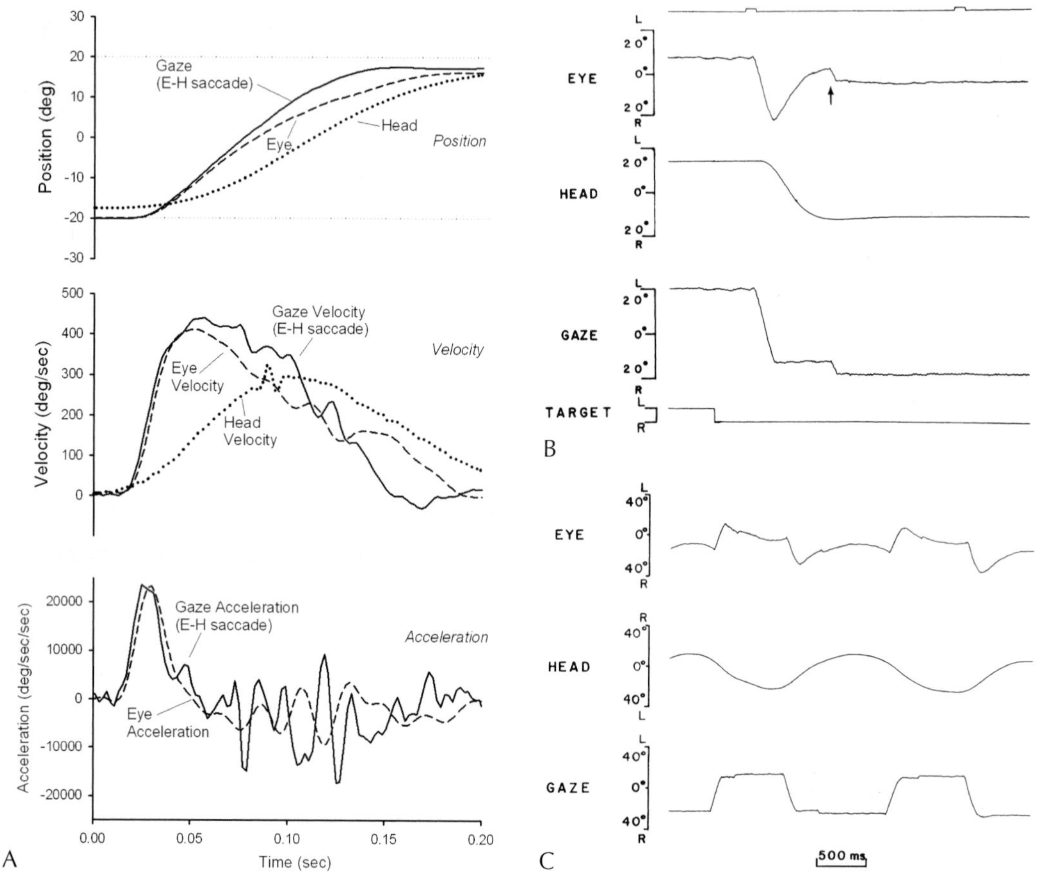

Figure 7–2. (A) Comparison of a rightward eye-head saccade and ocular saccade of similar size with the head stationary made by the same subject. Channels labeled as gaze or head refer to the eye-head saccade, and eye refers to the ocular saccade. In the middle panel, note that the gaze and eye velocity are similar and both show skewed waveforms, whereas the head velocity waveform is symmetric. (B) A combined, eye-head saccade in response to the unexpected appearance of a visual target. About 200 ms after the appearance of the target, the eye commences a saccade. A head movement follows and causes the eye to rotate back, due to the vestibulo-ocular reflex. The sum of the eye and head movements is a saccadic gaze shift. The latter is followed by a corrective saccade, indicated by an arrow. L: left; R: right. Time mark, at top, indicates 1 second. (C) Combined eye-head saccadic refixations between two stationary targets. Note the smooth, slow, "predictive" pattern of head motion rather than the "ballistic" pattern shown in (A) that is associated with a suddenly appearing target. Eye = eye position in the orbit; Head = head position in space; Gaze = Eye + Head = eye position in space. Note inversion of head position axis. (Adapted from Zee, 1977,[229] with permission of Springer Science and Business Media.)

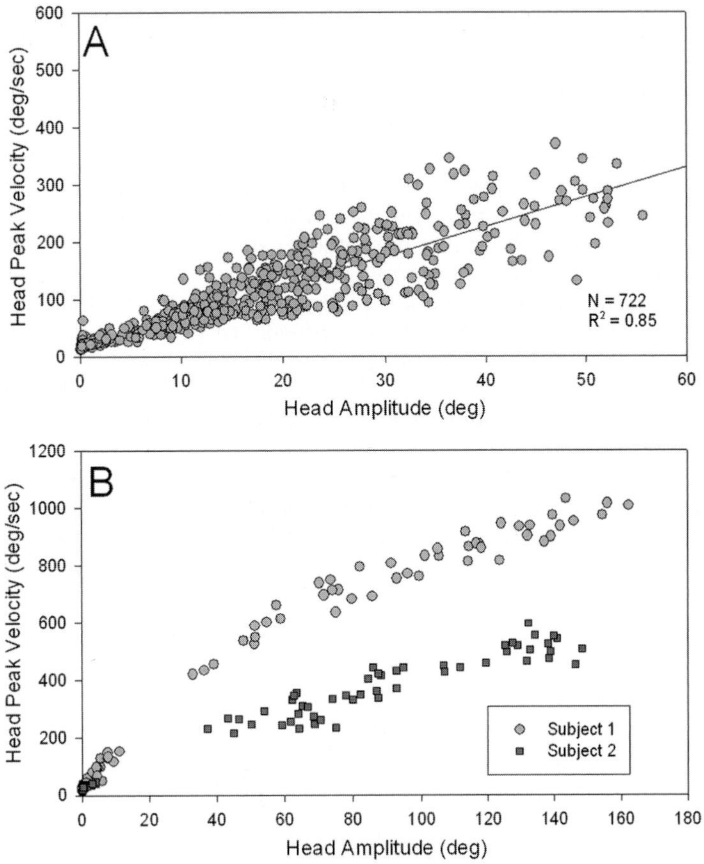

Figure 7–3. Main sequence plots for head components of eye-head saccades. (A) Plot of peak velocity versus amplitude for head saccades (n = 722) pooled from 10 normal subjects. The relationship is linear (R^2 = 0.85). (B) Comparison of large head saccades made by two subjects. Note that although their data differ in slope, both sets of data are fairly linear. (Adapted from Liao et al,[126] with permission of the New York Academy of Sciences.)

head velocity and gaze velocity (or eye velocity for head-stationary saccades) are different. Whereas large saccades show skewing of the velocity waveform (Fig. 7–2A), the head component of eye-head saccades does not.[126] When two visual targets are briefly presented in succession, the ocular response to this double-step stimulus is towards the second target whereas the head moves towards the first.[175] When eye-head saccades are made in response to diagonal target jumps, the trajectories of eye and head differ.[207,208] If a visual target is presented with a distracting stimulus, some eye-head saccades will be preceded by head movements that are initially in the wrong direction.[35,36] The countermanding task, which requires subjects to cancel a planned movement, also may dissociate ocular and head component responses of eye-head saccades.[34] Finally, when monkeys make large eye-head saccades, the eye velocity profile may show transient decelerations giving the appearance of two peaks.[64a,67] Taken together, these examples of dissociated properties of the eye and head components of eye-head saccades suggest that there are independent generators of eye and head components, a topic discussed further in the section Neural Substrate for Rapid Eye-Head Gaze Shifts.

THE PROPENSITY TO MAKE HEAD MOVEMENTS DURING EYE-HEAD SACCADES

The accuracy of gaze shifts during eye-head saccades is similar to eye saccades for gaze, but head position is less well controlled. Thus, we do not perceive the direction in which our head points as keenly as we perceive the direction of gaze.[10] The tendency to make an eye-head saccade, rather than a purely ocular saccade, varies substantially between subjects, but tends to remain quite constant for individual subjects. Thus, each subject shows *an eye-only range,* within which gaze shifts are not accompanied by head movements, and a *cus-*

tomary ocular motor range that corresponds to the width of region within which the eye is likely to be found at the end of eye-head saccades 90% of the time (ranging from about 20 to 60 degrees);[192] examples are shown in Figure 7–4. The variability of eye-only and customary ocular ranges between different subjects cannot be related to the properties of an individual's eye movements in eccentric gaze.[194] Thus, even though ocular motor palsies may have a substantial impact on head movements (as discussed in Chapter 9), in normals, the variability of the eye-only and customary ocular motor ranges cannot be ascribed to mechanical or geometric factors imposed by an individual's head and orbits.[194]

If visual targets are presented within the current ocular motor range, the tendency to make an eye-head saccade is influenced by an expectation of how eccentric the eye will be in the orbit at the end of the gaze shift.[151] Thus, subjects are more likely to make head movements when they expect the target to move more than once in the same direction, or be held longer in an eccentric position.[151] Each subject's idiosyncratic behavior is generally preserved whether the target is visual or auditory, a finding that has suggested that the propensity to make an eye-head saccade is determined in a common reference framework for these two sensory modalities.[81] It appears that central, rather than peripheral factors determine whether some individuals ("head-movers") are more prone to make eye-head saccades while others ("non-movers") tend not to.[71] Furthermore, these results implicate areas such as the frontal lobes in determining when a head movement will be made, since they are known to be important in determining predictive behaviors.[151,151a] If however, visual

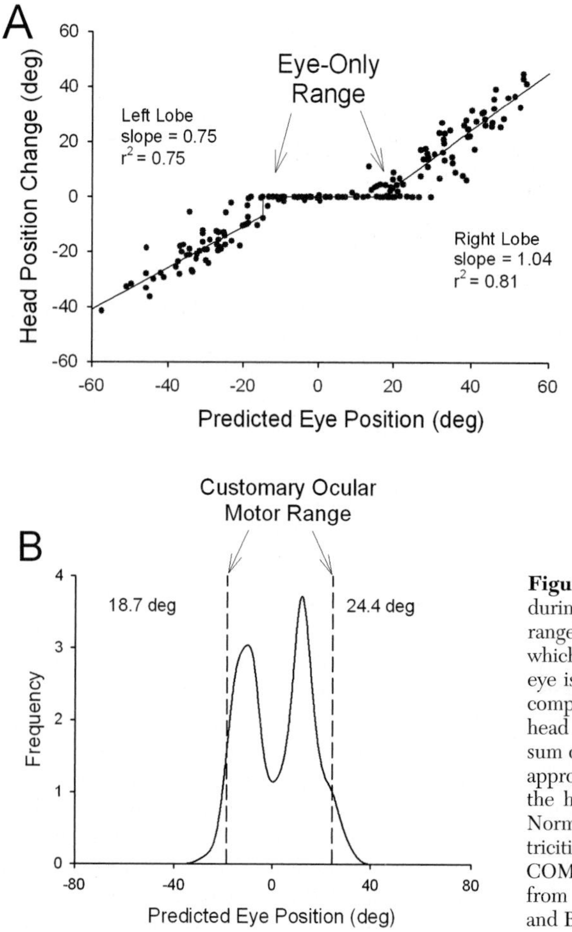

Figure 7–4. Eye-head saccade behavior of one subject during one experimental session showing the eye-only range, and the customary ocular motor range (COMR), which is defined as orbital eccentricity within which the eye is likely to be found with a probability of 90% at the completion of a gaze-shifting movement. (A) Change in head position versus predicted eye position, which is the sum of the gaze shift and initial eye position, and which is approximately equal to target eccentricity with respect to the head. Solid lines indicate a piecewise linear fit. (B) Normalized distribution of orbital postsaccadic eye eccentricities versus predicted eye position, with boundaries of COMR indicated by cursors. (Adapted, with permission from Stahl 1999,[192] with permission of Springer Science and Business Media.)

demands change, for example by restricting head movements with a collar, or wearing goggles with blinkers, both the propensity to make head movements and the customary ocular motor range change,[143,193] implying that eye-head saccades, like ocular saccades, are capable of adaptive plastic behavior.

EYE-HEAD SACCADES TO UNEXPECTED AND EXPECTED TARGET PRESENTATIONS

When the movement is toward a target that *unexpectedly* appears in the periphery, the saccadic eye movement usually starts 200 ms after the target appears and precedes the head movement by about 20 ms to 50 ms (Fig.7–2).[86,209,217] However, measurements of neck electromyographic (EMG) activity have shown that the neck command may precede the saccadic eye movements.[37] In response to auditory stimuli, gaze shifts are made at shorter latency, and head movement components are larger than in response to visual stimuli.[82]

A different pattern of eye-head coordination appears when the subject can *anticipate* the time and location of the next visual stimulus.[15] In this "predictive" mode of tracking, the head begins to move several hundred milliseconds before the saccade (Fig. 7–2B), and both begin before the stimulus moves. When self-paced and repetitive gaze shifts are required, eye and head components are more closely synchronized than in response to non-predictable target jumps.[119,166] This behavior is advantageous in everyday life and, for example, during natural locomotion around corners, head and eyes are directed towards the future direction.[85] When subjects use combined eye-head movements during manual tasks, the latency and velocity of the eye movement are influenced by both gaze shift and hand movements.[190]

As noted above, rapid gaze shifts achieved by a combined eye-head movement are capable of *adaptation* to novel conditions. Thus, if subjects wear goggles with an aperture that restricts the effective ocular motor range to a few degrees, they adapt by making more use of head movements that are specific for the residual ocular motor range,[42,143,193] along with changes in the preferred axis of head rotation.[41] Adaptive changes of eye-head saccades to new visual demands partly transfer to eye-only saccades, suggesting that the substrate for adaptation lies upstream of the site where separate eye and head commands are programmed, perhaps depending on cortical drives.[33,165]

BEHAVIORAL STUDIES OF THE INTERACTION BETWEEN THE SACCADIC COMMAND AND VESTIBULO-OCULAR DURING RAPID EYE-HEAD GAZE SHIFTS

During rapid eye-head gaze shifts, the saccadic command interacts with the mechanisms that act to hold gaze steady. In normal subjects, the VOR is of prime importance in holding gaze steady. The cervico-ocular reflex (COR), which depends upon proprioceptive afferents from neck muscles to the vestibular nucleus,[62,111] makes little contribution to the stabilization of gaze in humans,[5,8181] unless vestibular function has been lost.[22,29,108] What is the nature of the interaction between the saccadic command and the VOR during eye-head saccades?

Bizzi and colleagues[15] initially proposed that, during eye-head saccades, there is a linear summation of the saccadic command and the VOR. Thus, the VOR would negate the effect of the head rotation and the gaze shift would be determined solely by the saccadic command. One prediction of this hypothesis is that the speed and accuracy of eye-head saccades would be independent of the head movement. This is not the case for *large* eye-head gaze shifts. In both humans and monkeys, during large eye-head saccades, gaze velocity and duration are clearly influenced by head velocity (Fig. 7–5).[122] Thus, if the subject deliberately moves the head slower, gaze velocity is reduced. This is strong evidence against the linear summation hypothesis. Furthermore, if the head is abruptly perturbed during large eye-head saccades, the eye movements produced indicate that the VOR is partially disabled.[48,95,122,157,199,202,203] However, linear summation of the saccadic command and VOR can account for *small* eye-head saccades (i.e., within the ocular motor range).[95,157,201] Such small shifts of gaze bring objects to the fovea that have already been seen and lie within the current ocular motor range. Thus, these small saccades may represent a different class of eye movement than large eye-head saccades.

Despite behavioral evidence that the VOR is not working fully during large eye-head gaze

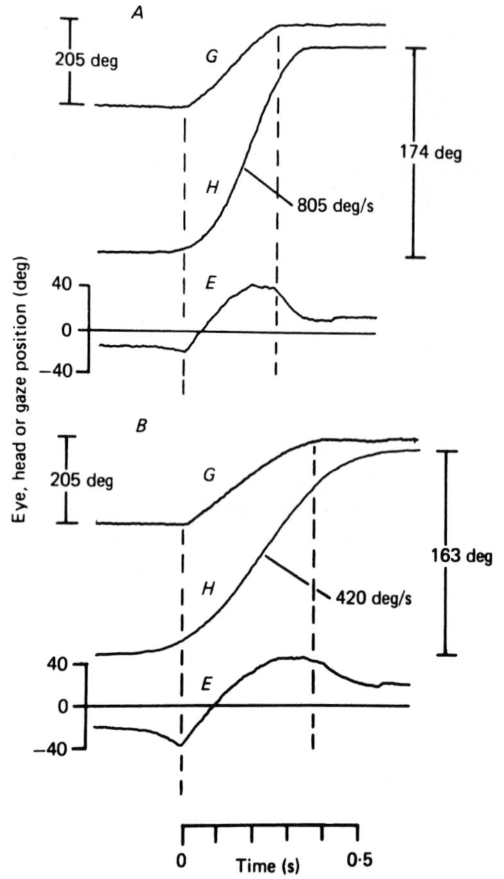

Figure 7–5. Demonstration of how the duration of an eye-head saccade can be influenced by the speed of the head movement. The behavior of eye, E, head, H, and gaze, G, are shown during eye-head saccades between targets 205 degrees apart. In (B), the subject deliberately moved his head more slowly than in (A). In (A), the duration (vertical dashed lines) was 250 ms; in (B), 380 ms. (From Laurutis and Robinson,[122] with permission of Blackwell Publishing.)

shifts, and a degree of independence of the contributions that eyes and head may make,[166] a mechanism appears to monitor head movements so that the accuracy of the eye-head saccade is guaranteed.[122,157,183] So, for example, if the head is unexpectedly perturbed during an eye-head saccade, gaze still lands on the target. This finding has lead to the proposal that head velocity information, although disconnected from the conventional VOR, is still available to control the duration of the saccadic burst neurons,[122] Electrophysiological evidence will be reviewed in the next section that provides a hypothesis to account for these behavioral findings.

Neural Substrate for Rapid Eye-Head Gaze Shifts

In trying to understand how eye and head movements are coordinated during eye-head saccades, we first compare structures projecting to ocular motoneurons versus to motoneurons in the cervical spinal cord that control voluntary head movements. Second, we consider how saccadic and vestibular signals could interact in the brainstem during rapid eye-head gaze shift. Third, we examine how the brainstem machinery for eye-head saccades is influenced by the superior colliculus, cerebellum, and cerebral cortex.

PROJECTIONS TO SPINAL MOTONEURONS CONCERNED WITH HEAD MOVEMENTS

The major projections to the cervical cord (C2) are from the brainstem reticular formation, including the head movement region in the nucleus reticularis gigantocellularis (see next section), the paramedian pontine reticular formation (PPRF), the mesencephalic reticular formation adjacent to the interstitial nucleus of Cajal, and the rostral interstitial nucleus of the medial longitudinal fasciculus (riMLF) (see Fig. 6–3, Chapter 6).[173] In addition, vestibular and fastigial nuclei (see Box 6–13) project to these cervical areas, but the superior colliculus does not directly.

THE GIGANTOCELLULAR HEAD-MOVEMENT REGION

Anatomical and electrophysiological studies in monkeys have defined neurons within the nucleus reticularis gigantocellularis (see. Fig 6–2) that are important for generating head movements during eye-head gaze shifts.[38,39,171,173] This region lies in the rostral medulla, between the posterior aspect of the abducens nucleus rostrally and the rostral third of the hypoglossal nucleus caudally. It lies caudal and ventral to the physiologically defined PPRF. Electrical stimulation here evokes head movements at a latency of about 30 ms. These evoked movements are usually ipsilaterally directed horizontal (yaw) rotations; sometimes pitch or roll movements are evoked. The size and speed of the induced head rotation is determined by the frequency and duration of the electrical stimulus.[171] Electrical stimulation in the gigantocellular head-movement region during eye-saccades increases the head component, reduces eye velocity, and produces hypermetric gaze shifts; counter-rotational eye movements that occur during stimulation are attributed to the vestibulo-ocular reflex.[65] These findings have been interpreted as evidence that ocular saccadic dynamics are influenced by the head movement command.[64,65] Neurotoxic damage to this area in cats abolishes spontaneous head movements.[197]

The gigantocellular head-movement region receives a major input from the posterior part of the superior colliculus, and afferents from the mesencephalic reticular formation surrounding the riMLF and interstitial nucleus of Cajal, the medial pontine reticular formation, and the fastigial and vestibular nuclei (see Fig. 6–3, Chapter 6).[39] It projects to the upper cervical cord, via the anterolateral funiculus and the medial longitudinal fasciculus, to terminate in lateral parts of the ventral horn. Here axons contact cervical interneurons that also receive vestibulospinal inputs. These interneurons project to motoneurons that innervate rectus capitus, obliquus capitus, and splenius capitus muscles. It has been suggested that the gigantocellular head-movement region contributes to a variety of behaviors such as feeding, as well as eye-head gaze shifts. Since electrical stimulation here does not produce gaze shifts, it appears that synchronization of movements of the eyes and head must occur upstream. The frontal eye fields do not appear to project directly to the gigantocellular premotor area, and thus, inputs from the superior colliculus seem crucial for programming eye-head gaze saccades.

THE ROLE OF THE PARAMEDIAN PONTINE RETICULAR FORMATION AND VESTIBULAR NUCLEUS NEURONS IN EYE-HEAD SACCADES

Two classes of burst neurons in the PPRF of alert monkeys have been defined: those with discharge activity related to the size of the eye-in-orbit movement (ocular burst neurons) and others that discharge in relation to the size of the eye-in-space movement (gaze burst neurons).[46,47,52,224] It has been suggested that the different properties of these two classes of neurons reflect the effects of vestibular (head velocity) projections to ocular, but not gaze, burst neurons.[201]

During eye-head gaze shifts, neurons in the VOR pathway change their discharge relationships.[52] For example, position-vestibular pause (PVP) neurons in the vestibular nucleus and nucleus prepositus hypoglossi, which play an important role in the VOR and project to abducens motoneurons, attenuate their discharge by 75% or more during head-free saccades.[68a,136,177] Nonetheless, the vestibular head velocity signal is apparently available to burst neurons so that an accurate gaze shift can be achieved. Abducens motoneurons discharge similarly during ocular saccades or eye-head saccades.[45] Therefore either the gaze-burst neurons in the PPRF must project to a separate location than the ocular motoneurons, or their head contribution must be canceled out at the level of the ocular motoneurons.

THE MESENCEPHALIC RETICULAR FORMATION, ROSTRAL INTERSTITIAL NUCLEUS OF THE MEDIAL LONGITUDINAL FASCICULUS, AND EYE-HEAD SACCADES

Several parts of the mesencephalic reticular formation project to the cervical cord region. One is the area ventrolateral to the interstitial nucleus of Cajal, and stimulation in this area may induce the ocular tilt reaction (see Chapter 11).[222] The central mesencephalic reticular formation (cMRF), which has reciprocal connections with the superior colliculus, may contribute to both horizontal and vertical gaze.[215] Pharmacological inactivation of the cMRF caused a head tilt, but this may have been due to spread to the adjacent interstitial nucleus of Cajal.[216] In addition, cells within the riMLF project to the cervical cord,[173] and—like the pontine reticular formation for horizontal eye-head saccades—may coordinate vertical movements.

THE SUPERIOR COLLICULUS AND EYE-HEAD SACCADES

In monkeys, electrical stimulation of the intermediate layers of the rostral two-thirds of the superior colliculus evokes saccadic eye movements (see Fig. 3–3, Chapter 3). Stimulation at more caudal sites in the superior colliculus produces combined eye-head gaze shifts at an average latency of 40 ms; both eye and head movements are directed contralaterally to the side stimulated.[38] In fact, the distinction between an "eye-only" rostral zone and an "eye-head" caudal zone of the superior colliculus is probably artificial, since EMG studies suggest that the neck muscles are activated for most voluntary gaze shifts.[37] The relationship between the timing and size of eye and head components of these electrically evoked gaze shifts is not tight; such studies indicate that superior colliculus neurons encode desired gaze direction in retinal coordinates.[114]

Current evidence supports a scheme in which the superior colliculus projects separately to the saccadic burst generator and premotor centers for head movements. First, single neuron activity in the ventral layers of the superior colliculus during experiments that independently controlled gaze, head, and eye-in-head movements indicates that these neurons are concerned with gaze displacement, and that separate eye and head displacement signals are decomposed downstream from the colliculus.[66] Second, stimulation of omnipause neurons just prior to eye-head saccades prevents the eye component but does not slow the head movement.[191] Third, if human subjects are presented with a distracting stimulus (visual or auditory) in addition to a visual target, they may make a wrongly directed head movement prior to the gaze shift.[36]

A further insight into the role played by the superior colliculus in guiding eye-head saccades comes from the behavior of cats, who may respond to a visual stimulus by making a multistep series of hypometric gaze shift. In this case, the superior colliculus neurons encode the total movement rather than the size of each component.[14] This suggests that the superior colliculus is important for target selection rather than in feedback guidance of eye-head saccades, although the issue is still debated.[134,152] The role of the superior colliculus in the control of ocular saccades is discussed in Chapter 3.

THE FRONTAL LOBES AND EYE-HEAD SACCADES

The *frontal eye field* (FEF, see Fig. 6–8, Chapter 6) contains a class of neurons that discharge in relation to head movements.[16] In patients who are about to undergo surgery for intractable epilepsy, per-operative stimulation causes ocular saccades directed contralaterally, sometimes accompanied by a head movement.[19] Experimental lesions of the FEF acutely cause a contralateral neglect during which the monkey tends not to look at targets in the contralateral hemifield and, when it does so, generates eye-head saccades that are hypometric.[211] Effects of FEF lesions on eye saccades are summarized in Chapter 3; no changes in the timing of eye and head contributions to eye-head saccades are reported. With recovery, the contribution of head movements to eye-head saccades tends to increase.[211]

Electrical stimulation of the *supplementary eye fields* (SEF) also produces eye-head movements that are directed contralaterally and have similar dynamic properties to natural eye-head saccades.[132] The SEF appear to play an important role in coordinating eye-head movements, since the effects of microstimulation vary according to stimulation site, ranging from eye-centered to body-centered behavior.[131] The descending pathway from the FEF for eye-head saccades is probably similar to that for eye saccades (see Fig. 6–9, Chapter 6) and differs from the pathways mediating voluntary control of the limbs.[189] Stimulation within the brainstem also elicits head movements and, as is the case for eye movements, there appears to be a midbrain decussation for the direction of elicited head movement.[13]

In humans, functional imaging has been used to compare cerebral areas that are activated during eye-head saccades versus ocular saccades.[164] During eye-head saccades, the frontal and supplementary eye fields were activated along with other areas reported with ocular saccades. An additional region that was activated during combined eye-head gaze shifts, but not with ocular saccades, consisted of the posterior part of the planum temporale and the parieto-insular vestibular cortex (PIVC). This area corresponds to that activated using caloric stimulation,[61] and therefore probably reflects vestibular stimulation that occurs during eye-head saccades Transcranial stimulation over motor cortex in humans evokes electromyographic responses in the contralateral sternocleidomastoid, trapezius and splenius capitis muscles at short (6–12 ms) latency.[72]

Smooth Tracking with Head and Eyes

BEHAVIORAL PROPERTIES

We may choose to visually track a smoothly moving target with the eyes alone (i.e., head stationary—smooth pursuit) or using a combination of eye and head movements—gaze pursuit. In general, normal subjects track equally well under either condition.[7,124] During combined eye-head tracking, the VOR must be negated in order for gaze to follow the movement of the target smoothly. Behavioral studies suggest that two separate mechanisms act to negate the VOR during eye-head tracking: cancellation of the VOR by a smooth-pursuit signal, and a partial, parametric reduction of VOR gain (VOR suppression).

One experimental strategy to determine whether the VOR is still operating during eye-head tracking is to perturb the subject's head and measure the short-latency (< 15 ms) vestibulo-ocular response before visually mediated eye movements have time to act (> 80 ms). This is the basis for the head-brake experiment, in which the head is suddenly stopped during eye-head pursuit (Fig. 7–6).[121] In normal subjects, ocular smooth pursuit is initiated too promptly for it to be in response to target motion after the head stops. Since there is insufficient time to initiate pursuit after the head is braked, it follows that the smooth pursuit system must have been operative during combined eye-head tracking, and it seems likely that this signal is being used to cancel the VOR. If the head-brake experiment is performed in patients who have lost their vestibular function (Fig 7–6, bottom), smooth pursuit does not commence promptly after their heads stop, but takes about 100 ms to be generated. An explanation for this result is that patients who have lost their vestibular function have no VOR to cancel during eye-head pursuit; therefore an ocular smooth pursuit signal is not needed. Some of these patients show better performance during eye-head tracking than during smooth pursuit with the head stationary (Fig.7–6, bottom), and this result could be because, with no VOR to cancel, fewer demands are made of the pursuit system.[124] Cancellation by a smooth-pursuit signal appears to be the main mecha-

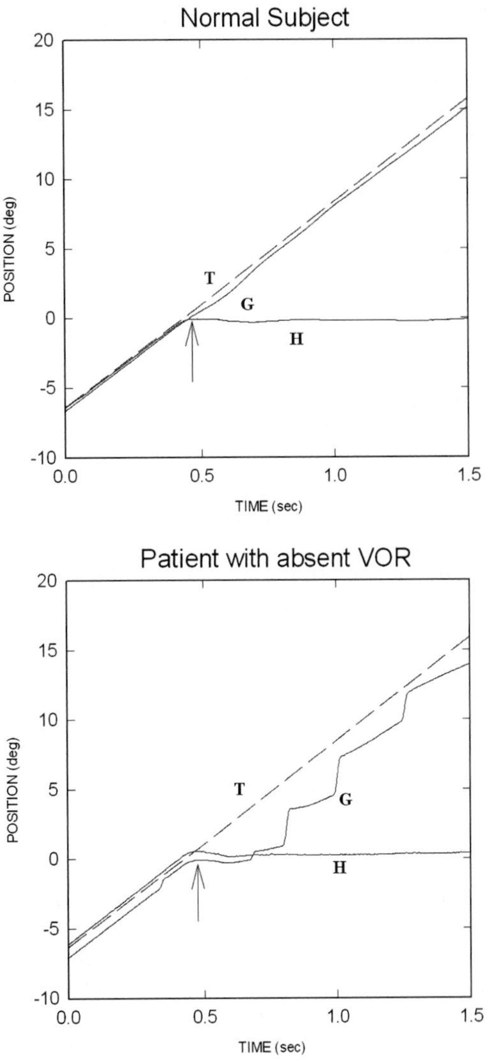

Figure 7–6. The head brake experiment. Typical responses from a normal subject (top) and a patient who had lost vestibular function (bottom) G: gaze; H: head; T: target. At the beginning of each record, the subject is visually tracking a head-fixed target that moves with the vestibular chair in which they are sitting (eye-head tracking). At the arrow, the chair is suddenly and unexpectedly stopped (head brake) while the visual target continues to move. The normal subject continues to generate a smooth tracking eye movement, implying that the smooth pursuit system was already active during the prior eye-head tracking. In contrast, after the onset of the head brake, the patient with no VOR temporarily stopped tracking the target: G fell behind T, and only recommenced tracking with saccades and pursuit after about 200 ms. This implied that the smooth pursuit system was not active during the prior combined eye-head tracking. Also note that the patient, but not the normal subject, showed superior eye-head tracking to smooth pursuit.

nism by which the VOR is negated during eye-head tracking, especially when head movements are made actively,[9,218] or if the subject is walking.[54] Several lines of behavioral evidence suggest that a second mechanism—parametric reduction of VOR gain or VOR suppression—may contribute during eye-head pursuit. For example, by visually fixing upon a head-fixed target during roll head rotations (around the naso-occipital axis), it is possible to cancel the torsional VOR, and yet there is no torsional smooth pursuit and only a weak torsional optokinetic response.[123] Studies of the way that the VOR and smooth pursuit obey Listing's law during three-dimensional head rotations indicate that VOR gain is reduced if subjects fixate a target that moves with the head.[142] Certain patients with cerebellar or brainstem disorders may show disparate defects of smooth pursuit and combined eye-head tracking (Fig. 7–9).[28,84,172] Barbiturate drugs impair cancellation of the VOR more profoundly than they impair smooth pursuit.[129] Some normal subjects may show combined eye-head tracking during passive rotation in the horizontal plane that is superior to their ocular smooth pursuit.[137] However, performance during head-free gaze tracking is usually similar to that of smooth pursuit (Fig. 7–5, top).[9] Finally, the ability to visually "enhance" the VOR when the target is stationary and head moves also appears to depend on more than a simple summation of vestibular and visual signals.[53] Thus, behavioral evidence is suggestive of more than one mechanism to negate the VOR during eye-head pursuit. Firmer evidence comes from electrophysiological studies.

NEURAL SUBSTRATE FOR SMOOTH EYE-HEAD PURSUIT

Semicircular canal nerve afferents show no modulation of their discharge due to visual stimulation,[27] and show similar discharge properties during either passive or active horizontal head rotations.[49,51] Thus, vestibular signals from the periphery must be negated centrally during eye-head pursuit. The premotor neurons concerned with *horizontal* eye-head tracking mainly lie in the vestibular nuclei and nucleus prepositus hypoglossi. Three types of vestibular nucleus neurons appear to contribute to eye-head tracking: position-vestibular-pause (PVP) neurons, vestibular-only (VO) neurons, and eye-head (EH) neurons.[52,68,204] As detailed in Chapter 2, PVP neurons encode contralaterally directed eye position, ipsilateral directed head velocity, and pause their discharge during saccades or quick phases of nystagmus. Most PVP neurons send an excitatory projection to motoneurons in the contralateral abducens nucleus (Fig. 6-1, Chapter 6). If monkeys view a head-fixed target while they are passively rotated, the discharge of PVP neurons is attenuated by about 30% compared with passive rotation in darkness (VOR).[50,176] During active, head-free smooth pursuit, attenuation of PVP neurons increases to about 50%.[177]

In contrast, VO neurons appear to be more concerned with the vestibulo-collic reflex (VCR) and vestibulospinal reflexes.[75] They also receive inputs from vestibular afferents and encode head velocity, but not eye movements and, consequently, do not directly contribute to the VOR.[50] An important property of VO neurons is that during active eye-head movements, whether saccadic or pursuit, their head velocity signal is reduced by about 70% compared with during passive rotation.[74,76] This corresponds to a reduction of the VCR that would be a hindrance to active head movements. It seems unlikely that neck proprioception makes a substantial contribution to the reduction of VO neurons discharge during active head movements.[52]

The third group of neurons concerned with eye-head tracking, EH neurons may correspond to flocculus target neurons,[127] and relay a gaze velocity signal to abducens motoneurons during combined eye-head pursuit. EH neurons also receive inputs from vestibular afferents, and seem to be the site of summation of pursuit and vestibular signals required for cancellation of the VOR during smooth eye-head tracking.[177] How might these three neuronal types account for the two mechanisms identified by behavioral studies as contributing to modulation of the VOR during smooth eye-head tracking?

First, recall that if a subject's head is perturbed during eye-head pursuit, a reduced response is evident at a latency of less than 100 ms, indicating a reduction of vestibular responses rather than any visually mediated mechanism.[49,98,103] It seems that this VOR reduction can be attributed to attenuation of discharge of PVP neurons, perhaps due to inhibition from the vestibular cerebellum,[177] or dorsal vermis.[188] The cue to generate a cancellation signal might be when neck proprioceptive signals match those expected on the basis of the neck motor command.[178] During visual cancellation of the translational VOR, the relationship with smooth pursuit is even more non-linear, also suggesting a switching mechanism.[140]

Second, behavioral evidence indicates that a more important mechanism consists of cancellation of the residual vestibular signal by an oppositely directed ocular smooth-pursuit signal.[44] The EH or flocculus target neurons in the medial vestibular and prepositus nuclei seem well suited for this function since they modulate their discharge during smooth pursuit and eye-head tracking, but not during the VOR. These neurons probably receive a pursuit signal from the vestibulocerebellum, which is derived from a descending pursuit pathway (Fig. 6–7, Chapter 6). Some Purkinje cells in the flocculus and ventral paraflocculus encode a gaze velocity signal during ocular and eye-head pursuit, but do not modulate their discharge during the VOR.[141] However, most of these Purkinje cells seem more concerned with smooth ocular pursuit rather than either smooth or saccadic eye-head tracking.[11,12] Thus, pharmacological inactivation of the flocculus compromises smooth ocular pursuit but has much less effect on eye-head tracking with the head free.[11] In contrast, the dorsal vermis of the cerebellum contains Purkinje cells that more faithfully encode gaze velocity during eye-head tracking.[188]

In the *vertical plane*, the y-group (see Box 6–8) may play a key role by relaying a gaze-velocity signal from the vestibulocerebellar to ocular motoneurons; this signal could then cancel the head velocity signal that projects from vertical PVP neurons to ocular motoneurons in the oculomotor and trochlear nuclei.[30,204,231]

Rostral to the brainstem and cerebellum, cortical areas concerned with smooth pursuit also contribute to eye-head tracking, such as the medial superior temporal (MST) visual area,[60] and the frontal eye fields,[69,70] as well as pontine nuclei to which they project.[150] The contributions of these cortical areas to smooth tracking are discussed in Chapter 4.

EXAMINATION OF EYE-HEAD MOVEMENTS

Head movements can be examined at the bedside using a similar approach to that used for eye movements. First note any spontaneous head tilt, turn, tremor, or other adventitious movement when the patient is at rest and when walking. Then instruct the patient to rapidly move the head from one target to another on command ("quickly, point your nose at the target"), so that the velocity, accuracy, and latency of head saccades can be noted. During eye-head saccades, note if the eye movement continues after the head movement is complete—a finding in some patients with slow saccades (see Video Display: Acquired Ocular Motor Apraxia).

To assess head pursuit, instruct the patient to track a slowly moving target, using the head and eyes together ("keep your nose pointed at the target"). A useful clinical test is to rotate the patient's head while he or she fixates a head-fixed target.[59,230] In this way, the eye is held near to central position and smooth tracking can be evaluated without contamination from gaze-evoked nystagmus (see Video Display: Disorders of Smooth Pursuit). Patients who have muscle weakness can be rotated in a wheelchair while fixating a pointer that rotates with the chair. The rotation of the chair should be gentle at first. If eye-head pursuit is inadequate (impaired cancellation of the VOR), the eyes will be continually taken off target by slow phases of the VOR and corrective saccades will be made. For example, deficient smooth pursuit to the right will usually be accompanied by deficient cancellation of the VOR on rotation to the right. In patients in whom smooth pursuit is impaired (lower tracking gain) compared with combined eye-head tracking, one should suspect an inadequate VOR; if there is no VOR to cancel, eye-head tracking is superior to smooth pursuit.[124]

Head nystagmus or tonic head deviation due to the vestibulo-collic reflex can be detected by rotating the patient in an office chair with the head free to move (see Video Display: Parkinsonian Disorders).[153] Some normal individuals, mainly children, may show head nystagmus during low-frequency sinusoidal body rotation either in the dark or light. In the latter case, head nystagmus reflects a combined vestibular and visual (optokinetic) input.

LABORATORY EVALUATION OF EYE-HEAD MOVEMENTS

In many laboratories, routine testing of combined, eye-head movements consists of measurement of cancellation of the VOR during passive rotation in a vestibular chair to which a fixation light is attached. Measurement of "VOR suppression" offers the means to test visually mediated tracking eye movements in patients in whom either a limited ocular motor range or gaze-evoked nystagmus prevents reliable measurement of smooth pursuit with the head stationary. When the intent is to compare combined eye-head tracking with smooth pursuit, it is essential to test the VOR (Fig 7–9).

Either sinusoidal or velocity-step stimuli (e.g., sudden onset of rotation at 20 degrees per second) can be used. For each stimulus, the peak eye velocity is measured ($\dot{E}_C$). Then the procedure is repeated in darkness, while the subject attempts to fixation a remembered target location (provided by an intermittently flashed light-emitting diode), to obtain the peak velocity of unsuppressed vestibular eye movements ($\dot{E}_V$). Comparison of the two ($1 - [\dot{E}_C/\dot{E}_V]$) enables calculation of the gain of VOR cancellation. Some normal subjects may show greater gain values for VOR cancellation during passive rotation than for smooth pursuit with the head stationary.[116,137] Like smooth pursuit, combined eye-head tracking changes during development and aging,[154,214] and each laboratory should establish its range of normal values.

Fixation suppression of nystagmus induced by caloric stimulation is a less precise measure of the ability to use visual signals to modulate vestibular responses, partly because cold or warm-water stimulation of one ear causes vertigo. The amount of suppression depends upon whether a small or large-field visual target is viewed,[101] and the attention of the subject. Severe impairment of visual fixation suppression of caloric nystagmus often implies a disorder of the central nervous system,[100,101,109] especially pathways mediating smooth pursuit, such as the vestibulocerebellum.[200] The properties of visual fixation are discussed in the first part of Chapter 4.

Testing eye-head saccades may also provide useful information, especially in patients with ocular motor apraxia (see Video Displays: Congenital Ocular Motor Apraxia and Acquired Ocular Motor Apraxia), or slow saccades due to degenerative conditions (see Video Display: Disorders of Saccades).

Quantitative testing of active eye-head movements can be achieved by a number of simple methods. Head movements can be measured using a light, snugly fitting helmet attached to a potentiometer, angular rate sensor, or accelerometer. Best results are probably obtained using the magnetic search coil method, which allow the head to move freely (see Appendix B). Eye movements can be measured using electro-oculography, head-fixed video eye trackers, or the search coil method, but infrared reflection techniques are not well suited because of their limited range of linear operation.

Rotating the subject in a vestibular chair can test stability of the head and gaze during perturbations of the body. The stimuli should ideally be of high frequency (0.5–5.0 Hz) and non-predictable (either "pseudorandom" or non-predictable transient rotations), to simulate the perturbations that occur during locomotion (Fig. 7–1). Eye-head saccades or smooth pursuit can be tested with visual stimuli similar to those used to test ocular saccades (Chapter 3) and measure smooth pursuit (Chapter 4).

During testing of combined eye-head movements, it is important to remember that changes in gaze must be related to the proximity of the target being viewed. If the subject views distant targets, then changes in gaze (eye in space) are simply the sum of the eye-in-orbit and head rotations. For near targets, however, the relationship is more complicated because the eyes are not located at the center of rotation of the head; they lie about 10 cm in front of the axis of head rotation. As an example, consider a head rotation during fixation of a near, earth-fixed target; during this head rotation, the eyes are displaced (translated) laterally and either anteriorly or posteriorly. Consequently, an additional rotation of the globes is required above what is needed to compensate for the head rotation, if the line of sight is to be held upon the target. Thus, the gain of the VOR should ideally be 1.0 when viewing distant targets, but greater than 1.0 when viewing near targets. The situation is even more complicated if both eyes are considered, since they are separated from each other and must therefore rotate by different

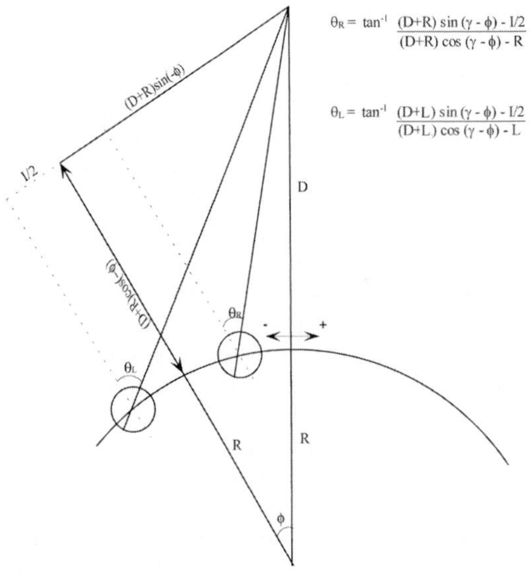

Figure 7–7. Geometric relationships between the angle of head rotation φ, the radius of head rotation (R), the distance of the target from the center of head rotation (R+D), interocular distance (I), target eccentricity (γ), and the rotation of the right eye (θ_R) required to main target fixation during viewing of a stationary near target.[97,212] (Reproduced with permission of the American Physiological Society.)

amounts. The geometric solution of this problem has been discussed by several authors,[18,97,212] and is summarized in Figure 7–7. Neglecting the separation between the eyes, and assuming head rotations are relatively small, an equation that approximately relates eye and head rotations, and the viewing distance of the target is:

$$E_O = [1 + R/(R+D)] * -H$$

where E_O = eye rotation in orbit, H = head rotation (the negative sign indicates that eye and head rotations are in different directions), R = radius of rotation of eyes in head (i.e., distance from center of rotation of head to the eyes, typically about 10 cm), and (R+D) = distance from center of rotation of head to target.

DISORDERS OF EYE-HEAD MOVEMENT

In this section, we will first deal with conditions that disrupt stability of head and gaze and then discuss disordered voluntary control of eye-head movements.

Disorders of Head and Gaze Stabilization

EFFECTS OF VESTIBULAR DISTURBANCES ON EYE-HEAD STABILITY

Abnormalities of head posture and gaze may be caused by disturbance of vestibular function. Thus, acute *unilateral loss of vestibular function* due to a peripheral process may cause an ipsilesional head tilt as part of an ocular tilt reaction (see Video Display: Disorders of the Vestibular System).[96] Following experimental labyrinthectomy, eye-head saccades are reduced in size, speed, and accuracy.[148] In patients with chronic unilateral labyrinthine loss, sudden perturbations of the trunk (applied by rotating the chair in which they sit) cause greater head oscillations and diminished head stability in space when they are rotated towards the lesioned side.[162]

Patients who have *bilateral loss of vestibular function* show two main changes in the control of head stability during locomotion.[169] First, they lose the ability to sustain a steady angle of head orientation in the sagittal (pitch) plane. Second, they lose the normal pattern of pitch rotations that compensate for vertical translations and point the naso-occipital axis at the object of regard.[169] However, patients who have lost vestibular function seldom complain about problems of head stability, partly because the passive mechanical of the head and neck provide some head stability at higher frequencies,[90] and partly because some patients develop adaptive head postures.[169] Their main complaint is oscillopsia (illusory movement of the visual world), during head movements, particularly those movements that occur during locomotion,[63,106] or riding in an automobile.[31] These visual symptoms appear with head perturbation (rotations or translations) above about 1.5 Hz, when visually mediated eye movements cannot compensate for loss of the VOR.[90,125] Thus, the main disability of such patients is due to loss of the VOR rather than loss of head stability.[55,90] Head movements made while subjects surveyed traffic prior to crossing a busy road were no different in patients with unilateral loss of vestibular function compared with controls.[17]

A number of adaptive strategies are employed by to labyrinthine-defective patients

Table 7–1. **Summary of Adaptive Strategies to Compensate for Loss of Vestibular Function***

- Substitution of small saccades and quick phases in the direction opposite head rotation to augment inadequate compensatory slow phases
- Potentiation of the cervico-ocular reflex
- Preprogramming of compensatory slow eye movements in anticipation of a head movement
- Decreased saccadic gain (saccade amplitude/target amplitude) during active, combined eye-head movements, to prevent gaze overshoot
- Extension of the range of frequencies over which the visual-following reflexes (pursuit) perform adequately
- Perceptual adaptations so that oscillopsia can be ignored
- Restriction of movement of the head so as not to challenge an inadequate vestibulo-ocular reflex
- Use of the effort of spatial localization to increase the gain of compensatory slow phases.

*References:[22,23,57,58,89,108,147,160,161,198,210]

so that they can stabilize gaze in the absence of a functioning VOR. These are summarized in Table 7–1. Perhaps most important of these is the development of rapid gaze position corrections. Such movements are difficult to study because of their variable temporal profile but, by studying patients with unilateral vestibular loss, and by making phase-place plots of gaze velocity versus gaze position, a strong case has been made that they are saccades.[160,161] An example is provided in the Video Display: Disorders of the Vestibular System.

CENTRAL NEUROLOGIC DISORDERS AFFECTING HEAD STABILITY

Disease of the central nervous system may affect head stability in a number of ways. For example, multisystem atrophy may limit the development of adaptive strategies, such as potentiation of the cervico-ocular reflex.[24,220] Paradoxically, one patient with a cerebellar tumor was reported to show an increase in the normal low gain of the cervico-ocular reflex.[22] Lesions affecting the central otolithic pathways—either in the vestibular nuclei, medial longitudinal fasciculus, or interstitial nucleus of Cajal—may cause the ocular tilt reaction,[20] which is discussed in Chapter 11.

Tremors of the head due to essential tremor or Parkinson's disease seldom interfere with steady gaze, because an adequate VOR is maintained. However, cerebellar disease causing titubation also frequently involves central vestibular connections and disturbs gaze either due to spontaneous ocular oscillations or to an abnormal VOR. Patients who have a head tremor *and* a deficient VOR may complain of oscillopsia and be mistakenly diagnosed as having nystagmus.[21] Oscillopsia brought on by head movements may also be caused by disease of the central nervous system, such as in internuclear ophthalmoplegia, when the VOR is deficient.[89] Observation with an ophthalmoscope is a useful clinical method of evaluating the stability of gaze during head tremor.

Patients with *Parkinson's disease and progressive supranuclear palsy* frequently show rigidity of the neck. In Parkinson's disease, muscle tone may be reduced by levodopa so that compensatory head movements increase during rotational perturbations of the body.[221] The vestibulo-collic reflex, which is vestigial in normal subjects,[153] may become clinically evident in patients with certain degenerative disorders. For example, patients with progressive supranuclear palsy, and some patients with dementia,[107] lose the corrective phase of head nystagmus during whole-body rotation with the head free. The vestibulo-collic reflex elicits a slow phase of head nystagmus in an attempt to stabilize the position of the head in space, but no corrective quick phase is made to maintain head alignment on the body. As a result, the head tonically deviates in the direction opposite to body rotation (see Video Display: Parkinsonian Disorders). If the quick phase of eye nystagmus is also absent, the eyes are also tonically deviated in the direction opposite to body rotation.

Several studies have addressed the relationship between *spasmodic torticollis* and a possible underlying vestibular imbalance. In response to head rotations in roll, both increases and decreases of the gain of counter-rolling have been demonstrated, without directional asymmetries or torsional nystagmus.[3,56] Other studies have investigated horizontal vestibular responses in darkness, and reported asymmetries[25] and hyperactivity of responses.[104]

Eye-head saccades show smaller head, and larger eye, components opposite to the direction of the torticollis;[135] these findings have been interpreted as adaptations to the abnormal head posture. Whether vestibular abnormalities are the root cause or simply a secondary effect of spasmodic torticollis—due, for example, to reduced neck motion—has not been settled,[26,104,196] but there might be a subgroup of patients in whom spasmodic torticollis is precipitated by vestibular disease.[26] In any case, patients with spasmodic torticollis show changes in their perceptions of the subjective visual vertical and straight ahead.[1,2]

Patients with *Wallenberg's syndrome (lateral medullary infarction)* occasionally show abnormal eye-head coordination.[117] Their head and their eyes may tonically deviate towards the side of the lesion, and occasionally they have spontaneous head nystagmus. These abnormalities probably reflect lesions in vestibulospinal and reticulospinal projections to cervical motoneurons.

CONGENITAL DISORDERS

Two infantile disorders characterized by head tremor and disturbance of gaze are spasmus nutans (see Box 10–13) and congenital nystagmus (Box 10–11); both conditions are discussed in Chapter 10, and examples are shown in the Video Display: Congenital Forms of Nystagmus. Children with the bobble-head doll syndrome show arrhythmic, to-and-fro, flexion-extension, bobbing of the head and, occasionally, the trunk.[80,155] In one patient, electromyography of the neck extensor muscle showed contractions at 2 Hz–3 Hz.[180] Such patients often have a slowly growing mass near or in the anterior part of the third ventricle, or aqueductal stenosis. The mechanism for this oscillation is unknown, but the movements cease following treatment of the hydrocephalus.

Disorders of Voluntary Head and Gaze Control

PARALYSIS OF VOLUNTARY HEAD TURNING

Paresis of voluntary head turning occurs as a component of conjugate gaze paresis following an acute lesion of one cerebral hemisphere: the head and eyes are turned toward the side of the lesion (see Box 12–18). Head turning depends upon both the sternocleidomastoid muscle (SCM) and the splenius capitis muscle. The splenius capitis receives contralateral cortical innervation, but the SCM appears to receive both contralateral and ipsilateral input.[72] Patients who have suffered a unilateral cerebral lesion often show some weakness of the SCM ipsilateral to the side of the cerebral lesion (recall that the SCM turns the head to the contralateral side). Thus, a right hemispheric lesion might produce gaze palsy to the left, involving head and eye movements; the right SCM would be weak, but there would be a left hemiplegia, with involvement of the left trapezius muscle. This finding suggests that the descending pathways to SCM are either uncrossed[4] or undergo a double decussation.[77] In support of the latter hypothesis, it has been reported that brainstem lesions may cause SCM weakness and hemiparesis on the same side,[133] presumably because the lesions are below the first decussation for SCM but above the second. The site of the second decussation for SCM is unknown. It might occur in the high cervical cord because, hemisection of the cord at C1 on the right, causes a flaccid right hemiparesis that spares the right SCM but causes left SCM weakness.[105] Furthermore, lesions at C4 may cause paralysis of the trapezius and quadriparesis but spare the SCM.[130,144] It seems likely that the brainstem pathways to the SCM, and perhaps to the splenius capitis muscle, lie in the tegmentum, because ventral pontine infarction that causes quadriparesis and trapezius weakness may spare the SCM.[130] An important consequence of this is that patients who are in the locked-in or deefferented state due to ventral pontine infarction often recover voluntary eye and head movements, which may be important for communication.[179]

HEAD TURNING IN EPILEPSY

Involuntary head turning is a common feature of focal motor epileptic seizures. Head turning away from the side of the seizure focus is called adversive or contraversive; head turning towards the side of the seizure focus is called ipsiversive. Although both adversive and ipsiversive head turning may occur with seizures, certain associated features may help with localization of the seizure focus. If the patient remains conscious during the attack, then head turning at the onset is generally, but not always, away from the side of the seizure focus, which is usually frontal.[138] A contralateral focus is also likely in patients who show forceful, sustained, and unnatural lateral positioning of their head and eyes.[225,226] In patients who are unconscious, whose seizures generalize, or who show milder deviations of the head and eyes, about half manifest ipsiversive movements of the head.[78,149] The site of the seizure focus may be in any lobe, but frontal and temporal are the most common. Contraversive eye deviation often accompanies the head turning, and may be followed by nystagmus; this issue is discussed further under Eye Movements during Epileptic Seizures, in Chapter 12

EYE-HEAD STRATEGIES IN PATIENTS WITH ABNORMAL SACCADES

Disordered Eye-Head Co-ordination in Ocular Motor Apraxia

Prominent head movements (thrusts) are a prominent feature of ocular motor apraxia. This term is commonly applied to patients who show an impaired ability to generate saccades on command. Apraxia is often defined as the lack of learned, skilled movements despite an intact, innate neurophysiological substrate for performing such movements. Ocular motor apraxia, therefore, should refer to a condition in which voluntary eye movements are impaired but reflexly induced saccades and quick phases are intact. In fact, the term has been applied to deficits of voluntary saccades that either spare,[185] or involve,[167] saccades made reflexively to visual targets. In either case, a cardinal feature of ocular motor apraxia is that quick phases of vestibular nystagmus are preserved. Acquired ocular motor apraxia occurs with bilateral parieto-frontal lesions (see Video Display: Acquired Ocular Motor Apraxia). Congenital forms of ocular motor apraxia include Cogan's idiopathic form, and in a number of genetic disorders that also cause ataxia (see Video Display: Congenital Ocular Motor Apraxia).

Patients with ocular motor apraxia are more easily able to voluntarily shift their gaze when they make an eye-head movement rather than a saccade with the head stationary. This pattern of behavior is similar to that of afoveate animals, that are unable to make voluntary gaze shifts without a head movement. Other eye-head strategies, such as turning the head past the target to carry along the eye in far lateral gaze, are sometimes employed. Theses are discussed further in Chapter 12.

Eye-Head Movements in Patients with Slow or Inaccurate Saccades

In patients with *slow ocular saccades* (see Table 12–4), the saccadic eye movements may outlast the head movements, even if saccadic latency is not prolonged (see Video Display: Disorders of Saccades). In some patients, head movements (also made with a blink) may increase the range of voluntary gaze shifts (Fig. 7–8), but without substantially increasing peak velocity. This is a quite different behavior from patients with ocular motor apraxia, who make few spontaneous saccades but, when they do, are of normal velocity.

In patients with *cerebellar disease* causing saccadic dysmetria, the accuracy of head movements and eye-head saccades may be also be affected.[187,229] The pattern of saccadic gaze dysmetria may vary depending on whether or not a head movement occurs with the gaze shift. Furthermore, the influence of the cerebellum on the ocular and head components of a combined movement probably differs, since transcranial magnetic stimulation over the cerebellum decreases the latency of saccade onset, but delays the start of the head component.[146] Pharmacological inactivation of the cerebellar fastigial nucleus (see Box 12–4, Chapter 12) causes ipsilateral hypermetria and contralateral hypometria of eye-head gaze shifts.[79,156] These findings are similar to the pattern of dysmetria of eye saccades following fastigial inactivation.[174] Patients with cerebellar disease also show impaired smooth tracking of the head, requiring "catch-up" head movements to keep up with the target.[229]

Huntington's disease causes difficulties in initiating saccades, which may be slow. Such patients often use a combined head thrust and blink to generate voluntary gaze shifts (see Video Display: Parkinsonian Disorders). Patients with Parkinson's disease may show delayed, small,

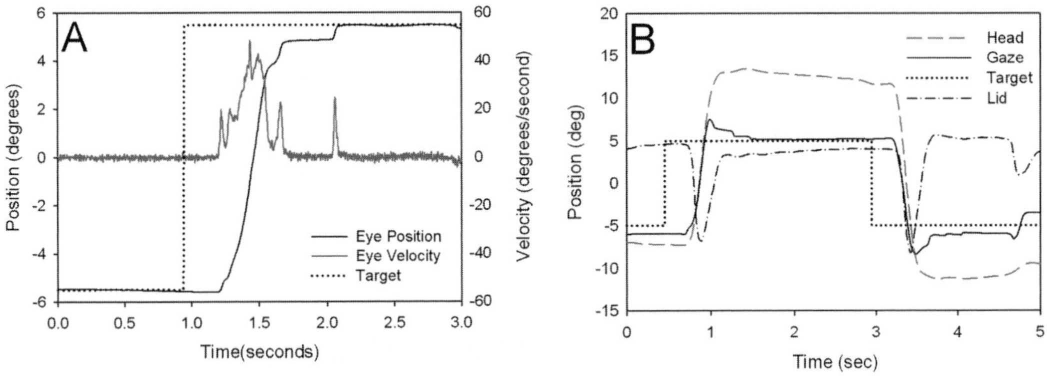

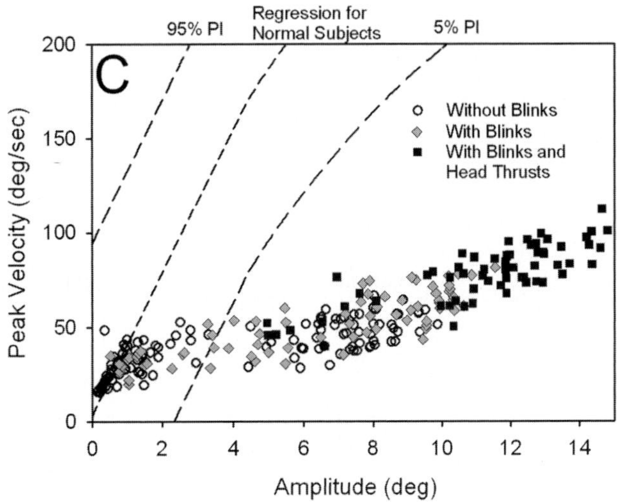

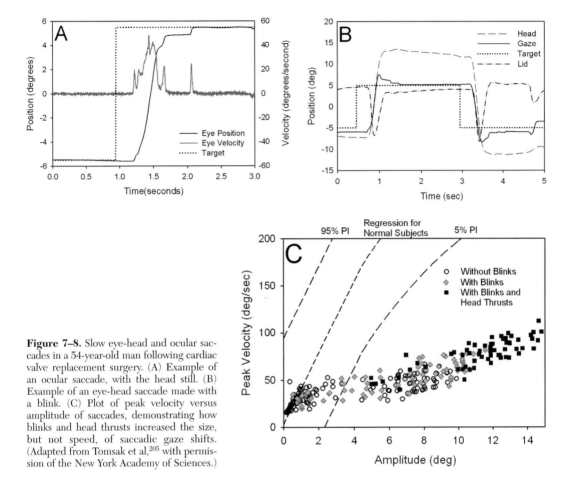

Figure 7–8. Slow eye-head and ocular saccades in a 54-year-old man following cardiac valve replacement surgery. (A) Example of an ocular saccade, with the head still. (B) Example of an eye-head saccade made with a blink. (C) Plot of peak velocity versus amplitude of saccades, demonstrating how blinks and head thrusts increased the size, but not speed, of saccadic gaze shifts. (Adapted from Tomsak et al,[205] with permission of the New York Academy of Sciences.)

and slow head movements during head-free tracking of step displacements of targets.[223]

Eye-Head Movements in Patients with Restricted Ocular Motor Range

Patients with ocular motor palsies, disease of the neuromuscular junction, or of the extraocular muscles all may show an increased range of head movements to compensate for their ocular deficit.[120] This is especially prominent in children with congenital ophthalmoplegia.[182] In affected individuals head saccades are bigger, slower, and less frequent than eye saccades in normals; they may also use slow head movements to scan the environment. With such adaptive strategies, normal activities, such as making a cup of tea, are performed as efficiently as by controls.[120] At least some patients rapidly learn to substitute head movements following loss of eye movements.[73] Head turns and tilts in patients with restricted ocular motility are discussed in Chapter 9.

SMOOTH HEAD TRACKING DISORDERS

As a general rule, disorders that impair smooth ocular pursuit—including drugs such as sedatives (see Table 12–11, Chapter 12)—also affect eye-head tracking. Like smooth pursuit, eye-head tracking deteriorates with age.[112] When there is a disparity, eye-head pursuit is usually superior,[84] perhaps reflecting the two mechanisms by which the VOR is negated during eye-head pursuit (see Smooth Tracking with Head and Eyes, above). So, for example, unilateral lesions affecting secondary visual areas concerned with motion analysis impair both smooth ocular pursuit and eye-head tracking as the patient follows targets moving towards the side of the lesion,[28,186] but eye-

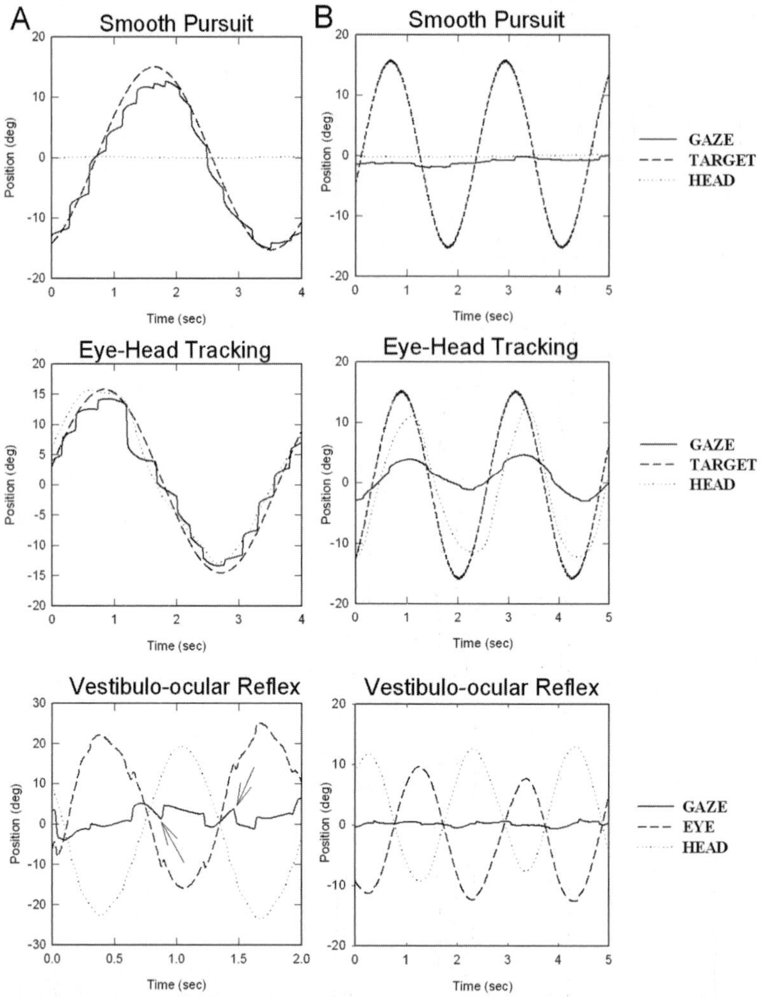

Figure 7–9. Comparison of smooth ocular pursuit and eye-head tracking (A) in the horizontal plane in a patient with cerebellar degeneration, and (B) in the vertical plane in a patient with progressive supranuclear palsy (PSP). The cerebellar patient shows better smooth pursuit (gain 0.38) than eye-head tracking (gain 0.29); the difference is partly explained by her visually assisted VOR, which was hyperactive (gain 1.11), necessitating "back-up" saccades (indicated by arrows). The patient with PSP showed superior combined eye-head tracking to that during smooth pursuit. Some of the difference reflected the inability to generate vertical catch-up saccades to foveate the moving target; such saccades were less necessary during combined eye-head tracking. However, preservation of the mechanism by which VOR gain is reduced during combined eye-head tracking may account for the difference. TARG: target.

head pursuit is superior in some patients.[102] Other disorders that impair smooth pursuit, such as cerebellar disease, multiple sclerosis,[184] Parkinson's disease,[223] and progressive supranuclear palsy, frequently also affect eye-head tracking, and this can be detected clinically during passive chair rotation.

When smooth ocular pursuit and head-free eye-head pursuit deficits are compared in patients with brainstem and cerebellar disease, in the horizontal and sagittal planes, combined eye-head tracking is usually, but not always, superior (Fig. 7–9).[84,219] In the torsional (roll) plane, in which optokinetic responses are weak in normals and patients, combined eye-head tracking is invariably better. In patients who have bilateral loss of vestibular function, combined eye-head tracking is often superior to smooth pursuit (Fig. 7–6, bottom),[124] perhaps because such patients have little VOR to cancel during combined eye-head tracking. Similarly, patients with deficient vestibular function can more accurately fixate upon a head-fixed target during locomotion than can normal subjects.[55] Conversely, patients with an increased VOR gain (due, for example, to cerebellar disease) may show better smooth pursuit than eye-head tracking (Fig. 7–9A).

SUMMARY

1. During natural behavior, eye and head movements usually occur together—a linkage reflected in a number of behavioral, anatomic, and physiologic similarities between the cephalomotor and ocular motor control systems. Primates have evolved a high degree of independent voluntary control over both eye and head movements.
2. During natural activities such as locomotion, the head is held relatively steady, with velocities generally below 100 degrees per second (Fig. 7–1). The frequency range of rotational head perturbations that occur during locomotion ranges between 0.5 and 5.0 Hz. The stability of the head during such perturbations is mainly due to the vestibulo-collic reflex, the mass of the head, and the visco-elastic properties of the neck. The vestibulo-collic and cervico-collic reflexes may prevent head oscillations in pitch and roll during locomotion.
3. The head component of eye-head saccades shows some dynamic differences from eye saccades, such as lack of skewing of the velocity waveform (Figs. 7–2 and 7–3). The propensity to make an eye-head, rather than an ocular, saccade is variable between subjects, but quite consistent for each individual (Fig. 7–4), and can be related to central, not peripheral, factors. During large gaze shifts to reorient the head and eyes in space (eye-head or gaze saccades; Fig. 7–5), the vestibulo-ocular reflex is, at least in part, disconnected. During smaller eye-head saccades in response to visual stimuli within the field of vision, a linear addition of the saccade command and the vestibulo-ocular reflex may occur. The head component of eye-head saccades is generated by neurons in the nucleus reticularis gigantocellularis in the pons.
4. During combined, smooth eye-head tracking (Fig. 7–4), the vestibulo-ocular reflex is canceled by an internal smooth pursuit signal and, in addition, the VOR gain may be reduced during smooth eye-head tracking. Vestibular nucleus neurons encode signals that could account for both mechanisms.
5. Disorders of eye-head coordination may be conceptualized as abnormalities of head stability or posture, and abnormalities of gaze shifting by either eye-head saccades or smooth eye-head tracking. Proper evaluation of disorders of eye-head tracking requires separate evaluation of the vestibulo-ocular reflex (Fig. 7–9). Certain patterns of head movements observed in patients with impaired VOR, ocular saccades, or smooth pursuit are adaptive and help stabilize or change gaze as necessary.

REFERENCES

1. Anastasopoulos D, Bhatia K, Marsden CD, Gresty MA. Perception of spatial orientation in spasmodic torticollis. Part 2: the visual vertical. Movement Disorders 12, 709–714, 1997.
2. Anastasopoulos D, Nasios G, Psilas K, et al. What is straight ahead to a patient with torticollis? Brain 121, 91–101, 1998.
3. Averbuch-Heller L, Rottach KG, Zivotofsky AZ, et al. Torsional eye movements in patients with skew deviation and spasmodic torticollis: responses to static and dynamic head roll. Neurology 48, 506–514, 1997.
4. Balagura S, Katz RG. Undecussated innervation to the sternocleidomastoid muscle: a reinstatement. Ann Neurol 7, 84–85, 1980.
5. Barlow D, Freedman W. Cervico-ocular reflex in the normal adult. Acta Otolaryngol (Stockh) 89, 487–496, 1980.
6. Barnes GR. Vestibulo-ocular function during coordinated head and eye movements to acquire visual targets. J Physiol (Lond) 287, 127–147, 1979.
7. Barnes GR. Head-eye co-ordination: visual and non-visual mechanisms of vestibulo-ocular reflex slow-phase modification. Prog Brain Res 76, 319–328, 1988.
8. Barnes GR, Forbat LN. Cervical and vestibular afferent control of oculomotor response in man. Acta Otolaryngol (Stockh) 88, 79–87, 1979.
9. Barnes GR, Lawson JF. Head-free pursuit in the human of a visual target moving in a pseudo-random manner. J Physiol (Lond) 410, 137–155, 1989.
10. Becker W, Saglam H. Perception of angular head position during attempted alignment with eccentric visual objects. Exp Brain Res 138, 185–192, 2001.
11. Belton T, Mccrea RA. Contribution of the cerebellar flocculus to gaze control during active head movements. J Neurophysiol 81, 3105–3109, 1999.

12. Belton T, Mccrea RA. Context contingent signal processing in the cerebellar flocculus and ventral paraflocculus during gaze saccades. J Neurophysiol 92, 797–807, 2004.
13. Bender MB, Shanzer S, Wagman IH. On the physiologic decussation concerned with head turning. Confin Neurol 24, 169–181, 1964.
14. Bergeron A, Matsuo S, Guitton D. Superior colliculus encodes distance to target, not saccade amplitude, in multi-step gaze shifts. Nat Neurosci 6, 404–413, 2003.
15. Bizzi E. Eye-head coordination. In Brooks VB (ed). Handbook of Physiology. The Nervous System. Section 1, Volume 2, Part 2. American Physiological Society, Bethesda, MD,1981 pp 1321–1336.
16. Bizzi E, Schiller PH. Single unit activity in the frontal eye fields of unanesthetized monkeys during eye and head movement. Exp Brain Res 10, 151–158, 1970.
17. Black RA, Halmagyi GM, Curthoys IS, Thurtell MJ, Brizuela AE. Unilateral vestibular deafferentation produces no long-term effects on human active eye-head coordination. Exp Brain Res 122, 362–366, 1998.
18. Blakemore C, Donaghy M. Co-ordination of head and eyes in the gaze changing behavior of cats. J Physiol (Lond) 300, 317–335, 1980.
19. Blanke O, Seeck M. Direction of saccadic and smooth eye movements induced by electrical stimulation of the human frontal eye field: effect of orbital position. Exp Brain Res 150, 174–183, 2003.
20. Brandt T, Dieterich M. Vestibular syndromes in the roll plane: topographic diagnosis from brain stem to cortex. Ann Neurol 36, 337–347, 1994.
21. Bronstein AM, Gresty MA, Mossman SS. Pendular pseudonystagmus arising as a combination of head tremor and vestibular failure. Neurology 42, 1527–1531, 1992.
22. Bronstein AM, Hood JD. The cervico-ocular reflex in normal subjects and patients with absent vestibular function. Brain Res 373, 399–408, 1986.
23. Bronstein AM, Hood JD. Oscillopsia of peripheral vestibular origin. Central and cervical compensatory mechanisms. Acta Otolaryngol (Stockh) 104, 307–314, 1987.
24. Bronstein AM, Mossman S, Luxon LM. The neck-eye reflex in patients with reduced vestibular and optokinetic function. Brain 114, 1–11, 1991.
25. Bronstein AM, Rudge P. Vestibular involvement in spasmodic torticollis. J Neurol Neurosurg Psychiatry 49, 290–295, 1986.
26. Bronstein AM, Rudge P, Beechey AH. Spasmodic torticollis following unilateral VIII nerve lesions: neck EMG modulation in response to vestibular stimuli. J Neurol Neurosurg Psychiatry 50, 580–586, 1987.
27. Büttner U, Waespe W. Vestibular nerve activity in the alert monkey during vestibular and optokinetic nystagmus. Exp Brain Res 41, 310–315, 1981.
28. Chambers BR, Gresty MA. The relationship between disordered pursuit and vestibulo-ocular reflex suppression. J Neurol Neurosurg Psychiatry 46, 61–66, 1983.
29. Chambers BR, Mai M, Barber HO. Bilateral vestibular loss, oscillopsia, and the cervico-ocular reflex. Otolaryngol Head Neck Surg 93, 403–407, 1985.
30. Chubb MC, Fuchs AF. Contribution of y group of vestibular nuclei and dentate nucleus of cerebellum to generation of vertical smooth eye movements. J Neurophysiol 48, 75–99, 1982.
31. Clack TD, Milburn WO, Graham MD. Ear-eye reflexes while riding in a car. Laryngoscope 95, 182–185, 1985.
32. Collewijn H. Eye- and head movements in freely moving rabbits. J Physiol (Lond) 266, 471–498, 1977.
33. Constantin AG, Wang H, Crawford JD. Role of superior colliculus in adaptive eye-head coordination during gaze shifts. J Neurophysiol 92, 2168–2184, 2004.
34. Corneil BD, Elsley JK. Countermanding eye-head gaze shifts in humans: marching orders are delivered to the head first. J Neurophysiol 94, 883–895, 2005.
35. Corneil BD, Hing CA, Bautista DV, Munoz DP. Human eye-head gaze shifts in a distractor task. I. Truncated gaze shifts. J Neurophysiol 82, 1390–1405, 1999.
36. Corneil BD, Munoz DP. Human eye-head gaze shifts in a distractor task. II. Reduced threshold for initiation of early head movements. J Neurophysiol 82, 1406–1421, 1999.
37. Corneil BD, Olivier E, Munoz DP. Visual responses on neck muscles reveal selective gating that prevents express saccades. Neuron 42, 831–841, 2004.
38. Cowie RJ, Robinson DL. Subcortical contributions to head movements in macaques. 1. Contrasting effects of electrical stimulation of a medial pontomedullary region and the superior colliculus. J Neurophysiol 72, 2648–2664, 1994.
39. Cowie RJ, Smith MK, Robinson DL. Subcortical contributions to head movements in macaques. 2. Connections of a medial pontomedullary head-movement region. J Neurophysiol 72, 2665–2682, 1994.
40. Crane BT, Demer JL. Human gaze stabilization during natural activities: translation, rotation, magnification, and target distance effects. J Neurophysiol 78, 2129–2144, 1997.
41. Crawford JD, Ceylan MZ, Klier EM, Guitton D. Three-dimensional eye-head coordination during gaze saccades in the primate. J Neurophysiol 81, 1760–1782, 1999.
42. Crawford JD, Guitton D. Primate head-free saccade generator implements a desired (post-VOR) eye position command by anticipating intended head motion. J Neurophysiol 78, 2811–2816, 1997.
43. Crawford JD, Medendorp WP, Marotta JJ. Spatial transformations for eye-hand coordination. J Neurophysiol 92, 10–19, 2004.
44. Cullen KE, Chen-Huang C, Mc Crea RA. Firing behavior of brain stem neurons during voluntary cancellation of the horizontal vestibuloocular reflex. 2. Eye movement related neurons. J Neurophysiol 70, 844–856, 1993.
45. Cullen KE, Galiana HL, Sylvestre PA. Comparing extraocular motoneuron discharges during head-restrained saccades and head-unrestrained gaze shifts. J. Neurophysiol 83, 630–637, 2000.
46. Cullen KE, Guitton D. Analysis of primate IBN spike trains using system identification techniques. II. Relationship to gaze, eye, and head movement dynamics during head-free gaze shifts. J Neurophysiol 78, 3283–3306, 1997.
47. Cullen KE, Guitton D. Analysis of primate IBN spike trains using system identification techniques. III.

Relationship to motor error during head-fixed saccades and head-free gaze shifts. J Neurophysiol 78, 3307–3322, 1997.
48. Cullen KE, Huterer M, Braidwood DA, Sylvestre PA. Time course of vestibuloocular reflex suppression during gaze shifts. J Neurophysiol 92, 3408–3422, 2004.
49. Cullen KE, McCrea RA. Firing behavior of brain stem neurons during voluntary cancellation of the horizontal vestibuloocular reflex. 1. Secondary vestibular neurons. J Neurophysiol 70, 828–843, 1993.
50. Cullen KE, McCrea RA. Firing behavior of brain stem neurons during voluntary cancellation of the horizontal vestibuloocular reflex. I. Secondary vestibular neurons. J Neurophysiol 70, 828–843, 1993.
51. Cullen KE, Minor LB. Semicircular canal afferents similarly encode active and passive head-on-body rotations: implications for the role of vestibular efference. J Neurosci 22, RC226, 2002.
52. Cullen KE, Roy JE. Signal processing in the vestibular system during active versus passive head movements. J Neurophysiol 91, 1919–1933, 2004.
53. Das VE, DiScenna AO, Feltz A, Yaniglos SS, Leigh RJ. Tests of a linear model of visual-vestibular interaction using the technique of parameter estimation. Biol Cybern 78, 183–195, 1998.
54. Das VE, Leigh RJ, Thomas CW, et al. Modulation of high-frequency vestibulo-ocular reflex during visual tracking in humans. J Neurophysiol 74, 624–632, 1995.
55. Das VE, Zivotofsky AZ, DiScenna AO, Leigh RJ. Head perturbations during walking while viewing a head-fixed target. Aviat Space Environ Med 66, 728–732, 1995.
56. Diamond SG, Markham CH, Baloh RW. Ocular counterrolling abnormalities in spasmodic torticollis. Arch Neurol 45, 164–169, 1988.
57. Dichgans J, Bizzi E, Morasso P, Tagliasco V. Mechanisms underlying recovery of eye-head coordination following bilateral labyrinthectomy in monkeys. Exp Brain Res 18, 548–562, 1973.
58. Dichgans J, Bizzi E, Morasso P, Tagliasco V. The role of vestibular and neck afferents during eye-head coordination in the monkey. Brain Res 71, 225–232, 1974.
59. Dichgans J, von Reutern GM, Rommelt U. Impaired suppression of vestibular nystagmus by fixation in cerebellar and non-cerebellar patients. Archiv Psychiat Nervenkr 226, 183–199, 1978.
60. Dicke PW, Their P. The role of cortical area MST in a model of combined smooth eye-head pursuit. Biol Cybern 80, 71–84, 1999.
61. Dieterich M, Bense S, Lutz S, et al. Dominance for vestibular cortical function in the non-dominant hemisphere. Cereb Cortex 13, 994–1007, 2003.
62. Edney DP, Porter JD. Neck muscle afferent projections to the brainstem of the monkey: implications for the neural control of gaze. J Comp Neurol 250, 389–398, 1986.
63. Ford FR, Walsh FB. Clinical observations upon the importance of the vestibular reflexes in ocular movements. The effects of section of one or both vestibular nerves. Bull Johns Hopkins Hosp 58, 80–88, 1936.
64. Freedman EG. Interaction between eye and head control signals can account for movement kinematics. Biol Cybern 84, 453–462, 2001.
64a. Freedman EG. Head-eye interactions during vertical gaze shifts made by rhesus monkeys. Exp Brain Res 167, 557–570, 2005.
65. Freedman EG, Quessy S. Electrical stimulation of rhesus monkey nucleus reticularis gigantocellularis. II. Effects on metrics and kinematics of ongoing gaze shifts to visual targets. Exp Brain Res 156, 357–376, 2004.
66. Freedman EG, Sparks DL. Activity of cells in the deeper layers of the superior colliculus of the rhesus monkey: evidence for a gaze displacement command. J Neurophysiol. 78, 1669–1690, 1997.
67. Freedman EG, Sparks DL. Coordination of the eyes and head: movement kinematics. Exp Brain Res 131, 22–32, 2000.
68. Fuchs AF, Kim J. Unit activity in vestibular nucleus of the alert monkey during horizontal angular acceleration and eye movement. J Neurophysiol 38, 1140–1161, 1975.
68a. Fuchs AF, Ling L, Phillips JO. Behavior of the position vestibular pause (PVP) interneurons of the vestibuloocular reflex during head-free gaze shifts in the monkey. J Neurophysiol 94, 4481–4490, 2005.
69. Fukushima K, Akao T, Kurkin S, Fukushima J. Role of vestibular signals in the caudal part of the frontal eye fields in pursuit eye movements in three-dimensional space. Ann N Y Acad Sci 1039, 272–282, 2005.
70. Fukushima K, Sato T, Fukushima J, Shinmei Y, Kaneko CR. Activity of smooth pursuit-related neurons in the monkey periarcuate cortex during pursuit and passive whole-body rotation. J Neurophysiol 83, 563–587, 2000.
71. Fuller JH. Head movement propensity. Exp Brain Res 92, 152–164, 1992.
72. Gandevia SC, Applegate C. Activation of neck muscles from the human motor cortex. Brain 111, 801–813, 1988.
73. Gaymard B, Siegler I, Rivaud-Pechoux S, et al. A common mechanism for the control of eye and head movements in humans. Ann Neurol 47, 819–822, 2000.
74. Gdowski GT, Belton T, McCrea RA. The neurophysiological substrate for the cervico-ocular reflex in the squirrel monkey. Exp Brain Res 140, 253–264, 2001.
75. Gdowski GT, McCrea RA. Integration of vestibular and head movement signals in the vestibular nuclei during whole-body rotation. J Neurophysiol 82, 436–449, 1999.
76. Gdowski GT, McCrea RA. Neck proprioceptive inputs to primate vestibular nucleus neurons. Exp Brain Res 135, 511–526, 2000.
77. Geschwind N. Nature of the decussated innervation of the sternomastoid muscle. Ann Neurol 10, 495, 1981.
78. Gloor P, Quesney F, Ives J, Ochs R, Olivier A. Significance of direction of head turning during seizures. Neurology 37, 1092, 1987.
79. Goffart L, Pelisson D, Guillaume A. Orienting gaze shifts during muscimol inactivation of caudal fastigial nucleus in the cat. II. Dynamics and eye-head coupling. J Neurophysiol 79, 1959–1976, 1998.
80. Goikhman I, Zelnik N, Peled N. Bobble-head doll syndrome: A surgically treatable condition manifested as a rare movement disorder. Movement Disorders 13, 192–194, 1998.

81. Goldring JE, Dorris MC, Cornell BD, Ballantyne PA, Munoz DP. Combined eye-head gaze shifts to visual and auditory targets in humans. Exp Brain Res 111, 68–78, 1996.
82. Goossens HH, Van Opstal AJ. Human eye-head coordination in two dimensions under different sensorimotor conditions. Exp Brain Res 114, 542–560, 1997.
83. Goossens HH, Van Opstal AJ. Influence of head position on the spatial representation of acoustic targets. J Neurophysiol 81, 2720–2736, 1999.
84. Grant MP, Leigh RJ, Seidman SH, Riley DE, Hanna JP. Comparison of predictable smooth ocular and combined eye-head tracking behaviour in patients with lesions affecting the brainstem and cerebellum. Brain 115, 1323–1342, 1992.
85. Grasso R, Prevost P, Ivanenko YP, Berthoz A. Eye-head coordination for the steering of locomotion in humans: an anticipatory synergy. Neurosci Lett 253, 115–118, 1998.
86. Gresty MA. Coordination of head and eye movements to fixate continuous and intermittent targets. Vision Res 14, 395–403, 1974.
87. Gresty MA. Stability of the head: studies in normal subjects and in patients with labyrinthine disease, head tremor, and dystonia. Movement Disorders 2, 165–185, 1987.
88. Gresty MA. Stability of the head in pitch (neck flexion-extension): studies in normal subjects and patients with axial rigidity. Movement Disorders 4, 233–248, 1989.
89. Gresty MA, Hess K, Leech J. Disorders of the vestibulo-ocular reflex producing oscillopsia and mechanisms compensating for loss of labyrinthine function. Brain 100, 693–716, 1977.
90. Grossman GE, Leigh RJ. Instability of gaze during locomotion in patients with deficient vestibular function. Ann Neurol 27, 528–532, 1990.
91. Grossman GE, Leigh RJ, Abel LA, Lanska DJ, Thurston SE. Frequency and velocity of rotational head perturbations during locomotion. Exp Brain Res 70, 470–476, 1988.
92. Grossman GE, Leigh RJ, Bruce EN, Huebner WP, Lanska DJ. Performance of the human vestibuloocular reflex during locomotion. J Neurophysiol 62, 264–272, 1989.
93. Guitton D, Kearney RE, Wereley N, Peterson BW. Visual, vestibular and voluntary contributions to human head stabilization. Exp Brain Res 64, 59–69, 1986.
94. Guitton D, Munoz DP, Galiana HL. Gaze control in the cat: studies and modelling of the coupling between orienting eye and head movements in different behavioral tasks. J Neurophysiol 64, 509–531, 1997.
95. Guitton D, Volle M. Gaze control in humans: eye-head coordination during orientating movements to targets within and beyond the oculomotor range. J Neurophysiol 58, 427–459, 1987.
96. Halmagyi GM, Gresty MA, Gibson WPR. Ocular tilt reaction with peripheral vestibular lesion. Ann Neurol 6, 80–83, 1979.
97. Han Y, Somers JT, Kim JI, Kumar AN, Leigh RJ. Ocular responses to head rotations during mirror viewing. J Neurophysiol 86, 2323–2329, 2001.
98. Han YH, Kumar AN, Reschke MF, et al. Vestibular and non-vestibular contributions to eye movements that compensate for head rotations during viewing of near targets. Exp Brain Res 165, 294–304, 2005.
99. Hirasaki E, Moore ST, Raphan T, Cohen B. Effects of walking velocity on vertical head and body movements during locomotion. Exp Brain Res 127, 117–130, 1999.
100. Hood JD, Korres S. Vestibular suppression in peripheral and central vestibular disorders. Brain 102, 785–804, 1979.
101. Hood JD, Waniewski E. Influence of peripheral vision upon vestibulo-ocular reflex suppression. J Neurol Sci 63, 27–44, 1984.
102. Huebner WP, Leigh RJ, Seidman SH, Billian C. An investigation of horizontal combined eye-head tracking in patients with abnormal vestibular and smooth pursuit eye movements. J Neurol Sci 116, 152–164, 1993.
103. Huebner WP, Leigh RJ, Seidman SH, et al. Experimental tests of a superposition hypothesis to explain the relationship between the vestibuloocular reflex and smooth pursuit during horizontal combined eye-head tracking in humans. J Neurophysiol 68, 1775–1792, 1992.
104. Huygen PLM, Verhagen WIM, van Hoof JJM, Horstink MWIM. Vestibular hyperreactivity in patients with idiopathic spasmodic torticollis. J Neurol Neurosurg Psychiatry 52, 782–785, 1989.
105. Iannone AM, Gerber AM. Brown-Sequard syndrome with paralysis of head turning. Ann Neurol 12, 116, 1982.
106. JC. Living without a balancing mechanism. N Engl J Med 246, 458–460, 1952.
107. Jenkyn LR, Walsh DB, Walsh BT, Culver CM, Reeves AG. The nuchocephalic reflex. J Neurol Neurosurg Psychiatry 38, 561–566, 1975.
108. Kasai T, Zee DS. Eye-head coordination in labyrinthine-defective human beings. Brain Res 144, 123–141, 1978.
109. Katsarkas A, Kirkham TH. Failure of suppression of post-caloric nystagmus by fixation. J Otolaryngol 11, 57–59, 1982.
110. Keshner EA, Cromwell RL, Peterson BW. Mechanisms controlling human head stabilization. II. Head-neck characteristics during random rotations in the vertical plane. J Neurophysiol 73, 2302–2312, 1995.
111. Khalsa SBS, Tomlinson RD, Schwarz DWF. Secondary vestibular and neck position signals in the vestibular nuclei of alert rhesus monkeys performing active head movements. Acta Otolaryngol (Stockh) 106, 269–275, 1988.
112. Kim JS, Sharpe JA. The vertical vestibulo-ocular reflex, and its interaction with vision during active head motion: effects of aging. J Vestib Res 11, 3–12, 2001.
113. King OS, Seidman SH, Leigh RJ. Control of head stability and gaze during locomotion in normal subjects and patients with deficient vestibular function. In Berthoz A, Graf W, Vidal PP (eds). Second Symposium on Head-Neck Sensory-Motor System. Oxford University Press, New York,1990, pp 568–570.
114. Klier EM, Wang H, Crawford JD. The superior colliculus encodes gaze commands in retinal coordinates. Nat Neurosci 4, 627–632, 2001.
115. Klier EM, Wang H, Crawford JD. Three-dimensional eye-head coordination is implemented

downstream from the superior colliculus. J Neurophysiol 89, 2839–2853, 2003.
116. Koenig E, Dichgans J, Dengler W. Fixation suppression of the vestibulo-ocular reflex (VOR) during sinusoidal stimulation in humans as related to the performance of the pursuit system. Acta Otolaryngol (Stockh) 102, 423–431, 1986.
117. Kommerell G, Hoyt WF. Lateropulsion of saccadic eye movements. Electro-oculographic studies in a patient with Wallenberg's syndrome. Arch Neurol 28, 313–318, 1973.
118. Kopinska A, Harris LR. Spatial representation in body coordinates: evidence from errors in remembering positions of visual and auditory targets after active eye, head, and body movements. Can J Exp Psychol 57, 23–37, 2003.
119. Land MF. Predictable eye-head coordination during driving. Nature 359, 318–320, 1992.
120. Land MF, Furneaux SM, Gilchrist ID. The organization of visually mediated actions in a subject without eye movements. Neurocase 8, 80–87, 2002.
121. Lanman J, Bizzi E, Allum J. The coordination of eye and head movement during smooth pursuit. Brain Res 153, 39–53, 1978.
122. Laurutis VP, Robinson DA. The vestibulo-ocular reflex during human saccadic eye movements. J Physiol (Lond) 373, 209–233, 1986.
123. Leigh RJ, Maas EF, Grossman GE, Robinson DA. Visual cancellation of the torsional vestibulo-ocular reflex in humans. Exp Brain Res 75, 221–226, 1989.
124. Leigh RJ, Sharpe JA, Ranalli PJ, Thurston SE, Hamid MA. Comparison of smooth pursuit and combined eye-head tracking in human subjects with deficient labyrinthine function. Exp Brain Res 66, 458–464, 1987.
125. Lempert T, Gianna CC, Gresty MA, Bronstein AM. Effect of otolith dysfunction: impairment of visual acuity during linear head motion in labyrinthine defective subjects. Brain 120, 1005–1113, 1997.
126. Liao K, Kumar AN, Han YH, et al. Comparison of velocity waveforms of eye and head saccades. Ann N Y Acad Sci 1039, 477–479, 2005.
127. Lisberger SG, Pavelko TA, Broussard DM. Responses during eye movements of brain stem neurons that receive monosynaptic inhibition from the flocculus and ventral paraflocculus in monkeys. J Neurophysiol 72, 909–927, 1994.
128. Macdougall HG, Moore ST. Marching to the beat of the same drummer: the spontaneous tempo of human locomotion. J Appl Physiol 99, 1164–1173, 2005.
129. Mai M, Dayal VS, Tomlinson RD, Farkashidy J. Study of pursuit and vestibulo-ocular cancellation. Otolaryngol Head Neck Surg 95, 589–591, 1986.
130. Manon-Espaillat R, Ruff RL. Dissociated weakness of sternocleidomastoid and trapezius muscles with lesions in the CNS. Neurology 38, 796–797, 1988.
131. Martinez-Trujillo JC, Medendorp WP, Wang H, Crawford JD. Frames of reference for eye-head gaze commands in primate supplementary eye fields. Neuron 44, 1057–1066, 2004.
132. Martinez-Trujillo JC, Wang H, Crawford JD. Electrical stimulation of the supplementary eye fields in the head-free macaque evokes kinematically normal gaze shifts. J Neurophysiol 89, 2961–2974, 2003.
133. Mastaglia FL, Knezevic W, Thompson PD. Weakness of head turning in hemiplegia: a quantitative study. J Neurol Neurosurg Psychiatry 49, 195–197, 1986.
134. Matsuo S, Bergeron A, Guitton D. Evidence for gaze feedback to the cat superior colliculus: discharges reflect gaze trajectory perturbations. J Neurosci 24, 2760–2773, 2004.
135. Maurer C, Mergner T, Lucking CH, Becker W. Adaptive changes of saccadic eye-head coordination resulting from altered head posture in torticollis spasmodicus. Brain 124, 413–426, 2001.
136. McCrea RA, Gdowski GT. Firing behaviour of squirrel monkey eye movement-related vestibular nucleus neurons during gaze saccades. J Physiol 546, 207–224, 2003.
137. McKinley PA, Peterson BW. Voluntary modulation of the vestibuloocular reflex in humans and its relation to smooth pursuit. Exp Brain Res 60, 454–464, 1985.
138. McLachlan RS. The significance of head and eye turning in seizures. Neurology 37, 1617–1619, 1987.
139. Melvill Jones G. Predominance of anticompensatory oculomotor response during rapid head rotation. Aerospace Med 35, 965–968, 1964.
140. Meng H, Green AM, Dickman JD, Angelaki DE. Pursuit-vestibular interactions in brainstem neurons during rotation and translation. J Neurophysiol 93, 3418–3433, 2005.
141. Miles FA, Fuller JH. Visual tracking and the primate flocculus. Science 189, 1000–1002, 1975.
142. Misslisch H, Tweed D, Fetter M, Dichgans J, Vilis T. Interaction of smooth pursuit and vestibuloocular reflex in three dimensions. J Neurophysiol 75, 2520–2532, 1996.
143. Misslisch H, Tweed D, Vilis T. Neural constraints on eye motion in human eye-head saccades. J Neurophysiol 79, 859–869, 1998.
144. Modi G, Bill PLA, Hoffman MW. Sternocleidomastoid and trapezius dissociation. Neurology 39, 454–455, 1989.
145. Moore ST, Hirasaki E, Cohen B, Raphan T. Effect of viewing distance on the generation of vertical eye movements during locomotion. Exp Brain Res 129, 347–361, 1999.
146. Nagel M, Zangemeister WH. The effect of transcranial magnetic stimulation over the cerebellum on the synkinesis of coordinated eye and head movements. J Neurol Sci 213, 35–45, 2003.
147. Nakamura T, Bronstein AM. The perception of head and neck angular displacement in normal and labyrinthine-defective subjects—A quantitative study using a 'remembered saccade' technique. Brain 118, 1157–1168, 1995.
148. Newlands SD, Hesse SV, Haque A, Angelaki DE. Head unrestrained horizontal gaze shifts after unilateral labyrinthectomy in the rhesus monkey. Exp Brain Res 140, 25–33, 2001.
149. Ochs R, Gloor P, Quesney F, Ives J, Olivier A. Does head-turning during a seizure have lateralizing or localizing significance? Neurology 34, 884–890, 1984.
150. Ono S, Das VE, Mustari MJ. Gaze-related response properties of DLPN and NRTP neurons in the rhesus macaque. J Neurophysiol 91, 2484–2500, 2004.
151. Oommen BS, Smith RM, Stahl JS. The influence of future gaze orientation upon eye-head coupling during saccades. Exp Brain Res 155, 9–18, 2004.

151a. Oommen BS, Stahl JS. Overlapping gaze shifts reveal timing of an eye-head gate. Exp Brain Res 167, 276–286, 2005.
152. Optican LM. Sensorimotor transformation for visually guided saccades. Ann N Y Acad Sci 1039, 132–148, 2005.
153. Outerbridge JS, Melvill Jones G. Reflex vestibular control in head movement in man. Aerospace Med 42, 935–940, 1971.
154. Paige GD. Senescence of human visual-vestibular interactions: smooth pursuit, optokinetic, and vestibular control of eye movements with aging. Exp Brain Res 98, 355–372, 1994.
155. Parizek J, Nemeckova J, Sercl M. Bobble-head doll syndrome associated with the III ventricular cyst. Three cases in children 7 years after CVP or CVA shunting. Childs Nerv Syst 5, 241–245, 1989.
156. Pelisson D, Goffart L, Guillaume A. Contribution of the rostral fastigial nucleus to the control of orienting gaze shifts in the head-unrestrained cat. J Neurophysiol 80, 1180–1196, 1998.
157. Pelisson D, Prablanc C, Urquizar C. Vestibuloocular reflex inhibition and gaze saccade control characteristics during eye-head orientation in humans. J Neurophysiol 59, 997–1013, 1988.
158. Peng GC, Hain TC, Peterson BW. A dynamical model for reflex activated head movements in the horizontal plane. Biol Cybern 75, 309–319, 1996.
159. Peng GC, Hain TC, Peterson BW. Predicting vestibular, proprioceptive, and biomechanical control strategies in normal and pathological head movements. IEEE Trans Biomed Eng 46, 1269–1280, 1999.
160. Peng GC, Minor LB, Zee DS. Gaze position corrective eye movements in normal subjects and in patients with vestibular deficits. Ann N Y Acad Sci 1039, 337–348, 2005.
161. Peng GC, Zee DS, Minor LB. Phase-plane analysis of gaze stabilization to high acceleration head thrusts: a continuum across normal subjects and patients with loss of vestibular function. J Neurophysiol 91, 1763–1781, 2004.
162. Peng GCY, Minor LB, Zee DS. Coupled asymmetries of the vestibulo-ocular (VOR) and vestibulocollic (VCR) reflexes in patients with unilateral vestibular loss (UVL). Soc Neurosci Abstr 23, 1294, 1997.
163. Peterson BW, Choi H, Hain T, Keshner E, Peng GC. Dynamic and kinematic strategies for head movement control. Ann N Y Acad Sci 942, 381–393, 2001.
164. Petit L, Beauchamp MS. Neural basis of visually guided head movements studied with fMRI. J Neurophysiol 89, 2516–2527, 2003.
165. Phillips JO, Fuchs AF, Ling L, IwamotoY, Votaw S. Gain adaptation of eye and head movement components of simian gaze shifts. J Neurophysiol 78, 2817–2821, 1997.
166. Phillips JO, Ling L, Fuchs AF, Siebold C, Plorde JJ. Rapid horizontal gaze movement in monkey. J Neurophysiol 73, 1632–1652, 1995.
167. Pierrot-Deseilligny C, Gautier J-C, Loron P. Ocular motor paresis versus apraxia. Ann Neurol 25, 209–210, 1989.
168. Pozzo T, Berthoz A, Lefort L. Head stabilization during various locomotor tasks in humans. I. Normal subjects. Exp Brain Res 82, 97–106, 1990.
169. Pozzo T, Berthoz A, Lefort L, Vitte E. Head stabilization during various locomotor tasks in humans. II. Patients with bilateral vestibular deficits. Exp Brain Res 85, 208–217, 1991.
170. Pulaski PD, Zee DS, Robinson DA. The behavior of the vestibulo-ocular reflex at high velocities of head rotation. Brain Res 222, 159–165, 1981.
171. Quessy S, Freedman EG. Electrical stimulation of rhesus monkey nucleus reticularis gigantocellularis. I. Characteristics of evoked head movements. Exp Brain Res 156, 342–356, 2004.
172. Ranalli PJ, Sharpe JA. Vertical vestibulo-ocular reflex, smooth pursuit and eye-head tracking dysfunction in internuclear ophthalmoplegia. Brain 111, 1299–1317, 1988.
173. Robinson FR, Phillips JO, Fuchs AF. Coordination of gaze shifts in primates: brainstem inputs to neck and extraocular motoneuron pools. J Comp Neurol 346, 43–62, 1994.
174. Robinson FR, Straube A, Fuchs AF. Role of the caudal fastigial nucleus in saccade generation. II. Effects of muscimol inactivation. J Neurophysiol 70, 1741–1758, 1993.
175. Ron S, Berthoz A, Gur S. Saccade-vestibular-ocular reflex co-operation and eye-head uncoupling during orientation to flashed targets. J Physiol (Lond) 464, 595–611, 1993.
176. Roy JE, Cullen KE. A neural correlate for vestibulo-ocular reflex suppression during voluntary eye-head gaze shifts. Nat Neurosci 1, 404–410, 1998.
177. Roy JE, Cullen KE. Vestibuloocular reflex signal modulation during voluntary and passive head movements. J Neurophysiol 87, 2337–2357, 2002.
178. Roy JE, Cullen KE. Dissociating self-generated from passively applied head motion: neural mechanisms in the vestibular nuclei. J Neurosci 24, 2102–2111, 2004.
179. Ruff RL, Leigh RJ, Wiener SN, et al. Long-term survivors of the "locked-in" syndrome: patterns of recovery and potential for rehabilitation. J Neuro Rehab 1, 31–42, 1987.
180. Russo RH, Kindt GW. A neuroanatomical basis for the bobble-head doll syndrome. J Neurosurg 41, 720–723, 1974.
181. Sawyer RN, Thurston SE, Becker KR, et al. The cervico-ocular reflex of normal human subjects in response to transient and sinusoidal trunk rotations. J Vestib Res 4, 245–249, 1994.
182. Schmidt D. Congenitale Augenmuskelparesen. Albrecht von Graefes Arch Klin Exp Ophthalmol 192, 285–312, 1974.
183. Segal BN, Katsarkas A. Goal-directed vestibulo-ocular function in man: gaze stabilization by slow-phase and saccadic eye movements. Exp Brain Res 70, 26–32, 1988.
184. Sharpe JA, Goldberg HJ, Lo AW, Herishanu Y. Visual-vestibular interaction in multiple sclerosis. Neurology 31, 427–433, 1981.
185. Sharpe JA, Johnston JL. Ocular motor paresis versus apraxia. Ann Neurol 25, 209, 1989.
186. Sharpe JA, Lo AW. Voluntary and visual control of the vestibulo-ocular reflex after cerebral hemidecortication. Ann Neurol 10, 164–172, 1981.

187. Shimizu N, Naito M. Eye-head co-ordination in patients with parkinsonism and cerebellar ataxia. J Neurol Neurosurg Psychiatry 44, 509–515, 1981.
188. Shinmei Y, Yamanobe T, Fukushima J, Fukushima K. Purkinje cells of the cerebellar dorsal vermis: simple-spike activity during pursuit and passive whole-body rotation. J Neurophysiol 87, 1836–1849, 2002.
189. Shinoda Y, Sugiuchi Y, Izawa Y, Hata Y. Long descending motor tract axons and their control of neck and axial muscles. In Büttner-Ennever JA (ed). Neuroanatomy of the Oculomotor System. Prog Brain Res 151, 533–550, 2006.
190. Smeets JB, Hayhoe MM, Ballard DH. Goal-directed arm movements change eye-head coordination. Exp Brain Res 109, 434–440, 1996.
191. Sparks DL, Barton EJ, Gandhi NJ, Nelson J. Studies of the role of the paramedian pontine reticular formation in the control of head-restrained and head-unrestrained gaze shifts. Ann N Y Acad Sci 956, 85–98, 2002.
192. Stahl JS. Amplitude of human head movements associated with horizontal saccades. Exp Brain Res 126, 41–54, 1999.
193. Stahl JS. Adaptive plasticity of head movement propensity. Exp Brain Res 139, 201–208, 2001.
194. Stahl JS. Eye-head coordination and the variation of eye-movement accuracy with orbital eccentricity. Exp Brain Res 136, 200–210, 2001.
195. Stark L, Zangemesiter WH, Edwards J, et al. Head rotation trajectories compared with eye saccades by main sequence relationships. Invest Ophthalmol Vis Sci 19, 986–988, 1980.
196. Stell R, Bronstein AM, Marsden CD. Vestibulo-ocular abnormalities in spasmodic torticollis before and after botulinum toxin injections. J Neurol Neurosurg Psychiatr 52, 57–62, 1989.
197. Suzuki SS, Siegal JM, Wu M-F. Role of pontomedullary reticular formation neurons in horizontal head movements: an ibotenic acid lesion study in the cat. Brain Res 484, 78–93, 1989.
198. Tabak S, Collewijn H. Human vestibulo-ocular responses to rapid, helmet-driven head movements. Exp Brain Res 102, 367–378, 1994.
199. Tabak S, Smeets JBJ, Collewijn H. Modulation of the human vestibuloocular reflex during saccades: probing by high-frequency oscillation and torque pulses of the head. J Neurophysiol 76, 3249–3263, 1996.
200. Takemori S, Cohen B. Loss of visual suppression of vestibular nystagmus after flocculus lesions. Brain Res 72, 213–224, 1974.
201. Tomlinson RD. Combined eye-head gaze shifts in the primate. III. Contributions to the accuracy of gaze saccades. J Neurophysiol 64, 1873–1891, 1990.
202. Tomlinson RD, Bahra PS. Combined eye-head gaze shifts in the primate. I. Metrics. J Neurophysiol 56, 1542–1557, 1986.
203. Tomlinson RD, Bahra PS. Combined eye-head gaze shifts in the primate. II. Interactions between saccades and the vestibuloocular reflex. J Neurophysiol 56, 1558–1570, 1986.
204. Tomlinson RD, Robinson DA. Signals in vestibular nucleus mediating vertical eye movements in the monkey. J Neurophysiol 51, 1121–1136, 1984.
205. Tomsak RL, Volpe BT, Stahl JS, Leigh RJ. Saccadic palsy after cardiac surgery: visual disability and rehabilitation. Ann N Y Acad Sci 956, 430–433, 2002.
206. Tweed D. Three-dimensional model of the human eye-head saccadic system. J Neurophysiol 77, 654–666, 1997.
207. Tweed D, Glenn B, Vilis T. Eye-head coordination during large gaze shifts. J Neurophysiol 73, 766–779, 1995.
208. Tweed D, Haslwanter T, Fetter M. Optimizing gaze control in three dimensions. Science 281, 1363–1366, 1998.
209. Uemara T, Arai Y, Shimazaki C. Disturbances of eye-head coordination during lateral gaze in labyrinthine disease. Ann N Y Acad Sci 374, 571–578, 1981.
210. Uemura T, Arai Y, Shimazaki C. Eye-head coordination during lateral gaze in normal subjects. Acta Otolaryngol (Stockh) 90, 191–198, 1980.
211. Van der Steen J, Russell IS, James GO. Effects of unilateral frontal eye-field lesions on eye-head coordination in monkey. J Neurophysiol 55, 696–714, 1986.
212. Viirre E, Tweed D, Milner K, Vilis T. A reexamination of the gain of the vestibuloocular reflex. J Neurophysiol 56, 439–450, 1986.
213. Vliegen J, Van Grootel TJ, Van Opstal AJ. Dynamic sound localization during rapid eye-head gaze shifts. J Neurosci 24, 9291–9302, 2004.
214. Von Hofsten C, Rosander K. The development of gaze control and predictive tracking in young infants. Vision Res 36, 81–96, 1996.
215. Waitzman DM, Silakov VL, Cohen B. Central mesencephalic reticular formation (cMRF) neurons discharging before and during eye movements. J Neurophysiol 75, 1546–1572, 1996.
216. Waitzman DM, Silakov VL, Palma-Bowles S, Ayers AS. Effects of reversible inactivation of the primate mesencephalic reticular formation. I. Hypermetric goal-directed saccades. J Neurophysiol 83, 2260–2284, 2000.
217. Warabi T. The reaction time of eye-head coordination in man. Neuroscience Letters 6, 47–51, 1977.
218. Waterston JA, Barnes GR. Visual-vestibular interaction during head-free pursuit of pseudorandom target motion in man. J Vestib Res 2, 71–88, 1992.
219. Waterston JA, Barnes GR, Grealy MA. A quantitative study of eye and head movements during smooth pursuit in patients with cerebellar disease. Brain 115, 1348–1358, 1992.
220. Waterston JA, Barnes GR, Grealy MA, Luxon LM. Coordination of eye and head movements during smooth pursuit in patients with vestibular failure. J Neurol Neurosurg Psychiatry 55, 1125–1131, 1992.
221. Weinrich M, Bhatia R. Abnormal eye-head coordination in Parkinson's disease patients after administration of levodopa: a possible substrate of levodopa-induced dyskinesia. J Neurol Neurosurg Psychiatry 49, 785–790, 1986.
222. Westheimer G, Blair SM. Synkinesis of head and eye movements evoked by brainstem stimulation in the alert monkey. Exp Brain Res 24, 89–95, 1975.
223. White OB, Saint-Cyr JA, Tomlinson RD, Sharpe JA. Ocular motor deficits in Parkinson's disease. III. Coordination of eye and head movements. Brain 111, 115–129, 1988.
224. Whittington DA, Lestienne F, Bizzi E. Behavior of

preoculomotor burst neurons during eye-head coordination. Exp Brain Res 55, 215–222, 1984.
225. Wyllie E, Luders H, Morris HH, Lesser RP, Dinner DS. The lateralizing significance of versive head and eye movements during epileptic seizures. Neurology 36, 606–611, 1986.
226. Wyllie E, Luders H, Morris HH, et al. Ipsilateral forced head and eye turning at the end of the generalized tonic-clonic phase of versive seizures. Neurology 36, 1212–1217, 1986.
227. Zambarbieri D, Schmid R, Versino M, Beltrami G. Eye-head coordination toward auditory and visual targets in humans. J Vestib Res 7, 251–263, 1997.
228. Zangemeister WH, Jones A, Stark L. Dynamics of head movement trajectories: Main sequence relationship. Exp Neurology 71, 76–91, 1981.
229. Zee DS. In Brooks BA, Bajandas FJ (eds). Eye Movements. Plenum Press, New York,1977 pp 9–39.
230. Zee DS. Suppression of vestibular nystagmus. Ann Neurol 1, 207, 1977.
231. Zhang Y, Partsalis AM, Highstein SM. Properties of superior vestibular nucleus flocculus target cells in squirrel monkey. I. General properties in comparison with flocculus projecting neurons. J Neurophysiol 73, 2261–2278, 1997.

Chapter 8

Vergence Eye Movements

THE PURPOSE OF VERGENCE EYE MOVEMENTS

In previous chapters, we have discussed the control of ocular movements as if the brain were directing a single eye between targets lying in different directions. Since the two eyes are separate by several centimeters, it is necessary to control the rotation of each eye separately when we view near objects. This chapter and the next will discuss how such binocular movements are coordinated. Under natural conditions, gaze is shifted between targets lying *both* at different distances and in different directions. This requires that vergence and conjugate movements be coordinated, an issue also addressed in this chapter.

In some lower species (e.g., the chameleon), the two eyes may be aimed independently, although reflex eye movements (vestibular, optokinetic) remain conjugate.[118,259] In primates, who have foveae and frontally directed eyes, all eye movements are binocularly coordinated. The reasons for this "uniform motion" of our eyes were already appreciated by Porterfield in his 1759 Treatise on the Eye:

> The final cause is … that the sight might thence be rendered more strong and perfect: for since each eye apart impresses the mind with an idea of the same object, the impression must be more strong and lively when both eyes concur, than when only one: and consequently the mind must receive a strong, lively and perfect idea of the object in view, as is agreeable to experience: and that both may concur it is necessary that they move uniformly. … A second advantage that we reap from the uniform motion of our eyes, which is yet more considerable than the former, consists in our being thereby enabled to judge with more certainty of the distance of objects. There is yet another advantage … that is thought to arise from the uniform motion of our eyes, and that is, the single appearance of objects seen with both eyes. [269]

Although monocular cues such as motion parallax and overlay of contours can be used to derive a sense of an object's distance, stereoscopic vision is necessary for an accurate perception of the third dimension, especially in the space around us in which we use our hands. Both stereopsis and bifoveal fixation of a single object of interest require precise alignment of the visual axes. This onus falls upon the vergence system. Unless we are viewing objects located at a great distance (optical infinity), disconjugate (eyes rotate by different amounts) and sometimes even disjunctive (oppositely directed) components must be incorporated into all normal eye movements. Otherwise, we would see double and be unable to calculate the correct location of objects with respect to our bodies.

Because of the horizontal separation of the orbits, each eye receives a slightly different image of an object. These dissimilar retinal images allow creation of a three-dimensional (3-D) percept, stereopsis. For single vision to be derived from the inputs of the two eyes, however, the images of an object of interest must fall on corresponding retinal points, allowing for sensory fusion, the perception of an object seen by both eyes as single.[351,352] The visual angle over which images can be separated, and still be perceived as one, is called Panum's area. Such corresponding retinal elements also allow a subjective sense of visual direction, based on the concept of an imaginary, third, cyclopean eye.[75,123,126,255] If the two images of an object fall on non-corresponding retinal areas in each eye, then that object is simultaneously localized in two separate visual directions, causing double vision, or diplopia. Alternatively, two different objects may be localized to the same position in space and appear to overlap, causing visual confusion. In normal circumstances, because of our horizontal vergence system, foveal retinal disparity is short-lived, and we seldom experience diplopia or visual confusion. A pioneer in the field, Maddox, identified disparity of retinal images as one drive to vergence, along with the state of focus (accommodation), visual cues of the proximity of objects, tonic vergence, and psychic or voluntary factors.[203]

Some terms commonly used to describe aspects of vergence movements and binocular vision are summarized in Table 8–1. For more detailed treatment of binocular vision, stereopsis, and accommodation, the reader is referred to textbooks by Regan,[285] Howard and Rogers,[142] and Schor and Ciuffreda.[306]

STIMULI TO VERGENCE MOVEMENTS

There are two primary stimuli to disjunctive eye movements: the *disparity* between the location of images on the two retinas, which produces diplopia and leads to fusional vergence movements, and *retinal blur* (defocused images), which leads to a loss of sharpness of perceived images and accommodation-linked vergence movements. Other cues, such as awareness of the proximity of targets, based on cues such as perspective,[74,370] changes in size (looming),[221] and monocular cues derived from motion parallax,[51,285,289] may evoke vergence. Voluntary, attentional factors can modulate vergence movements by influencing which of many disparities from a complex visual scene are selected to provide the stimulus for depth.[81,336]

There is also an underlying resting level of vergence tone—*tonic vergence*—about which changes in vergence induced by new sensory cues take place.[260] Vergence movements are under a degree of voluntary control. However, vergence movements are mainly performed

Table 8–1. **Glossary of Terms Used to Describe Aspects of Vergence Eye Movements**

Term	Definition
AC/A ratio	The synkinetic relationship between accommodative-linked convergence and accommodation, which is expressed in prism diopters/sphere diopters (see text: Interactions Between Accommodation And Vergence and measurement by the heterophoria method).
Accommodation	The process by which the refractive power of the lens of the eye is altered to diminish retinal blur and to obtain clear vision of a near object. Accommodation is measured in sphere diopters (D). (See text: The Near Triad)
CA/C ratio	The synkinetic relation between convergence-linked accommodation and convergence which is expressed in sphere diopters/prism diopters (see AC/A ratio).
Corresponding retinal elements	Those points of the two retinas that, during binocular vision, give rise to localization of seen objects in the same subjective visual direction. If images from a single object do not fall upon corresponding retinal elements, retinal disparity is present and serves as the stimulus to fusional vergence and stereopsis.
Depth perception	A sense of an object's distance that depends upon stereopsis and monocular cues (e.g., motion parallax, overlay of contours).
Fusion	A cortical phenomenon, wherein the two retinal images are perceived as one.
Near triad	The synkinesis of accommodation, convergence, and pupillary constriction. (See text: the Near Triad)
Phoria	The relative deviation of the visual axes during monocular viewing of a single target. This is a latent ocular misalignment, since fusional vergence mechanisms maintain alignment during binocular viewing.
Prism diopter (△)	One prism diopter is the strength of a prism that deviates a light ray 1 cm, measured tangentially at 1 m; 1 prism diopter (Δ) corresponds to approximately 1/2 degree.
Sphere diopter (D)	One sphere diopter is the amount of accommodation that occurs when the fixation distance (d) is 1 m. (In general, $D = 1/d$).
Stereopsis	The ability to visually perceive the third dimension, which depends on each eye receiving a slightly different image of the same object.
Tropia	The relative deviation of the visual axes during binocular viewing of a single target. This is a manifest ocular misalignment, which fusional vergence cannot correct: Exotropia (deviation out), Esotropia (deviation in), Hypertropia (vertical deviation—e.g., right hypertropia = right eye higher).
Vergence or disjunctive movements	Movements that rotate the eyes simultaneously in opposite directions: Convergence, Divergence, Incyclovergence (upper poles to nose), Excyclovergence (lower poles to nose). The two main types of vergence movements are fusional (disparity) and accommodative (blur).
Versions or conjugate movements	Movements that rotate the eyes in the same direction by the same amount. (Movements are disconjugate if they do not rotate the eyes in the same direction by the same amount.)

without our being aware of them, in much the same way that we unconsciously shift our line of sight across the visual field.

Under natural circumstances, retinal blur, retinal disparity, and other stimuli that act as clues to the distance of a target combine to elicit appropriate vergence eye movements. Early studies of vergence emphasized testing of responses to each of these stimuli separately. A more recent trend has been to use stimuli that combine disparity and blur stimuli, sometimes in a natural visual environment. Therefore, we will first briefly review the effects of disparity and blur stimuli alone on vergence eye movements, and then consider aspects of their interaction. Thereafter, in our general discussion of the dynamic properties of vergence eye movements, we will point out when pure disparity or blur stimuli have been applied.

Fusion or Disparity-Induced Vergence

Fusional or disparity-induced vergence may be studied independently of the effects of retinal blur and its attendant accommodation, if the subject views the test object through optical pinholes. This procedure ensures a large depth of focus so that the image is sharp on the retina, irrespective of the lens power of the eye or the distance of the object. One can then study disparity-driven vergence alone by, for example, placing a wedge prism before one eye. This shifts the position of the image on the retina of that eye and thereby induces a retinal disparity that can serve as a stimulus for vergence. Although peripheral visual cues can drive fusional vergence, most potent stimuli for vergence lie within the central 5 degrees of the visual field.[6] The change in disparity may be large and abrupt, as would occur when changing one's line of sight from near to far. In this case, a single, relatively rapid vergence movement is made, which, in some ways, is analogous to the rapid shift of conjugate gaze that occurs with a saccade. On the other hand, the change in disparity may be smooth and slow, as would occur with a target moving slowly in depth. In this case, a smooth vergence movement is made, which, in some ways, is analogous to the smooth change of conjugate gaze during tracking of a target with pursuit.

Blur-Induced Vergence

Accommodative vergence responses may be studied independently of the effects of retinal disparity by covering one eye. In the classic experiment of Müller,[236] when the seeing eye changed fixation from a distant to a near target along the visual axis of that eye, the eye under cover converged (see Fig. 8–1 and Video Display: Disorders of Vergence). The seeing eye seemed not to move, although sensitive recording methods show that it is not always perfectly still, and may make small vergence movements with corrective saccades (Fig. 8–1).[64,78,170]

Fusional vergence movements reduce the stimulus that produces them—retinal disparity—to a minimum; that is, they use negative visual feedback. However, the vergence movements associated with accommodation have no direct effect upon the retinal blur stimulus that evokes them. They are open-loop responses. Thus, in the Müller experiment, once accommodation is adequate and retinal blur is quelled, accommodative vergence tone is held steady irrespective of whether or not the eye under cover points at the target. (Of course, under normal binocular viewing conditions, fusional vergence movements will precisely direct the lines of sight.)

Interactions between Accommodation and Vergence

The synkinetic relationship between accommodation (A) of the lens and accommodation-linked convergence (AC) can be expressed as a ratio (AC/A, expressed in prism diopters/sphere diopters). This ratio would be close to 6.0 (the average interpupillary distance in centimeters), if the amount of vergence linked to accommodation were equal to that required for binocular fixation at all viewing distances. In fact, the AC/A ratio is usually smaller (about 3.5). Hence, during binocular viewing of near objects, disparity-induced vergence must also be enlisted to align the visual axes correctly.

Not only is convergence (C) causally linked to accommodation but, likewise, accommodation is linked to vergence (convergence-linked accommodation [CA]). The CA/C ratio—the amount of accommodation in sphere diopters induced per prism diopter of convergence—is typically about 0.08 to 0.15, being higher in younger subjects.[84,174,228,244] This ratio should be about 0.16 if the amount of convergence-linked accommodation were just equal to that required for clear vision at all viewing distances.

Under normal conditions of binocular viewing, accommodative and fusional drives work

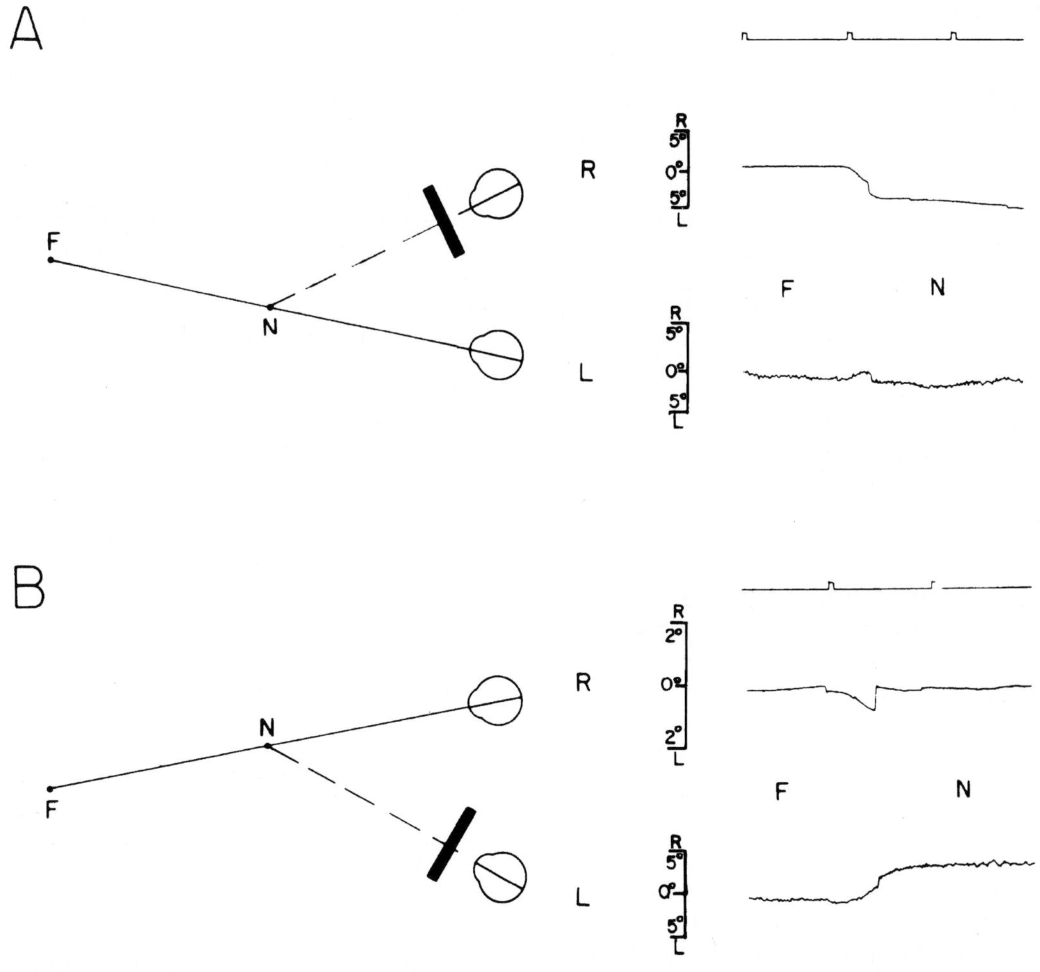

Figure 8–1. Accommodative vergence movements induced in a manner similar to the classic experiment of Müller. On the left, the experimental conditions are shown; on the right, the corresponding eye movements are presented. Movements of the right eye were recorded using the magnetic search coil method; movements of the left eye were recorded by electro-oculography. The time scale at the top is in seconds. In each condition—A and B—the subject changed fixation from a far target (F) to a near target (N), aligned along the line of sight of the viewing eye. (A) With the left eye viewing and the right eye under cover, both eyes began to converge toward the target, but the amplitude of the right eye's movement was larger. The left eye was taken off target by the convergent movement and a corrective saccade was made. (B) With the right eye viewing and the left eye under cover, the vergence movements of the right eye are evident at the higher sensitivity of recording (note different calibration setting). A saccade enabled the right eye to reacquire the target.

together to enable clear, single vision of close or distant objects. Maddox[203] believed that the accommodative stimulus was the main contributor to vergence and that disparity-induced fusional vergence was a supplement. Current evidence, however, suggests that fusional vergence is the more important contributor to ocular alignment.[142,157] In other words, accommodation of the lens is more strongly linked to disparity (vergence) than is vergence to blur (accommodation).[64,84,225,228] According to this view, the role of blur is to serve as the stimulus for the fine-tuning of accommodation. Some of the other stimuli that contribute to a sense of nearness, including size, texture, and looming, are also important for stimulating vergence under conditions of natural viewing. The interactions between vergence and accommodation have been addressed in models that explicitly incorporate cross-coupling between accommodation and vergence (see Phoria Adaptation).[146,296,305]

The Near Triad

Vergence is one part of the near triad.[317] A second component is a change in the shape of the lens of the eye, *accommodation*. When the lens is focused to view objects at optical infinity, the lens is stretched by its attachments. To focus on close objects, the ciliary muscle contracts to reduce the tension on the suspensory ligaments of the lens. The lens then becomes more spherical and is accommodated for near vision. Accommodation is measured in sphere diopters (D), which are related to the reciprocal of the viewing distance (Table 8–1). The third component of the near triad is *pupillary constriction*. Although it probably plays only a minor role in focusing near objects, the degree of pupillary constriction is a useful clinical sign.

DYNAMIC PROPERTIES OF VERGENCE EYE MOVEMENTS

Horizontal Vergence

THE RESPONSE TIME (LATENCY) OF HORIZONTAL VERGENCE

In response to regular, *predictable target jumps* of a visual target between far and near locations, most subjects make vergence drifts in anticipation of target jumps (Fig. 8–2).[190,382] Such anticipatory responses are probably based on a memory of prior stimuli. When stimulus presentation is *unpredictable,* the reaction time for blur-driven vergence movements is about 200 ms. The reaction time for a disparity-driven vergence movement is about 160 ms when the task is to change fixation from one depth to another. However, there are differences between the reaction times to convergence and divergence. On the one hand, the latency to onset of divergence depends on the starting vergence angle, being smaller if the eyes are converged when the stimulus is presented. On the other hand, the latency to onset of convergence is fairly independent of the starting angle of vergence.[7]

Much smaller latencies are reported (<100 ms) when the visual stimulus is full-field in size and the disparity small in amplitude.[33] Such responses can be induced by presenting stimuli to each eye that are anticorrelated (a black dot in one eye corresponds to a white dot in the other) and do not induce a perception of depth; thus, this "pre-attentive" behavior is probably due to local matching of binocular features in primary visual cortex.[205] These early responses are best elicited in the wake of a saccade, which is when they would be needed most to restore clear vision after a change in fixation.[39]

Vergence latencies are decreased by manipulation of the timing of turning off the fixation target relative to the appearance of a new target at a different depth (gap stimulus—Fig. 3–2, Chapter 3, but not to the same degree as are saccade latencies. For example, in one study, a decrease in reaction time of 17 ms for vergence occurred, compared to 41 ms for saccades, when the fixation target was extin-

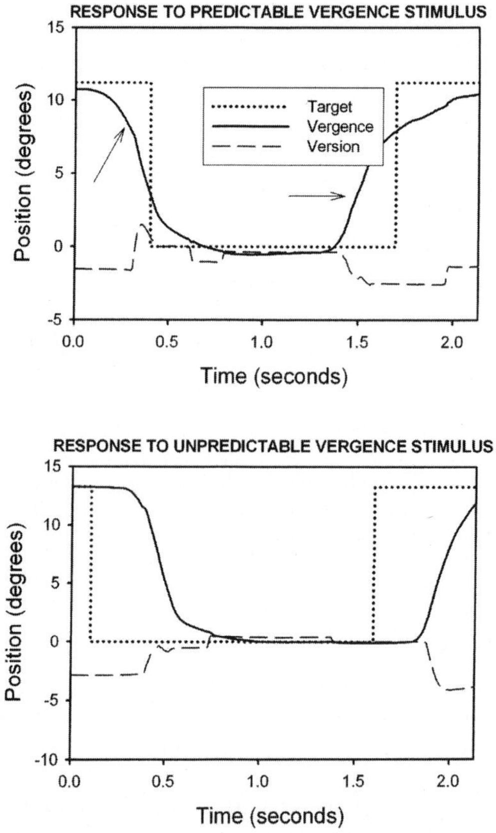

Figure 8–2. Prediction and vergence responses. Top panel: Responses to a regular stepping vergence stimulus at 0.4 Hz. Note how the vergence responses precede the target jumps (arrows). Bottom panel: Responses to a vergence stimulus that stepped with unpredictable timing. Vergence responses follow the target jumps. Positive values indicate convergence or rightward version (conjugate) movements. (Adapted from Kumar et al., 2002,[190] with permission of the American Physiological Society.)

guished 75 ms to 200 ms before the target light came on.[340] Both adults and children, who are more likely to generate express saccades, show a more prominent effect for divergence than convergence, movements.[31,60] Vergence movements made in conjunction with saccades show an "express" latency distribution, similar to that for saccades;[60] saccade-vergence interactions are discussed below. For smooth vergence tracking, latency decreases when the motion of the target is predictable.[83,181]

THE PRECISION OF HORIZONTAL VERGENCE

The horizontal fusional vergence system maintains correspondence of images on the retina with precision, but not perfection. The remaining disparity is known as *fixation disparity*.[89] This residual disparity leads to a steady-state vergence error that is presumably the "feedback" signal that is required by the fusional vergence system to sustain its motor command. The smallest range of disparities that can be fused is at the fovea, where horizontal retinal disparities of more than 10 minutes of arc may cause diplopia. This is called Panum's area of single binocular vision. Panum's area is under some degree of dynamic control, so that somewhat larger disparities, such as those that occur during head movements, can be tolerated without diplopia.[56] Under natural viewing conditions, normal subjects may make vergence movements that do not point both foveae at the target, and report no diplopia, perhaps because of multiple disparities presented by a rich visual environment.[59,204]

DYNAMIC PROPERTIES OF HORIZONTAL VERGENCE

The *waveform* of an isolated vergence movement, stimulated by a sudden, *step* change in retinal disparity or blur, approximates a negative exponential with a time constant in the range of the orbital plant (about 150 to 200 ms) (see Figs. 8–2, and 5–1,Chapter 5). This might suggest that the command signal for pure vergence movements is approximately a step (or tonic) change in innervation to the extraocular muscles.[290] If the change in retinal disparity is relatively large, the vergence response can be separated into *two components*: initiation and completion.[155,369] Initiation reflects a coarse, transient, "trigger" mechanism, which can respond to large retinal disparities of images that can be quite dissimilar.[142] Completion reflects a slower, feature-sensitive, "fusion-lock" mechanism, which sustains vergence at the level necessary for fusion. Analysis of such vergence waveforms—using, for example, the phase plane plot (eye position versus eye velocity)—confirm that there is an initial fast, "open-loop" or "preprogrammed" response, usually complete within several hundred milliseconds, which is followed by a slower response that completes the vergence movement and brings the image of the target to both foveae.[134,166,317] Occasionally, two rapid vergence responses will occur to a single disparity, the second response being similar to a corrective saccade strategy in the conjugate system;[8] the second response occurs at shorter latency than could be accounted for by visual feedback.[10]

Vergence movements to *ramp* stimuli also may show what appear to be two types of vergence responses: step-like to large disparities and ramp-like to small disparities.[318] Whether these reflect different control modes comparable to "saccadic" and "pursuit" vergence, or processing of disparity of different sizes by different channels, is debatable.[265]

The *peak velocity* of vergence can be related to its amplitude in the same way as the peak velocity of saccades is related its amplitude, using a main sequence plot. There is some disagreement in the literature as to whether convergence movements are faster than divergence.[148,190,384] In fact, divergence peak velocity is influenced by the starting angle of convergence; if the eyes start very converged, then the divergence velocity is faster.[7] Convergence movements, however, do not appear to show this dependence on starting vergence angle,[7] which may account for the apparent discrepancies between convergence versus divergence velocities in prior reports.

INFLUENCE OF DEVELOPMENT AND AGING ON VERGENCE

Development and aging both have effects on vergence dynamics. Neonates commonly show ocular misalignment that resolves as vergence develops during the first two months of life.[136] By age three months, most infants can make appropriate vergence movements, although appropriate accommodative responses to blur occur later.[117,348] The dynamic properties of vergence responses are similar from age about 8 years until the mid-forties,[273] although they are more variable than those of saccades.[9] However, once the presence or absence of associated saccades (including vertical saccades) and blinks are taken into account, and the analysis is restricted to the early "preprogrammed" component of the vergence response, much of the variability disappears.[145] In response to a sudden change in target disparity, older subjects generate vergence responses at increased latency and with decreased peak velocity and acceleration compared to younger subjects.[280] However, responses to ramp disparity stimuli (corresponding to usual bedside testing) are similar in older and younger subjects. Conversely, in response to monocular, mainly accommodative stimuli, older subjects generate similar initial responses to younger subjects, but show a decreased response to ramp disparity stimuli.[280] The decrease in steady-state response to accommodative stimuli may be because of presbyopia. Thus, elderly subjects show diminution in convergence associated with a given accommodative stimulus,[128,129] and this may lead to compensatory adaptation in the linkage between convergence and accommodation.[292,293]

ASYMMETRIC VERGENCE RESPONSES

When targets are slightly displaced from the midline, and the task is to look from far to near, some subjects can make asymmetric, smooth adducting movements, with the dynamic properties of slow vergence.[78] If the target is aligned on the visual axis of one eye, markedly asymmetric eye movements may be made that brings both eyes to the target (Fig. 8–3).[76] Both of these responses question the validity of an important corollary of Hering's Law of equal innervation. Hering's Law itself states that the yoking of the eyes arises because both eyes get their innervation from a single "conjugate" command. An alternative interpretation is that seemingly independent movements of the eyes are actually produced by summation of a pure vergence (disjunctive) command and a pure versional (conjugate) command. Several lines of evidence support this view. First, when subjects carried out prolonged smooth tracking of targets moving in both direction and depth, the vergence component deteriorated before the pursuit component.[284] Second, when monkeys tracked step-ramp targets moving along the visual axis of one eye, pursuit and fusional vergence components can be temporally separated, indicating that vergence and pursuit work in parallel.[176] Third, during smooth pursuit of a target aligned on one eye, it has been possible to confirm that vergence and pursuit movements were being summed by "tagging" vergence responses with a vertical component induced by training.[210]

During saccade-vergence interactions, which are discussed further in the next section, it is more difficult to tease out whether there are separate saccade and vergence commands

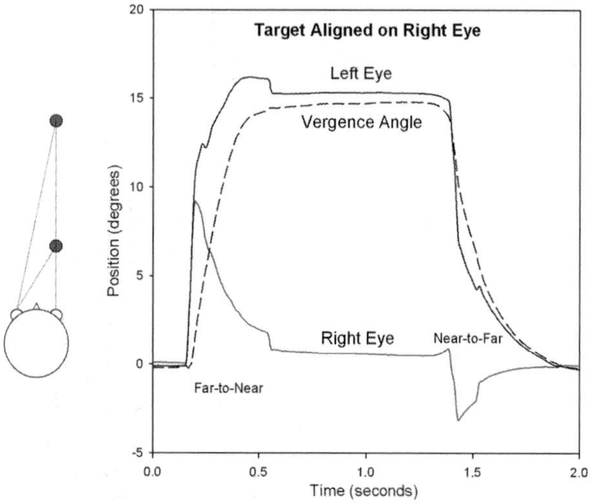

Figure 8–3. Asymmetric vergence movement in response to viewing near and far targets aligned on the visual axis of the right eye. Note that although the right eye does not need to move, during convergence, it makes a saccade to the right and then a vergence movement to the left. Positive values indicate convergence or rightward version (conjugate) movements.

or disjunctive saccades are being programmed. Behavioral evidence has supported Hering's law,[274] whereas electrophysiological studies provide evidence for independent programming of the movements of each eye.[213,338,390] Furthermore, measured forces in the horizontal rectus muscles show decreases during convergence, which is not consistent with increased motoneuron activity during convergence.[229] Thus, the relationship between motoneuron activity and muscle forces during convergence requires clarification.

In contrast to convergence, when a pure divergence is called for, it is usually accompanied by a saccade that initially brings one eye (usually the dominant one) closer to the target.[53,76,78,79,384] Such a strategy would allow rapid identification (albeit primarily based on information from one eye) of an object suddenly appearing in the visual field beyond a near point of regard.

Vertical Vergence and Cyclovergence

Vertical and torsional fusional movements are also possible, but their properties differ from those of the horizontal system, primarily in their slow speed and restricted range of amplitudes.[138,139,175,322] *Vertical fusional movements* to a step of disparity, for example, take seconds for completion, and usually cannot overcome disparities of more than a degree or two. They are more robust for near viewing,[121] and are improved by a visual background that is in the same plane as that of the fusional stimulus.[5] Responses to transient visual stimuli indicate that vertical vergence responds only to first-order (luminance-defined) and not second-order (feature-defined) stimuli;[324,335] these differences of visual following, which are discussed further in Chapter 4, may account for the distinctive properties of vertical vergence and, perhaps, some unusual abnormalities (such as the Heimann-Bielschowsky phenomenon, discussed in Chapter 10, which consists of monocular vertical drifts of a blind eye while the seeing eye holds fixation; see Video Display: Nystagmus and Visual Disorders). In some patients with a vertical muscle imbalance, however, the vertical fusional range may be strikingly increased,[235] and in normal adults, as discussed below, the vertical fusional range can be increased with training.[110] Some individuals with strabismus who lack horizontal vergence maintain vertical vergence responses.[375]

Cyclodisparities elicit torsional fusional movements—*cyclovergence*—but, just as for vertical vergence, they are slow and of limited range.[133,143,175,359] During fixation, cyclovergence is more tightly controlled than the torsional position of each eye alone (i.e., cycloversion).[154,268,360] This finding suggests that the relative alignment of the two eyes around the visual axis plays a role in certain types of depth perception, such as determining the slant of objects toward or away from the subject.[141] So, for example, disturbances of the perception of slant accompany the cyclodeviation of superior oblique palsy, and can be used as a diagnostic test.[201] For a vertical bar, the top will appear closer to the subject. For a horizontal bar, the two images will be slanted with respect to each other, with the apparent intersection of the lines pointing toward the side of the affected, excylodeviated eye. Slant cues presented without horizontal disparity can induce vergence responses.[325] However, other cues, such as vertical size ratio contribute to perception of slant.[16]

Changes in the relative torsional alignment of the eyes also occur in normal subjects with near viewing; there is relative intorsion on upgaze and extorsion on downgaze.[223,230,358] This finding can also be related to the orientation of Listing's plane. With convergence, there is a relative temporal rotation of Listing's plane in each eye that is independent of orbital eye position,[334] but is dependent on the visual stimulus being used to induce vergence.[160] These changes in torsion with near viewing might be implemented by movement of the pulleys, which define the functional points of origin of the extraocular muscles (see Chapter 9).[69,180] In patients with intermittent exotropia, the added convergence needed to overcome the inherent exophoria is also associated with an increased temporal rotation of Listing's plane.[354]

Vergence Responses to Natural Stimuli

As we move forward through our environment, a radial optic flow of images occurs on the retina. At the same time, if the point of fixation remains on a single object, the vergence angle must increase, and vergence responses may occur at short latency in response to radial-flow stimuli.[35,226,374] Sudden changes of the size of a visual stimulus induce radial flow and constitute a looming stimulus; short-latency vergence responses are induced.[152] However, the stimulus necessary for a sensation of motion in depth (stereomotion), which occurs as we move forward through our environment, is not always the same as that which elicits vergence eye movements.[27,34,51,285] Thus, the sensation of motion in depth requires a change in the *relative disparity* of one target with respect to another, but neither target need be at the fixation point. A change in *absolute disparity* (the disparity of an object point with respect to the fixation point) need not elicit a sense of motion in depth, but can induce a change in vergence (for example, a single target moving on a featureless background). As a general rule, relative disparities provide the basis for stereovision and binocular perception; absolute disparities are used for control of vergence eye movements.

Properties of Vergence Made in Conjunction with Other Eye Movements

INTERACTION OF VERGENCE WITH GAZE-STABILIZING (VESTIBULAR) EYE MOVEMENTS

During natural behaviors, whenever the eyes are converged for near viewing, there must be adjustments of the properties of both the rotational and translational vestibulo-ocular reflexes; these interactions are discussed in Chapters 2 and 7 (Fig. 7–7). One issue addressed here is whether or not it is the vergence angle that sets the gain of the rotational vestibulo-ocular reflex (VOR) to an appropriate level. Because the eyes (i.e., the orbits) do not lie at the center of head rotation, VOR gain must be greater than 1.0 (eye rotations exceed head rotations) during viewing of a near target. In both humans and monkeys, when the eyes are converged, a sudden head rotation produces a VOR gain greater than 1.0 at a latency too short to be accounted for by visual tracking.[63,330,363] During sinusoidal rotation, studies in humans suggest that rather than vergence angle per se, it is the context of viewing a near target that sets VOR gain. For example, when a subject views the image of her nose in a mirror a few centimeters from her face, VOR gain is not increased, even at high frequencies of rotation, as it would be if the target for fixation were an earth-fixed near target requiring a similar vergence angle.[119] Furthermore, if subjects are converged while viewing a near target during sinusoidal head rotations, and the head is unexpectedly perturbed, VOR gain is not increased.[120] If vergence is linked repetitively to head movements, it is possible to train monkeys to make combined vergence-vestibular movements at short latency.[1] Finally, if head perturbations are applied during the course of a vergence movement made by a monkey, the adjustment of VOR occurs prior to attainment of the required vergence angle, suggesting that it is the signal driving vergence rather than vergence angle itself that determines modulation of VOR gain.[332] Likewise for the translational VOR; the gain of the reflex can be set based on knowledge of the location of the target in depth and the upcoming context— "Will my eyes have to fix upon a target moving with the head, or one stationary in the environment."[277] Vergence angle may also determine the VOR gain in animals, although the mental set of experimental animals cannot be readily determined.[11,367] Taken together, these studies suggest that it is not vergence angle itself that sets the VOR gain to an appropriate level during near viewing, but rather the context and stimulus conditions employed during testing. Thus, the VOR gain during near viewing appears to depend on expectations of where the eyes must point as well as the temporal nature of the stimulus (unpredictable transient or predictable sine wave), and the species being tested.

INTERACTION OF VERGENCE WITH GAZE-SHIFTING EYE (SACCADIC) MOVEMENTS AND BLINKS

Behavioral Findings

In a 3-D world, most shifts of the point of fixation are between targets lying at different distances and in different directions, requiring a combination of vergence and saccades. Thus, during natural behavior, saccades are almost invariably accompany vergence movements,[147] and the same 3-D visual input is used to program both components.[44,340] The ability to make combined saccade-vergence responses develops during childhood.[376]

It has been classically taught that vergence eye movements are slow, taking as long as a second for completion.[284,290] This is the case when vergence movements are tested in a laboratory setting, such as by presenting isolated disparity stimuli under dichoptic viewing conditions (each eye sees a different image). However, vergence movements are much faster when tested under natural conditions, using real targets or having the subject move toward a stationary target.[83] Specifically, vergence movements are speeded up by saccades (Fig. 8–4),[384] even if the vergence movement is horizontal and the saccadic movement is vertical.[73] In addition, saccades made with vergence movements are slowed down compared with similar-size conjugate movements.[53] The degree to which the change in alignment appears to be incorporated into the saccade depends upon the distance of the target[355] and the size of the change in realignment; smaller disparities can be overcome entirely during the saccade.[40] Interestingly, accommodation, like vergence, is also speeded up when it occurs in association with saccades.[310]

Blinks also affect vergence, but their effects are somewhat complicated by a transient vergence that occurs with blinks alone (see Chapter 3). Generally, if they occur later during the eye movement, blinks tend to slow convergence, divergence, and saccades,[283] and impose a transient change in velocity of smooth vergence movements directed opposite to the movements (e.g., a convergence transient during divergence).[281] A transient, small, stereotyped divergence oscillation commonly occurs at the onset of vergence movements made in conjunction with saccades, and may be due to orbital properties rather than central factors.[339] Nevertheless, blinks frequently accompany attempts to fuse disparities, and are probably part of a strategy to facilitate disparity driven vergence.

Possible Mechanisms for Vergence-Saccade Interactions

The mechanism for facilitation of vergence by saccades and blinks is not settled. One hypothesis suggests that the same pontine neurons (omnipause neurons) that gate activity of saccadic burst neurons also gate vergence activity.[384] During the time that pause-cell inhibition is lifted, not only can saccades occur but vergence would also be facilitated (Fig. 8–5A). There is electrophysiological support

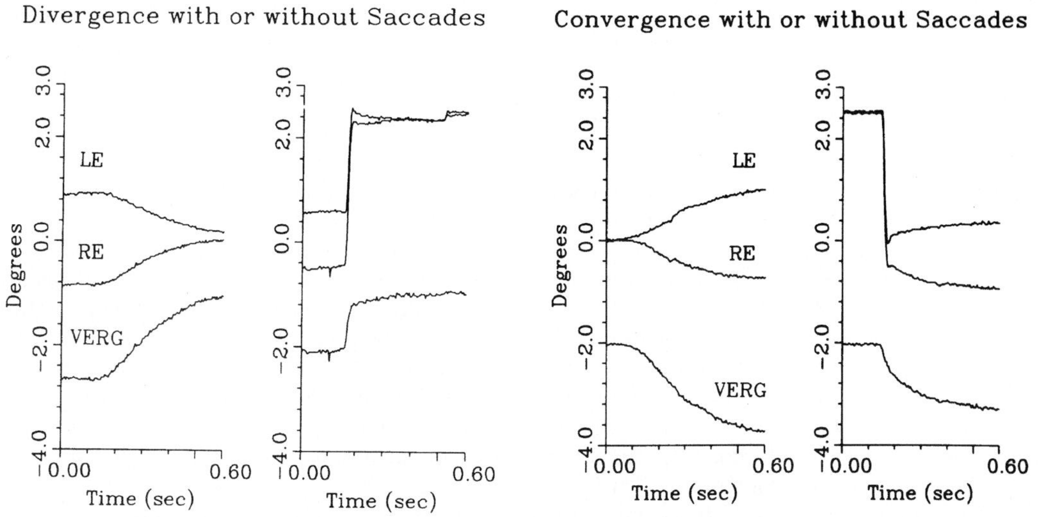

Figure 8–4. Vergence changes with or without an accompanying saccade, shown using binocular search coil recordings in a Rhesus monkey. LE = left eye, RE = right eye, VERG = vergence change. Vergence traces (obtained by subtracting the right and left eye position signals) are offset for clarity. Convergence is negative. Note the increase in vergence speed when a saccade is conjoined with vergence. The facilitation is greater for divergence, probably because of the inherent divergence associated with horizontal saccades.

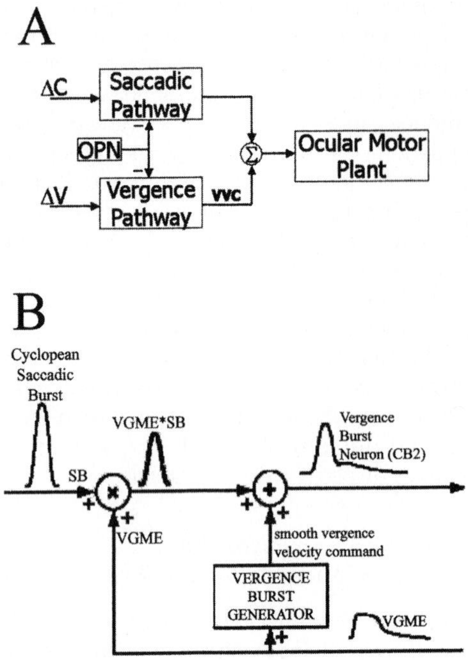

Figure 8–5. Model of saccade-vergence interaction. (A) Schematic summary of a model of Zee, FitzGibbon and Optican,[384] which proposes that when vergence is made with a saccade, the increased speed of the vergence velocity command (VVC) is due to synchronous removal of inhibition (−) by omnipause neurons (OPN) from both the saccadic and vergence pathways (burst neurons). ΔC is desired change in conjugate position; ΔV is desired change in vergence. (B) Alternative model of Busettini and Mays,[38] which proposes increased vergence velocity is due to current vergence motor error signal (VGME) being multiplied by the cyclopean saccadic burst command (SB). Thus a subpopulation of vergence burst neurons (CB2 cells) carries the sum of a smooth vergence velocity command and vergence motor error multiplied by the cyclopean burst. Redrawn with permission of the authors and the American Physiological Society.

for this hypothesis; stimulation of omnipause neurons slows ongoing vergence.[215] Omnipause cells also cease discharging during blinks, and this too would account for facilitation of vergence by blinks.[256,264]

However, there is evidence against this omnipause neuron hypothesis for saccade-vergence interaction. First, at least in monkeys, vergence peak velocity increases with saccadic peak velocity, which would not be predicted if only the omnipause neurons linked activity in the two systems.[37] Second, positioning the near target above the far target (which is less common than the converse in nature) causes the saccadic and vergence components to become temporally dissociated (the saccade peak velocity leads the vergence peak velocity by up to 100 ms) and, when this happens, the vergence movement becomes less skewed.[189] This finding, taken with similar prior studies,[356] suggests that the vergence and saccadic systems act separately, but interact with each other whenever they occur at the same time. It has been suggested that this interaction could be a multiplication of the vergence motor error by the saccadic system (Fig. 8–5B).[38] Alternatively, the saccadic burst might enhance the discharge of the vergence burst neurons.[189]

Other hypotheses to explain saccade-vergence interaction, not necessarily mutually exclusive, include programming of saccades of different sizes in each eye,[40,54,76,355,390] and nonlinear interactions between version and vergence at the level of the ocular motoneurons or in the eye muscles themselves.[171] A more radical proposal, based on electrophysiological studies, is that some saccadic premotor burst neurons generate monocular saccades, thereby generating fast disjunctive movements independently of vergence commands.[177,390]

Other findings that must be considered in interpreting saccade-vergence interaction include the transient change in vergence (usually divergence in adults) that occurs even when saccades are made between targets on an isovergence array (calling for no change in vergence).[52,163,206,384] In contrast, children younger than 10 years of age usually show a transient convergence during saccades.[86] It has been suggested that these changes in alignment during and immediately after saccades in normal subjects are a byproduct of inherent asymmetries in the mechanical characteristics of the ocular plant (muscles and orbital tissues), and the adaptive processes that attempt to compensate for them.[86]

As noted above, saccades associated with vergence are generally slower than saccades made without vergence; an exception is for the eye that is abducting and diverging.[53,54,274] The mechanism for this saccadic slowing is also uncertain and, for example, transient suppression of omnipause neuron prior to saccades cannot account for the observed behavior.[36]

Interaction of Asymmetric Horizontal Vergence and Vertical Saccades

Because the eyes are horizontally separated, they must also rotate by different amounts when making vertical saccades between near targets that are separated vertically and off to one side (i.e., closer to one eye than the other). Even saccades made in darkness to the remembered locations of vertically displaced targets are disconjugate to nearly the same degree as if the visual targets were actually present.[379] When vertical disparities are induced artificially, with a prism or dichoptic display, the vertical saccades become more disconjugate when the stimuli appear to be close.[355,379] When a subject is asked to wear a vertically oriented prism in front of just one part of the visual field of one eye (for example, the lower field) for a day, there is an adaptive change in the vertical yoking of the eyes such that the degree of disconjugacy is appropriate to the visual demands created by the prism.[379] These findings suggest that the brain develops a 3-D map (horizontal, vertical, depth) for vertical saccade yoking. This map is used to preprogram automatically the relative excursions of the eyes during vertical saccades, based upon the point of regard before and after the change in gaze. Other factors, related to the relative pulling directions of the vertical muscles in the orbit, may also contribute to this automatic disconjugacy,[70,77] but central mechanisms, subject to adaptive modification, are clearly important.[379] A facilitation of vertical vergence by horizontal saccades does not consistently occur in normal subjects,[379] but has been postulated in the syndrome of dissociated vertical deviation (DVD).[115,327] As discussed above, when vertical saccades are combined with horizontal vergence, the two components are synchronized when the far target is low, but the vergence component is delayed if the near target is higher.[189] This behavior provides a means to further test interactions between vertical saccades and horizontal vergence.

Effects of Visual Processing of Combined Vergence-Saccade Movements

Whether the images seen by the two eyes are processed in the same or different cerebral hemispheres also influences how saccades and vergence are combined.[85] For saccades, when the images of the targets seen by the left eye and the right eye are in the same hemifield and processed by the same hemisphere, the resulting averaging saccade is made to a position nearly between the two targets ("global effect"). When the images are in opposite hemifields, and processed by opposite hemispheres, the saccade is directed to just one of the targets. Saccade latencies are also influenced by hemispheric localization.[85] If in the same hemisphere, saccade latency increases by about 2.5 ms per degree of disparity, with a baseline of 215 ms. If in opposite hemispheres, there is a different relationship. Latency is about 260 ms, with no dependence on disparity. Because of the relatively small distance between the pupils, most naturally occurring saccades will be to targets that are seen by the same hemisphere. Hence it has been argued that the global averaging effect on saccades, when they are combined with vergence, would allow for a *symmetric* vergence movement to complete any necessary change in alignment when the "cyclopean" (average between the two eyes) saccade was completed.[85]

Finally, there is behavioral evidence that fusional vergence movements require that visual information from each eye reach the same hemisphere. Thus, Westheimer and Mitchell studied vergence movements in a split-brain patient who had undergone section of the corpus callosum and anterior commissure.[369] A near-target light located on either side of the sagittal plane induced vergence eye movements, but a near target located exactly in the midsagittal plane did not. In this latter circumstance, images lay on the temporal retina of each eye, and therefore did not gain access to the same cerebral hemisphere.

NEURAL SUBSTRATE OF VERGENCE MOVEMENTS

Ocular Motoneurons and Vergence

The medial rectus motoneurons are of prime importance for horizontal vergence. Studies of the oculomotor nucleus have shown that medial rectus motoneurons do not lie in one discrete location; the cells are segregated into different groups. Three distinct aggregates of medial rectus motoneurons have been identified: subgroup A, located ventral and rostral; subgroup B, located dorsal and caudal; and subgroup C, located dorso-medial and rostral (see Fig. 9–9). Subgroup C is composed of the smallest cell bodies and can be labeled independently of the other subgroups by selective injections of tracer near the muscle attachments to the globe, where there are non-twitch fibers.[41] The subgroup C receives inputs from pretectal nuclei concerned with the near response.[366] Thus, extraocular muscle fibers supplied by subgroup C may be involved in generating slower eye movements, such as vergence; non-twitch fibers, which are adjacent to palisade ending, might play a role in a proprioceptive feedback mechanism.[41] Abducens motoneurons and internuclear neurons may also contribute to horizontal vergence, and their role is discussed further below.

Neurophysiologic studies in monkeys have shown that most oculomotor neurons subserving the medial rectus and most neurons in the abducens nucleus discharge for both conjugate (version) and disjunctive (vergence) eye movements (Fig. 8–6).[168,169,216] Medial rectus motoneurons show a velocity-position (phasic-tonic) change in discharge rate during vergence, as is the case for conjugate movements.[101] Even though most of the motoneurons subserving the lateral and medial recti carry both version and vergence signals, the sensitivity of individual neurons to changes in eye position varies according to whether the eye position is reached by a version or a vergence movement. In other words, there is evidence that different neurons play relatively smaller or larger roles in conjugate versus vergence eye movements.[338]

Premotor Commands for Vergence in the Midbrain

The midbrain houses neurons involved specifically in the control of vergence that appear to project to ocular motoneurons.[214,388] These cells lie in the mesencephalic reticular formation, 1 to 2 mm dorsal and dorsolateral to the oculomotor nucleus,[158,212,217] a region that has been called the supraoculomotor area.[100] Three main types of neurons can be found: those that discharge in relation to vergence angle (vergence tonic cells), to vergence velocity (vergence burst cells), and to both vergence angle and velocity (vergence burst-tonic cells). Many of these neurons also discharge with accommodation, although when vergence and accommodation are experimentally dissociated and pitted against each other, some remain predominantly related to vergence.[158,389]

Most *vergence tonic cells* increase their discharge directly in relation to the angle of convergence; they change their firing rate 10 ms to 30 ms before any detectable eye movements.

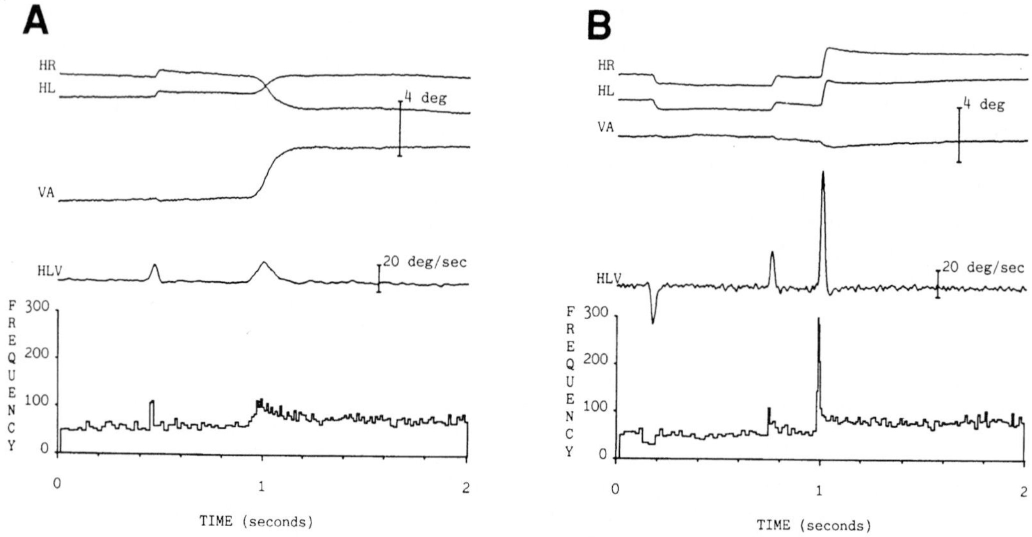

Figure 8–6. Neural activity of a medial rectus motoneuron during convergence and during a rightward saccade. During convergence (A), the neuron discharges in relation to both the eye velocity (HLV, horizontal left eye velocity) and the vergence angle (VA). Likewise, during saccades (B) the discharge frequency is proportional to both eye velocity and (conjugate) eye position. HR = horizontal position of right eye; HL = horizontal position of left eye (Courtesy of L.E. Mays and based upon Gamlin and Mays,[101] with permission of the American Physiological Society.)

A second, smaller group of cells increases the rate of discharge with divergence. The activity of both of these types of cells is unaffected by the direction of conjugate gaze.

Before and during vergence, *vergence burst cells* exhibit a burst of activity that is linearly related to the velocity of the vergence movement (Fig. 8–7).[217] For most of these cells, the number of spikes within each burst (i.e., the integral of the rate of discharge) is correlated with the amplitude of the movement. These vergence burst neurons are analogous to the saccadic burst neurons that discharge in relation to saccade velocity. There are both convergence and divergence burst neurons, with convergence neurons being more abundant.

Vergence burst-tonic cells combine vergence position and vergence velocity information in their output: the burst is related to vergence velocity and the tonic firing rate to vergence angle. Most of these cells are located next to the dorsolateral portion of the oculomotor nucleus.

Premotor Commands for Vergence in the Pons

The role of *abducens internuclear neurons* (see Box 6–1 and Fig. 6–1, Chapter 6) and *oculomotor internuclear neurons* in generating the vergence command is not well understood. Each of these interneurons has projections to the other nucleus, presumably via the medial longitudinal fasciculus (MLF). Clinically, lesions in the MLF (internuclear ophthalmoplegia (INO)—see Box 12–7, Chapter 12) do not impair the ability to make vergence movements. The MLF does, however, carry activity related to vergence.[97] Furthermore, monkeys with an acute lidocaine-induced internuclear ophthalmoplegia show an *increased* AC/A ratio, implying that the MLF carries signals that inhibit vergence.[48,98] Likewise, increased convergence tone is shown by some patients with no internuclear ophthalmoplegia.[14] One possible source of additional vergence inputs

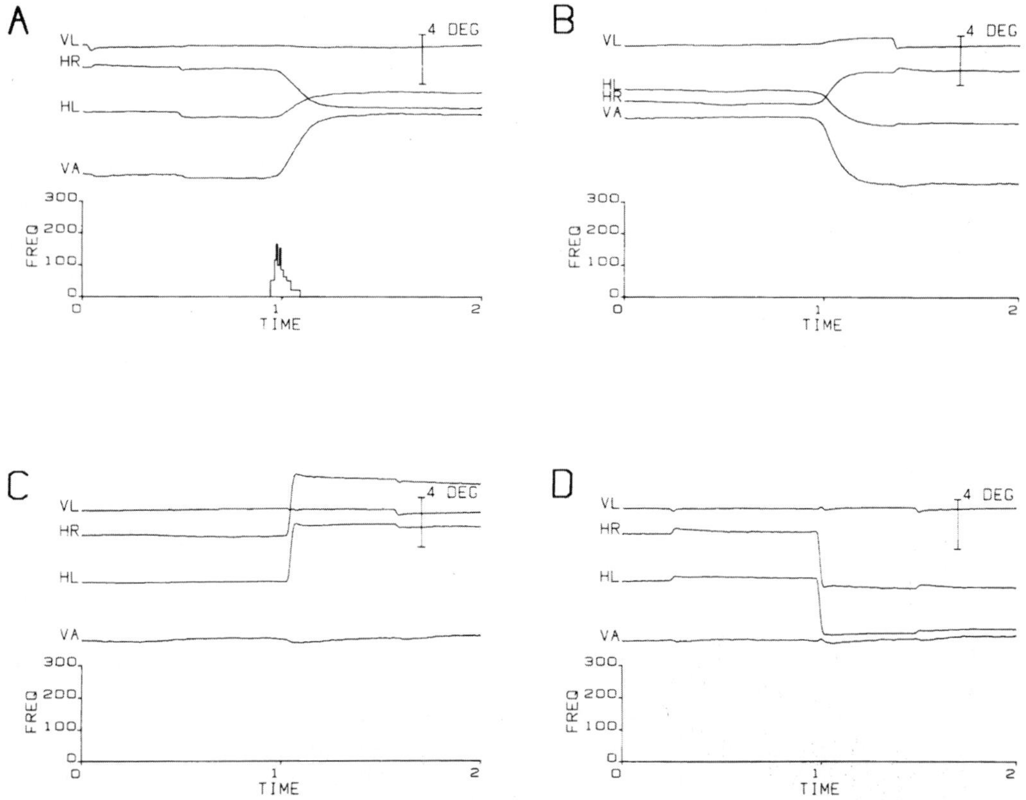

Figure 8–7. Vergence burst neuron. The neuron only discharges ("bursts") during convergence (A), and its frequency of discharge (bottom trace) can be correlated with vergence velocity. (B) Divergence; (C) rightward saccade; (D) leftward saccade. VL = vertical position of left eye, HR = horizontal position of right eye, HL = horizontal position of left eye, VA = vergence angle. (From Mays et al.,[217] with permission of the American Physiological Society.)

to the abducens nucleus is the pontine nuclei, which are discussed next.

Vergence-related cells lie close to other neurons in the *nucleus reticularis tegmenti pontis (NRTP)* that discharge either with saccades (located more caudally in NRTP) or smooth pursuit (located more rostrally in NRTP—see sections in Chapters 3 and 4 on pontine nuclei). Electrical stimulation sometimes produces saccades combined with vergence. Hence, NRTP may mediate some aspects of saccade-vergence and, possibly, saccade-pursuit interactions. The NRTP projects to the oculomotor vermis of the cerebellum (lobules VI and VII), the interposed and fastigial nuclei, and the cerebellar flocculus, and could therefore be a source of vergence (and disparity) information to the cerebellum. The NRTP receives projections from many structures, including the frontal lobes; this may be one source of premotor vergence commands to the NRTP and cerebellum (see next section).[103] Patients have been described with disturbance of slow vergence with lesions affecting NRTP,[279] and involvement of fast vergence with more rostral pontine lesions (Fig. 8–10).[282] More studies are required to define better the role of NRTP and other pontine nuclei in the generation of vergence movements made in combination with saccades or pursuit.[193]

Although conventionally thought of as part of the saccadic system, there is evidence that the *superior colliculus* also contributes to vergence. First, neurons in the *superior colliculus* that discharge for saccades modulate (increase or decrease) their activity during combined saccade-vergence movements.[365] Second, stimulation of the rostral pole of the superior colliculus partially suppresses vergence as well as saccades.[46] Third, a patient with a presumed demyelinating lesion affecting the rostral superior colliculus was reported to show paralysis of vergence and accommodation.[250]

Since the rostral pole of the superior colliculus projects to *omnipause neurons*,[42] it seems possible that this circuit concerns not just saccades, but also vergence, especially during combined saccade-vergence movements. Consistent with this hypothesis, stimulating omnipause neurons slows down ongoing vergence movements.[215] Convergence, in turn, decreases the discharge of omnipause neurons,[36] but it is unclear whether this could provide a means of inhibiting omnipause neurons until the vergence movement is completed (a vergence "latch" circuit, analogous to the saccadic latch circuit, which keeps neurons from resuming their discharge until the saccade is finished).

Influence of the Cerebellum on Vergence

Historically, two lines of evidence have implicated the cerebellum in the control of vergence. First, based on clinical observations, Holmes[131] described a weakness of convergence in patients with acute cerebellar lesions. Subsequent studies have demonstrated a range of abnormalities of binocular alignment in patients with cerebellar disorders, including paralysis of convergence, esodeviations during viewing of a far target, vertical skew deviations that sometimes alternate on right and left horizontal gaze, and disconjugate saccadic dysmetria, with impaired yoking of the eyes during and after saccades.[233,251,361,383] Functional imaging studies in humans show activation of the cerebellar hemispheres and vermis during the near response.[288]

The second line of evidence comes from studies in monkeys. Westheimer and Blair showed that acute ablation of the cerebellum in the monkey leads to a transient paralysis of vergence.[368] The *cerebellar flocculus* has neurons that discharge in relation to the vergence angle.[227] However, it seems possible that these neurons are more concerned with adjustment of the gain of the vestibulo-ocular reflex as a function of target distance,[120,227,331] than with other aspect of vergence, since monkeys with floccular lesions still appeared able to undergo adaptive changes in ocular alignment and the AC/A ratio.[156]

The *posterior interposed nucleus*—corresponding to the posterior globose and emboliform nuclei in humans) and the posterior portion of the *fastigial nucleus* (FOR or fastigial oculomotor region) have cells that discharge in relation to vergence (and accommodation).[100,386,387] The FOR and posterior interposed nucleus have reciprocal anatomic connections with the midbrain areas that contain neurons that convey premotor vergence commands to the oculomotor nuclei.[211] Neurons in the posterior interposed nucleus seem related to a far response (divergence), and those in the FOR to a near response (convergence). The projection from the deep nuclei is predominantly contralateral, whereas the projection to the deep nuclei is predominantly ipsilateral. Pharmacological inactivation of the FOR interferes with convergence.[100,104]

The *dorsal vermis*, which projects to the FOR and posterior interposed nuclei, may also play a role in vergence. Thus, surgical lesions of the dorsal vermis in monkeys cause an esodeviation, variation of ocular alignment with orbital position (incomitancy), disconjugacy of saccades, and defects in phoria adaptation.[342] In humans, positron emission tomography (PET) shows an increase in activity in the cerebellar vermis in humans performing a binocularity discrimination task.[114]

Cerebral Control of Vergence

A number of areas of cerebral cortex contribute to vergence movements. In general, posterior visual areas are concerned with sensory processing and generation of more reflexive, stimulus-bound movements, whereas frontal cortex is more concerned with volitional, self-initiated movements.[99,100] This is a comparable organization to the cerebral control of saccades and pursuit.

PRIMARY VISUAL CORTEX (V1)

Some neurons in monkey *primary visual cortex* (V1) respond to disparate inputs from each eye appropriately to signal the depth of the stimulus.[271,349] Consistent with this electrophysiology, impaired stereopsis (tested with random-dot stereograms) can be induced by repetitive magnetic stimulation of occipital cortex in humans.[344] Functional image studies show activation of striate cortex with blur cues.[288] Other neurons in V1 may play a role in the generation of the ultra short-latency (60 ms–85 ms) vergence responses to small disparities in a large field of view.[34,205]

MIDDLE TEMPORAL (MT) AND MEDIAL SUPERIOR TEMPORAL (MST) VISUAL AREAS

Neurons in secondary visual cortex, such as the *middle temporal area (MT, V5)*,[68] and area V3A in humans,[17] seem important for perception of stereoscopic depth. Furthermore, neurons in the adjacent *medial superior temporal visual area (MST)* may signal self motion and be concerned with the initiation of vergence.[345] Although individual units in MST show variable responses to disparity stimuli, the population of neurons in MST has been shown to encode signals necessary for generating the initial vergence responses.[345,346] As discussed in Chapter 4, neurons in dorsal MST are important for analyzing the optic flow induced during locomotion,[261] and may thus generate short-latency vergence responses to sudden changes in radial flow due to a looming stimulus. Other neurons in MST also discharge during either purely vergence smooth tracking or combined pursuit-vergence.[2]

PARIETAL LOBE

Some neurons in the *lateral intraparietal area (LIP)*, on the lateral bank of the intraparietal sulcus (see Box 6–17), encode a signal related to retinal disparity that changes with fixation distance, implying that this population of cells contributes to a transformation of visual signals from retinal to body-centered coordinates, so that objects can be located in 3-D space.[105] Neurons in area LIP also discharge not only for saccades but also when a saccade is combined with a vergence movement to take the eyes to a particular depth plane.[106] In addition, neurons in the caudal part of the lateral bank and fundus of the intraparietal cortex discharge in relationship to the three-dimensional orientation or motion of objects.[50,326] Functional imaging has shown that the left inferior parietal lobule, as well as bilateral temporal-occipital areas are activated during vergence eye movements in humans.[122] Transcranial magnetic stimulation (TMS) over the right parietal cortex increases the latency for vergence movements, but this effect is context dependent.[165]

FRONTAL LOBE

In the *frontal eye field (FEF)* there are neurons that discharge for convergence or divergence eye movements made in response to step displacements of a target in depth,[102] and during smooth pursuit of a target that moves in depth.[94,95] These vergence neurons lie just in front of the saccade-related FEF area, in the anterior bank of the arcuate sulcus. Microstimulation of this region also induces vergence eye movement.[102]

In the *supplementary eye field (SEF)s*, there are neurons that modulate their discharge during pursuit of a target moving in depth, and which might contribute to predictive vergence tracking.[93] There is also indirect evidence that the *dorsolateral prefrontal cortex (DLPC)* influences vergence. TMS over dorsolateral prefrontal cortex decreases the latency of convergence movements made with or without a saccade.[61] Thus, like its effects on saccades, TMS may release the superior colliculus from frontal lobe inhibition.[238] Conversely, TMS stimulation over right parietal cortex increases vergence latency.[164]

The widely distributed nature of processing of information about three-dimensional space is reflected in PET studies of humans performing binocular disparity discrimination. There are increases in blood flow in the polar striate and neighboring peristriate cortex, the parietal lobe, the dorsal lateral and medial prefrontal cortex, and the cerebellar vermis.[114]

CONCEPTUAL MODELS OF SUPRANUCLEAR CONTROL OF VERGENCE

The organization of vergence premotor neurons has many parallels with that of the saccadic system, and it is useful to compare the functional roles of these various types of neurons in the generation of saccadic and vergence movements. Likewise, smooth tracking of targets moving slowly in depth is in some ways comparable to smooth pursuit of targets moving across the visual field. Accordingly, we will use a conceptual framework for the supranuclear control of vergence analogous to current ideas about the control of saccades and pursuit. Although this scheme is speculative, we believe it useful for understanding vergence. A number of models have been offered to account for various features of vergence eye movements.[38,184,263,305,311,381,384]

Vergence Integrator

Both the saccadic system and the vergence system must provide the appropriate position-coded information to *hold* the eyes steady at the end of each movement. This involves maintaining the eyes in a particular orbital position after saccades and at a particular vergence angle after vergence. Because the eyes are held in position reasonably well even in darkness, immediate visual feedback cannot account for the perseveration of tonic activity in the dark. One way to obtain the necessary position information is to integrate (in the mathematical sense) the prior velocity command that brought the eyes to their present position. Models for generating conjugate eye movements incorporate such a velocity-to-position integrator (see The Need for a Neural Integrator of Ocular Motor Signals in Chapter 5). Models of the vergence system have also incorporated an integrator to explain vergence input-output relationships.[184] Electrophysiological evidence suggests that the nucleus reticularis tegmenti pontis makes a major contribution to the vergence integrator.[100] This vergence position integrator is conceptually distinct from the conjugate position integrator, though there is experimental evidence for shared conjugate and vergence signals distributed over a network of neurons.[62,220,337]

Commands for "Saccadic" Vergence Movements

One source of input to the vergence integrator may be vergence burst cells.[217] Vergence tonic cells may then carry the output of the vergence integrator, and vergence burst-tonic cells seem to combine both vergence velocity and vergence position information. A parsimonious interpretation of these observations—analogous to the premotor commands for conjugate eye movements—is that the vergence system uses a direct (velocity) pathway from vergence burst neurons, in parallel with a vergence integrator (position) pathway; the combined signal may be the input to the ocular motoneurons. The finding that ocular motoneurons discharge not only in relation to the angle of vergence but also to the velocity of vergence is consistent with this idea.[101] However, it is not settled whether a desired vergence position, or a desired *change* in vergence position (analogous to the change in eye position signals that drives saccades), is the critical input signal to the premotor vergence generator.[188]

What determines when vergence burst neurons cease discharging? A scheme analogous to that for saccades (see Fig. 3–9, Chapter 3), using internal signals proportional to desired vergence position, actual vergence position (based on efference copy), and vergence motor error, has been proposed.[385] Vergence motor error would serve as the necessary error signal to drive the vergence burst neurons to provide the appropriate vergence velocity command for the correct duration.

It seems probable that when a combined saccade-vergence is initiated, this is a synchronized event in the frontal eye field. Downstream, however, their respective trigger signals must diverge, since each can be influenced separately by the conditions of fixation (see, for example, the "gap" effect discussed above).[340] Parallel saccadic and vergence pathways, both controlled by omnipause neurons have been postulated to account for the interaction between saccades and vergence during combined shifts of gaze that move the point of regard both across the visual field and in depth (Fig. 8–5A).[384] Alternatively, to account for the finding that vergence peak velocity is influenced by saccadic peak velocity,[37] it has been proposed that a vergence motor error signal may be multiplied by the saccadic signals when saccades and vergence movements are synchronized (Fig. 8–5B).[38] Eye dominance,[356] and synchronous timing of saccadic and vergence components,[189] influence the dynamic features of the vergence response. The latter finding has suggested that when the saccadic and vergence responses are synchronized the saccadic drive amplifies the vergence response.

Commands for "Pursuit" Vergence Movements

One can also propose a scheme, analogous to models of smooth pursuit (see Chapter 4), for *pursuit vergence* tracking of slower, smoothly moving stimuli. In this case, a desired *vergence velocity* would be recreated and used to generate a vergence velocity error signal and, in turn, a vergence acceleration command. Thus, we speculate that there may be separate vergence premotor networks for generating *saccadic* and *pursuit* vergence. This notion is supported by electrophysiological findings from frontal cortex that are reviewed in the prior section.[94] One can envision that both systems work in concert, just as for pursuit and saccades in the conjugate system. One movement brings images to the fovea, and the other attempts to keep them there. In fact, such a combination of saccadic and pursuit vergence has been reported when the velocity of the disparity change is high.[319] Pontine lesions in humans are reported to have differential effects on fast and slow vergence responses.[279,282]

One implication of this scheme for vergence is that it has been possible to classify vergence disorders in a way similar to that for disorders of saccades, pursuit and conjugate gaze-holding. For example, selective deficits of vergence responses to step,[282] and ramp,[279] stimuli have been described in patients with pontine lesions (Fig. 8–10). Furthermore, some subjects may show impaired ability to hold positions of convergence, with consequent divergent drift (Fig. 8–11). This would be analogous to the impaired holding of eccentric positions of conjugate gaze after saccades, with consequent centripetal drift. Instability of the conjugate integrator leads to slow phases with an *increasing* velocity waveform. Similarly, the vergence integrator might become unstable, leading to excessive convergence and convergence spasm (see Abnormalities of Vergence).

ADAPTIVE MECHANISMS TO MAINTAIN OCULAR ALIGNMENT

As has been emphasized in previous chapters dealing with the conjugate eye movement systems, a robust and versatile adaptive capability is essential if an organism is to maintain optimal visuomotor function throughout its life. Most research has focused on *conjugate* adaptive mechanisms, especially those of the saccade and vestibular systems. Usually, however, muscle weakness is unilateral and asymmetric, so that many of the needed adaptive corrections are *disconjugate* and may have to vary with the position of the eye in the orbit. Such a capability implies that Hering's Law of equal innervation is not immutable, though the exact mechanisms by which this adaptation takes place are unknown.

Phoria Adaptation

BEHAVIORAL PROPERTIES OF PHORIA ADAPTATION

Phoria is the relative deviation of the visual axes when a single target is viewed with one eye, and reflects tonic vergence, in the absence of disparity. Phoria adaptation is an adaptation of the tonic vergence component. Thus, if a disparity is introduced by placing a wedge prism in front of one eye, the subject's phoria changes by an amount equal to the strength of the prism. Tropia, the relative deviation of the visual axes when the target is viewed binocularly, does not occur if the new disparity is within the range in which fusional mechanisms can cope, but the residual fixation disparity, or steady-state vergence error during binocular viewing, is increased. In seconds to minutes, however, the subject undergoes phoria adaptation, so that both the phoria and the fixation disparity (measured with the prism on) revert to their pre-prism values. Thus, there has been a resetting of the alignment of the two visual axes by an amount equivalent to the prismatic demand.[43,57,90,191,202,225,247,249,303,305,321]

Phoria adaptation can also be achieved by simply by sustaining a vergence effort for over 30 seconds.[380] After a sustained period of convergence, vergence dynamics as well as static vergence angle are affected, such as the peak velocity of the initial vergence response.[237,320] Like saccades, the dynamic properties of vergence can be adapted using double-step stimuli.[341] Vertical and cyclovergence responses can also be adapted to visual demands using dove prisms or artificially induced cyclodisparity with dichoptic viewing.[209,262,311,347]

Other forms of vergence adaptation have been described. For example, vergence adaptation can also be linked to other eye movements, such as the VOR; in this case, head rotation can determine a context for adaptation of vergence.[301] Conversely, vergence angle can determine a context for adaptation of the VOR.[197] Dynamic vergence adaptation can be induced by artificially altering the position of the target, using visual feedback, to make each initial vergence movement of incorrect amplitude (similar to the method used to induce adaptation of saccades).[80] After a training period, the vergence response is adjusted to correct for the artificially induced dysmetria.[316]

An adaptive mechanism has also been demonstrated for *accommodation*. By opening the visual feedback loop, one can measure the *tonic* level of accommodation (i.e., the accommodative phoria). Using appropriate lenses, one can demonstrate that the tonic level of accommodation can be adaptively readjusted, independent of a change in disparity.[222,245,294]

CLINICAL IMPLICATIONS OF PHORIA ADAPTATION

Certain aspects of phoria adaptation are pertinent to clinical practice.[57] Thus, short-term phoria adaptation influences measures of the range of divergence and convergence as tested with base-in or base-out prisms; this influence varies with viewing distance.[247,295] Conversely, to fully appreciate the baseline phoria in a symptomatic patient, one must eliminate binocular cues for hours to days, allowing phoria adaptation to dissipate.[132,149,240] Normal subjects, too, commonly show a change in phoria after prolonged monocular occlusion, often in the pattern of an oblique muscle imbalance, with excyclophoria.[109,199,239] Rarely, a symptomatic tropia may emerge after prolonged patching of one eye, requiring treatment with prisms or even surgery.[32] Wearing prisms for a few hours to neutralize diplopia in patients with ocular motor nerve palsies may bring out the amount of adaptation that normally contributes to their ocular alignment.[253] A robust phoria adaptation mechanism might act to limit the efficacy of prismatic therapy for ocular motor imbalance. Such patients "eat up the prism," as their phoria adaptation overcomes the effect of the prism and defeats its purpose. Elderly individuals show decreased phoria adaptation, but this has the advantage that they often accept a prismatic correction more readily than younger patients.[372] Children show greater vergence adaptation ability than adults.[373] Individuals with convergence insufficiency, a condition described under Abnormalities of Vergence, may show impaired prism adaptation in the horizontal, but not in the vertical, plane.[25,26]

MECHANISMS FOR PHORIA ADAPTATION

It has been suggested that the reduction in fixation disparity after prolonged wearing of a prism is accomplished by a *slow fusional adaptive mechanism*.[249,305,306] The output of the slow fusional mechanism resets the level of tonic vergence so as to reduce fixation disparity. This relieves the stress from the increased disparity demands of the prism on the fast fusional mechanism (or what we commonly think of as disparity-induced vergence).

These ideas have been developed into formal models for phoria adaptation that incorporate both accommodation and vergence (Fig. 8–8).[146,305] The fast fusional system uses *retinal image disparity*, and the slow fusional adaptive system uses the *motor output* of the fast fusional system as its error signal. The fast fusional vergence system appears to use a slightly imperfect, *leaky integrator* with a time constant of 10 to 15 seconds. This is the vergence position integrator previously described. The slow fusional adaptive system also uses a leaky integrator but with a much longer time constant (minutes or more). In fact, there are probably multiple mechanisms that subserve phoria adaptation, with different capabilities, degrees of permanency, and time courses of action. In time, the slow fusional mechanism takes over much of the load of keeping the eyes aligned, by resetting the level of tonic vergence. Thus, phoria adaptation resets the resting position of the eyes toward the original phoria, and thereby restores the dynamic range (or fusional reserve) in which fast fusional vergence can function. Similar considerations apply to the accommodation system. The fast accommodative system uses retinal blur and the slow accommodative system adjusts tonic accommodation using the output of the fast system as its error signal. One unresolved issue is the stage of central processing at which voluntary vergence and accommodation interject their influences on phoria adaptation.[71,222]

One may ask if the AC/A or CA/C ratios are *genetically* fixed, or if they can be modified by environmental factors. If subjects wear periscopic spectacles, to simulate an increase in the interocular separation, both the AC/A and the CA/C ratios may change.[24,88,159,228] Such a mechanism would be necessary, for example, to optimize visual function as the interpupillary distance increased during growth, or to assure an accurate response when accommodation or vergence fatigues.[225] Some disorders of binocular ocular motor function (e.g., vergence excess or vergence insufficiency) may have their basis in alterations in the strength of the cross-linkages between accommodation and convergence and/or in the sensitivity of the slow adaptive mechanisms for vergence and accommodation (see Abnormalities of Vergence).

The anatomic substrate underlying phoria adaptation is incompletely known. Electrophysiological recordings in primates indicate that some but not all of the phoria adaptation signal is carried by midbrain vergence-related neurons.[232] Patients with cerebellar lesions occasionally show a decrease in phoria adaptation,[183,224] but in many cases it is normal.[116] Monkeys with floccular lesions may still be able

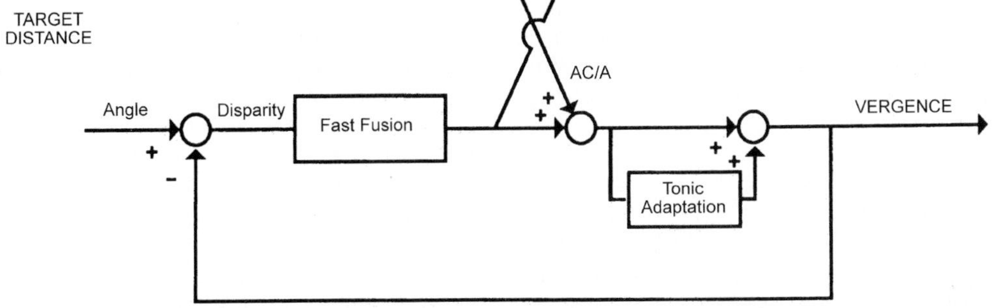

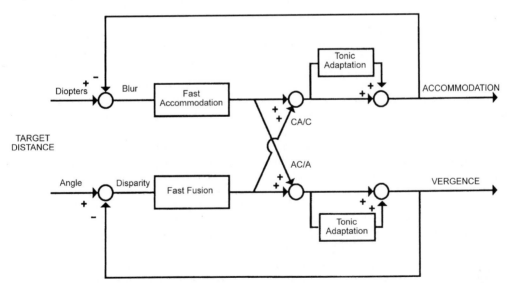

Figure 8–8. Model of vergence-accommodation interaction. Note the cross-links producing accommodation-linked convergence (AC/A) and convergence-linked accommodation (CA/C). The fast system provides the immediate (hundreds of milliseconds), phasic response to a change in disparity (angle) or blur (diopters). The tonic adaptation (slow) system uses the motor output of the fast system to provide a slower (seconds) adjustment in tonic level of accommodation or vergence. (Reproduced with permission from Schor CM. Influence of accommodative and vergence adaptation on binocular motor disorders. Am J Optom Physiol Opt 65, 464–475, 1988, copyright American Academy of Optometry.)

to undergo phoria adaptation.[156] However, surgical lesions of the dorsal vermis in monkeys induce defects in phoria adaptation.[342]

Disconjugate Adaptation

PROPERTIES OF DISCONJUGATE ADAPTATION

A special case of phoria adaptation is illustrated by the response to wearing an anisometropic spectacle correction.[124,321] Anisometropia is a difference in the anterior-posterior dimensions of the two eyes and requires a corrective lens of a different power for each eye. Corrective spectacle lenses have a prismatic effect that results in the relative displacement of an image of an object from its actual position. This is also known as the rotational magnification effect because it changes the amount the eye must rotate to fix upon a target located at a given point in space.[297] (The linear magnification effect, on the other hand, describes the relative size of an image of an object. Contact lenses have a linear but not a rotational magnification effect.) The prismatic effect of a spectacle lens is roughly proportional to both its power and the distance from its optical center. This effect will increase continuously toward the lens periphery. With an anisometropic correction, the prismatic effect of each spectacle lens is different. Therefore, the retinal disparity between the images of a given object will change as a function of gaze position. Accordingly, ocular alignment must undergo disconjugate adaptation to produce a new pattern of innervation, as a function of orbital position. When subjects begin wearing an anisometropic spectacle correction, their phoria (as measured while wearing their spectacle correction) soon reverts to the pre-adaptation state in all positions of gaze (i.e., the resting ocular alignment appropriately varies as a function of orbital position).[124] This is the way to assure concomitance while wearing glasses; ocular alignment becomes correct in all orbital positions. However, to achieve fusion promptly upon changing gaze, a subject wearing an anisometropic spectacle correction also must be able to change the alignment of the visual axes *during* the saccade.

The most frequent circumstance to which a disconjugate adaptive mechanism must respond is asymmetry in the strengths of the eye muscles themselves. This may occur either during natural development and aging, or after trauma or disease of the ocular motor nerves or orbital contents. Such asymmetries lead to a noncomitant deviation and consequent diplopia if the disparity-driven fusional mechanisms cannot overcome it. It is due to this visuomotor problem that our disconjugate adaptation mechanisms evolved, certainly not from a need to wear corrective spectacles!

Disconjugate adaptation has been extensively investigated, using a number of techniques, and covering time frames of adaptation ranging from minutes to days.[55] These paradigms include having anisometropic subjects wear newly fitted corrective spectacles,[82,195,258] or having emmetropic subjects wear optical devices that simulate a spectacle-corrected anisometropia, such as a contact-lens–spectacle combination[124,385] or an afocal magnifier.[194,308] Other techniques used to elicit disconjugate adaptation include wearing displacing prisms in front of one eye in just one part of the visual field,[13,257,379,385] presenting different-sized images (aniseikonia) of a target to each eye,[161,162,355] and dissociating the images seen by each eye at the end of a saccade.[4,72,162,308] In experimental animals, surgically or botulinum-induced asymmetrical muscle weakness elicits disconjugate adaptation.[151,362] Human patients with strabismus have also been a model group for studying disconjugate adaptation.[28,72,150]

IMPLICATIONS OF DISCONJUGATE ADAPTATION

What have we learned from these many experiments? First, clinical experience indicates that the degree to which the innervation to the two eyes can be selectively adjusted to overcome a noncomitant deviation is limited. If the relative degree of weakness is large, disconjugate mechanisms may be overwhelmed. Another factor may the degree of ocular dominance. Patients who strongly prefer to fix with one eye (even with both eyes viewing) may undergo no adaptation at all if the preferred eye is the strong one. If the preferred eye is the weak one, they may undergo conjugate adaptation, which increases the innervation to both eyes.

Second, in some individuals, especially some patients with a long-standing requirement for a disconjugate correction, disconjugate adaptation can be remarkably robust. As an example, consider the recordings shown from a subject who had been wearing spectacles to correct a large degree of anisometropia (Fig. 8–9). It is important to note that the intrasaccadic and postsaccadic changes in alignment occurred under *both* binocular and monocular viewing conditions. In other words, the subject learned to preprogram intrasaccadic and postsaccadic disconjugate movements independent of any immediate disparity cues.

Third, and even more remarkable, is the finding that subjects may have more than one motor program of disconjugate innervation, which can be gated in and out on the basis of context.[258] Both the phoria and the yoking of the eyes can be trained to specific combinations of eye positions, both across the visual field and in depth.[45,312,313,379] Even the angle of head tilt can be a contextual clue for gating in different adaptive changes in phoria.[207,208] The degree of context specificity does have some limits. If two different eye positions used as contextual cues are too close to each other, adaptation at each will interfere with adaptation at the other.[257,308] These types of interactions can be successfully simulated using neural network models.[218,219] Disconjugate

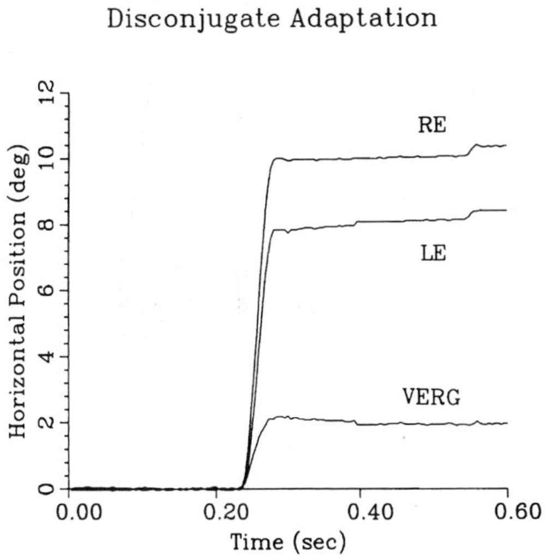

Figure 8–9. Search coil recordings showing disconjugate adaptation to spectacle-corrected anisometropia.[258] The subject habitually wore a spectacle-correction of about −10 diopters (myopic correction) in front of the left eye and −0.5 diopters in front of the right eye. (This correction calls for divergence on right gaze and convergence on left gaze.). For this recording the right eye only was viewing the target (i.e., there were no disparity cues). Note the change in vergence during the saccade and the corresponding change in phoria at the end of the saccade. RE = right eye position, LE = left eye position, Verg = vergence angle, obtained by subtracting the right and left eye position traces.

adaptation also can be made selective to one type of conjugate eye movement (e.g., pursuit) and not to another (e.g., saccades).[305] Disconjugate pursuit adaptation and phoria adaptation can be trained together, leaving saccade conjugacy unchanged.[307] This last finding suggests that the velocity ("pulse") and position ("step") components of conjugate innervation to each eye may be differentially adapted.

The exact mechanisms underlying both the static and dynamic changes in ocular alignment that occur with disconjugate adaptation are not known.[13,72,161,194,195,257,258,307,355] Presumably, the retinal disparity that occurs at the end of conjugate eye movements, or perhaps the disparity-driven vergence effort to overcome it, is the necessary error signal used to readjust the relative innervation to the eyes during and after eye movements. Afferent cues from orbital proprioceptors may also be important.[198] Disconjugate adaptation to fourth nerve palsy is affected by deafferentation of orbital proprioceptors.[198] Patients with microstrabismus and lack of bifoveal fixation can still undergo disconjugate adaptation, but only if some degree of binocular function is present.[28] The beneficial effect of corrective surgery in childhood strabismus is aided by disconjugate adaptive mechanisms that may come into play once some binocular function is restored.[87,150]

With respect to the motor learning itself, there could be an adjustment of the innervation to the two eyes independently, or it could perhaps reflect a modification of the normal interaction between saccade and vergence eye movements.[13] Recall that even under normal circumstances, changes in ocular alignment are facilitated when vergence movements are combined with an ongoing saccade (see Fig. 8–4). Whatever the precise mechanisms, such a disconjugate adaptive capability is exceedingly important. It will make adjustments not only for acquired abnormalities, but also for the small, inherent asymmetries in ocular muscle strength and in other orbital mechanical properties that exist in all humans.

EXAMINATION OF VERGENCE MOVEMENTS

As with the interpretation of all ocular motor function, it is important, first, to measure the corrected visual acuity of each eye, for both near and far viewing. In addition, it is important to measure stereopsis as a prelude to evaluating vergence. It has been suggested than stereoacuity can be used as an index of vergence accuracy during testing.[187] Appendix A contains a summary of the examination.

Vergence Induced by Combined Disparity-Accommodation Stimuli

Conventionally, the examiner tests fusional and accommodative vergence together by asking the patient to fix upon an accommodative target (one that requires bringing its image into focus) as it is slowly brought in along the sagittal plane to the bridge of the nose. It is also important to test vergence movements made as the patient alternatively shifts the point of fixation between a far target (at optical infinity) and a near target (see Video Display: Disorders of Vergence). Such testing usually induces vergence movements combined with saccades, but the latter can be minimized if the near and far stimuli are aligned on the patient's midsagittal plane at eye level. In testing horizontal vergence in patients with a vertical ocular misalignment, it is helpful to use a pencil orientated up and down, which eliminates the vertical disparity. More quantitative estimates of a near point of convergence can be made using both objective and subjective tests. Such measurements are helpful in evaluating patients with visual fatigue (asthenopia) or horizontal diplopia due to convergence insufficiency. The neurologist should always keep in mind that presbyopia, the loss of accommodation that becomes symptomatic when humans reach their early forties, is often the cause of a number of visual complaints, and decompensation of long-standing, even congenital strabismus. These symptoms include episodic diplopia, visual fatigue, and difficulty with reading.

Testing Vergence Responses to Disparity Stimuli

The fusional vergence system may be tested directly by asking the patient to fix upon a distant target. Insertion of a horizontal prism before one eye will then induce a fusional vergence movement, often in combination with a saccade. By slowly and progressively increasing the amplitude of the prism (for example, using a rotary prism) until diplopia occurs (the break point of vergence), one can gain a measure of the range of fusional amplitudes for both convergence and divergence. Fusional capabilities depend upon the stimulus. Thus, disparities presented to the central retina are most powerful,[140,267] but stimuli seen in the periphery aid fusion of central targets.[155] Measures of fusional vergence amplitudes can only be properly interpreted if the patient's underlying phoria is known. The recovery point of vergence (when fusion is restored as the prism strength is decreased) is also an important measure, and may be different from the break point in patients with, for example, intermittent deviations (see Von Noorden and Campos,[364] for a discussion of these testing techniques).

Testing Vergence Responses to Accommodative Stimuli

The accommodative vergence system may be tested using the procedure of the Müller experiment (the heterophoria method, Fig. 8–1). One eye is covered and the other eye changes fixation from a far to a near target, both of which lie along the visual axis of the viewing eye. A convenient method is to use a Spielmann semi opaque occluder (easily made, for example, with semi opaque slide-holder material), which permits the examiner to view the eye under cover without the patient being able to see the visual target (see Video Display, Disorders of Vergence).[333] Alternatively, a plus or a minus lens may be placed in front of the viewing eye to change the depth of focus. The vergence movement of the covered eye is recorded or measured using prisms when the occluder is switched to the other, uncovered eye. This procedure is often used to measure the AC/A (accommodative convergence/accommodation) ratio. Conventionally, measurements of the phoria are made when viewing a distant target and one at 33 cm. Then, the AC/A ratio is given by the equation:

$$AC/A = IPD + (phoria[n] - phoria[d])/d$$

where IPD is the interpupillary distance (cm); phoria[n] is the phoria in prism diopters (exodeviations are negative, esodeviations are positive) when viewing the near target; phoria[d] is the phoria when viewing the distant target, and d is the fixation distance of the near target in sphere diopters (in this case, 3.0).

The dynamic aspects of vergence eye movements can be judged at the bedside by asking the patient to change fixation abruptly between near and far targets aligned along the midsagittal plane ("saccadic vergence"), and to follow a target moving slowly in depth ("pursuit vergence"). Combined saccade-vergence movements can also be elicited by slightly offsetting the distant or near target. The dynamic responses of vergence movements elicited by pure disparity or pure accommodation stimuli can be elicited with prisms and lenses, as already described.

Vergence movements, which are characteristically slow, should be differentiated from abnormal rapid disjunctive movements, such as the quick phases of convergent or divergent nystagmus. Eye movement recordings can often help make the distinction. Nystagmus that has a vergence component can often best be appreciated at the bedside by looking at the bridge of the patient's nose, but focusing attention on the phase relationship between the motions of the two eyes.

LABORATORY TESTING OF VERGENCE EYE MOVEMENTS

Vergence eye movements can be studied in the laboratory applying disparity or blur stimuli separately.[306] Dichoptic viewing devices consist of mirrors arranged so that each eye views a different image, such as a visual display on two computer monitors. A number of software packages now provide the ability to present visual stimuli with a range of depth, disparity, and motion cues.[324] Vergence responses to combined disparity-accommodation stimuli can be tested using an array of light-emitting diodes (LEDs) fixed at different distances to a horizontal sheet of plastic; if the room is otherwise dark, this provides the ability to measure the latency to onset of vergence responses as the LEDs are turned on. Finally, targets such as small black crosses drawn on a white background that are mounted at different viewing distances, and viewed in room lighting, provide natural stimuli to vergence movements.

Horizontal vergence movements can be monitored using infrared reflection or video-based eye movement monitors. However, the magnetic search coil techniques provide the ability to measure 3-D eye rotations (including cyclotorsional responses) with precision. More details are provided in Appendix B.

ABNORMALITIES OF VERGENCE

Development Disorders of Vergence

Inborn defects of the vergence mechanisms are common. Abnormalities of the accommodative-convergence synkinesis (high AC/A ratio) accompany some forms of childhood strabismus (see Diagnosis of Concomitant Strabismus in Chapter 9),[364] and experimental models for strabismus.[350] Common disorders of binocular function include convergence insufficiency, convergence excess, divergence insufficiency, and divergence excess.[291] In these conditions, "excess" refers to a high AC/A ratio, and "insufficiency" refers to a low ratio; "convergence" and "divergence" refer to the viewing distance (near or far) at which the largest phoria exists.

The cause of these disorders may be related to an inability to adjust correctly the level of tonic vergence and tonic accommodation, as well as the values of the cross-links between accommodation and convergence, as reflected in the AC/A and CA/C ratios.[246,304,309] Specifically, patients with unusually high AC/A ratios (vergence excess) usually have a poor ability to adaptively adjust their level of tonic accommodation. Patients with unusually low AC/A ratios (vergence insufficiency) usually have a poor ability to adaptively adjust their level of tonic vergence. High AC/A ratios are associated with low CA/C ratios, and vice versa.

Children who complain of vertigo, but have a normal vestibular examination, have been reported to show abnormal vergence movements, which are slow, made at longer latency and hypometric compared with controls.[29,30] It is postulated that their complaints of dizziness are caused by inadequate vergence responses, perhaps due to impaired modulation of the VOR for near viewing. Orthoptic exercises, which are designed to restore normal vergence-accommodation interactions,[113] improve these children's vergence movements.[29]

The neurologist is sometimes asked to evaluate patients with diplopia due to *convergence insufficiency*. This is a common disorder among teenagers and college students (often those with an increased visual workload and stress), the elderly, and individuals who have suffered even mild head trauma.[186] Affected individual may show impaired phoria adaptation to prisms.[25] Convergence insufficiency is usually treated by orthoptic exercises or prism therapy.[96,112,302,357] Anecdotal reports attest to the efficacy of orthoptic exercises in treating disorders of fusional convergence following head trauma and cerebral ischemia.[172,173]

Acquired Disorders of Vergence

REDUCED VERGENCE RESPONSES

Many acquired neurologic disorders impair vergence responses but, in older patients, it is important to take into account the reduced responses especially to accommodative stimuli.[280] Furthermore, a wide range of sedative drugs, including alcohol and anticonvulsants, impair vergence ability.[286]

When judged clinically by observing responses to the examiner's finger brought towards the patient's nose, vergence is commonly impaired in parkinsonian disorders, including idiopathic Parkinson's disease,[287] and especially progressive supranuclear palsy (PSP). Midbrain lesions causing impaired vertical gaze also may impair vergence but, more characteristically, there is evidence of excessive vergence tone; this is discussed in the next section.

Laboratory studies have provided further insights into the nature of vergence eye movements in patients with brainstem lesions. Thus, in patients with PSP, decreased vergence velocities have been demonstrated during saccade-vergence movements between far and near targets.[21,179] More important, specific disorders of fast or slow vergence have been defined in patients with pontine infarctions. Thus, in one study, two patients showed selective defects of vergence tracking of a target moving slowly in depth, but preserved fast vergence responses to targets that were stepped between different distances.[279] Their lesions were in the more caudal pons and included NRTP. In a second study, two patients showed slowing of vergence responses when they were asked alternate rapidly switch their fixation point between far and near targets (Fig. 8–10); in one patient, slowing of these vergence movements was evident clinically.[282] Although these vergence movements were made in combination with small saccades, in neither patient could the slowing of vergence be attributed to slow saccades. Both patients also showed a mild impairment of vergence tracking of a target moving slowly in depth. These patient's lesions lay more rostral in the pons (Fig. 8–10). Although correlation with animal studies of NRTP and other pontine nuclei is not yet possible, these reports clearly show that vergence disorders can arise with pontine lesions.

Occasionally, acquired cerebral lesions (especially of the nondominant cerebral hemisphere and probably the parietal lobe) may lead to both impaired stereopsis and poor fusional vergence.[19,91,252,353]

The ability to sustain a converged position of the eyes is not routinely tested, but is similar to testing sustained eccentric conjugate gaze. Some normal subjects develop divergent drifts of the eyes with convergence quick phases (Fig. 8–11), evidence of a leaky vergence integrator, and this deserves more systematic study in normals and patients.

Divergence Insufficiency

The terms divergence insufficiency and divergence paralysis have long been used in the clinical literature to describe a heterogeneous group of patients with esotropia during far viewing that could not be ascribed to a specific extraocular muscle weakness. Such cases should be differentiated from bilateral sixth nerve palsy. Bielschowsky[23] defined the diagnostic criteria for divergence paralysis: an esotropia with uncrossed diplopia during fixation of a distant object; single vision during fixation of objects located at about 10 to 20 inches; crossed diplopia with fixation closer than about 10 to 20 inches (due to associated convergence insufficiency); horizontal motion of the eyes that may be normal; and diplopia that, on lateral, gaze is unchanged or may even disappear. To these should be added another more modern criterion: normal amplitude and speed of horizontal saccades, to exclude bilateral weakness or restriction of the lateral recti. In fact, few reported patients with divergence insufficiency have undergone reliable measurement of horizontal saccades to determine if their movements lie on the normal main sequence (Fig. 3–3, Chapter 3).[178,200]

With this caveat in mind (and the possibility of excessive convergence—see below), divergence paralysis has been reported with a variety of neurologic diseases associated with raised intracranial pressure (such as tumor, pseudotumor, intracranial hematoma, or head trauma),[185] with tumors in the midbrain,[192] craniocervical-junction anomalies,[3,144,196,342,343,361] and in spinocerebellar ataxia type 3.[254] It

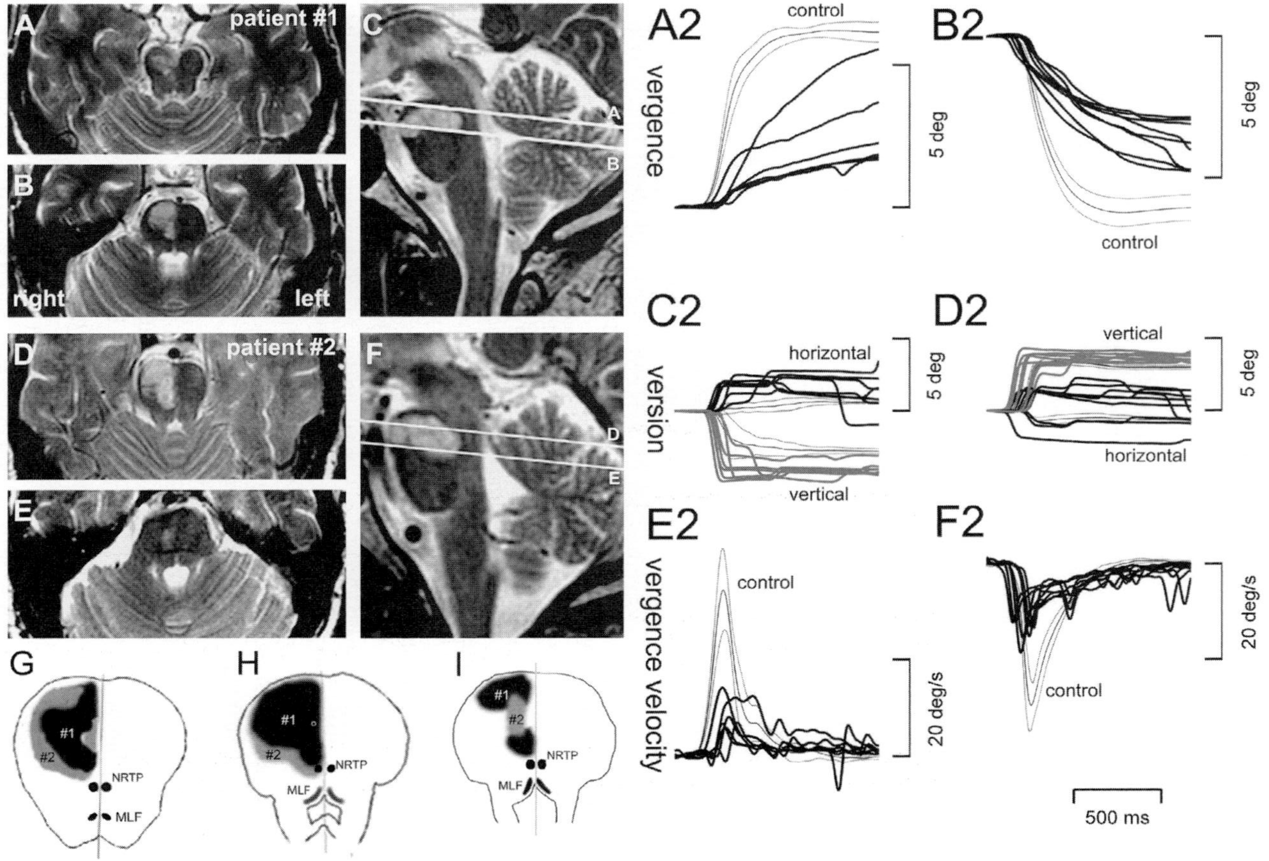

Figure 8–10. Selective impairment of fast vergence due to pontine infarction in two patients. Left panel: Axial MRI slices (T2-weighted) of Patient 1 (A–C) and Patient 2 (D–F) and the anatomic reconstruction (G–I) are shown. The lines (C and F) indicate the appropriate level of the axial slices. The gray areas in (G–I) indicate the extent of the lesions (black: Patient 1; gray: Patient 2), and the black areas indicate the nucleus reticularis tegmenti pontis (NRTP) (circles) or the medial longitudinal fascicle (MLF) (ovals). The lesion in both patients involves in part the NRTP but spares the MLF, the omnipause neurons, and the midbrain. Right panel: In A2 to F2, "fast" vergence eye position (A2, B2) and velocity (E2, F2) are superimposed for convergence (A2, E2) and divergence (B2, F2) for Patient 2. The horizontal (black solid line) and vertical (gray solid line) version components (small saccades) are shown in (C2, D2). Horizontal and vertical saccades were similar to control subjects. The mean of the control subjects (thin solid line) ±1 SD (dotted lines) are superimposed for comparison. "Fast" vergence is clearly decreased in the convergence and divergence direction. (Reproduced with permission of Lippincott Williams and Wilkins, from Rambold et al.[282])

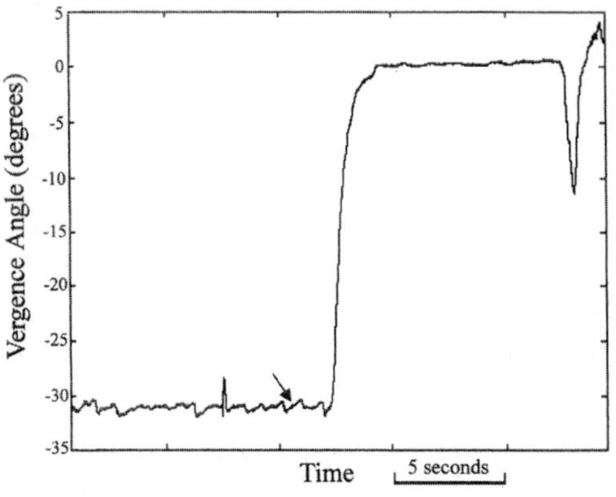

Figure 8–11. An example of convergence-induced nystagmus in a normal subject who has been viewing a near target (light-emitting diode in a dark room) for over 30 seconds. Note that the slow phases are divergence (positive–see arrow) with convergent quick phases.

may also occur with intracranial hypotension (the "low-pressure syndrome"),[135,231] as the initial sign of the Miller Fisher syndrome,[92] and in association with diazepam.[12]

INCREASED VERGENCE RESPONSES

Spasm of Convergence

Spasm of convergence (or spasm of the near triad) may be a sign of an organic lesion or of a functional disorder. The organic form occurs most commonly with disease at the diencephalic-mesencephalic junction—*thalamic esotropia*, characterized by "eyes peering at the nose";[108,130] this is associated with thalamic hemorrhage, pineal tumors, and midbrain strokes.[47] Convergence spasm also occurs with lower brainstem and cerebellar disorders. Thus, Cogan[49] described convergence spasm, elicited by extending the neck, in a patient who had downbeat nystagmus, and it is also reported with Wernicke-Korsakoff syndrome,[127] occipitoatlantal instability with vertebrobasilar ischemia,[58] Chiari malformations and other posterior fossa lesions,[65,125,266] multiple sclerosis,[270] and metabolic disturbances.[234] Convergence spasm must be distinguished from substitution of vergence for versional movements in patients with horizontal gaze palsies (see Chapter 9).[298]

In practice, convergence spasm in association with neurological disease is uncommon whereas it occurs commonly in patients with psychological disorders. In this regard, it is interesting to note that some normal subjects show sustained vergence tone after converging for 10 to 20 seconds, and thus, convergence spasm may constitute an idiosyncratic normal behavior in some otherwise normal subjects. The following is an example how convergence spasm, accompanied by pupillary constriction and accommodation, may be a manifestation of psychological disturbance.

CASE HISTORY: Functional Convergence Spasm

A 20-year-old woman presented to the emergency room complaining of headache and diplopia. Her headache had come on suddenly the previous evening. It had been getting worse, and on direct questioning, she agreed that it was "the worst headache of my life."

Despite her pain, she remained alert and oriented. Her vital signs were normal. In the emergency room, she developed a "noticeable esotropia.... her eye movements are full, but not conjugate." The patient's neck was supple, and her neurologic examination was otherwise normal.

She was thought to have had a subarachnoid hemorrhage, and so computed tomography and a spinal tap were performed; both test results were normal.

Her headache persisted and the nursing staff noted that she was "unable to focus her eyes well."

When seen in consultation, she was emotionally upset. Her corrected near visual acuity was 20/30 when each eye was tested separately. Ocular ductions (movements with one eye viewing) were full. With both eyes viewing (versions), there was a characteristic limitation in movement of the abducting eye: as it crossed the midline there were shimmering, small to-and-fro movements associated with varying constriction of the pupils.

It eventually emerged that the patient had been summarily dismissed from her job the afternoon before admission.

Comment: This case history illustrates features typical of spasm of the near triad.[107] It is frequently misdiagnosed as bilateral sixth nerve palsy (leading to inappropriate tests and procedures).[49,111,300] Careful examination of the eye movements allows the diagnosis to be made. There is often a full range of movements and less pupillary constriction with only one eye viewing.[242] With both eyes viewing, the patient limits abduction by imposing a strong convergence command (voluntary vergence) that causes accommodation and, most importantly, miosis. On lateral gaze, there may be dissociated nystagmus, greater in the abducting eye.[182]

Convergence spasms typically come and go, but some patients can sustain them for long periods. They may cause ocular pain. Rapid, passive head-turns (the doll's-head maneuver) elicit a full range of eye movements. Treatment is best directed toward the underlying psychological factors,[300,315] although cycloplegic eye drops and refractive measures (positive or negative lenses) may be effective.[300,328] Another example of convergence spasm is included in the Video Display: Disorders of Vergence.

Convergence Retraction Nystagmus

This disorder often occurs as a component of the dorsal midbrain syndrome, which is discussed in Chapter 10 (see Video Display: Disorders of Vergence). There is controversy about whether convergence-retraction nystagmus consists of asynchronous, opposed saccades,[248] or is a disorder primarily of the vergence system.[278] Evidence for both possibilities has been reported, and it seems that both mechanisms may contribute to the syndrome. Affected patients may show other evidence of excessive convergence drives, such as pseudo-abducens palsy, in which the abducting eye moves slower than the adducting eye (see Video Display: Disorders of Vergence).[20,66,272,371] This disorder often leads patients with pretectal lesions to complain of difficulty in reading because of the break of fusion that occurs when changing lines. Pretectal pseudobobbing, another disorder of saccades associated with lesions in the midbrain, is nonrhythmic, rapid, combined downward and adducting movements, often preceded by a blink; each movement is followed by a slow return toward the midline.[167]

VERGENCE OSCILLATIONS

Various forms of *pendular nystagmus* may have a convergence-divergence component. These include pendular nystagmus associated with multiple sclerosis, oculopalatal tremor, and Whipple's disease. In some patients with pendular nystagmus, in whom the oscillations are about 180 degrees out of phase in the horizontal and torsional planes (excyclovergence with horizontal convergence) but conjugate in the vertical plane, an oscillation affecting the vergence system itself seems possible, since these 3-D relationship are similar to those occurring during normal vergence movements.[15]

An important example of pendular vergence oscillations occurs in *Whipple's disease* of the central nervous system, when the nystagmus is associated with contractions of the masticatory muscles. This is called oculomasticatory myorhythmia.[314] The ocular oscillations are characterized by smooth, pendular, convergent-divergent movements, occurring at a frequency of 0.8 Hz–1.2 Hz (see Video Display: Acquired Pendular Nystagmus). Oculomasticatory myorhythmia is pathognomonic of Whipple's disease. Such patients commonly have a vertical saccadic palsy and a picture that might suggest progressive supranuclear palsy. Somnolence and intellectual deterioration are associated features.

Divergence nystagmus (nystagmus with divergent quick phases) may occur in patients with hindbrain anomalies (e.g., Arnold–Chiari malformation) who also have downbeat nystagmus.[377] Upbeat nystagmus may also have a divergent component (see Fig. 10–3, Chapter 10). These patients have slow phases of nystagmus that are directed upward or downward and inward. Divergent nystagmus may be an inappropriate manifestation of an otolithic response; normal individuals may show it during forward linear acceleration of the head.[329] In the rabbit, the projections from the flocculus to the vestibular nuclei inhibit only the adduction component of the horizontal vestibulo-ocular reflex.[153] A flocculus lesion might then lead to excessive adduction and divergence nystagmus. The convergence excess that often occurs with hindbrain anomalies may also be related to divergence nystagmus in such patients.

Repetitive divergence has been reported in a patient comatose due to hepatic encephalopathy.[243] The eyes slowly diverged to extreme bilateral abduction and then rapidly returned to the primary position. A similar abnormality was reported in a neonate in association with abnormalities of the electroencephalogram, perhaps related to seizures.[241]

EFFECTS OF CONVERGENCE ON CONJUGATE FORMS OF NYSTAGMUS

Convergence often damps or stops *congenital nystagmus* (see Video Display: Congenital Forms of Nystagmus), and this is the basis for treating such patients with spectacles that incorporate base-out prisms, which induce convergence (see Chapter 10). The mechanism by which convergence suppresses nystagmus is not clear. One hypothesis was that co-contraction of the medial and lateral rectus muscles might mechanically damp the oscillations in orbit. However, measurements of muscle forces using transducers embedded in the horizontal rectus muscles indicate that co-contraction of the horizontal rectus muscles does not occur during convergence.[229] Thus, the suppressive effects of convergence on nystagmus are probably centrally mediated. Occasionally, convergence increases congenital nystagmus, although this phenomenon is more common with acquired nystagmus (Fig. 10–16, Chapter 10).

Downbeat nystagmus may be brought out or accentuated by convergence. In some patients, convergence suppresses or changes the direction of the nystagmus, so that it becomes upbeat nystagmus (see Video Display: Downbeat, Upbeat, Torsional Nystagmus). Upbeat and torsional nystagmus may also be suppressed by convergence. In some patients, a convergent-divergent form of pendular nystagmus may be induced by convergence (for example, in patients with multiple sclerosis).[15,18,323]

Lid nystagmus may be affected by convergence tone. Thus, a patient with lateral medullary infarction (Wallenberg's syndrome) showed synchronous lid and ocular nystagmus that was suppressed by convergence.[67] Pure lid nystagmus, induced by convergence, has also been described.[299]

Convergence often induces small, high-frequency, conjugate ocular oscillations in normal subjects.[384] This is especially the case if a large vergence movement is made with a small saccade.[276] Some normal subjects can induce *voluntary flutter* as a party trick;[137,378] in fact, these movements are saccadic oscillations that are often induced with a convergence effort (see Video Display: Saccadic Oscillations and Intrusions).[275] In patients with pathological flutter or opsoclonus, combined saccadic-vergence movements can often bring out the oscillations.[22] The possible mechanism for these saccadic oscillations is discussed in Chapter 3.

SUMMARY

1. Vergence movements rotate the eyes in opposite directions to enable binocular fixation of a single object. Vergence movements occur in response to several distinct stimuli. Fusional (disparity) vergence movements are stimulated when images from one object fall on noncorresponding retinal elements in the two eyes. Accommodative vergence movements are stimulated by retinal blur. Another important stimulus for vergence is the sense of nearness (proximal vergence), which may be abstracted from cues such as size and motion. These stimulus-induced changes of vergence are superimposed upon an underlying level of vergence tone (tonic vergence). Vergence is also under a degree of voluntary control. Under normal circumstances, fusional and accommodative vergence are tightly coupled, each affecting the other through neural cross-linkage. Vergence movements occur synkinetically with accommodation of the lens and pupillary constriction (the near triad).
2. When performed without accompanying saccades, vergence movements are slow and show an approximately negative exponential waveform. In most natural circumstances, however, vergence movements are used in combination with saccades, to place the images of an object on both foveae, or with pursuit, to keep the images of a moving object on both foveae. When vergence is combined with saccades, the change in relative alignment is much faster than with vergence movements made alone (Fig. 8–4).
3. During a vergence movement from a far to a near target, ocular motoneurons show a phasic-tonic (velocity-position) change in innervation (Fig. 8–6). Premotor vergence neurons of three major types lie in the midbrain, dorsal and lateral to the oculomotor nuclei. They encode vergence velocity, vergence position, or a combination of both signals.
4. The maintenance of both static and dynamic ocular alignment is under long-term adaptive control to ensure that with every change of gaze, the lines of sight of both eyes are promptly brought to the fixation target, and kept there (Fig. 8–9).
5. Abnormal vergence eye movements should be differentiated from disorders of conjugate eye movements induced by convergence. Midbrain disorders that impair vertical gaze may also show ver-

gence abnormalities, especially convergence spasm, convergence-retraction nystagmus, and pseudo-abducens palsy. Selective impairment of fast or slow vergence responses may occur with pontine lesions. Divergence nystagmus (slow phases convergent, quick phases divergent) may be a sign of lesions at the craniocervical junction. Bilateral sixth nerve palsies must be differentiated from divergence palsy and from voluntary spasm of the near reflex, which is recognized by the accompanying miosis and full range of movement during monocular viewing or vestibulo-ocular testing.

REFERENCES

1. Akao T, Kurkin S, Fukushima K. Latency of adaptive vergence eye movements induced by vergence-vestibular interaction training in monkeys. Exp Brain Res 158, 129–132, 2004.
2. Akao T, Mustari MJ, Fukushima J, Kurkin SA, Fukushima K. Discharge characteristics of pursuit neurons in the MST during vergence eye movements. J Neurophysiol 93, 2415–2434, 2004.
3. Akman S, Dayanir V, Sanac A, Kansu T. Acquired esotropia as presenting sign of cranio-cervical junction anomalies. Neuro-ophthalmol 15, 311–314, 1995.
4. Albano JE, Marrero JA. Binocular interactions in rapid saccadic adaptation. Vision Res 35, 3439–3450, 1995.
5. Allison RS, Howard IP, Fang X. Depth selectivity of vertical fusional mechanisms. Vision Res 40, 2985–2998, 2000.
6. Allison RS, Howard IP, Fang X. The stimulus integration area for horizontal vergence. Exp Brain Res 156, 305–313, 2004.
7. Alvarez TL, Semmlow JL, Pedrono C. Divergence eye movements are dependent on initial stimulus position. Vision Res 45, 1847–1855, 2005.
8. Alvarez TL, Semmlow JL, Yuan W. Closely spaced, fast dynamic movements in disparity vergence. J Neurophysiol 79, 37–44, 1998.
9. Alvarez TL, Semmlow JL, Yuan W, Munoz P. Dynamic details of disparity convergence eye movements. Ann Biomed Eng 27, 380–390, 1999.
10. Alvarez TL, Semmlow JL, Yuan W, Munoz P. Disparity vergence double responses processed by internal error. Vision Res 40, 341–347, 2000.
11. Angelaki DE. Eyes on target: what neurons must do for the vestibuloocular reflex during linear motion. J Neurophysiol 92, 20–35, 2004.
12. Arai M, Fujii S. Divergence paralysis associated with the ingestion of diazepam. J Neurol 237, 45–46, 1990.
13. Averbuch-Heller L, Lewis RF, Zee DS. Disconjugate adaptation of saccades: contribution of binocular and monocular mechanisms. Vision Res 39, 341–352, 1999.
14. Averbuch-Heller L, Rottach KG, Zivotofsky AZ, et al. Torsional eye movements in patients with skew deviation and spasmodic torticollis: responses to static and dynamic head roll. Neurology 48, 506–514, 1997.
15. Averbuch-Heller L, Zivotofsky AZ, Remler BF, et al. Convergent-divergent pendular nystagmus: possible role of the vergence system. Neurology 45, 509–515, 1995.
16. Backus BT, Banks MS, van Ee R, Crowell JA. Horizontal and vertical disparity, eye position, and stereoscopic slant perception. Vision Res 39, 1143–1170, 1999.
17. Backus BT, Fleet DJ, Parker AJ, Heeger DJ. Human cortical activity correlates with stereoscopic depth perception. J Neurophysiol 86, 2054–2068, 2001.
18. Barton JJ, Cox TA, Digre KB. Acquired convergence-evoked pendular nystagmus in multiple sclerosis. J Neuro-ophthalmol 19, 34–38, 1999.
19. Benton AL, Hacaen H. Stereoscopic vision in patients with unilateral cerebral disease. Neurology 20, 1084–1088, 1970.
20. Bernstein R, Bernardini GL. Abnormal vergence with upper brainstem infarcts: pseudoabducens palsy. Neurology 56, 424–425, 2001.
21. Bhidayasiri R, Riley DE, Somers JT, et al. Pathophysiology of slow vertical saccades in progressive supranuclear palsy. Neurology 57, 2070–2077, 2001.
22. Bhidayasiri R, Somers JT, Kim JI, et al. Ocular oscillations induced by shifts of the direction and depth of visual fixation. Ann Neurol 49, 24–28, 2001.
23. Bielschowsky A. Lectures on motor anomalies. Dartmouth College Publications, Hanover, NH, 1943.
24. Bobier WR, McRae M. Gain changes in the accommodative convergence cross-link. Ophthalmic Physiol Opt 16, 318–325, 1996.
25. Brautaset RL, Jennings JA. Distance vergence adaptation is abnormal in subjects with convergence insufficiency. Ophthal Physiol Opt 25, 211–214, 2005.
26. Brautaset RL, Jennings JA. Horizontal and vertical prism adaptation are different mechanisms. Ophthal Physiol Opt 25, 215–218, 2005.
27. Brenner W, Van den Berg AV, Van Damme WJ. Perceived motion in depth. Vision Res 36, 699–706, 1996.
28. Bucci MP, Kapoula Z, Eggert T, Garraud L. Deficiency of adaptive control of the binocular coordination of saccades in strabismus. Vision Res 37, 2767–2777, 1997.
29. Bucci MP, Kapoula Z, Yang Q, Bremond-Gignac D, Wiener-Vacher S. Speed-accuracy of saccades, vergence and combined eye movements in children with vertigo. Exp Brain Res 157, 286–295, 2004.
30. Bucci MP, Kapoula Z, Yang Q, Wiener-Vacher S, Bremond-Gignac D. Abnormality of vergence latency in children with vertigo. J Neurol 251, 204–213, 2004.
31. Bucci MP, Pouvreau N, Yang Q, Kapoula Z. Influence of gap and overlap paradigms on saccade latencies and vergence eye movements in seven-year-old children. Exp Brain Res 164, 48–57, 2005.
32. Burke JP, Firth AY. Temporary prism treatment of acute esotropia precipitated by fusion disruption. Br J Ophthalmol 79, 787–788, 1995.
33. Busettini C, FitzGibbon EJ, Miles FA. Short-latency disparity vergence in humans. J Neurophysiol 85, 1129–1152, 2001.
34. Busettini C, Masson GS, Miles FA. A role for stereoscopic depth cues in the rapid visual stabilization of the eyes. Nature 380, 342–345, 1996.
35. Busettini C, Masson GS, Miles FA. Radial optic flow induces vergence eye movements with ultra-short latencies. Nature 390, 512–515, 1997.

36. Busettini C, Mays LE. Pontine omnipause activity during conjugate and disconjugate eye movements in macaques. J Neurophysiol 90, 3838–3853, 2003.
37. Busettini C, Mays LE. Saccade-vergence interactions in macaques. I.Test of the omnipause multiply model. J Neurophysiol 94, 2295–2311, 2005.
38. Busettini C, Mays LE. Saccade-vergence interactions in macaques. II. Vergence enhancement as the product of a local feedback vergence motor error and a weighted saccadic burst. J Neurophysiol 94, 2312–2330, 2005.
39. Busettini C, Miles FA, Krauzlis RJ. Short-latency disparity vergence responses and their dependence on a prior saccadic eye movement. J Neurophysiol 75, 1392–1410, 1996.
40. Bush GA, Van der Steen J, Miles FA. When the two eyes see patterns of unequal size they produce saccades of unequal amplitude. In Delgado-García JM, Godaux E, Vidal P-P (eds). Information Processing Underlying Gaze Control. Pergamon Press, 1994, pp 261–267.
41. Büttner-Ennever JA, Horn AK, Graf W, Ugolini G. Modern concepts of brainstem anatomy: from extraocular motoneurons to proprioceptive pathways. Ann N Y Acad Sci 956, 75–84, 2002.
42. Büttner-Ennever JA, Horn AK, Henn V, Cohen B. Projections from the superior colliculus motor map to omnipause neurons in monkey. J Comp Neurol 413, 55–67, 1999.
43. Carter DB. Fixation disparity and heterophoria following prolonged wearing of prism. J Optom 42, 141–151, 1965.
44. Chaturvedi V, Gisbergen JA. Shared target selection for combined version-vergence eye movements. J Neurophysiol 80, 849–862, 1998.
45. Chaturvedi V, Van Gisbergen JA. Specificity of saccadic adaptation in three-dimensional space. Vision Res 37, 1367–1382, 1997.
46. Chaturvedi V, Van Gisbergen JA. Stimulation in the rostral pole of monkey superior colliculus: effects on vergence eye movements. Exp Brain Res 132, 72–78, 2000.
47. Choi KD, Jung DS, Kim JS. Specificity of "peering at the tip of the nose" for a diagnosis of thalamic hemorrhage. Arch Neurol 61, 417–422, 2004.
48. Clendaniel RA, Mays LE. Characteristics of antidromically identified oculomotor internuclear neurons during vergence and versional eye movements. J Neurophysiol 71, 1111–1127, 1994.
49. Cogan DG, Freese CG. Spasm of the near reflex. Arch Ophthalmol 54, 752–759, 1955.
50. Colby CL, Duhamel JR, Goldberg ME. Ventral intraparietal area of the macaque: anatomic location and visual response properties. J Neurophysiol 69, 902–914, 1993.
51. Collewijn H, Erkelens CJ. Binocular eye movements and the perception of depth. In Kowler E (ed). Eye movements and their role in visual and cognitive processes. Elsevier, Amsterdam, 1990, pp 213–261.
52. Collewijn H, Erkelens CJ, Steinman RM. Binocular co-ordination of human horizontal saccadic eye movements. J Physiol (Lond) 404, 157–182, 1988.
53. Collewijn H, Erkelens CJ, Steinman R.M. Voluntary binocular gaze-shifts in the plane of regard: dynamics of version and vergence. Vision Res 35, 3335–3358, 1995.
54. Collewijn H, Erkelens CJ, Steinman RM. Trajectories of the human binocular fixation point during conjugate and non-conjugate gaze-shifts. Vision Res 37, 1049–1069, 1997.
55. Collewijn H, Kapoula Z. Binocular oculomotor coordination and plasticity. Vision Res 35, 3207–3540, 1995.
56. Collewijn H, Steinman RM, Erkelens CJ, Regan D. Binocular fusion, stereopsis and stereoacuity with a moving head. In Regan D (ed). Vision and Visual Dysfunction. MacMillan, London, 1991, pp 121–136.
57. Cooper J. Clinical implications of vergence adaptation. Optom Vis Sci 69, 300–307, 1992.
58. Coria F, Rebollo M, Quintana F, Polo J, Berciano J. Occipitoatlantal instability and vertebrobasilar ischemia: case report. Neurology 32, 303–305, 1982.
59. Cornell ED, MacDougall HG, Predebon J, Curthoys IS. Errors of binocular fixation are common in normal subjects during natural conditions. Optom Vis Sci 80, 764–771, 2003.
60. Coubard O, Daunys G, Kapoula Z. Gap effects on saccade and vergence latency. Exp Brain Res 154, 368–381, 2004.
61. Coubard O, Kapoula Z, Muri R, Rivaud-Pechoux S. Effects of TMS over the right prefrontal cortex on latency of saccades and convergence. Invest Ophthalmol Vis Sci 44, 600–609, 2003.
62. Cova A, Galiana HL. Providing distinct vergence and version dynamics in a bilateral oculomotor network. Vision Res 35, 3359–3371, 1995.
63. Crane BT, Demer JL. Human horizontal vestibulo-ocular reflex initiation: effects of acceleration, target distance, and unilateral deafferentation. J Neurophysiol 80, 1151–1166, 1998.
64. Cumming BG, Judge SJ. Disparity-induced and blur-induced convergence eye movements and accommodation in the monkey. J Neurophysiol 55, 896–914, 1986.
65. Dagi LR, Chrousos GA, Cogan DG. Spasm of the near reflex associated with organic disease. Am J Ophthalmol 103, 582–585, 1987.
66. Daroff RB, Hoyt WF. Supranuclear disorders of ocular control systems in man: Clinical, anatomical and physiological correlations. In Bach-y-Rita P, Collins CC, Hyde JE (eds). The Control of Eye Movements. Academic Press, New York, 1971, pp 175–236.
67. Daroff RB, Hoyt WF, Sanders MD, Nelson LR. Gaze-evoked eye-lid and ocular nystagmus inhibited by the near reflex: unusual ocular motor phenomena in a lateral medullary syndrome. J Neurol Neurosurg Psychiatry 31, 362–367, 1968.
68. DeAngelis GC, Cumming BG, Newsome WT. Cortical area MT and the perception of stereoscopic depth. Nature 394, 677–680, 1998.
69. Demer JL. Ocular kinematics, vergence, and orbital mechanics. Strabismus 11, 49–57, 2003.
70. Demer JL, Clark CH, Howard TD, Miller JM. The oculomotor plant simplifies binocular yoking during vertical gaze shift [abstract]. Invest Ophthalmol Vis Sci 37, B699, 1996.
71. Ebenholtz SM, Citek K. Absence of adaptive plasticity after voluntary vergence and accommodation. Vision Res 35, 2773–2783, 1995.
72. Eggert T, Kapoula Z. Position dependency of rapidly induced saccade disconjugacy. Vision Res 35, 3493–3503, 1995.
73. Enright JT. Changes in vergence mediated by saccades. J Physiol 350, 9–31, 1984.

74. Enright JT. Perspective vergence: oculomotor responses to line drawings. Vision Res 27, 1513–1526, 1987.
75. Enright JT. The cyclopean eye and its implications: vergence state and visual direction. Vision Res 28, 925–930, 1988.
76. Enright JT. The remarkable saccades of asymmetrical vergence. Vision Res 32, 2261–2276, 1992.
77. Enright JT. Unexpected role of the oblique muscles in the human vertical fusional reflex. J Physiol (Lond) 451, 279–293, 1992.
78. Enright JT. Slow-velocity asymmetrical convergence: a decisive failure of "Hering's law". Vision Res 36, 3667–3684, 1996.
79. Enright JT. Monocularly programmed human saccades during vergence changes? J Physiol (Lond) 512, 235–250, 1998.
80. Erkelens CJ. Adaptation of ocular vergence to stimulation with large disparities. Exp Brain Res 66, 507–516, 1987.
81. Erkelens CJ, Collewijn H. Control of vergence: gating among disparity inputs by voluntary target selection. Exp Brain Res 87, 671–678, 1991.
82. Erkelens CJ, Collewijn H, Steinman RM. Asymmetrical adaptation of human saccades to anisometropia spectacles. Invest Ophthalmol Vis Sci 30, 1132–1145, 1989.
83. Erkelens CJ, van der Steen SJ, Steinman RM, Collewijn H. Ocular vergence under natural conditions. I. Continuous changes of target distance along the median plane. Proc R Soc Lond B Biol Sci 236, 417–440, 1989.
84. Fincham EF, Walton J. The reciprocal actions of accommodation and convergence. J Physiol (Lond) 137, 488–508, 1957.
85. Findlay JM, Harris LR. Horizontal saccades to dichoptically presented targets of differing disparities. Vision Res 33, 1001–1010, 1993.
86. Fioravanti F, Inchingolo P, Pensiero S, Spanio M. Saccadic eye movement conjugation in children. Vision Res 35, 3217–3238, 1995.
87. Firth AY. The role of vergence adaptation in recovery of binocular single vision (BSV) following sensory strabismus. Strabismus 7, 237–240, 1999.
88. Fisher SK, Ciuffreda KJ. Adaptation to optically increased interocular separation under naturalistic viewing conditions. Perception 19, 171–180, 1990.
89. Fogt N, Jones R. Comparison of the monocular occlusion and a direct method for objective measurement of fixation disparity. Optom Vis Sci 74, 43–50, 1997.
90. Fogt N, Toole AJ. The effect of saccades and brief fusional stimuli on phoria adaptation. Optom Vis Sci 78, 815–824, 2001.
91. Fowler S, Munro N, Richardson A, Stein J. Vergence control in patients with lesions of the posterior parietal cortex. J Physiol (Lond) 417, 92p, 1989.
92. Friling R, Yassur Y, Merkin L, Herishanu O. Divergence paralysis versus bilateral sixth nerve palsy in an incomplete Miller-Fisher syndrome. Neuro-ophthalmol 4, 215–217, 1993.
93. Fukushima J, Akao T, Takeichi N, et al. Pursuit-related neurons in the supplementary eye fields: discharge during pursuit and passive whole body rotation. J Neurophysiol 91, 2809–2825, 2004.
94. Fukushima K, Yamanobe T, Shinmei Y, Fukushima J, Kurkin S. Role of the frontal eye fields in smooth-gaze tracking. Prog Brain Res 143, 391–401, 2004.
95. Fukushima K, Yamanobe T, Shinmei Y, et al. Coding of smooth eye movements in three-dimensional space by frontal cortex. Nature 419, 157–162, 2002.
96. Gallaway M, Scheiman M, Malhotra K. The effectiveness of pencil pushups treatment for convergence insufficiency: a pilot study. Optom Vis Sci 79, 265–267, 2002.
97. Gamlin PD, Gnadt JW, Mays LE. Abducens internuclear neurons carry an inappropriate signal for ocular convergence. J Neurophysiol 62, 70–81, 1989.
98. Gamlin PD, Gnadt JW, Mays LE. Lidocaine-induced unilateral internuclear ophthalmoplegia: effects on convergence and conjugate eye movements. J Neurophysiol 62, 82–95, 1989.
99. Gamlin PDR. Subcortical neural circuits for ocular accommodation and vergence in primates. Ophthalmic Physiol Opt 19, 81–89, 1999.
100. Gamlin PDR. Neural mechanisms for the control of vergence eye movements. Ann N Y Acad Sci 956, 264–272, 2002.
101. Gamlin PDR, Mays LE. Dynamic properties of medial rectus motoneurons during vergence eye movements. J Neurophysiol 67, 64–74, 1992.
102. Gamlin PDR, Yoon K. An area for vergence eye movement in primate frontal cortex. Nature 407, 1003–1007, 2000.
103. Gamlin PDR, Yoon K, Zhang H. The role of cerebro-ponto-cerebellar pathways in the control of vergence eye movements. Eye 10, 167–171, 1996.
104. Gamlin PDR, Zhang HY. Effects of muscimol blockade of the posterior fastigial nucleus on vergence and ocular accommodation in the primate. Soc Neurosci Abst 22, 1034, 1996.
105. Genovesio A, Ferraina S. Integration of retinal disparity and fixation-distance related signals toward an egocentric coding of distance in the posterior parietal cortex of primates. J Neurophysiol 91, 2670–2684, 2004.
106. Gnadt JW, Mays LE. Neurons in monkey parietal area LIP are tuned for eye-movement parameters in three-dimensional space. J Neurophysiol 73, 280–297, 1995.
107. Goldstein JH, Schneekloth BB. Spasm of the near reflex: a spectrum of anomalies. Surv Opthalmology 40, 269–278, 1996.
108. Gomez CR, Gomez SM, Selhorst JB. Acute thalamic esotropia. Neurology 38, 1759–1762, 1988.
109. Graf EW, Maxwell JS, Schor CM. Changes in cyclotorsion and vertical eye alignment during prolonged monocular occlusion. Vision Res 42, 1185–1194, 2002.
110. Green JF. Plasticity of the vergence system. Transactions of the VIII International Orthoptics Conference 3–14, 1995.
111. Griffin JF, Wray SH, Anderson DP. Misdiagnosis of spasm of the near reflex. Neurology 26, 1018–1020, 1976.
112. Grishham JD. Visual therapy results for convergence insufficiency. Am J Optom Physiol Opt 65, 448–454, 1988.
113. Grishham JD, Bowman MC, Owyang LA., Chan C.L. Vergence orthoptics: validity and persistence of the training effect. Optom Vis Sci 68, 441–451, 1991.
114. Gulyás B, Roland PE. Binocularity disparity discrimination in human cerebral cortex: Functional

anatomy by positron emission tomography. Proc Natl Acad Sci 91, 1239–1243, 1994.
115. Guyton DL. Dissociated vertical deviation: etiology, mechanism, and associated phenomena. Costenbader Lecture. J AAPOS 4, 131–144, 2000.
116. Hain TC, Luebke AE. Phoria adaptation in patients with cerebellar dysfunction. Invest Ophthalmol Vis Sci 31, 1394–1397, 1990.
117. Hainline L, Riddell PM. Development of accommodation and convergence in infancy. Vision Res 35, 3229–3236, 1995.
118. Haker H, Misslisch H, Ott M, et al. Three-dimensional vestibular eye and head reflexes of the chameleon: characteristics of gain and phase and effects of eye position on orientation of ocular rotation axes during stimulation in yaw direction. J Comp Physiol 189, 509–517, 2003.
119. Han Y, Somers JT, Kim JI, Kumar AN, Leigh RJ. Ocular responses to head rotations during mirror viewing. J Neurophysiol 86, 2323–2329, 2001.
120. Han YH, Kumar AN, Reschke MF, et al. Vestibular and non-vestibular contributions to eye movements that compensate for head rotations during viewing of near targets. Exp Brain Res 165, 295–304, 2005.
121. Hara N, Steffen H, Roberts DC, Zee DS. Effects of horizontal vergence on the motor and sensory components of vertical fusion. Invest Ophthalmol Vis Sci 39:2268–2276, 1998.
122. Hasebe H, Oyamada H, Kinomura S, et al. Human cortical areas activated in relation to vergence eye movements—a PET study. Neuroimage 10, 200–208, 1999.
123. Helmholtz Hv. Treatise on Physiological Optics (1910). Dover, New York, 1962.
124. Henson DB, Dharamshi BG. Oculomotor adaptation to induced heterophoria and anisometropia. Invest Ophthalmol Vis Sci 22, 234–240, 1982.
125. Hentschel SJ, Yen KG, Lang FF. Chiari I malformation and acute acquired comitant esotropia: case report and review of the literature. J Neurosurg 102, 407–412, 2005.
126. Hering E. Die Lehre Vom binocularen Sehen (1868, Leipzig, Engelmann). Plenum Press, New York, 1977.
127. Herman P. Convergence spasm. Mt Sinai J Med 44, 501–509, 1977.
128. Heron G, Charman WN, Schor C. Dynamics of the accommodation response to abrupt changes in target vergence as a function of age. Vision Res 41, 507–519, 2001.
129. Heron G, Charman WN, Schor CM. Age changes in the interactions between the accommodation and vergence systems. Optom Vis Sci 78, 754–762, 2001.
130. Hertle RW, Bienfang DC. Oculographic analysis of acute esotropia secondary to a thalamic hemorrhage. J Clin Neuro-ophthalmol 10, 21–26, 1990.
131. Holmes G. Clinical symptoms of cerebellar disease and their interpretation (Croonian lectures III.). Lancet ii, 59–65, 1922.
132. Holmes JM, Kaz KM. Recovery of phorias following monocular occlusion. J Pediatr Ophthalmol Strabismus 31, 110–113, 1994.
133. Hooge IT, Van den Berg AV. Visually evoked cyclovergence and extended listing's law. J Neurophysiol 83, 2757–2775, 2000.
134. Horng JL, Semmlow JL, Hung GK, Ciuffreda KJ. Dynamic asymmetries in disparity convergence eye movements. Vision Res 38, 2761–2768, 1998.
135. Horton JC, Fishman RA. Neurovisual findings in the syndrome of spontaneous intracranial hypotension from dural cerebrospinal fluid leak [abstract]. Ophthalmology 101, 244–251, 1994.
136. Horwood A. Neonatal ocular misalignments reflect vergence development but rarely become esotropia. Br J Ophthalmol 87, 1146–1150, 2003.
137. Hotson JR. Convergence-initiated voluntary flutter: a normal intrinsic capability in man. Brain Res 294, 299–304, 1984.
138. Houtman WA, Roze JH, Scheper W. Vertical vergence movements. Doc Ophthalmol 51, 199–207, 1981.
139. Howard IP, Allison RS, Zacher JE. The dynamics of vertical vergence. Exp Brain Res 116, 153–159, 1997.
140. Howard IP, Fang X, Allison RS, Zacher JE. Effects of stimulus size and eccentricity on horizontal and vertical vergence. Exp Brain Res 130, 124–132, 2000.
141. Howard IP, Ohmi M, Sun L. Cyclovergence: a comparison of objective and psychophysical measurements. Exp Brain Res 97, 349–355, 1993.
142. Howard IP, Rogers BJ. Seeing in Depth. I. Porteous, Toronto, 2002.
143. Howard IP, Sun L, Shen X. Cycloversion and cyclovergence: the effects of the area and the position of the visual display. Exp Brain Res 100, 509–514, 1994.
144. Hoyt CS, Good WV. Acute onset comcomitant esotropia: when is it a sign of serious neurological disease? Br J Ophthalmol 79, 498–501, 1995.
145. Hung GC, Ciuffreda KJ, Semmlow JL, Horng J-L. Vergence eye movements under natural viewing conditions. Invest Ophthalmol Vis Sci 35, 3486–3492, 1994.
146. Hung GK. Adaptation model of accommodation and vergence. Ophthalmic Physiol Opt 12, 319–326, 1992.
147. Hung GK. Saccade-vergence trajectories under free- and instrument-space environments. Curr Eye Res 17, 159–164, 1998.
148. Hung GK, Zhu H, Ciuffreda KJ. Convergence and divergence exhibit different response characteristics to symmetric stimuli. Vision Res 37, 1197–1205, 1997.
149. Hwang JM, Guyton DL. The Lancaster red-green test before and after occlusion in the evaluation of incomitant strabismus. J AAPOS 3, 151–156, 1999.
150. Inchingolo P, Accardo A, Da Pozzo S, Pensiero S, Perissutti P. Cyclopean and disconjugate adaptive recovery from post-saccadic drift in strabismic children before and after surgery. Vision Res 36, 2897–2913, 1996.
151. Inchingolo P, Optican LM, FitzGibbon EJ, Goldberg ME. Adaptive mechanisms in the monkey saccadic system. In Schmid R, Zambarbieri D (eds). Oculomotor Control and Cognitive Processes. Elsevier, Amsterdam, pp 147–162, 1991.
152. Inoue Y, Takemura A, Suehiro K, Kodaka Y, Kawano K. Short-latency vergence eye movements elicited by looming step in monkeys. Neurosci Res 32, 185–188, 1998.
153. Ito M, Nisimaru N, Yamamoto M. Specific patterns of neuronal connexions involved in the control of the rabbit's vestibulo-ocular reflexes by the cerebellar flocculus. J Physiol (Lond) 265, 833–854, 1977.

154. Ivins JP, Porrill J, Frisby JP. Instability of torsion during smooth asymmetric vergence. Vision Res 39, 993–1009, 1999.
155. Jones R, Stephens GL. Horizontal fusional amplitudes—Evidence for disparity tuning. Invest Ophthalmol Vis Sci 30, 1638–1642, 1989.
156. Judge SJ. Optically-induced changes in tonic vergence and AC/A ratios in normal monkeys and monkeys with lesions of the flocculus and the ventral paraflocculus. Exp Brain Res 66, 1–9, 1987.
157. Judge SJ. Vergence. In Carpenter RHS (ed). Eye Movements. MacMillan Press, London, 1991, pp 157–174.
158. Judge SJ, Cumming BG. Neurons in the monkey midbrain with activity related to vergence eye movements and accommodation. J Neurophysiol 55, 915–930, 1986.
159. Judge SJ, Miles FA. Changes in the coupling between accommodation and vergence eye movements induced in human subjects by altering the effective interocular separation. Perception 14, 617–629, 1985.
160. Kapoula Z, Bernotas M, Haslwanter T. Listing's plane rotation with convergence: role of disparity, accommodation, and depth perception. Exp Brain Res 126, 175–186, 1999.
161. Kapoula Z, Eggert T, Bucci MP. Immediate saccade amplitude disconjugacy induced by unequal images. Vision Res 35, 3505–3518, 1995.
162. Kapoula Z, Eggert T, Bucci MP. Disconjugate adaptation of the vertical ocular motor system. Vision Res 36, 2735–2745, 1996.
163. Kapoula Z, Hain TC, Zee DS, Robinson DA. Adaptive changes in post-saccadic drift induced by patching one eye. Vision Res 27, 1299–1307, 1987.
164. Kapoula Z, Yang Q, Coubard O, Daunys G, Orssaud C. Transcranial magnetic stimulation of the posterior parietal cortex delays the latency of both isolated and combined vergence-saccade movements in humans. Neurosci Lett 360, 95–99, 2004.
165. Kapoula Z, Yang Q, Coubard O, Daunys G, Orssaud C. Contextual influence of TMS on the latency of saccades and vergence. Neurosci Lett 376, 87–92, 2005.
166. Kawata H, Ohtsuka K. Dynamic asymmetries in convergence eye movements under natural viewing conditions. Jpn J Ophthalmol 45, 437–444, 2001.
167. Keane JR. Pretectal pseudobobbing. Five patients with 'V'-pattern convergence nystagmus. Arch Neurol 42, 592–594, 1985.
168. Keller EL. Accommodative vergence in the alert monkey. Vision Res 13, 1565–1575, 1973.
169. Keller EL, Robinson DA. Abducens unit behavior in the monkey during vergence eye movements. Vision Res 12, 369–382, 1972.
170. Kenyon RV, Ciuffreda KJ, Stark L. Binocular eye movements during accommodative vergence. Vision Res 18, 545–555, 1978.
171. Kenyon RV, Ciuffreda KJ, Stark L. Unequal saccades during vergence. Am J Optom Physiol Opt 57, 586–594, 1980.
172. Kerkhoff G, Stögerer E. Behandlung von Fusionsstörungen bei Patienten nach Hirnschädigung. Klin Monatsbl Augenheilkd 205, 70–75, 1994.
173. Kerkhoff G, Stögerer E. Recovery of fusional convergence after systematic practice. Brain Injury 8, 15–22, 1994.
174. Kersten D, Legge GE. Convergence accommodation. J Opt Soc Am 73, 332–338, 1983.
175. Kertesz AE. Vertical and cycloversional disparity vergence. In Schor CM, Ciuffreda KJ (eds). Vergence Eye Movements: Basic and Clinical Aspects. Butterworths, Woburn, MA, 1983, pp 317–348.
176. King WM, Zhou W. Initiation of disjunctive smooth pursuit in monkeys: evidence that Hering's law of equal innervation is not obeyed by the smooth pursuit system. Vision Res 35, 3389–3400, 1995.
177. King WM, Zhou W. Neural basis of disjunctive eye movements. Ann N Y Acad Sci 956, 273–283, 2002.
178. Kirkham TH, Bird AC, Sander MD. Divergence paralysis with raised intracranial pressure. Br J Ophthalmol 56, 776–782, 1972.
179. Kitthaweesin K, Riley DE, Leigh RJ. Vergence disorders in progressive supranuclear palsy. Ann N Y Acad Sci 956, 504–507, 2002.
180. Koene A, Erkelens C. Mechanical interdependence of version and vergence eye movements. Strabismus 11, 221–227, 2003.
181. Koken P, Erkelens CJ. Short delays of vergence eye movements in man during pursuit tasks in light and dark conditions. In d'YDewalle G, van Rinsbergen J (eds). Studies in Visual Information Processing, III. North-Holland, Amsterdam,1992.
182. Kommerell G, Jaedicke S. Dissoziierter Nystagmus als Symptom des Naheinstellungsspasmus. 1972. Munchen, JF Bergmann. Bericht über die 71. usammenkunft der Deutschen Ophthalm. Gesellschaft in Heidelberg1971.
183. Kono R, Hasebe S, Ohtsuki H, Kashihara K, Shiro Y. Impaired vertical phoria adaptation in patients with cerebellar dysfunction. Invest Ophth Vis Sci 43, 673–678, 2002.
184. Krishnan VV, Stark L. Models of the disparity vergence system. In Schor CM, Ciuffreda KJ (eds). Vergence Eye Movements: Basic and Clinical Aspects. Butterworths, Woburn, MA, 1983, pp 349–371.
185. Krohel GB, Kristan RW, Simon JW, Barrows NA. Divergence paralysis. Am J Ophthalmol 94, 506–510, 1982.
186. Krohel GB, Kristan RW, Simon JW, Barrows NA. Posttraumatic convergence insufficiency. Ann Ophthalmol 18, 101–104, 1986.
187. Kromeier M, Schmitt C, Bach M, Kommerell G. Stereoacuity versus fixation disparity as indicators for vergence accuracy under prismatic stress. Ophthalmic Physiol Opt 23, 43–49, 2003.
188. Krommenhoek KP, Van Gisbergen JA. Evidence for nonretinal feedback in combined version-vergence eye movements. Exp Brain Res 102, 95–109, 1994.
189. Kumar AN, Han Y, Dell'osso LF, Durand DM, Leigh RJ. Directional asymmetry during combined saccade-vergence movements. J Neurophysiol 93, 2797–2808, 2004.
190. Kumar AN, Han Y, Garbutt S, Leigh RJ. Properties of anticipatory vergence responses. Invest Ophthalmol Vis Sci 43, 2626–2632, 2002.
191. Larson WL, Faubert J. An investigation of prism adaptation latency. Optom Vis Sci 71, 38–42, 1994.
192. Lee SA, Sunwoo IN, Kim KW. Divergence paralysis due to a small hematoma in the tegmentum of the brainstem. Yonsei Med J 28, 326–328, 1987.
193. Leigh RJ. Throwing a glance: fast vergence eye movements. Neurology 64, 179, 2005.

194. Lemij HG, Collewijn H. Long-term nonconjugate adaptation of human saccades to anisometropic spectacles. Vision Res 31, 1939–1953, 1991.
195. Lemij HG, Collewijn H. Short-term nonconjugate adaptation of human saccades to anisometropic spectacles. Vision Res 31, 1955–1966, 1991.
196. Lewis AR, Kline LB, Sharpe JA. Acquired esotropia due to Arnold-Chiari I Malformation. J Neuro-ophthalmol 16, 49–54, 1996.
197. Lewis RF, Clendaniel RA, Zee DS. Vergence-dependent adaptation of the vestibulo-ocular reflex. Exp Brain Res 152, 335–340, 2003.
198. Lewis RF, Zee DS, Gaymard B, Guthrie B. Extraocular muscle proprioception functions in the control of ocular alignment and eye movement conjugacy. J Neurophysiol 71, 1028–1031, 1994.
199. Liesch A, Simonsz HJ. Up- and downshoot in adduction after monocular patching in normal volunteers. Strabismus 1, 25–36, 1993.
200. Lim L, Rosenbaum AL, Demer JL. Saccadic velocity analysis in patients with divergence paralysis. J Pediatr Ophthalmol Strabismus 32, 76–81, 1995.
201. Lindblom B, Westheimer G, Hoyt WF. Torsional diplopia and its perceptual consequences. Neuro-ophthalmol 18, 105–110, 1997.
202. Luu CD, Abel L. The plasticity of vertical motor and sensory fusion in normal subjects. Strabismus 11, 109–118, 2003.
203. Maddox EE. The Clinical Use of Prisms: and the Decentering of Lenses. John Wright & Sons, Bristol, England, 1893.
204. Malinov IV, Epelboim J, Herst AN, Steinman RM. Characteristics of saccades and vergence in two kinds of sequential looking tasks. Vision Res 40, 2083–2090, 2000.
205. Masson GS, Busettini C, Miles FA. Vergence eye movements in response to binocular disparity without depth perception. Nature 389, 283–286, 1997.
206. Maxwell JS, King WM. Dynamics and efficacy of saccade-facilitated vergence eye movements in monkeys. J Neurophysiol 68, 1248–1260, 1992.
207. Maxwell JS, Schor CM. Adaptation of vertical eye alignment in relation to head tilt. Vision Res 36, 1195–1205, 1996.
208. Maxwell JS, Schor CM. Head-position-dependent adaptation of non-concomitant vertical skew. Vision Res 37, 441–446, 1997.
209. Maxwell JS, Schor CM. Adaptation of torsional eye alignment in relation to head roll. Vision Res 39, 4192–4199, 1999.
210. Maxwell JS, Schor CM. Symmetrical horizontal vergence contributes to the asymmetrical pursuit of targets in depth. Vision Res 44, 3015–3024, 2004.
211. May PJ, Porter JD, Gamlin PDR. Interconnections between the cerebellum and midbrain near response regions. J Comp Neurol 315, 98–116, 1992.
212. Mays LE. Neural control of vergence eye movements: convergence and divergence neurons in the midbrain. J Neurophysiol 51, 1091–1108, 1984.
213. Mays LE. Has Hering been hooked? Nature Med 4, 889–890, 1998.
214. Mays LE, Gamlin PD. Neuronal circuitry controlling the near response. Curr Opin Neurobiol 5, 763–768, 1995.
215. Mays LE, Gamlin PDR. A neural mechanism subserving saccade-vergence interactions. In Findlay JM, Walker R, Kentridge RW (eds). Eye Movement Research: Mechanisms, Processes and Applications. Elsevier, Amsterdam, 1995, pp 215–223.
216. Mays LE, Porter JD. Neural control of vergence eye movements: activity of abducens and oculomotor neurons. J Neurophysiol 52, 743–761, 1984.
217. Mays LE, Porter JD, Gamlin PD, Tello CA. Neural control of vergence eye movements: neurons encoding vergence velocity. J Neurophysiol 56, 1007–1021, 1986.
218. McCandless JW, Schor CM. A neural net model of the adaptation of binocular vertical alignment. Network: Comput Neural Syst 8, 55–70, 1997.
219. McCandless JW, Schor CM. An association matrix model of context-specific vertical vergence adaptation. Network: Comput Neural Syst 8, 239–258, 1997.
220. McConville K, Tomlinson RD, King WM, Paige G, Na EQ. Eye position signals in the vestibular nuclei: consequences for models of integrator function. J Vestib Res 4, 391–400, 1994.
221. McLin LN, Schor CM. Changing size (looming) as a stimulus to accommodation and vergence. Vision Res 28, 883–896, 1988.
222. McLin LN, Schor CM. Voluntary effort as a stimulus to accommodation and vergence. Invest Ophthalmol Vis Sci 29, 1739–1746, 1988.
223. Mikhael S, Nicolle D, Vilis T. Rotation of Listing's plane by horizontal, vertical and oblique prism-induced vergence. Vision Res 35, 3243–3254, 1995.
224. Milder DG, Reinecke RD. Phoria adaptation to prisms: a cerebellar-dependent response. Arch Neurol 40, 339–342, 1983.
225. Miles FA. Adaptive regulation in the vergence and accommodation control systems. Rev Oculomot Res 1, 81–94, 1985.
226. Miles FA. Short-latency visual stabilization mechanisms that help to compensate for translational disturbances of gaze. Ann N Y Acad Sci 871, 260–271, 1999.
227. Miles FA, Fuller JH, Braitman DJ, Dow BA. Long-term adaptive changes in primate vestibuloocular reflex. III. Electrophysiological investigations in flocculus of normal monkeys. J Neurophysiol 43, 1437–1476, 1980.
228. Miles FA, Judge SJ, Optican LM. Optically induced changes in the couplings between vergence and accommodation. J Neurosci 7, 2576–2589, 1987.
229. Miller JM, Bockisch CJ, Pavlovski DS. Missing lateral rectus force and absence of medial rectus co-contraction in ocular convergence. J Neurophysiol 87, 2421–2433, 2002.
230. Minken AWH, Van Gisbergen JAM. Dynamical version-vergence interactions for a binocular implementation of Donders' law. Vision Res 36, 853–867, 1996.
231. Mokri B. Low cerebrospinal fluid syndromes. Neurol Clin 22, 55–74, 2004.
232. Morley JW, Judge SJ, Lindsey JW. Role of monkey midbrain near-response neurons in phoria adaptation. J Neurophysiol 67, 1475–1492, 1992.
233. Mossman S, Halmagyi GM. Partial ocular tilt reaction due to unilateral cerebellar lesion. Neurology 49, 491–493, 1997.
234. Moster ML, Hoenig EM. Spasm of the near reflex associated with metabolic encephalopathy. Neurology 38, 150, 1989.
235. Mottier CO, Mets MB. Vertical fusional vergence in patients with superior oblique muscle palsies. Am Orthopt J 40, 88–93, 1990.

236. Müller J. Elements of Physiology. Taylor & Walton, London, 1843.
237. Munoz P, Semmlow JL, Yuan W, Alvarez TL. Short term modification of disparity vergence eye movements. Vision Res 39, 1695–1705, 1999.
238. Müri RM, Rivaud S, Gaymard B, et al. Role of the prefrontal cortex in the control of express saccades. A transcranial magnetic stimulation study. Neuropsychologia 37, 199–206, 1999.
239. Neikter B. Effects of diagnostic occlusion on ocular alignment in normal subjects. Strabismus 2, 67–77, 1994.
240. Neikter B. Horizontal and vertical deviations after prism neutralization and diagnostic occlusion in intermittent exotropia. Strabismus 2, 13–22, 1994.
241. Nelson KR, Brenner RP, Carlow T. Divergent-convergence eye movements and transient eye lid opening associated with an EEG burst-suppression pattern. J Clin Neuro Ophthalmol 6, 43–46, 1986.
242. Newman NJ, Lessell S. Pupillary dilatation with monocular occlusion as a sign of nonorganic oculomotor dysfunction. Am J Ophthalmol 108, 461–462, 1989.
243. Noda S, Ide K, Umezaki H, Itoh H, Yamamoto K. Repetitive divergence. Ann Neurol 21, 109–110, 1987.
244. Nonaka F, Hasebe S, Ohtsuki H. Convergence accommodation to convergence (CA/C) ratio in patients with intermittent exotropia and decompensated exophoria. Jpn J Ophthalmol 48, 300–305, 2004.
245. North R, Henson DB. Adaptation to lens-induced heterophorias. Am J Optom Physiol Opt 62, 774–780, 1985.
246. North RV, Henson DB. The effect of orthoptic treatment upon the vergence adaptation mechanism. Optom Vis Sci 69, 294–299, 1992.
247. North RV, Sethi B, Owen K. Prism adaptation and viewing distance. Ophthal Physiol Opt 10, 81–85, 1990.
248. Ochs AL, Stark L, Hoyt WF, D'Amico D. Opposed adducting saccades in convergence-retraction nystagmus. A patient with sylvian aqueduct syndrome. Brain 102, 479–508, 1979.
249. Ogle KN, Prangen A. Observations on vertical divergences and hyperphorias. Arch Ophthalmol 49, 313–334, 1953.
250. Ohtsuka K, Maeda S, Oguri N. Accommodation and convergence palsy caused by lesions in the bilateral rostral superior colliculus. Am J Ophthalmol 133, 425–427, 2002.
251. Ohtsuka K, Maekawa H, Sawa M. Convergence paralysis after lesions of the cerebellar peduncles. Ophthalmologica 206, 143–148, 1993.
252. Ohtsuka K, Maekawa H, Takeda M, Uede N, Chiba S. Accommodation and convergence insufficiency with left middle cerebral artery occlusion. Am J Ophthalmol 106, 60–64, 1988.
253. Ohtsuki H, Hasabe S, Furuse T, et al. Contribution of vergence adaptation to difference in vertical deviation between distance and near viewing in patients with superior oblique palsy. Am J Ophthalmol 134, 252–260, 2002.
254. Ohyagi Y, Yamada T, Okayama A, et al. Vergence disorders in patients with spinocerebellar ataxia 3/Machado-Joseph disease: a synoptophore study. J Neurol Sci 173, 120–123, 2000.
255. Ono H. Binocular visual direction of an object when seen as single or double. In Regan D (ed). Binocular Vision. MacMillan Press, London, 1991, pp 1–18.
256. Oohira A. Vergence eye movements facilitated by saccades. Jpn J Ophthalmol 37, 400–413, 1993.
257. Oohira A, Zee DS. Disconjugate ocular motor adaptation in rhesus monkey. Vision Res 32, 489–497, 1992.
258. Oohira A, Zee DS, Guyton DL. Disconjugate adaptation to long-standing, large-amplitude, spectacle-corrected anisometropia. Invest Ophthalmol Vis Sci 32, 1693–1703, 1991.
259. Ott M. Chameleons have independent eye movements but synchronize both eyes during saccadic prey tracking. Exp Brain Res 139, 173–179, 2001.
260. Owens DA, Leibowitz HW. Perceptual and motor consequences of tonic vergence. In Schor CM, Ciuffreda KJ (eds). Vergence Eye Movements: Basic and Clinical Aspects. Butterworths, Boston, 1983, pp 25–74.
261. Page WK, Duffy CJ. Heading representation in MST: sensory interactions and population encoding. J Neurophysiol 89, 1994–2013, 2003.
262. Patel N, Firth AY. Vertical vergence adaptation does improve with practice. Optom Vis Sci 80, 316–319, 2003.
263. Patel SS, Ogmen H, White JM, Jiang BC. Neural network model of short-term horizontal disparity vergence dynamics. Vision Res 37, 1383–1399, 1997.
264. Peli E, McCormack G. Blink vergence in an antimetropic patient. Am J Optom Physiol Opt 63, 981–984, 1986.
265. Pobuda M, Erkelens CJ. The relationship between absolute disparity and ocular vergence. Biol Cybern 68, 221–228, 1993.
266. Pokharel D, Siatkowski RM. Progressive cerebellar tonsillar herniation with recurrent divergence insufficiency esotropia. J AAPOS 8, 286–287, 2005.
267. Popple AV, Smallman HS, Findlay JM. The area of spatial integration for initial horizontal disparity vergence. Vision Res 38, 319–326, 1998.
268. Porrill J, Ivins JP, Frisby JP. The variation of torsion with vergence and elevation. Vision Res 39, 3934–3950, 1999.
269. Porterfield W. A Treatise on the Eye, the Manner and Phenomena of Vision. Hamilton and Balfour, Edinburgh, 1759.
270. Postert TH, Büttner TH, McMonagle U, Przuntek H. Spasm of the near reflex: case report and review of the literature. Neuro-ophthalmology 17, 149–152, 1997.
271. Prince SJ, Pointon AD, Cumming BG, Parker AJ. The precision of single neuron responses in cortical area V1 during stereoscopic depth judgments. J Neurosci 20, 3387–3400, 2000.
272. Pullicino P, Lincoff N, Truax BT. Abnormal vergence with upper brainstem infarcts: pseudoabducens palsy. Neurology 55, 352–358, 2000.
273. Qing Y, Kapoula Z. Saccade-vergence dynamics and interaction in children and in adults. Exp Brain Res 156, 212–223, 2004.
274. Ramat S, Das VE, Somers JT, Leigh RJ. Tests of two hypotheses to account for different-sized saccades during disjunctive gaze shifts. Exp Brain Res 129, 500–510, 1999.

275. Ramat S, Leigh RJ, Zee DS, Optican LM. Ocular oscillations generated by coupling of brainstem excitatory and inhibitory saccadic burst neurons. Exp Brain Res, 2004.
276. Ramat S, Somers JT, Das VE, Leigh RJ. Conjugate ocular oscillations during shifts of the direction and depth of visual fixation. Invest Ophthalmol Vis Sci 40, 1681–1686, 1999.
277. Ramat S, Straumann D, Zee DS. The interaural translational VOR: suppression, enhancement and cognitive control. J Neurophysiol 94, 2391–2402, 2005.
278. Rambold H, Kompf D, Helmchen C. Convergence retraction nystagmus: a disorder of vergence? Ann Neurol 50, 677–681, 2001.
279. Rambold H, Neumann G, Helmchen C. Vergence deficits in pontine lesions. Neurology 62, 1850–1853, 2004.
280. Rambold H, Neumann G, Sander T, Helmchen C. Age-related changes of vergence under natural viewing conditions. Neurobiol Aging 27, 163–172, 2005.
281. Rambold H, Neumann G, Sprenger A, Helmchen C. Blink effect on slow vergence. NeuroReport 13, 2041–2044, 2002.
282. Rambold H, Sander T, Neumann G, Helmchen C. Palsy of "fast" and "slow" vergence by pontine lesions. Neurology 64, 338–340, 2005.
283. Rambold H, Sprenger A, Helmchen C. Effects of voluntary blinks on saccades, vergence eye movements, and saccade-vergence interactions in humans. J Neurophysiol 88, 1220–1233, 2002.
284. Rashbass C, Westheimer G. Disjunctive eye movements. J Physiol (Lond) 159, 339–360, 1961.
285. Regan D. Depth from motion and motion-in-depth. In Regan D (ed). Binocular Vision. MacMillan Press, London, 1991, pp 137–169.
286. Remler BF, Leigh RJ, Osorio I, Tomsak RL. The characteristics and mechanisms of visual disturbance associated with anticonvulsant therapy. Neurology 40, 791–796, 1990.
287. Repka MX, Claro MC, Loupe DN, Reich SG. Ocular motility in Parkinson's disease. J Pediatr Ophthalmol Strabismus 33, 144–147, 1996.
288. Richter HO, Costello P, Sponheim SR, Lee JT, Pardo JV. Functional neuroanatomy of the human near/far response to blur cues: eye-lens accommodation/vergence to point targets varying in depth. Eur J Neurosci 20, 2722–2732, 2004.
289. Ringach DL, Hawken MJ, Shapley R. Binocular eye movements caused by the perception of three-dimensional structure from motion. Vision Res 36, 1479–1492, 1996.
290. Robinson DA. The mechanics of human vergence eye movements. J Pediatr Ophthalmol 3, 31–37, 1966.
291. Roper-Hall G. Clinical dysfunction of the vergence system. In Schor CM, Ciuffreda KJ (eds). Vergence Eye Movements: Clinical and Basic Aspects. Butterworths, Woburn, MA, 1983, pp 671–698.
292. Rosenfield M, Ciuffreda KJ. Accommodative convergence and age. Ophthal Physiol Opt 10, 403–404, 1990.
293. Rosenfield M, Ciuffreda KJ, Chen HW. Effect of age on the interaction between the AC/A and CA/C ratios. Ophthalmic Physiol Opt 15, 451–455, 1995.
294. Rosenfield M, Ciuffreda KJ, Ong E, Azimi A. Proximally induced accommodation and accommodative adaptation. Invest Ophth Vis Sci 31, 1163–1167, 1990.
295. Rosenfield M, Ciuffreda KJ, Ong E, Super S. Vergence adaptation and the order of clinical vergence range testing. Optom Vis Sci 72, 219–223, 1995.
296. Rosenfield M, Gilmartin B. The effect of vergence adaptation on convergent accommodation. Ophthalmic Physiol Opt 8, 172–177, 1988.
297. Rubin ML. Optics for Clinicians. Triad Publishing, Gainesville, FL, 1974.
298. Safran AB, Roth A, Gauthier G. Le syndrome des spasmes de convergence. Plus Klin Mbl Augenheilk 180, 471–473, 1982.
299. Sanders MD, Hoyt WF, Daroff RB. Lid nystagmus evoked by ocular convergence: an ocular electromyographic study. J Neurol Neurosurg Psychiatry 31, 368–371, 1968.
300. Sarkies NJC, Sander MD. Convergence spasm. Trans Ophthalmol UK 104, 782–786, 1985.
301. Sato F, Akao T, Kurkin S, Fukushima J, Fukushima K. Adaptive changes in vergence eye movements induced by vergence-vestibular interaction training in monkeys. Exp Brain Res 156, 164–173, 2004.
302. Scheiman M, Mitchell GL, Cotter S, et al. A randomized clinical trial of treatments for convergence insufficiency in children. Arch Ophthalmol 123, 14–24, 2005.
303. Schor CM. Fixation disparity and vergence adaptation. In Schor CM, Ciuffreda KJ (eds). Vergence Eye Movements: Basic and Clinical Aspects. Butterworths, Woburn, MA, 1983, pp 465–516.
304. Schor CM. Influence of accommodative and vergence adaptation on binocular motor disorders. Am J Optom Physiol Opt 65, 464–475, 1988.
305. Schor CM. A dynamic model of cross-coupling between accommodation and convergence: simulations of step and frequency responses. Optom Vis Sci 69, 258–269, 1992.
306. Schor CM, Ciuffreda KJ. Vergence Eye Movements: Basic and Clinical Aspects. Butterworths, London, 1983.
307. Schor CM, Gleason G, Lunn R. Interactions between short-term vertical phoria adaptation and nonconjugate adaptation of vertical pursuits. Vision Res 33, 55–63, 1993.
308. Schor CM, Gleason G, Maxwell JS, Lunn R. Spatial aspects of vertical phoria adaptation. Vision Res 33, 73–84, 1993.
309. Schor CM, Horner D. Adaptive disorders of accommodation and vergence in binocular dysfunction. Ophthal Physiol Opt 9, 264–268, 1989.
310. Schor CM, Lott LA, Pope D, Graham AD. Saccades reduce latency and increase velocity of ocular accommodation. Vision Res 39, 3769–3795, 1999.
311. Schor CM, Maxwell JS, McCandless J, Graf E. Adaptive control of vergence in humans. Ann N Y Acad Sci 956, 297–305, 2002.
312. Schor CM, McCandless JW. Distance cues for vertical vergence adaptation. Optom Vis Sci 72, 478–486, 1995.
313. Schor CM, McCandless JW. Context-specific adaptation of vertical vergence to correlates of eye position. Vision Res 37, 1929–1937, 1997.
314. Schwartz MA, Selhorst JB, Ochs AL, et al. Oculomasticatory myorhythmia: a unique movement disorder occurring in Whipple's Disease. Ann Neurol 20, 677–683, 1986.
315. Schwartze GM, McHenry LC, Proctor RC. Conver-

gence spasm—treatment by Amytal interview. J Clin Neuro-ophthalmol 3, 123–125, 1983.
316. Semmlow JL, Abdel-Wahed S, Hung GK, Ciuffreda KJ. Adaptive response dynamics in disparity vergence. Sixth annual frontiers of medicine conference (IEEE), 1984, pp 492–494, Los Angeles, CA.
317. Semmlow JL, Hung G. The near response: theories of control. In Schor CM, Ciuffreda KJ (eds). Vergence Eye Movements: Basic and Clinical Aspects. Butterworths, Woburn, MA, 1983, pp 175–195.
318. Semmlow JL, Hung GK, Ciuffreda KJ. Quantitative assessment of disparity vergence components. Invest Ophthalmol Vis Sci 27, 558–564, 1986.
319. Semmlow JL, Hung GK, Horng JL, Ciuffreda KJ. Disparity vergence eye movements exhibit preprogrammed motor control. Vision Res 34, 1335–1343, 1994.
320. Semmlow JL, Yuan W. Adaptive modification of disparity vergence components: an independent component analysis study. Invest Ophthalmol Vis Sci 43, 2189–2195, 2002.
321. Sethi B. Vergence adaptation: a review. Doc Opthalmol 63, 247–263, 1986.
322. Sharma K, Abdul-Rahim AS. Vertical fusional amplitude in normal adults. Am J Ophthalmol 114, 636–637, 1992.
323. Sharpe JA, Hoyt WF, Rosenfield MA. Convergence-evoked nystagmus. Arch Neurol 32, 191–194, 1975.
324. Sheliga BM, Chen KJ, FitzGibbon EJ, Miles FA. Short-latency disparity vergence in humans: evidence for early spatial filtering. Ann N Y Acad Sci 1039, 252–259, 2005.
325. Sheliga BM, Miles FA. Perception can influence the vergence responses associated with open-loop gaze shifts in 3D. J Vis 3, 654–676, 2003.
326. Shikata E, Tanaka Y, Nakamura H, Taira M, Sakata H. Selectivity of the parietal visual neurons in 3D orientation of surface of stereoscopic stimuli. NeuroReport 7, 2389–2394, 1996.
327. Simonsz HJ, Van Rijn LJ. Facilitation of vertical vergence by horizontal saccades, found in a patient with dissociated vertical deviation. Strabismus 2, 143–146, 1994.
328. Smith JL. Accommodative spasm versus spasm of the near reflex. J Clin Neuro-ophthalmol 7, 132–134, 1987.
329. Smith R. Vergence eye-movement response to whole-body linear acceleration stimuli in man. Ophthal Physiol Opt 5, 303–311, 1985.
330. Snyder LH, King WM. Effect of viewing distance and location of the axis of head rotation on the monkey's vestibuloocular reflex. I. Eye movement responses. J Neurophysiol 67, 861–874, 1992.
331. Snyder LH, King WM. Behavior and physiology of the macaque vestibulo-ocular reflex response to sudden off-axis rotation: computing eye translation. Brain Res Bull 40, 293–301, 1996.
332. Snyder LH, Lawrence DM, King WM. Changes in vestibulo-ocular reflex (VOR) anticipate changes in vergence angle in monkey. Vision Res 32, 569–575, 1992.
333. Spielmann A. A translucent occluder for studying eye position under unilateral or bilateral cover test. Am Orthop J 36, 65–74, 1986.
334. Steffen H, Walker MF, Zee DS. Rotation of Listing's plane with convergence: independence from eye position. Invest Ophthalmol Vis Sci 41, 715–721, 2000.
335. Stevenson SB. Visual processing in disparity vergence control. Ann N Y Acad Sci 956, 492–494, 2002.
336. Stevenson SB, Lott LA, Yang J. The influence of subject instruction on horizontal and vertical vergence tracking. Vision Res 37, 2891–2898, 1997.
337. Sylvestre PA, Choi JT, Cullen KE. Discharge dynamics of oculomotor neural integrator neurons during conjugate and disjunctive saccades and fixation. J Neurophysiol 90, 739–754, 2003.
338. Sylvestre PA, Cullen KE. Dynamics of abducens nucleus neuron discharges during disjunctive saccades. J Neurophysiol 88, 3452–3468, 2002.
339. Sylvestre PA, Galiana HL, Cullen KE. Conjugate and vergence oscillations during saccades and gaze shifts: implications for integrated control of binocular movement. J Neurophysiol 87, 257–272, 2002.
340. Takagi M, Frohman EM, Zee DS. Gap-overlap effects on latencies of saccades, vergence and combined vergence-saccades in humans. Vision Res 35, 3373–3388, 1995.
341. Takagi M, Oyamada H, Abe H, et al. Adaptive changes in dynamic properties of human disparity-induced vergence. Invest Ophthalmol Vis Sci 42, 1479–1486, 2001.
342. Takagi M, Tamargo R, Zee DS. Effects of lesions of the cerebellar oculomotor vermis on eye movements in primate: binocular control. Prog Brain Res 142, 19–33, 2003.
343. Takagi M, Trillenberg P, Zee DS. Adaptive control of pursuit, vergence and eye torsion in humans: basic and clinical implications. Vision Res 41, 3331–3344, 2001.
344. Takayama Y, Sugishita M. Astereopsis induced by repetitive magnetic stimulation of occipital cortex. J Neurol 241, 522–525, 1994.
345. Takemura A, Inoue Y, Kawano K, Quaia C, Miles FA. Single-unit activity in cortical area MST associated with disparity-vergence eye movements: evidence for population coding. J Neurophysiol 85, 2245–2266, 2001.
346. Takemura A, Kawano K, Quaia C, Miles FA. Population coding in cortical area MST. Ann N Y Acad Sci 956, 284–296, 2002.
347. Taylor MJ, Roberts DC, Zee DS. Effect of sustained cyclovergence on eye alignment: rapid torsional phoria adaptation. Invest Ophthalmol Vis Sci 41, 1076–1083, 2000.
348. Thorn F, Gwiazda J, Cruz AAV, Bauer JA, Held R. The development of eye alignment, convergence, and sensory binocularity in young infants. Invest Ophthalmol Vis Sci 35, 544–553, 1994.
349. Trotter Y, Celebrini S, Durand JB. Evidence for implication of primate area V1 in neural 3-D spatial localization processing. J Physiol Paris 98, 125–134, 2004.
350. Tychsen L, Scott C. Maldevelopment of convergence eye movements in macaque monkeys with small- and large-angle infantile esotropia. Invest Ophthalmol Vis Sci 44, 3358–3368, 2003.
351. Tyler CW. Cyclopean vision. In Regan D (ed). Binocular Vision. MacMillan Press, London, 1991, pp 38–74.
352. Tyler CW. The horopter and binocular vision. In Regan D (ed). Binocular Vision. MacMillan Press, London, 1991, pp 19–37.

353. Vaina VL. Selective impairment of visual motion interpretation following lesions of the right occipitoparietal area in humans. Biol Cybern 61, 347–359, 1989.
354. Van Den Berg A, Van Rijn LJ, Defaber J. Excess cyclovergence in patients with intermittent exotropia. Vision Res 35, 3265–3278, 1995.
355. Van der Steen J, Bruno P. Unequal amplitude saccades produced by aniseikonic patterns: effects of viewing distance. Vision Res 35, 3459–3471, 1995.
356. van Leeuwen AF, Collewijn H, Erkelens CJ. Dynamics of horizontal vergence movements: interaction with horizontal and vertical saccades and relation with monocular preferences. Vision Res 38, 3943–3954, 1998.
357. van Leeuwen AF, Westen MJ, van der Steen SJ, de Faber JT, Collewijn H. Gaze-shift dynamics in subjects with and without symptoms of convergence insufficiency: influence of monocular preference and the effect of training. Vision Res 39, 3095–3107, 1999.
358. Van Rijn LJ, Van den Berg AV. Binocular eye orientation during fixations: Listing's law extended to include eye vergence. Vision Res 33, 691–708, 1993.
359. Van Rijn LJ, Van der Steen J, Collewijn H. Visually-induced cycloversion and cyclovergence. Vision Res 32, 1875–1883, 1992.
360. Van Rijn LJ, Van der Steen J, Collewijn H. Instability of ocular torsion during fixation: cyclovergence is more stable than cycloversion. Vision Res 34, 1077–1087, 1994.
361. Versino M, Hurko O, Zee DS. Disorders of binocular control of eye movements in patients with cerebellar dysfunction. Brain 119, 1933–1950, 1996.
362. Viirre ES, Cadera W, Vilis T. Monocular adaptation of the saccadic system and vestibuloocular reflex. Invest Ophth Vis Sci 29, 1339–1347, 1988.
363. Viirre ES, Tweed D, Milner K, Vilis T. A reexamination of the gain of the vestibuloocular reflex. J Neurophysiol 56, 439–450, 1986.
364. Von Noorden GK, Campos EC. Binocular Vision and Ocular Motility. Mosby, St. Louis, 2001.
365. Walton MM, Mays LE. Discharge of saccade-related superior colliculus neurons during saccades accompanied by vergence. J Neurophysiol 90, 1124–1139, 2003.
366. Wasicky R, Horn AK, Buttner-Ennever JA. Twitch and nontwitch motoneuron subgroups in the oculomotor nucleus of monkeys receive different afferent projections. J Comp Neurol 479, 117–129, 2004.
367. Wei M, DeAngelis GC, Angelaki DE. Do visual cues contribute to the neural estimate of viewing distance used by the oculomotor system? J Neurosci 23, 8340–8350, 2003.
368. Westheimer G, Blair SM. Oculomotor defects in cerebellectomized monkeys. Invest Ophthalmol 12, 618–620, 1973.
369. Westheimer G, Mitchell DE. The sensory stimulus for disjunctive eye movements. Vision Res 9, 749–755, 1969.
370. Wick B, Bedell HE. Magnitude and velocity of proximal vergence. Invest Ophthalmol Vis Sci 30, 755–760, 1989.
371. Wiest G. Abnormal vergence with upper brainstem infarcts: pseudoabducens palsy. Neurology 56, 424–425, 2001.
372. Winn B, Gilmartin B, Sculfor DL, Bamford JC. Vergence adaptation and senescence. Optom Vis Sci 71, 797–800, 1994.
373. Wong LC, Rosenfield M, Wong NN. Vergence adaptation in children and its clinical significance. Binocul Vis Strabismus Q 16, 29–34, 2001.
374. Yang D, FitzGibbon EJ, Miles FA. Short-latency vergence eye movements induced by radial optic flow in humans: dependence on ambient vergence level. J Neurophysiol 81, 945–949, 1999.
375. Yang DS, FitzGibbon EJ, Miles FA. Short-latency disparity-vergence eye movements in humans: sensitivity to simulated orthogonal tropias. Vision Res 43, 431–443, 2003.
376. Yang Q, Bucci MP, Kapoula Z. The latency of saccades, vergence, and combined eye movements in children and in adults. Invest Ophthalmol Vis Sci 43, 2939–2949, 2002.
377. Yee RD, Baloh RW, Honrubia V, Lau CG, Jenkins HA. Slow build-up of optokinetic nystagmus associated with downbeat nystagmus. Invest Ophthalmol Vis Sci 18, 622–629, 1979.
378. Yee RD, Spiegel PH, Yamada T, Abel LA, Zee DS. Voluntary saccadic oscillations resembling ocular flutter and opsoclonus. J Neuro-ophthalmology 14, 95–101, 1994.
379. Ygge J, Zee DS. Control of vertical eye alignment in three-dimensional space. Vision Res 35, 3169–3181, 1995.
380. Ying SH, Zee DS. Phoria adaptation after sustained convergence: influence of saccades. Exp Brain Res In Press, 2005.
381. Yuan W, Semmlow JL, Muller-Munoz P. Model-based analysis of dynamics in vergence adaptation. IEEE Trans Biomed Eng 48, 1402–1411, 2001.
382. Yuan W, Semmlow JL, Munoz P. Effects of prediction on timing and dynamics of vergence eye movements. Ophthalmic Physiol Opt 20, 298–305, 2000.
383. Zee DS. Considerations on the mechanisms of alternating skew deviation in patients with cerebellar lesions. J Vestib Res 6, 1–7, 1996.
384. Zee DS, FitzGibbon EJ, Optican LM. Saccade-vergence interactions in humans. J Neurophysiol 68, 1624–1641, 1992.
385. Zee DS, Levi L. Neurological aspects of vergence eye movements. Rev Neurol (Paris) 145, 613–620, 1989.
386. Zhang H, Gamlin PD. Neurons in the posterior interposed nucleus of the cerebellum related to vergence and accommodation. I. Steady-state characteristics. J Neurophysiol. 79, 1255–1269, 1998.
387. Zhang HY, Gamlin PDR. Single-unit activity within the posterior fastigial nucleus during vergence and accommodation in the alert primate [abstract]. Soc Neurosci Abstr 22, 2034, 1996.
388. Zhang Y, Gamlin PDR, Mays LE. Antidromic identification of midbrain near response cells projecting to the oculomotor nucleus. Exp Brain Res 84, 525–528, 1991.
389. Zhang Y, Mays LE, Gamlin PD. Characteristics of near response cells projecting to the oculomotor nucleus. J Neurophysiol 67, 944–960, 1992.
390. Zhou W, King WM. Premotor commands encode monocular eye movements. Nature 393, 692–695, 1998.

PART **2**

THE DIAGNOSIS OF DISORDERS OF EYE MOVEMENTS

In Chapters 9 to 12, we describe clinical features of disorders of ocular motility, referring to the video-based presentations on the accompanying compact disc. After describing cardinal features of each disorder, we will draw on anatomic, physiologic, and pharmacological principles developed in previous sections of the book to provide a pathophysiological explanation whenever this is possible. The reader should be aware that, at the bedside, these pathophysiologic hypotheses might fall short of explaining clinical findings. When they do so, we hope that they may encourage a re-evaluation of the assumptions that are used in clinical diagnosis. The advantage of this strategy was commented upon by William James,[386] who noted: "*...how few facts 'experience' will discover unless some prior interest, born of theory, is already awakened in the mind.*"

Chapter 9

Diagnosis of Peripheral Ocular Motor Palsies and Strabismus

A PATHOPHYSIOLOGICAL APPROACH TO DIPLOPIA

The most common symptom caused by abnormal eye movements is double vision (diplopia). Diplopia is usually due to misalignment of the visual axes—strabismus (Table 9–1). The clinical evaluation of diplopia or strabismus may be challenging, especially in young or uncooperative patients, and requires an organized and systematic approach. Recognizing this problem, Alfred Bielschowsky (1871–1940) commented:

> In examining and treating motor anomalies (of the eyes), one never loses an uneasy feeling of incompetence until he has become thoroughly familiar with the physiologic fundamentals from which the signs and symptoms of those anomalies are to be derived.[72]

Those physiologic fundamentals had been established by the nineteenth century European pioneers, and Bielschowsky played an impor-

Table 9–1. **A Glossary of Terms Related to Strabismus**

Term	Definition
Cardinal or diagnostic positions of gaze	Primary, secondary, and tertiary positions, which are defined separately, below (total of nine).
Central position	The position of the eye when looking straight ahead; the visual axis is parallel to the midsagittal plane of the head.
Concomitant or comitant deviation	Misalignment of the visual axes that does not change in different positions of gaze with either eye fixating (for diagnosis, see text).
Crossed diplopia	Double vision caused by exotropia. The false image is displaced to the side opposite to the paralyzed eye (e.g., due to medial rectus palsy).
Cyclodeviation	Misalignment of the eyes in the torsional plane (eye rotations around the visual axis). With both eyes viewing, such misalignment causes a cyclodisparity, which stimulates cyclovergence. Incyclodeviation: relative intorsion of the eyes (increased separation of lower poles of eyes). Excyclodeviation: relative extorsion of the eyes (increased separation of upper poles of eyes).
Duction	Rotation of one eye while it alone is viewing: Adduction (horizontally towards the nose); Abduction (horizontally away from the nose); Supraduction or Sursumduction (elevation); Infraduction or Deorsumduction (depression); Incycloduction (intorsion, upper pole nasalward); Excycloduction (extorsion, upper pole templeward).
Non-concomitant deviation	Misalignment of the visual axes that varies with position of gaze and changes according to which eye is fixating. Most non-concomitant deviations are paralytic in origin.
Orthophoria	Maintained alignment of the visual axes while viewing a distant target with one eye, when disparity-induced vergence is prevented.
Orthotropia	Alignment of the visual axes while viewing a distant target with both eyes.
Paralytic strabismus	Non-concomitant deviation due to extraocular muscle weakness from disease of the nerve, neuromuscular junction, or muscles.
Phoria (or Heterophoria)	The relative deviation of the visual axes during monocular viewing of a single target. This is a latent ocular misalignment, since fusional vergence mechanisms maintain alignment during binocular viewing.
Primary deviation	The deviation of the paretic eye under cover while the normal eye is fixating (for mechanism of primary and secondary deviation see text).
Primary position	The position of the eye from which pure horizontal or vertical rotations will be associated with zero torsional component. (See Listing's law in text.)
Secondary deviation	The deviation of the normal eye under cover while the paretic eye is fixating (for mechanism of primary and secondary deviation see text).
Secondary position	The position of the eye in adduction, abduction, elevation, or depression.

Table 9–1. *(continued)*

Term	Definition
Strabismus	A misalignment or deviation of the visual axes.
Tertiary position	The position of the eye after combined horizontal and vertical movement away from the central position (e.g., adduction and elevation).
Tropia (or Heterotropia)	The relative deviation of the visual axes during binocular viewing of a single target. This is a manifest ocular misalignment, which fusional vergence cannot correct: Exotropia (deviation out), Esotropia (deviation in), Hypertropia (vertical deviation—e.g., right hypertropia = right eye higher).
Uncrossed diplopia:	Double vision caused by esotropia. The false image is displaced on the same side as the paralyzed eye (e.g., due to lateral rectus palsy).
Vergence	Movements that rotate the eyes simultaneously in opposite directions: Convergence, Divergence, Incyclovergence (upper poles to nose), Excyclovergence (lower poles to nose). The two main types of vergence movements are fusional (disparity) and accommodative (blur).
Version	Movements that rotate the eyes in the same direction by the same amount: Dextroversion, Levoversion, Sursumversion (elevation), Deorsumversion (depression), Dextrocycloversion (upper poles to subject's right), Levocycloversion (upper poles to subject's left).
Visual axis	The line connecting the fovea with the fixation point.

tant role in bringing them to the New World. One pioneer worthy of special note was Ewald Hering (1834–1918), who taught Bielschowsky. When Hering published his *Theory of Binocular Vision* in 1868,[343] it was widely held that coordinated movement of the eyes was an acquired skill. Hering challenged this view in his treatise, stating that "one and the same impulse of will drives both eyes simultaneously as we can direct a pair of horses with single reins." Although recent research has questioned the mechanisms by which equal innervation reaches each eye,[955] the idea that the brain controls the globes as a single organ—"the Double Eye"—still forms the basis for our understanding of ocular alignment.

ANATOMY OF THE ORBITAL FASCIA AND THE EXTRAOCULAR MUSCLES

The eyeball is suspended in the cone-shaped orbit by a fibrous sac of fascia called Tenon's capsule, which is attached anteriorly to the conjunctiva behind the corneal limbus and posteriorly to the orbital fat surrounding the optic nerve. Tenon's capsule has a tough peripheral part, which is penetrated by the rectus extraocular muscles, and a thin, delicate central region, which is penetrated by the optic nerve, posterior ciliary nerves, and ciliary vessels. The attachments of Tenon's capsule, between the anterior circumference of the eyeball (behind the corneal limbus) and the orbital rim, effectively suspend the eye in a "drumhead" that mechanically governs its freedom of rotation (Fig. 9–1).[201] The thin, central part of Tenon's capsule allows the optic nerve and the ciliary vessels and nerves to move with the eye. One other important fascial connection is between the superior surface of the superior rectus muscle sheath and the lower surface of the levator palpebrae superioris.[889]

Six muscles rotate each eye: four rectus muscles and two oblique muscles (Fig. 9–1 and Table 9–2). The four recti and the superior oblique arise from the apex of the orbit (the annulus of Zinn, Fig. 9–2). The inferior oblique muscle arises from the inferior nasal aspect of the orbit and in 10% of subjects is double-bellied.[188] The four rectus muscles insert into the sclera *anterior* to the equator of the globe: the medial rectus muscle on the nasal side, the lateral rectus muscle on the temporal side, the superior rectus muscle on the superior side, and the inferior rectus muscle on the inferior side. The insertions of the medial and lateral rectus contain muscle tissue connecting directly with the sclera.[385] The superior and inferior oblique muscles approach the globe from its anterior and medial aspect and insert *posterior* to the equator of the globe. The superior oblique muscle

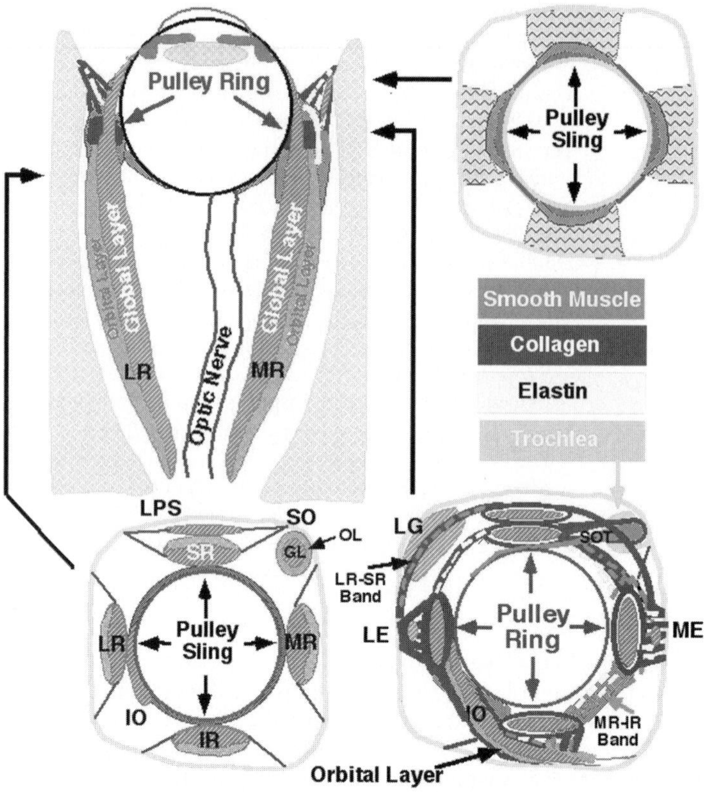

Figure 9–1. Schematic representation of orbital connective tissues. GL: global layer; IR: inferior rectus; LPS: levator palpebrae superioris; LR: lateral rectus; MR: medial rectus; OL: orbital layer; SO: superior oblique; SOT: superior oblique tendon; SR: superior rectus. The three coronal views correspond to the levels indicated by arrows in the horizontal section. In the horizontal section, note the attachment of the globe to the orbit by the anterior part of Tenon's capsule (collagen and elastin) through which the extraocular muscles pass in sleeves, which serve as pulleys. Note also bands of smooth muscle and collagen between the LR and SR, and between the MR and IR. A color version of this figure may be found on the compact disc. (Reproduced, with permission, from Demer JL. Anatomy of strabismus. In Taylor D, Hoyt C (eds). Pediatric Ophthalmology and Strabismus, third edition. London: Elsevier, 2005, pp 849–861.)

first passes through the trochlea (a fibrous, cartilaginous, U-shaped ring that lies just inside the superior medial orbital rim) before inserting on the superior side of the globe. The inferior oblique inserts on the temporal side of the globe.

Each rectus muscle has an outer orbital layer and an inner global layer, each with dif-

Table 9–2. **Actions of the Extraocular Muscles with the Eye in Central Position**

Muscle	Primary Action	Secondary Action	Tertiary Action
Medial Rectus	Adduction	—	—
Lateral Rectus	Abduction	—	—
Superior Rectus	Elevation	Intorsion	Adduction
Inferior Rectus	Depression	Extorsion	Adduction
Superior Oblique	Intorsion	Depression	Abduction
Inferior Oblique	Extorsion	Elevation	Abduction

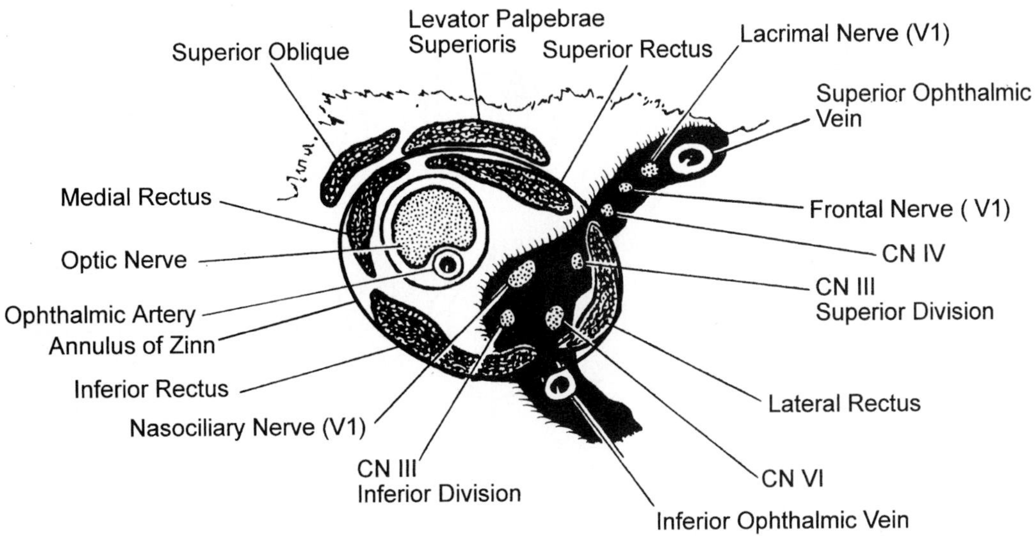

Figure 9–2. Posterior aspect of the right orbit showing the relationship of the sites of extraocular muscle attachment (which define the annulus of Zinn) and adjacent neurovascular structures. (Redrawn from von Noorden.[889])

ferent fiber types, which are discussed in the following sections. Although the global muscle layer inserts on the globe of the eye, the orbital layer does not; it inserts into a fascial component of Tenon's capsule.[197,723] Thus, the tendons of the rectus extraocular muscles, which emanate from the inner global layer, pass through sleeve-like *fibromuscular pulleys* that lie within peripheral Tenon's capsule. These pulleys lie several millimeters posterior to the equator of the globe (Fig. 9–1), approximately 10 mm behind the insertion sites of the muscles. Each rectus pulley consists of an encircling ring of collagen, located near the equator of the eyeball in Tenon's capsule. The pulleys are attached to the wall of the orbit, adjacent extraocular muscles and Tenon's fascia by sling-like bands containing collagen, elastin, and smooth muscle.[203] The orbital layer of the inferior oblique muscle inserts into the inferior rectus and lateral rectus pulleys. The orbital layer of the superior oblique muscle inserts into the superior rectus pulley.[460] What is the functional significance of this anatomy, which has undergone a conceptual revolution in the past decade?

It is generally agreed that one important function of the fibromuscular pulleys is to limit sideslip movement of the rectus muscles during eye rotations. For example, during horizontal rotations with the eyes in upgaze, the lateral rectus muscle and its tendon do not slide over the surface of the eye ball; this has been confirmed by MRI.[154,567] Thus, the pulleys effectively change the point of origin of the rectus muscles, just as the trochlea changes the functional point of origin of the superior oblique muscle. Some forms of congenital strabismus have been ascribed to congenital misplacement of pulleys,[155] although evidence from experimentally induced strabismus in monkeys suggests that disordered processing of sensorimotor information may sometimes be the main factor.[182] It may be that the insertion of the orbital muscle layer into the pulleys assists in ocular rotation by overcoming the resistance posed by the connective tissues surrounding the globe.[723] J. L. Demer has argued that the fibromuscular pulleys play an active role in determining the kinematic properties of eye rotations,[197] an issue that we discuss next.

The Pulling Directions of the Extraocular Muscles and the Planes of Rotation of the Eye

The eyes rotate about three axes (Fig. 9–3); one current convention refers to these axes as X (parasagittal), Y (transverse), and Z (vertical). All axes pass through the center of rotation of the globe. Translations (linear movements) of the globe are small, owing to the properties of Tenon's capsule, which sus-

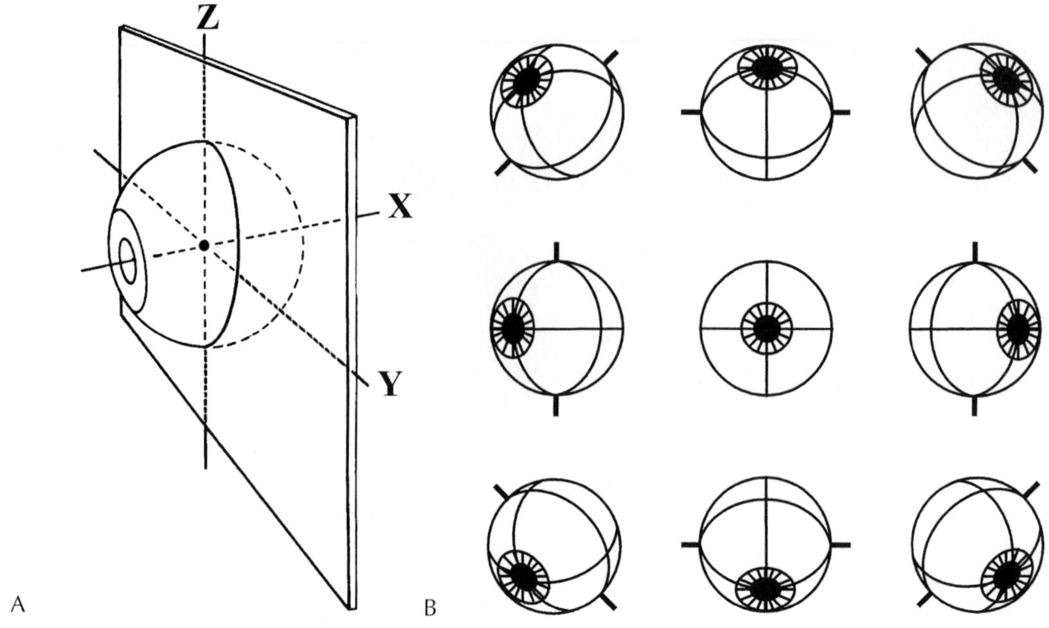

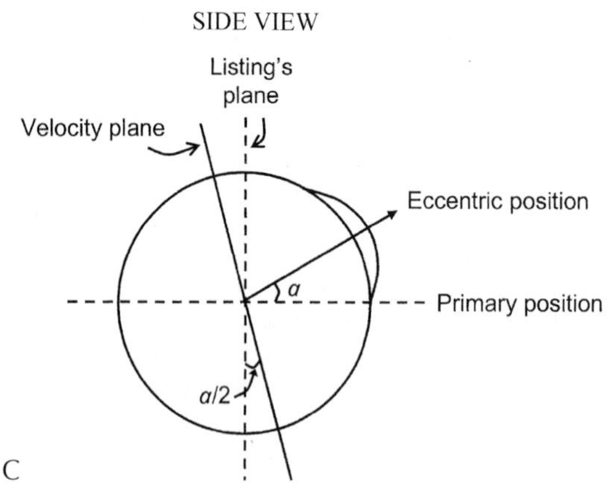

Figure 9–3. Three-dimensional aspects of eye rotations. (A) Listing's plane and the axes of rotation of the eye (X,Y,Z). (B) Orientations of the eye when they rotate to secondary and tertiary positions and obey Listing's law; in tertiary position, the eyes appear to rotate around the visual axis (cyclotorsion). (C) The half-angle rule, which states that when the eye starts to rotate from an eccentric position (which makes angle α with Listing's plane), it does so in a velocity plane that is rotated in the same direction as the movement but by only half as much (which makes angle α/2 with Listing's plane). Panels B and C are re-drawn from Wong,[919] with permission of Elsevier.

pends the eyeball. The pulling actions of the extraocular muscles are summarized in Table 9–2. The primary action of the muscle refers to the axis about which the eye principally rotates when that muscle contracts; the secondary and tertiary actions refer to the axes about which there are lesser rotations. The horizontal recti rotate the eye horizontally about the Z-axis, more or less irrespective of the vertical position of the globe. The superior recti are the main elevators of the eyes, and the inferior recti are the main depressors; these muscles also have smaller torsional and horizontal actions. The pulling actions of the oblique muscles are more torsional, but because they approach the eye from its medial aspect, their direction of pull is substantially affected by the horizontal position of gaze. For example, the superior oblique acts more as a depressor when the eye is adducted and more as an intorter when the eye is abducted (Fig. 9–4). The tertiary action of the oblique muscles is to abduct the eye.

Three-dimensional eye rotations pose certain computational problems for the brain. One important issue is that eye rotations are non-commutative. Thus, if a series of eye rotations are required as part of some behavior, the *order* of these rotations must be specified or else the eye may end up at the wrong orientation. Another issue is that during a series of eye movements, torsional rotations occur, and these must remain similar in each eye to hold

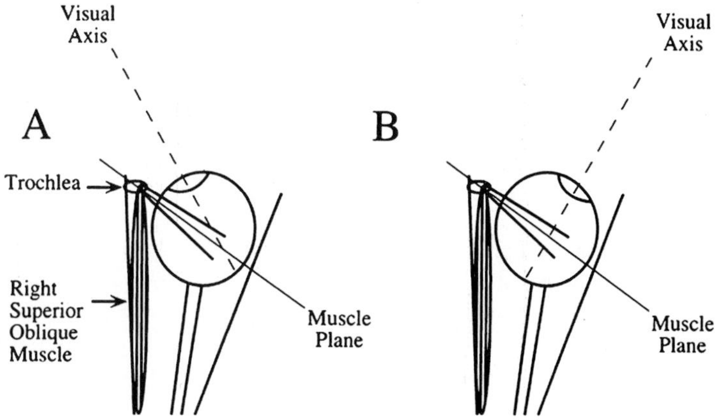

Figure 9–4. Schematic summarizing the pulling directions of the right superior oblique muscle, viewed from above. (A) When the eye is fully adducted, its depressing action is increased. (B) When the eye is fully abducted, its action is mainly intorsion.

torsional disparity constant, and they must not accumulate or the eye will be excessively twisted about the line of sight. How are 3-D eye movements controlled in order to avoid these problems?

Although in theory the eye could rotate about axes lying in any plane, in fact, the axes of rotation are confined to the equatorial or Listing's plane, which is perpendicular to the fixation line in primary position (Fig. 9–3A). Thus, Listing's law states that any eye position can be described by rotation of the eye from the primary position about a single axis lying in the equatorial plane.[337,919] One consequence of this scheme is that the vertical meridian of the eye, which is earth-vertical and parasagittal with the head upright and the eye in the primary position, remains vertical when the eye rotates to a secondary position but systematically tilts with respect to vertical in any tertiary position (Fig. 9–3B). Donders' law states that the angle of tilt in any tertiary position of gaze depends upon the horizontal and vertical gaze angles, irrespective of how the eye reached that position of gaze. In other words, the torsional orientation of the eye is fixed for a given horizontal and vertical position. Both Donders' and Listing's laws have been shown to apply approximately to saccadic and smooth-pursuit eye movements.[247,248,823] One geometric consequence of Listing's law is that primary position is now defined as the position from which purely horizontal or purely vertical rotations of the eye are unassociated with any torsion. Note that primary position may not correspond to looking straight ahead, which we call central position. The location of primary position is a simple way to describe Listing's plane, and its location can be a useful diagnostic tool, for example, in separating congenital and acquired superior oblique palsy.[822]

Another geometric property of eye rotations that follow Listing's law concerns the axis of rotation when the eye turns from one tertiary position to another. Under these circumstances, the eye rotates about an axis that is tilted half the angle between Listing's plane and the current direction of gaze (the half angle rule; Fig. 9–3C).[859] Experimental studies of eye kinematics commonly test whether Listing's law is being obeyed by determining whether the rotational *eye velocity* vector conforms to the half angle rule. During convergence eye movements, Listing's plane is rotated temporally through about one quarter of the angle of vergence.[577,869] There is evidence that this rotation is mediated by the superior oblique muscle.[565] During the rotational vestibulo-ocular reflex (rVOR), eye rotations do not obey Listing's law,[578] but show an approximate quarter-angle rule. During head rotations in roll (ear-to-shoulder) the eye counterrolls (torsional rotations), taking the eye out of Listing's plane even if gaze stays close to primary position. On the other hand, during the translational VOR, Listing's law is obeyed.[895]

What factors impose Listing's law on saccadic and smooth-pursuit eye movements? Since the eyeball is suspended in the "drumhead" of fascia provided by Tenon's capsule, and the fibromuscular pulleys determine the pulling directions of the extraocular muscles, it has been suggested that the pulleys partly enforce Listing's law, thereby making the 3-D computations easier for the brain.[197,694] Thus, each pulley is by displaced by contraction of fibers of orbital layer of the muscle, which insert onto it. The global layer fibers pass through the pulley and insert directly onto the eyeball, which they rotate. The displacement of the pulley then appears to play a role in determining the axis of eye rotations, and this mechanical system (the active pulley hypothesis) could solve the problem posed by the non-commutative property of rotations, thereby simplifying neural control.[197] However, for this to occur, the orbital and global layers of the rectus muscles must be able to contract independently, and some anatomical evidence argues against this.[723] Furthermore, not all anatomical evidence supports the active pulley hypothesis.[550a]

There is also evidence that Listing's law is imposed by central neural commands. First, some eye movements do not obey Listing's law, examples being the normal rotational vestibulo-ocular reflex,[578] and eye movements occurring after ingesting alcohol.[251,568] Second, if subjects view a near target aligned on one eye (asymmetric convergence), then the Listing's plane of that eye is altered even though its orbital position has not changed.[816] Third, inducing a change in vertical alignment of the visual axes by wearing a prism over one eye for three days induces a change in Listing's plane for that eye.[815] Fourth, if the eye is driven out of Listing's plane in a slow phase of torsional optokinetic nystagmus (induced by viewing a large visual display that rotates around the line of sight), then quick phases bring the eye back into Listing's plane.[492] Patients with strabismus also provide evidence for a neural implementation of Listing's law. Thus, in one patient with alternating strabismus, the orientation of Listing's plane depended on which eye the subject chose to view with.[561] Furthermore, surgical correction of strabismus may cause not only the operated, but also the non-operated eye, to change its 3-D rotational properties, suggesting that Listing's law must depend, at least partly, on active innervation.[92]

Electrophysiological studies provide some conflicting results. Thus, on the one hand, neurons in the nucleus reticularis tegmenti pontis show properties supporting the view that the brain takes into account deviations from Listing's law and corrects them.[867] On the other hand, motoneurons in the oculomotor and trochlear nerve nuclei do not modulate their discharge according to torsional movements that occur during pursuit movements between eccentric orbital positions, implying that these torsional movements are due to the orbital tissues.[285] Furthermore, direct stimulation of the abducens nerve induces eye movements that obey Listing's law (the half-angle rule), which is direct evidence that orbital mechanical factors impose this behavior.[443] Thus, at present, there is evidence that both central and orbital factors exert influences over the 3-D properties of eye rotations, and this field is likely to remain an active area of research.[24] For clinicians, some basic knowledge of 3-D eye rotations provides insights into the disorders of ocular alignment that we discuss in later sections.

STRUCTURE AND FUNCTION OF EXTRAOCULAR MUSCLE

Unique Characteristics of Extraocular Muscle

Extraocular muscles differ anatomically, physiologically, and immunologically from limb muscle.[678,680,944] Eye muscle fibers are smaller, more variable in size, and more richly innervated than limb muscle fibers. Some extraocular muscle fibers are amongst the fastest contracting and yet remain fatigue-resistant.[267] Motor unit size is the lowest known, being about 10 to 20 muscle fibers per motoneuron. Like limb muscles, the extraocular muscles contain twitch fibers that have a single end-plate per fiber and can generate an all-or-none propagating response (action potential). In addition, there are non-twitch fibers that cannot generate action potentials and show graded contractions to trains of electrical pulse stimuli; these are similar to the tonic fibers found in amphibians.[588,762] The global layer non-twitch fibers are unique in stretching the whole length of the muscle.[631] At their insertion into the muscle tendon, they are covered by axonal terminals called palisade endings, which may be proprioceptive in function.[722] Fibers with intermediate properties also exist; they have multiple nerve terminals on individual fibers, but still generate slow action potentials.[588]

Another difference from limb muscles is that extraocular muscles expresses virtually all known striated muscle isoforms of myosin heavy chain, including skeletal and cardiac, as well as embryonic isoforms in the proximal and distal portions of muscle fibers in the orbital layers (see following section).[681,803,944] This preservation of embryonic myosin may partly account for the different ways that extraocular muscles respond to changes in innervation and disease states.[677] In addition, expression of myosin may vary along the length of single muscle fibers, with "fast" forms being more prominent in the central region of most fibers, thereby accounting for the ability of both orbital and global fibers to contract quickly.[101]

Fibers with single and multiple nerve end plates have different antigens.[627] One factor in this antigenic difference may lie in the structure of the acetylcholine receptor. Both the embryonic $\alpha_2\beta\gamma\delta$ type and adult $\alpha_2\beta\epsilon\delta$ isoforms of the acetylcholine receptor are present on multiply innervated, and some singly innervated, adult extraocular muscle fibers. Adult skeletal muscle and the levator of the eyelid possess only the adult isoform.[355,400] The basement membranes of the extraocular muscles differ from skeletal muscle by showing different isoforms of laminins that are the major noncollagenous components.[441] Compared with gene expression in limb or jaw muscle, extraocular muscle is low in enzymes and regulators related to glycogen metabolism, a finding consistent with low glycogen content of extraocular muscle and pointing to important differences in energy metabolism.[677] Extraocular muscles show other biological differences from skeletal muscles, including transcriptional regulation, sarcomeric organization, excitation-contraction coupling, intermediary metabolism and the immune response.[803]

Extraocular muscle is more susceptible to some disease processes (e.g., myasthenia gravis)[403,405,678] and more resistant to others (e.g., Duchenne's dystrophy)[399,435,944] than skeletal muscles. One reason for this may be that the safety factor, which is the amount by which the endplate potential exceeds the threshold required to trigger an action potential, is smaller in extraocular than skeletal muscles due to less prominent synaptic folds and, possibly, less acetylcholine receptors on the post-synaptic membrane.[405] Another factor is that extraocular muscles express lower levels of decay accelerating factor, which is an inhibitor of complement mediated responses;[684] this might partly account for more severe involvement of extraocular muscles in myasthenia gravis.[402] When disease does involve extraocular muscle, the histopathologic changes may be quite unlike those observed in skeletal muscle affected by a similar condition. For example, experimental denervation of the extraocular muscles causes little muscle atrophy but with a mononuclear infiltrate.[682,682] Some of these findings would suggest a myopathic process if encountered in limb muscle.

Structure and Function of Extraocular Muscle Fiber Types

Each extraocular muscle has two distinct layers (Fig. 9–5).[803] Near the origin of each muscle, these lie in two concentric zones, but as the muscle is traced anteriorly, two parallel zones or layers are formed: a central global layer and a peripheral orbital layer. Each layer contains fibers more suited for either sustained contraction or brief rapid contraction. However, the orbital zone contains many fatigue-resistant twitch fibers. The two layers show transcription differences consistent with different roles postulated by the active pulley hypothesis (discussed above).[434] Using modern methods, six types of fibers have been defined in the extraocular muscles (Fig. 9–5).[680,681,801,801,802]

In the orbital layer, about 80% are singly innervated fibers, have fast-type myofibrillar ATPase, and high oxidative activity (with numerous mitochondria in dense clusters). These very fatigue-resistant fibers, which have an increased microvascular structure, are not found in skeletal muscle or the eyelid, and are probably the main contributors to sustained muscle tone.[202,680] They show predominant long-term effects after injection of botulinum toxin.[800] The remaining 20% of orbital fibers are multiply innervated. They have twitch capacity near the center of the fiber, and nontwitch activity proximal and distal to the end plate band.

In the global layer, about 33% of fibers are singly innervated, fast-twitch, and fatigue-resistant. About 33% are pale, singly innervated fibers with fast-twitch properties but low fatigue resistance. About 25% are singly innervated fibers with fast-twitch properties, numerous mitochondria, and an intermediate level of fatigue resistance. The remaining 10% are multiply innervated fibers, with synaptic endplate along their entire length, as well as at the myotendinous junction, where there are palisade organ proprioceptors.[217] Like amphibian muscle, these fibers show tonic properties, with slow, graded, non-propagated responses

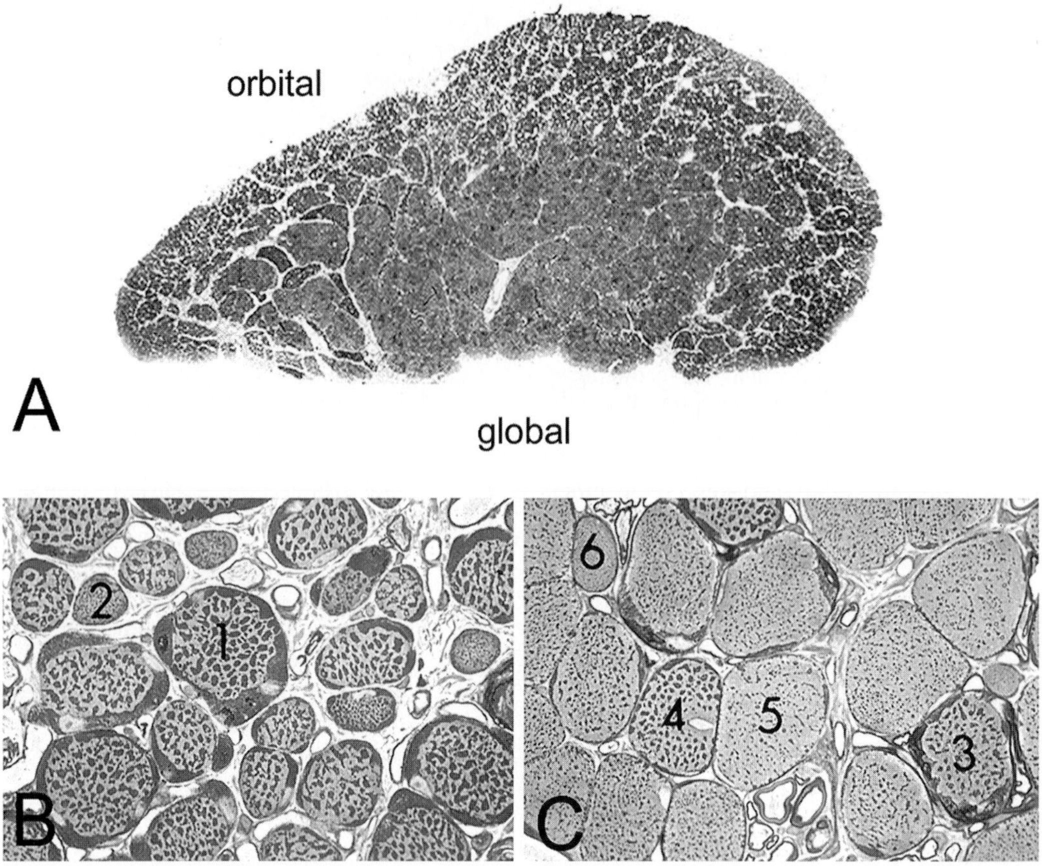

Figure 9–5. Histological profiles of the EOM layers (A) and fiber types (B,C) in the monkey lateral rectus muscle. Note general fiber type size differences, with the c-shaped orbital layer containing smaller diameter fibers. Profiles of the singly innervated fibers (SIFs) (1,3-5) and multiply innervated fibers (MIFs) (2,6) in the orbital (B) and global (C) layers are indicated. Phase contrast light photomicrographs of semithin (1 μm) sections highlight differences in mitochondrial content of different muscle fiber types. 1, orbital SIF; 2, orbital MIF; 3, global red SIF; 4, global intermediate SIF; 5, global white SIF; 6, global MIF. (Reproduced courtesy of Dr. John D. Porter,[803] with permission of Elsevier.)

to neural or pharmacological activation. Nontwitch fibers receive innervation from distinct groups of motoneurons that lie outside the confines of the conventional borders of the abducens, trochlear, and oculomotor nuclei.[121]

The levator palpebrae superioris contains the three singly innervated muscle types encountered in the global layer of the extraocular muscles, plus a true slow-twitch fiber type. The multiply innervated fiber types and the fatigue-resistant singly innervated type seen in the orbital layer are absent.

Although direct electrophysiological confirmation of the contribution of each fiber type to different types of eye movement is lacking, electromyographic studies by Scott and Collins, using miniature electrode needles with multiple recording sites, established a division of labor between global and orbital layers of extraocular muscle (Fig. 9–6).[749] They found that orbital fibers are active throughout nearly the entire range of movement, but during fixation, global fibers are recruited only as the eye is called into the field of action of that muscle. It seems likely, therefore, that the singly innervated, fatigue-resistant orbital fibers play a key role in sustaining eye position and maintaining extraocular muscle "tone" in any eye position. During saccades, both global and orbital fibers are activated, but the activity of global fibers subsequently may fall, whereas that of orbital fibers is sustained. These findings are consistent with the presence of more fatigue-resistant fibers in the orbital layers. Further, it has been shown experimentally that "fast fatigable" muscle fibers are the strongest,[762] so such global fibers may be best able to generate rapid eye movements. Thus, the order of recruitment of fibers appears to reflect mainly their fatigability; the less fatigue-resistant fibers of the global layers may only be activated during saccades. However, this order of recruitment may also be influenced by the attachment of the orbital layer to the pulley and the global layer to the eyeball.

A remaining problem is to resolve the range of electrophysiological activity in extraocular muscle with that of single ocular motoneurons in the abducens, trochlear, and oculomotor nuclei, which appear to discharge for all types of eye movements. One interpretation is that although each fiber can potentially contribute to all classes of eye movement, orbital, fatigue-resistant twitch fibers are most important for holding the eye in steady fixation, whereas global, pale, twitch fibers only become active when the eye is moved rapidly to a new orbital position. A special exception to this "common pathway" hypothesis is posed by the multiply innervated tonic fibers, which do not generate action potentials and thus cannot be monitored by electromyographic activity. Their motoneurons lie outside the confines of the classic boundaries of the abducens, trochlear, and

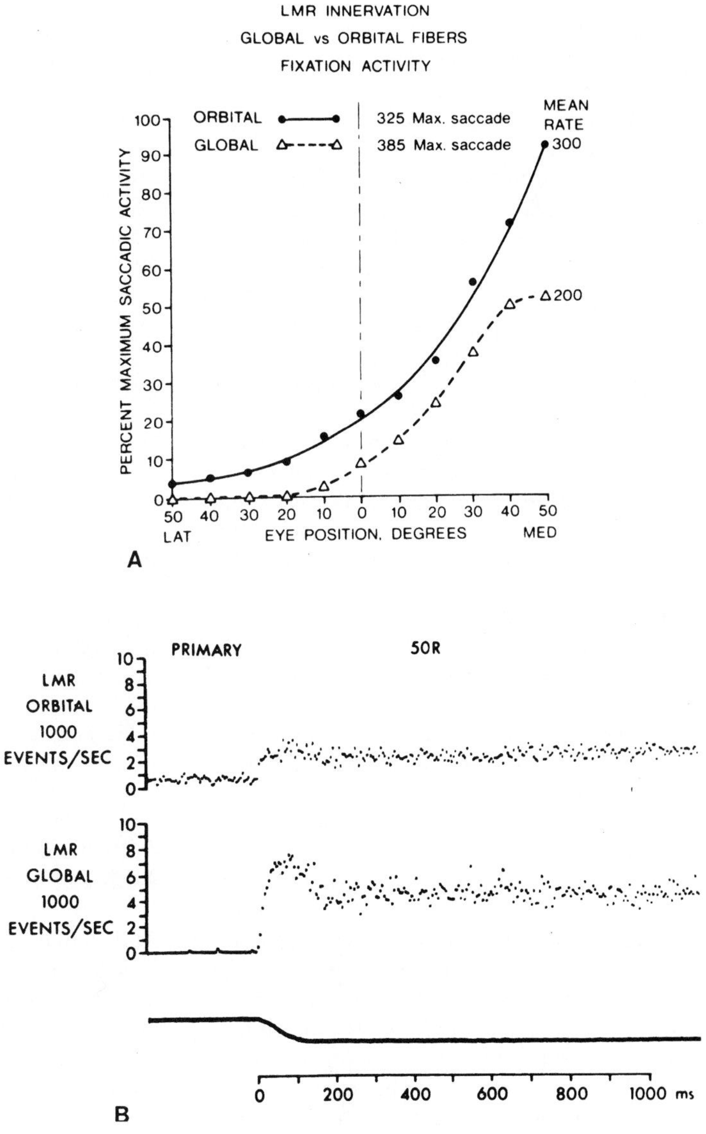

Figure 9–6. The relationship between discharge rate of extraocular muscle fibers and eye movements in human subjects. A miniature multi-electrode enabled simultaneous sampling of different fiber layers of the same muscle. (A) The relative contributions of orbital and global fibers of the left medial rectus muscle (LMR) are shown as the eye is held in various positions in the orbit. The orbital fibers progressively increase their activity as the fixation point is moved to the right. The global fibers, however, appear to saturate as the medial rectus is called upon to sustain stronger contractions during fixation into the far right field. (B) The integrated electromyographic activity in outer orbital and inner global layers of the left medial rectus muscle is sampled during a saccade from primary position to 50 degrees to the right. (Eye position is on bottom trace.) The global fibers are maximally innervated during the saccade, but their activity falls when the eye reaches extreme rightward gaze. The orbital fibers, however, maintain their new level of activity to hold the eye in its new position. (From Collins,[165] with permission.)

oculomotor nuclei.[120] Non-twitch motoneurons receive inputs predominantly from the pretectal area and medullary structures concerned with gaze-holding suggesting these fibers are more concerned with vergence, gaze-holding, and, along with the pallisade endings, they may contribute to proprioceptive feedback of the extraocular muscles.[903]

Extraocular Proprioception

Although human extraocular muscles contain muscle spindles,[217,528,721] the palisade tendon organs seem most important for ocular proprioception (Fig. 9–9C),[122,221a,722] despite some evidence that they might have motor properties.[529,903] Afferents from these proprioceptors project via the ophthalmic branch of the trigeminal nerve and the Gasserian ganglion, to the spinal trigeminal nucleus (pars interpolaris and pars caudalis);[676] eyelid afferents take a similar route.[548] Proprioceptive inputs may also project centrally via the ocular motor nerves.[282] From the trigeminal nucleus, proprioceptive information is distributed widely to structures involved in ocular motor control—the superior colliculus, vestibular nuclei, nucleus prepositus hypoglossi, cerebellum, and frontal eye fields—as well as to structures involved in visual processing—the lateral geniculate body, pulvinar, and visual cortex. The palisade endings are mainly associated with distal myotendinous junctions of the global, multiply innervated fiber. This fiber type, which only accounts for about 10% of global fibers, is innervated by a separate pool of motoneurons;[121] it is absent from the eyelid and might function similarly to the intrafusal fibers of skeletal muscle.[119]

What purpose could proprioception play in the normal control of eye movements? After all, vision provides continuous sensory feedback by which the brain can monitor the precision of gaze. Furthermore, no external loads are applied to the extraocular muscles (as they may be to skeletal muscles), and the extraocular muscles appear to lack a stretch reflex.[430] After the trigeminal proprioceptors are severed, monkeys make normal eye movements,[512] and they can still aim their eyes accurately after they are perturbed by electrical stimulation while in darkness.[312] This evidence suggests that the brain monitors an efference copy or corollary discharge of ocular motor commands rather than relying on proprioception for the moment-to-moment control of eye movements.

Extraocular proprioception may play a role in programming eye movements when visual cues are impoverished.[20,872,873] Thus, if one eye is artificially displaced with a suction contact lens and the subject views with the other eye, spatial localization is perturbed in the direction of forced eye rotation.[277] Spatial localization is also impaired in patients who have undergone trigeminal nerve thermocoagulation for tic douloureux.[875] Studies of a patient with a congenital oculomotor-trigeminal nerve synkinesis, who could adduct one eye by moving her jaw, also provide evidence that extraocular proprioception could contribute to spatial localization.[510] Thus, when this patient viewed with her normal eye, but adducted her covered, abnormal eye by moving her jaw, she mislocalized targets opposite to the direction of eye rotation, consistent with the effects of active contraction of the left medial rectus on palisade tendon organs.

It has also been suggested that proprioception may play a role in maintaining correct ocular alignment.[278,502] There is also evidence that proprioception plays a role in the normal development of binocularity.[111] Furthermore, if trochlear nerve palsy is induced experimentally in monkeys, proprioceptive deafferentation of the paretic eye produces gradual worsening of both static alignment and saccadic conjugacy.[511] However, bilateral proprioceptive deafferentation had no effect on eye movements in otherwise normal monkeys, and did not influence saccadic adaptation to novel visual demands.[512] Thus, in summary, current evidence indicates that proprioception may influence some long-term control over eye movements when visual cues are compromised.

ANATOMY OF OCULAR MOTOR NERVES AND THEIR NUCLEI

The ocular motor nuclei are located in the brainstem, close to the midline.[802] They lie adjacent to the medial longitudinal fasciculus and reticular formation, ventral to the aqueduct of Sylvius and fourth ventricle. The intracranial courses of the ocular motor nerves are shown in Figure 9–7.

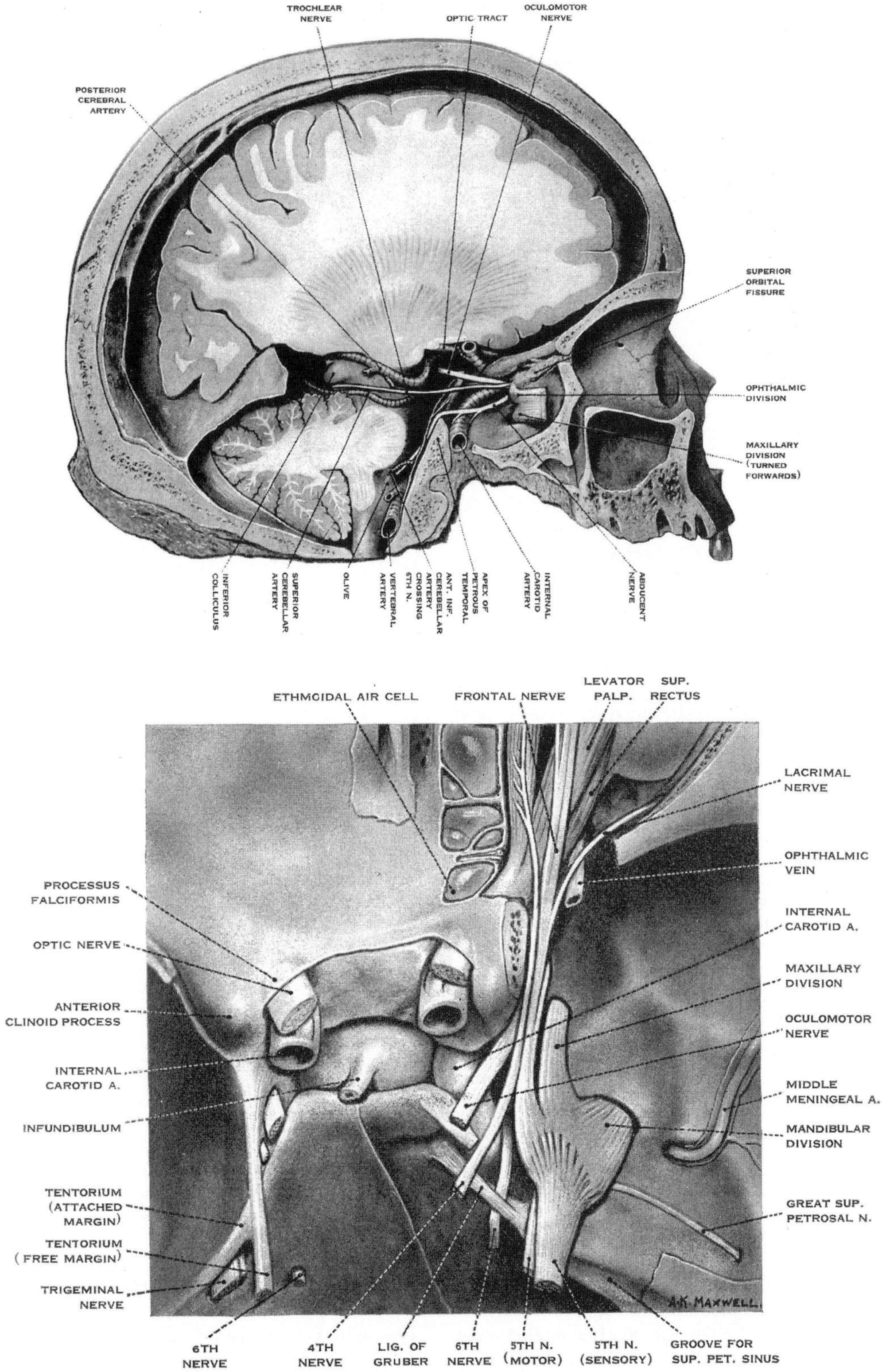

Figure 9–7. The intracranial courses of the third, fourth, and sixth cranial nerves. (Top) Parasagittal view. (Bottom) Superior view. Lig. of Gruber: petroclinoid ligament. (From Warwick R: Wolff's Anatomy of the Eye and Orbit, ed 7. WB Saunders, Philadelphia, 1976, pages 281 and 295, with kind permission of Springer Science and Business Media.)

Anatomy of the Abducens Nerve

The abducens nucleus lies in the floor of the fourth ventricle, in the lower pons (see Fig. 6–1, Chapter 6).[117] It is capped by the genu of the facial nerve. The abducens nucleus houses motor neurons, which innervate the lateral rectus muscle, and internuclear neurons, which innervate contralateral medial rectus motoneurons via the medial longitudinal fasciculus. Thus, the neurons of the abducens nucleus contain the neural signals responsible for conjugate horizontal eye movements. From the medial aspect of the nucleus, fibers destined for the ipsilateral lateral rectus muscle course ventrally, laterally, and caudally, passing through the pontine tegmentum and medial lemniscus, to emerge at the caudal border of the pons. Here the abducens nerve lies close to the anterior inferior cerebellar artery. In some individuals, the nerve consists of several trunks that eventually fuse within the cavernous sinus.[19,611,650] The nerve then courses nearly vertically along the clivus, through the prepontine cistern, and close to the inferior petrosal sinus. It then rises to the petrous crest, where it bends acutely forward to penetrate the dura,[326,862,864] medial to the trigeminal nerve, and passes under the petroclinoid ligament in Dorello's canal. It courses forward in the body of the cavernous sinus, where it lies lateral to the internal carotid artery and medial to the ophthalmic division of the trigeminal nerve (Fig. 9–8). For a few millimeters, pupillosympathetic fibers run with the sixth nerve as they leave the carotid artery to reach the first division of the trigeminal nerve.[531,531] The abducens nerve then enters the orbit through the superior orbital fissure,[612] and passes through the annulus of Zinn to innervate the lateral rectus on the inner surface of the muscle.

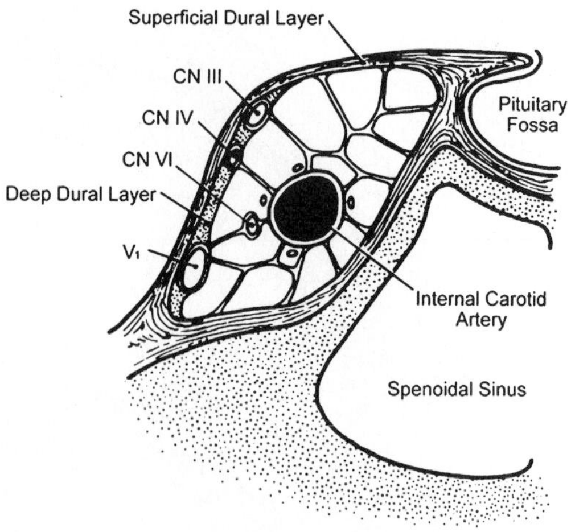

Figure 9–8. Diagram of transverse section of the cavernous sinus, showing superficial and deep layers, and the relationships of the oculomotor (III), trochlear (IV), abducens (VI), and ophthalmic division of the trigeminal nerve (V_1). (Redrawn from Umansky and Nathan.[863])

Anatomy of the Trochlear Nerve

The trochlear nerve is the longest and thinnest of all cranial nerves, which makes it susceptible to trauma. Each trochlear nucleus sends axons to supply the contralateral superior oblique muscle. The trochlear nucleus lies at the ventral border of the central, periaqueductal gray matter, dorsal to the medial longitudinal fasciculus, at the level of the inferior colliculus.[117] Its fibers pass dorsolaterally and caudally around the central gray matter, and decussate completely in the anterior medullary velum (the roof of the aqueduct). The trochlear nerve emerges, as one or more rootlets,[611] from the dorsal aspect of the brainstem, caudal to the inferior colliculus, and close to the tentorium cerebelli. The nerve passes laterally around the upper pons, lying between the superior cerebellar and posterior cerebral arteries, to reach the prepontine cistern. During its cisternal course, the trochlear nerve receives its blood supply from branches of the superior cerebellar artery.[536] It then runs forward on the free edge of the tentorium for 1 to 2 cm before penetrating the dura of the tentorial attachment and entering the cavernous sinus. Within the lateral wall of the sinus (Fig. 9–8), the fourth nerve lies below the third nerve and above the ophthalmic division of the fifth nerve, with which it shares a connective tissue coat. It then crosses over the oculomotor nerve to enter the superior orbital fissure above the annulus of Zinn,[612] passing to the medial aspect of the orbit to supply the superior oblique muscle.[724]

Anatomy of the Oculomotor Nerve

The oculomotor nucleus is a paired structure that lies at the ventral border of the periaqueductal grey matter; it extends rostrally to the level of the posterior commissure and caudally to the trochlear nucleus (Fig. 9–9).[117] It sends efferent fibers to the medial rectus, superior rectus, inferior rectus, and inferior oblique muscles; the levator palpebrae superioris; the pupillary constrictor muscle; and the ciliary body. Warwick's anatomic scheme[902] for the oculomotor nucleus of the rhesus monkey, which is shown in Figure 9–9A, has undergone substantial revisions.[118,903] Specifically, neurons supplying the medial rectus muscle are distributed into three areas of the oculomotor nucleus, designated A, B, and C (Fig. 9–9B). Neurons from area C project to non-twitch fibers in the medial and inferior rectus muscles. In addition, neurons from midline area S project to non-twitch fibers in the inferior oblique and superior rectus muscles. Such fibers seem most suited for sustained contraction, such as during convergence and gaze-holding; they may also contribute to a proprioceptive mechanism.[119,121,903] Neurons from areas A, B, and C all receive inputs from the contralateral abducens nucleus, via the medial longitudinal fasciculus (Fig. 9–9B). The neurons innervating each superior rectus muscle lie next to each other, and their axons decussate in the caudal portion of this nucleus.[73] The caudal nucleus, supplying both levator palpebrae superioris muscles, is a single structure. All projections from the oculomotor nucleus are ipsilateral save for those to the superior rectus, which are totally crossed, and those to the levator palpebrae superioris, which are both crossed and uncrossed. Parasympathetic innervation for the pupil originates in the Edinger-Westphal nucleus.[466] The closely coordinated movements of the superior rectus and levator palpebrae superioris is due to common inputs from the M-group of neurons, which lies rostral to the interstitial nucleus of Cajal.[353]

The fascicles of the oculomotor nerve originate from the entire rostral-caudal extent of the nucleus and pass ventrally through the medial longitudinal fasciculus, the red nucleus, the substantia nigra, and the medial part of the cerebral peduncle. As they pass through the red nucleus, the fascicles fan out, to converge again before exiting the midbrain. Attempts have been made to identify the topographic organization of the oculomotor fascicles, based on clinicoradiologic and clinicopathologic findings. One scheme proposes that from lateral to medial, the order is inferior oblique, superior rectus, medial rectus and levator palpebrae, inferior rectus, and pupil.[140,276] However, selective involvement of the levator and superior rectus with some ventral midbrain lesions has suggested that, even at this stage, the organization corresponds to the superior and inferior branching of the oculomotor nerve that occurs in the orbit.[473]

The third nerve emerges from the interpeduncular fossa as several rootlets, which then fuse to form a single trunk. The nerve then runs between the posterior cerebral artery and superior cerebellar artery, passing forward, downward, and laterally through the basal cistern.[11] It passes lateral to the posterior communicating artery and below the temporal lobe uncus, where it runs over the petroclinoid ligament, medial to the trochlear nerve and just lateral to the posterior clinoid process. During its subarachnoid course, parasympathetic pupillary fibers lie peripherally in the dorsomedial part of the nerve.[432,826] Segregation of fibers into those that will supply superior and inferior branches of the oculomotor nerve in the orbit may already have occurred.[317] As the oculomotor nerve pierces the dura, it lies close to the free edge of the tentorium cerebelli. Within the cavernous sinus, the third nerve lies initially above the trochlear nerve, and here it receives sympathetic fibers from the carotid artery (Fig. 9–8). As it leaves the cavernous sinus, it is crossed superiorly by the trochlear and abducens nerves and divides into a superior and inferior ramus. These pass through the superior orbital fissure,[612] and enter the orbit within the annulus of Zinn (Fig. 9–2). The superior oculomotor ramus or division runs lateral to the optic nerve and ophthalmic artery and supplies the superior rectus and levator palpebrae muscles. The larger inferior oculomotor ramus or division branches in the posterior orbit and supplies the medial rectus, inferior rectus, and inferior oblique muscles, and the ciliary ganglion.[724] The blood supply of the intracranial portion of the oculomotor nerve from its emergence from the brainstem until it passes the posterior cerebral artery originates from thalamoperforating branches.[124] From this point until the nerve enters the cavernous sinus, it receives no nutrient arterioles from adjacent arteries. The part of the oculomotor nerve within the cavernous sinus receives branches from the inferior cavernous sinus artery and from a tentorial artery arising from the meningohypophyseal trunk.

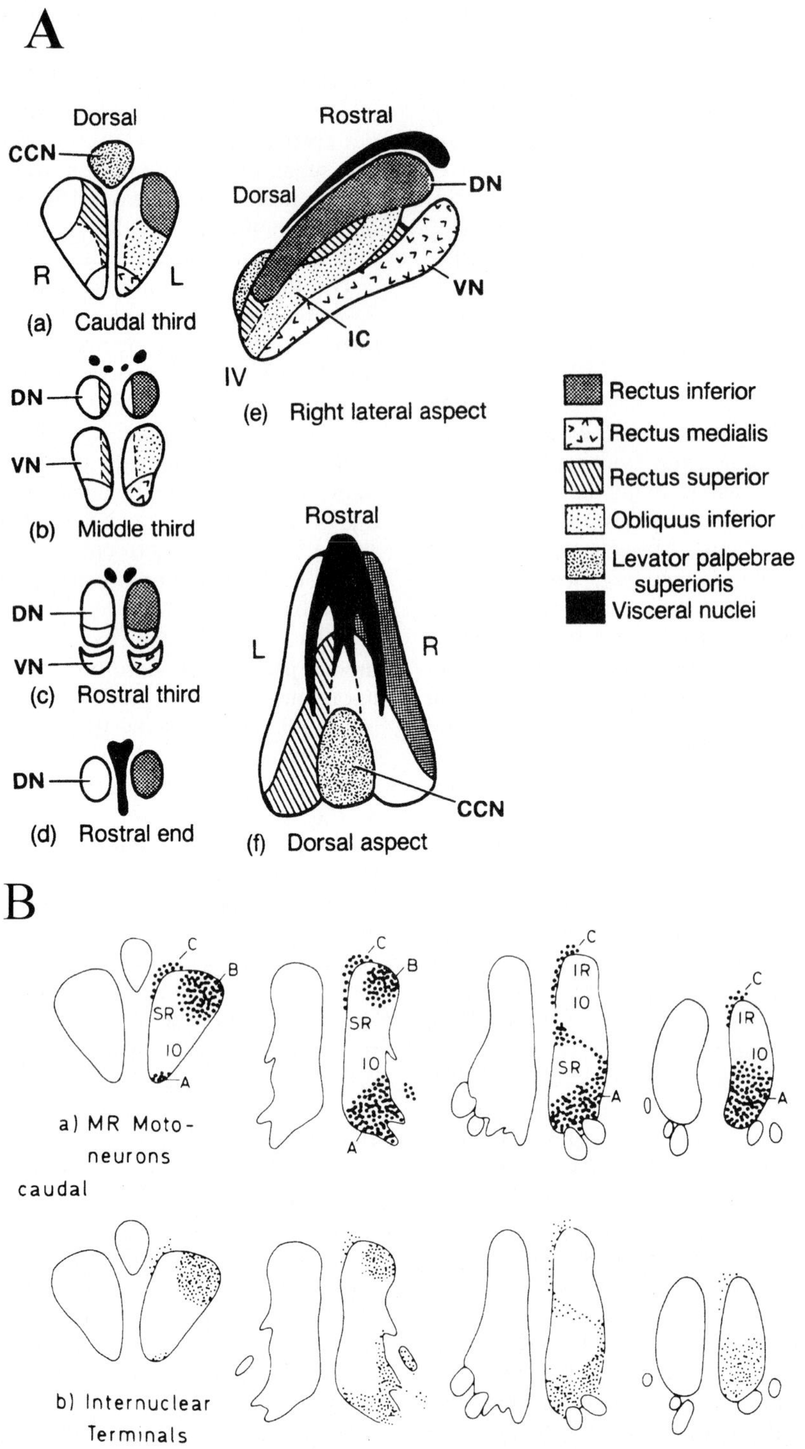

Figure 9–9. The anatomy of the oculomotor complex in the rhesus monkey. (A) Warwick's scheme, based on retrograde denervation studies. CCN = caudal central nucleus; DN = dorsal nucleus; IC = intermediate nucleus; IV = trochlear nucleus; VN = ventral nucleus; R = right; L = left. (Adapted from Warwick,[902] with permission of John Wiley and Sons, Inc.) (B) Scheme of Büttner-Ennever and Akert, based on radioactive tracer techniques. Top: the medial rectus (MR) motoneurons, identified by injecting isotope into medial rectus muscle, lie in three groups, A, B, and C. IO = inferior oblique; IR = inferior rectus; SR = superior rectus. Bottom: These same three areas also receive inputs from abducens internuclear neurons as demonstrated by injecting isotope into the contralateral sixth nerve nucleus. (From Büttner-Ennever and Akert,[118] with permission of John Wiley and Sons, Inc.)

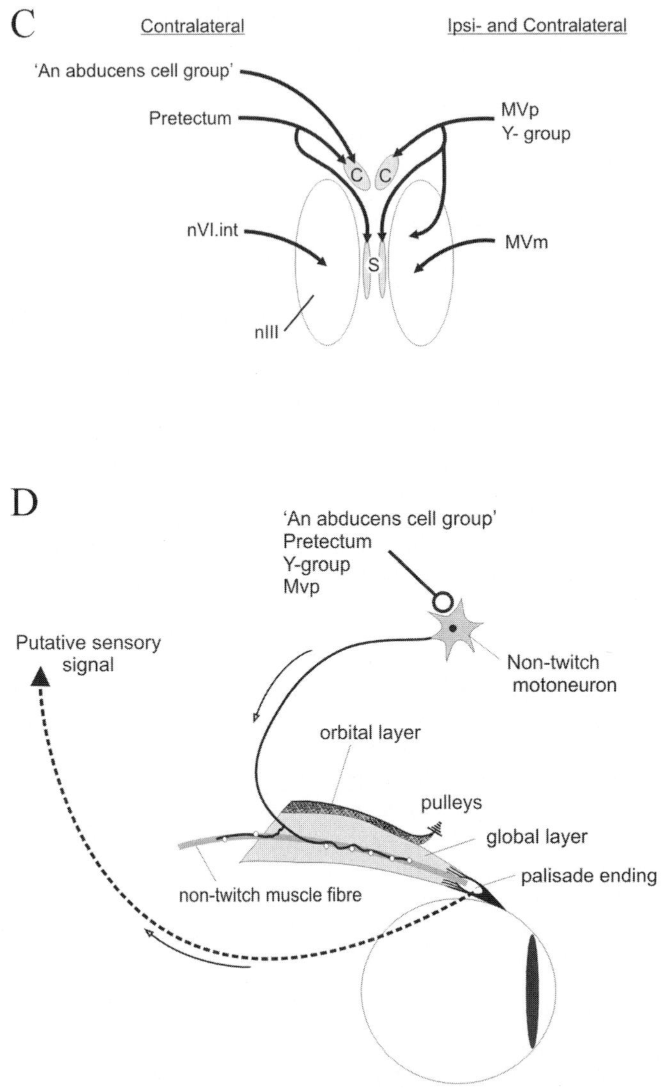

Figure 9–9. *(Continued)* (C) Summary of the different afferents to the twitch motoneurons in nIII and to the nontwitch motoneurons in the C and S groups. MVm = magnocellular medial vestibular nucleus; MVp = parvocellular medial vestibular nucleus. (D) Schematic drawing of a current hypothesis on the function of nontwitch motoneurons. Only the nontwitch muscle fibers of the global layer are associated with palisade endings at the myotendinous junction. Nontwitch muscle fibers are suited to tonic activity and could also modulate a proprioceptive feedback signal from the palisade endings. (From Wasicky et al., [903] with permission of John Wiley and Sons, Inc.)

PHYSIOLOGIC BASIS FOR CONJUGATE MOVEMENTS: YOKE MUSCLE PAIRS

Law of Reciprocal Innervation

Sherrington proposed that whenever an agonist muscle (e.g., the lateral rectus) receives a neural impulse to contract, an equivalent inhibitory impulse is sent to the motor neurons supplying the antagonist muscle of the same eye (e.g., the medial rectus) so that it will relax—the law of reciprocal innervation.[769] In fact, the extraocular muscles maintain a constant state of tension that implies some co-contraction, which may be necessary to linearize the relationship between innervation and muscle force.[166] Sherrington postulated that this reciprocal innervation was due to a stretch reflex in extraocular muscle.[769] Although, as reviewed above, the extraocular muscles do possess proprioceptors, neurophysiologic evidence in monkeys argues against the existence of a classic stretch reflex. Thus, when a trained monkey fixates a target with one eye, perturbation of the other, covered eye, using a suction contact lens, produces no change in the discharge of neurons in the abducens nucleus corresponding to the perturbed eye.[430] Moreover, bilateral section of the ophthalmic division of the trigeminal nerve, which conveys extraocular proprioceptive inputs,[683] does not affect the ability of the brain to program saccadic eye movements accurately.[312] In summary, although the mechanisms proposed by Sherrington require some revision, the principle of push-pull control of the extraocular muscles remains an important concept of the way that the brain could linearize the control of eye movements.

Law of Motor Correspondence

A second physiological principle is that for the eyes to move together requires a coordination or yoking of pairs of muscles, one from each eye. For example, to produce a horizontal movement to the left requires that the left lateral rectus and right medial rectus muscles contract together. These muscles are a yoke pair, as are the left medial rectus and right lateral rectus, which relax during the same movement. Implicit in the concept of a yoke pair is that corresponding muscles of each eye (e.g., left lateral rectus and right medial rectus) receive equal innervation so that the eyes move together. This is the simplest statement of Hering's law of motor correspondence.[343] Conventionally, vertically acting muscles are also conceptualized as being arranged in yoke pairs (e.g., the right superior rectus and the left inferior oblique), a concept that has received experimental support.[595] In fact, the way in which the extraocular muscles interact is complicated and all the extraocular muscles probably contribute force during even a simple horizontal movement. Furthermore, recent studies suggest that premotor neurons encode monocular eye movement signals.[955] Nonetheless, the concept of "yoke muscle pairs" is valuable in interpreting the results of clinical testing.

Deviations of the Visual Axes

Many normal subjects develop a deviation of the visual axes when sensory fusional mechanisms are temporarily interrupted by covering one eye. This is a *phoria* or latent deviation of the visual axes (Table 9–1). The deviation is usually constant in all directions of gaze and is called concomitant (or comitant). A deviation of the visual axis with both eyes viewing is called a *tropia.* Often the size of a tropia will change according to the direction of gaze; this is called a non-concomitant deviation, and may be due to extraocular muscle weakness or mechanical hindrance. Note that long-standing muscle palsies may become concomitant, due to changes in innervation and muscle properties, so that concomitant deviations do not exclude neurological disease.[520]

During saccadic eye movements made by normal subjects, the eyes do not move exactly together.[164] In addition, the yoking mechanism is not fixed, but can undergo some limited, adaptive changes to partially compensate for mild degrees of extraocular muscle weakness.[643] This capability can also be shown to adjust the relative innervation to the eyes in response to wearing spectacles in which the strength of the correction is different between the eyes, thereby imposing different-sized images to each eye,[644] an issue discussed further in Chapter 8 (Disconjugate Adaptation).

CLINICAL TESTING IN DIPLOPIA

The prerequisite for accurate diagnosis of diplopia and strabismus is a clear understanding of underlying anatomy and physiology. One should also record the results of each part of the examination, heeding Darwin's advice that "it is a fatal fault to reason while observing, though so necessary beforehand and so useful afterwards."

History: The Symptomatology of Strabismus

Misalignment of the visual axes—strabismus—causes the two images of a seen object to fall on noncorresponding areas of the two retinas (Fig. 9–10). This usually causes diplopia—the

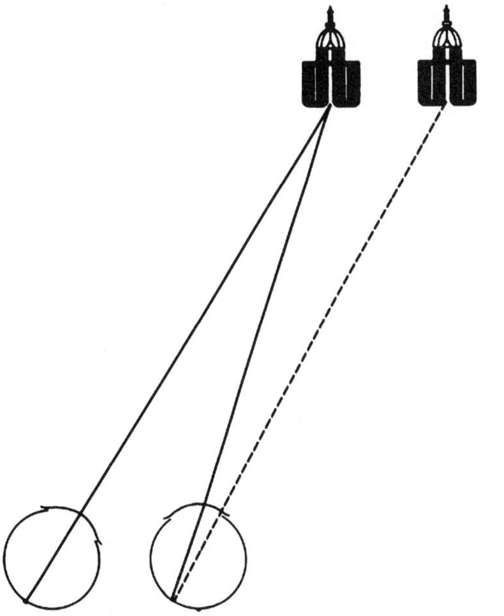

Figure 9–10. Disparate retinal images. The image of a distant object lies on the fovea of the left eye but, because of an esotropia in the right eye (due to a right lateral rectus weakness, for instance), the image lies medial to the fovea. Each retinal element corresponds to a specific subjective visual direction. Consequently, the subject localizes the same object in two different directions and experiences diplopia. The broken line indicates the perceived direction of the false image.

sensation of seeing an object at two different locations in space. In addition, the two foveae are simultaneously presented different images, so that occasionally two different objects are perceived at the same point in space. This is called visual confusion.

At an early point in the evaluation, it should be determined whether the diplopia is binocular or monocular. Covering one eye can make the distinction. Monocular diplopia is most commonly caused by astigmatism or spherical refractive errors,[158,927] incipient cataract, corneal irregularity,[345] lens dislocation, or eye trauma. Such patients may report that the two images differ in brightness or that there are more than two images. Monocular diplopia caused by lens or corneal abnormality can be improved by pinhole vision. Monocular diplopia can be a psychiatric symptom. Sometimes, retinal disorders that effectively displace the macula can lead to binocular diplopia.[58] In the dragged-fovea diplopia syndrome, central, but not peripheral, diplopia diminishes when the patient views illuminated optotypes in a dark room.[187] Thus, ophthalmoscopy, slit-lamp examination, and other special testing may be necessary to identify ocular disorders causing diplopia. Rarely, diplopia is reported with cerebral disorders.[554,728]

Patients who complain of little or no visual disturbance despite an obvious ocular misalignment usually have had their strabismus from early in life. Thus, it is important to enquire about any history of strabismus, eye patching, or abnormal head posture; old photographs may be of help. It is also worthwhile asking about prior visits to ophthalmologists and optometrists. On occasion, patients with strabismus (especially children) present with an abnormal head posture but without any visual complaints.[130] Occasionally patients with a large acquired exotropia will not complain of diplopia because the images are so far apart.

Ask about the type of diplopia (horizontal, vertical, torsional), in what direction of gaze it is most marked, if it is worse for near or distant viewing, and if it is affected by head posture. For example, a lateral rectus weakness leads to horizontal diplopia that is typically worse on looking ipsilaterally and at distant objects and is less troublesome if the head is turned toward the side of the palsy.

Other symptoms caused by misalignment of the visual axes include blurred vision, vertigo, and oscillopsia; the last two complaints relate to inadequate compensatory movements of the eyes during head rotation.[234,916] Patients with acquired strabismus tend to close one eye. Some patients who have brainstem disease or who are confused may even keep one eye closed and yet deny double vision.[254]

The Examination in Strabismus

Certain essential preliminaries should precede ocular motor testing. These include measurement of corrected visual acuity in each eye, tests for stereopsis, and a simple confrontation assessment of the central and the peripheral visual fields. In certain patients, especially children and some young adults, refraction is necessary. Note any abnormal head posture, such as a tilt or turn. These observations completed, the examination consists of four parts: assessment of the range of eye movements, subjective diplopia testing, cover testing, and, with vertical deviations, the Bielschowsky head-tilt test. Appendix A contains a summary of this testing.

RANGE OF EYE MOVEMENTS

Ask the patient to follow a small target through the full range of movement, including the nine cardinal or diagnostic positions of gaze (Table 9–1). First test one eye at a time with the other covered, movements referred to as ductions. Then test both eyes together, movements referred to as versions or conjugate movements. Note any limitation of eye movement that persists despite vigorous encouragement. A simple, approximate method to evaluate ocular alignment during versional movements is to ask the patient to fixate on a penlight and to note the position of the corneal reflection of the light in the nine cardinal positions. Rather than moving the penlight, move the patient's head so that the examiner's eye stays aligned with the penlight. If the images from the two corneas appear centered, then the visual axes are usually correctly aligned. This method is especially valuable when facial asymmetries, such as hypertelorism, ptosis, or epicanthic folds, give the false impression of strabismus. Epicanthic folds simulate esotropia in young children. However, some individual may appear to be exotropic because there is a medial displacement of the reflected images within the pupils. This is due to a positive angle kappa, which defines the geometric relationship between the pupillary and visual axes; it is more common in albinism, a finding possibly related to the anomalous crossed visual decussation of axons from temporal retina in this condition.[107] Semiquantitative methods of measuring range of eye movements are available that are helpful in clinical studies, such as drug trials in myasthenia gravis.[477]

When the range of movement is limited, it is important to determine whether the limitation is due to muscle weakness or mechanical restriction. For this purpose, a forced duction test may be of value. After applying topical anesthesia, an attempt is made to move the eye into the direction of action of the paretic muscle. This can be done using ophthalmic forceps or by simply pressing a cotton-tipped applicator against the limbus of the cornea. First ask the patient to attempt to look in the direction of action of the weak muscle. If it is possible for the examiner to move the eye into the paretic field, this implies weakness of that muscle. Restriction to passive movement constitutes a positive passive forced duction test and indicates mechanical restriction. Second, ask the patient to attempt to look in the direction of action of the paretic muscle while the examiner's forceps actively opposes this movement. Resistance to the forceps constitutes a positive active forced duction test (or force generation test) and suggests that muscle strength is intact and that the loss of ocular motility is due to mechanical restriction. High-resolution MRI techniques often allow precise diagnosis in such patients.

In any patient with a reduced range of voluntary eye movements, it is important to exclude myasthenia gravis; usually an edrophonium (Tensilon) test is performed (see below).

SUBJECTIVE DIPLOPIA TESTING

When the patient is cooperative, subjective tests of diplopia may reliably indicate the disparity between retinal images. When strabismus is due to extraocular muscle weakness (non-concomitant or paralytic strabismus), the patient can view, with the fovea of the nonparetic eye, targets in all directions of gaze. The eye with the paretic muscle, however, will not be able to bring to the fovea the image of a target located in the field of weakened action; consequently, the image will be projected onto extrafoveal retina (Fig. 9–10). In other words, the patient will interpret the object to be displaced in the direction of the paralysis (or opposite to the direction of the deviation). When the image is on the nasal retina, the patient thinks the object is in the temporal field of vision. This is uncrossed diplopia and is typical of esotropia (e.g., due to lateral rectus palsy). When the image is projected onto the temporal retina, the patient thinks the object is located nasally. This is crossed diplopia and is typical of exotropia (e.g., due to medial rectus palsy).

Two further principles are important in this type of diplopia testing: (1) the two images are maximally separated when the patient looks into the direction of action of the paretic muscle, and (2) the target seen by the paretic eye is usually projected more peripherally, particularly as the patient looks into the paretic field. One can determine which image comes from the paretic eye by transiently occluding either eye and asking the patient to report to which eye the most remotely located image belongs.

The use of a red glass or Maddox rod (Fig. 9–11) usually aids examination. A Maddox rod consists of small glass rods with a red filter; it may be oriented according to the desired plane of testing—horizontal or vertical. When the Maddox rod is held before the right eye and a penlight is viewed with both eyes, the patient sees a white spot of light with the left eye and, through the Maddox rod, a red line. Since the Maddox rod can be rotated 90 degrees, the horizontal and vertical components of diplopia can be evaluated separately. Ask the patient to follow the penlight as the eyes are taken into the nine cardinal positions. For each position, the patient reports how far the white light and red line are separated and where the white light is located in relation to the red line. The image from the eye with the weakened muscle (whether it be the white light or the red line) will be projected furthest into the paretic field of gaze. Note that the Maddox rod prevents disparity-driven vergence because the images are so dissimilar. Therefore, it primarily tests for phorias and latent palsies that may not be apparent under binocular viewing conditions. Normal individuals commonly have a phoria, so that small, concomitant deviations detected during Maddox rod testing may be normal. If a phoria is non-concomitant, however, an extraocular muscle may be weak or restricted. The Maddox rod test is most useful for evaluating small deviations. Larger deviations may cause image displacements that make the test difficult for the patient to understand, and are therefore best evaluated with cover tests (described in the next section). Two Maddox rods (one white, one red) can be used to evaluate torsional disparity between the two eyes, although careful interpretation of the results is necessary. Other methods, such as fundus photography,[889] and scanning laser ophthalmoscopy,[224] are sometimes indicated.

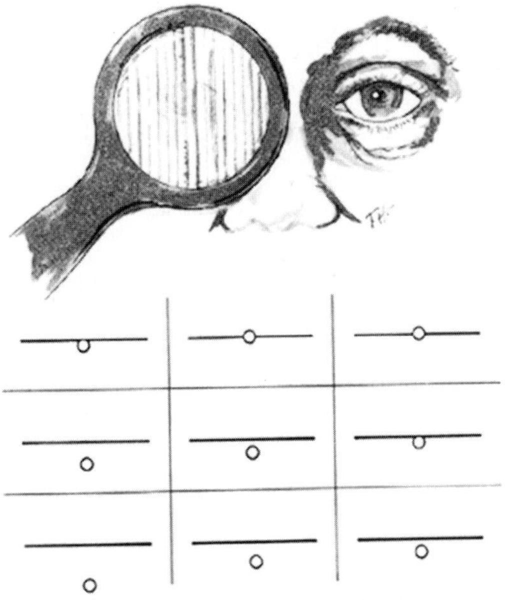

Figure 9–11. The Maddox rod test. Because the Maddox rod breaks fusional vergence, it tests for both phorias and tropias. (See text for explanation.) This patient has a left superior oblique weakness. The separation of images is greatest when the patient looks down and to the right.

Other subjective tests that dissociate the images seen by the two eyes include the Hess screen test and the Lancaster red-green test.[488] In the Lancaster test, the patient wears goggles with a red filter in front of the right eye and a green filter in front of the left. Thus, the patient can see the image of a red light with one eye and the image of a green light with the other. The test prevents disparity-driven vergence. The examiner holds one flashlight and the patient holds the other. The separation of the red and green images on a screen, in each of the nine cardinal positions of gaze, is measured and represents the deviation of the visual axes. An alternative method is to measure the separation of red and green lights at various points on the horizontal and vertical meridians;[952] the inferred positions of the right and left eyes can then be plotted on a graph. The deviation of such a curve from the line for orthophoria can be used to compare relative strengths of yoke muscles and to determine whether the deviation is concomitant or nonconcomitant (paralytic). The Lancaster red-green test can be performed with simple, inexpensive portable equipment.[810]

Hess screens are another standard way to graphically display the ocular deviation at different gaze angles. Rather than plotting vertical versus horizontal position, a modified Hess screen plots pairs of the three rotational vectors of each eye (X, Y, Z) and also allows visualization of Listing's plane (see Video Display: Diplopia and Strabismus).[822]

COVER TESTS

Cover tests demand less cooperation on the part of the patient than do the red glass and Maddox rod tests, so they are more suitable for examining young or inattentive patients. Moreover, cover tests can be used in patients without binocular vision, provided they can fixate with the fovea. Cover tests depend upon the principle that, when one eye is required to fix upon an object, it will do so with the fovea. (Certain exceptions to this rule, due to eccentric fixation and anomalous retinal correspondence, occur in some patients with congenital strabismus.)[889] If the principal visual axis is not directed toward the object, then an eye movement (saccade) will be necessary to move the image of the object onto the fovea. It is the detection and estimation of the size of this corrective saccade (*movement of redress*) that provides the clinician with an indication of misalignment of the visual axes.

The *cover test* (Fig. 9–12) reveals *heterotropia* (or *tropia*)—a misalignment of the visual axes when both eyes are viewing a single target (see Video Display: Diplopia and Strabismus). A target that requires visual discrimination (e.g., an "E") should be used to ensure a fixed accommodative state. This fixation target should ideally be at a distance of 6 meters (20 ft). Testing with a near target at 35 cm (14 in) is also necessary. First with the eyes in the central position (Fig. 9–12A), cover the right eye and look for any movement of the uncovered left eye—the movement of redress. If no movement of the left eye is detected (Fig. 9–12B), remove the cover (Fig. 9–12C) and then cover the left eye, looking for a movement of redress of the right eye (Fig. 9–12D) (see Video Display: Diplopia and Strabismus). Repeat this test with the eyes brought to the nine cardinal positions of gaze, by rotating the patient's head while the eyes fix upon the same target. The test should then be repeated with a near target.

Note that during the cover test only the uncovered eye is observed. When the cover is removed from the other eye, it may also rotate to reacquire the target, if it is the preferred eye for fixation (Fig. 9–12E). If, however, neither eye is preferred (*alternate fixation*), then no movement occurs when the cover is removed (Fig. 9–12F). Movements of an eye that occur when the cover is removed from it—the *cover-uncover test* may indicate either a tropia or phoria. Therefore, the cover test must first be performed to determine if a tropia is present; if it is not, then movement of the eye when the cover is removed indicates a phoria. Use of a translucent occluder, which is opaque to the

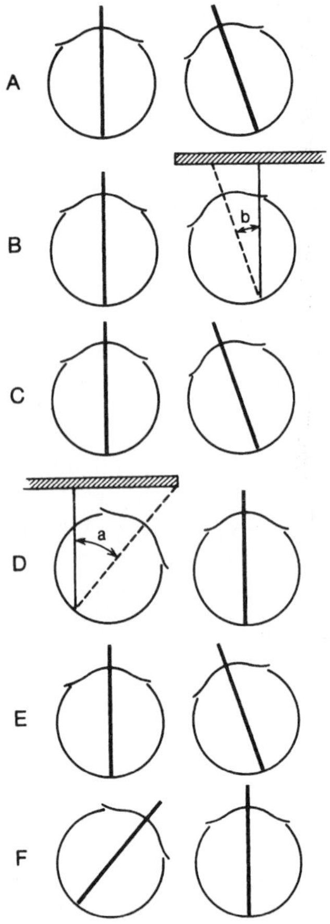

Figure 9–12. The cover test. (A) Initially, with both eyes viewing, there is an esotropia (right eye turned in). (B) When the cover is placed before the non-fixating right eye, no movement occurs; nor does it occur when (C) the cover is removed. (D) When the left eye is covered, the right eye must fixate the target and a movement of redress occurs. Note that the deviation of the sound eye under cover (the secondary deviation—a) is greater than that of the paretic eye under cover (primary deviation—b). When the cover is removed, either (E) the left eye again takes up fixation, or (F) the paretic eye continues to fixate, if the patient is an "alternate fixator."

patient but transparent to the examiner, allows movements of the eye under cover to be observed.[805]

In order to bring out the maximal deviation—whether tropia or phoria—the *alternate cover test* should be used. As the occluder is quickly transferred from one eye to the other (to prevent binocular viewing), any movement of redress is noted (see Video Display: Diplopia and Strabismus). Each eye must be covered for several seconds, to allow the eyes to acquire their new resting position, before switching the cover. Deviations may grow over 10 to 20 seconds. An example of the use of the alternate cover test in diagnosing a right sixth nerve palsy is shown in Figure 9–13. Because the deviation varies according to the direction of gaze, the strabismus is non-concomitant and probably paralytic. During the alternate cover test, the detection of a larger movement of redress in one eye than the other also helps identify the weak member of a yoke muscle pair. The deviation of the paretic eye under cover while the normal eye is fixating is referred to as the *primary deviation*; the deviation of the normal eye under cover while the paretic eye is fixating is called the *secondary deviation*. The secondary deviation is greater than the primary deviation (see below). When the cover is moved from the paretic eye to the normal eye, the difference between the primary and secondary deviations can be observed (see Fig. 9–12 and Fig. 9–13). On the other hand, with concomitant strabismus, the movement of redress is equal in both eyes. It is often helpful to perform the alternate cover test during fixation of both near and far targets; sixth nerve palsy may only become evident while viewing far targets.

Performing the *alternate cover test with prisms* is a convenient way to measure the deviation. Place a prism before the viewing eye and then alternate the cover to establish whether there is any change in the size of the movement of redress. For esodeviations, the prism should be placed base out; for exodeviations, base in; for left hyperdeviation, base down in front of the left eye; and for right hyperdeviation, base down in front of the right eye. (Generally, this may be stated, "The apex of the prism points toward the deviation.") The strength of the prism is increased until the movement of redress is absent or just reverses (e.g., esotropia becomes exotropia). The prism strength at this point then indicates the magnitude of the deviation. This procedure is simple (it may be performed at the bedside) and often aids in the diagnosis and documentation of a change in the strabismus.

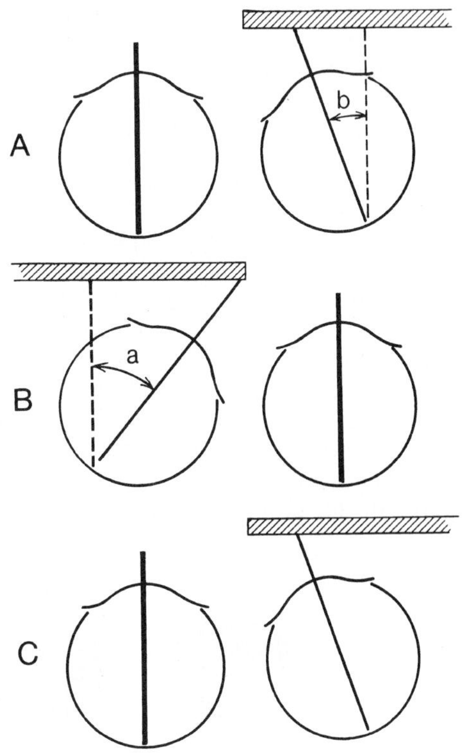

Figure 9–13. The alternate cover test. This test prevents fusional vergence and thus tests for phorias and tropias. Any movement of the eyes, as the cover is quickly transferred (to prevent binocular vision), is noted. In this example, there is an esodeviation caused by a right lateral rectus weakness. The secondary deviation (a) of the sound, left eye under cover (shown in B) is greater than the primary deviation (b) of the paretic, right eye under cover (shown in A and C).

DIAGNOSIS OF VERTICAL OCULAR MOTOR DEVIATION: THE BIELSCHOWSKY HEAD-TILT TEST

Testing of a vertical deviation is best performed as a four-stage procedure: First, determine the side of the hypertropia. Second, determine whether the deviation is greater in right or left gaze. Third, determine whether the deviation is greater in up or down gaze. Finally, measure the size of the deviation with head tilt to the right or left shoulder (the Bielschowsky head-tilt test, see Video Display: Diplopia and Strabismus).

Consider a patient with an acute left superior oblique weakness (Fig. 9–14). First, with the eyes in central position, use the cover-uncover test to reveal the tropia. The alternate cover test confirms a left hyperdeviation (Fig. 9–14A). (By convention, all vertical deviations are described as hyperdeviations.) This means that either the depressors of the left eye or elevators of the right eye are weak. Second, ask the patient to look to the right and to the left and, in both positions, use the alternate cover test to determine the effect on the vertical deviation. In our patient, the left hyperdeviation is more marked on gaze to the right (Fig. 9–14B). In this position of gaze, the oblique muscles become more important for control of the vertical position of the left eye and the vertical recti become more important for the right eye. Thus, either the left superior oblique or the right superior rectus must be weak. Third, ask the patient to look up and down in right gaze (Fig. 9–14C). The left hyperdeviation will be more marked in gaze down (the field of action of the left superior oblique), pinpointing the weakness to the left superior oblique muscle. Finally, the head is tilted first to the left and then to the right, performing the alternate cover test in each position (Fig. 9–14D). It is important to maintain the eyes close to central position during this part of the testing. With a left superior oblique palsy, the left hyperdeviation becomes more marked on tilt of the head to the left shoulder (positive Bielschowsky

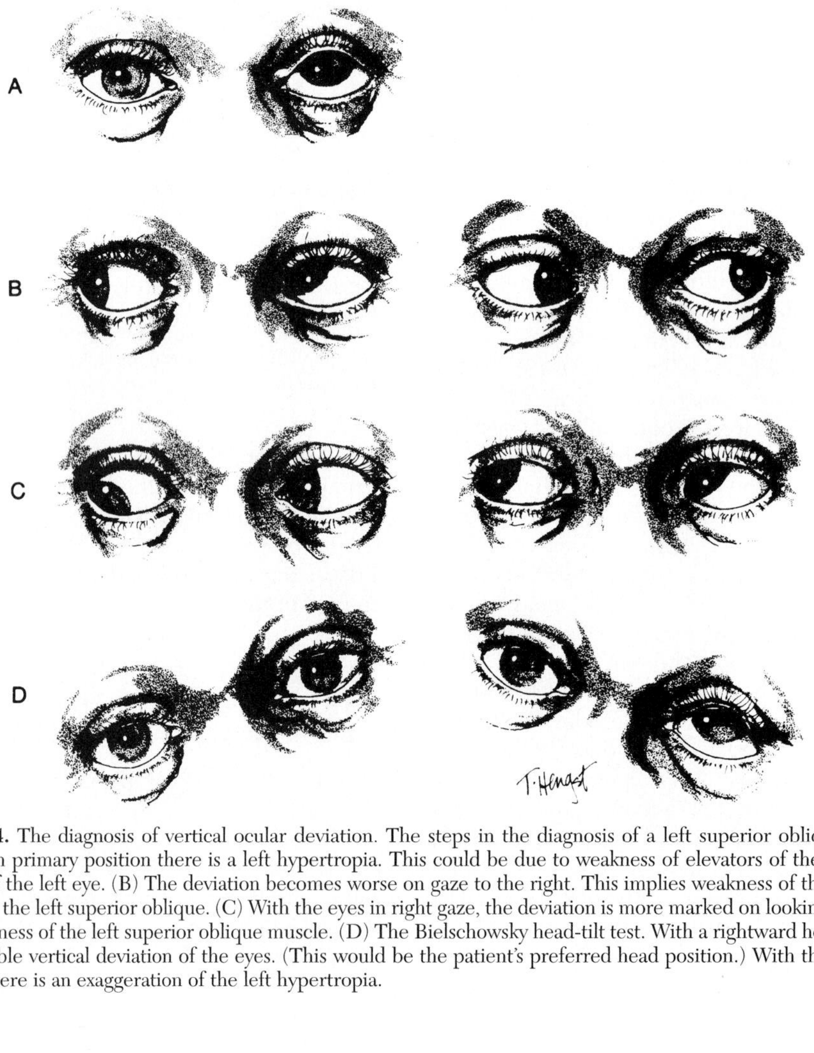

Figure 9–14. The diagnosis of vertical ocular deviation. The steps in the diagnosis of a left superior oblique palsy are shown. (A) In primary position there is a left hypertropia. This could be due to weakness of elevators of the right eye or depressors of the left eye. (B) The deviation becomes worse on gaze to the right. This implies weakness of the right superior rectus or the left superior oblique. (C) With the eyes in right gaze, the deviation is more marked on looking down. This implies weakness of the left superior oblique muscle. (D) The Bielschowsky head-tilt test. With a rightward head tilt, there is no detectable vertical deviation of the eyes. (This would be the patient's preferred head position.) With the head tilted to the left, there is an exaggeration of the left hypertropia.

head-tilt test). The reason for this is that normally a small (about 5 degree) counter-rolling movement about the visual axis occurs when the head is tilted 45 degrees to either shoulder. This ocular counter-rolling reflex is accomplished by the concerted action of the superior rectus and superior oblique of one eye and by the inferior rectus and inferior oblique of the other eye. When the action of the superior oblique muscle is lacking on one side, only the superior rectus will contract on that side, and it elevates and intorts the eye. In some patients with fourth nerve palsy, dynamic head rolling may induce vertical nystagmus rather than the torsional nystagmus that normally occurs.[452]

With acute muscle palsy, the first three tests usually give the diagnosis. With time, deviations that were originally paralytic in type may become equal in all directions of gaze (so-called spread of concomitance); patients may variably recruit the vertical recti or oblique muscles to gain motor fusion.[600] In long-standing superior oblique palsy, the deviation may even become greater on up gaze. This may be due to a change in innervational pattern as well as due to mechanical factors. Occluding one eye for 24 to 48 hours—a diagnostic occlusion test—may bring out the maximum deviation. Alternatively, when a muscle paresis affects a strongly dominant eye, the innervation to the other eye may appear to be affected. Consider a patient with a left superior oblique palsy, who habitually fixates with the left eye. To elevate the adducted left eye requires less innervation for the left inferior oblique muscle. By Hering's law, the innervation to the right superior rectus (to which the left inferior oblique is yoked) will also be less and so the depressed right eye may falsely suggest a paresis of the right superior rectus muscle.[207,887] This may make steps 1 and 2 inconclusive,[654] but step 3 will still show that the deviation is greater in down gaze and the Bielschowsky head-tilt test results usually will be positive, the left hypertropia being maximized on left head tilt.

The head-tilt test is positive in most cases of superior oblique muscle palsy, and the vertical deviation often increases with time.[781] The test results are positive less frequently with palsies of the vertical recti, inferior oblique, or restrictive ophthalmopathy.[480] Bielschowsky thought that a vertical deviation combined with a negative head-tilt test result usually indicated a vertical rectus palsy.[72]

The *physiologic basis* of the head-tilt test rests with the pattern of innervation to the extraocular muscles during a head tilt to either shoulder, when stimulation of the vestibular otoliths induces ocular counter-rolling. In this situation, the vertical eye muscles no longer are driven in their usually yoked pairs. Instead, the otolithic reflex causes compensatory cyclorotation of the eyes by co-innervation of the ipsilateral (to the side of the tilt) superior oblique and superior rectus muscles, producing intorsion, and of the contralateral inferior oblique and inferior rectus muscles, producing extorsion. Weakness of any one of these muscles leads to both a cyclodeviation and a vertical deviation of the eyes. Nevertheless, the deviation that occurs following superior oblique palsy is often larger than can be accounted for simply by weakness of this muscle. Quantitative analysis indicates that such deviations must be due to overaction of the superior rectus of the same eye.[708] This increase in the deviation, which tends to become greater with time, may be due to an increase in the gain (i.e., hyperactivity) of ocular counter-rolling,[454,635,781] or to a "tight" or contracted superior rectus.

PATHOPHYSIOLOGY OF SOME COMMONLY ENCOUNTERED SIGNS IN STRABISMUS

Primary and Secondary Deviation

Testing of the movements of each eye viewing alone (ductions) may not reveal minimal muscle weakness that the patient can overcome by effort. Observing the movements of both eyes at the same time (conjugate movements or versions), however, will often reveal a subtle muscle paresis. The hallmark of strabismus due to muscle paresis is incomitance—the deviation varies as a function of the angle of gaze. During alternate cover testing, the deviations of the two eyes (as judged by the movement of redress) may differ. Most patients normally fixate with their good eye, and the paretic eye deviates a certain amount from the line of sight: this is the primary deviation. If, by briefly covering the good eye, the weak eye is forced to fixate a target located within its paretic field of action, then a larger deviation of the good eye under cover occurs: the secondary deviation

(Fig. 9–12 and Fig. 9–13) (see Video Display: Diplopia and Strabismus). The discrepancy between the size of the primary and secondary deviations forms the basis of a widely accepted clinical dictum used to differentiate paralytic from nonparalytic strabismus. The secondary deviation (the angle between the visual axes of the eyes when the paretic eye fixates a given target) is greater than the primary deviation (the angle between the visual axes when the normal eye fixates the same target).

The explanation of this phenomenon is mainly related to the change in the position of the eyes within the orbits when either one eye or the other takes up fixation of the same target. When a single given muscle is paretic, the deviation between the two eyes is proportional to the difference between the forces generated by the paretic muscle and its normal yoke muscle. Furthermore, the amount of force contributed by a given muscle toward holding the eye in a given orbital position increases as the eye is moved into the direction of action of that muscle. Therefore, as the eyes move in the direction of action of the paretic muscle, the difference in forces generated by the normal and paretic yoke muscles increases, thus increasing the deviation between the two eyes—the hallmark of a paralytic or noncomitant strabismus.

Why is secondary deviation evident when the paretic eye is fixating? In this case, the affected eye is held in an orbital position further in the direction of action of the paretic muscle than when the nonparetic eye is fixating the same target (Fig. 9–12 and Fig. 9–13). Therefore, the secondary deviation is greater than the primary deviation, mainly because of the change in the positions of both eyes toward the direction of action of the paretic muscle. In addition, if the paretic eye is unable to foveate a target that lies in its paretic field of action, then the inability to decrease the retinal error (difference between the location of the image of the target on the retina and the fovea) precludes normal, negative feedback (see Chapter 4). This open-loop stimulation may lead to an increase in the innervation sent to the extraocular muscle and the secondary deviation is made even larger. The fundamental reason for the phenomenon, however, relates to where both eyes are located in the orbits, and the forces that must keep them there.

Past-Pointing and Disturbance of Egocentric Localization

Patients who have an acute paralytic strabismus may mislocalize objects (e.g., an examiner's finger) when rapidly reaching in the direction of the field of action of the paretic extraocular muscle. The phenomenon is more easily demonstrated if the patient's pointing arm is hidden from his or her view by, for example, being held under a table. Alternatively, the patient is asked to look at the target and then point with the eyes closed. For example, a patient with a left lateral rectus palsy, when viewing with the left eye and reaching into the left field, will tend to past-point to the left of the target. Although past-pointing is usually thought of as a sign of paralytic strabismus, it has been encountered occasionally with concomitant deviations when sight, long deprived from one eye, is suddenly restored.[21]

The explanation of past-pointing is controversial. It could occur because, for example, with a left lateral rectus palsy, the image of the examiner's finger lies nasal to the fovea of the paretic eye, and hence the patient incorrectly localizes the object in the temporal field. This explanation, however, does not account for the persistence of past-pointing after the image of the target has been brought to the fovea of the paretic eye.[658,888] Another explanation for past-pointing is that it reflects what Helmholtz called the "intensity of the effort of will,"[341] or efference copy, which is sent to the paretic muscle (as evidenced by the large deviation of the normal eye under cover).

It has also been suggested that a mismatch between extraocular proprioception and the neural signal being sent to these muscles may contribute to the phenomenon of past-pointing. Recall that the extraocular proprioceptors are probably the palisade organs that lie at the musculotendinous junctions.[119,217,722] It is reported that if patients who have undergone correction of strabismus are tested the instant the bandage is removed from their operated eye, they pointed accurately to targets, provided that the musculotendinous junction was not involved in the operation. If, however, surgery has disrupted the musculotendinous junction, pointing is inaccurate.[817,818] These results have not always been confirmed, however.[84] Other evidence to support a role for proprioception comes from the report that patients with herpes zoster ophthalmicus,[131] or those who have undergone thermocoagulation of the trigeminal nerve,[875] may show past-pointing. This may be due to dysfunction of the proprioceptive inputs that run in the first division of the trigeminal nerve. Experimental proprioceptive denervation of the extraocular muscles in monkeys does not impair pointing accuracy, implying that efference copy is important.[509] Finally, enucleation in infancy may lead to esotropia of the remaining eye,[342] implying that afferent information from a blind eye is important for the alignment of the fellow eye. Thus, the relative roles of inflow and outflow in past-pointing in patients with strabismus have yet to be agreed upon, but this common clinical sign remains an important method for studying the ways that the brain constructs an accurate internal map of extrapersonal space.

Head Tilts and Turns

Commonly, patients with strabismus turn or tilt their heads to minimize diplopia. Indeed, these findings suggest a paralytic deviation of the eyes.[130] Head turns are frequently associated with paresis of the horizontal extraocular muscles, most typically lateral rectus palsy, in which case the head is turned toward the side of the weakness. They also occur in patients with congenital nystagmus, when the nystagmus is reduced by keeping the eyes in an eccentric (null) position in the orbit. Rarely, a continuous change of horizontal head position occurs in periodic alternating nystagmus. Head turns with nystagmus are discussed in Chapter 10.

Patients with weakness of the vertical recti may carry their heads flexed or extended to keep the eye out of the field of action of the paretic muscle. Similarly, patients whose horizontal diplopia is made worse in elevation or depression of the eyes—A-pattern and V-pattern—may elevate or depress their chin (see Clinical Features and Diagnosis of Concomitant Strabismus, below).

Head tilts (ear to shoulder) are most common with paresis of the oblique muscles, but also occur with restrictive ophthalmopathy. With a superior oblique palsy, the head is characteristically turned and tilted away from the side of the weakness and the chin may be depressed. The tilted posture of the head with a superior oblique palsy is usually adopted to lessen diplopia. In some patients, the head is habitually tilted toward the side of the lesion; in this situation, the deviation is actually greater, but presumably this makes it easier for the patient to ignore one image. In general, however, patients adopt abnormal head postures that keep the eye out of the field of action of the paretic muscle. Compensatory ocular head tilt should be differentiated from the ocular tilt reaction (Chapter 11), and from spasmodic torticollis of other cause.

Dynamic Properties of Eye Movements in Paralytic Strabismus

Clinical testing of strabismus emphasizes examination of static deviations of the eyes, since these are relatively easy to quantify and compare. Nonetheless, paralytic strabismus invariably leads to changes in dynamic properties of the various classes of eye movement.

Four different types of abnormalities are encountered in patients with paralytic strabismus. First, weakness of an extraocular muscle causes slowing and restriction of all classes of eye movements made into the field of action of that muscle, although the specific pattern of weakness will depend upon the innervational command (see below). Second, if the patient views with the paretic eye but the movements of the covered, normal eye are measured, then as the patient persists in attempts to look at a target in the paretic field of action, larger movements of the normal eye will occur. This latter effect is referred to as an open-loop response since the paretic eye is not able to foveate the desired target and the inability to decrease the retinal error precludes normal negative feedback (for discussion, see Chapter 4). This phenomenon may contribute to development of a secondary deviation. Third, if the patient chooses to habitually view with the paretic eye (for example, by patching the normal eye), then plastic-adaptive changes will occur; specifically, the brain will increase innervation conjugately in an attempt to improve the accuracy of movements of the paretic eye. These adaptive changes affect saccades,[4,456,646] smooth pursuit,[646] the vestibulo-ocular reflex,[765,880,921] and even the yoking mechanism itself. The last is only amenable to a relatively small range of adaptive change, which may nevertheless be adequate to compensate for partial muscle palsies.[643] Fourth, depending on the muscle that is paretic, eye movements may not obey Listing's law in the acute phase, but may do so after time to adapt to chronic lesions, which is evidence that this law is implemented neurally.[920,923] However, in chronic ocular motor palsies, Listing's plane may be still be shifted.[822] A fuller discussion of these adaptive changes may be found in chapters dealing with each class of eye movements, but here we present findings from a patient to illustrate some key points.

The patient was a 70-year-old diabetic man who suffered a left abducens palsy 1 month previously. At the time of eye movement recording, the patient had been habitually fixating with his normal, right eye. With the sound eye covered, the patient was able to look about 8 degrees left into the field of action of the paretic lateral rectus muscle.

SACCADES IN PARALYTIC STRABISMUS

With the *sound right eye viewing*, the patient was asked to alternately refixate targets located 8 degrees to the right and to the left of the midline in the horizontal plane (Fig. 9–15A). Leftward saccades, made by the paretic eye, were slow and hypometric, with onward post-saccadic drifts that slowed as the eye moved into the left field of gaze. The initial part of these saccades, from right gaze to the central position, was faster because of the elastic restoring forces, which helped the eye to the midline. Rightward saccades, made by the left eye, were, in contrast, rapid and only mildly hypometric. The saccades of the normal, right eye showed only mild hypometria.

With the *paretic left eye viewing*, a series of slow, leftward saccades occurred in that eye, as the patient attempted to foveate the leftward target. During refixations from the target located at right 8 degrees to that at left 8 degrees, an initial saccadic command for a

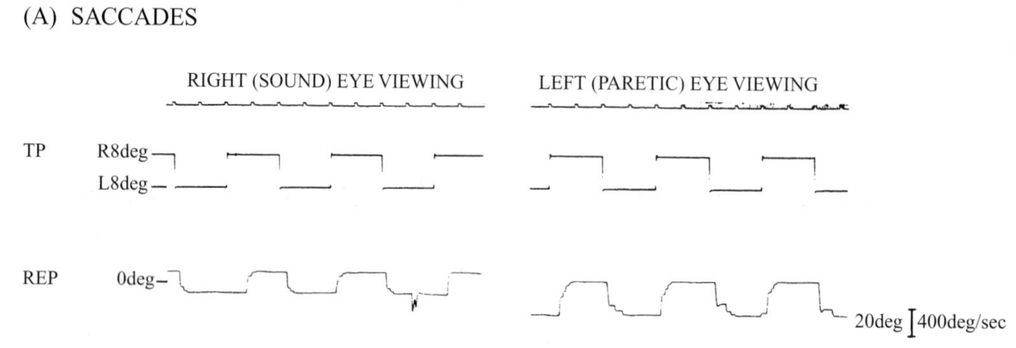

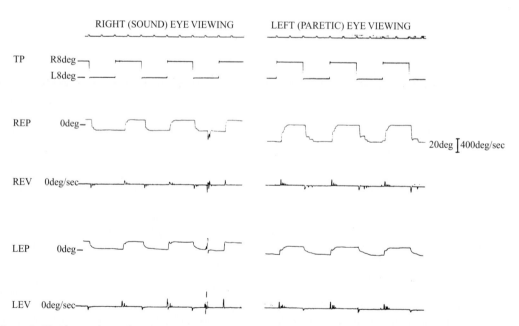

Figure 9–15. Abnormalities of versional eye movements in a patient with a left sixth nerve palsy. Eye movements were recorded by infrared oculography. (A) Saccades between two targets located 8 degrees to the right and left of the midline. With the sound right eye viewing, leftward saccades made by the right eye were of normal velocity and only mildly hypometric, whereas leftward saccades made by the left eye were slow and hypometric. With the paretic left eye viewing, leftward saccades made by the left eye were slow and hypometric, whereas leftward saccade made by the right eye were hypermetric, reflecting the neural command sent to both eyes.

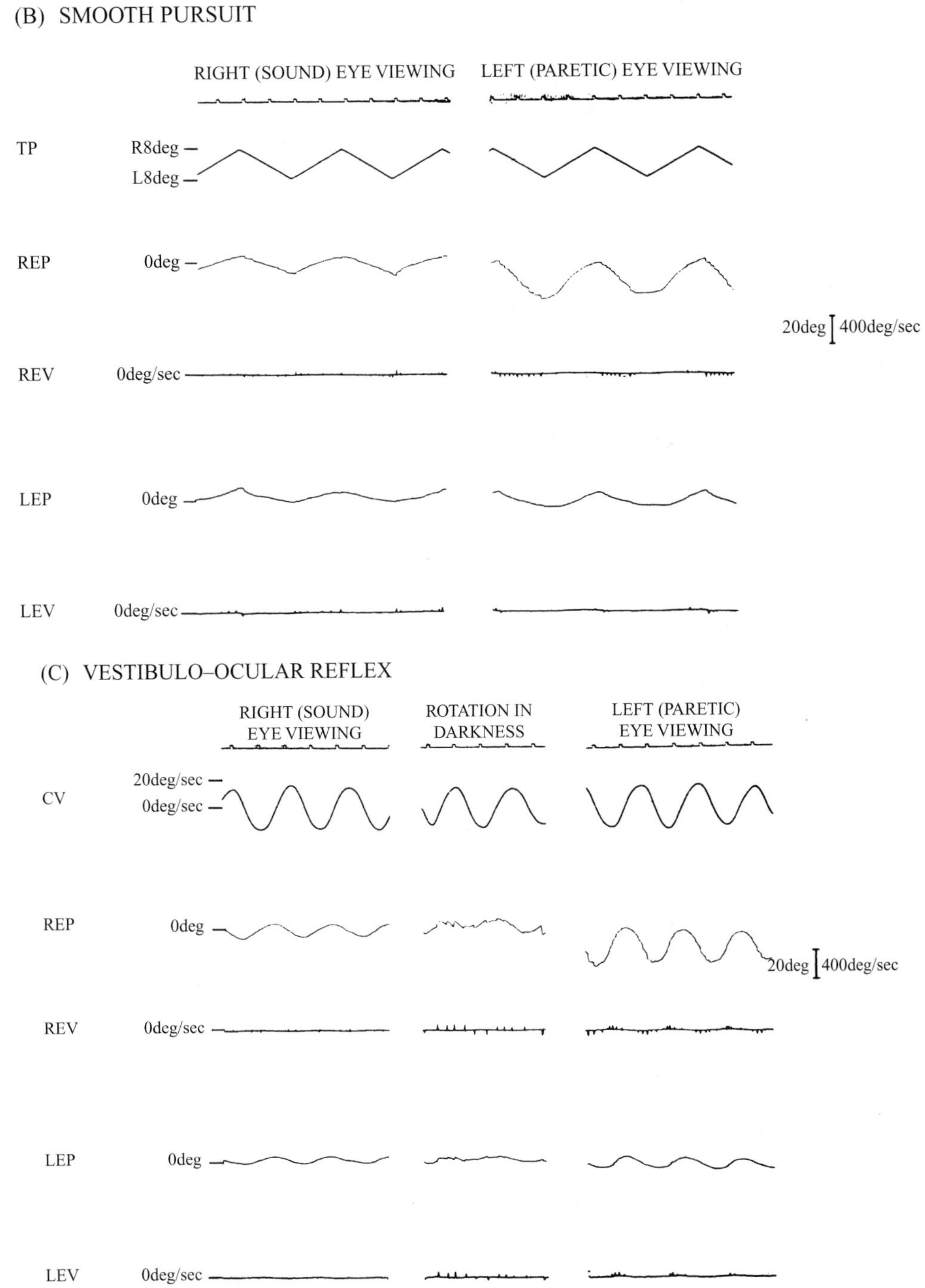

Figure 9–15. *(Continued)* (B) Smooth pursuit. With the sound right eye viewing, the right eye made smooth pursuit with some catch-up saccades; corresponding movements in the left eye were of smaller amplitude. With the paretic left eye viewing, the left eye appeared to make smooth following movements. The right eye, however, showed a series of small saccades, especially when tracking to the left, and a larger range of tracking movements, indicating the neural commands being sent to both eyes. (C) Vestibulo-ocular reflex. During rotation in darkness, asymmetry of movements was evident in the left eye, due to the lateral rectus paresis; similar findings occurred during visual fixation with the sound right eye. During fixation with the paretic left eye, the range of movements in the covered right eye increased, due partly to saccades, reflecting the neural signals being sent to both eyes. CV: chair (head) velocity; LEP: left eye position; LEV: left eye velocity; REP: right eye position; REV: right eye velocity; TP: target position. Time marks at top are in seconds. Upward deflections indicate rightward movements.

movement of about 16 degrees was sent out. This is revealed by the movements of the sound right eye under cover, which reflect the neural command sent to both eyes (Hering's law). The paretic eye, however, fell short of the target, and the persistent retinal error stimulated a corrective saccadic command. In this way, the paretic eye made a series of saccades until the target was placed on the fovea. When this was achieved, the sound eye under cover was deviated to the left of the desired eye position, a secondary deviation.

By contrast, rightward saccades made by the viewing, paretic left eye were rapid, though hypometric. Each of these rightward saccades was followed by backward drift of the eye, which necessitated small corrective saccades. The corresponding movements of the sound eye under cover consisted of an initial rightward saccade of about 14 degrees, followed by a series of smaller saccades.

The *drifts* of the paretic eye that follow saccades can be attributed to at least three factors. First, although the two horizontal extraocular muscles in each eye contribute reciprocally to eye movements, the relative contributions of each depend upon orbital position. Second, the amount by which the force of the agonist increases and antagonist decreases can be related to the pulse-step innervation program for saccades (see Fig. 1–3 of Chapter 1). Saccades need much larger agonist forces than do slower movements such as pursuit. Relaxation of antagonist forces can contribute relatively little to the pulse portion of saccades, since incremental forces in the agonist must be so much higher compared to the possible forces from a decrement in activity in the antagonist. The *step* portion of saccades, however, does depend upon contributions from a muscle both when it is acting as the agonist (an increase in force) and as the antagonist (a decrease in force). Hence, saccades made by the affected eye, in the direction of action of the paretic muscle, usually show a postsaccadic drift in the direction of the movement, owing to the decrement in antagonist forces. Third, the backward drift following saccades made into the normal field of movement by the paretic eye may reflect a loss of the decrement in antagonist forces of the weak eye for the step of innervation (i.e., the paretic muscle cannot be normally relaxed). Alternatively, these backward drifts that follow saccades made into the normal field of movement by the paretic eye may reflect a central misrepresentation of the position of the paretic eye by the gaze-holding network (neural integrator). This would be a consequence of the series of saccades required to attain leftward gaze.[953]

SMOOTH PURSUIT IN PARALYTIC STRABISMUS

With the *sound right eye viewing*, tracking by the right eye was probably normal for the patient's age, with some catch-up saccades evident (Fig. 9–15B). The paretic eye, under cover, made similar movements through a smaller range, due to the lateral rectus weakness. With the *paretic left eye viewing*, the left eye appeared to make smooth following movements, especially to the right. The movements of the sound eye, under cover, however, showed that the patient was tracking target movement to the left mainly with a series of small saccades. The total amplitude of the movements in the right eye was much greater than those in the left (partly because of open-loop stimulation—see Chapter 4).

VESTIBULAR RESPONSES IN PARALYTIC STRABISMUS

Sinusoidal rotation during fixation of a stationary target by the *sound eye*, or *in darkness*, demonstrated a slightly asymmetric reflex caused by the left lateral rectus weakness (Fig. 9–15C); gain may be reduced in both directions.[922] This reduced range of vestibular eye movements probably accounts for the complaints of oscillopsia, vertigo, or "dizziness" by some patients with paralytic strabismus.[821,916] With the *paretic eye viewing*, the amplitude of movements of the sound right eye under cover were increased, owing partly to saccades.

CLINICAL FEATURES AND DIAGNOSIS OF CONCOMITANT STRABISMUS

A common diagnostic problem for the neurologist is to determine whether or not strabismus is paralytic. Sometimes a history of strabismus since childhood will settle the matter; lack of diplopia in such patients is due to suppression of images from one eye. In other patients, the demonstration of associated findings such as the lack of stereoacuity or the presence of latent nystagmus (see Box 10–12, Chapter 10) help identify a longstanding strabismus. Occasionally adults with a history of strabismus since childhood will develop diplopia if a new pair of spectacles encourages fixation with their nondominant eye.[481] This "fixation switch diplopia" can be remedied with refraction that encourages fixation with their dominant eye.

Most nonparalytic *horizontal* deviations of the optic axes are relatively concomitant; that is, the deviation remains approximately the same for all fields of gaze, whichever eye is fixating. Most normal individuals have small concomitant phorias when the fusional mechanism is interrupted by covering one eye. Concomitant tropias (deviations that the fusional mechanism cannot correct) or "strabismus" is associated with a variety of factors.[889] These include refractive errors (especially hypermetropia) and abnormalities of the accommodation-convergence synkinesis (see Abnormalities of Vergence in Chapter 8).

The acute onset of strabismus and diplopia later in life need not be paralytic; sometimes, nonspecific illness, head injury, or eye injury disrupts the fusional mechanisms that maintain orthotropia. These may present as convergence insufficiency or divergence weakness (see Chapter 8). If, however, the acute onset of a concomitant tropia occurs without history of previous strabismus, monocular visual loss, or myopia, and if nystagmus or other neurological abnormalities are present, imaging studies are warranted.[358] Thus, certain acquired, central, neurologic problems such as tumors or the Arnold-Chiari malformation occasionally present with onset or worsening of strabismus.[76,295,780,913]

In some nonparalytic forms of horizontal strabismus, the deviation is vertically nonconcomitant; that is, the horizontal deviation of the visual axes varies according to the vertical position of the eyes. These have been called A-pattern (e.g., esotropia that increases in upward gaze, or exotropia that increases in downward gaze) and V-pattern (e.g., esotropia that increases in downward gaze, or exotropia that increases in upward gaze). Such patterns are encountered in patients with craniosynostosis with hypertelorism,[146] and in some cases is due to congenital misplacement of the fibromuscular pulleys in the coronal plane.[197] Occasionally these patterns are encountered in paralytic strabismus, the best example being a V-pattern esotropia in bilateral trochlear nerve palsy. V-patterns also occur in craniofacial anomalies and with lesions of the dorsal midbrain.[610]

Asymptomatic *vertical* phorias may occur in some normal individuals in the periphery of gaze.[789] A commonly encountered, nonconcomitant, nonparalytic form of strabismus is dissociated vertical deviation (DVD, also called alternating sursumduction). It is characterized by upward deviation of whichever eye is under cover.[868] In some patients it manifests without covering one eye. The phenomenon is unexplained,[93] but usually coexists with esotropia and latent nystagmus (see Box 10–12, Chapter 10).[108] It has been postulated that DVD might represent a mechanism to suppress the small torsional-vertical component of latent nystagmus.[318,371] Alternatively, DVD might reflect the action of the phylogenetically old dorsal light reflex that attempts to restore vertical orientation of the eye if a tilt of the body is perceived during monocular viewing.[105]

Another nonparalytic vertical deviation is so-called overactivity of the inferior oblique muscle.[106] This causes a hyperdeviation of whichever eye is adducted (also called upshoot in adduction or unilateral sursumduction), but no deviation in central position.[782] Differentiation from fourth nerve palsy depends upon demonstrating that the deviation is greatest in up gaze rather than in down gaze, though the two may coexist. Skew deviation is a vertical tropia that may vary in right and left gaze, and is due to disturbance of prenuclear, otolithic inputs. It is usually part of the ocular tilt reaction and is associated with other signs of brainstem dysfunction (see Chapter 11).

When strabismus is associated with either amblyopia or acquired visual loss, abnormal dynamic properties of eye movements may coexist, which reflect changes in visual cortical areas.[246,362,860] During attempted fixation, gaze is unstable in the eye with poor vision (Fig. 10–8B).[153,499,809] This is evident as low-frequency, bidirectional drifts that are more prominent vertically, and unidirectional drifts with nystagmus that are more evident horizontally; the latter often conform to the pattern of latent nystagmus.[108] Instability of gaze is probably due to the poor vision rather than strabismus. Saccades in patients with poor vision in one eye are disconjugate, with post-saccadic drifts, implying that normal vision is required to calibrate the yoking mechanism.[369,499,547] Surgery to correct childhood strabismus may improve the conjugacy of the saccadic pulse, but not the subsequent drift.[110] Saccadic latency is increased if the visual stimulus is presented to the amblyopic eye.[152] Amblyopia may be associated with temporal-nasal asymmetry of monocular optokinetic responses, which is discussed in Chapter 4.

CLINICAL FEATURES OF OCULAR NERVE PALSIES

Our approach in discussing palsies of the ocular motor nerves will be: (1) to review the typical clinical features; (2) to comment on the differential diagnosis; (3) to discuss features that aid in topological diagnosis; and (4) to summarize the clinical management. Some laboratory tests that often aid the evaluation of palsies of the ocular motor nerves are summarized in Table 9–3. The differential diagnosis of palsies of CN III, IV, and VI are summarized in Table 9–4. Diagnosis has been aided by MRI and MRA of the head,[149] with special views of the ocular motor nerves,[236] and by the application of surface coils to visualize individual extraocular muscles, orbital vessels, and nerves.[79,199,235,556,771] Nonetheless, even with modern imaging and laboratory testing, the cause of ocular nerve palsy is not determined in 20% to 35% of patients.[63,70,702,841] For example, transient diplopia in the setting of stress or exercise may be a manifestation of migraine, although careful evaluation and follow-up are required to exclude more serious causes.[409] Some drugs causing diplopia are summarized in Table 12–11 in Chapter 12.

Table 9–3. **Laboratory Evaluation of Palsies of CN III, IV, VI**

Complete blood count with differential and platelet count
Erythrocyte sedimentation rate, C-reactive protein, fibrinogen
Tests for diabetes, thyroid disorder, syphilis, Lyme disease
Chest X-ray
Nasopharyngeal examination*
Consider CT, MRI with gadolinium enhancement,† MRA
Consider spinal tap
Edrophonium (Tensilon) test for painless and subtle deficits

*Especially with abducens palsy and facial pain.
†Especially in patients older than 50 years.[149]

Table 9–4. **Differential Diagnosis of Ocular Motor Nerve Palsies**

Concomitant strabismus, with or without a history of eye muscle surgery
Disorders of vergence, especially spasm of the near triad
Brainstem disorders causing abnormal prenuclear inputs (e.g., skew deviation and internuclear ophthalmoplegia)
Miller Fisher syndrome
Myasthenia gravis
Botulism
Restrictive ophthalmopathies (e.g., Brown's superior oblique tendon sheath syndrome)
Trauma (e.g., blowout fracture of the orbit)
Ophthalmic Graves' disease
Orbital metastases
Orbital pseudotumor
Orbital infections (e.g., trichinosis)
Disease affecting extraocular muscle (e.g., oculopharyngeal dystrophy)
Kearns-Sayre syndrome

Abducens Nerve Palsy

CLINICAL FEATURES OF ABDUCENS NERVE PALSY

Abducens nerve palsy is the most common ocular motor paralysis. It causes horizontal diplopia, which is greatest when viewing distant objects and when looking ipsilaterally; the two images are uncrossed. Abduction is restricted or slowed (see Video Display: Diplopia and Strabismus), and there is an esotropia (or in mild cases, only an esophoria) that is greatest on looking toward the side of the lesion (Fig. 9–12 and Fig. 9–13). With the Maddox rod, some patients may show small, associated, vertical deviations.[784,924]

Abducens palsy should be differentiated

from other causes of impaired abduction (Table 9–4). Differentiation from long-standing esotropia can sometimes be difficult, but old photographs often will help. Stereopsis, impaired in strabismus, is usually preserved in patients with acquired abducens palsy. Duane syndrome, discussed below, is associated with retraction of the globe on adduction. Functional convergence spasm is sometimes confused with sixth nerve palsy, but careful observation of the pupils and of ductions (range of movement with one eye covered) will help identify this psychogenic cause of reduced abduction. Restrictive ophthalmopathies, such as that due to thyroid ophthalmopathy, are identified by a forced duction test and orbital ultrasound. Myasthenia gravis can usually be diagnosed by the edrophonium (Tensilon) test. Causes of abducens palsy are summarized in Table 9–5.

DISORDERS AFFECTING THE ABDUCENS NUCLEUS

Acquired Horizontal Gaze Palsies

Sixth nerve palsy should be differentiated from the effects of lesions of the abducens nucleus (see Box 12–5, in Chapter 12). The latter contains abducens motor neurons that supply the lateral rectus muscle, and abducens internuclear neurons that project, via the medial longitudinal fasciculus, to the medial rectus subdivision of contralateral oculomotor nucleus (see Fig. 6–1, Chapter 6). Thus, lesions of the abducens nucleus cause an ipsilateral, conjugate gaze palsy, with defective abduction in the ipsilateral eye and defective adduction in the contralateral eye (see Video Display: Pontine Syndromes).[67,558,573,603] An ipsilateral, peripheral facial nerve palsy is a common but not invariable accompaniment,[573] because of the proximity of the fascicles of this nerve to the abducens nucleus. Larger lesions may also affect the ventral pons and pyramidal tracts; for example, Foville's syndrome consists of an ipsilateral, horizontal gaze palsy, ipsilateral facial palsy, and contralateral hemiparesis.

Möbius Syndrome and Failure of Development of the Abducens Nucleus

The abducens nucleus is susceptible to abnormalities of development or injury in early life. Möbius syndrome consists of a congenital disturbance of conjugate horizontal gaze and facial diplegia.[136,569] It may be accompanied by atrophy of the tongue, deformities of the head and face, endocrine abnormalities, and malformations of the chest, great vessels, and extremities. Although Möbius syndrome can be an hereditary disorder,[468,656] environmental insult to the fetus is probably a more common cause.[136,230,517] Other musculoskeletal anomalies are associated, and there is an overlap with other congenital disorders of gaze, which are discussed below.[571]

Horizontal Gaze Palsy with Progressive Scoliosis (HGPPS)

The syndrome of congenital paralysis of horizontal gaze associated with progressive scoliosis but mild or absent facial weakness has been recognized for over 30 years,[472,957] some cases being familial.[764,937] All horizontal conjugate saccadic, pursuit, optokinetic and vestibular eye movements are absent (see Video Display: Diplopia and Strabismus).[91] Horizontal convergence is relatively preserved, and some patients can substitute vergence for absent conjugate gaze shifts (see below). Some patients have esotropia or vertical deviations. Vertical eye saccades are preserved but vertical smooth pursuit may be deficient. Some patients show small amplitude, horizontal or elliptical pendular nystagmus at about 2 Hz, sometimes accompanied by head shaking, and which may be influenced by caloric stimulation.[671] Intermittent slow blinking of one or both eyes has been noted. Visual function may be normal with stereopsis. The scoliosis is progressive and disabling.[91]

Magnetic resonance imaging findings have revealed pontine hypoplasia, absence of the facial genu, deep pontine cleft, and medullary hypoplasia,[666,714] and absence of the pyramidal decussation, which may account for the scoliosis.[390] Linkage studies have localized a mutation of the ROBO3 gene on chromosome11q23, which is important for hindbrain midline axon crossing.[389,390] Other major sensory pathways may also lack the normal crossing of axons in the brainstem.[777]

Patients with congenital absence of horizontal, conjugate eye movements may adopt several adaptive strategies to compensate for their deficit (see Video Display: Diplopia and

Table 9–5. **Etiology of Abducens Nerve Palsy**[70,273,415,449,496,660,702,737,841]

Nuclear (characterized by horizontal gaze palsy)

Möbius syndrome[136,468,517,569,656]
Other congenital or hereditary gaze palsies[472,764,937] including horizontal gaze palsy with scoliosis[91]
Duane syndrome (most cases)[204,357,357,601]
Infarction[67,603]
Tumor[558]
Wernicke-Korsakoff syndrome[160]
Trauma[171]
Histiocytosis X[667]

Fascicular (nucleus to exit from brainstem)

Infarction[216,268,415,429]
Demyelination[51,415,596]
Tumor*[415]
Inflammation[543]
Wernicke-Korsakoff syndrome[160]

Subarachnoid

Compression by arteriosclerotic or anomalous vessels or aneurysm (anterior inferior cerebellar artery, posterior inferior cerebellar artery, or basilar artery)[83,177,634]
Subarachnoid hemorrhage*[415]
Trauma[415]
Meningitis (infectious—including syphilis and Lyme disease),[45,421,616,788] neoplastic,[145,688] idiopathic hypertrophic,[479] and in association with HIV[69,421,605]
Wegener's granulomatosis[618]
Clivus tumor[327,886]
Cerebellopontine angle tumors[415]
Trigeminal tumor,[693] or hemangioma,[98] or following radiofrequency rhizolysis[332]
Abducens nerve tumors[7,540,607,637]
Neurosurgical complication[940]

Petrous

Infection of mastoid or tip of petrous bone[186]
Thrombosis of inferior petrosal sinus[829]
Trauma[25,504,606]
Downward displacement of brainstem by supra-tentorial mass (e.g., tumor, pseudotumor cerebri)[469,716]
Following lumbar puncture, myelography, spinal or epidural anesthesia, ventriculo-atrial shunt, spinal traction, or trauma[66,233,622,669,730]
Spontaneous intracranial hypotension[28,250,354]
Aneurysm, arteriovenous malformation, or persistent trigeminal artery[590,857]

Cavernous Sinus and Superior Orbital Fissure

Carotid aneurysm[2,313] or dissection[743]
Cavernous sinus thrombosis[211,896]
Carotid-cavernous fistula: direct and dural[338,431,464,508,758]
Tumor: pituitary adenoma, nasopharyngeal carcinoma, meningioma, other[148,176,328,367,368,524,613]
Dental anesthesia[535,894]
Sphenoidal mucocele,[10,602,691] or tumor[193]

Table 9–5. *(continued)*

Tolosa-Hunt syndrome[128]
Herpes zoster[29]
Abducens nerve tumor[522]
Nerve infarction

Orbital†

Tumor, and other infiltrates
Following arterial ligation for epistaxis[169,382]

Localization Uncertain

Nerve infarction (associated with diabetes, hypertension or arteritis)[751]
Migraine[657]
In association with viral and other infections, immunization, and the idiopathic form of childhood[77,86,162,445,899,908,956]
Transient palsy in newborns[270,507]
Toxic side effect of drugs[192,645,825,844,876]

*Common causes of bilateral abducens palsy.
†May cause paresis by involvement of nerve or extraocular muscle.

Strabismus). They substitute rapid head movements (head saccades) for eye saccades to change gaze rapidly.[744] When the head is restrained, they may use their intact vergence system to move both eyes into adduction and then cross-fixate, using the right eye to view objects seen on the left and vice versa. Such substitution of vergence for versional movements also has been reported in patients with a variety of gaze and muscle palsies.[113,114,911] In some patients, retraction of the nonfixing eye occurs during such vergence movements.[957]

Duane Retraction Syndrome

Definition and Classification

This syndrome occurs in three forms,[889] each of which are characterized by a narrowing of the palpebral fissure on adduction secondary to retraction of the eye. Type I, the most common, is characterized by limitation of abduction but full adduction. In type II, the eye abducts well but adduction is incomplete. Type-III patients show limitation of both abduction and adduction.[954]

Clinical Features

The key to clinical diagnosis of Duane syndrome is identification of retraction of the eyeball, evident as narrowing of the palpebral fissure, on adduction. This phenomenon is brought out during horizontal saccades (see Video Display: Diplopia and Strabismus), or by observing the affected eye from the side during nystagmus induced by optokinetic stimulation. In addition to limitation of horizontal movement (usually abduction), there may also be abnormal "upshoot" or "downshoot" movements as the patient attempts to shift horizontal gaze.[80] Duane syndrome is more common in female patients, affects the left eye more than the right, and may be bilateral. It may be familial,[346,656] and a number of associated congenital abnormalities have been reported.[204,538,555,766] Patients with Duane syndrome seldom complain of diplopia; in fact, they usually have binocular, single vision with good stereopsis and fusion when the eyes are in the field of intact movement.[852] Occasionally, diplopia may develop later in life, making differential diagnosis from abducens palsy difficult. In such patients, ocular retraction during adduction provides a useful diagnostic clue.

Anatomy of the Disorder

Most cases of Duane retraction syndrome are due to a congenital anomaly of innervation, with failure to develop normal innervation of the lateral rectus muscle.[204] This view was initially based on electromyographic evidence,[360,363,539] and has been confirmed subsequently by clinicopathologic studies. Neuropathologic examination of one patient with a unilateral left-sided type-I Duane syndrome showed an absent left abducens nerve, which accounted for the abduction deficit.[574] Aberrant branches from the inferior division of the oculomotor nerve innervated the left lateral rectus. Thus, retraction of the globe on adduction was brought about by co-contraction of the horizontal recti. The brainstem of this patient showed a normal right abducens nucleus but the left abducens nucleus contained less than half as many neurons as the right; these remaining cells were thought to be abducens internuclear neurons, since the medial longitudinal fasciculi were intact. Similar autopsy findings were reported in a patient with familial, unilateral Duane type-III syndrome.[601] Another patient who had bilateral type-III Duane syndrome lacked both abducens nuclei and nerves.[357] Therefore, the limitation of horizontal movement in most cases of Duane syndrome can be ascribed to an agenesis of abducens motoneurons (see Fig. 6–1, Chapter 6). Failure of abduction is due to lack of innervation of the lateral rectus by the abducens nerve. Absence of the abducens nerve in type I and type III Duane syndrome has been demonstrated by MRI.[437,655]

Pathophysiology of the Disorder of Eye Movements

It is possible to draw on the results of these anatomical studies in combination with studies of eye movements to develop hypotheses to account for the disturbances of gaze in Duane syndrome. Retraction of the globe on adduction is brought about by co-contraction of the horizontal recti, which is the consequence of aberrant innervation of the lateral rectus muscle by the oculomotor nerve. When there is limited adduction of the eye, this could also be due to co-contraction of the lateral and medial recti. Similarly, adducting saccades made by the affected eye are slower and smaller than in the normal eye, possibly due to co-contraction of the medial and lateral rectus muscles.[948] Conversely, adducting saccades of the normal eye of patients with a unilateral type-I Duane syndrome usually have normal velocities or only slight slowing.[303, 934,948] This finding supports the notion that the abducens internuclear neurons are preserved and project to the medial rectus subnucleus of the unaffected side. Some patients show hypermetria of the normal eye for centrifugal saccades toward the sound side, which could represent limited ability to adapt the saccadic pulse command for disconjugate movements, although there is some variability between patients depending on factors such as eye dominance.[948] The upshoot and downshoot of the eye that occurs during horizontal movements in Duane syndrome may be because of side-slip of the horizontal recti, brought about by weakening of the horizontal recti due to chronic cocontraction.[201] Alternatively, certain patients may have anomalous innervation of vertically acting muscles.

Etiologies of the Disorder

The occurrence of Duane syndrome in patients with thalidomide embryopathy suggested that the disturbance in development occurs between about 21 and 26 days.[570] It appears than several genetic mutations may be found in families with Duane syndrome, with some overlap with other forms of infantile esotropia.[167] Linkage studies in one family with Duane retraction syndrome localized a gene on chromosome 2q31,[27] whereas other studies have identified a region on chromosome 8q13.[127] Mutant mouse models are being developed that fail to develop oculomotor and trochlear motoneurons and show aberrant innervation of extraocular muscles.[678,679]

Case reports of patients also suggest other forms of congenital anomalous innervation of extraocular muscles, such as abduction twitch on attempted up gaze (Fig. 9–16),[453] upshot on adduction,[642] or synkinesis of the levator and lateral rectus, with eyelid elevation occurring on attempted abduction.[604] Another reported anomaly is restricted up gaze and exotropia in up gaze due to the persistence of a retractor bulbi muscle, which, in rodents, retracts the globe.[866] Congenital fibrosis of the extraocular muscles, discussed at the end of this chapter, has also been shown to comprise a spectrum of

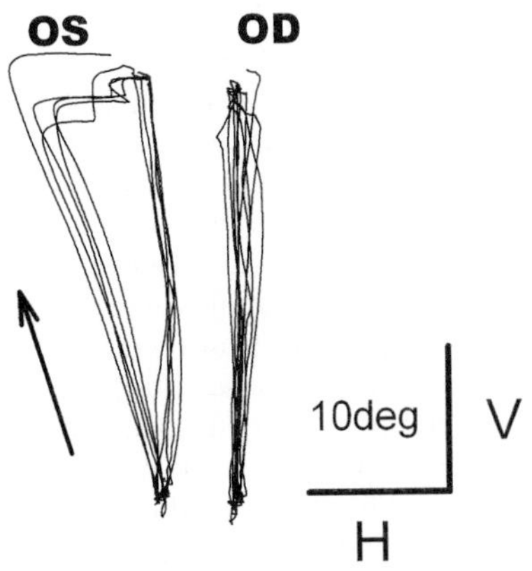

Figure 9–16. Probable congenital synkinesis of superior rectus and lateral rectus, causing abduction with upward movements. The patient was a 27-year-old woman who had no visual complaints but was noted to have a diagonal trajectory for upward, but not downward, saccades. This difference was more marked when she made vertical saccades in right gaze. Rapid vestibular movements were similarly affected. OD: movements of right eye; OS: movements of left eye. The arrow indicates the direction of upward saccades in the left eye.

genetic disorders characterized by failure of development of ocular motoneurons.[230]

Although most cases of Duane syndrome are congenital, a similar clinical syndrome can occur with acquired disease of the extraocular muscles or of the orbit (e.g., fibrosis or inflammation of muscle or fascia)[288,812,889] Furthermore, Duane syndrome can be mimicked by other processes such as skull base tumor, and MRI is indicated in patients with unusual findings.[778]

DISORDERS AFFECTING THE ABDUCENS FASCICLES

As the abducens nerve fascicles course through the medial pons to gain the ventral surface, they pass next to the pyramidal tract. Hence, infarction of the ventral paramedian pons may produce ipsilateral abducens palsy, contralateral hemiplegia, and ipsilateral facial weakness, Millard-Gubler syndrome. Sixth nerve palsy accompanied only by contralateral hemiplegia constitutes Raymond's syndrome. Other important causes of nuclear and fascicular sixth nerve lesions include both pontine and cerebellar tumors, Wernicke's encephalopathy, and multiple sclerosis. Demyelination causes bilateral sixth nerve palsy as commonly as unilateral. Rarely, isolated sixth nerve palsy may be due to a fascicular lesion.[216]

DISORDERS AFFECTING THE SUBARACHNOID PORTION OF THE ABDUCENS NERVE

After emerging from the brainstem, the nerve may fall prey to infectious or neoplastic meningitis and may be compressed by vascular structures such as an enlarged dolichoectatic basilar artery.[294] As the nerve ascends to the petrous ridge, it may be compressed by clivus tumor, such as chordoma or meningioma; such tumors may produce bilateral, isolated sixth nerve palsy. The abducens nerve is fixed where it pierces the dura, so that any downward displacement of the brainstem caused by a supratentorial mass lesion may produce either unilateral or bilateral sixth nerve palsy. Although oculomotor nerve palsy is a more useful diagnostic sign of acute transtentorial herniation, abducens palsy is more common when such a process evolves slowly. Diplopia caused by lateral rectus weakness sometimes develops after otherwise uncomplicated lumbar puncture, with or without accompanying increased intracranial pressure, after halopelvic traction for neck injury, and with intracranial hypotension. In such cases, traction on the subarachnoid portion of the abducens nerve seems the likely mechanism.

DISORDERS AFFECTING THE PETROUS PORTION OF THE ABDUCENS NERVE

After leaving the subarachnoid space, the nerve rests upon the petrous bone and its crest. Here it is susceptible to trauma (temporal bone fractures) and spread of infections from the underlying mastoid process. These infections can cause petrositis or thrombosis of the inferior petrosal sinus, both of which may affect function in the adjacent fifth and sixth cranial nerves, with consequent diplopia and facial (usually supraorbital) pain. The combination of pain in the distribution of the first trigeminal division and impaired abduction (often accompanied by deafness) constitutes Gradenigo's syndrome. This syndrome is now uncommon with infection,[768,881] but is encountered in patients with cancer.

DISORDERS AFFECTING THE CAVERNOUS PORTION OF THE ABDUCENS NERVE

After the sixth nerve passes forward into the cavernous sinus, it lies lateral to the internal carotid artery, where the oculosympathetic fibers are located (Fig. 9–8). Aneurysms of the internal carotid artery and tumors or infection in the cavernous sinus may cause weakness of the ipsilateral lateral rectus muscle and, rarely, an associated ipsilateral Horner's syndrome.[2,313,824] Tumor, inflammation, or carotid-cavernous fistula may compromise the abducens nerve as it passes through the cavernous sinus and superior orbital fissure. Tumor arising from the base of the skull, particularly nasopharyngeal carcinoma, may compress the sixth nerve. This occurs because most nasopharyngeal tumors arise in the fossa of Rosenmuller, immediately beneath the foramen lacerum. Extension of the tumor up through the foramen lacerum brings it into contact with the fifth and sixth cranial nerves.[368,712] Thus, the combination of facial pain and diplopia is a common presentation of nasopharyngeal carcinoma. Serous otitis media is a frequent accompaniment because of blockage of the eustachian tube. Infarction of the abducens nerve, in association with diabetes or hypertension, may also occur within its cavernous portion.

BILATERAL ABDUCENS NERVE PALSY

Compared with unilateral palsies, bilateral abducens nerve palsy more commonly occurs with tumors, demyelination, subarachnoid hemorrhage, meningitis, Wernicke's encephalopathy, and increased intracranial pressure.[415] Associated abnormalities, such as other cranial nerve deficits and long tract signs, usually help make the diagnosis. Bilateral abducens palsy must be differentiated from functional convergence spasm and divergence paresis; these entities are discussed in Chapter 8.

ABDUCENS NERVE PALSY IN CHILDREN

Sixth nerve palsy in children up to age 3 years seldom causes a complaint of double vision; a head turn to the involved side is the most prominent finding. Certain childhood disorders commonly cause abducens palsy.[331,428,449,496] Thus, abduction weakness, sometimes transient, may be the first sign of tumor of the posterior fossa.[409] In these cases, a coexistent horizontal gaze palsy may suggest a pontine glioma. Coexistent cerebellar signs usually indicate astrocytoma, ependymoma, or medulloblastoma. Less commonly, supratentorial mass lesions present with lateral rectus weakness, usually with papilledema. Sixth nerve palsy in childhood may also occur in association with viral illness or vaccination (see Video Display: Diplopia and Strabismus).[86,162,445,908] If diplopia is the only symptom, and imaging studies, spinal fluid examination, and myasthenia gravis test results are normal, the child usually recovers; relapse is rare.[445] Gradenigo's syndrome may be due to middle ear infection, though if hearing is preserved, a tumor may be the cause.

In infants, sixth nerve palsy must be differentiated from Duane syndrome or congenital esotropia with crossfixation. The latter may occur in association with latent nystagmus as part of the infantile squint syndrome.[195] In a patient who cross-fixates, the lateral rectus can be shown to be intact by the doll's head maneuver or, if necessary, by patching one eye for several days. Patching forces the child to abduct the eye to see laterally. Any child who suddenly develops an ocular deviation must be carefully evaluated for loss of vision in the deviating eye, which may be due to tumors in the retina or anterior visual pathways.

MANAGEMENT OF ABDUCENS NERVE PALSY

Patients presenting with abduction weakness may have a variety of disorders other than sixth nerve palsy (Table 9–4). After these differential diagnoses are excluded, certain routine tests are usually indicated to identify the site and cause of the palsy (Table 9–3). Most patients have abducens palsy in association with diabetes or hypertension ("medical sixth") and although some initial worsening is the rule,[377] over 75% show some recovery within 6 months.[438] These patients usually require little work-up at the time of their presentation. However, young adults,[660] children, and older individuals who do not have diabetes or hypertension merit fuller investigation, including brain imaging. Although sixth nerve palsy associated with diabetes usually resolves,[732] it may not in patients in whom hypertension is implicated or if no other cause is found. Abducens nerve palsy that persists for more than 6 months and is unaccompanied by other symptoms or signs may sometimes be due to intracavernous aneurysms, tumors such as meningioma, or metastases.[273,438] Unilateral abducens nerve palsy following head injury often shows spontaneous recovery, whereas bilateral palsy often does not, and often requires prisms or surgical therapy.[348-350] Studies of the dynamic properties of eye movements indicate that in patients with fascicular abducens nerve palsies, there is little recovery of saccade speed or movement range; however, with peripheral abducens palsies, speed improves although range may remain restricted.[763] Abnormalities of the vestibulo-ocular reflex may also persist.[922]

Trochlear Nerve Palsy

CLINICAL FEATURES OF TROCHLEAR NERVE PALSY

Trochlear nerve palsy accounts for most cases of acquired vertical strabismus. Most patients with unilateral trochlear nerve palsy complain of vertical and torsional diplopia that is typically worse when looking down, such as when descending a flight of stairs. Disturbances of the perception of slant also occur, due to the cyclodeviation.[515] Thus, if the patient views a vertical bar, the top will appear closer. When viewing a horizontal bar, the two images will be slanted with respect to each other, with the apparent intersection of the lines pointing toward the side of the affected, excylodeviated eye.

Trochlear nerve palsy causes a hypertropia of the affected eye, which is increased during adduction and depression. A common finding is head tilt away from the side of the lesion. The most reliable clinical test to diagnose fourth nerve palsy is the head-tilt test (Fig. 9–14) (see Video Display: Diplopia and Strabismus). The hypertropia is maximized as the head is tilted toward the side of the lesion and minimized on contralateral head tilt. It may also increase on attempted down gaze and with ipsilateral head turn (contralateral gaze). In a patient who has a third nerve palsy and who is unable to adduct, the action of the superior oblique muscle can be best evaluated by looking for intorsion of the abducted eye on attempted downward gaze. Clinical features of bilateral trochlear nerve palsy are summarized in the case history below. Measurement of eye movements in patients with trochlear nerve palsy has shown that vertical saccadic velocities may be normal, but downward saccades are hypometric.[813,840]

The main differential diagnoses of trochlear nerve palsy are skew deviation, thyroid and other restrictive ophthalmopathies,[837] and overaction of the inferior oblique muscle. With skew deviation, the head-tilt test is usually negative. Accompanying brainstem findings, such as internuclear ophthalmoplegia, are common with skew deviation but rare with trochlear nerve palsy.[870] Typically, the hypertropic eye in fourth nerve palsy is extorted, whereas with skew deviation it is intorted; these differences are relatively small, however, and may fall within the range shown by normal subjects.[208] Perhaps the key differentiating feature is the direction of torsion: intorsion of the elevated eye occurs in skew deviation (along with extorsion of the other eye) whereas extorsion of the elevated eye occurs in superior oblique palsy. Restrictive ophthalmopathies are diagnosed by a forced duction test and imaging of the orbit. Certain patients with nonparetic strabismus since childhood may have clinical findings that mimic fourth nerve palsy;[782] these have been referred to by the terms upshoot in adduction or unilateral sursumduction. Since the deviation is greatest in adduction and up gaze, overaction of the inferior oblique muscle may be the mechanism. Such patients show large vertical fusional abilities that have been developed to compensate for their muscle weakness. Old photographs, showing a longstanding head tilt, may help make the diagnosis. In diagnosing fourth nerve palsy, it should be noted that some normal individuals may show small hyperdeviations, as revealed with the Maddox rod.[789] Causes of trochlear palsy are summarized in Table 9–6. The superior oblique is amenable to MRI, using surface coils, to demonstrate size and contractility.[200]

DISORDERS AFFECTING THE TROCHLEAR NUCLEUS AND FASCICLES

The trochlear nucleus may be congenitally absent or hypoplastic. In addition, it may be damaged by brainstem infarction, hemorrhage,

Table 9–6. **Etiology of Trochlear Nerve Palsy**[70,351,422,449,533,702,841,891]

Nuclear and Fascicular	
Aplasia[136]	
Mesencephalic hemorrhage or infarction[90,597,831,870]	
Tumor and other mass lesion[52,418,470,633]	
Arteriovenous malformation[314]	
Trauma[418]	
Demyelination[381,941]	
Neurosurgical complication[422]	
Subarachnoid	
Trauma,[383,422,504] including shaking injury in infancy[123]	
Tumor: pineal tumors, tentorial meningioma, ependymoma, metastases, trochlear nerve tumors, others[283,374,422,733,738,795,858]	
Aneurysm of the superior cerebellar artery,[13] posterior cerebral artery,[319] or posterior communicating artery[770]	
Hydrocephalus[316]	
Neurosurgical procedure[163,384,940]	
Meningitis (infectious, neoplastic, idiopathic hypertrophic) [139,422,479,688,725]	
Superficial siderosis[772]	
Following lumbar puncture or spinal anesthesia[439]	
Cavernous Sinus and Superior Orbital Fissure	
Tumor[446] including pituitary tumor[659]	
Tolosa-Hunt syndrome*	
Herpes zoster[29,491,701]	
Internal carotid aneurysm[30] or dissection[743]	
Carotid-cavernous sinus dural fistula[755,783]	
Orbit†	
Trauma	
Tumor and other infiltrates[597,718]	
Localization Uncertain	
Nerve infarction (associated with diabetes or hypertension)[702]	
Congenital, including absence on MRI[34,142,333,449]	
Idiopathic[702]	
Tetanus[647]	
In association with familial periodic ataxia[41]	
Sjögren's syndrome[151]	

*More commonly accompanied by other ocular motor nerve palsies (see Table 9–9).

†May cause paresis by involvement of nerve, tendon, trochlea, or extraocular muscle.

trauma, or tumor. Congenital fourth nerve palsy is quite common,[351] and some cases may be part of the spectrum of failure of embryogenesis of the cranial nerve nuclei. Since the fascicles of the trochlear nerve lie so close to the nucleus, it is usually impossible to differentiate nuclear from fascicular lesions. When fourth nerve palsy is associated with a Horner's syndrome on the side opposite to the palsy, however, a brainstem location affecting fibers prior to their decussation may be present.[314] Lesions that affect both the trochlear nucleus and adjacent structures may lead to associated brainstem signs such as upbeat nystagmus.[531a]

TROCHLEAR NERVE PALSY DUE TO HEAD TRAUMA

The most frequently diagnosed cause of fourth nerve palsy is head trauma, especially blunt frontal injury (e.g., that caused by motorcycle accidents). Occasionally, mild head trauma may cause a superior oblique weakness, especially if there is an underlying disorder, such as an arteriovenous malformation.[383] With bilateral trochlear nerve palsies, the lesions are likely to be in the anterior medullary velum, where the nerves emerge together. Contrecoup forces transmitted to the brainstem by the free tentorial edge may injure the nerves at this site. The following case is typical.

CASE HISTORY: Bilateral Trochlear Nerve Palsy

A 35-year-old man, who had just been released from jail, drank a large quantity of beer and decided to spend his first evening of freedom sleeping on the roof of a garage "underneath the stars." He awoke the next morning lying on the ground with a headache and double vision. When evaluated in the emergency room he complained of vertical diplopia. With the red glass before his right eye, in central position, he reported the white light to be above the red one. On looking down and to the left, the images separated further, but the white light was still above the red one. On looking down and to the right, the images were also separated, but now the white light was below the red one.

Cover testing revealed right hypertropia and a small esotropia in the central position. The right hypertropia increased on left lateral gaze and reversed to a left hypertropia on right gaze. On tilting the head to the right, there was a right hypertropia; on tilting the head to the left, there was a left hypertropia. The impression was that the patient had a bilateral fourth nerve palsy secondary to trauma.

Comment: This case illustrates the cardinal diagnostic features of a bilateral superior oblique paresis: an alternating hyperdeviation depending on the direction of horizontal gaze and, in asymmetric cases, tilt of the head. Both subjective and objective tests of superior oblique function in the diagnostic positions of gaze, and the head-tilt test, brought out the bilateral weakness of the superior oblique muscles. Other features of bilateral superior oblique palsy include a large degree of excyclotropia that may be evident during ophthalmoscopy (elevated position of the disc in relation to the macula) and a V-pattern esotropia (i.e., esotropia that is worse on looking down).[493,673,887,891] It is important to differentiate fourth nerve palsy secondary to head trauma from orbital blow-out fracture (see below).

OTHER COMMON CAUSES OF TROCHLEAR NERVE PALSY

The second most commonly diagnosed cause of trochlear palsy is ischemic neuropathy, often associated with diabetes ("medical fourth"). Unlike third nerve palsy, no clinicopathologic correlation of this process has been made. The prognosis of medical fourth is better than that following head trauma. Pressure from hydrocephalus or adjacent diseased vascular structures may cause fourth nerve palsy. When an intracavernous carotid aneurysm compresses the trochlear nerve, the oculomotor nerve is usually also affected. Certain tumors (Table 9–6) and neurosurgical procedures may cause trochlear palsy, as may hydrocephalus. Herpes zoster ophthalmicus may affect any of the ocular motor nerves,[29] but fourth nerve palsy may be more commonly associated with zoster because the ophthalmic trigeminal division and the trochlear nerve share the same connective tissue sheath. When only the trochlear nerve is involved, the palsy may be caused by a local granulomatous angiitis, which originates in the ophthalmic division and spreads upward; postmortem examination in one patient with total, unilateral ophthalmoplegia revealed inflammation and demyelination of the trochlear nerve within the cavernous sinus.[491] Orbital disease may cause weakness of the superior oblique muscle, but in most of these cases, damage to the muscle, the trochlea, or the tendon is more likely than a lesion of the fourth cranial nerve.

CONGENITAL TROCHLEAR NERVE PALSY

Many patients with congenital superior oblique "palsy" may actually have a normal appearing muscle on orbital imaging and at surgery. They may, however, have an abnormality of the superior oblique tendon that leads to a pattern of strabismus similar to that of a superior oblique palsy.[889] The distinction between congenital and acquired superior oblique palsy may be difficult unless there is a clear history of acute onset of vertical diplopia in the setting of trauma or in a patient with risk factors for ischemic lesions. Furthermore, many patients with presumed congenital superior oblique palsy only develop symptoms well into adulthood, often in association with presbyopia. An important clue to the origin of the palsy early in life in these patients is a longstanding head tilt, often seen in old family pictures. Traditionally, patients with congenital superior oblique palsy were thought to be distinguished by having larger ocular deviations often with a considerable deviation on up as well as down gaze, larger vertical fusional amplitudes, and facial asymmetries. None of these criteria, however, can be used to reliably exclude an acquired superior oblique palsy though when the ocular deviation is *greater* in up gaze than in down gaze in a patient with an otherwise typical pattern of superior oblique palsy, the etiology is likely congenital.[142,155,822,874]

MANAGEMENT OF TROCHLEAR NERVE PALSY

Patients presenting with vertical diplopia usually have trochlear nerve palsy or skew deviation,[96] but consideration should be given to other disorders that are summarized in Table 9–4. Some patients may have congenital palsies that have decompensated later in life and cause vertical diplopia. Consideration should also be given to the syndrome of overaction of the inferior oblique.[782,889] In patients who lack a history of head trauma, MRI may show relevant brainstem lesions, and gadolinium enhancement usually demonstrates infiltrative or inflammatory processes involving the long course of the fourth nerve.[283] Often the cause of fourth nerve palsy cannot be ascertained.[702] Isolated superior oblique palsy with no apparent cause is only rarely caused by tumor or aneurysm. If the results of imaging of the head and orbit are normal, and test results for diabetes and myasthenia are negative, then the outcome is usually favorable. Although some improvement of dynamic properties occurs during recovery,[920,921] many patients with fourth nerve palsy are left with permanent, disabling vertical diplopia and, in them, muscle surgery may improve conjugacy.[513]

BROWN'S SYNDROME

Brown's syndrome is characterized by limited elevation of the adducted eye because the movements of the superior oblique tendon are restricted in the trochlea.[269] When congenital, the superior oblique tendon may be short or tethered.[322,761] When acquired, the tendon may be prevented from passing through the trochlea by tendosynovitis, adhesions, metastases,[787] or trauma,[42,563] which may cause the muscle itself to become entrapped in the roof of the orbit.[46] Paradoxically, sometimes trauma to the trochlea leads to hypertropia rather than impaired elevation in adduction.[497] Rarely, Brown's syndrome may occur in the absence of an intact superior oblique muscle,[330] making the point that limited ability to evaluate the eye in adduction can be caused by other abnormal orbital tissues. When Brown's syndrome occurs in association with rheumatological disorders, anti-inflammatory drugs are usually effective.[269]

Occasionally, the clinical appearance may alternate between that of Brown's syndrome and a superior oblique palsy. When the patient attempts to look up there is initially restriction but, sometimes after an audible click, the eye does eventually elevate (see Video Display: Diplopia and Strabismus). Subsequently there may be initial limitation of downgaze. In some patients with this superior oblique click syndrome, a tumor has been demonstrated on the superior oblique tendon that hindered movement through the trochlea.[909]

SUPERIOR OBLIQUE MYOKYMIA

Patients with superior oblique myokymia typically complain of brief, recurrent episodes of monocular blurring of vision, or tremulous sensations in one eye.[97,359,501] Some also report vertical or torsional diplopia or oscillopsia. Attacks usually last less than 10 seconds, but may occur many times per day. The attacks may be brought on by looking downward, by tilting the head towards the side of the affected eye, and by blinking. Most patients with superior oblique myokymia have no underlying disease, though cases have been reported following trochlear nerve palsy, head injury, possible demyelination or brainstem stroke, and with cerebellar tumor. Another possible pathogenesis is neurovascular compression at the root entry zone.[336,359,410,593,839,943]

The eye movements of superior oblique myokymia are often difficult to appreciate on gross examination, but the spasms of torsional-vertical rotations can sometimes be detected by looking for the movement of a conjunctival vessel, as the patient announces the onset of symptoms (see Video Display: Diplopia and Strabismus). They are more easily detected during examination with an ophthalmoscope or slit lamp. Measurement of the movements of superior oblique myokymia using the magnetic search coil technique has demonstrated an initial intorsion and depression of the affected eye, followed by irregular oscillations of small amplitude (Fig. 9–17).[501,593,828,839] The frequency of these oscillations is variable; some resemble jerk nystagmus at frequencies of 2 Hz–6 Hz, but superimposed upon these oscillations are low-amplitude, irregular oscillations with frequencies ranging up to 50 Hz.

Electromyographic recordings from superior oblique muscles affected by the disorder have revealed abnormal discharge from some muscle fibers, either spontaneous or following contraction of the muscle.[359,451,457] These discharge abnormalities include prolonged duration, increased amplitude, and a polyphasic pattern, with a spontaneous discharge rate of approximately 45 Hz. Spontaneous activity is only absent with large saccades in the "off" (upward) direction. Those fibers having an irregular discharge following muscle contraction subside to a regular discharge of about 35 Hz. These findings have been interpreted as indicating neuronal damage and subsequent regeneration, leading to desynchronized contraction of muscle fibers. Experimental lesions of the trochlear nerve have demonstrated regenerative capacities such that the remain-

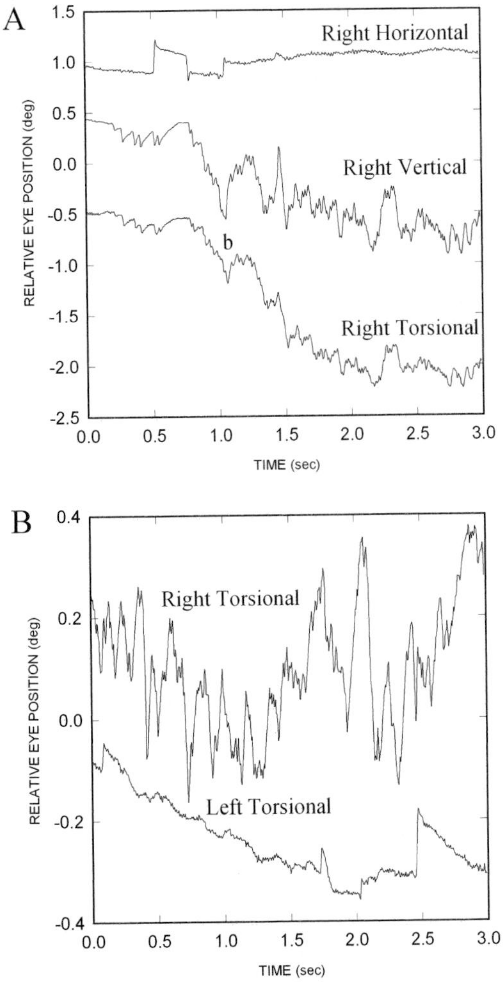

Figure 9–17. Superior oblique myokymia (see Video Display: Diplopia and Strabismus). Panel A shows a typical attack affecting the right eye, which the patient induced by blinking (b). The affected right eye depressed and intorted, and high frequency oscillations were superimposed. Panel B compares the torsional position of the right eye and left; note that the high frequency oscillations of superior oblique myokymia are only present in the right eye; the left eye shows some drift and nystagmus that is typical in the torsional plane for normal subjects during fixation. Upward deflections indicate rightward, upward, or clockwise rotations, from the point of view of the subject. Eye position is relative, individual records having been offset to aid clarity of display.

ing motor neurons increase their number of axons to hold the total constant.[366,893] Patients with superior oblique myokymia usually do not report a prior episode of diplopia, but MRI studies sometimes show atrophy of the superior oblique muscle,[556] and it seems possible that mild damage to the trochlear nerve could trigger the regeneration mechanism for maintaining a constant number of axons in the nerve;[495,501] some of these cases might be predisposed to superior oblique myokymia.

No treatments for superior oblique myokymia are consistently effective, but individual patients may respond to carbamazepine, baclofen, gabapentin,[410,848] and systemically or topically administered beta blockers. In some patients, superior oblique myokymia spontaneously resolves,[97] but in others the symptoms are so troublesome that surgical treatment is considered, and a modification of the Harada-Ito procedure—nasal transposition of the anterior portion of the superior oblique tendon, to weaken cyclorotation—has been beneficial.[463] In patients diagnosed with vascular compression of the trochlear nerve, decompression of the nerve at the root exit zone has stopped the oscillations.[731,741]

Oculomotor Nerve Palsy

CLINICAL FEATURES OF OCULOMOTOR NERVE PALSY

The third cranial nerve supplies four extraocular muscles (medial, superior and inferior recti, and inferior oblique) and the levator of the lid, and contains parasympathetic fibers that supply the sphincter of the pupil and the ciliary body. Complete, peripheral third nerve palsy is easily recognized by ptosis, a fixed, dilated pupil, and a resting eye position that is "down and out" (see Video Display: Diplopia and Strabismus). Incomplete third nerve palsies, however, are more common, and characteristic patterns of loss of function can be correlated with lesions at various sites along the course of the nerve from nucleus to muscle. It is necessary to differentiate such patterns of muscle weakness from a variety of restrictive ophthalmopathies, and from myasthenia gravis (Table 9–4).

Accurate diagnosis of the site and cause of oculomotor palsy is important, since some underlying conditions—notably aneurysms—require prompt therapy (Table 9–7). MRI often helps to confirm the underlying cause.[75,78]

NUCLEAR OCULOMOTOR NERVE PALSY

Lesions of the nucleus of the third nerve are rare. When they occur, they usually also

Table 9–7. **Etiology of Oculomotor Nerve Palsy**[70,449,702,841]

Nuclear

Congenital hypoplasia[321,370,689]
Infarction or hemorrhage[280,281,447,458]
Tumor[150,425,692]
Trauma[843]
Infection[26,752,851]

Fascicular

Infarction[140,473,598]
Hemorrhage[258,419,473]
Demyelination[271,861]
Syphilis[885]
Trauma[43,423]

Subarachnoid

Aneurysm (typically posterior communicating artery; occasionally basilar artery)[14,306,307,424,594,871,897,918]
Meningitis (infectious, syphilitic, granulomatous, Lyme, neoplastic, and idiopathic hypertrophic)[64,329,396,479,572,640,736,851]
Nerve infarction (associated with diabetes)[905]
Tumors of the oculomotor nerve[3,413,516,617,665,700,933]
Neurosurgical complication[572,940]
Trauma[423]
Spontaneous intracranial hypotension,[94,250] or following lumbar puncture[260]

At the Tentorial Edge

Uncal herniation[672,711]
Pseudotumor cerebri[550]
Hydrocephalus[720]
Trauma[471]

Cavernous Sinus and Superior Orbital Fissure

Aneurysm of internal carotid artery[54,440,625]
Carotid-cavernous fistula[9,431,476,579]
Cavernous sinus thrombosis[896]
Internal carotid artery stenosis,[44] or dissection[129,172]
Tumor: pituitary adenoma, meningioma, nasopharyngeal carcinoma, lymphoma, metastases, angioma, arachnoid cyst, other[1,50,102,272,414,446,532,624,630]
Pituitary infarction (apoplexy)[566,699,715]
Nerve infarction (associated with diabetes, hypertension, or arteritis)[32,220,713,836] or hemorrhage[580]
Sphenoidal sinusitis and mucocele[12,393,691]
Herpes zoster[29]
Tolosa-Hunt syndrome[35]
In association with monoclonal gammopathy and Waldenström's macroglobulinemia[89,487]

Orbit*

Trauma[504]
Mucormycosis and other fungal infections[696]
Tumor, hemorrhage, and other infiltrates of the nerve[391,767]
Frontal or sphenoidal sinus mucocele[223,759,814]

Localization Uncertain

In association with viral and other infections, and following immunization[126,141,427,754]
In association with cancer chemotherapy,[796] cocaine,[564] and sildenafil[215]
Nerve infarction[184,323]
Migraine[649,819,926]
Following dental[662] or retrobulbar anesthesia[189]

*May cause paresis by involvement of nerve or extraocular muscle.

involve structures important for vertical conjugate gaze. Based on current knowledge of the anatomic organization of the oculomotor nucleus (Fig. 9–9), it is possible to set certain criteria for diagnosis of nuclear third nerve palsy;[178] these are summarized in Table 9–8. However, it is important to recognize that, in this small area of the midbrain, the nuclei and fascicles of the oculomotor nerve lie in close proximity, and both may be affected to varying degrees. Thus, some caution is required in relying on MRI findings to differentiate between nuclear and fascicular lesions.[88,518, 584,690]

When nuclear lesions affect the superior rectus subnucleus, elevation of both eyes is impaired.[109,281] This is because axons from one superior rectus subnucleus cross and pass through the fellow subnucleus of the opposite side.[73,950] Thus, a lesion of one superior rectus subnucleus is effectively a bilateral lesion. It follows that in those case reports when only one superior rectus muscle—either ipsilateral or contralateral to the side of the lesion—is involved,[484] the lesion probably involved the superior rectus nerve fascicles (i.e., axons after they have left the nucleus).[484]

Table 9–8. **Diagnosis of Nuclear Oculomotor Nerve Palsy*[178,281]**

Obligatory Lesions
Unilateral third nerve palsy with contralateral superior rectus paresis and bilateral partial ptosis
Bilateral third nerve palsy associated with spared levator function (internal ophthalmoplegia may be present or absent)
Possible Nuclear Lesions
Bilateral total third nerve palsy
Bilateral ptosis
An isolated weakness of any single muscle except the levator, superior rectus, and medial rectus muscles
Conditions that are Unlikely to be due to Nuclear Lesions
Unilateral third nerve palsy, with or without internal involvement, associated with normal contralateral superior rectus function
Unilateral internal ophthalmoplegia
Unilateral ptosis
Isolated unilateral or bilateral medial rectus weakness

* In the absence of pupillary involvement, ocular myasthenia must always be ruled out.

Similarly, when lesions affect the central caudal nucleus, the result is bilateral ptosis. This is because of the unpaired nature of the central caudal subnucleus that supplies both levator muscles (Fig. 9–9). Since the central caudal nucleus sits at the bottom of the oculomotor nuclear complex, it may be selectively affected and bilateral ptosis may be the only manifestation of the nuclear palsy. The "plus-minus" lid syndrome of unilateral ptosis and contralateral eyelid retraction has been reported in association with nuclear third lesions,[280] and adjacent mesencephalon.[15] If raising the ptotic lid does not abolish the contralateral lid retraction (which would be expected according to Hering's law of the eyelids),[37] and if the lesion is acute (i.e., there has not been time for aberrant reinnervation), then the eye lid retraction in such cases is most probably due to loss of inhibition of the levator. The origin of this inhibition is undetermined, but it appears to depend on the mesencephalic M-group of neurons before their axons reach the central caudal nucleus.[353] Since ptosis is unilateral, the lesion cannot be localized to the central caudal nucleus (even though other parts of the oculomotor nucleus are), and the ptosis is fascicular in origin.

The medial rectus neurons lie at three locations within the nucleus and so it would seem unlikely for medial rectus paralysis (unilateral or bilateral) to be the sole manifestation of a nuclear third nerve palsy. Similarly, because the visceral nuclei are spread throughout the rostral half of the nucleus, unilateral internal ophthalmoplegia is unlikely to be the sole manifestation of a lesion of the oculomotor nucleus. Involvement of the pupil with midbrain third nerve lesion suggests a rostral site in the nucleus.[726]

The third-nerve nucleus also houses oculomotor internuclear neurons, which project to the contralateral abducens nucleus. Experimental studies indicate that they play a role in coordinating conjugate eye movements, and that pharmacological inactivation of these internuclear neurons with lidocaine causes a contralateral abduction weakness.[156] We have observed abduction weakness with esotropia in a patient with a midbrain multiple sclerosis plaque (see Video-Display: Midbrain Syndromes).

Paralysis of the inferior rectus or inferior oblique muscles in isolation is theoretically possible, but is usually associated with conjugate vertical gaze disorders. Patients reported to have impaired depression of one eye associated with impaired elevation of the other, with or without adduction paresis of the higher eye,[190,237,334,901] may have skew deviation rather than nuclear oculomotor palsy.[791] Disruption of saccadic inputs from the riMLF has sometimes been invoked to account for vertical disconjugacy in patients with lesions involving the oculomotor nucleus. However, the demonstration of axon collaterals from upward saccadic burst neurons in the riMLF (see Fig. 6–5), which contact yoke muscle pairs in the oculomotor nucleus,[595] means that violations of Hering's law for upward saccades must reflect lesions within or close to the motoneurons. This issue is discussed further in Chapter 12 (see Box 12–10).

CONGENITAL OCULOMOTOR NERVE PALSY

Congenital palsies of the third nerve are usually incomplete and unilateral; aberrant reinnervation is a common associated finding (see below).[47,321,747] The location of the lesion is variable, and may be associated with other developmental anomalies.[227,296,321] Rarely, congenital oculomotor weakness may alternate with periodic spasms of third nerve overactivity, such as esotropia or miosis; this is called oculomotor palsy with cyclic spasms.[262,523] This syndrome sometimes occurs with acquired oculomotor palsies;[455,856] its pathogenesis is unknown, but it is reported in adults following skull base irradiation.[575]

Ophthalmoplegic migraine usually has its onset in childhood.[40] The oculomotor palsy is usually complete, but rarely just the superior ramus is affected.[411] The palsy typically lasts for days or weeks after the headache has resolved. Rarely, patients are reported with congenital limitation of ocular motility that suggests anomalous innervation of muscles normally supplied by the oculomotor nerve. One example is a syndrome of congenital, unilateral adduction palsy; when the patient attempts to look into the field of action of the weak medial rectus muscle, the affected eye abducts rather than adducts (synergistic divergence). Electromyographic studies suggest a pattern of anomalous innervation, which is analogous to the abnormality in Duane retraction syndrome (see above).[173,892] Slowly progressive third nerve palsy in childhood may, in some cases, be due to schwannoma of the nerve sheath that can be detected with imaging studies,[3] but, in others, no cause can be found.[449,581] Rarely, cerebrovascular malformations can cause third nerve palsy in infants.[833]

DISORDERS AFFECTING THE FASCICLES OF THE OCULOMOTOR NERVE

As the fascicles of the oculomotor nerve traverse the midbrain, they pass through important structures that enable precise localization of third nerve palsies.[519] If the oculomotor nerve is involved as it traverses the cerebral peduncle, a contralateral hemiparesis will result, called Weber's syndrome.[779] Involvement of the oculomotor fascicles, red nucleus, and superior cerebellar peduncle causes Claude's syndrome: oculomotor palsy (often partial), contralateral ataxia, asynergy, and dysdiadochokinesis (see Video Display: Diplopia and Strabismus).[103,756] More extensive lesions may affect the third nerve fascicles, cerebral peduncle, and adjacent red nucleus and substantia nigra, causing Benedikt's syndrome: oculomotor palsy, contralateral hemiparesis, and contralateral involuntary movements or tremor.[15] Dorsal midbrain lesions that involve the oculomotor nucleus and produce a combination of nuclear and supranuclear gaze limitation with ataxia have been called Nothnagel's syndrome.[519] The third nerve may also be affected by hemorrhages caused by downward herniation of the brainstem. Small midbrain lesions may selectively involve the fascicles of the oculomotor nerve, causing paresis of one or more of the extraocular muscles with no associated neurologic deficits.[140,276,361,473,474,727] The pattern of involvement of the third nerve has been used to advance theories for the topographic organization of the oculomotor fascicles (see Anatomy of the Oculomotor Nerve, above).

DISORDERS AFFECTING THE SUBARACHNOID PORTION OF THE OCULOMOTOR NERVE

After its exit from the brainstem, the third nerve runs in the subarachnoid space and is susceptible to meningeal processes (infection, tumor, blood) and compression by arterial aneurysm, even if they are small.[264] Basilar artery aneurysms can cause oculomotor nerve palsy,[855] but the internal carotid–posterior communicating arterial junction is the more common site. With both types of aneurysm, it is unusual for the pupil to be affected alone; ptosis and external ophthalmoplegia usually coexist. With posterior communicating aneurysms, third nerve palsy may occur in the setting of subarachnoid hemorrhage, but another presentation is of acute diplopia with facial or orbital pain but without subarachnoid hemorrhage. Occasionally, minor head trauma may precipitate oculomotor nerve palsy due to aneurysms or tumors.[897]

A common clinical challenge is to differentiate third nerve compression due to aneurysm from nerve infarction in association with diabetes or hypertension (see below), in which cerebral arteriography is not indicated. The presence of pupillary involvement can generally be relied on to identify those patients that harbor an aneurysm. Initially, however, the pupil may be spared,[14,54,440,625] so pupil-sparing third nerve palsy requires careful observation for a week before a decision can be made about arteriography. After a week, third nerve palsy with complete pupillary sparing is rarely due to aneurysm.[416] Cases of complete extraocular palsy with normal pupils due to aneurysm are rare.[530] Partial pupillary involvement may be grounds for an arteriogram,[444] although mild involvement of the pupil may occur with non-compressive processes.[81] About one third of patients with diabetic third nerve palsy show anisocoria, but this is usually only about 1 mm.[378] Pleocytosis in the cerebrospinal fluid may occur with aneurysm.[424,467] Spontaneous resolution of an oculomotor paresis does not necessarily mean that aneurysm is excluded.[306] Another factor that should be weighed when considering arteriography for acute oculomotor palsy is the patient's age: individuals between 20 and 50 years of age are more likely to have an aneurysm,[853] whereas children younger than 11 years almost never do.[918] MRI, MRA, or CT often help to differentiate nerve infarction from compressive or brainstem lesions,[78,925] and gadolinium enhancement of the cisternal portion of the oculomotor nerve is a sensitive index of neoplastic or inflammatory processes, including migraine.[819]

COMPRESSION OF THE OCULOMOTOR NERVE AT THE TENTORIAL EDGE

The third nerve may also be compressed against the tentorial edge, petroclinoid ligament, or clivus by the uncus of the temporal lobe during transtentorial herniation.[672] Alternatively, the third nerve may be stretched by displacement of the midbrain.[711] Classically, the pupillary fibers are affected first and mydriasis results. When the pupil becomes fixed, extraocular muscle weakness also appears. Rarely, upward herniation of a posterior fossa mass lesion may cause a third nerve palsy.

DISORDERS AFFECTING THE CAVERNOUS PORTION OF THE OCULOMOTOR NERVE

Within the cavernous sinus (Fig. 9–8), the oculomotor nerve may be compressed by aneurysm or tumor. Intracavernous (infraclinoid) aneurysms are less common than posterior communicating (supraclinoid) aneurysms and seldom rupture. The typical presentation of intracavernous aneurysms is progressive ophthalmoplegia and ptosis, often with signs of aberrant reinnervation.[537] About half of all patients suffer pain in the face. Often the abducens and trochlear nerves are also affected. Symptoms are usually slowly progressive and may suggest tumor. Sparing of the pupil is more common with aneurysms involving the cavernous sinus than with posterior communicating aneurysms, probably because the inferior division of the oculomotor nerve, which contains the pupillomotor fibers, is less frequently involved in the latter.[853] An alternative explanation is that sympathetic paresis and parasympathetic paresis coexist. Rarely, the aneurysm ruptures and creates a carotid-cavernous fistula (see below). Current evidence suggests that patients with cavernous sinus aneurysms have a better prognosis with endovascular surgery than no treatment.[293]

Tumors arising near the cavernous sinus, including meningioma, pituitary adenomas, and lymphomas, may cause third nerve palsy; usually other nerves in the cavernous sinus are also affected. Typically, the tumors grow slowly without producing any pain. Sometimes, the diagnosis only becomes evident with serial MRIs. Occasionally, hemorrhage occurs into a pituitary tumor, causing the syndrome of pituitary apoplexy as in the following case history (see Video Display: Diplopia and Strabismus).

CASE HISTORY: Pituitary Apoplexy

A 56-year-old man suddenly developed nausea and vomiting, which lasted for 24 hours and then resolved. The next day, he noticed a mild headache; several hours later, he suddenly developed diplopia and a left, partial ptosis. On examination, he had normal visual acuity and full visual fields. His left pupil diameter was 6 mm and his right was 5 mm. There was a left exotropia and hypotropia; testing showed weakness of all extraocular muscles supplied by the left oculomotor nerve, but sparing of the lateral rectus and superior oblique. He was hypertensive, but had no neck stiffness, and results of the general neurologic examination were normal. CT showed possible enlargement of the sella turcica. A carotid arteriogram showed no aneurysm.

A spinal tap revealed a protein of 57 mg/dL, glucose of 54 mg/dL, 200 red cells/mm^3, and 4 white cells/mm^3. MRI showed a pituitary tumor that extended laterally on the left to compress the oculomotor nerve (Fig. 9–18). The patient was treated with corticosteroids and underwent a successful transsphenoidal resection of his tumor. Histological examination demonstrated hemorrhage in a chromophobe adenoma.

Comment: This case illustrates several features of pituitary apoplexy: sudden onset of headache (usually severe), variable degrees of ophthalmoparesis (which may be bilateral and complete), and subarachnoid hemorrhage. Visual loss and endocrine insufficiency may also occur. CT or MRI confirms the diagnosis. Prompt transsphenoidal neurosurgical intervention, preceded by massive corticosteroid administration, is usually required.[661,699,906]

Septic thrombosis of the cavernous sinus is now rare,[206] but low-grade inflammatory processes may cause oculomotor nerve palsy as part of the Tolosa-Hunt syndrome (see below).

INFARCTION OF THE OCULOMOTOR NERVE

Solitary third nerve palsy may be due to infarction, usually in association with diabetes or hypertension ("medical third"). It is also reported in association with collagen vascular disease or giant cell arteritis.[184] The pupil is usually spared or only minimally involved, though it may occasionally be fixed to light.[287] Patients often complain of facial or orbital pain that usually precedes the muscle palsy and disappears when diplopia or ptosis develops. The onset of diplopia is sudden, but the muscle paresis may evolve for up to 2 weeks.[380] Recovery is usually the rule within 3 months.[132] Although it generally occurs in diabetic patients who already have evidence of small-vessel disease in other organs, third nerve palsy may be the presenting symptoms of the disease and has been reported in children with diabetes.[311] Pathologic examination of the third

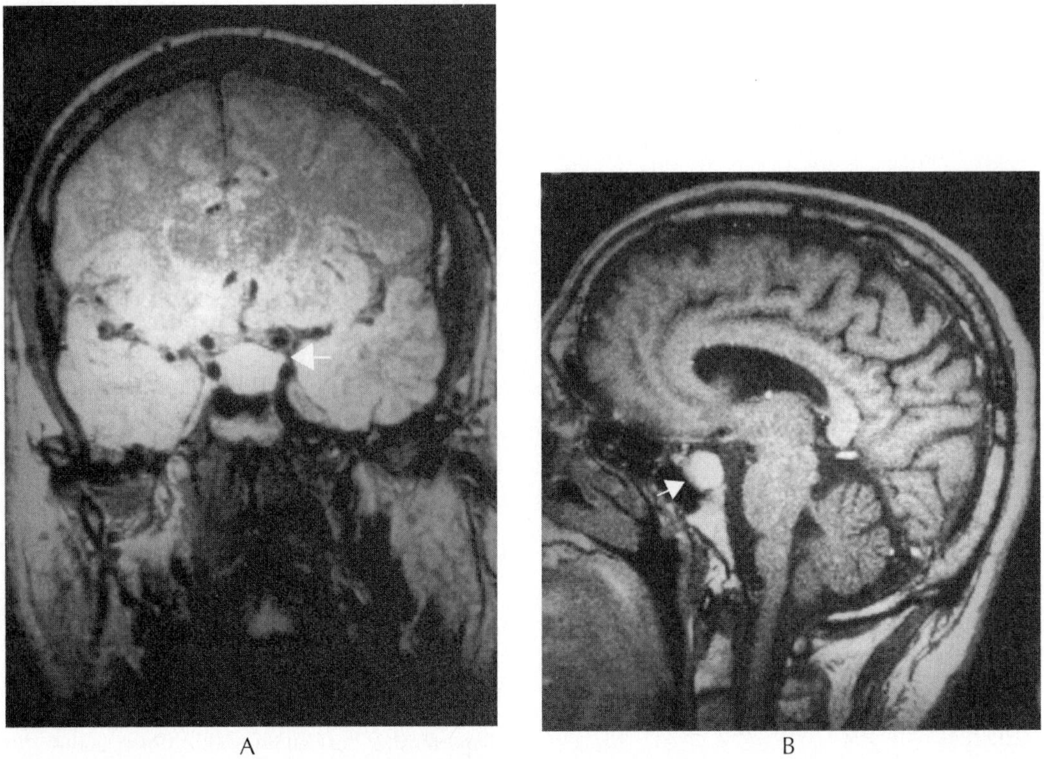

A B

Figure 9–18. Magnetic resonance images of a patient who presented with a left third nerve palsy due to infarction of a pituitary tumor (see Case History: Pituitary apoplexy and Video Display: Diplopia and Strabismus). (A) Sagittal view, showing tumor (arrow). (B) Coronal view, showing encroachment on left cavernous sinus by the tumor (arrow).

nerve in diabetic patients has shown infarction of the nerve in the intracavernous[32,220] or subarachnoid portions.[905] The core of the nerve is most severely involved, thus sparing the peripherally located pupillary fibers. The oculomotor nerves of diabetics who have not suffered third nerve palsy show microfasciculation of edge fibers and changes in the distribution of fiber size.[790] Other studies, however, suggest that a common site of nerve infarction in diabetics is within the brainstem.[297] Coexistent involvement of the oculomotor nerve and the trochlear nerve, or of all three ocular motor nerves and the ophthalmic division of the trigeminal nerve, probably implies occlusion of branches of the inferolateral trunk that arises from the intracavernous carotid artery.[490] Mucormycosis must always be considered in the diabetic patient who develops ocular muscle palsies.

OCULOMOTOR NERVE PALSY DUE TO TRAUMA

In most large series of patients with oculomotor nerve palsy, trauma is an important cause. The head injury usually causes fracture or loss of consciousness; only rarely does palsy follow mild trauma, and then other diagnoses, such as tumors at the base of the skull, should be considered.[239] The third nerve may be injured as it emerges from the brainstem (root avulsion), in its subarachnoid course as it attaches to the dura, or by fractures at the supraorbital fissure. Penetrating injuries to the orbit or brain may also cause third nerve palsy.[423]

ABERRANT REGENERATION OF THE OCULOMOTOR NERVE

A common sequel of oculomotor nerve palsy is aberrant regeneration. Ramon y Cajal first showed that after experimental transection of the oculomotor nerve, the regenerating fibers no longer follow their previous paths, but innervate different muscles supplied by the third nerve.[695] Other studies have confirmed such misrouting of axons.[249,775,776] This cannot be the mechanism in every case, however, since anomalous synkinesis can occur transiently after an acute third nerve palsy.[505,775,776] Anomalous synkinesis has also been reported following a mesencephalic lesion affecting the oculomotor fascicles.[562]

The clinical signs of aberrant regeneration include abnormal lid movements. Most commonly the lid elevates during adduction or depression of the eye. Other common patterns include depression of the lid on abduction, and pupillary constriction on adduction or depression of the eye, but absent direct pupillary light reaction. All these combined movements are due to co-contraction of muscles innervated by the third nerve. Rarely, the lid of the other eye may be affected with elevation on down gaze.[315] Acquired oculomotor-abducens synkinesis has also been reported.[395]

Aberrant reinnervation of the oculomotor nerve may occur after trauma,[750] aneurysm,[785,871] congenital third nerve palsy,[47] migraine,[74] and as a complication of neurosurgery.[373] If aberrant regeneration is encountered without a history of preceding oculomotor palsy, then slowly growing intracavernous meningioma[87,742] or carotid aneurysm[170] is likely, though sometimes no cause can be found.[485] Aberrant regeneration almost never occurs with diabetic third nerve palsy. Aberrant regeneration in which misdirected fibers of the abducens nerve came to innervate the pupil has been proposed as the explanation of miosis with abduction in a patient who suffered palsies of CN III, IV, and VI following head trauma.[663]

PARTIAL OCULOMOTOR NERVE PALSY

As the oculomotor nerve passes through the cavernous sinus, it divides into superior and inferior rami or divisions. The superior oculomotor division supplies the superior rectus and levator palpebrae superioris; the inferior oculomotor division supplies the medial and inferior rectus and inferior oblique, the pupil, and the ciliary body. Isolated lesions of these branches occur.[99,174,226,304,632,735,814] The pattern of weakness encountered with a superior division lesion can be produced, however, by lesions located in the more proximal portions of the nerve,[317] or even within the brainstem.[473] Less commonly, individual muscles supplied by the third cranial nerve may be paralyzed.[140,599,692,890] In patients with isolated ptosis or paralysis of individual muscles, myasthenia gravis should be considered. Rarely, double-elevator palsy, with no tropia in primary position, is due to a brainstem lesion (see Chapter 12).

MANAGEMENT OF OCULOMOTOR NERVE PALSY

Complete oculomotor palsy is easily diagnosed, but with partial involvement, consideration should be given to whether the patient has another condition (Table 9–4). In adults, a common challenge is to determine whether the palsy is due to nerve infarction in association with diabetes or hypertension, or due to a compressive lesion, such as arterial aneurysm. If the pupil is completely fixed to light, the chance of aneurysm is high, and angiography is usually indicated. Patients with partial involvement of the pupil and complete involvement of the extraocular muscles and lid should undergo MRI -MRA, and be closely observed. MRA will reveal some, but not all, aneurysms compressing CN III. It is wise to closely observe all patients who have developed a third nerve palsy for several days, since their signs may evolve and cerebral angiography may become indicated. Anisocoria of greater than 2 mm may be considered grounds for an arteriogram.[854] An MRI may also demonstrate brainstem infarction or hemorrhage, and gadolinium enhancement may demonstrate inflammation or infiltration affecting the oculomotor nerve throughout its course.[78] Oculomotor nerve palsy in children is less likely to be due to aneurysm, but if there has been no antecedent trauma, cerebral tumors should be sought with MRI.[449]

Multiple Ocular Motor Nerve Palsies

The principal culprits causing combined third, fourth, and sixth nerve palsies are brainstem stroke, lesions within the cavernous sinus or superior orbital fissure (where the three nerves lie near each other), trauma, and generalized neuropathies (Table 9–9). Any of these processes can lead to complete ophthalmoplegia.[417] Other causes to be considered in the patient with complete ophthalmoplegia include neuromuscular disorders (myasthenia gravis, Miller Fisher syndrome, and botulism), drug intoxications (see Table 12–11), and Wernicke's encephalopathy.

Table 9–9. **Etiology of Multiple Ocular Motor Nerve Palsies[70,417,449,504,702,841]**

Brainstem
Tumor[720]
Infarction or hemorrhage[417,847,928]
Encephalitis[297]
Subarachnoid
Meningitis (infectious and neoplastic)[521,688]
Trauma[420,504,534]
Clivus tumor
Aneurysm and dolichoectasia[221]
Cavernous Sinus and Superior Orbital Fissure
Aneurysm of internal carotid artery[256,537]
Occlusion of internal carotid artery[279,914]
Tumor: meningioma, pituitary adenoma with apoplexy, cavernous angioma or hemangiopericytoma, nasopharyngeal carcinoma, lymphoma, myeloma, Waldenström's macroglobulinemia, other[33,196,344,486,525,549,608,674,699,757,827]
Pseudotumor cerebri[489]
Cavernous sinus thrombosis[211,896]
Sphenoid sinus tumor[125]
Tolosa-Hunt syndrome[35,128,290,365]
Neurosurgical complication[940]
Herpes zoster[29]
Nerve infarction (associated with diabetes or arteritis)[183,465,560]
Carotid-cavernous fistula[301,431,508]
Orbital*
Mucormycosis and other infections[175,392,498,696,949]
Trauma[546]
Tumor and other infiltrates[459]
Aneurysm of the ophthalmic artery[232]
Localization Uncertain
Generalized neuropathies, especially post-inflammatory type (Guillain-Barré and Miller Fisher syndromes)[255,559]
Sjögren's syndrome[544]
Toxins[830]
Behçet's disease[626]

*May cause paresis by involvement of nerve or extraocular muscle.

BRAINSTEM LESIONS CAUSING OPHTHALMOPLEGIA

Infarction or hemorrhage of the brainstem, especially the midbrain, may limit both horizontal and vertical eye movements;[417,928] diagnostic features are described in Chapter 12. A combination of ocular motor nerve palsies, with brainstem lesions, is encountered in some patients with HIV infection.[324,421,605] The nuclei of the ocular motor nerves are usually spared in amyotrophic lateral sclerosis (ALS), with only rare documentation of pathological involvement in advanced cases,[582,638] although other brainstem nuclei may be involved.[36] This rarity of involvement has been related to the low concentrations of glycinergic and muscarinic cholinergic receptors of these nuclei, when compared with other cranial nerve nuclei or the spinal cord.[910] Abnormalities of eye movements in ALS are discussed in Chapter 12. Limitation of eye movements has been described in some forms of spinal muscular atrophy.[310,651]

CAVERNOUS SINUS AND SUPERIOR ORBITAL FISSURE SYNDROMES

Within the cavernous sinus (Fig. 9–8), a variety of processes may affect the ocular motor nerves. To differentiate cavernous sinus from orbital apex lesions, associated findings are helpful.[95] Involvement of the first two sensory divisions of the trigeminal nerve suggests disease of the cavernous sinus; if all three divisions are involved, a retrocavernous process may be present. If trigeminal function is normal but vision is impaired, then the process is probably in the orbit. The ocular motor deficit may be complete if disease occurs in either the cavernous sinus or orbit, but with a more anterior location, the pupil and muscles supplied by the inferior division of the oculomotor nerve tend to be spared.[855] Tumors (particularly meningioma, pituitary adenoma, and nasopharyngeal carcinoma) are common causes of combined ophthalmoparesis. Meningioma and pituitary adenoma are slow growing, but hemorrhage into a pituitary adenoma, as already discussed, produces the distinctive clinical syndrome of pituitary apoplexy. Combined ocular motor palsies may also be due to nerve infarction in the cavernous sinus.[490]

CAROTID-CAVERNOUS FISTULA

This abnormal communication between the carotid arterial system and the cavernous sinus is of two types: direct and dural. *Direct fistulae* are caused by tears in the intracavernous portion of the internal carotid artery arising from severe head trauma or from rupture of a preexisting aneurysm. These are high-flow fistulae, characterized by sudden onset of pulsatile proptosis, bruit, and impaired vision; they lie anteriorly in the cavernous sinus and drain forward into the orbit.[508] *Dural fistulae* are due to rupture of thin-walled meningeal branches of the internal or external carotid arteries within the cavernous sinus; such rupture may occur spontaneously, especially in elderly, hypertensive patients, and following minor head trauma or straining. These low-flow fistulae present more subtly, with subjective bruit, mild proptosis, chemosis, conjunctival redness, and glaucoma; they lie posteriorly in the cavernous sinus and tend to drain posteriorly to the inferior petrosal sinus rather than into the superior ophthalmic vein. Occasionally, the presentation is one of painful ophthalmoplegia without chemosis or exophthalmos.[9,338,464] Thrombosis of the superior ophthalmic vein may produce temporary worsening of symptoms followed by spontaneous remission.[758]

Diplopia is common with both direct and dural fistulae; abduction weakness is frequent and all eye movements may be affected. It is thought that while all three ocular motor nerves may be affected, a more common cause of the restricted ocular motility is hypoxic, congested extraocular muscles.[503] Embolization is an effective treatment for many patients with carotid-cavernous fistula.[431,476,508,576] Some dural shunts spontaneously resolve.

TOLOSA-HUNT SYNDROME AND PAINFUL OPHTHALMOPLEGIA

Almost any process causing ophthalmoplegia can be painful, with the possible exceptions of myasthenia gravis and chronic progressive external ophthalmoplegia.[35] The physician should always be concerned about infections and tumors. However, there are patients who present with painful, combined ophthalmoplegia due to a granulomatous inflammatory process that affects the cavernous sinus, extending forward to the superior orbital fissure and orbital apex. Called the Tolosa-Hunt syndrome, this is usually a disease of middle or later life that may spontaneously remit and relapse. The presenting complaints are steady, retro-orbital pain and diplopia. The third, fourth, or sixth nerves, or a combination of ocular motor nerves, may be affected. Visual impairment occurs in some patients.[365,845] There is some overlap with orbital pseudotumor. Sensation supplied by the ophthalmic and maxillary trigeminal divisions may be impaired. The pupil may be constricted if the sympathetic innervation is involved, or dilated if parasympathetic innervation is involved. Pathologic examination has shown a low-grade, non-caseating, granulomatous, inflammatory response in the cavernous sinus encroaching on the carotid artery and nerves of passage.[128,290]

Diagnosis is by gadolinium-enhanced MRI, which demonstrates soft-tissue infiltration in the cavernous sinus, sometimes with extension into the orbit apex, but without erosion of bone.[300,394] The infiltrate is either hypointense on T1-weighted images and isointense on T2-weighted images,[942] or hyperintense on T1-weighted and intermediate-weighted images.[300] Angiography may show narrowing of the carotid siphon, occlusion of the superior orbital vein, and non-visualization of the cavernous sinus.

It has been suggested that the Tolosa-Hunt syndrome is a variant of a larger syndrome of recurrent multiple cranial neuropathies.[49,397,865] There is also an association with other forms of vasculitis, such as lupus or Wegener's granulomatosis.[183,585] Patients with the Tolosa-Hunt syndrome usually respond promptly to corticosteroid treatment. However, caution is required in attributing diagnostic value to a positive response, because tumors in the cavernous region may respond similarly to steroids [799] or even resolve spontaneously.[272] Thus, serial MRIs to monitor such patients are advisable.[300,394,483,615,838,942]

The differential diagnosis of Tolosa-Hunt syndrome includes the entities described in Table 9–9. Orbital myositis may usually be distinguished by swelling and erythema of the eyes.[112,583,786,808] The combination of painful palsies of the ocular motor nerves associated with Horner's syndrome is called Raeder's paratrigeminal syndrome,[308] and usually reflects coexistent involvement of the oculosympathetic fibers in the cavernous sinus, commonly due to mass lesions. Ophthalmoplegic migraine is reported to affect each of the ocular motor nerves and sometimes is difficult to distinguish from Tolosa-Hunt syndrome.[180,820]

HEAD TRAUMA AND OPHTHALMOPLEGIA

Multiple ocular motor nerve palsies occurring with trauma are usually due to severe head injury, with fractures of the orbital, sphenoid, or petrous temporal bones. Blow-out fracture of the orbit may be confused with ocular motor palsies. It is caused by a blunt impact to the globe or infraorbital rim that fractures the orbital floor.[115,433,753,917] Prolapse of the inferior rectus muscle through the bony defect mechanically restricts upward gaze. There may also be enophthalmos, and injury to the globe may seriously disturb vision and pupillary reactions. Diagnosis is suggested by a history of painful vertical diplopia following trauma and is confirmed by resistance to forced duction of the eye, and by CT, which shows herniation of soft tissue through the fracture.[546]

NEUROPATHIES CAUSING OPHTHALMOPLEGIA

Guillain-Barré and Miller Fisher Syndromes

The oculomotor, abducens, and trochlear nerves may be involved in Guillain-Barré syndrome, which is now viewed as a group of distinct disorders.[31] Thus, acute inflammatory demyelinating neuropathy, acute motor axonal neuropathy, and acute motor-sensory axonal neuropathy may all involve eye movements.[243,709] However, it is the Miller Fisher syndrome that most frequently affects ocular motility, and which has also provided many insights into this spectrum of disorders.

Miller Fisher syndrome comprises ophthalmoplegia (external and sometimes internal), areflexia, and ataxia of the limbs or gait;[255] facial weakness, ptosis and mydriasis are also reported.[589] The degree of ophthalmoparesis varies, but certain patterns might suggest involvement of either the peripheral or central nervous system.[17,557,734] For example, the ophthalmoplegia may resemble a horizontal or vertical gaze palsy or internuclear ophthalmoplegia. Ptosis is often absent even in the presence of significant ophthalmoparesis. Bell's phenomenon may also be preserved even when vertical eye movements are otherwise absent. Rebound nystagmus, impairment of smooth pursuit, optokinetic nystagmus, and suppression (cancellation) of the vestibulo-ocular reflex point to cerebellar dysfunction.[951] As with myasthenia gravis, some of these findings might be due the effects of central adaptation to peripheral weakness. Other findings, however, such as the confusion that some patients suffer, the dissociated involvement of the levator palpebrae superioris and superior rectus, and the MRI findings in some cases, point to central involvement—an encephalitic component.[78,710,951] C. Miller Fisher himself was impressed by the symmetry of the ocular motor deficit and by ataxia unaccompanied by sensory loss, and "reluctantly interpreted" the clinical signs "as manifestations of an unusual and unique disturbance of peripheral neurons."[255]

Immunological evidence has clarified the relationship of Miller Fisher syndrome to Guillain-Barré syndrome and involvement of the central nervous system. First, anti-GQ1b IgG autoantibodies have been detected in over 85% of patients with the acute phase of Miller Fisher syndrome, and provide a useful diagnostic test.[147,623,652] Antibodies against the ganglioside GQ1b have also been detected in those patients with Guillain-Barré syndrome who have involvement of their eye movements, and also in patients with Bickerstaff's brainstem encephalitis.[16,629] The latter is characterized by ophthalmoplegia and ataxia, but also by pyramidal and sensory tract findings and cerebrospinal fluid pleocytosis.[946]

Consistent with this immunopathologic hypothesis, immunotherapy (plasmapheresis or intravenous immunoglobulin, IVIG) is reported to improve both Bickerstaff's encephalitis and Miller Fisher syndrome.[218,398, 620,945] In a mouse model, anti-GQ1b antibodies induce increased frequency of miniature end-plate potential (due to quantal acetylcholine release) at the neuromuscular junction, followed by transmission block.[376] Intravenous immunoglobulin (IVIG) stops anti-GQ1b antibodies from binding to GQ1b ganglioside receptors and thereby prevents the electrophysiological effects.[376] Neuropathologic examination of two patients with Miller Fisher syndrome showed a normal central nervous system.[191,664] Autopsy of a patient who had Bickerstaff's encephalitis in association with Guillain-Barré syndrome and anti-GQ1b antibodies showed a normal brainstem but demyelination of the ocular motor and spinal nerves.[947] Other studies have shown staining of the molecular layer of the cerebellum by anti-GQ1b antibodies, which is evidence for a central origin of the ataxia—and probably some of the eye movement disorders—in Miller Fisher syndrome.[461]

Thus, evidence suggests that anti-GQ1b antibodies play a key role in producing the disturbance of eye movements in Miller Fisher syndrome, Guillain-Barré syndrome, and Bickerstaff's encephalitis.[620] As in Guillain-Barré syndrome, Campylobactor jejuni may be the responsible trigger, since anti-GQ1b antibodies bind to surface epitopes on this organism, and its lipopolysaccharide fraction may molecularly mimic the ganglioside.[23,375] Furthermore, different strains of this organism may specifically trigger either Miller Fisher or Guillain-Barré syndrome.[832] It has also been suggested that Haemophilus influenza may be the triggering infection in some patients.[450] Some patients with chronic ophthalmoplegia and positive anti-GQ1b antibodies have been reported; one responded to immunotherapy.[698]

Recurrent Neuropathies Causing Ophthalmoplegia

Certain patients with chronic relapsing neuropathies, such as chronic inflammatory demyelinating neuropathy (CIDP), may have involvement of the extraocular muscles. Ocular palsies may precede the development of the neuropathy by weeks.[214,259] Motor symptoms may be slight[407] and some patients appear to have "relapsing Fisher's syndrome."[740,884] In the future, immunological studies are likely to clarify these entities. Rarely, recurrent ocular motor palsies may be part of a familial disorder that is characterized principally by recurrent Bell's palsy.[18]

OCULAR NEUROMYOTONIA

This rare disorder is characterized by episodes of diplopia that are usually precipitated by holding the eyes in eccentric gaze, often sustained adduction.[240,265,619,938] In most cases, these episodes of diplopia are caused by involuntary, occasionally painful, contraction of one or more muscles innervated by one oculomotor nerve. One patient with bilateral oculomotor nerve involvement has been described,[592] and another with involvement of the lateral rectus muscle.[53] Many reported patients have undergone radiation therapy to the parasellar region,[263] but idiopathic cases have also been reported,[265] and the phenomenon is reported in association with vascular compression.[842,877a]

One reported patient showed ocular neuromyotonia in the muscles supplied by his right oculomotor nerve.[265] There was no diplopia or misalignment of the visual axes in primary gaze. Following sustained left gaze, he developed horizontal diplopia and an esotropia (see Video Display: Diplopia and Strabismus), but following sustained right gaze, no diplopia or deviation occurred. Following sustained down gaze, he developed diplopia and left hypertropia, and following sustained up gaze, he developed diplopia and a right hypertropia. The metrics of his saccades indicated a defect of both relaxation and maximal contraction of affected muscles.

The mechanism responsible for ocular neuromyotonia is unknown. Both ephaptic neural transmission and changes in the pattern of neuronal transmission following denervation have been suggested,[265] because spontaneous activity has been observed in the ocular electromyograph of affected patients.[653,704] Axonal hyperexcitability due to dysfunction of potassium channels has also been implicated by analogy with systemic neuromyotonia.[240,621]

The episodic nature of the diplopia often suggests myasthenia gravis, but anticholinergic medicines are ineffective. Carbamazepine, however, is often effective treatment. Some patients can control their attacks by sustaining gaze opposite to the direction that causes symptoms.[729] Other differential diagnoses are superior oblique myokymia, thyroid ophthalmopathy, cyclic oculomotor palsy, and rippling muscle disease.[462] The specific relationship of the onset symptoms following sustained attempts to hold eccentric gaze points to the diagnosis, and this should be specifically looked for during the examination of patients with evanescent, unexplained diplopia.

DISORDERS OF THE NEUROMUSCULAR JUNCTION

Several diseases affecting the neuromuscular junction at either presynaptic or postsynaptic sites may cause abnormalities of eye movements. Acute poisoning with organophosphate anticholinesterases (insecticides), can also cause ophthalmoparesis, ptosis or other abnormal eye movements as part of a picture of generalized weakness.[514,541]

Systemic Botulism

The neurotoxin of *Clostridium botulinum* blocks release of acetylcholine from nerve terminals. Botulism may be caused by ingested toxin in contaminated food, intestinal production of toxin in infants, wound infection, and in subcutaneous heroin abuse.[339,340,542,697,850] In any of these forms, varying degrees of internal and external ophthalmoplegia may occur. In patients with complete ophthalmoplegia, the differential diagnosis includes brainstem stroke, drug intoxications (see Table 12–11 in Chapter 12), Wernicke's encephalopathy, pituitary apoplexy, myasthenia gravis, and Guillain-Barré and Miller Fisher syndromes.[417]

Residual eye movements in two patients with systemic botulism were reported to show hypometric, multistep saccades. These saccades were followed by backward drifts that gave the appearance of quivering movements similar to those encountered in myasthenia gravis.[340] This finding might reflect a greater sensitivity of the orbital, singly innervated muscle fibers to botulinum toxin.[800] These fibers are continuously active and appear to be important for holding the eye steady after a saccade has ended.[681] Another patient who was studied six days after mild systemic botulism showed slow horizontal and vertical saccades with centripetal post-saccadic drift (see Figure 9–19 and Video Display: Diplopia and Strabismus).[811] Edrophonium (Tensilon) may produce some improvement of saccadic velocity and increased range of movement.[38]

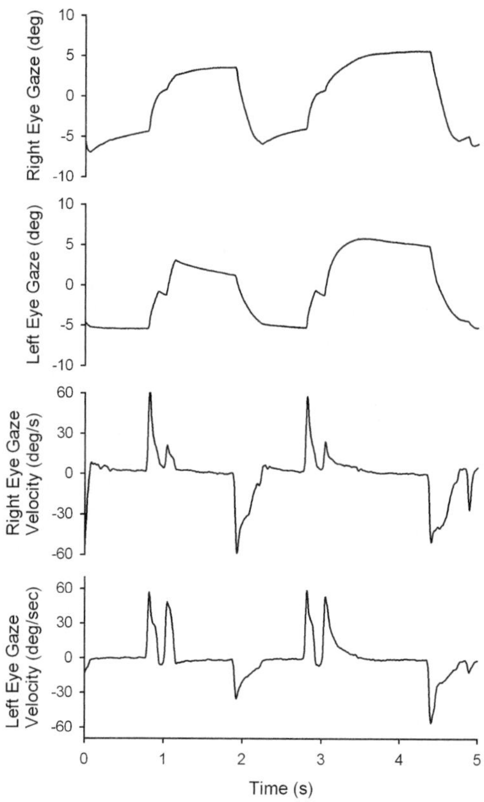

Figure 9–19. Slow saccades due to botulism (see Video Display: Diplopia and Strabismus). Eye movements of a 39-year-old man with botulism. Measurements of his horizontal eye movements made on day six of his illness show slow saccades. Note also that abducting saccades are slower than adducting saccades, causing a transient convergence at the end of each horizontal gaze shift. The top two traces are position plots and the bottom two traces are corresponding velocity plots for the right eye (OD) and left eye (OS).

Botulinum Toxin as Therapy for Abnormal Eye Movements

Alan B. Scott introduced botulinum A toxin as therapy for congenital or acquired strabismus.[748] It is a helpful adjunct in the management of childhood strabismus,[553,804] and some cases of paralytic strabismus.[8,494] Botulinum A toxin has also been used to reduce or abolish acquired nystagmus by injecting it either into selected extraocular muscles or into the retrobulbar space (see Fig. 10–17 in Chapter 10).[500,849] Botulinum toxin is an effective treatment for facial spasms and blepharospasm; occasionally, transient diplopia may occur after such therapy.[811,932]

The Lambert-Eaton Myasthenic Syndrome

Lambert-Eaton myasthenic syndrome (LEMS) is due to impaired release of acetylcholine secondary to an autoimmune disorder affecting P/Q voltage-gated calcium channels.[305] LEMS is usually associated with carcinoma, which may be occult, but it may also be a primary autoimmune disorder, especially in patients under age 45 years, and who never smoked cigarettes. Typical symptoms are weakness and fatigability of the proximal limb muscles, along with autonomic dysfunction. Ptosis or diplopia may be accompanied by bulbar symptoms, suggesting a diagnosis of myasthenia gravis.[116,717] Measurements of eye movements may demonstrate characteristic hypometric, closely-spaced saccades.[172,194] Some patients also show slow saccades. The characteristic facilitation of muscle power with repeated efforts can sometimes be observed as hypometria gives way to hypermetria during repetitive saccades. Occasionally, the edrophonium (Tensilon) test may be positive, causing saccadic hypermetria.[194]

Myasthenia Gravis

CLINICAL FEATURES OF MYASTHENIA GRAVIS

Myasthenia gravis is a disease of post-synaptic neuromuscular junction that is characterized by fatigable muscle weakness.[402,882,883] It commonly affects the extraocular muscles. Half of all patients present with ocular symptoms and more than 90% eventually develop eye movement abnormalities.[793] Of those patients who present with ocular symptoms, half persist with purely ocular myasthenia. Of those who generalize, most do so within 2 years of the onset of the disease.[71,478]

Transient neonatal myasthenia gravis, which is due to transfer of antibody from the mother, tends to spare eye movements.[275] Congenital myasthenia constitutes a heterogeneous group of genetic disorders affecting neuromuscular transmission that presents in the first year of life, mainly produces ptosis, and usually has a benign course.[225] Juvenile myasthenia, which is similar to adult myasthenia apart from its early age of onset, presents with ocular symptoms in more than half of all cases.[275] In general, younger patients tend to have a more benign course, though relapses may occur.[65,551] In the elderly, ocular myasthenia affects men more commonly, and is associated with thyroid disease, progression of symptoms, but absence of thymoma and good response to medical therapy.[907] Rarely, ocular myasthenia occurs as a reversible complication of penicillamine therapy.[412]

Muscle fatigue is the hallmark of myasthenia gravis and may affect the lids, eye movements, or both. Lid abnormalities include progressive and often asymmetric ptosis, brought out by attempting sustained upward gaze. If there is a small, asymmetric ptosis, instruct the patient to fix upon an object with the eye showing less ptosis and observe the ptotic eye behind a cover; over the course of a minute, worsening of the ptosis may become evident. Ptosis in myasthenia may be improved by applying an ice pack over the closed eye for 2 minutes.[760] Transient eyelid retraction occurs during refixations from down to straight ahead, called Cogan's eyelid twitch sign (see Video Display: Diplopia and Strabismus).[159] This sign is not pathognomonic, however, and may occur with brainstem or oculomotor disorders.[586] Patients with unilateral ptosis and contralateral lid retraction demonstrate "Hering's law of equal eyelid innervation." Thus, when the ptotic lid is manually raised, the contralateral lid falls to a normal position, since a large innervation is no longer required (see Video Display: Diplopia and Strabismus).[37] Ptosis is often relieved after a short nap.[628] Attempted forceful eyelid closure is commonly impaired in myasthenia.

The more common abnormalities of myasthenia are summarized in Table 9–10. Myasthenia gravis characteristically causes intermittent diplopia, due to variable extraocular muscle weakness. Such weakness is often asymmetric and may mimic third, fourth, or sixth nerve palsy, gaze paresis, internuclear ophthalmoplegia, one-and-a-half syndrome (Chapter 12) or strabismus. The pseudo-internuclear ophthalmoplegia of myasthenia gravis is sometimes associated with depression or down-shoot of the adducting eye.[387] Fatigue, during sustained attempts to hold lateral or upward gaze, is manifest as centripetal drift or increasing fatigue nystagmus (Fig. 9–20A), which may be followed by rebound nystagmus.

Perhaps the earliest and most sensitive signs of extraocular involvement are abnormalities of saccades and quick phases of nystagmus. Examples are shown in Figure 9–20. Large saccades may be hypometric and small saccades may be hypermetric. For large saccades, the eye may start off rapidly, but slow in midflight and creep up to the desired eye position. A characteristic quiver movement consists of an initial, small saccadic movement followed by a rapid drift backward (Fig. 9–20B). The relationship between the peak velocity and amplitude of saccades (the main-sequence relationship) is more variable than that of normal subjects.[62] The duration of saccades is decreased[61] and the velocity of smaller saccades may be increased.[60] During prolonged optokinetic nystagmus, quick phases may become slow. Injection of edrophonium (Tensilon) often reverses extraocular muscle weakness and causes saccades to become hypermetric. Sometimes the patient is not able to hold steady fixation because of repetitive hypermetric saccades that overshoot the target in both directions—macrosaccadic oscillations (see Video Display: Diplopia and Strabismus).

Table 9–10. **Ocular Manifestations of Myasthenia Gravis**

Ptosis
Peek-a-boo sign: prolonged eyelid closure leading to involuntary eye opening
Lid twitch[159]
Gaze-evoked centripetal drift,[648] or nystagmus[253]
Diplopia: due to single or multiple extraocular muscle weaknesses, which may simulate oculomotor, trochlear,[719] abducens,[252] or combined palsies; internuclear ophthalmoplegia;[289,372,668] gaze palsy; one-and-a-half syndrome[48,185,807]
Saccades: hypometria of large saccades, hypermetria of small saccades, quiver movements, and "hyperfast" saccades[161,242,641,745,746,792,798,936,939]
After edrophonium: saccadic hypermetria, macrosaccadic oscillations

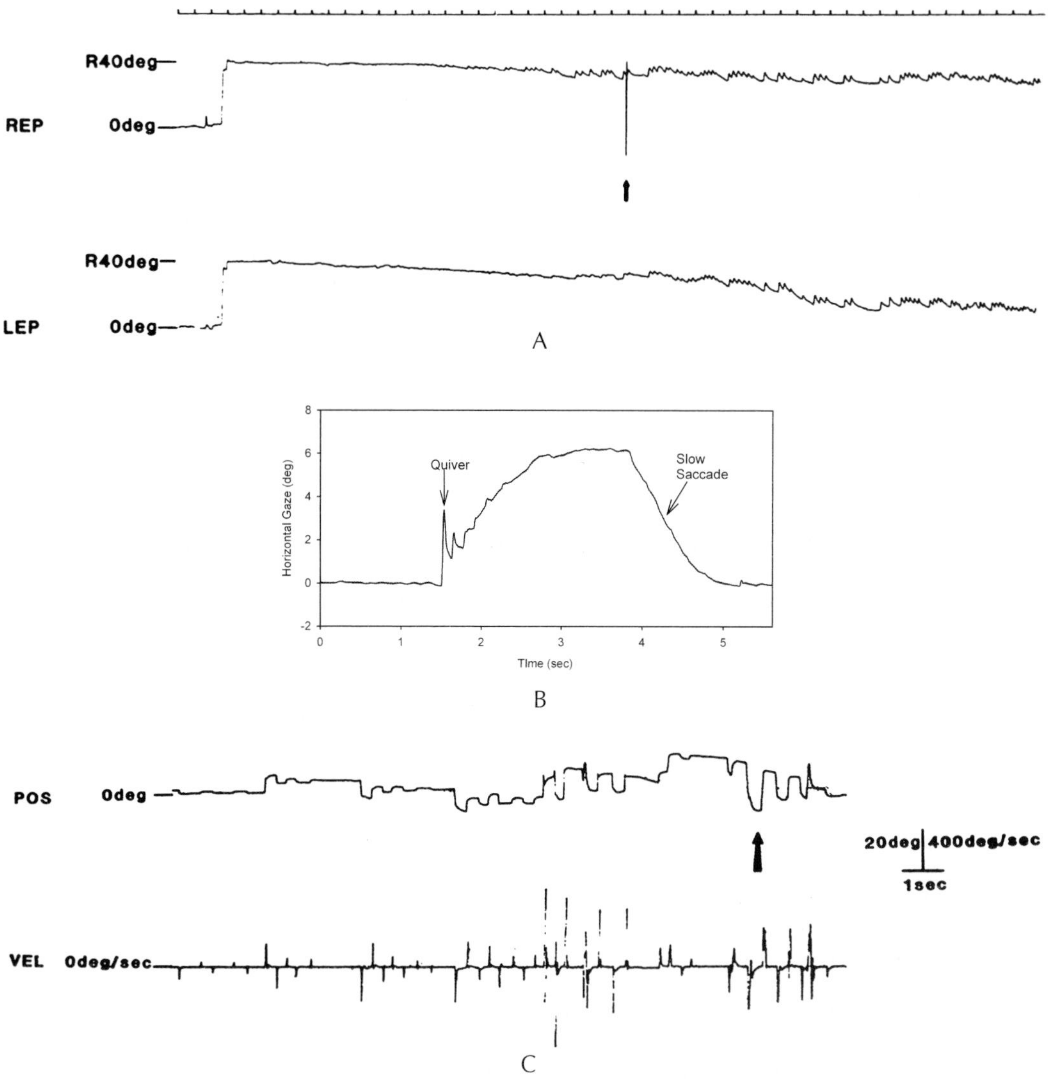

Figure 9–20. Myasthenia gravis. Fatigue of extraocular muscles causing eye movement abnormalities in myasthenia gravis. (A) Development of gaze-evoked nystagmus during attempts to sustain lateral gaze. After about 15 seconds, the patient developed a centripetal drift, more marked in the adducting, left eye, and gaze-evoked nystagmus. (Arrow indicates artifact.) (B) Two quiver movements (see Video Display: Diplopia and Strabismus) and one slow saccade prior to edrophonium. (C) Effects of edrophonium. The patient is asked to make saccades between fixed target lights located at 0 degrees, and 5 degrees to the right and left. However, as the effects of the edrophonium become manifest, he finds this impossible to do and begins to develop oscillations about the target located at 0 degrees (indicated at arrow). These square wave oscillations reflect the increase in saccadic gain due to central adaptive changes and the effects of edrophonium (see Video Display: Diplopia and Strabismus). LEP; left eye position; REP right eye position; POS: position; VEL: velocity.

PATHOPHYSIOLOGY OF OCULAR MOTOR FINDINGS IN MYASTHENIA GRAVIS

Two separate factors account for the various ocular motor findings in myasthenia gravis: failure of neuromuscular transmission and central adaptive mechanisms.

Failure of Neuromuscular Transmission

During repetitive activation of motor nerves, the amount of acetylcholine released at the nerve terminals declines to a plateau value that depends upon the firing frequency. In myasthenia, neuromuscular transmission is tenuous, since the number of functioning postsynaptic acetylcholine receptors is reduced. A small decrease in the amount of released neurotransmitter reduces the probability that an endplate potential will be generated and so predisposes to failure of neuromuscular transmission. Factors that may predispose the extraocular muscles to frequent involvement in myasthenia gravis include their higher discharge rates, differences in complement inhibitor proteins, and the lack of action potentials in the tonic fibers.[404,405] Though failure of neuromuscular transmission affects both global and orbital extraocular muscle fibers, the more constant activity of the latter makes them more susceptible to fatigue.

The fundamental process in myasthenia gravis is probably an autoimmune response against the acetylcholine receptor.[364,882] Thus, over 80% of patients with generalized myasthenia and about 50% with the pure ocular form have anti-acetylcholine–receptor antibodies in their sera. Rarely, antibodies to other components of muscle, such as muscle-specific receptor tyrosine kinase, have been reported in ocular myasthenia (anti-MuSK).[134] It had been suggested that antibodies specifically directed against the fetal form of the acetylcholine receptor, which may be found at synapses on extraocular but not skeletal muscles, may be an important factor that predisposes the extraocular muscles to involvement by myasthenia.[400,403,406] However, myasthenia also affects the levator of the lids, which does not have synaptic fetal acetylcholine receptors.[401] Another factor that might predispose to more severe involvement of the extraocular muscles in myasthenia is the lower level of expression of decay accelerating factor, which is an inhibitor of complement mediated responses.[402,404,684]

Saccades that start off at high velocities but slow in midflight and creep up to the target (Fig. 9–20B) probably reflect intrasaccadic fatigue; muscle fibers are unable to sustain the vigorous muscular contraction required for the duration of the saccadic pulse of innervation. The saccadic step of innervation then carries the eye slowly to its final position. The peak velocity of such saccades may be normal but the duration is prolonged. Early in the disease, subtle changes in the waveform of saccades, best detected in velocity traces, may be noted with a characteristic deceleration that varies from saccade to saccade. Normal subjects only show these changes for large saccades.[5]

Later in the disease, patients with little residual ocular motility may seem to make super-fast saccades within their limited range of motion. The peak velocity of these movements is often greater than would be expected for the size of the saccade.[641] Though central adaptive changes may be partly responsible (see below), this cannot be the whole explanation; adaptive increases in saccadic innervation that occur in other types of muscle palsies do not produce super-fast saccades.[646] A more likely explanation is that the global (predominantly fast-twitch) fibers of the agonist muscle, which are relatively inactive and rested during fixation, can start the saccade with a normal pulse of activity. So tenuous is neuromuscular transmission, however, that fatigue develops rapidly, aborting the pulse. Since the orbital (predominantly tonic) fibers may also become fatigued during the saccade, the eye stops and may even begin to drift backward. When the tonic fibers are completely fatigued, the step is absent. Then the mechanical forces of the orbit pull the eye rapidly back towards the central position, causing a glissade. The combination of the aborted saccade and oppositely directed glissade constitutes the quiver movement (Fig. 9–20B). The presence of such rapid movements in patients with restricted ocular motility should always suggest myasthenia; such movements are absent in patients who have slow or restricted movements due to disease of the central nervous system. Occasionally, a quiver-like movement may be followed by a slow continuation of the saccade; presumably the fatigued pulse is followed, after a brief period of electrical silence, by either a renewed step from tonic fibers or another corrective saccadic pulse (Fig. 9–20B).

The ability to hold the eye steadily after a saccade may be affected by postsaccadic fatigue. Depending upon whether the pulse or step is more affected, the resulting pulse-step mismatch causes onward or backward postsaccadic drift. Often sustained eccentric gaze will bring out nystagmus (Fig. 9–20A), with slow-phase waveforms that follow a linear or negative exponential time course. This has been called fatigue nystagmus, or muscle-paretic nystagmus[746] and probably occurs when the orbital fibers are fatigued. This nystagmus differs from gaze-evoked nystagmus due to cerebellar disease, which often diminishes with sustained effort. The global fibers are relatively spared, since they only discharge vigorously during saccades or quick phases. Occasionally, when nystagmus develops with sustained eccentric gaze, the amplitude (as well as the velocity) is more marked in the abducting eye. This dissociated nystagmus mimics internuclear ophthalmoplegia.[807]

Adaptation and the Effects of Edrophonium in Myasthenia Gravis

Not all features of myasthenic eye movements can be ascribed to neuromuscular block. As discussed in Chapter 3, the brain monitors the accuracy of saccades and makes adaptive changes of innervation to optimize ocular motor performance. When myasthenia causes paretic saccades, central adaptation is stimulated if the patient habitually views with the paretic eye. These mechanisms can be applied to the pulse-step pattern of innervation that normally produces fast, accurate saccades. Large saccades often fall short of the target; they are hypometric. Smaller saccades, however, made around the central position, are often orthometric or even overshoot the target. Why should saccades become hypermetric in myasthenia gravis? The answer is apparent from the observation of the effects of edrophonium (Tensilon). During the edrophonium test, saccade size increases. Many saccades become too large, and occasionally an extreme degree of hypermetria produces continuous, to-and-fro saccadic movements about the target known as macrosaccadic oscillations (Fig. 9–20C) (see Video Display: Diplopia and Strabismus). Saccade hypermetria occurs because the central nervous system has adaptively increased the size of the saccadic pulse in an attempt to overcome the myasthenic weakness. The central changes are revealed by edrophonium, which transiently removes the peripheral neuromuscular blockade, exposing the increased saccadic innervation. If the brain had been standing idly by, edrophonium would merely have caused refixations to become orthometric.

EYE MOVEMENTS AND THE DIAGNOSIS OF MYASTHENIA GRAVLS

When ocular motility is minimally affected, careful study of eye movements—preferably measurements of saccades—before and during the edrophonium (Tensilon) test or the neostigmine test may be particularly useful.[57] Before edrophonium, an early finding is variability of saccadic trajectory and main-sequence relationships.[62] Edrophonium is best given in small (0.2-mg) increments to avoid missing a positive response owing to cholinergic excess. Neostigmine (0.5 mg, given intramuscularly with atropine, 0.5 mg) is also useful, because it allows more time to make both clinical observations and quantitative measurements. It is important to examine and record at 15- to 20-minute intervals for about 45 minutes to look for a positive response, which includes changes in saccadic accuracy and especially the production of hypermetria. Such effects are probably diagnostic of myasthenia gravis. The duration of saccades, especially larger movements, tends to shorten.[60] The velocity, especially of larger saccades, tends to increase.[60] In contrast, normal subjects or patients with ocular motor palsies show increased duration and slowing of saccades after edrophonium.[60,61] These changes in normal subjects and in patients with non-myasthenic strabismus illustrate the dangers in not measuring the nature of the changes produced by edrophonium. Furthermore, some non-myasthenic ocular deviations get worse after edrophonium, if one muscle is more susceptible to the effects of the drug than the others. In particular, subjective tests such as the red glass, Maddox rod, or Lancaster red-green test must be interpreted cautiously, as they may give misleading results. Only the direct observation of a weak muscle becoming stronger after edrophonium is reliable evidence of myasthenia.[179] Even then, the diagnosis depends on the full clinical picture; false-positive test results have been reported with central structural lesions, and myasthenia can coexist with intracranial lesions.[209,586] If the Tensilon test is negative, the longer-acting agent, neostigmine (given with atropine), may help make the diagnosis by providing the examiner with more time to detect a change in ocular alignment or saccade metrics, although its rate of absorption after intramuscular injection varies.

In patients with purely ocular manifestations, single-fiber EMG of the superior rectus and levator muscles may contribute to the diagnosis by showing jitter,[707] but are difficult to administer. Single-fiber EMG of the orbicularis oculi is currently the most sensitive test for ocular myasthenia and, coupled with standard EMG, usually distinguishes myasthenia from other disorders such as mitochondrial myopathy or oculopharyngeal dystrophy.

Late in the course of myasthenia gravis, all ocular motility may become restricted and the patient may be refractory to edrophonium or neostigmine testing. Imaging studies show atrophied extraocular muscles.[639] If a clear history is unavailable, differentiation from the syndrome of chronic progressive external ophthalmoplegia may be difficult.

TREATMENT OF OCULAR MYASTHENIA

Anticholinesterase drugs, such as pyridostigmine are often used as first-line therapy for ocular myasthenia,[687] although they may be less effective for the treatment of diplopia and ptosis than for other symptoms.[238] Because of the variability of ocular deviations, prisms are not usually helpful and surgery is only considered if there is troublesome diplopia in patients who are otherwise in remission.[636] Most patients who present with ocular myasthenia will generalize within a two-year period; in retrospective studies, oral prednisone has been shown to reduce the rate of generalization.[478] Treatment with a short course of prednisone and long-term azathioprine is reported to reduce the risk and severity of generalized symptoms and to promote remission of the disease.[479a,794] Thymectomy, prompted by abnormal appearances on chest CT, is reported to provide no advantage over medical treatment for ocular symptoms.[59,794] Simple measures such as dark glasses to reduce the discomfort of diplopia, prisms to correct for stable ocular deviations, and "lid-crutches" for ptosis are often appreciated by selected patients.[793] Occasional patients benefit from surgery to correct strabismus.[591]

CHRONIC PROGRESSIVE EXTERNAL OPHTHALMOPLEGIA AND RESTRICTIVE OPHTHALMOPATHIES

The syndrome of chronic progressive external ophthalmoplegia (CPEO), characterized by progressive limitation of eye movements and ptosis, but usually without diplopia, occurs in many disease states (Table 9–11). In most patients the orbicularis oculi is also involved, but the pupils are spared. Saccades in CPEO are characteristically slow throughout the remaining range of movement, unlike those in myasthenia, in which initial saccadic velocity is often normal. Depending on the etiology, MR imaging of the orbit may show small extraocular muscles.[135]

The peculiar histological features of the extraocular muscles and their unusual responses to disease have complicated attempts to identify separate disease entities (see section on Struc-

Table 9–11. **Differential Diagnosis of Chronic Progressive Ophthalmoplegia**

Oculopharyngeal dystrophy[675]
Autosomal recessive myopathy with external ophthalmoplegia[526]
Disorders of Mitochondrial DNA: Kearns-Sayre syndrome, MELAS*, MERRF†[552]
Myotonic dystrophy[22,878]
Congenital myopathies[291]
Congenital fibrosis of the extraocular muscles and genetic disorders of cranial nerve nucleus development (see Table 9-13)[230]
Progressive brainstem disorders (e.g., progressive supranuclear palsy)
Bassen-Kornzweig syndrome (abetalipoproteinemia)[935]
Endocrine ophthalmoparesis (ophthalmic Graves' disease)[837]
Orbital pseudotumor[284]
Myasthenia gravis[59]

*MELAS, mitochondrial encephalopathy, lactic acidosis, and stroke.
†MERRF, myoclonic epilepsy and ragged red fibers.

ture and Function of Extraocular Muscle). Because of this difficulty in reliably discerning distinct nosologic entities, the term ophthalmoplegia plus has been used to describe CPEO accompanied by a variety of other findings.[219] However, modern genetic techniques have defined distinct defects of nuclear or mitochondrial DNA in a growing number of these disorders.[475,552]

Involvement of the Extraocular Muscles in Muscular Dystrophies

DUCHENNE'S DYSTROPHY

Duchenne's and Becker's dystrophies, which are due to allelic abnormalities of genetic expression of the protein dystrophin, lead to severe weakness of the limbs and trunk but, remarkably, spare the extraocular muscles in most patients. Thus, for example, patients with advanced disease may have normal-velocity saccades,[399] except for larger movements.[527] One patient with Becker's dystrophy and saccadic slowing is described.[739] Immunohistochemical studies have confirmed that the extraocular muscles are preserved,[435] which led to the speculation that they are better able to manage the massive calcium influx that accompanies the dystrophin defect.[678,685] Other hypotheses are that the extraocular muscles may be protected by endogenous upregulation of a dystrophin analog, utrophin,[686] or the presence of additional laminin isoforms in the basement membranes of the extrasynaptic sarcolemmal of extraocular versus limb muscle.[441] Eye movements are also reported to be normal in patients with fascioscapulohumeral dystrophy.[877]

MYOTONIC DYSTROPHY

Myotonic dystrophy, an autosomal dominant condition due to trinucleotide repeats, has widespread manifestations including ptosis and defects in ocular motility that are usually mild, but occasionally conform to the syndrome of CPEO.[506] Saccades may be slow, hypometric, and made at increased latency.[22,448,835] Both smooth pursuit and suppression of the vestibulo-ocular reflex during eye-head tracking are impaired, but the vestibulo-ocular reflex is normal.[22] There is debate as to whether these defects in eye movements can be ascribed to central involvement by the disease process or involvement of the extraocular muscles by the myotonic process. Impaired suppression of the vestibulo- ocular reflex suggests central involvement.[22] However, there is also some evidence for myotonia directly affecting the extraocular muscles. Thus, the saccadic velocity profile may be influenced by the length of the prior fixation (myotonic effect).[878] Moreover, if repetitive saccades are tested after a rest period, their amplitude and peak velocity progressively increase ("warm-up" effect).[325,878]

OCULOPHARYNGEAL DYSTROPHY

Autosomal dominant oculopharyngeal dystrophy has been described in several ethnic groups,[82,614,675,879,915] with linkage on chromosome 14q. The symptoms usually begin after age 40 years, and consist of ptosis, limitation and slowing of saccadic eye movements, weakness of the facial and proximal limb muscles, and dysphagia. Pharyngeal symptoms are most prominent and bulbar dysfunction may lead to the death of the patient. Surgical treatment (cricopharyngeal myotomy) is reported to help.[212] Ptosis is generally more prominent than restricted ocular motility. Weakness of neck or limb muscles may develop but is usually mild. Biopsy of limb muscles has shown characteristic red-rimmed vacuoles and nuclear inclusions.[82,212 846] The onset of symptoms is earlier, and the findings are more severe, in patients who are homozygous for the disorder.[82]

AUTOSOMAL RECESSIVE MYOPATHY WITH EXTERNAL OPTHALMOPLEGIA

This recently described disorder affected eight highly inbred Arab families in Israel.[526] Mean age of diagnosis was 27 years, but onset was almost certainly earlier, probably in childhood or the early teen years. A detailed description of the disturbance of eye movements was provided by Lea Averbuch-Heller and her colleagues. The findings were fairly stereotyped. Ocular alignment was normal and none complained of diplopia. Eye movements were limited, especially upgaze. Saccades were slow. Pursuit was smooth and cancellation of the vestibulo-ocular reflex (eye-head tracking) was preserved within the remaining range of movement. Convergence was impaired. Rapid head rotations did not induce rapid eye movements or increase the range of movement. Patients often employed head movements to voluntarily shift gaze shifts. Forced duction testing showed no resistance to passive movement. There was no ptosis or pupillary abnormality. In addition there was symmetric involvement of face (including orbicularis oculi) and neck muscles (especially flexors), giving the appearance of a long thin face. Speech was nasal but there was no dysphagia. Limb weakness was mild, proximal, and greater in the arms; reflexes were preserved. Scapular winging and scoliosis was present in more severely affected individuals. Orbital MRI scans showed atrophy of extraocular muscles with fatty replacement, especially the superior rectus. Myosin immunohistochemistry of limb muscles showed marked type 1 muscle fiber predominance with core-like formations. Linkage studies identified markers on chromosome 17p13.1-p12, an interval to which several genes for sarcomeric heavy chain map. It is possible that this syndrome is related to other type 1 fiber myopathies, central core myopathy, or other disorders of myosin heavy chains that occur in both extraocular and limb muscles.[442]

CONGENITAL MYOPATHIES

This is a rare and heterogeneous group of disorders,[705] which is undergoing re-evaluation as a result of the genetic revolution.[291] It includes myotubular myopathy (or centronuclear myopathy), which is characterized by ptosis, progressive limitation of ocular motility, and weakness of facial muscles, neck flexors, and the limbs.[85,388,806] Limb muscle biopsy shows small type-1 fibers and the presence of central nuclei.[706] Extraocular muscles in this condition also have central nuclei, and type 1 fiber predominance.[388,706] Nemaline myopathy also may rarely present with ptosis and limitation of eye movements.[931] Ptosis and impaired range of eye movements may also be present in patients with central core myopathy and multicore disease.[85,475]

Kearns-Sayre Syndrome and Disorders of Mitochondrial DNA

It has been established that one cause of chronic progressive ophthalmoplegia, the Kearns-Sayre syndrome,[181,426] is due, in most cases, to deletions or duplications of mitochondrial DNA.[104,266,436,552,587,773,834,912] A sporadic single deletion at base pair 4977 is the commonest cause of CPEO.[552] Rare cases are reported in which there appears to be a defect of communication between nuclear and mitochondrial genomes.[137,774] Mitochondrial DNA mutations appear to be more common in tissues with higher oxidative metabolism, and this is true of the extraocular muscles.[944]

This multisystem disorder is characterized by progressive ophthalmoparesis beginning in childhood or adolescence, atypical pigmentary degeneration of the retina, and heart block. Contrary to prior reports, some patients complain of diplopia and many have exotropia.[703] Both the cardiac and endocrine complications of Kearns-Sayre syndrome may be life threatening. The associated abnormalities are summarized in Table 9–12. Ultrastuctural analysis

Table 9–12. **Features of the Kearns-Sayre Syndrome**[68,181,205,274,309,356,426]

Chronic progressive ophthalmoplegia*
Retinal pigmentary deposition
Heart block*
Small stature
Hearing loss (vestibular disturbance)
Cerebellar ataxia
Pendular nystagmus
Corticospinal tract signs
Impaired intellect
Cranial muscle weakness (face, palate, neck)
Peripheral neuropathy
"Myopathy" affecting skeletal muscles (ragged-red fibers)
Corneal clouding
Scrotal tongue
Spinal fluid abnormalities (elevated protein)
Basal ganglion calcification
Slowed electroencephalogram
Endocrine abnormalities (hypoparathyroidism; diabetes; hypogonadism)
Elevated serum glutamic oxaloacetic transaminase, creatinine phosphokinase, lactic dehydrogenase, altered lactate-pyruvate metabolism

*For diagnosis of Kearns-Sayre syndrome, these features should be present before 20 years of age.

of extraocular muscle from one patient with a mitochondrial DNA deletion and complete bilateral ptosis and non-restrictive exotropia showed a selective vacuolization of some muscle fibers, with abnormal mitochondria.[138]

Some patients show clinical features that overlap Kearns-Sayre syndrome and other mitochondrially inherited disorders, including MELAS (mitochondrial encephalopathy, lactic acidosis, and stroke), and MERRF (myoclonic epilepsy and ragged red fibers).[143] An uneven distribution of deletions of mitochondrial DNA in different tissues may account for the different phenotypic expressions. Pathologically, both limb and extraocular muscles often show ragged-red fibers with trichrome stains; this appearance is due to increased numbers of abnormal sarcolemmal mitochondria. Limb muscle also shows a mosaic of cytochrome c oxidase (COX) deficient fibers and mitochondrial DNA deletions or point mutations. The brain shows a spongy degeneration that results in cerebral and cerebellar atrophy.[104,181,930] Therapy with vitamins and agents such as Coenzyme Q10 aims to improve respiratory chain activity,[100] but their clinically efficacy is unproven.[552]

Thyroid Ophthalmopathy

Thyroid disease is an important cause of restrictive ophthalmopathy.[55,379] Orbital abnormalities encountered in patients with thyroid disorders include chemosis, periorbital congestion, lid retraction and lid lag, proptosis (exophthalmos), ophthalmoparesis, and optic neuropathy.[55,56] Exophthalmos and periorbital edema usually precede the development of impaired ocular motility, though diplopia may be the first symptom. Patients with thyroid ophthalmopathy often complain of diplopia, unlike most forms of CPEO. In contrast to myasthenia, symptoms are usually worse in the morning. Lid retraction and lid lag on downward gaze are common signs.

The most common abnormalities of eye movements are impaired elevation, and extorsion of the abducted eye. Abduction and downward movements may also be impaired. These deficits reflect preferential involvement of the inferior rectus, followed in order by the medial rectus, superior rectus, lateral rectus and superior oblique.[837] The limitation of movement reflects a restrictive ophthalmopathy, which can usually be confirmed by the forced duction test. The velocity and amplitude of saccadic eye movements is reduced in some patients,[929] and the development of these abnormalities may correlate with progression of orbital disease.[244,545]

The primary process underlying Graves' ophthalmopathy appears to be due to an immune attack on orbital fibroblasts,[39] which share common epitopes with thyroid.[402] Patients with Graves' disease who show ophthalmic involvement tend to show different autoantibody profiles, with higher thyroid-stimulating immunoglobulin.[292] Enlargement of the extraocular muscles in Graves' disease (Fig. 9–21) is due to abnormal accumulation of glycosaminoglycans in the connective tissue of the endomysium and in the orbital fat. The ligament of Lockwood, to which the inferior rectus and inferior oblique muscles are attached, is involved by the inflammatory changes, and contributes to impaired upward movements. The disturbances of eye movements in Graves' disease have been partly ascribed to the effects of increased tissue volume within the orbit.[245]

In many patients with thyroid ophthalmopathy, symptoms and signs are minimal and diagnosis may sometimes be difficult.[797] As many as 20% of patients are euthyroid. In this group, a thyrotropin releasing hormone (TRH) stimulation test or antibody studies (antithyroglobulin and antimicrosomal antibodies) may help confirm the diagnosis. Also of great value is orbital imaging and ultrasound, which can provide evidence of extraocular muscle enlargement (Fig. 9–21) and provide a reliable index of the presence and progression of disease.[320,904] In patients with small tropias due to thyroid ophthalmopathy, prisms may alleviate diplopia. Periocular injection of triamcinolone is reported to be effective for treatment of diplopia in ophthalmic Graves' disease of recent onset without side effects.[222] Surgery that is performed to decompress the orbit when vision is threatened may exacerbate ocular misalignment.[6] Operative treatment to realign the eyes is best attempted during the quiescent phase of the disease, although it may be successful in selected patients during the acute period.[157] With chronic tropias, surgical recessions may be successful in restoring single, binocular vision in primary and reading

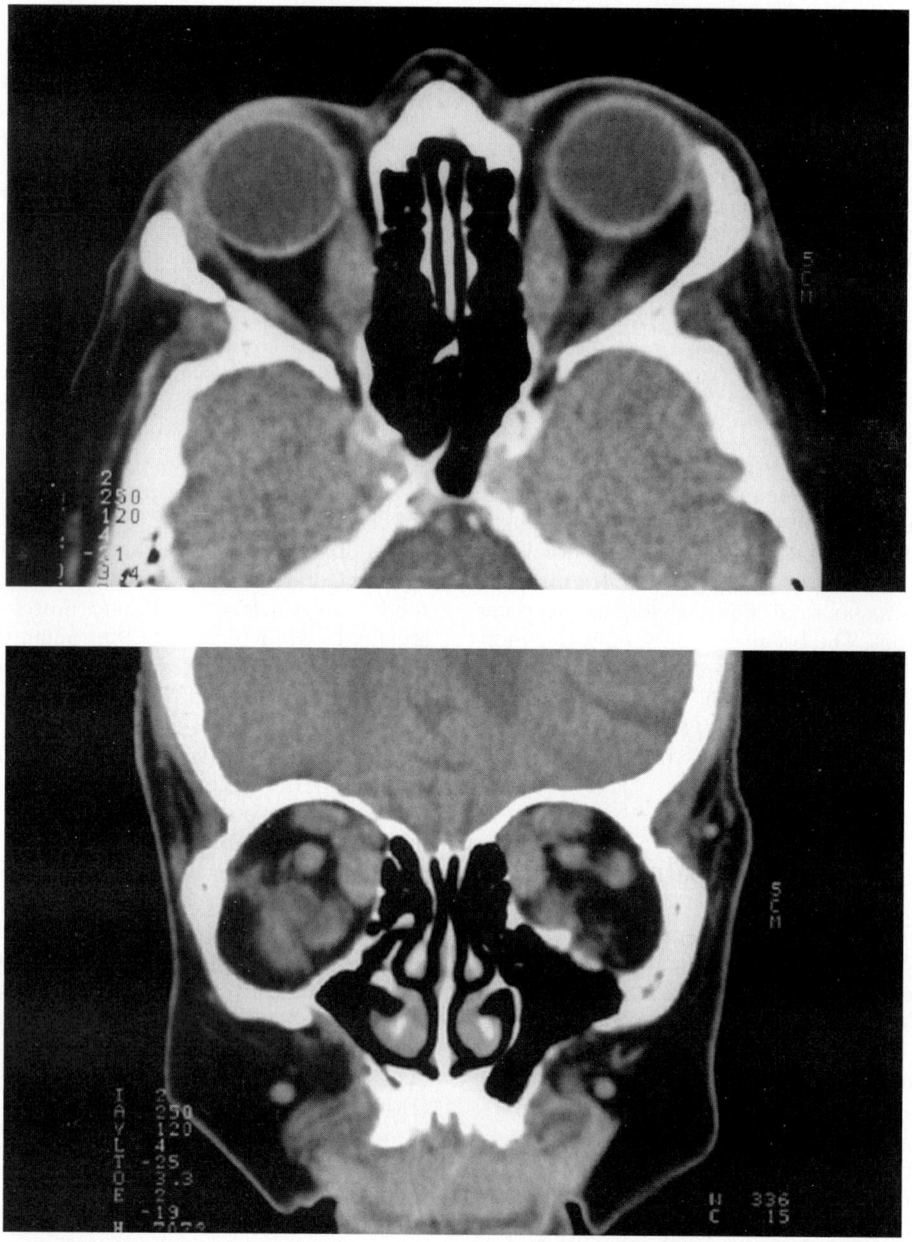

Figure 9–21. CT of the orbits showing enlarged extraocular muscles in a 76-year-old woman with Graves ophthalmopathy and myasthenia gravis, a reported association.[482] On examination she had bilateral ptosis, worse on the left. Horizontal range of motion was moderately restricted, and forced duction tests of the right eye indicated restriction of the inferior rectus. (Courtesy Dr. Henry J. Kaminski.)

positions,[257,889] but a normal, conjugate range of eye movements is achieved less often. Radiotherapy to the orbit in Graves' disease has been reported to have little therapeutic effect,[298,299] but is still used in selected patients.

Restrictive Ophthalmopathy and Congenital Fibrosis of the Extraocular Muscles

A variety of other conditions are reported to restrict eye movements. In some, extraocular muscles appear enlarged on computed tomography; these include metastatic tumor deposits,[133,144,206,241,261,335,347] amyloid,[352] sarcoid,[168] parasites,[408] carotid-cavernous fistula (see above), orbital myositis, and orbital pseudotumor.[284,583,898] Some patients with giant-cell arteritis or Wegener's granulomatosis develop nearly complete ophthalmoplegia due to muscle ischemia.[210 670]

Congenital Disorders of Eye Movements Attributable to Failure of Neurological Embryogenesis

Progress in genetics has provided insights into a number of congenital diseases affecting ocular motility (see Table 9–13). Thus, it has been possible to identify several distinct disorders that had previously been lumped under the term *congenital fibrosis of the extraocular muscles* (CFEOM). At least some of these have been shown to be due to failure of embryogenesis of ocular motor subnuclei supplying specific muscles, or tracts connecting them,[227,228] and some patients show aberrant regeneration of cranial nerves.[302]

Thus, CFEOM1 results from maldevelopment of the superior division of the oculomotor nerve and the motoneurons, which normally supply axons to the levator palpebrae superioris and superior rectus; these findings have been confirmed at autopsy.[229] This analysis revealed absence of the superior division of the oculomotor nerves and the corresponding motoneurons, and atrophy of the levator and superior rectus muscles, which contained connective tissue and fat. Magnetic resonance imaging can identify similar deficits in affected individuals.[198] Consequently, there is bilateral ptosis and the eyes are deviated down. Strabismus is the rule, but diplopia is usually absent due to the ability to suppress images from either eye. Associated defects, including mild facial diplegia, may be present. Affected family members show a chin-up head posture, with ptosis and the eyes fixed in down gaze. Eye movements are limited, especially vertically, with substitution of vergence for versional movements, convergence on upgaze, and the appearance of pendular nystagmus and ocular retraction during attempted gaze shifts. Those patients with the severest limitation may completely substitute head movements for eye movements.[286] CFEOM1 maps to the centromere of chromosome 12.[231]

Table 9–13. **Genetic Disorders of Cranial Nucleus Development Causing Abnormal Eye Movements**

Cranial Nerve Nucleus	Syndrome Name*	Gene/Chromosome	Major Clinical Features
Oculomotor (CNIII)	CFEOM1	FEOM1/12cen	Bilateral or unilateral ptosis; eyes deviated down; chin-up posture; ptosis
Oculomotor (CNIII)	CFEOM3	FEOM3/16qter	Eyes deviated down and out; bilateral or unilateral ptosis
Oculomotor (CNIII)	Congenital Ptosis	PTOSIS1/1p34-p32 PTOSIS2/Xq24-q27.1	Bilateral ptosis
Oculomotor (CNIII) and Trochlear (CNIV)	CFEOM2	FEOM2, ARIX/11q13	Bilateral ptosis, with eyes fixed in extreme abduction
Abducens (CNVI)	Duane syndrome	DURS1/8q13 DUR2/2q31 HOXA1/7p15.2	Retraction of eye on adduction with limitation of either abduction (type1), adduction (type2), or both (type 3; HOXA1 syndrome)[842a]
Abducens (CNVI)+	Horizontal gaze palsy with scoliosis	ROBO3/11q23	Absent conjugate horizontal gaze; preservation of vergence and some vertical movements

*CFEOM: Congenital fibrosis of the extraocular muscles. Adapted from Engle and Leigh.[230]

CFEOM2 is characterized from birth by bilateral ptosis, with the eyes fixed in extreme abduction, and is caused by an autosomal recessive defect that maps to the CFEOM2 locus on chromosome 11q13.[609,900] CFEOM3 causes maldevelopment of all muscles supplied by the oculomotor nerve, and maps to chromosome 16q24; the phenotypic features are variable, but the eyes of severely affected individuals are deviated down and out.[213] Failure of development of individual muscles is also reported.[428]

What remains unexplained about such patients is the absence of aberrant innervation to the superior rectus and levator palpebrae superioris from the intact abducens nucleus, unlike the situation in Duane syndrome, in which the lateral rectus gains some innervation from the oculomotor nerve. Development of genetic models for this group of disorders is likely to clarify how the normal embryology of the extraocular muscles can go awry.[230,679,680]

REFERENCES

1. Aaberg TM Jr., Kay M, Sternau L. Metastatic tumors to the pituitary. Am J Ophthalmol 119, 779–785, 1995.
2. Abad JM, Alvarez F, Blazquez MG. An unrecognized neurological syndrome: sixth-nerve palsy and Horner's syndrome due to traumatic intracavernous carotid aneurysm. Surg Neurol 16, 140–144, 1981.
3. Abdul-Rahim AS, Savino PJ, Zimmerman RA, Sergott RC, Bosley, TM. Cryptogenic oculomotor nerve palsy. The need for repeated neuroimaging studies. Arch Ophthalmol 107, 387–390, 1989.
4. Abel LA, Schmidt D, Dell'Osso LF, Daroff RB. Saccadic system plasticity in humans. Ann Neurol 4, 313–318, 1978.
5. Abel LA, Traccis S, Troost BT, Dell'Osso LF. Saccadic trajectories change with amplitude, not time. Neuro-ophthalmology 7, 309–314, 1987.
6. Abramoff MD, Kalmann R, de Graaf ME, Stilma JS, Mourits MP. Rectus extraocular muscle paths and decompression surgery for Graves orbitopathy: mechanism of motility disturbances. Invest Ophthalmol Vis Sci 43, 300–307, 2002.
7. Acharya R, Husain S, Chhabra SS, et al. Sixth nerve schwannoma: a case report with literature review. Neurol Sci 24, 74–79, 2003.
8. Acheson JF, Bentley CR, Shallo-Hoffmann J, Gresty MA. Dissociated effects of botulinum toxin chemodenervation on ocular deviation and saccade dynamics in chronic lateral rectus palsy. Br J Ophthalmol 82, 67–71, 1998.
9. Acierno MD, Trobe JD, Cornblath WT, Gebarski SS. Painful oculomotor palsy caused by posterior-draining dural carotid cavernous fistulas. Ann Ophthalmol 113, 1045–1049, 1995.
10. Ada M, Kaytaz A, Tuskan K, Guvenc MG, Selcuk H. Isolated sphenoid sinusitis presenting with unilateral VIth nerve palsy. Int J Pediatr Otorhinolaryngol 68, 507–510, 2004.
11. Adler DE, Milhorat TH. The tentorial notch: anatomical variation, morphometric analysis, and classification in 100 human autopsy cases. J Neurosurg 96, 1103–1112, 2002.
12. Aeumjaturapat S, Wadwongtham W. Sphenoid sinus mucocele presenting with isolated oculomotor nerve palsy. J Med Assoc Thai 84, 1340–1343, 2001.
13. Agostinis C, Caverni L, Moschini L, Rottoli MR, Foresti C. Paralysis of the fourth cranial nerve due to superior cerebellar artery aneurysm. Neurology 42, 457–458, 1992.
14. Ajtai B, Fine EJ, Lincoff N. Pupil-sparing painless compression of the oculomotor nerve by expanding basilar artery aneurysm: a case of ocular pseudomyasthenia. Arch Neurol 61, 1448–1450, 2004.
15. Akdal G, Kutluk K, Men S, Yaka E. Benedikt and "plus-minus lid" syndromes arising from posterior cerebral artery branch occlusion. J Neurol Sci 228, 105–107, 2005.
16. Al-Din ASN, Anderson M, Bickerstaff ER, Harvey I. Brainstem encephalitis and the syndrome of Miller Fisher. Brain 105, 481–495, 1982.
17. Al-Din SN, Anderson M, Eeg-Olofsson O, Trontelj JV. Neuro-ophthalmic manifestations of the syndrome of ophthalmoplegia, ataxia and areflexia: a review. Acta Neurol Scandinav 89, 157–163, 1994.
18. Aldrich MS, Beck RW, Albers JW. Familial recurrent Bell's palsy with ocular motor palsies. Neurology 37, 1369–1371, 1987.
19. Alkan A, Sigirci A, Ozveren MF, et al. The cisternal segment of the abducens nerve in man: three-dimensional MR imaging. Eur J Radiol 51, 218–222, 2004.
20. Allin F, Velay JL, Bouquerel A. Shift in saccadic direction induced in humans by proprioceptive manipulation: a comparison between memory-guided and visually guided saccades. Exp Brain Res 110, 473–481, 1996.
21. Ambrose PS, von Noorden GK. Past pointing in comitant strabismus. Arch Ophthalmol 94, 1896–1898, 1976.
22. Anastasopoulos D, Kimmig H, Mergner T, Psilas K. Abnormalities of ocular motility in myotonic dystrophy. Brain 119, 1923–1932, 1996.
23. Ang CW, Laman JD, Willison HA, et al. Structure of Campylobacter jejuni lipopolysaccharides determines antiganglioside specificity and clinical features of Guillain-Barre and Miller Fisher patients. Infect Immun 70, 1202–1208, 2002.
24. Angelaki DE, Hess BJM. Control of eye orientation: where does the brain's role end and the muscle's begin? Eur J Neurosci 19, 1–10, 2004.
25. Antoniades K, Karakasis D, Taskos N. Abducent nerve palsy following transverse fracture of the middle cranial fossa. J Cranio-Maxillo-Facial Surg 21, 172–175, 1993.
26. Antworth MV, Beck RW. Third nerve palsy as a presenting sign of acquired immune deficiency syndrome. J Clin Neuro-Ophthalmol 7, 125–128, 1987.
27. Appukuttan B, Gillanders E, Juo SH, et al. Localization of a gene for Duane retraction syndrome to

chromosome 2q31. Am J Hum Genet 65, 1639–1646, 1999.
28. Apte RS, Bartek W, Mello A, Haq A Spontaneous intracranial hypotension. Am J Ophthalmol 127, 482–485, 1999.
29. Archambault P, Wise JS, Rosen J, Polomeno RS, Auger N. Herpes zoster ophthalmoplegia. Report of six cases. J Clin Neuro-Ophthalmol 8, 185–191, 1988.
30. Arruga J, DeRivas P, Espinet HL, Conesa G. Chronic isolated trochlear nerve palsy produced by intracavernous internal carotid artery aneurysm. J Clin Neuro-Ophthalmol 11, 104–108, 1991.
31. Asbury AK. New concepts of Guillain-Barre syndrome. J Child Neurol 15, 183–191, 2000.
32. Asbury AK, Aldredge H, Hershberg R, Fisher CM. Oculomotor palsy in diabetes mellitus: a clinicopathological study. Brain 93, 555–566, 1970.
33. Ashworth B, Gordon A. Ophthalmoplegia due to chondrosarcoma in the cavernous sinus. Neuro-ophthalmology 6, 145–151, 1986.
34. Astle WF, Rosenbaum AL. Familial congenital fourth cranial nerve palsy. Arch Ophthalmol 103, 532–535, 1985.
35. Averbuch-Heller L, Daroff RB. Headache. In Goadsby PJ, Silberstein SD (eds). Blue Books of Practical Neurology. Volume 17. Butterworth-Heinemann, London, 1997, pp 285–297.
36. Averbuch-Heller L, Helmchen C, Horn AKE, Leigh RJ, Büttner-Ennever JA. Slow vertical saccades in amyotrophic lateral sclerosis: correlation of structure and function. Ann Neurol, 44, 641–648, 1998.
37. Averbuch-Heller L, Poonyathalang A, von Maydell RD, Remler BF. Hering's law for eyelids: still valid. Neurology 45, 1781–1782, 1995.
38. Averbuch-Heller L, von Maydell RD, Poonyathalang A, Kori AA, Remler BF. 'Inverse Argyll Robertson pupil' in botulism: late central manifestation. Neuro-Ophthalmolgy 16, 351–354, 1996.
39. Bahn RS, Heufelder AE. Pathogenesis of Graves' ophthalmopathy. N Engl J Med 329, 1468–1475, 1993.
40. Bailey TD, O'Connor PS, Tredici TJ, Shacklett DE. Ophthalmoplegic migraine. J Clin Neuro-Ophthalmol 4, 225–228, 1984.
41. Bain PG, Larkin GBR, Calver DM, O'Brien MD. Persistent superior oblique paresis as a manifestation of familial periodic cerebellar ataxia. Br J Ophthalmol 75, 619–621, 1991.
42. Baker RS, Conklin JD. Acquired Brown's syndrome from blunt orbital trauma. J Pediatr Ophthalmol Strabismus 24, 17–21, 1987.
43. Balcer LJ, Galetta SL, Bagley LJ, Pakola SJ. Localization of traumatic oculomotor nerve palsy to the midbrain exit site by magnetic resonance imaging. Am J Ophthalmol 122, 437–439, 1996.
44. Balcer LJ, Galetta SL, Yousem DM, Golden MA, Asbury AK. Pupil-involving third-nerve palsy and carotid stenosis: rapid recovery following endarterectomy. Ann Neurol 41, 273–276, 1997.
45. Balcer LJ, Winterkorn JMS, Galetta SL. Neuro-ophthalmic manifestations of Lyme disease. J Neuro-Ophthalmology 17, 108–121, 1997.
46. Baldwin L, Baker RS. Acquired Brown's syndrome in a patient with an orbital roof fracture. J Clin Neuro-Ophthalmol 8, 127–130, 1988.
47. Balkan R, Hoyt CS. Associated neurological abnormalities in congenital third nerve palsies. Am J Ophthalmol 97, 319, 1984.
48. Bandini F, Faga D, Simonetti S. Ocular myasthenia mimicking a one-and-a-half syndrome. J Neuro-Ophthalmol 21, 210–211, 2001.
49. Barontini F, Maurri S, Marrapodi E. Tolosa-Hunt syndrome versus recurrent cranial neuropathy. Report of two cases with prolonged follow-up. J Neurol 234, 112–115, 1987.
50. Barr D, Kupersmith MJ, Pinto R, Turbin R. Arachnoid cyst of the cavernous sinus resulting in third nerve palsy. J Neuro-Ophthalmol 19, 249–251, 1999.
51. Barr D, Kupersmith MJ, Turbin R, Bose S, Roth R. Isolated sixth nerve palsy: an uncommon presenting sign of multiple sclerosis. J Neurol 247, 701–704, 2000.
52. Barr DB, McFadzean RM, Hadley D, et al. Acquired bilateral superior oblique palsy: a localising sign in the dorsal midbrain. Eur J Ophthalmol 7, 271–276, 1997.
53. Barroso L, Hoyt WF. Episodic exotropia from lateral rectus neuromyotonia—appearance and remission after radiation therapy for a thalamic glioma. J Ped Ophthalmol Strabismus 30, 56–57, 1993.
54. Bartleson JD, Trautmann JC, Sundt TM, Jr. Minimal oculomotor nerve paresis secondary to unruptured intracranial aneurysm. Arch Neurol 43, 1015–1020, 1986.
55. Bartley GB. The epidemiologic characteristics and clinical course of ophthalmopathy associated with autoimmune thyroid disease in Olmsted County Minnesota. Trans Am Ophthalmol Soc 92, 477–458, 1994.
56. Bartley GB, Fatourechi V, Kadrmas EF, et al. Clinical features of Graves' ophthalmopathy in an incidence cohort. Am J Ophthalmol 121, 284–290, 1996.
57. Barton JJ. Quantitative ocular tests for myasthenia gravis: a comparative review with detection theory analysis. J Neurol Sci 155, 104–114, 1998.
58. Barton JJ. "Retinal diplopia" associated with macular wrinkling. Neurology 63, 925–927, 2004.
59. Barton JJ, Fouladvand M. Ocular aspects of myasthenia gravis. Semin Neurol 20, 7–20, 2000.
60. Barton JJS, Huaman AG, Sharpe JA. Effects of edrophonium on saccadic velocity in normal subjects and myasthenic and nonmyasthenic ocular palsies. Ann Neurol 36, 585–594, 1994.
61. Barton JJS, Jama A, Sharpe JA. Saccadic duration and intrasaccadic fatigue in myasthenic and non-myasthenic ocular palsies. Neurology 45, 2065–2072, 1995.
62. Barton JJS, Sharpe JA. "Saccadic jitter" is a quantitative ocular sign in myasthenia gravis. Invest Ophthalmol Vis Sci 36, 1566–1572, 1995.
63. Batocchi AP, Evoli A, Majolini L, et al. Ocular palsies in the absence of other neurological or ocular symptoms: analysis of 105 cases. J Neurol 244, 639–645, 1997.
64. Beck RW, Janssen RS, Smiley ML, et al. Melioidosis and bilateral third-nerve palsies. Neurology 34, 105–107, 1984.
65. Beekman R, Kuk JB, Oosterhuis HJ. Myasthenia gravis: diagnosis and follow-up of 100 consecutive patients. J Neurology 244, 112–118, 1997.
66. Bell JA, McIllwaine GG, O'Neill D. Iatrogenic lateral

rectus palsies. A series of five postmyelographic cases. J Neuro-Ophthalmology 14, 205–209, 1994.
67. Bennett AH, Savill T. A case of permanent conjugate deviation of the eyes and head the result of a lesion limited to the sixth nucleus; with remarks on associated lateral movements of the eyeballs and rotation of the head and neck. Brain 12, 102–116, 1889.
68. Berenberg RA, Pellock JM, DiMauro S, et al. Lumping or splitting? "Ophthalmoplegia-plus" or Kearns-Sayre syndrome? Ann Neurol 1, 37–54, 1977.
69. Berger JR, Flaster M, Schatz S, et al. Cranial neuropathy heralding otherwise occult AIDS-related large cell lymphoma. J Clin Neuroophthalmol 13, 113–118, 1993.
70. Berlit P. Isolated and combined pareses of cranial nerves III, IV and VI A retrospective study of 412 patients. J Neurol Sci 103, 10–15, 1991.
71. Bever CT, Aquino AV, Penn AS, Lovelace RE, Rowland LP. Prognosis of ocular myasthenia. Ann Neurol 14, 516–519, 1983.
72. Bielschowsky A. Lectures on Motor Anomalies. Dartmouth College Publications, Hanover New Hampshire, 1940.
73. Bienfang DC. Crossing axons in the third nerve nucleus. Invest Ophthalmol 14, 927–931, 1975.
74. Biller J, Shapiro R, Evans LS, Haag JR, Fine M. Oculomotor nuclear complex infarction. Clinical and radiological correlation. Arch Neurol 41, 985–987, 1984.
75. Biousse V, Newman NJ. Third nerve palsies. Semin Neurol 20, 55–74, 2000.
76. Biousse V, Newman NJ, Petermann SH, Lambert SR. Isolated comitant esotropia and Chiari I malformation. Am J Ophthalmol 130, 216–220, 2000.
77. Bixenman WW, von Noorden GK. Benign recurrent VI nerve palsy in childhood. J Ped Ophthalmol Strabismus 18, 29–34, 1981.
78. Blake PY, Mark AS, Kattah J, Kolsky M. MR of oculomotor nerve. Am J Neuroradiol 16, 1665–1672, 1995.
79. Bloom JN, Cadera W, Heiberg E, Karlik S. A magnetic resonance imaging study of horizontal rectus muscle palsies. J Ped Ophthalmol Strabismus 30, 296–300, 1993.
80. Bloom JN, Gravis ER, Mardelli PG. A magnetic resonance imaging study of the upshoot-downshoot phenomenon of Duane's retraction syndrome. Am J Ophthalmol 111, 548–554, 1991.
81. Blumen SC, Feiler-Ofry V, Korczyn AD. Does pupillary sparing oculomotor nerve palsy really spare the pupil? J Clin Neuroophthalmol 11, 92–94, 1991.
82. Blumen SC, Sadeh M, Korczyn AD, et al. Intranuclear inclusions in oculopharyngeal muscular dystrophy among Bukhara Jews. Neurology 46, 1324–1328, 1996.
83. Blumenthal EZ, Gomori JM, Dotan S. Recurrent abducens nerve palsy caused by dolichoectasia of the cavernous internal carotid artery. Am J Ophthalmol 124, 255–257, 1997.
84. Bock O, Kommerell G. Visual localization after strabismus surgery is compatible with the "outflow" theory. Vision Res 26, 1825–1829, 1986.
85. Bodensteiner JB. Congenital myopathies. Muscle and Nerve 17, 131–144, 1994.
86. Boger WPI, Puliafito CA, Magoon EH, et al. Recurrent isolated sixth nerve palsy in children. Ann Ophthalmol 16, 237–244, 1984.
87. Boghen D, Chartrand JP, Laflamme P, et al. Primary aberrant third nerve regeneration. Ann Neurol 6, 415–418, 1979.
88. Bogousslavsky J, Maeder P, Regli F, Meuli R. Pure midbrain infarction: clinical syndromes MRI, and etiologic patterns. Neurology 44, 2032–2040, 1994.
89. Bogousslavsky J, Steck AJ. Bilateral third nerve palsy and anterior ischemic optic neuropathy. Neuro-ophthalmology 6, 117–120, 1986.
90. Bolzani W, Rognone F, Savoldi F, Montalbetti L. Colliculus hemorrhage. Rev Neurol (Paris) 152, 548–551, 1996.
91. Bosley TM, Slaih MA, Jen JC, et al. Neurologic features of horizontal gaze palsy and progressive scoliosis with mutations in ROBO3. Neurology 64, 1196–1203, 2005.
92. Bosman J, ten Tusscher MP, de JI, Vles JS, Kingma H. The influence of eye muscle surgery on shape and relative orientation of displacement planes: indirect evidence for neural control of 3D eye movements. Strabismus 10, 199–209, 2002.
93. Boylan C, Clement RA, Howrie A. Normal visual pathway routing in dissociated vertical deviation. Invest Ophthalmol Vis Sci 29, 1165–1167, 1988.
94. Brady-McCreery KM, Speidel S, Hussein MA, Coats DK. Spontaneous intracranial hypotension with unique strabismus due to third and fourth cranial neuropathies. Binocul Vis Strabismus Q 17, 43–48, 2002.
95. Bray WH, Giangiacomo J, Ide CH. Orbital apex syndrome. Surv Ophthalmol 32, 136–140, 1987.
96. Brazis PW, Lee AG. Binocular vertical diplopia. Mayo Clin Proc 73, 55–66, 1998.
97. Brazis PW, Miller NR, Henderer JD, Lee AG. The natural history and results of treatment of superior oblique myokymia. Neuroophthalmology 12, 1063–1067, 1994.
98. Brazis PW, Wharen RE, Czervionke LF, Witte RJ, Jones AD. Hemangioma of the mandibular branch of the trigeminal nerve in the Meckel cave presenting with facial pain and sixth nerve palsy. J Neuro-ophthalmol 20, 14–16, 2000.
99. Bregman DK, Harbour R. Diabetic superior division oculomotor nerve palsy. Arch Opthalmol 106, 1169–1170, 1988.
100. Bresolin N, Bet L, Binda A, et al. Clinical and biochemical correlations in mitochondrial myopathies treated with coenzyme Q10. Neurology 38, 892–899, 1988.
101. Briggs MM, Schachat F. The superfast extraocular myosin (MYH13) is localized to the innervation zone in both the global and orbital layers of rabbit extraocular muscle. J Exp Biol 205, 3133–3142, 2002.
102. Bristol R, Santora A, Fantozzi L, Delfini R. Cavernoma of the cavernous sinus: case report. Surg Neurol 48, 160–163, 1997.
103. Broadley SA, Taylor J, Waddy HM, Thompson PD. The clinical and MRI correlate of ischaemia in the ventromedial midbrain: Claude's syndrome. J Neurol 248, 1087–1089, 2001.
104. Brockington M, Alsanjari N, Sweeney MG, et al. Kearns-Sayre syndrome associated with mitochondrial DNA deletion or duplication: a molecular genetic and pathological study. J Neurol Sci 131, 78–87, 1995.
105. Brodsky MC. Dissociated vertical divergence: perceptual correlates of the human dorsal light reflex. Arch Ophthalmol 120, 1174–1178, 2002.

106. Brodsky MC, Donahue SP. Primary oblique muscle overaction: the brain throws a wild pitch. Arch Ophthalmol 119, 1307–1314, 2001.
107. Brodsky MC, Fray KJ. Positive angle kappa: a sign of albinism in patients with congenital nystagmus. Am J Ophthalmol 137, 625–629, 2004.
108. Brodsky MC, Tusa RJ. Latent nystagmus: vestibular nystagmus with a twist. Arch Ophthalmol 122, 202–209, 2004.
109. Bryan JS, Hamed LM. Levator-sparing nuclear oculomotor palsy. Clinical and magnetic resonance imaging findings. J Clin Neuroophthalmol 12, 26–30, 1992.
110. Bucci MP, Kapoula Z, Yang Q, Roussat B, Bremond-Gignac D. Binocular coordination of saccades in children with strabismus before and after surgery. Invest Ophthalmol Vis Sci 43, 1040–1047, 2002.
111. Buisseret P. Influence of extraocular muscle proprioception on vision. Physiol Rev 75, 323, 1995.
112. Bullen CL, Younge BR. Chronic orbital myositis. Arch Ophthalmol 100, 1749–1751, 1982.
113. Burian HM, Cahill JE. Congenital paralysis of medial rectus muscle with unusual synergism of the horizontal muscles. Trans Am Ophthalmol Soc 50, 87–102, 1952.
114. Burian HM, Van Allen MW, Sexton RR, Baller RS. Substitution phenomena in congenital and acquired supranuclear disorders of eye movement. Trans Am Acad Ophthalmol Otolaryngol 69, 1106–1114, 1965.
115. Burm JS, Chung CH, Oh SJ. Pure orbital blowout fracture: new concepts and importance of medial orbital blowout fracture. Plast Reconstr Surg 103, 1839–1849, 1999.
116. Burns TM, Russell JA, LaChance DH, Jones HR. Oculobulbar involvement is typical with Lambert-Eaton myasthenic syndrome. Ann Neurol 53, 270–273, 2003.
117. Büttner-Ennever JA. The extraocular motor nuclei. In Büttner-Ennever JA (ed). Neuroanatomy of the Oculomotor System. Prog Brain Res 151, 95–125, 2006.
118. Büttner-Ennever JA, Akert K. Medial rectus subgroups of the oculomotor nucleus and their abducens internuclear input in monkey. J Comp Neurol 197, 17–27, 1981.
119. Büttner-Ennever JA, Horn AK. The neuroanatomical basis of oculomotor disorders: the dual motor control of extraocular muscles and its possible role in proprioception. Curr Opin Neurol 15, 35–43, 2002.
120. Büttner-Ennever JA, Horn AK, Graf W, Ugolini G. Modern concepts of brainstem anatomy: from extraocular motoneurons to proprioceptive pathways. Ann N Y Acad Sci 956, 75–84, 2002.
121. Büttner-Ennever JA, Horn AK, Scherberger H, D'Ascanio P. Motoneurons of twitch and nontwitch extraocular muscle fibers in the abducens trochlear and oculomotor nuclei of monkeys. J Comp Neurol 438, 318–335, 2001.
122. Büttner-Ennever JA, Konakci KZ, Blumer R. Sensory control of extraocular muscles. In Büttner-Ennever JA (ed). Neuroanatomy of the Oculomotor System. Prog Brain Res 151, 2006.
123. Cackett P, Fleck B, Mulhivill A. Bilateral fourth-nerve palsy occurring after shaking injury in infancy. J AAPOS 8, 280–281, 2004.
124. Cahill M, Bannigan J, Eustace P. Anatomy of the extraneural blood supply to the intracranial oculomotor nerve. Br J Ophthalmol 80, 177–181, 1996.
125. Cakmak O, Ergin NT, Aydin MV. Isolated sphenoid sinus adenocarcinoma: a case report. Eur Arch Otorhinolaryngol 259, 266–268, 2002.
126. Caksen H, Acar N, Odabas D, et al. Isolated left oculomotor nerve palsy following measles. J Child Neurol. 17, 784–785, 2002.
127. Calabrese G, Telvi L, Capodiferro F, et al. Narrowing the Duane syndrome critical region at chromosome 8q13 down to 40 kb. Eur J Hum Genet 8, 319–324, 2000.
128. Campbell RJ, Okazaki H. Painful ophthalmoplegia (Tolosa-Hunt variant): autopsy findings in a patient with necrotizing intracavernous carotid vasculitis and inflammatory disease of the orbit. Mayo Clin Proc 62, 520–526, 1987.
129. Campos CR, Massaro AR, Scaff M. Isolated oculomotor nerve palsy in spontaneous internal carotid artery dissection: case report. Arq Neuropsiquiatr 61, 668–670, 2003.
130. Campos EC. Ocular torticollis. Intl Ophthalmol 6, 49–53, 1983.
131. Campos EC, Chiesi C, Bolzani R. Abnormal spatial localization in patients with herpes zoster ophthalmicus. Arch Ophthalmol 104, 1176–1177, 1986.
132. Capo H, Warren F, Kupersmith MJ. Evolution of oculomotor nerve palsies. J Clin Neuroophthalmol 12, 21–25, 1992.
133. Capone A Jr., Slamovits TL. Discrete metastasis of solid tumors to extraocular muscles. Arch Ophthalmol 108, 237–243, 1990.
134. Caress JB, Hunt CH, Batish SD. Anti-MuSK myasthenia gravis presenting with purely ocular findings. Arch Neurol 62, 1002–1003, 2005.
135. Carlow TJ, Depper MH, Orrison WW Jr. MR of extraocular muscles in chronic progressive external ophthalmoplegia. Am J Neuroradiol 19, 95–99, 1998.
136. Carr MM, Ross DA, Zuker RM. Cranial nerve defects in congenital facial palsy. J Otolaryngol 26, 80–87, 1997.
137. Carrozzo R, Hirano M, Fromenty B, et al. Multiple mtDNA deletions in autosomal dominant and recessive diseases suggest distinct pathogeneses. Neurology 50, 99–106, 1998.
138. Carta A, D'Adda T, Carrara F, Zeviani M. Ultrastructural analysis of extraocular muscle in chronic progressive external ophthalmoplegia. Arch Ophthalmol 118, 1141–1145, 2000.
139. Carter N, Miller NR. Fourth nerve palsy caused by Ehrlichia chaffeensis. J Neuroophthalmology 17, 47–50, 1997.
140. Castro O, Johnson LN, Mamourian AC. Isolated inferior oblique paresis from brain-stem infarction. Perspective on oculomotor fascicular organization in the ventral midbrain tegmentum. Arch Neurol 47, 235–237, 1990.
141. Chan CC, Sogg RL, Steinman L. Isolated oculomotor palsy after measles immunization. Am J Ophthalmol 89, 446–448, 1980.
142. Chan TK, Demer JL. Clinical features of congenital absence of the superior oblique muscle as demonstrated by orbital imaging. J AAPOS 3, 143–150, 1999.
143. Chang TS, Johns DR, Walker D, et al. Ocular clinicopathologic study of the mitochondrial encephalomyopathy overlap syndromes. Arch Ophthalmol 111, 1254–1262, 1993.
144. Char DH, Miller T, Kroll S. Orbital metastases: diag-

nosis and course. Br J Ophthalmol 81, 386–390, 1997.
145. Chen KS, Hung IJ, Lin KL. Isolated abducens nerve palsy: an unusual presentation of leukemia. J Child Neurol 17, 850–851, 2002.
146. Cheng H, Burdon MA, Shun-Shin GA, Czypionka S. Dissociated eye movements in craniosynostosis: a hypothesis revived. Br J Ophthalmol 77, 563–568, 1993.
147. Chiba A, Kusonoki S, Obata H, Machinami R, Kanazawa I. Serum anti-GQ1b IgG antibody is associated with ophthalmoplegia in Miller-Fisher syndrome and Guillain-Barré syndrome: clinical and immunohistochemical studies. Neurology 43, 1911–1917, 1993.
148. Cho DY, Wang YC, Ho WL. Primary intrasellar mixed germ-cell tumor with precocious puberty and diabetes insipidus. Childs Nervous System 13, 42–46, 1997.
149. Chou KL, Galetta SL, Liu GT, et al. Acute ocular motor mononeuropathies: prospective study of the roles of neuroimaging and clinical assessment. J Neurol Sci 219, 35–39, 2004.
150. Chou TM, Demer JL. Isolated inferior rectus palsy caused by a metastasis to the oculomotor nucleus. Am J Ophthalmol 126, 737–740, 1998.
151. Chu K, Kang DW, Song YW, Yoon BW. Trochlear nerve palsy in Sjogren's syndrome. J Neurol Sci 177, 157–159, 2000.
152. Ciuffreda KJ, Kenyon RV, Stark L. Increased saccadic latencies in amblyopic eyes. Invest Ophthalmol Vis Sci 17, 697–702, 1978.
153. Ciuffreda KJ, Kenyon RV, Stark L. Increased drift in amblyopic eyes. Br J Ophthalmol 64, 7–14, 1980.
154. Clark RA, Miller JM, Demer JL. Location and stability of rectus muscle pulleys: muscle paths as a function of gaze. Invest Ophthalmol Vis Sci 38, 227–240, 1997.
155. Clark RA, Miller JM, Rosenbaum AL, Demer JL. Heterotopic muscle pulleys or oblique muscle dysfunction? J AAPOS 2, 17–25, 1998.
156. Clendaniel RA, Mays LE. Characteristics of antidromically identified oculomotor internuclear neurons during vergence and versional eye movements. J Neurophysiol 71, 1111–1127, 1994.
157. Coats DK, Paysse EA, Plager DA, Wallace DK. Early strabismus surgery for thyroid ophthalmopathy. Ophthalmology 106, 324–329, 1999.
158. Coffeen P, Guyton DL. Monocular diplopia accompanying ordinary refractive errors. Am J Ophthalmol 105, 451–459, 1988.
159. Cogan DG. Myasthenia gravis. A review of the disease and a description of lid twitch as a characteristic sign. Arch Ophthalmol 74, 217–221, 1965.
160. Cogan DG, Victor M. Ocular signs of Wernicke's disease. Arch Ophthalmol 51, 204–211, 1954.
161. Cogan DG, Yee RD, Gittinger J. Rapid eye movements in myasthenia gravis. I Clinical observations. Arch Ophthalmol 94, 1083–1085, 1976.
162. Cohen HA, Nussinovitch M, Ashkenazi A, Straussberg R, Kaushansky A. Benign abducens nerve palsy of childhood. Pediatr Neurol 9, 394–395, 1993.
163. Cohen-Gadol AA, Leavitt JA, Lynch JJ, Marsh WR, Cascino GD. Prospective analysis of diplopia after anterior temporal lobectomy for mesial temporal lobe sclerosis. J Neurosurg 99, 496–499, 2003.
164. Collewijn H, Erkelens CJ, Steinman RM. Binocular coordination of human horizontal saccadic eye movements. J Physiol (Lond) 404, 157–182, 1988.
165. Collins CC. The human oculomotor control system. In Lennerstrand G, Bach-y-Rita P (eds). Basic Mechanisms of Ocular Motility and their Clinical Implications. Pergamon, Oxford, 1975, pp 145–180.
166. Collins CC, O'Mera D, Scott AB. Muscle tension during unrestrained human eye movements. J Physiol (Lond) 245, 351–369, 1975.
167. Connell B, Wilkinson RM, Barbour JM, et al. Are Duane syndrome and infantile esotropia allelic? Ophthalmic Genet 25, 189–198, 2004.
168. Cornblath WT, Elner V, Rolfe M. Extraocular muscle involvement in sarcoidosis. Ophthalmology 100, 501–505, 1993.
169. Couch JM, Somer ME, Gonzalez C. Superior oblique muscle dysfunction following anterior ethmoidal artery ligation for epistaxis. Ann Ophthalmol 108, 1110–1113, 1990.
170. Cox TA, Wurster JB, Godfrey WA. Primary aberrant oculomotor regeneration due to intracranial aneurysm. Arch Neurol 36, 570–571, 1979.
171. Crouch ER, Urist MJ. Lateral rectus muscle paralysis associated with closed-head trauma. Am J Ophthalmol 79, 990–996, 1975.
172. Cruciger MP, Brown B, Denys EH, et al. Clinical and subclinical oculomotor findings in the Eaton-Lambert syndrome. J Clin Neuroophthalmol 3, 19–22, 1983.
173. Cruysberg JRM, Mtanda AT, Duinkerke-Eerola KU, Huygen PLM. Congenital adduction palsy and synergistic divergence: a clinical and electro-oculographic study. Br J Ophthalmol 73, 68–75, 1989.
174. Cunningham ET Jr., Good WV. Inferior branch oculomotor nerve palsy: a case report. J Neuro-ophthalmology 14, 21–23, 1994.
175. Currie JN, Coppeto JR, Lessell S. Chronic syphilitic meningitis resulting in superior orbital fissure syndrome and posterior fossa gumma. A report of two cases followed for 20 years. J Clin Neuroophthalmol 8, 145–155, 1988.
176. Currie JN, Lubin JH, Lessell S. Chronic isolated abducens paresis from tumors at the base of the brain. Arch Neurol 40, 226–229, 1983.
177. Cushing H. Strangulation of the nerve abducentes by lateral branches of the basilar artery in cases of brain tumor. With an explanation of some obscure palsies on the basis of arterial constriction. Brain 33, 204–235, 1919.
178. Daroff RB. Ocular motor manifestations of brainstem and cerebellar dysfunction. In Smith JL (ed). Neuro-Ophthalmology. Volume 5. Huffman, Hallandale Florida, 1970, pp 104–118.
179. Daroff RB. The office tensilon test for ocular myasthenia gravis. Arch Neurol 43, 843–844, 1986.
180. Daroff RB. The eye and headache. Headache Quart 6, 89–96, 1995.
181. Daroff RB, Solitaire GB, Pincus JH, Glaser GH. Spongioform encephalopathy with chronic progressive external ophthalmoplegia. Central ophthalmoplegia mimicking ocular myopathy. Neurology 16, 161–169, 1966.

182. Das VE, Fu LN, Mustari MJ, Tusa RJ. Incomitance in monkeys with strabismus. Strabismus 13, 33–41, 2005.
183. Davalos A, Matias-Guiu J, Codina A. Painful ophthalmoplegia in systemic lupus erythematosus. J Neurol Neurosurg Psychiatry 47, 323–324, 1984.
184. Davies GE, Shakir RA. Giant cell arteritis presenting as oculomotor nerve palsy with pupillary dilatation. Postgrad Med J 70, 298–299, 1994.
185. Davis TL, Lavin PJM. Pseudo one-and-a-half syndrome with ocular myathenia. Neurology 39, 1553, 1989.
186. De Graaf J, Cats H, de Jager AEJ. Gradenigo's syndrome: a rare complication of otitis media. Clin Neurol Neurosurg 90, 237–239, 1988.
187. De Pool ME, Campbell JP, Broome SO, Guyton DL. The dragged-fovea diplopia syndrome. Clinical characteristics, diagnosis, and treatment. Ophthalmology 112, 1455–1462, 2005.
188. Deangelis DD, Kraft SP. The double-bellied inferior oblique muscle: clinical correlates. J AAPOS 5, 76–81, 2001.
189. deFaber J-THN, von Noorden GK. Inferior rectus muscle palsy after retrobulbar anesthesia for cataract surgery. Am J Ophthalmol 112, 209–211, 1991.
190. Dehaene I, Marchau M, Vanhooren G. Nuclear oculomotor nerve paralysis. Neuroophthalmology 7, 219–222, 1987.
191. Dehaene I, Martin JJ, Geens K, Cras P. Guillain-Barre syndrome with ophthalmoplegia: clinicopathological study of the central and peripheral nervous systems including the oculomotor nerves. Neurology 36, 851–854, 1986.
192. Delany C, Jay WM. Papilledema and abducens nerve palsy following ethylene glycol ingestion. Semin Ophthalmol 19, 72–74, 2004.
193. Deleu D, Lagopoulos M, al Moundhry M, Katchy K. Isolated bilateral abducens nerve palsy in primary sphenoidal sinus non-Hodgkin lymphoma. Acta Neurol Belg 100, 103–106, 2000.
194. Dell'Osso LF, Ayyar DR, Daroff RB, Abel LA. Edrophonium test in Eaton-Lambert syndrome: quantitative oculography. Neurology 33, 1157–1163, 1983.
195. Dell'Osso LF, Ellenberger C Jr., Abel LA, Flynn JT. The nystagmus blockage syndrome. Congenital nystagmus, manifest latent nystagmus, or both? Invest Ophthalmol Vis Sci 24, 1580–1587, 1983.
196. Delpassand ES, Kirkpatrick JB. Cavernous sinus syndrome as the presentation of malignant lymphoma: case report and review of the literature. Neurosurgery 23, 501–504, 1988.
197. Demer JL. Pivotal role of orbital connective tissues in binocular alignment and strabismus: the Friedenwald lecture. Invest Ophthalmol Vis Sci 45, 729–738, 2004.
198. Demer JL, Clark RA, Engle EC. Magnetic resonance imaging evidence for widespread orbital dysinnervation in congenital fibrosis of extraocular muscles due to mutations in KIF21A. Invest Ophthalmol Vis Sci 46, 530–539, 2005.
199. Demer JL, Kerman BM. Comparison of standardized echography with magnetic resonance imaging to measure extraocular muscle size—Reply. Am J Ophthlmol 119, 383–384, 1995.
200. Demer JL, Miller JM. Magnetic resonance imaging of the functional anatomy of the superior oblique muscle. Invest Ophthalmol Vis Sci 36, 906–913, 1995.
201. Demer JL, Miller JM, Poukens V, Vinters HV, Glasgow BJ. Evidence for fibromuscular pulleys of the recti extraocular muscles. Invest Ophthalmol Vis Sci 36, 1125–1136, 1995.
202. Demer JL, Oh SY, Poukens V. Evidence for active control of rectus extraocular muscle pulleys. Invest Ophthalmol Vis Sci 41, 1280–1290, 2000.
203. Demer JL, Poukens V, Miller JM, Micevych P. Innervation of extraocular pulley smooth muscle in monkeys and humans. Invest Ophthalmol Vis Sci 38, 1774–1785, 1997.
204. DeRespinis PA, Caputo AR, Wagner RS, Guo S. Duane's retraction syndrome. Surv Ophthalmol 38, 257–288, 1993.
205. Dewhurst AG, Hall D, Schwartz MS, McKeran RO. Kearns-Sayre syndrome hypoparathyroidism and basal ganglia calcification. J Neurol Neurosurg Psychiatry 49, 1323–1324, 1986.
206. DiBernardo C, Pacheco EM, Hughes JR, Iliff WJ, Byrne SF. Echographic evaluation and findings in metastatic melanoma to extraocular muscles. Ophthalmology 103, 1794–1797, 1996.
207. Dickey CF, Scott WE, Cline RA. Oblique muscle palsies fixating with the paretic eye. Surv Ophthalmol 33, 97–107, 1988.
208. Dieterich M, Brandt T. Ocular torsion and perceived vertical in oculomotor trochlear and abducens nerve palsies. Brain 116, 1095–1104, 1993.
209. Diir LY, Donofrio PD, Patton JF, Troost BT. A false-positive edrophonium test in a patient with a brainstem glioma. Neurology 39, 865–867, 1989.
210. Dimant J, Grob D, Brunner NG. Ophthalmoplegia ptosis and miosis in temporal arteritis. Neurology 30, 1054–1058, 1980.
211. DiNubile MJ. Septic thrombosis of the cavernous sinuses. Arch Neurol 45, 567–572, 1988.
212. Dobrowski JM, Zajtchuk JT, LaPiana FG, Hensley SD. Oculopharyngeal muscular dystrophy: clinical and histopathologic correlations. Otolaryngol Head Neck Surg 95, 131–142, 1986.
213. Doherty EJ, Macy ME, Wang SM, et al. CFEOM3: a new extraocular congenital fibrosis syndrome that maps to 16q24.2–q24.3. Invest Ophthalmol Vis Sci 40, 1687–1694, 1999.
214. Donaghy M, Earl CJ. Ocular palsy preceding chronic relapsing polyneuropathy by several weeks. Ann Neurol 17, 49–50, 1985.
215. Donahue SP, Taylor RJ. Pupil-sparing third nerve palsy associated with sildenafil citrate (Viagra). Am J Ophthalmol 126, 476–477, 1998.
216. Donaldson D, Rosenberg NL. Infarction of abducens nerve fascicle as cause of isolated sixth nerve palsy related to hypertension. Neurology 38, 1654, 1988.
217. Donaldson IM. The functions of the proprioceptors of the eye muscles. Philos Trans R Soc Lond B Biol Sci 355, 1685–1754, 2000.
218. Donofrio PD. Immunotherapy of idiopathic inflammatory neuropathies. Muscle Nerve 28, 273–292, 2003.
219. Drachman DA. Ophthalmoplegia plus: the neurodegenerative disorders associated with progressive

external ophthalmoplegia. Arch Neurol 18, 654–674, 1968.
220. Dreyfus PM, Hakim S, Adams RD. Diabetic ophthalmoplegia. Report of case with postmortem study and comments on vascular supply of human oculomotor nerve. Arch Neurol Psychiatry 77, 337–349, 1957.
221. Durand JR, Samples JR. Dolichoectasia and cranial nerve palsies. J Clin Neuroophthalmol 9, 249–253, 1989.
221a. Eberhorn AC, Horn AK, Eberhorn N, et al. Palisade endings in extraocular eye muscles revealed by SNAP-25 immunoreactivity. J Anat 206, 307–315, 2005.
222. Ebner R, Devoto MH, Weil D, et al. Treatment of thyroid associated ophthalmopathy with periocular injections of triamcinolone. Br J Ophthalmol 88, 1380–1386, 2004.
223. Ehrenpreis SJ, Biedlingmaier JF. Isolated third-nerve palsy associated with frontal sinus mucocele. J Neuroophthalmol 15, 105–108, 1995.
224. Ehrt O, Boergen KP. Scanning laser ophthalmoscope fundus cyclometry in near-natural viewing conditions. Graefes Arch Clin Exp Ophthalmol 239, 678–682, 2001.
225. Engel AG, Ohno K, Bouzat C, Sine SM, Griggs RC. End-plate acetylcholine receptor deficiency due to nonsense mutations in the e subunit. Ann Neurol 40, 810–817, 1996.
226. Engelhardt A, Cedzich C, Kömpf D. Isolated superior branch palsy of the oculomotor nerve in influenza A. Neuroophthalmology 9, 233–235, 1989.
227. Engle EC. Applications of molecular genetics to the understanding of congenital ocular motility disorders. Ann N Y Acad Sci 956, 55–63, 2002.
228. Engle EC. The molecular basis of the congenital fibrosis syndromes. Strabismus 10, 125–128, 2002.
229. Engle EC, Goumnerov BC, McKeown CA, et al. Oculomotor nerve and muscle abnormalities in congenital fibrosis of the extraocular muscles. Ann Neurol 41, 314–325, 1997.
230. Engle EC, Leigh RJ. Genes, brainstem development and eye movements. Neurology 59, 304–305, 2002.
231. Engle EC, Marondel I, Houtman WA, et al. Congenital fibrosis of the extraocular muscles (autosomal dominant congenital external ophthalmoplegia): genetic homogeneity, linkage refinement, and physical mapping on chromosome 12. Am J Hum Genet 57, 1086–1094, 1995.
232. Ernemann U, Freudenstein D, Pitz S, Naegele T. Intraorbital aneurysm of the ophthalmic artery: a rare cause of apex orbitae compression syndrome. Graefes Arch Clin Exp Ophthalmol 240, 575–577, 2002.
233. Espinosa JA, Giroux M, Johnston K, Kirkham T, Villemure JG. Abducens palsy followin shunting for hydrocephalus. Can J Neurol Sci 20, 123–125, 1993.
234. Estanol B, Lopez-Rios G. Looking with a paralysed eye: adaptive plasticity of the vestibulo-ocular reflex. J Neurol Neurosurg Psychiatry 47, 799–804, 1984.
235. Ettl A, Kramer J, Daxer A, Koornneef L. High resolution magnetic resonance imaging of neurovascular orbital anatomy. Ophthalmology 104, 869–877, 1997.
236. Ettl A, Salomonowitz E. Visualization of the oculomotor cranial nerves by magnetic resonance imaging. Strabismus 12, 85–96, 2004.
237. Eustace P. Partial nuclear third nerve palsies. Neuroophthalmology 5, 259–262, 1985.
238. Evoli A, Tonali P, Bartoccioni E, Lo M. Ocular myasthenia: diagnostic and therapeutic problems. Acta Neurol Scand 77, 31–35, 1988.
239. Eyster EF, Hoyt WF, Wilson CB. Oculomotor palsy from minor head trauma. An initial sign of basal intracranial tumor. JAMA 220, 1083–1086, 1972.
240. Ezra E, Spalton D, Sanders MD, Graham EM, Plant GT. Ocular neuromyotonia. Br J Ophthalmol 80, 350–355, 1996.
241. Fekrat S, Miller NR, Loury MC. Alveolar rhabdomyosarcoma that metastasized to the orbit. Ann Ophthalmol 111, 1662–1664, 1993.
242. Feldon SE, Stark L, Lehman SL, Hoyt WF. Oculomotor effects of intermittent conduction block in myasthenia gravis and Guillain-Barre syndrome. Arch Neurol 39, 497–503, 1982.
243. Feldon SE, Stark L, Lehman SL, Hoyt WF. Oculomotor effects of intermittent conduction block in myasthenia gravis and Guillain-Barre syndrome. An oculographic study with computer simulations. Arch Neurol 39, 497–503, 1982.
244. Feldon SE, Unsold R. Graves' ophthalmopathy evaluated by infrared eye-movement recordings. Arch Ophthalmol 100, 324–328, 1982.
245. Fells P, Kousoulides L, Pappa A, Munro P, Lawson J. Extraocular muscle problems in thyroid eye disease. Eye 8, 497–505, 1994.
246. Fenstemaker SB, Kiorpes L, Movshon JA. Effects of experimental strabismus on the architecture of macaque monkey striate cortex. J Comp Neurol 438, 300–317, 2001.
247. Ferman L, Collewijn H, Van den Berg AV. A direct test of Listing's law—I Human ocular torsion measured in static tertiary positions. Vision Res 27, 929–938, 1987.
248. Ferman L, Collewijn H, Van den Berg AV. A direct test of Listing's law—II Human ocular torsion measured under dynamic conditions. Vision Res 27, 939–951, 1987.
249. Fernandez E, Pallini R, Gangitano C, et al. Oculomotor nerve regeneration in rats. Functional, histological, and neuroanatomical studies. J Neurosurg 67, 428–437, 1987.
250. Ferrante E, Savino A, Brioschi A, et al. Transient oculomotor cranial nerves palsy in spontaneous intracranial hypotension. J Neurosurg Sci 42, 177–179, 1998.
251. Fetter M, Bork T, Haslwanter T. Effect of alcohol on Listing's law. Soc Neurosci Abstr 23, 1298, 1997.
252. Feuer H, Jagoda A. Myasthenia gravis presenting as a unilateral abducens nerve palsy. Am J Emerg Med 19, 410–412, 2001.
253. Finelli PF, Hoyt WF. Myasthenic abduction nystagmus in a patient with hyperthyroidism. Neurology 26, 589–590, 1976.
254. Fisher CM. Some neuro-ophthalmological observations. J Neurol Neurosurg Psychiatry 30, 383–392, 1967.
255. Fisher M. An unusual variant of acute idopathic polyneuritis (syndrome of ophthalmoplegia ataxia and areflexia. N Engl J Med 255, 57–65, 1956.
256. FitzSimon JS, Toland J, Phillips J, Logan P, Eustace

P. Giant aneurysms in the cavernous sinus. Neuroophthalmol 15, 59–65, 1995.
257. Flanders M, Hastings M. Diagnosis and surgical management of strabismus associated with thyroid-related orbitopathy. J Pediatr Ophthalmol Strabismus 34, 333–340, 1997.
258. Fleet WS, Rapcsak SZ, Huntley WW, Watson RT. Pupil-sparing oculomotor palsy from midbrain hemorrhage. Ann Ophthalmol 20, 345–346, 1988.
259. Fleet WS, Valenstein E. Ocular palsy preceding chronic relapsing polyneuropathy. Ann Neurol 19, 413–414, 1986.
260. Follens I, Godts D, Evens PA, Tassignon MJ. Combined fourth and sixth cranial nerve palsy after lumbar puncture: a rare complication. A case report. Bull Soc Belge Ophtalmol 29–33, 2001.
261. Freedman MI, Folk JC. Metastatic tumors to the eye and orbit. Patient survival and clinical characteristics. Arch Ophthalmol 105, 1215–1219, 1987.
262. Frenkel REP, Brodsky MC, Spoor TC. Adult-onset cyclic esotropia and optic atrophy. J Clin Neuro-ophthalmol 6, 27–30, 1986.
263. Fricke J, Neugebauer A, Kirsch A, Russmann W. Ocular neuromyotonia: a case report. Strabismus 10, 119–124, 2002.
264. Friedman JA, Piepgras DG, Pichelmann MA, et al. Small cerebral aneurysms presenting with symptoms other than rupture. Neurology 57, 1212–1216, 2001.
265. Frohman EM, Zee DS. Ocular neuromyotonia: clinical features, physiological mechanisms, and response to therapy. Ann Neurol 37, 620–626, 1995.
266. Fromenty B, Carrozzo R, Shanske S, Schon EA. High proportions of mtDNA duplications in patients with Kearns-Sayre syndrome occur in the heart. Am J Med Genet 71, 443–452, 1997.
267. Fuchs AF, Binder MD. Fatigue resistance of human extraocular muscles. J Neurophysiol 49, 28–34, 1983.
268. Fukutake T, Hirayama K. Isolated abducens nerve palsy from pontine infarction in a diabetic patient. Neurology 42, 2226, 1992.
269. Fuller GN, Matthews TD, Maini RN, Kennard C. An unusual cause for diplopia: acquired Brown's syndrome. J Neurol Neurosurg Psychiatry 58, 506–507, 1995.
270. Galbraith RS. Incidence of neonatal sixth nerve palsy in relation to mode of delivery. Am J Obstet Gynecol 170, 1158–1159, 1994.
271. Galer BS, Lipton RB, Weinstein S, Bello L, Solomon S. Apoplectic headache and oculomotor nerve palsy. Neurology 40, 1465–1466, 1990.
272. Galetta SL, Sergott RC, Wells GB, Atlas SW, Bird SJ. Spontaneous remission of a third-nerve palsy in meningeal lymphoma. Ann Neurol 32, 100–102, 1992.
273. Galetta SL, Smith JL. Chronic isolated sixth nerve palsies. Arch Neurol 46, 79–82, 1989.
274. Gallastegui J, Hariman RJ, Handler B, Lev M, Bharati S. Cardiac involvement in the Kearns-Sayre syndrome. Am J Cardiology 60, 385–388, 1987.
275. Gamio S, Garcia-Erro M, Vaccarezza MM, Minella JA. Myasthenia gravis in childhood. Binocul Vis Strabismus Q 19, 223–231, 2004.
276. Gauntt CD, Kashii S, Nagata I. Monocular elevation paresis by an oculomotor fascicular impairment. J Neuroophthalmol 15, 11–14, 1995.
277. Gauthier GM, Nommay D, Vercher J-L. Ocular muscle proprioception and visual localization of targets in man. Brain 113, 1857–1871, 1990.
278. Gauthier GM, Vercher J-L, Zee DS. Changes in ocular alignment and pointing accuracy after sustained passive rotation of one eye. Vision Res 34, 2613–2627, 1994.
279. Gautier JC, Awanda A, Majdalani A. Ophthalmoplegia with contralateral hemiplegia. Occlusion of the internal carotid artery due to thrombosis of an intracavernous aneurysm. Stroke 17, 1321–1322, 1986.
280. Gaymard B, Lafitte C, Gelot A, deToffol B. Plus-minus lid syndrome. J Neurol Neurosurg Psychiatry 55, 846–848, 1992.
281. Gaymard B, Larmande P, deToffol B, Autret A. Reversible nuclear oculomotor nerve paralysis. Eur Neurol 30, 128–131, 1990.
282. Gentle A, Ruskell G. Pathway of the primary afferent nerve fibers serving proprioception in monkey extraocular muscles. Ophthalmic Physiol Optics 17, 225–231, 1997.
283. Gentry LR, Mehta RC, Appen RE, Weinstein JM. MR imaging of primary trochlear nerve neoplasms. Am J Neuroradiol 12, 707–713, 1991.
284. George J-L, Algan M, Lesure P. Oculomotor disturbances due to idiopathic inflammatory orbital pseudotumor. Orbit 8, 117–122, 1989.
285. Ghasia FF, Angelaki DE. Do motoneurons encode the noncommutativity of ocular rotations? Neuron 47, 1–13, 2005.
286. Gilchrist ID, Brown V, Findlay JM. Saccades without eye movements. Nature 390, 130–131, 1997.
287. Gilmore PC, Carlow TJ. Diabetic oculomotor paresis with pupil fixed to light. Neurology 30, 1229–1230, 1980.
288. Gittinger JW Jr., Hughes JP, Suran EL. Medial orbital wall blow-out fracture producing an acquired retraction syndrome. J Clin Neuroophthalmol 6, 153–156, 1986.
289. Glaser JS. Myasthenic pseudo-internuclear ophthalmoplegia. Arch Ophthalmol 75, 363–366, 1966.
290. Goadsby PJ, Lance JW. Clinicopathological correlation in a case of painful ophthalmoplegia: Tolosa-Hunt syndrome. J Neurol Neurosurg Psychiatry 52, 1290–1293, 1989.
291. Goebel HH. Congenital myopathies at their molecular dawning. Muscle and Nerve 27, 527–548, 2003.
292. Goh SY, Ho SC, Seah LL, Fong KS, Khoo DH. Thyroid autoantibody profiles in ophthalmic dominant and thyroid dominant Graves' disease differ and suggest ophthalmopathy is a multiantigenic disease. Clin Endocrinol (Oxf) 60, 600–607, 2004.
293. Goldenberg-Cohen N, Curry C, Miller NR, Tamargo RJ, Murphy KP. Long term visual and neurological prognosis in patients with treated and untreated cavernous sinus aneurysms. J Neurol Neurosurg Psychiatry 75, 863–867, 2004.
294. Goldenberg-Cohen N, Miller NR. Noninvasive neuroimaging of basilar artery dolichoectasia in a patient with an isolated abducens nerve paresis. Am J Ophthalmol 137, 365–367, 2004.
295. Goldstein JH, Wolintz AH, Stein SC. Concomitant strabismus as a sign of intracranial disease. Ann Ophthalmol 15, 53–55, 1983.
296. Good WV, Barkovich AJ, Nickel BL, Hoyt CS. Bilateral congenital oculomotor nerve palsy in a

patient with brain anomalies. Am J Ophthalmol 111, 555–558, 1991.
297. Gordon CR, Leveton-Kriss S, Gutman I, Zoldan J, Gadoth N. Brainstem encephalitis due to herpes simplex causing permanent external ophthalmoplegia. Neuroophthalmol 7, 273–277, 1987.
298. Gorman CA. Radiotherapy for Graves' ophthalmopathy: results at one year. Thyroid 12, 251–255, 2002.
299. Gorman CA, Garrity JA, Fatourechi V, et al. The aftermath of orbital radiotherapy for graves' ophthalmopathy. Ophthalmology 109, 2100–2107, 2002.
300. Goto Y, Hosokawa S, Goto I, Hirakata R, Hasuo K. Abnormality in the cavernous sinus in three patients with Tolosa-Hunt syndrome: MRI and CT findings. J Neurol Neurosurg Psychiatry 53, 231–234, 1990.
301. Goto Y, Yamabe K, Aiko Y, Kuromatsu C, Fukui M. Cavernous hemangioma in the cavernous sinus. Neurochirurgia 36, 93–95, 1993.
302. Gottlob I, Jain S, Engle EC. Elevation of one eye during tooth brushing. Am J Ophthalmol 134, 459–460, 2002.
303. Gourdeau A, Miller N, Zee D, Morris J. Central ocular motor abnormalities in Duane's retraction syndrome. Arch Ophthalmol 99, 1809–1810, 1981.
304. Gray LG, Galetta SL, Hershey B, Winkelman AC, Wulc A. Inferior division third nerve paresis from an orbital dural arteriovenous malformation. J Neuroophthalmol 19, 46–48, 1999.
305. Greenberg DA. Calcium channels in neurological disease. Ann Neurol 42, 275–282, 1997.
306. Greenspan BN, Reeves AG. Transient partial oculomotor nerve paresis with posterior communicating artery aneurysm. A case report. J Clin Neuroophthalmol 10, 56–58, 1990.
307. Griffiths PD, Gholkar A, Sengupta RP. Oculomotor nerve palsy due to thrombosis of a posterior communicating artery aneurysm following diagnostic angiography. Neuroradiology 36, 614–615, 1994.
308. Grimson BS, Thompson HS. Raeder's syndrome. A clinical review. Surv Ophthalmol 24, 199–210, 1980.
309. Groothuis DR, Schulman S, Wollman R, Frey J, Vick NA. Demyelinating radiculopathy in the Kearns-Sayre syndrome: a clinicopathological study. Ann Neurol 8, 373–380, 1980.
310. Gruber H, Zeitlhofer J, Prager J, Pils P. Complex oculomotor dysfunctions in Kugelberg-Welander disease. Neuroophthalmol 3, 125–128, 1983.
311. Grunt JA, Destro RL, Hamtil LW, Baska RE. Ocular palsies in children with diabetes mellitus. Diabetes 25, 459–462, 1976.
312. Guthrie BL, Porter JD, Sparks DL. Corollary discharge provides accurate eye position information to the oculomotor system. Science 221, 1193–1195, 1983.
313. Gutman I, Levartovski S, Goldhammer Y, Tadmor R, Findler G. Sixth nerve palsy and unilateral Horner's syndrome. Ophthalmology 93, 913–916, 1986.
314. Guy JR, Day AL, Mickle JP, Schatz NJ. Contralateral trochlear nerve paresis and ipsilateral Horner's syndrome. Am J Ophthalmol 107, 73–76, 1989.
315. Guy JR, Engel HM, Lessner AM. Acquired contralateral oculomotor synkinesis. Arch Neurol 46, 1021–1023, 1989.
316. Guy JR, Friedman WF, Mickle JP. Bilateral trochlear nerve paresis in hydrocephalus. J Clin Neuroophthalmol 9, 105–111, 1989.
317. Guy JR, Savino PJ, Schatz NJ, Cobbs WH, Day AL. Superior division paresis of the oculomotor nerve. Ophthalmology 92, 777–784, 1985.
318. Guyton DL. Dissociated vertical deviation: etiology, mechanism, and associated phenomena. Costenbader Lecture. J AAPOS 4, 131–144, 2000.
319. Hall JK, Jacobs DA, Movsas T, Galetta SL. Fourth nerve palsy, homonymous hemianopia and hemisensory deficit caused by a proximal posterior cerebral artery aneurysm. J Neuroophthalmol 22, 95–98, 2002.
320. Hallin E, Feldon S. Graves' ophthalmopathy: II Correlation of clinical signs with measures derived from computed tomography. Br J Ophthalmol 72, 678–682, 1988.
321. Hamed LM. Associated neurologic and ophthalmologic findings in congenital oculomotor nerve palsy. Ophthalmology 98, 708–714, 1991.
322. Hamed LM. Bilateral Brown syndrome in three siblings. J Ped Ophthalmol Strabismus 28, 306–309, 1991.
323. Hamed LM, Guy JR, Moster ML, Bosley T. Giant cell arteritis in the ocular ischemic syndrome. Am J Ophthalmol 113, 702–705, 1992.
324. Hamed LM, Schatz NJ, Galetta SL. Brainstem ocular motility defects and AIDS Am J Ophthalmol 106, 437–442, 1988.
325. Hansen HC, Lueck CJ, Crawford TJ, Kennard C, Zangemeister WH. Evidence for the occurence of myotonia in the extraocular musculature in patients with dystrophia myotonica. Neuroophthalmol 13, 17–24, 1993.
326. Hanson RA, Ghosh S, Gonzalez-Gomez I, Levy ML, Gilles FH. Abducens length and vulnerability? Neurology 62, 33–36, 2004.
327. Harada T, Ohashi T, Ohki K, et al. Clival chordoma presenting as acute esotropia due to bilateral abducens palsy. Ophthalmologica 21, 109–111, 1997.
328. Harbison JW, Lessell S, Selhorst JB. Neuro-ophthalmology of sphenoid sinus carcinoma. Brain 107, 855–870, 1984.
329. Hardenack M, Volker A, Schroder JM, Gilsbach JM, Harders AG. Primary eosinophilic granuloma of the oculomotor nerve. Case report. J Neurosurg 81, 784–787, 1994.
330. Hargrove RN, Fleming JC, Kerr NC. Brown's Syndrome in the absence of an intact superior oblique muscle. J AAPOS 8, 507–508, 2004.
331. Harley R. Paralytic strabismus in children. Etiologic incidence and management of the third, fourth and sixth nerve palsies. Ophthalmology 87, 24–43, 1980.
332. Harrigan MR, Chandler WF. Abducens nerve palsy after radiofrequency rhizolysis for trigeminal neuralgia: case report. Neurosurgery 43, 623–625, 1998.
333. Harris DJ, Memmen JE, Katz NNK, Parks MM. Familial congenital superior oblique palsy. Ophthalmology 93, 88–90, 1986.
334. Harrison AR, Wirtschafter JD. Isolated inferior rectus paresis secondary to a mesencephalic cavernous angioma. Am J Ophthalmol 127, 617–619, 1999.
335. Hashimoto M, Ohtsuka K, Suzuki T, Nakagawa T. Orbital granular cell tumor developing in the inferior oblique muscle. Am J Ophthalmol 124, 404–406, 1998.
336. Hashimoto M, Ohtsuka K, Suzuki Y, Minamida Y, Houkin K. Superior oblique myokymia caused by

vascular compression. J Neuroophthalmol 24, 237–239, 2004.
337. Haslwanter T. Mathematics of three-dimensional eye rotations. Vision Res 35, 1727–1739, 1995.
338. Hawke SHB, Mullie MA, Hoyt WF, Hallinan JM, Halmagyi GM. Painful oculomotor nerve palsy due to dural-cavernous sinus shunt. Arch Neurol 46, 1252–1255, 1989.
339. Hayes MT, Lev MH, Ruoff KL, et al. Case records of the Massachusetts General Hospital. Weekly clinicopathological exercise. Case 22–1997. A 58–year-old woman with multiple cranial neuropathies. N Engl J Med 337, 184–190, 1997.
340. Hedges TR, Jones A, Stark L, Hoyt WF. Botulin ophthalmoplegia. Clinical and oculographic observations. Arch Ophthalmol 101, 211–213, 1983.
341. Helmholtz H. Physiological Optics. Translated by Southall PC. Dover Press, New York, 1962.
342. Helveston EM, Pinchoff B, Ellis FD, Miller K Unilateral esotropia after enucleation in infancy. Am J Ophthalmol 100, 96–99, 1985.
343. Hering E. The Theory of Binocular Vision. Plenum Press, New York, 1977.
344. Herishanu YO, Tovi F, Hertzanu Y, Goldstein J. Painful ophthalmoplegia with lymphoid hyperplasia of the nasopharynx. Neuroophthalmol 15, 9–14, 1995.
345. Hirst LW, Miller NR, Johnson RT. Monocular polyopia. Arch Neurol 40, 756–757, 1983.
346. Hofmann RJ. Monozygotic twins concordant for bilateral Duane's retraction syndrome. Am J Ophthalmol 99, 563–566, 1985.
347. Holland D, Maune S, Kovacs G, Behrendt S. Metastatic tumors of the orbit: a retrospective study. Orbit 22, 15–24, 2003.
348. Holmes JM, Beck RW, Kip KE, Droste PJ, Leske DA. Predictors of nonrecovery in acute traumatic sixth nerve palsy and paresis. Ophthalmology 108, 1457–1460, 2001.
349. Holmes JM, Droste PJ, Beck RW. The natural history of acute traumatic sixth nerve palsy or paresis. J AAPOS 2, 265–268, 1998.
350. Holmes JM, Leske DA. Long-term outcomes after surgical management of chronic sixth nerve palsy. J AAPOS 6, 283–288, 2002.
351. Holmes JM, Mutyala S, Maus TL, et al. Pediatric third, fourth, and sixth nerve palsies: a population-based study. Am J Ophthalmol 127, 388–392, 1999.
352. Holmstrom GE, Nyman KG. Primary orbital amyloidosis localised to an extraocular muscle. Br J Ophthalmol 71, 32–33, 1987.
353. Horn AK, Buttner-Ennever JA, Gayde M, Messoudi A. Neuroanatomical identification of mesencephalic premotor neurons coordinating eyelid with upgaze in the monkey and man. J Comp Neurol 420, 19–34, 2000.
354. Horton JC, Fishman RA. Neurovisual findings in the syndrome of spontaneous intracranial hypotension from dural cerebrospinal fluid leak. Ophthalmology 101, 244–251, 1994.
355. Horton RM, Manfredi AA, Conti-Tronconi BM. The "embryonic" gamma subunit of the nicotinic acetylcholine receptor is expressed in adult extraocular muscle. Neurology 43, 983–986, 1993.
356. Horwitz SJ, Roessmann U. Kearns-Sayre syndrome with hypoparathyroidism. Ann Neurol 3, 513–518, 1978.
357. Hotchkiss MG, Miller NR, Clark AW, Green WR. Bilateral Duane's retraction syndrome. Arch Ophthalmol 98, 870–874, 1980.
358. Hoyt CS, Good WV. Acute onset of concomitant esotropia: when is it a sign of serious neurological disease? Br J Ophthalmol 79, 498–501, 1995.
359. Hoyt WF, Keane JR. Superior oblique myokymia. Report and discussion on five cases of benign intermittent uniocular microtremor. Arch Ophthal 84, 461–467, 1970.
360. Hoyt WF, Nachtigaller H. Anomalies of ocular motor nerves. Neuroanatomic correlates of paradoxical innervation in Duane's syndrome and related congenital ocular motor disorders. Am J Ophthalmol 60, 443–448, 1965.
361. Hriso E, Masdeu JC, Miller A. Monocular elevation weakness and ptosis: an oculomotor fascicular syndrome? J Clin Neuroophthalmol 11, 111–113, 1991.
362. Hubel DH, Wiesel TN. Brain and visual perception. Oxford University Press, New York, 2005.
363. Huber A, Esslen E, Kloti R, Martenet AC. Zum Problem des Duane-Syndrom. Graefe's Arch Clin Exp Ophthalmol 167, 169–191, 1964.
364. Hughes BW, Moro De Casillas ML, Kaminski HJ. Pathophysiology of myasthenia gravis. Semin Neurol 24, 21–30, 2005.
365. Hunt WE, Meagher JN, LeFever HE, Zemen W. Painful ophthalmoplegia. Its relation to indolent inflammation of the cavernous sinus. Neurology 11, 56–62, 1961.
366. Iannuzzelli PG, Murray M, Murphy EH. Regenerative axonal sprouting in the cat trochlear nerve. J Comp Neurol 354, 229–240, 1995.
367. Ikezaki K, Toda K, Abe M, Tabuchi K. Intracavernous epidermoid tumor presenting with abducens nerve paresis—case report. Neurologia Medico-Chirurgica 32, 360–364, 1992.
368. Ilhan O, Sener EC, Ozyar E. Outcome of abducens nerve paralysis in patients with nasopharyngeal carcinoma. Eur J Ophthalmol 12, 55–59, 2002.
369. Inchingolo P, Accardo A, DaPozzo S, Pensiero S, Perissutti P. Cyclopean and disconjugate adaptive recovery from post-saccadic drift in strabismic children before and after surgery. Invest Ophthalmol Vis Sci 36, 2897–2913, 1996.
370. Ing EB, Sullivan TJ, Clarke MP, Buncic JR. Oculomotor nerve palsies in children. J Ped Ophthalmol Strabismus 29, 331–336, 1992.
371. Irving EL, Goltz HC, Steinbach MJ, Kraft SP. Vertical latent nystagmus component and vertical saccadic asymmetries in subjects with dissociated vertical deviation. J AAPOS 2, 344–350, 1998.
372. Ito K, Mizutani J, Murofushi T, Mizuno M. Bilateral pseudo-internuclear ophthalmoplegia in myasthenia gravis. ORL J Otorhinolaryngol Relat Spec 59, 122–126, 1997.
373. Iwabuchi T, Suzuki M, Nakaoka T, Suzuki S. Oculomotor nerve anastomosis. Neurosurgery 10, 490–491, 1982.
374. Jackowski A, Weiner G, O'Reilly G. Trochlear nerve schwannoma: a case report and literature review. Br J Neurosurg 8, 219–223, 1994.

375. Jacobs BC, Endtz H, van der Meche FG, et al. Serum anti-GQ1b IgG antibodies recognize surface epitopes on Campylobacter jejuni from patients with Miller Fisher syndrome.Ann Neurol 37, 260–264, 1995.
376. Jacobs BC, O'Hanlon GM, Bullens RW, et al. Immunoglobulins inhibit pathophysiological effects of anti-GQ1b-positive sera at motor nerve terminals through inhibition of antibody binding. Brain 126, 2220–2234, 2003.
377. Jacobson DM. Progressive ophthalmoplegia with acute ischemic abducens palsies. Am J Ophthalmol 122, 278–279, 1996.
378. Jacobson DM. Pupil involvement in patients with diabetes-associated oculomotor nerve palsy. Arch Ophthalmol 116, 723–727, 1998.
379. Jacobson DM. Dysthyroid orbitopathy. Semin Neurol 20, 43–54, 2000.
380. Jacobson DM, Broste SK. Early progression of ophthalmoplegia in patients with ischemic oculomotor nerve palsies. Arch Ophthalmol 113, 1535–1537, 1995.
381. Jacobson DM, Moster ML, Eggenberger ER, Galetta SL, Liu GT. Isolated trochlear nerve palsy in patients with multiple sclerosis. Neurology 53, 877–879, 1999.
382. Jacobson DM, Pesicka GA. Transient superior oblique palsy following arterial ligation for epistaxis. Ann Ophthalmol 109, 320–321, 1991.
383. Jacobson DM, Warner JJ, Choucair AK, Ptacek LJ. Trochlear nerve palsy following minor head trauma. A sign of structural disorder. J Clin Neuroophthalmol 8, 263–268, 1988.
384. Jacobson DM, Warner JJ, Ruggles KH. Transient trochlear nerve palsy following anterior temporal lobectomy for epilepsy. Neurology 45, 1465–1468, 1995.
385. Jaggi GP, Laeng HR, Müntener M, Killer HE. The anatomy of the muscle innervation (scleromuscular junction) of the lateral and medial rectus muscle in humans. Invest Ophthalmol Vis Sci 46, 2258–2263, 2005.
386. James W. The sense of dizziness in deaf-mutes. Am J Otol 4, 239–254, 1882.
387. Jay WM, Nazarian SM, Underwood DW. Pseudo-internuclear ophthalmoplegia with downshoot in myasthenia gravis. J Clin Neuroophthalmol 7, 74–76, 1987.
388. Jeannet PY, Bassez G, Eymard B, et al. Clinical and histological findings in autosomal centronuclear myopathy. Neurology 11, 1484–1490, 2004.
389. Jen J, Coulin CJ, Bosley TM, et al. Familial horizontal gaze palsy with progressive scoliosis maps to chromosome 11q23–25. Neurology 59, 432–435, 2002.
390. Jen JC, Chan WM, Bosley TM, et al. Mutations in a human ROBO gene disrupt hindbrain axon pathway crossing and morphogenesis. Science 304, 1509–1513, 2004.
391. Jinnai K, Hayashi Y. Hemorrhage in the oculomotor nerve as a complication of leukemia. Neuropathology. 21, 241–244, 2001.
392. Johnson EV, Kline LB, Julian BA, Garcia JH. Bilateral cavernous sinus thrombosis due to mucormycosis. Arch Neurol 106, 1089–1092, 1988.
393. Johnson LN, Hepler RS, Yee RD, Batzdorf U. Sphenoid sinus mucocele N (anterior clinoid variant) mimicking diabetic ophthalmoplegia and retrobulbar neuritis. Am J Ophthalmol 102, 111–115, 1986.
394. Johnston JL. Parasellar syndromes. Curr Neurol Neurosci Rep 2, 423–431, 2002.
395. Jordan DR, Miller DG, Anderson RL. Acquired oculomotor-abducens synkinesis. Can J Ophthalmol 25, 148–151, 1990.
396. Jordan K, Marino J, Damast M. Bilateral oculomotor paralysis due to neurosyphilis. Ann Neurol 3, 90–93, 1978.
397. Juncos JL, Beal MF. Idiopathic cranial polyneuropathy. A fifteen-year experience. Brain 110, 197–211, 1987.
398. Kambara C, Matsuo H, Fukudome T, Goto H, Shibuya N. Miller Fisher syndrome and plasmapheresis. Ther Apher 6, 450–453, 2002.
399. Kaminski HJ, Al-Hakim M, Leigh RJ, Katirji B, Ruff RL. Extraocular muscles are spared in advanced Duchenne dystrophy. Ann Neurol 32, 586–588, 1992.
400. Kaminski HJ, Kusner LL, Block CH. Expression of acetylcholine receptor isoforms at extraocular muscle endplates. Invest Ophthalmol Vis Sci 37, 345–351, 1996.
401. Kaminski HJ, Kusner LL, Nash KV, Ruff RL. The g-subunit of the acetylcholine receptor is not expressed in the levator palpebrae superioris. Neurology 45, 516, 1995.
402. Kaminski HJ, Li Z, Richmonds C, Ruff RL, Kusner L. Susceptibility of ocular tissues to autoimmune diseases. Ann N Y Acad Sci 998, 362–374, 2003.
403. Kaminski HJ, Maas E, Spiegel P, Ruff RL. Why are the eye muscles frequently involved in myasthenia gravis. Neurology 40, 1663–1669, 1990.
404. Kaminski HJ, Richmonds C, Lin F, Medof ME. Complement regulators in extraocular muscle and experimental autoimmune myasthenia gravis. Exp Neurol 189, 333–342, 2004.
405. Kaminski HJ, Richmonds CR, Kusner LL, Mitsumoto H. Differential susceptibility of the ocular motor system to disease. Ann N Y Acad Sci 956, 42–54, 2002.
406. Kaminski HJ, Ruff RL. Ocular muscle involvement by myasthenia gravis. Ann Neurol 41, 419–420, 1997.
407. Kaplan JG, Schaumburg HH, Sumner A. Relapsing ophthalmoparesis-sensory neuropathy syndrome. Neurology 35, 595–596, 1985.
408. Kars Z, Kansu T, Ozcan OE, Erbengi A. Orbital echinococcosis. J Clin Neuroophthalmol 2, 197–199, 1982.
409. Kashani S, Madil S, Tan C, Riordan-Eva P. Exercise-induced diplopia. Eye, In Press, 2005.
410. Kattah JC, FitzGibbon EJ. Superior oblique myokymia. Curr Neurol Neurosci Rep 3, 395–400, 2003.
411. Katz B, Rimmer S. Ophthalmoplegic migraine with superior ramus oculomotor paresis. J Clin Neuroophthalmol 9, 181–183, 1989.
412. Katz LJ, Lesser RL, Merikangas JR, Silverman JP. Ocular myasthenia gravis after D-penicillamine adminstration. Br J Ophthalmol 73, 1015–1018, 1989.
413. Kawasaki A. Oculomotor nerve schwannoma associated with ophthalmoplegic migraine. Am. J Ophthalmol 128, 658–660, 1999.
414. Kawase T, Shiobara R, Ohira T, Toya S. Developmen-

tal patterns and characteristic symptoms of petroclival meningiomas. Neurologia Medico-Chirurgica 36, 1–6, 1996.
415. Keane JR. Bilateral sixth nerve palsy. Analysis of 125 cases. Arch Neurol 33, 681–683, 1976.
416. Keane JR. Aneurysms and third nerve palsies. Ann Neurol 14, 696–697, 1983.
417. Keane JR. Acute bilateral ophthalmoplegia: 60 cases. Neurology 36, 279–281, 1986.
418. Keane JR. Trochlear nerve pareses with brainstem lesions. J Clin Neuroophthalmol 6, 242–246, 1986.
419. Keane JR. Isolated brain-stem third nerve palsy. Arch Neurol 45, 813–814, 1988.
420. Keane JR. Neurologic eye signs following motorcycle accidents. Arch Neurol 46, 761–762, 1989.
421. Keane JR. Neuro-ophthalmological signs of AIDS: 50 patients. Neurology 41, 841–845, 1991.
422. Keane JR. Fourth nerve palsy: historical review and study of 215 inpatients. Neurology 43, 2439–2443, 1993.
423. Keane JR. Third-nerve palsy due to penetrating trauma. Neurology 43, 1523–1527, 1993.
424. Keane JR. Aneurysmal third-nerve palsy presenting with pleocytosis. Neurology 48, 1176, 1996.
425. Keane JR, Zaias B, Itabashi HH. Levator-sparing oculomotor nerve palsy caused by a solitary midbrain metastasis. Arch Neurol 41, 210–212, 1984.
426. Kearns TP, Sayre GP. Retinitis pigmentosa, external ophthalmoplegia and complete heart block. Arch Ophthalmol 60, 280–289, 1958.
427. Keith CG. Oculomotor nerve palsy in childhood. Austr N Z J Ophthalmol 15, 181, 1987.
428. Keith CG, Webb G, Roger JG. Absence of a lateral rectus muscle associated with duplication chromosome segment 7q32–>q34. J Med Genetics 25, 122–127, 1988.
429. Kellen RI, Burde RM, Hodges FJ, Roper-Hall G. Central bilateral sixth nerve palsy associated with a unilateral preganglionic Horner's syndrome. J Clin Neuroophthalmol 8, 179–184, 1988.
430. Keller EL, Robinson DA. Absence of a stretch reflex in extraocular muscles of the monkey. J Neurophysiol 34, 908–919, 1971.
431. Keltner JL, Satterfield D, Dublin AB, Lee BCP. Dural and carotid cavernous sinus fistulas. Diagnosis, management and complications. Ophthalmology 94, 1585–1600, 1987.
432. Kerr FWL, Hollowell OW. Location of pupillomotor and accommodation fibres in the oculomotor nerve: experimental observations on paralytic mydriasis. J Neurol Neurosurg Psychiatry 27, 473–481, 1964.
433. Kersten RC. Blowout fracture of the orbital floor with entrapment caused by isolated trauma to the orbital rim. Am J Ophthalmol 103, 215–220, 1987.
434. Khanna S, Cheng G, Gong B, Mustari MJ, Porter JD. Genome-wide transcriptional profiles are consistent with functional specialization of the extraocular muscle layers. Invest Ophthalmol Vis Sci 45, 3055–3066, 2005.
435. Khurana TS, Prendergast RA, Alameddine HS, et al. Absence of extraocular pathology in Duchenne's muscular dystrophy: role for calcium homeostasis in extraocular muscle sparing. J Exp Med 182, 467–475, 1995.
436. Kiechl S, Horvath R, Luoma P, et al. Two families with autosomal dominant progressive external ophthalmoplegia. J Neurol Neurosurg Psychiatry 75, 1125–1128, 2004.
437. Kim JH, Hwang JM. Presence of the abducens nerve according to the type of Duane's retraction syndrome. Ophthalmology 112, 109–113, 2005.
438. King AJ, Stacey E, Stephenson G, Trimble RB. Spontaneous recovery rates for unilateral sixth nerve palsies. Eye 9, 476–478, 1995.
439. King RA, Calhoun JH. Fourth cranial nerve palsy following spinal anesthesia. J Clin Neuroophthalmology 7, 20–22, 1987.
440. Kissel JT, Burde RM, Klingele TG, Zeiger HE. Pupil-sparing oculomotor palsies with internal carotid-posterior communicating artery aneurysms. Ann Neurol 13, 149–154, 1983.
441. Kjellgren D, Thornell LE, Virtanen I, Pedrosa-Domellof F. Laminin isoforms in human extraocular muscles. Invest Ophthalmol Vis Sci 45, 4233–4239, 2004.
442. Kjellgren D, Thornwell L-E, Andersen J, Pedrosa-Domellof F. Myosin heavy chain isoforms in human extraocular muscles. Invest Ophthalmol Vis Sci 44, 1419–1425, 2003.
443. Klier EM, Meng H, Angelaki DE. Abducens nerve/nucleus stimulation produces knematically correct three-dimensional eye movement. Soc Neurosci Abstr 475.4, 2005.
444. Klingele TG, Burde RM, Kissel JT, Zeiger HE. Pupil sparing oculomotor palsy. Ann Neurol 14, 698, 1983.
445. Knapp CM, Gottlob I. Benign recurrent abducens (6th) nerve palsy in two children. Strabismus 12, 13–16, 2004.
446. Knosp E, Perneczky A, Koos WT, Fries G, Matula C. Meningiomas of the space of the cavernous sinus. Neurosurgery 38, 434–442, 1996.
447. Kobayashi S, Mukuno K, Tazaki Y, Ishikawa S, Okada K. Oculomotor nerve nuclear complex syndrome. A case with clinicopathological correlation. Neuro-ophthalmology 6, 55–59, 1986.
448. Koca MR, Horn F, Korth M. Alterations of saccadic eye movements in myotonic dystrophy. Graefe's Arch Clin Exp Ophthalmol 230, 437–441, 1992.
449. Kodsi SR, Younge BR. Acquired oculomotor, trochlear, and abducent cranial nerve palsies in pediatric patients. Am J Ophthalmol 114, 568–574, 1992.
450. Koga H, Gilbert M, Li J, et al. Antecedent infections in Fisher Syndrome. A common pathogenesis of molecular mimicry. Neurology 64, 1605–1611, 2005.
451. Komai K, Mimura O, Vyama J, et al. Neuro-ophthalmological evaluation of superior oblique myokymia. Neuroophthalmology 12, 135–140, 1992.
452. Kommerell G. The dynamic head-tilt test and the concept of a supranuclear trochlear palsy. Germ J Ophthalmol 3, 186–188, 1994.
453. Kommerell G, Bach M. A new type of Duane's syndrome. Twitch abduction on attempted upgaze and V-incomitance due to misinnervation of the lateral rectus by superior rectus neurons. Neuro-ophthalmology 6, 159–164, 1986.
454. Kommerell G, Klein U. Adaptive changes of the otolith-ocular reflex after injury to the trochlea. Neuroophthalmology 6, 101–107, 1986.
455. Kommerell G, Mehdorn E, Ketelsen UP, Vollrath-Junger C. Oculomotor palsy with cyclic spasms. Electromyographic and electron microscopic evi-

dence of chronic peripheral neuronal involvement. Neuroophthalmology 8, 9–21, 1988.
456. Kommerell G, Olivier D, Theopold H. Adaptive programming of phasic and tonic components in saccadic eye movements. Investigations in patients with abducens palsy. Invest Ophthalmol Vis Sci 15, 657–660, 1976.
457. Kommerell G, Schaubele G. Superior oblique myokymia. An electromyographical analysis. Trans Ophthal Soc U K 100, 504–506, 1980.
458. Kömpf D, Erbguth F, Kreiten K, Druschky K-F, Hacke W. Bilateral third nerve palsy in basilar vertebral artery disease. Neuroophthalmology 7, 355–362, 1987.
459. Konishi T, Saida T, Nishitani H. Orbital apex syndrome caused by rheumatoid nodules. J Neurol Neurosurg Psychiatry 49, 460–462, 1986.
460. Kono R, Poukens V, Demer JL. Superior oblique muscle layers in monkeys and humans. Invest Ophthalmol Vis Sci 46, 2790–2799, 2005.
461. Kornberg AJ, Pestronk A, Blume GM, et al. Selective staining of the cerebellar molecular layer by serum IgG in Miller-Fisher and related syndromes. Neurology 47, 1317–1320, 1996.
462. Kosmorsky G, Mehta N, Mitsumoto H, Prayson R. Intermittent esotropia associated with rippling muscle disease. J Neuroophthalmology 15, 147–151, 1995.
463. Kosmorsky GS, Ellis BD, Fogt N, Leigh RJ. The treatment of superior oblique myokymia utilizing the Harada-Ito procedure. J Neuropphthalmology 15, 142–146, 1995.
464. Kosmorsky GS, Hanson MR, Tomsak RL. Carotid-cavernous fistula presenting as painful ophthalmoplegia without external ocular signs. J Clin Neuroophthalmol 8, 131–135, 1988.
465. Kosmorsky GS, Tomsak RL. Ischemic ("diabetic") cavernous sinus syndrome. J Clin Neuroophthalmol 6, 96–99, 1986.
466. Kourouyan HD, Horton JC. Transneuronal retinal input to the primate Edinger-Westphal nucleus. J Comp Neurol 381, 68–80, 1997.
467. Kraus RR, Kattah J, Bortolotti C, Lanzino G. Oculomotor palsy from an unruptured posterior communicating artery aneurysm presenting with cerebrospinal fluid pleocytosis and enhancement of the third cranial nerve. Case report. J Neurosurg. 101, 352–353, 2004.
468. Kremer H, Kuyt LP, van den Helm B, et al. Localization of a gene for Möbius syndrome to chromosome 3q by linkage analysis in a Dutch family. Hum Mol Genet 5, 1367–1371, 1996.
469. Krishna R, Kosmorsky GS, Wright KW. Pseudotumor cerebri sine papilledema with unilateral sixth nerve palsy. J Neuroophthalmol 18, 53–55, 1998.
470. Krohel GB, Mansour AM, Petersen WL, Evenchik B. Isolated trochlear nerve palsy secondary to a juvenile pilocytic astrocytoma. J Clin Neuroophthalmol 2, 119–123, 1982.
471. Kruger M, Noel P, Ectors P. Bilateral primary traumatic oculomotor nerve palsy. J Trauma 26, 1151–1153, 1986.
472. Kruis JA, Houtman WA, van Weerden TW. Congenital absence of conjugate horizontal eye movements. Doc Ophthalmol 67, 13–18, 1987.
473. Ksiazek SM, Repka MX, Maguire A, et al. Divisional oculomotor nerve paresis caused by intrinsic brainstem disease. Ann Neurol 26, 714–718, 1989.
474. Ksiazek SM, Slamovits TL, Rosen CE, Burde RM, Parisi F. Fascicular arrangement in partial oculomotor paresis. Am J Ophthalmol 118, 97–103, 1994.
475. Kuncl RW, Hoffman PN. In Miller NR, Newman NJ (eds). Walsh and Hoyt's Clinical Neuro-ophthalmology. Vol. 1. 5th edition. Williams and Wilkins, Baltimore, 1998, pp 1351–1460.
476. Kupersmith MJ, Berenstein A, Flamm E, Ransohoff J. Neuroopthalmologic abnormalities and intravascular therapy of traumatic carotid cavernous fistulas. Ophthalmology 93, 906–912, 1986.
477. Kupersmith MJ, Fazzone HE. Comparing ocular muscle limitation tests for clinical trial use. Arch Ophthalmol 122, 347–348, 2004.
478. Kupersmith MJ, Latkany R, Homel P. Development of generalized disease at 2 years in patients with ocular myasthenia gravis. Arch Neurol 60, 243–248, 2003.
479. Kupersmith MJ, Martin V, Heller G, Shah A, Mitnick HJ. Idiopathic hypertrophic pachymeningitis. Neurology 62, 686–694, 2004.
479a. Kupersmith MJ, Ying G. Ocular motor dysfunction and ptosis in ocular myasthenia gravis: effects of treatment. Br J Ophthalmol 89, 1330–1334, 2005.
480. Kushner BJ. Simulated superior oblique palsy. Ann Ophthalmol 13, 337–343, 1981.
481. Kushner BJ. Fixation switch diplopia. Arch Ophthalmol 113, 896–899, 1995.
482. Kusuhara T, Nakajima M, Imamura A. Ocular myasthenia gravis associated with euthyroid ophthalmopathy. Muscle Nerve 28, 764–766, 2003.
483. Kwan ESK, Wolpert SM, Hedges TR, Laucella M. Tolosa-Hunt syndrome revisited: not necessarily a diagnosis of exclusion. AJR Am J Roentgenol 150, 413–418, 1988.
484. Kwon JH, Kwon SU, Ahn HS, Sung KB, Kim JS. Isolated superior rectus palsy due to contralateral midbrain infarction. Arch Neurol 60, 1633–1635, 2003.
485. Laguna JF, Smith MS. Aberrant regeneration in idiopathic oculomotor nerve palsy. J Neurosurg 52, 854–856, 1980.
486. Lam S, Margo CE, Beck R, Pusateri TJ, Pascucci S. Cavernous sinus syndrome as the initial manifestation of multiple myeloma. J Clin Neuroophthalmol 7, 135–138, 1987.
487. Lamarca J, Casquero P, Pou A. Mononeuritis multiplex in Waldenstrom's macroglobulinemia. Ann Neurol 22, 268–272, 1987.
488. Lancaster WB. Detecting, measuring, plotting and interpreting ocular deviations. Arch Ophthalmol 22, 867–880, 1939.
489. Landan I, Policheria H, McLaurin J. Complete external ophthalmoplegia in a case of pseudotumor cerebri. Headache 27, 573–574, 1987.
490. Lapresle J, Lasjaunias P. Cranial nerve ischemic arterial syndromes. A review. Brain 109, 207–215, 1986.
491. Lavin PJM, Younkin SG, Kori SH. The pathology of ophthalmoplegia in herpes zoster ophthalmicus. Neuroophthalmology 4, 75–80, 1984.
492. Lee C, Zee DS, Straumann D. Saccades from torsional offset positions back to listing's plane. J Neurophysiol 83, 3241–3253, 2000.

493. Lee J, Flynn JT. Bilateral superior oblique palsies. Br J Ophthalmol 69, 508–513, 1985.
494. Lee J, Harris S, Cohen J, et al. Results of a prospective randomized trial of botulinum toxin therapy in acute unilateral sixth nerve palsy. J Ped Ophthalmol Strabismus 31, 283, 1994.
495. Lee JP. Superior oblique myokymia. A possible etiologic factor. Arch Ophthalmol 102, 1178–1179, 1984.
496. Lee MS, Galetta SL, Volpe NJ, Liu GT. Sixth nerve palsies in children. Pediatr Neurol 20, 49–52, 1999.
497. Legge RH, Hedges TRI, Anderson M, Reese PD. Hypertropia following trochlear trauma. J Ped Ophthalmol Strabismus 29, 163–166, 1992.
498. Leigh RJ, Good EF, Rudy RP. Ophthalmoplegia due to actinomycosis. J Clin Neuroophthalmol 6, 157–159, 1986.
499. Leigh RJ, Thurston SE, Tomsak RL, Grossman GE, Lanska DJ. Effect of monocular visual loss upon stability of gaze. Invest Ophthalmol Vis Sci 30, 288–292, 1989.
500. Leigh RJ, Tomsak RL, Grant MP, et al. Effectiveness of botulinum toxin administered to abolish acquired nystagmus. Ann Neurol 32, 633–642, 1992.
501. Leigh RJ, Tomsak RL, Seidman SH, Dell'Osso LF. Superior oblique myokymia. Quantitative characteristics of the eye movements in three patients. Arch Ophthalmol 109, 1710–1713, 1991.
502. Lennerstrand G, Tian S, Han Y. Effects of eye muscle proprioceptive activation on eye position in normal and exotropic subjects. Graefe's Arch Clin Exp Ophthalmol 235, 63–69, 1997.
503. Leonard TJK, Moseley IF, Sanders MD. Ophthalmoplegia in carotid cavernous sinus fistula. Br J Ophthalmol 68, 128–134, 1984.
504. Lepore FE. Disorders of ocular motility following head trauma. Arch Neurol 52, 924–926, 1995.
505. Lepore FE, Glaser JS. Misdirection revisited. A critical appraisal of acquired oculomotor nerve synkinesis. Arch Ophthalmol 98, 2206–2209, 1980.
506. Lessell S, Coppeto J, Samet S. Opthalmoplegia in myotonic dystrophy. Am J Ophthalmol 71, 1231–1235, 1971.
507. Leung AKC. Transient sixth cranial nerve palsy in newborn infants. Br J Clin Pract 41, 717–718, 1987.
508. Lewis AI, Tomsick TA, Tew JM Jr. Management of 100 consecutive direct carotid-cavernous fistulas: results of treatment with detachable balloons. Neurosurgery 36, 239–244, 1995.
509. Lewis RF, Gaymard BM, Tamargo RJ. Efference copy provides the eye position information required for visually guided reaching. J Neurophysiol 80, 1605–1608, 1998.
510. Lewis RF, Zee DS. Abnormal spatial localization with trigeminal-oculomotor synkinesis. Evidence for a proprioceptive effect. Brain 116, 1105–1118, 1993.
511. Lewis RF, Zee DS, Gaymard B, Guthrie B. Extraocular muscle proprioception functions in the control of ocular alignment and eye movement conjugacy. J Neurophysiol 71, 1028–1031, 1994.
512. Lewis RF, Zee DS, Hayman MR, Tamargo RJ. Oculomotor function in the rhesus monkey after deafferentation of the extraocular muscles. Exp Brain Res 141, 349–358, 2001.
513. Lewis RF, Zee DS, Repka MX, Guyton DL, Miller NR. Regulation of static and dynamic ocular alignment in patients with trochlear nerve paresis. Vision Res 35, 3255–3264, 1995.
514. Liang TW, Balcer LJ, Solomon D, Messe SR, Galetta SL. Supranuclear gaze palsy and opsoclonus after Diazinon poisoning. J Neurol Neurosurg Psychiatry 74, 677–679, 2003.
515. Lindblom B, Westheimer G, Hoyt WF. Torsional diplopia and its perceptual consequences. Neuro-ophthalmology 18, 105–110, 1997.
516. Lingawi SS. Oculomotor nerve schwannoma: MRI appearance. Clin Imaging 24, 86–88, 2000.
517. Lipson AH, Webster WS, Brown-Woodman PD, Osborn RA. Moebius syndrome: animal model - human correlations and evidence for a brainstem vascular etiology. Teratology 40, 339–350, 1989.
518. Liu GT, Carrazana EJ, Charness ME. Unilateral oculomotor palsy and bilateral ptosis from paramedian midbrain infarction. Arch Neurol 48, 983–986, 1991.
519. Liu GT, Crenner CW, Logigian EL, Charness ME, Samuels MA. Midbrain syndromes of Benedikt, Claude, and Nothnagel: setting the record straight. Neurology 42, 1820–1822, 1992.
520. Liu GT, Hertle RW, Quinn GE, Schaffer DB. Comitant esodeviation resulting from neurologic insult in children. J AAPOS 1, 143–146, 1997.
521. Liu GT, Kay MD, Byrne GE, Glaser JS, Schatz N. Ophthalmoparesis due to Burkitt's lymphoma following cardiac transplantation. Neurology 43, 2147–2149, 1993.
522. Lo PA, Harper CG, Besser M. Intracavernous schwannoma of the abducens nerve: a review of the clinical features, radiology and pathology of an unusual case. J Clin Neurosci 8, 357–360, 2001.
523. Loewenfeld IE, Thompson HS Oculomotor paresis with cyclic spasms. A critical review of the literature and a new case. Surv Ophthalmol 20, 81–124, 1975.
524. Lopez R, David NJ, Gargano F, Post JD. Bilateral sixth nerve palsies in a patient with massive pituitary adenoma. Neurology 31, 1137–1138, 1981.
525. Lossos A, Averbuch-Heller L, Reches A, Abramsky O. Complete unilateral ophthalmoplegia as the presenting manifestation of Waldenström's macroglobulinemia. Neurology 40, 1801–1802, 1990.
526. Lossos A, Baala L, Soffer D, Averbuch-Heller L, et al. A novel autosomal recessive myopathy with external ophthalmoplegia linked to chromosome 17p13.1–p12. Brain 128, 42–51, 2005.
527. Lui F, Fonda S, Merlini L, Corazza R. Saccadic eye movements are impaired in Duchenne muscular dystrophy. Doc Ophthalmol 103, 219–228, 2001.
528. Lukas JR, Aigner M, Blumer R, Heinzl H, Mayr R. Number and distribution of neuromuscular spindles in human extraocular muscles. Invest Ophthalmol Vis Sci 35, 4317–4327, 1994.
529. Lukas JR, Blumer R, Denk M, et al. Innervated myotendinous cylinders in human extraocular muscles. Invest Ophthalmol Vis Sci 41, 2422–2431, 2000.
530. Lustbader JM, Miller NR. Painless pupil-sparing but otherwise complete oculomotor nerve paresis caused by basilar artery aneurysm. Arch Ophthalmol 106, 583–584, 1988.
531. Lyon DB, Lemke BN, Wallow IH, Dortzbach RK. Sympathetic nerve anatomy in the cavernous sinus and retrobulbar orbit of the cynomolgus monkey. Ophthalmic Plastic Reconstr Surg 8, 1–12, 1992.

531a. Makki ML, Newman NJ. A trochlear stroke. Neurology 65, 1988, 2005.
532. Manabe Y, Kurokawa K, Kashihara K, Abe K. Isolated oculomotor nerve palsy in lymphoma. Neurol Res 22, 347–348, 2000.
533. Mansour AM, Reinecke RD. Central trochlear palsy. Surv Ophthalmol 30, 279–297, 1986.
534. Mariak Z, Mariak Z, Stankiewicz A. Cranial nerve II-VII injuries in fatal closed head trauma. Eur J Ophthalmol 7, 68–72, 1997.
535. Marinho RO. Abducent nerve palsy following dental local anesthesia. Br Dental J 179, 69–70, 1995.
536. Marinkovic S, Gibo H, Zelic O, Nikodijevic I. The neurovascular relationships and the blood supply of the trochlear nerve: surgical anatomy of its cisternal segment. Neurosurgery 38, 161–169, 1996.
537. Markwalder T-M, Meienberg O. Acute painful cavernous sinus syndrome in unruptured intracavernous aneurysms of the internal carotid artery. J Clin Neuroophthalmol 3, 31–35, 1983.
538. Marshman WE, Schalit G, Jones RB, et al. Congenital anomalies in patients with Duane retraction syndrome and their relatives. J AAPOS 4, 106–109, 2000.
539. Maruo T, Kubota N, Arimoto H, Kikuchi R. Duane's syndrome. Jap J Ophthalmol 23, 453–468, 1979.
540. Mascarenhas L, Magalhaes Z, Honavar M, et al. Schwannoma of the abducens nerve in the cavernous sinus. Acta Neurochir (Wien.) 146, 389–392, 2004.
541. Maselli R, Jacobsen JH, Spire J-P. Edrophonium: an aid in the diagnosis of acute organophosphate poisoning. Ann Neurol 19, 508–510, 1986.
542. Maselli RA, Ellis W, Mandler RN, et al. Cluster of wound botulism in California: clinical, electrophysiologic, and pathologic study. Muscle and Nerve 20, 1284–1295, 1997.
543. Mastrianni JA, Galetta SL, Raps EC, Liu GT, Volpe NJ. Isolated fascicular abducens nerve palsy and Lyme disease. J Neuroophthalmology 14, 2–5, 1994.
544. Matsukawa Y, Nishinarita S, Horie T. Abducent and trochlear palsies in a patient with Sjögren's syndrome. Br J Rheumatology 34, 484–485, 1995.
545. Mauri L, Meienberg O, Roth E, Konig MP. Evaluation of endocrine ophthalmopathy with saccadic eye movements. J Neurol 231, 182–187, 1984.
546. Mauriello JA Jr., Antonacci R, Mostafavi R, et al. Combined paresis and restriction of the extraocular muscles after orbital fracture: a study of 16 patients. Ophthalmic Plastic Reconstr Surg 12, 206–210, 1996.
547. Maxwell GF, Lemij HG, Collewijn H. Conjugacy of saccades in deep amblyopia. Invest Ophthalmol Vis Sci 36, 2514–2522, 1995.
548. May PJ, Porter JD. The distribution of primary afferent terminals from the eyelids of macaque monkeys. Exp Brain Res 123, 368–381, 1998.
549. McCall S, Wagenhorst BB. Painful ophthalmoplegia caused by hemangiopericytoma of the cavernous sinus. J Neuroophthalmology 15, 98–101, 1995.
550. McCammon A, Kaufman HH, Sears ES. Transient oculomotor paralysis in pseudotumor cerebri. Neurology 31, 182–184, 1981.
550a. McClung JR, Allman BL, Dimitrova DM, Goldberg SJ. Extraocular connective tissues: a role in human eye movements? Invest Ophthalmol Vis Sci 47, 202–205, 2006.
551. McCreery KM, Hussein MA, Lee AG, et al. Major review: the clinical spectrum of pediatric myasthenia gravis: blepharoptosis, ophthalmoplegia and strabismus. A report of 14 cases. Binocul Vis Strabismus Q 17, 181–186, 2002.
552. McFarland R, Taylor R, Turnbull D. The neurology of mitochondrial DNA disease. Lancet 1, 343–351, 2002.
553. McNeer KW, Tucker MG, Spencer RF. Botulinum toxin management of essential infantile esotropia in children. Arch Ophthalmol 115, 1411–1418, 1997.
554. Meadows JC. Observations on a case of monocular diplopia of cerebral origin. J Neurol Sci 18, 249–253, 1973.
555. Mehel E, Quere MA, Lavenant F, Pechereau A. Epidemiological and clinical aspects of Stilling-Turk-Duane syndrome. J Francais Ophthalmologie 19, 533–542, 1996.
556. Mehta AM, Demer JL. Magnetic resonance imaging of the superior oblique muscle in superior oblique myokymia. J Ped Ophthalmol Strabismus 31, 378–383, 1994.
557. Meienberg O. Lesion site in Fisher's syndrome. Arch Neurol 41, 250–251, 1984.
558. Meienberg O, Büttner-Ennever JA, Kraus-Ruppert R. Unilateral paralysis of conjugate gaze due to lesion of the abducens nucleus. Clinico-pathological case report. Neuroophthalmology 2, 47–52, 1981.
559. Meienberg O, Ryffel E. Supranuclear eye movement disorders in Fisher's syndrome of ophthalmoplegia, ataxia, and areflexia. Arch Neurol 40, 402–405, 1983.
560. Melen O, Cohen BA, Sharma L. Cavernous sinus syndrome and systemic lupus erythematosis. Neurology 42, 1842–1843, 1992.
561. Melis BJ, Cruysberg JR, van Gisbergen JA. Listing's plane dependence on alternating fixation in a strabismus patient. Vision Res 37, 1355–1366, 1997.
562. Messe SR, Shin RK, Liu GT, Galetta SL, Volpe NJ. Oculomotor synkinesis following a midbrain stroke. Neurology 57, 1106–1107, 2001.
563. Meyer E, Shauly Y, Goldsher D, Zonis S. Computerized tomographic radiography of traumatic simulated Brown syndrome. Binocular Vision 3, 135–140, 1988.
564. Migita DS, Devereaux MW, Tomsak RL. Cocaine and pupillary-sparing oculomotor nerve paresis. Neurology 49, 1466–1467, 1997.
565. Migliaccio AA, Cremer PD, Aw ST, et al. Vergence-mediated changes in the axis of eye rotation during the human vestibulo-ocular reflex can occur independent of eye position. Exp Brain Res 151, 238–248, 2003.
566. Milazzo S, Toussaint P, Proust F, Touzet G, Malthieu D. Ophthalmological aspects of pituitary apoplexy. Eur J Ophthalmol 6, 69–73, 1996.
567. Miller JM. Functional anatomy of normal human rectus muscles. Vision Res 29, 223–240, 1989.
568. Miller JM, Demer JL. New orbital constraints on eye rotations. In Fetter M, Haslwanter T, Misslisch H, Tweed D (eds). Three-Dimensional Kinematics of Eye, Head, and Limb Movements. Harwood Academic Publishing, The Netherlands, 1997.

569. Miller MT, Ray V, Owens P, Chen F. Möbius and Möbius-like syndromes. J Ped Ophthalmol Strabismus 26, 176–188, 1989.
570. Miller MT, Stromland K. Ocular motility in thalidomide embryopathy. J Ped Ophthalmol Strabismus 28, 47–54, 1991.
571. Miller MT, Stromland K. The mobius sequence: a relook. J AAPOS 3, 199–208, 1999.
572. Miller NR. Solitary oculomotor nerve palsy in childhood. Am J Ophthalmol 83, 106–111, 1977.
573. Miller NR, Biousse V, Hwang T, et al. Isolated acquired unilateral horizontal gaze paresis from a putative lesion of the abducens nucleus. J Neuro-ophthalmol 22, 204–207, 2002.
574. Miller NR, Kiel SM, Green WR, Clark AW. Unilateral Duane's retraction syndrome (Type 1). Arch Ophthalmol 100, 1468–1472, 1982.
575. Miller NR, Lee AG. Adult-onset acquired oculomotor nerve paresis with cyclic spasms: relationship to ocular neuromyotonia. Am J Ophthalmol 137, 70–76, 2004.
576. Miller NR, Monsein LH, Debrun GM, Tamargo RJ, Nauta HJ. Treatment of carotid-cavernous fistula using superior ophthalmic vein approach. J Neurosurg 83, 838–842, 1995.
577. Minken AW, van Gisbergen JA. A three-dimensional analysis of vergence movements at various levels of elevation. Exp Brain Res 101, 331–345, 1994.
578. Misslisch H, Tweed D, Fetter M, Sievering D, Koenig E. Rotational kinematics of the human vestibuloocular reflex .3. Listing's law. J Neurophysiol 72, 2490–2502, 1994.
579. Miyachi S, Negoro M, Handa T, Sugita K. Dural carotid cavernous sinus fistula presenting as isolated oculomotor nerve palsy. Surg Neurol 39, 105–109, 1993.
580. Miyao S, Takano A, Teramoto J, Fujitake S, Hashizume Y. Oculomotor nerve palsy due to intraneural hemorrhage in idiopathic thrombocytopenic purpura: a case report. Eur Neurol 33, 20–22, 1993.
581. Mizen TR, Burde RM, Klingele TG. Cryptogenic oculomotor nerve palsies in children. Am J Ophthalmol 100, 65–67, 1985.
582. Mizutani T, Aki M, Shiozzawa R, et al. Development of ophthalmoplegia in amyotrophic lateral sclerosis during long-term use of respirators. J Neurol Sci 99, 311–319, 1990.
583. Mombaerts I, Koornneef L. Current status in the treatment of orbital myositis. Ophthalmology 104, 402–408, 1997.
584. Moncayo J, Bogousslavsky J. Vertebro-basilar syndromes causing oculo-motor disorders. Curr Opin Neurol 16, 45–50, 2003.
585. Montecucco C, Caporali R, Pacchetti C, Turla M. Is Tolosa-Hunt syndrome a limited form of Wegener's granulomatosis? Report of two cases with anti-neutrophil cytoplasmic antibodies. Br J Rheumatol 32, 640–641, 1993.
586. Moorthy G, Behrens MM, Drachman DB, et al. Ocular pseudomyasthenia or ocular myasthenia "plus": a warning to clinicians. Neurology 39, 1150–1154, 1989.
587. Moraes C. Mitochondrial disorders. Curr Opin Neurol 9, 367–368, 1996.
588. Morgan DL, Proske U. Vertebrate slow muscle: its structure pattern of innervation and mechanical properties. Physiol Rev 64, 103–169, 1984.
589. Mori M, Kuwabara S, Fukutake T, Yuki N, Hattori T Clinical features and prognosis of Miller Fisher syndrome. Neurology 56, 1104–1106, 2001.
590. Morioka T, Matsushima T, Yokoyama N, et al. Isolated bilateral abducens nerve palsies caused by rupture of a vertebral artery aneurysm. J Clin Neuroophthalmol 12, 263–267, 1992.
591. Morris OC, O'Day J. Strabismus surgery in the management of diplopia caused by myasthenia gravis. Br J Ophthalmol 88, 832, 2004.
592. Morrow MJ, Kao GW, Arnold AC. Bilateral ocular neuromyotonia: oculographic correlations. Neurology 46, 264–266, 1996.
593. Morrow MJ, Sharpe JA, Ranalli PJ. Superior oblique myokymia associated with a posterior fossa tumor: oculographic correlation with an idiopathic case. Neurology 40, 367–370, 1990.
594. Moschner C, Moser A, Kömpf D. Bilateral oculomotor nerve palsy due to dolichoectasia of the basilar artery. Neuroophthalmology 17, 39–43, 1997.
595. Moschovakis AK, Scudder CA, Highstein SM. A structural basis for Hering's law: Projections to extraocular motoneurons. Science 248, 1118–1119, 1990.
596. Moster ML, Savino PJ, Sergott RC, Bosley TM, Schatz NJ. Isolated sixth-nerve palsies in younger adults. Arch Ophthalmol 102, 1328–1330, 1984.
597. Moulis H, Mamus SW. Isolated trochlear nerve palsy in a patient with Waldenstrom's macroglobinemia: complete recovery with combination therapy. Neurology 39, 1399, 1989.
598. Mrabet A, Fredj M, Gouider R. Claude syndrome caused by mesencephalic infarction: 2 cases. Rev Neurol (Paris) 151, 274–276, 1995.
599. Muchnick RS, Stoj M, Hornblass A. Traumatic inferior oblique muscle paresis. J Ped Ophthalmol Strabismus 22, 143–146, 1985.
600. Mudgil AV, Walker M, Steffen H, Guyton DL, Zee DS. Motor mechanisms of vertical fusion in individuals with superior oblique paresis. J AAPOS 6, 145–153, 2002.
601. Mulhern M, Keohane C, O'Connor G. Bilateral abducens nerve lesions in unilateral type 3 Duane's retraction syndrome. Br J Ophthalmol 78, 588–591, 1994.
602. Muneer A, Jones NS. Unilateral abducens nerve palsy: a presenting sign of sphenoid sinus mucocoeles. J Laryngology Otology 111, 644–646, 1997.
603. Müri RM, Chermann JF, Cohen L, Rivaud S, Pierrot-Deseilligny C. Ocular motor consequences of damage to the abducens nucleus area in humans. J Neuroophthalmology 16, 191–195, 1996.
604. Murray RI, Steven PSC. Congenital levator and lateral rectus muscle associated reflex. Neuroophthalmology 6, 29–31, 1986.
605. Mwanza JC, Nyamabo LK, Tylleskar T, Plant GT. Neuro-ophthalmological disorders in HIV infected subjects with neurological manifestations. Br J Ophthalmol 88, 1455–1459, 2004.
606. Nabors MW, McCrary ME, Fischer BA, Kobrine AI. Delayed abducens nerve palsies associated with cervical spine fractures. Neurology 37, 1565, 1987.
607. Nakagawa T, Uchida K, Ozveren MF, Kawase T.

Abducens schwannoma inside the cavernous sinus proper: case report. Surg Neurol 61, 559–563, 2004.
608. Nakamura M, Kaga K, Ohira Y. Metastatic hypopharyngeal carcinoma to the temporal bone. Eur Arch Oto-Rhino-Laryngol 253, 185–188, 1996.
609. Nakano M, Yamada K, Fain J, et al. Homozygous mutations in ARIX(PHOX2A) result in congenital fibrosis of the extraocular muscles type 2. Nat Genet 29, 315–320, 2001.
610. Nashold BS, Seaber JH. Defects of ocular motility after stereotactic midbrain lesions in man. Arch Ophthalmol 88, 245–248, 1972.
611. Nathan H, Goldhammer Y. The rootlets of the trochlear nerve. Acta Anat (Basel) 84, 590–596, 1973.
612. Natori Y, Rhoton AL Jr. Microscopical anatomy of the superior orbital fissure. Neurosurgery 36, 762–775, 1995.
613. Neel HBI. Nasopharyngeal carcinoma. Otolaryngol Clin North America 18, 479–490, 1985.
614. Neetens A, Martin JJ, Brais B, et al. Oculopharyngeal muscular dystrophy (OPMD). Neuroophthalmology 17, 189–200, 1997.
615. Neigel JM, Rootman J, Robinson RG, Durity FA, Nugent RA. The Tolosa-Hunt syndrome: computer tomographic changes and reversal after steroid therapy. Can J Ophthalmol 21, 287–290, 1986.
616. Nelson JA, Wolf MD, Yuh WTC, Peeples ME. Cranial nerve involvement with Lyme borreliosis demonstrated by magnetic resonance imaging. Neurology 42, 671–673, 1992.
617. Netuka D, Benes V. Oculomotor nerve schwannoma. Br J Neurosurg 17, 168–173, 2003.
618. Newman NJ, Slamovits TL, Friedland S, Wilson WB. Neuro-ophthalmic manifestations of meningocerebral inflamation from the limited form of Wegener's granulomtosis. Am J Ophthalmol 120, 613–621, 1995.
619. Newman SA. Gaze-induced strabismus. Surv Ophthalmol 38, 303–309, 1993.
620. Newsom-Davis J. Myasthenia gravis and the Miller-Fisher variant of Guillain-Barré syndrome. Curr Opin Neurol 10, 18–21, 1997.
621. Newsom-Davis J, Mills KR. Immunological associations of acquired neuromyotonia (Isaac's syndrome). Brain 116, 453–469, 1993.
622. Niedermuller U, Trinka E, Bauer G. Abducens palsy after lumbar puncture. Clin Neurol Neurosurg 104, 61–63, 2002.
623. Nishimoto Y, Odaka M, Hirata K, Yuki N. Usefulness of anti-GQ1b IgG antibody testing in Fisher syndrome compared with cerebrospinal fluid examination. J Neuroimmunol 148, 200–205, 2004.
624. North KN, Anthony JH, Johnston IH. Dermoid of cavernous sinus resulting in isolated oculomotor nerve palsy. Pediatr Neurol 9, 221–223, 1993.
625. O'Connor PS, Tredici TJ, Green RP. Pupil-sparing third nerve palsies caused by aneurysm. Am J Ophthalmol 95, 395–397, 1983.
626. O'Duffy JD, Goldstein NP. Neurological involvement in seven patients with Behcet's disease. Am J Med 61, 170–178, 1976.
627. Oda K, Shibasaki H. Antigenic differences of acetylcholine receptors between single and multiple form endplates of human extraocular muscle. Brain Res 449, 337–340, 1988.
628. Odel JG, Winterkorn JMS, Behrens M. The sleep test: a safe alternative to Tensilon. J Clin Neuro-ophthalmol 11, 288–292, 1991.
629. Ogawara K, Kuwabara S, Yuki N. Fisher syndrome or Bickerstaff brainstem encephalitis? Anti-GQ1b IgG antibody syndrome involving both the peripheral and central nervous systems. Muscle Nerve 26, 845–849, 2002.
630. Ogilvy CS, Pakzaban P, Lee JM. Oculomotor nerve cavernous angioma in a patient with Roberts syndrome. Surg Neurol 40, 39–42, 1993.
631. Oh SY, Poukens V, Demer JL. Quantitative analysis of rectus extraocular layers in monkey and humans. Invest Ophthalmol Vis Sci 42, 10–16, 2001.
632. Ohtsuka K, Hashimoto M, Nakamura Y. Enhanced magnetic resonance imaging in a patient with acute paralysis of the inferior division of the oculomotor nerve. Am J Ophthalmol 124, 406–409, 1997.
633. Ohtsuka K, Hashimoto M, Nakamura Y. Bilateral trochlear nerve palsy with arachnoid cyst of the quadrigeminal cistern. Am J Ophthalmol 125, 268–270, 1998.
634. Ohtsuka K, Sone A, Igarashi Y, Akiba H, Sakata M. Vascular compressive abducens nerve palsy disclosed by magnetic resonance imaging. Am J Ophthalmol 122, 416–419, 1996.
635. Ohtsuki H, Hasebe S, Kono R, et al. Large Bielschowsky head-tilt phenomenon and inconspicuous vertical deviation in the diagnostic positions in congenital superior oblique palsy. Am J Ophthalmol 130, 854–856, 2000.
636. Ohtsuki H, Hasebe S, Okano M, Furuse T. Strabismus surgery in ocular myasthenia gravis. Ophthalmologica 210, 95–100, 1996.
637. Okada Y, Shima T, Nishida M, Okita S. Large sixth nerve neuroma involving the prepontine region: case report. Neurosurgery 40, 608–610, 1997.
638. Okamoto K, Hirai S, Amari M, et al. Oculomotor nuclear pathology in amyotrophic lateral sclerosis. Acta Neuropathol 85, 458–462, 1993.
639. Okamoto K, Ito J, Tokiguchi S, Furusawa T. Atrophy of bilateral extraocular muscles. CT and clinical features of seven patients. J Neuroophthalmol 16, 286–288, 1996.
640. Olson ME, Chernik NL, Posner JB. Infiltration of the leptomeninges by systemic cancer. Arch Neurol 30, 122–137, 1974.
641. Oohira A, Goto K, Sato Y, Ozawa T. Saccades of supernormal velocity. Adaptive response to ophthalmoplegia in a patient with myasthenia gravis. Neuroophthalmology 7, 203–209, 1987.
642. Oohira A, Masuzawa K. A case of congenital oblique retraction syndrome with upshoot in adduction. Strabismus 10, 39–44, 2002.
643. Oohira A, Zee DS. Disconjugate ocular motor adaptation in rhesus monkey. Vision Res 32, 489–497, 1992.
644. Oohira A, Zee DS, Guyton DL. Disconjugate adaptation to long-standing, large-amplitude, spectacle-corrected anisometropia. Invest Ophthalmol Vis Sci 32, 1693–1703, 1991.
645. Openshaw H, Slatkin NE, Smith E. Eye movement disorders in bone marrow transplantation patients on cyclosporin and ganciclovir. Bone Marrow Transplant 19, 503–505, 1997.
646. Optican LM, Zee DS, Chu FC. Adaptive response to ocular muscle weakness in human pursuit and saccadic eye movements. J Neurophysiol 54, 110–122, 1985.
647. Orwitz JI, Galetta SL, Teener JW. Bilateral trochlear

nerve palsy and downbeat nystagmus in a patient with cephalic tetanus. Neurology 49, 894–895, 1997.
648. Osher RH, Glaser JS. Myasthenic sustained gaze fatigue. Am J Ophthalmol 89, 443–445, 1980.
649. Ostergaard JR, Moller HU, Christensen T. Recurrent ophthalmoplegia in childhood: diagnostic and etiologic considerations. Cephalalgia 16, 276–279, 1996.
650. Ozveren MF, Sam B, Akdemir I, et al. Duplication of the abducens nerve at the petroclival region: an anatomic study. Neurosurgery 52, 645–652, 2003.
651. Pachter BR, Pearson J, Davidowitz J, et al. Congenital total external ophthalmoplegia associated with infantile spinal muscular atrophy. Fine structure of extraocular muscle. Invest Ophthalmol 15, 320–324, 1976.
652. Paparounas K. Anti-GQ1b ganglioside antibody in peripheral nervous system disorders: pathophysiologic role and clinical relevance. Arch Neurol 61, 1013–1016, 2004.
653. Papst W. Zur Differentialdiagnose der okulären Neuromyotonie. Ophthalmologica 164, 252–263, 1972.
654. Parks MM. Isolated cyclovertical muscle palsy. Arch Ophthalmol 60, 1027–1035, 1958.
655. Parsa CF, Grant E, Dillon WP, Jr., du Lac S, Hoyt WF. Absence of the abducens nerve in Duane syndrome verified by magnetic resonance imaging. Am J Ophthalmol 125, 399–401, 1998.
656. Paul TO, Hardage LK. The heritability of strabismus. Ophthalmic Genetics 15, 1–18, 1994.
657. Peatfield RC. Recurrent VI nerve palsy in cluster headache. Headache 25, 325–327, 1985.
658. Perenin MT, Jeannerod M, Prablanc C. Spatial localization with paralyzed eye muscles. Opthalmologica 175, 206–214, 1977.
659. Petermann SH, Newman NJ. Pituitary macroadenoma manifesting as an isolated fourth nerve palsy. Am. J Ophthalmol 127, 235–236, 1999.
660. Peters GB, III, Bakri SJ, Krohel GB. Cause and prognosis of nontraumatic sixth nerve palsies in young adults. Ophthalmology 109, 1925–1928, 2002.
661. Petersen P, Lindholm J. Pituitary apoplexy, the Houssay phenomenon, and accelerated proliferative retinopathy. Am J Med 79, 385–388, 1985.
662. Petrelli EA, Steller RE. Medial rectus muscle palsy after dental anesthesia. Am J Ophthalmol 90, 422–424, 1980.
663. Pfeiffer N, Simonsz H, Kommerell G. Misdirected regeneration of abducens nerve neurons into the parasympathetic pupillary pathway. Graefe's Arch Clin Exp Ophthalmol 230, 150–153, 1992.
664. Phillips MS, Stewart S, Anderson JR. Neuropathological findings in Miller Fisher syndrome. J Neurol Neurosurg Psychiatry 47, 492–495, 1984.
665. Piatt JH, Campbell GA, Oakes WJ. Papillary meningioma involving the oculomotor nerve in an infant. J Neurosurg 64, 808–812, 1986.
666. Pieh C, Lengyel D, Neff A, Fretz C, Gottlob I. Brainstem hypoplasia in familial horizontal gaze palsy and scoliosis. Neurology 59, 462–463, 2002.
667. Pierrot-Deseilligny C, Goasguen J. Isolated abducens nucleus damage due to histiocytosis X Brain 107, 1019–1032, 1984.
668. Pierrot-Deseilligny C, Michelin T. Pseudo-ophthalmoplegie internucleaire myasthenique. Rev Neurol (Paris) 139, 527–528, 1983.
669. Pinches E, Thompson D, Noordeen H, Liasis A, Nischal KK. Fourth and sixth cranial nerve injury after halo traction in children: a report of two cases. J AAPOS 8, 580–585, 2004.
670. Pinchoff BS, Spahlinger DA, Bergstrom TJ, Sandall GS. Extraocular muscle involvement in Wegener's granulomatosis. J Clin Neuroophthalmol 3, 163–168, 1983.
671. Plaitakis A, Tzagournissakis M, Christodoulou P, Jen JC, Baloh RW. Vestibular modification of congenital pendular nystagmus in HGPPS with the ROBO3 mutation [abstract]. Neurology 64(Suppl 1), A33. 2005.
672. Plum F, Posner JB. The Diagnosis of Stupor and Coma. FA Davis, Philadelphia, 1981.
673. Pollard ZF. Bilateral superior oblique muscle palsy associated with Apert's syndrome. Am J Ophthalmol 106, 337–340, 1988.
674. Poon W, Ng JK, Wong K, South JR. Primary intrasellar germinoma presenting with cavernous sinus syndrome. Surg Neurol 30, 402–405, 1988.
675. Porschke H, Kress W, Reichmann H, Goebel HH, Grimm T. Oculopharyngeal muscular dystrophy in a northern German family linked to chromosome 14q and presenting carnitine deficiency. Neuromuscul Disord 7 Suppl 1, S57–S62, 1997.
676. Porter JD. Brainstem terminations of extraocular muscle primary afferent neurons in the monkey. J Comp Neurol 247, 133–143, 1986.
677. Porter JD. Extraocular muscle: cellular adaptations for a diverse functional repertoire. Ann N Y Acad Sci 956, 7–16, 2002.
678. Porter JD, Baker RS. Muscles of a different 'color': the unusual properties of the extraocular muscles may predispose or protect them in neurogenic and myogenic disease. Neurology 46, 30–37, 1996.
679. Porter JD, Baker RS. Absence of oculomotor and trochlear motoneurons leads to altered extraocular muscle development in the Wnt-1 null mutant mouse. Brain Res Dev Brain Res 100, 121–126, 1997.
680. Porter JD, Baker RS. Anatomy and embryology of the ocular motor system. In Miller NR, Newman NJ (eds). Walsh and Hoyt's Clinical Neuro-ophthalmology. Vol. 1. 5th ed. Williams and Wilkins, Baltimore, 1998, pp 1043–1099.
681. Porter JD, Baker RS, Ragusa RJ, Brueckner JK. Extraocular muscles: basic and clinical aspects of structure and function. Surv Ophthalmol 39, 451–484, 1995.
682. Porter JD, Burns LA, McMahon EJ. Denervation of primate extraocular muscle. A unique pattern of structural alterations. Invest Ophthalmol Vis Sci 30, 1894–1908, 1989.
683. Porter JD, Guthrie BL, Sparks DL. Innervation of monkey extraocular muscles: Localization of sensory and motor neurons by retrograde transport of horseradish peroxidase. J Comp Neurol 218, 208–219, 1983.
684. Porter JD, Khanna S, Kaminski HJ. Extraocular muscle is defined by a fundamentally distinct gene expression profile. Proc Natl Acad Sci U S A 98, 12062–12067, 2001.
685. Porter JD, Merriam AP, Khanna S, et al. Constitutive properties, not molecular adaptations, mediate extraocular muscle sparing in dystrophic mdx mice. FASEB J 17, 893–895, 2003.
686. Porter JD, Rafael JA, Ragusa RJ, et al. The sparing of extraocular muscle in dystrophinopathy is lost in

mice lacking utrophin and dystrophin. J Cell Sci 111 (Pt 13), 1801–1811, 1998.
687. Porter NC, Salter BC. Ocular myasthenia gravis. Curr Treat Options Neurol 7, 79–88, 2005.
688. Posner JB. Neurological Complications of Cancer. FA Davis, Philadelphia, 1995.
689. Prats JM, Monzon MJ, Zuazo E, Garaizar C. Congenital nuclear syndrome of oculomotor nerve. Pediatr Neurol 9, 476–478, 1993.
690. Pratt DV, Orengo-Nania S, Horowitz BL, Oram O. Magnetic resonance imaging findings in a patient with nuclear oculomotor palsy. Ann Ophthalmol 113, 141–142, 1995.
691. Prepageran N, Subramaniam KN, Krishnan GG, Raman R. Ocular presentation of sphenoid mucocele. Orbit 23, 45–47, 2004.
692. Pusateri TJ, Sedwick LA, Margo CE. Isolated inferior rectus muscle palsy from a solitary metastasis to the oculomotor nucleus. Arch Ophthalmol 105, 675–677, 1987.
693. Qasho R, Vangelista T, Rocchi G, Ferrante L, Delfini R. Abducens nerve paresis as first symptom of trigeminal neurinoma. Report of two cases and review of the literature. J Neurosurg Sci 43, 223–228, 1999.
694. Quaia C, Optican LM. Commutative saccadic generator is sufficient to control a 3–D ocular plant with pulleys. J Neurophysiol 79, 3197–3215, 1998.
695. Ramon y Cajal S. Degeneration and Regeneration of the Nervous System. Oxford University Press, London, 1928.
696. Rangel-Guerra R, Martinez HR, Saenz C. Mucormycosis. Report of 11 cases. Arch Neurol 42, 578–581, 1985.
697. Rapoport S, Watkins PB. Descending paralysis resulting from occult wound botulism. Ann Neurol 16, 359–361, 1984.
698. Reddel SW, Barnett MH, Yan WX, Halmagyi GM, Pollard JD. Chronic ophthalmoplegia with anti-GQ1b antibody. Neurology 54, 1000–1002, 2000.
699. Reid RL, Quigley ME, Yen SSC. Pituitary apoplexy. A Review. Arch Neurol 42, 712–719, 1985.
700. Reifenberger G, Bostrom J, Bettag M, et al. Primary glioblastoma multiforme of the oculomotor nerve. Case report. J Neurosurg 84, 1062–1066, 1996.
701. Reshef E, Greenberg SB, Jankovic J. Herpes zoster ophthalmicus followed by contralateral hemiparesis: report of two cases and review of literature. J Neurol Neurosurg Psychiatry 48, 122–127, 1985.
702. Richards BW, Jones FR, Younge BR. Causes and prognosis in 4,278 cases of paralysis of the oculomotor trochlear and abducens nerves. Am J Ophthalmol 113, 489–496, 1992.
703. Richardson C, Smith T, Schaefer A, Turnbull D, Griffiths P. Ocular motility findings in chronic progressive external ophthalmoplegia. Eye 19, 258–263, 2005.
704. Ricker VK, Mertens HG. Okuläre Neuromyotonie. Klin Monatsbl Augenheilkd 156, 837–842, 1970.
705. Riggs JE, Bodensteiner JB, Schochet SS Jr. Congenital myopathies/dystrophies. Neurol Clin 21, 779–794, 2003.
706. Ringel SP, Wilson WB, Barden MT. Extraocular muscle biopsy in chronic progressive external ophthalmoplegia. Ann Neurol 6, 326–339, 1979.
707. Rivero A, Crovetto L, Lopez L, Maselli R, Nogues M. Single fiber electromyography of extraocular muscles: a sensitive method for the diagnosis of ocular myasthenia gravis. Muscle and Nerve 18, 943–947, 1995.
708. Robinson DA. Bielschowsky head-tilt test—II Quantitative mechanics of the Bielschowsky head-tilt test. Vision Res 25, 1983–1988, 1985.
709. Ropper AH. Unusual clinical variants and signs in Guillain-Barre syndrome. Arch Neurol 43, 1150–1152, 1986.
710. Ropper AH. Three patients with Fisher's syndrome and normal MRI. Neurology 38, 1630–1631, 1988.
711. Ropper AH, Cole D, Louis DN. Clinicopathological correlation in a case of pupillary dilatation from cerebral hemorrhage. Arch Neurol 48, 1166–1169, 1991.
712. Rosenbaum HE, Seaman WB. Neurologic manifestations of nasopharyngeal tumors. Neurology 5, 868–874, 1955.
713. Rosenstein ED, Sobelman J, Kramer N. Isolated, pupil-sparing third nerve palsy as initial manifestation of systemic lupus erythematosus. J Clin Neuroophthalmol 9, 285–288, 1989.
714. Rossi A, Catala M, Biancheri R, Di CR, Tortori-Donati P. MR imaging of brain-stem hypoplasia in horizontal gaze palsy with progressive scoliosis. AJNR Am J Neuroradiol 25, 1046–1048, 2004.
715. Rossitch E Jr., Carrazana EJ, Black PM. Isolated oculomotor nerve palsy following of a pituitary adenoma. J Neurosurg Sci 36, 103–105, 1992.
716. Round R, Keane JR. The minor symptoms of increased intracranial pressure: 101 patients with benign intracranial hypertension. Neurology 38, 1461–1464, 1988.
717. Rousseaux M, Leys D, Dubois F, LaFitte J-J, Petit H. Bilateral external ophthalmoplegia revealing an Eaton-Lambert syndrome. Neuroophthalmology 5, 207–210, 1985.
718. Rush JA. Isolated superior oblique paralysis in progressive systemic sclerosis. Ann Ophthalmol 13, 217–220, 1981.
719. Rush JA, Shafrin F. Ocular myasthenia presenting as superior oblique weakness. J Clin Neuroophthalmol 2, 125–127, 1982.
720. Rush JA, Younge BR. Paralysis of cranial nerves III, IV, and VI. Cause and prognosis in 1,000 cases. Arch Opthalmol 99, 76–79, 1981.
721. Ruskell GL. The fine structure of human extraocular muscle spindles and their potential proprioceptive capacity. J Anat 167, 199–214, 1989.
722. Ruskell GL. Extraocular muscle proprioceptors and proprioception. Prog Retin Eye Res 18, 269–291, 1999.
723. Ruskell GL, Haugen I-BK, Bruenech JR, Van der Werf F. Double insertions of extraocular rectus muscles in humans and the pulley theory. J Anat 206, 295–306, 2005.
724. Sacks JG. Peripheral innervation of extraocular muscles. Am J Ophthalmol 95, 520–527, 1983.
725. Sadun F, De Negri AM, Santopadre P, Pivetti PP. Bilateral trochlear nerve palsy associated with cryptococcal meningitis in human immunodeficiency virus infection. J Neuroophthalmol 19, 118–119, 1999.
726. Saeki N, Murai N, Sunami K. Midbrain tegmental

lesions affecting or sparing the pupillar fibers. J Neurol Neurosurg Psychiatry 61, 401–402, 1997.
727. Saeki N, Yamaura A, Sunami K. Bilateral ptosis with pupil sparing because of a discrete midbrain lesion: magnetic resonance imaging evidence of topographic arrangement within the oculomotor nerve. J Neuroophthalmol 20, 130–134, 2000.
728. Safran AB, Kline LB, Glaser JS, Daroff RB. Television-induced formed visual hallucinations and cerebral diplopia. Br J Ophthalmol 65, 707–711, 1981.
729. Safran AB, Magistris M. Terminating attacks of ocular neuromyotonia. J Neuroophthalmol 18, 47–48, 1998.
730. Sam B, Ozveren MF, Akdemir I, et al. The mechanism of injury of the abducens nerve in severe head trauma: a postmortem study. Forensic Sci Int 140, 25–32, 2004.
731. Samii M, Rosahl SK, Carvalho GA, Krzizok T. Microvascular decompression for superior oblique myokymia: first experience. Case report. J Neurosurg 89, 1020–1024, 1998.
732. Sanders SK, Kawasaki A, Purvin VA. Long-term prognosis in patients with vasculopathic sixth nerve palsy. Am J Ophthalmol 134, 81–84, 2002.
733. Santoreneos S, Hanieh A, Jorgensen RE. Trochlear nerve schwannomas occurring in patients without neurofibromatosis: case report and review of the literature. Neurosurgery 41, 282–287, 1997.
734. Sato K, Yoshikawa H. Bilateral abducens nerve paresis associated with anti-GQ1b IgG antibody. Am J Ophthalmol 131, 816–818, 2001.
735. Saul RF, Selhorst JB. Traumatic inferior division oculomotor palsy. Neurology 36 (Suppl 1), 250, 1986.
736. Savas R, Sommer A, Gueckel F, Georgi M. Isolated oculomotor nerve paralysis in Lyme disease. Neuroradiology 39, 139–141, 1997.
737. Savino PJ, Hilliker JK, Casell GH, Schatz NJ. Chronic sixth nerve palsies. Are they really harbingers of serious intracranial disease? Arch Ophthalmol 100, 1442–1444, 1982.
738. Sawle GV, Sarkies NJC. Bilateral fourth nerve palsy due to cerebellar haemangioblastoma. J R Soc Med 82, 111–112, 1989.
739. Scelsa SN, Simpson DM, Reichler BD, Dai M. Extraocular muscle involvement in Becker muscular dystrophy. Neurology 46, 564–566, 1996.
740. Schapira AHV, Thomas PK. A case of recurrent idopathic opthalmoplegic neuropathy (Miller Fisher syndrome). J Neurol Neurosurg Psychiatry 49, 463–464, 1986.
741. Scharwey K, Krzizok T, Samii M, Rosahl SK, Kaufmann H. Remission of superior oblique myokymia after microvascular decompression. Ophthalmologica 214, 426–428, 2000.
742. Schatz NJ, Savino PJ, Corbett JJ. Primary aberrant oculomotor regeneration. A sign of intracavernous meningioma. Arch Neurol 34, 29–32, 1977.
743. Schievink WI, Mokri B, Garrity JA, Nichols DA, Piegras DG. Ocular motor nerve palsies in spontaneous dissections of the cervical internal carotid artery. Neurology 43, 1938–1941, 1993.
744. Schmidt D. Congenitale Augenmuskelparesen. Albrecht Von Graefes Arch Klin Exp Ophthalm 192, 285–312, 1974.
745. Schmidt D, Dell'Osso LF, Abel LA, Daroff RB. Myasthenia gravis: saccadic eye movement waveforms. Exp Neurol 68, 346–364, 1980.
746. Schmidt D, Dell'Osso LF, Daroff RB. Myasthenia gravis: dynamic changes in saccadic waveform, gain, and velocity. Exp Neurol 68, 365–377, 1980.
747. Schumacher-Feero LA, Yoo KW, Solari FM, Biglan AW. Third cranial nerve palsy in children. Am J Ophthalmol 128, 216–221, 1999.
748. Scott AB. Botulinum toxin injection of eye muscles to correct strabismus. Trans Am Ophthalmol Soc 74, 734, 1981.
749. Scott AB, Collins CC Division of labor in human extraocular muscle. Arch Ophthalmol 90, 319–322, 1973.
750. Sebag J, Sadun AA. Aberrant regeneration of the third nerve following orbital trauma. Arch Neurol 40, 762–764, 1983.
751. Sedwick LA, Margo CE. Sixth nerve palsie, temporal artery biopsy, and necrotizing vasculitis. J Clin Neuroophthalmol 9, 119–121, 1989.
752. Segovia JG, Montilla P, Jimenez-Escrig A, Corral I, Gobernado JM. Isolated palsy of the third nerve nuclear complex caused by cerebral toxoplasmosis. Eur J Neurol 1, 91–92, 1994.
753. Seiff SR, Good WV. Hypertropia and posterior blowout fracture: mechanism and management. Ophthalmology 103, 152–156, 1996.
754. Sekizawa T, Nakamura S, Kogure K, et al. Idiopathic third cranial nerve palsy associated with herpes simplex virus infection. Br Med J 295, 813, 1987.
755. Selky AK, Purvin VA. Isolated trochlear nerve palsy secondary to dural carotid-cavernous sinus fistula. J Neuroophthalmol 14, 52–54, 1994.
756. Seo SW, Heo JH, Lee KY, et al. Localization of Claude's syndrome. Neurology 57, 2304–2307, 2001.
757. Sepehrnia A, Tatagiba M, Brandis A, Samii M, Prawitz R-H. Cavernous angioma of the cavernous sinus: case report. Neurosurgery 27, 151–157, 1990.
758. Sergott RC, Grossman RI, Savino PJ, Bosley TM, Schatz NJ. The syndrome of parodoxical worsening of dural-cavernous sinus arteriovenous malformations. Ophthalmology 94, 205–212, 1987.
759. Sethi DS, Lau DP, Chan C. Sphenoid sinus mucocele presenting with isolated oculomotor palsy. J Laryngol Otol 111, 471–473, 1997.
760. Sethi KD, Rivner MH, Swift TR. Ice pack test for myasthenia gravis. Neurology 37, 1383–1385, 1987.
761. Sevel D. Brown's syndrome—a possible etiology explained embryologically. J Ped Ophthalmol Strabismus 18, 26–31, 1981.
762. Shall MS, Goldberg SJ. Extraocular motor units: type classification and motoneuron stimulation frequency-muscle unit force relationships. Brain Res 587, 291–300, 1992.
763. Sharpe JA, McReelis K, Wong AM. Recovery of peripheral versus central nerves identified by saccadic velocity after abducens neuropathy. Ann N Y Acad Sci 1039, 417–429, 2005.
764. Sharpe JA, Silversides JL, Blain RDG. Familial paralysis of horizontal gaze. Associated with pendular nystagmus, progressive scoliosis and facial contraction with myokymia. Neurology 25, 1035–1040, 1975.
765. Sharpe JA, Tweed D, Wong AM. Adaptations and deficits in the vestibulo-ocular reflex after peripheral

ocular motor palsies. Ann N Y Acad Sci 1004, 111–121, 2003.
766. Shauly Y, Weissman A, Meyer E. Ocular and systemic characteristics of Duane syndrome. J Ped Ophthalmol Strabismus 30, 178–183, 1997.
767. Shen WC, Yang DY, Ho WL, Ho YJ, Lee SK. Neurilemmoma of the oculomotor nerve presenting as an orbital mass: MR findings. Am J Neuroradiol 14, 1253–1254, 1993.
768. Sherman SC, Buchanan A. Gradenigo syndrome: a case report and review of a rare complication of otitis media. J Emerg Med 27, 253–256, 2004.
769. Sherrington CS. Experimental note on two movements of the eye. J Physiol (Lond) 17, 27–29, 1894.
770. Shimo-Oku M, Izaki A, Shim-myo A. Fourth nerve palsy as an initial sign of internal carotid-posterior communicating artery aneurysm. Neuroophthalmol 19, 185–190, 1998.
771. Shin GS, Demer JL. High resolution, dynamic, magnetic resonance imaging in complicated strabismus. J Ped Ophthalmol Strabismus 33, 282–290, 1996.
772. Shinmei Y, Harada T, Ohashi T, et al. Trochlear nerve palsy associated with superficial siderosis of the central nervous system. Jpn J Ophthalmol 41, 19–22, 1997.
773. Shoffner JM. Maternal inheritance and the evaluation of oxidative phosphorylation diseases. Lancet 348, 1283–1288, 1996.
774. Shoubridge EA. Autosomal dominant chronic progressive external ophthalmoplegia. Ann Neurol 40, 693–694, 1996.
775. Sibony PA, Lessell S. Transient oculomotor synkinesis in temporal arteritis. Arch Neurol 41, 87–88, 1984.
776. Sibony PA, Lessell S, Gittinger JW Jr. Acquired oculomotor synkinesis. Surv Ophthalmol 28, 382–390, 1984.
777. Sicotte NL, Plaitakas A, Salamon G, et al. Brainstem axon crossing defects in horizontal gaze palsy with progressive scoliosis assessed with diffusion tensor imaging and neurophysiological testing [abstract]. Neurology 64(Suppl 1), A2. 2005.
778. Silverberg M, Demer J. Duane's syndrome with compressive denervation of the lateral rectus muscle. Am J Ophthalmol 131, 146–148, 2001.
779. Silverman IE, Liu GT, Volpe NJ, Galetta SL. The crossed paralyses.The original brain-stem syndromes of Millard-Gubler, Foville, Weber, and Raymond-Cestan. Arch Neurol 52, 635–638, 1995.
780. Simon JW, Waldman JB, Couture KC. Cerebellar astrocytoma manifesting as isolated comitant esotropia in childhood. Am J Ophthalmol 121, 584–586, 1996.
781. Simonsz HJ, Crone RA, van der Meer J, Merckel-Timmer CF, van Mourik-Noordenbos A. Bielschowsky head-tilt test—I Ocular counterrolling and Bielschowsky head-tilt test in 23 cases of superior oblique palsy. Vision Res 25, 1977–1982, 1985.
782. Simonsz HJ, Kolling GH, Kaufmann H, Van Dijk B. The length-tension diagrams of human oblique muscles in trochlear palsy and strabismus sursoadductorius. Doc Ophthalmol 70, 227–236, 1988.
783. Slavin ML. Isolated trochlear nerve palsy secondary to cavernous sinus meningioma. Am J Ophthalmol 104, 433–434, 1987.
784. Slavin ML. Hyperdeviation associated with isolated unilateral abducens palsy. Ophthalmology 96, 512–516, 1989.
785. Slavin ML, Einberg KR. Abduction defect associated with aberrant regeneration of the oculomotor nerve after intracranial aneurysm. Am J Ophthalmol 121, 580–582, 1996.
786. Slavin ML, Glaser JS. Idiopathic orbital myositis. Report of six cases. Arch Ophthalmol 100, 1261–1265, 1982.
787. Slavin ML, Goodstein S. Acquired Brown's syndrome caused by focal metastasis to the superior oblique muscle. Am J Ophthalmol 103, 598–599, 1987.
788. Slavin ML, Haimovic I, Patel M. Sixth nerve palsy and ponto-cerebellar mass due to luetic meningoencephalitis. Arch Ophthalmol 110, 322, 1992.
789. Slavin ML, Potash SD, Rubin SE. Asymptomatic physiologic hyperdeviation in peripheral gaze. Ophthalmology 95, 778–781, 1988.
790. Smith BE, Dyck PJ. Subclinical histopathological changes in the oculomotor nerve in diabetes mellitus. Ann Neurol 32, 376–385, 1992.
791. Smith JL. The "nuclear third" question. J Clin Neuroophthalmol 2, 61–63, 1982.
792. Sollberger CE, Meienberg O, Ludin H-P. The contribution of culography to early diagnosis of myasthenia gravis. Eur Arch Psychiatr Neurol Sci 236, 102–108, 1986.
793. Sommer N, Melms A, Weller M, Dichgans J. Ocular myasthenia gravis. A critical review of clinical and pathophysiological aspects. Doc Ophthalmol 84, 309–333, 1993.
794. Sommer N, Sigg B, Memms A, et al. Ocular myasthenia gravis: response to long-term immunosuppressive treatment. J Neurol Neurosurg Psychiatry 62, 156–162, 1997.
795. Soontornniyomkij V, Schelper RI. Pontine neurocytoma. J Clin Pathol 49, 764–765, 1996.
796. Soysal T, Ferhanoglu B, Bilir M, Akman N. Oculomotor nerve palsy associated with vincristine treatment. Acta Hematologica 90, 209–210, 1993.
797. Spector RH, Carlisle JA. Minimal thyroid ophthalmopathy. Neurology 37, 1803–1808, 1987.
798. Spector RH, Daroff RB, Birkett JE. Edrophonium infrared optokinetic nystagmography in the diagnosis of myasthenia gravis. Neurology 25, 317–321, 1975.
799. Spector RH, Fiandaca MS. The "sinister" Tolosa-Hunt syndrome. Neurology 36, 198–203, 1986.
800. Spencer RF, McNeer KW. Botulinum paralysis of adult monkey extraocular muscle: structural alterations in the orbital, singly innervated muscle fibers. Arch Ophthalmol 105, 1703–1711, 1987.
801. Spencer RF, McNeer KW. Morphology of the extraocular muscles in relation to the clinical manifestations of strabismus. In Lennerstrand G, von Noorden GK, Campos EC (eds). Strabismus and Amblyopia. Plenum Press, New York, 1988, pp 37–45.
802. Spencer RF, McNeer KW. The peripheral extraocular muscles and motoneurons. In Carpenter RHS (ed). Eye Movements. Vol 8. Macmillan Press, London, 1991, pp 175–199.
803. Spencer RF, Porter JD. Biological organization of the extraocular muscles. Prog Brain Res 151, 43–79, 2006.
804. Spencer RF, Tucker MG, Choi RY, McNeer KW. Botulinum toxin management of childhood intermit-

tent exotropia. Ophthalmology 104, 1762–1767, 1997.
805. Spielmann A. A translucent occluder for studying eye position under unilateral or bilateral cover test. Am Orthop J 36, 65–74, 1986.
806. Spiro AJ, Shy GM, Gonatas NK. Myotubular myopathy. Arch Neurol 14, 1–14, 1966.
807. Spooner JW, Baloh RW. Eye movement fatigue in myasthenia gravis. Neurology 29, 29–33, 1979.
808. Spoor TC, Hartel WC. Orbital myositis. J Clin Neuroophthalmol 3, 67–74, 1983.
809. Srebro R. Fixation of normal and amblyopic eyes. Arch Ophthalmol 101, 214–217, 1983.
810. Stahl JS. A portable and affordable Lancaster red-green test. Neuroophthalmology 15, 321–322, 1995.
811. Stahl JS, Averbuch-Heller L, Remler BF, Leigh RJ. Clinical evidence of extraocular muscle fiber-type specificity of botulinum toxin. Neurology 51, 1093–1099, 1998.
812. Stamler JF, Nerad JA, Keech RV. Acquired pseudo-Duane's retraction syndrome secondary to acute orbital myositis. Binocular Vision 4, 103–108, 1989.
813. Stathacopoulos RA, Yee RD, Bateman JB. Vertical saccades in superior oblique palsy. Invest Ophthalmol Vis Sci 32, 1938–1943, 1991.
814. Stefanis L, Przedborski S. Isolated palsy of the superior branch of the oculomotor nerve due to chronic erosive sphenoid sinusitis. J Clin Neuroophthalmol 13, 229–231, 1993.
815. Steffen H, Walker M, Zee DS. Changes in Listing's plane after sustained vertical fusion. Invest Ophthalmol Vis Sci 43, 668–672, 2002.
816. Steffen H, Walker MF, Zee DS. Rotation of Listing's plane with convergence: independence from eye position. Invest Ophthalmol Vis Sci 41, 715–721, 2000.
817. Steinbach MJ, Kirshner EL, Arstikaitis MJ, Recession vs marginal myotomy surgery for strabismus: effects on spatial localization. Invest Ophthalmol Vis Sci 28, 1870–1872, 1987.
818. Steinbach MJ, Smith DR. Spatial localization after strabismus surgery: evidence for inflow. Science 213, 1407–1409, 1981.
819. Stommel EW, Ward TN, Harris RD. MRI findings in a case of ophthalmoplegic migraine. Headache 33, 234–237, 1993.
820. Straube A, Bandmann O, Büttner U, Schmidt H. A contrast enhanced lesion of the III nerve on MR of a patient with ophthalmic migraine as evidence for Tolosa-Hunt syndrome. Headache 33, 446–448, 1993.
821. Straube A, Paulis J, Quintern J, Brandt T. Visual ataxia induced by eye-movements: posturographic measurments in normals and patients with ocular motor disorders. Clin Vis Sci 4, 107–113, 1989.
822. Straumann D, Steffen H, Landau K, et al. Primary position and listing's law in acquired and congenital trochlear nerve palsy. Invest Ophthalmol Vis Sci 44, 4282–4292, 2003.
823. Straumann D, Zee DS, Solomon D, Kramer PD. Validity of Listing's Law during fixation, saccades, smooth pursuit eye movements and blinks. Exp Brain Res 112, 135–146, 1996.
824. Striph GG, Burde RM. Abducens nerve palsy and Horner's syndrome revisited. J Clin Neuroophthalmol 8, 13–17, 1988.
825. Strominger MB, Liu GT, Schatz NJ, Optic nerve swelling and abducens palsies associated with OKT3. Am J Ophthalmol 119, 664–665, 1995.
826. Sunderland S, Hughes ESR. The pupillo-constrictor pathway and the nerves to the ocular muscles in man. Brain 69, 301–309, 1946.
827. Supler ML, Friedman WA. Acute bilateral ophthalmoplegia secondary to cavernous sinus metastasis: a case report. Neurosurgery 31, 783–786, 1992.
828. Suzuki Y, Washio N, Hashimoto M, Ohtsuka K. Three-dimensional eye movement analysis of superior oblique myokymia. Am J Ophthalmol 135, 563–565, 2003.
829. Symonds CP. A discussion of cranial nerve palsies associated with otitis. Proc Royal Soc Med 37, 386–387, 1944.
830. Szlatenyi CS, Wang RY. Encephalopathy and cranial nerve palsies caused by intentional trichloroethylene inhalation. Am J Emerg Med 14, 464–466, 1996.
831. Tachibana H, Mimura O, Shiomi M, Oono T. Bilateral trochlear nerve palsies from a brainstem hematoma. J Clin Neuroophthalmol 10, 35–37, 1990.
832. Takahashi M, Koga M, Yokoyama K, Yuki N. Epidemiology of Campylobacter jejuni isolated from patients with Guillain-Barre and Fisher syndromes in Japan. J Clin Microbiol 43, 335–339, 2005.
833. Tamhankar MA, Liu GT, Young TL, Sutton LN, Hurst RW. Acquired, isolated third nerve palsies in infants with cerebrovascular malformations. Am J Ophthalmol 138, 484–486, 2004.
834. Taylor RW, Turnbull DM. Mitochondrial DNA mutations in human disease. Nat Rev Genetics 6, 389–402, 2005.
835. Ter Bruggen JP, Bastiaensen LAK, Tyssen CC, Gielen G. Disorders of eye movement in myotonic dystrophy. Brain 113, 463–473, 1990.
836. Teuscher AU, Meienberg O. Ischaemic oculomotor nerve palsy. Clinical features and vascular risk factors in 23 patients. J Neurol 232, 144–149, 1985.
837. Thacker NM, Velez FG, Demer JL, Rosenbaum AL. Superior oblique muscle involvement in thyroid ophthalmopathy. J AAPOS 9, 174–178, 2005.
838. Thomas DJB, Charlesworth MC, Afshar F, Galton DJ. Computerised axial tomography and magnetic resonance scanning in the Tolosa-Hunt syndrome. Br J Ophthalmol 72, 299–302, 1988.
839. Thurston SE, Saul RF. Superior oblique myokymia. Quantitative description of the eye movement. Neurology 35, 1518–1521, 1991.
840. Tian S, Lennerstrand G. Vertical saccadic velocity and force development in superior oblique palsy. Vision Res 34, 1785–1798, 1994.
841. Tiffin PA, MacEwen CJ, Craig EA, Clayton G Acquired palsy of the oculomotor trochlear and abducens nerves. Eye 10, 377–384, 1996.
842. Tilikete C, Vial C, Niederlaender M, Bonnier PL, Vighetto A. Idiopathic ocular neuromyotonia: a neurovascular compression syndrome? J Neurol. Neurosurg. Psychiatry 69, 642–644, 2000.
842a. Tischfield MA, Bosley TM, Salih MA, et al. Homozygous HOXA1 mutations disrupt human brainstem, inner ear, cardiovascular and cognitive development. Nat Genet 37, 1035–1037, 2005.
843. Tognetti F, Godano U, Galassi E. Bilateral trau

matic third nerve palsy. Surg Neurol 29, 120–124, 1988.
844. Toker E, Yenice O, Ogut MS. Isolated abducens nerve palsy induced by vincristine therapy. J AAPOS 8, 69–71, 2004.
845. Tolosa E. Periateritic lesions of the carotid siphon with the clinical features of a carotid infraclinoid aneurysm. J Neurol Neurosurg Psychiatry 17, 300–302, 1954.
846. Tomé FMS, Askanas V, Engel WK, Alvarez RB, Lee C-S. Nuclear inclusions in innervated cultured muscle fibers from patients with oculopharyngeal muscular dystrophy. Neurology 39, 926–932, 1989.
847. Tomecek FJ, Morgan JK. Ophthalmoplegia with bilateral ptosis secondary to midbrain hemorrhage. A case with clinical and radiological correlation. Surg Neurol 41, 131–136, 1994.
848. Tomsak RL, Kosmorsky GA, Leigh RJ. Gabapentin attenuates superior oblique myokymia. Am J Ophthalmol 133, 721–723, 2002.
849. Tomsak RL, Remler BF, Averbuch-Heller L, Chandran M, Leigh RJ. Unsatisfactory treatment of acquired nystagmus with retrobulbar botulinum toxin. Am J Ophthalmol 119, 489–496, 1995.
850. Townes JM, Cieslak PR, Hatheway CL, et al. An outbreak of type A botulism associated with a commercial cheese sauce. Ann Int Med 125–558, 1997.
851. Traboulsi E, Achram M, Fares B. Brainstem tuberculoma and isolated third nerve palsy. Neuroophthalmol 5, 43–45, 1985.
852. Tredici TD, von Noorden GK. Are anisometropia and amblyopia common in Duane's syndrome? J Ped Ophthalmol Strabismus 22, 23–25, 1985.
853. Trobe JD. Third nerve palsy and the pupil. Arch Ophthalmol 106, 601–602, 1988.
854. Trobe JD. Managing oculomotor nerve palsy. Arch Ophthalmol 116, 798, 1998.
855. Trobe JD, Glaser JS, Quencer RM. Isolated oculomotor paralysis. The product of saccular and fusiform aneurysms of the basilar artery. Arch Ophthalmol 96, 1236–1240, 1978.
856. Troost BT, Abel LA, Noreika J, Genovese FM. Acquired cyclic esotropia in an adult. Am J Ophthalmol 91, 8–13, 1981.
857. Tsuboi K, Shibuya F, Yamada T, Nose T. Giant aneurysm at the junction of the left internal carotid and persistent trigeminal arteries—case report. Neurologia Medico-Chirurgica 32, 778–781, 1992.
858. Ture U, Ozduman K, Elmaci I, Pamir MN. Infratentorial lateral supracerebellar approach for trochlear nerve schwannoma. J Clin Neurosci 9, 595–598, 2002.
859. Tweed D, Vilis T. Geometric relations of eye position and velocity vectors during saccades. Vision Res 30, 111–127, 1990.
860. Tychsen L, Wong AM, Burkhalter A. Paucity of horizontal connections for binocular vision in V1 of naturally strabismic macaques: cytochrome oxidase compartment specificity. J Comp Neurol. 474, 261–275, 2004.
861. Uitti RJ, Rajput AH. Multiple sclerosis presenting as isolated oculomotor nerve palsy. Can J Neurol Sci 13, 270–272, 1986.
862. Umansky F, Elidan J, Valarezo A. Dorello's canal: a microanatomical study. J Neurosurg 75, 294–298, 1991.
863. Umansky F, Nathan H. The lateral wall of the cavernous sinus: with special reference to the nerves related to it. J Neurosurg 56, 228–234, 1982.
864. Umansky F, Valarezo A, Elidan J. The microscopic anatomy of the abducens nerve in its intracranial course. Laryngoscope 102, 1285–1292, 1992.
865. Vallat JM, Vallat M, Julien J, Dumas M, Dany A. Painful ophthalmoplegia (Tolosa-Hunt) accompanied by facial paralysis. Ann Neurol 8, 645, 1980.
866. Valmaggia C, Zaunbauer W, Gottlob I. Elevation deficit caused by accessory extraocular muscle. Am J Ophthalmol 121, 444–445, 1996.
867. Van Opstal AJ, Hepp K, Suzuki Y, Henn V. Role of monkey nucleus reticularis tegmenti pontis in the stabilization of Listing's plane. J Neurosc 16, 7284–7296, 1996.
868. Van Rijn LJ, Simonsz HJ, ten Tusscher MPM. Dissociated vertical deviation and eye torsion: relation to disparity-induced vertical vergence. Strabismus 5, 13–20, 1997.
869. Van Rijn LJ, Van den Berg AV. Binocular eye orientation during fixations: Listing's law extended to include eye vergence. Vision Res 33, 691–708, 1993.
870. Vanooteghem P, Dehaene I, van Zandycke M, Casselman J. Combined trochlear nerve palsy and internuclear ophthalmoplegia. Arch Neurol 49, 108–109, 1992.
871. Varma R, Miller NR. Primary oculomotor synkinesis caused by an extracavernous intradural aneurysm. Am J Ophthalmol 118, 83–87, 1994.
872. Velay JL, Roll R, Demaria JL, Bouquerel A, Roll JP. Human eye muscle proprioceptive feedback is involved in target velocity perception during smooth pursuit. Vision Res 79–85, 1995.
873. Velay JL, Roll R, Lennerstrand G, Roll JP. Eye proprioception and visual localization in humans: influence of ocular dominance and visual context. Vision Res 34, 2169–2176, 1994.
874. Velez FG, Clark RA, Demer JL. Facial asymmetry in superior oblique muscle palsy and pulley heterotopy. J AAPOS 4, 233–239, 2000.
875. Ventre-Dominey J, Dominey PF, Sindou M. Extraocular proprioception is required for spatial localization in man. Neuroreport 7, 1531–1535, 1996.
876. Ventura GJ, Keating MJ, Castellanos AM, Glass JP. Reversible bilateral lateral rectus muscle palsy associated with high-dose cytosine arabinoside and mitoxantrone therapy. Cancer 58, 1633–1635, 1986.
877. Verhagen WI, Huygen PL, Padberg GW. The auditory vestibular and oculomotor system in fascioscapulohumeral dystrophy. Acta Otolaryngol (Stockh) Suppl 520, Part 1, 140–142, 1995.
877a. Versino M, Colnaghi S, Todeschini A, et al. Ocular neuromyotonia with both tonic and paroxysmal components due to vascular compression. J Neurol 252, 227–229, 2005.
878. Versino M, Rossi B, Beltrami G, Sandrini G, Cosi V. Ocular motor myotonic phenomenon in myotonic dystrophy. J Neurol Neurosurg Psychiatry 72, 236–240, 2002.
879. Victor M, Hayes R, Adams RD. Oculopharyngeal muscular dystrophy. A familial disease of late life characterized by dysphagia and progressive ptosis of the eyelids. N Engl J Med 267, 1267–1272, 1962.

880. Viirre E, Cadera W, Vilis T. Monocular adaptation of the saccadic system and vestibulo-ocular reflex. Invest Ophthalmol Vis Sci 29, 1339–1347, 1988.
881. Villa G, Lattere M, Rossi A, Di PP. Acute onset of abducens nerve palsy in a child with prior history of otitis media: a misleading sign of Gradenigo syndrome. Brain Dev. 27, 155–159, 2005.
882. Vincent A. Unravelling the pathogenesis of myasthenia gravis. Nat Rev Immunol 2, 797–804, 2002.
883. Vincent A, McConville J, Farrugia ME, Newsom-Davis J. Seronegative myasthenia gravis. Semin Neurol 24, 125–133, 2004.
884. Vincent FM, Vincent T. Relapsing Fisher's syndrome. J Neurol Neurosurg Psychiatry 49, 604–606, 1986.
885. Vogl T, Dresel S, Lochmuller H, et al. Third cranial nerve palsy caused by gummatous neurosyphilis: MR findings. Am J Neuroradiol 14, 1329–1331, 1993.
886. Volpe NJ, Liebach NJ, Munzenrider JE, Lessell S. Neuro-ophthalmological findings in chordoma and chondrosarcoma of the skull base. Am J Ophthalmol 115, 97–104, 1993.
887. von Noorden GK. Clinical and theoretical aspects of cyclotropia. J Pediatric Ophthalmol Strabismus 21, 126–132, 1984.
888. von Noorden GK, Awaya S, Romano PE. Past-pointing in paralytic strabismus. Am J Ophthalmol 71, 27–33, 1971.
889. von Noorden GK, Campos EC. Binocular Vision and Ocular Motility. Mosby, St. Louis, 2001.
890. von Noorden GK, Hansell R. Clinical characteristics and treatment of isolated inferior rectus paralysis. Ophthalmology 98, 253–257, 1991.
891. von Noorden GK, Murray E, Wong SY. Superior oblique paralysis. A review of 270 cases. Arch Ophthalmol 104, 1771–1776, 1986.
892. Wagner RS, Caputo AR, Frohman LP. Congenital unilateral adduction deficit with simultaneous abduction. A variant of Duane's retraction syndrome. Ophthalmology 94, 1049–1053, 1987.
893. Waldeck RF, Murphy EH, Pinter MJ. Properties of motor units after self-reinnervation of the cat superior oblique muscle. J Neurophysiol 74, 2309–2318, 1995.
894. Walker M, Drangsholt M, Czartoski TJ, Longstreth WT, Jr. Dental diplopia with transient abducens palsy. Neurology 63, 2449–2450, 2004.
895. Walker MF, Shelhamer M, Zee DS. Eye-position dependence of torsional velocity during interaural translation horizontal pursuit and yaw-axis rotation in humans. Vision Res 44, 613–620, 2004.
896. Walsh FB. Ocular signs of thrombosis of the intracranial venous sinuses. Arch Opthalmol 17, 46–65, 1937.
897. Walter KA, Newman NJ, Lessell S. Oculomotor palsy from minor head trauma: initial sign of intracranial aneurysm. Neurology 44, 148–150, 1994.
898. Wan WL, Cano MR, Green RL. Orbital myositis involving the oblique muscles. Ophthalmology 95, 1522–1528, 1988.
899. Wang CH, Chou ML, Huang CH. Benign isolated abducens nerve palsy in Mycoplasma pneumoniae infection. Pediatr Neurol 18, 71–72, 1998.
900. Wang SM, Zwaan J, Mullaney PB, et al. Congenital fibrosis of the extraocular muscles type 2, an inherited exotropic strabismus fixus, maps to distal 11q13. Am J Hum Genet 63, 517–525, 1998.
901. Warren W, Burde RM, Klingele TG, Roper-Hall G. Atypical oculomotor paresis. J Clin Neuroophthalmol 2, 13–18, 1982.
902. Warwick R. Representation of the extra-ocular muscles in the oculomotor nuclei of the monkey. J Comp Neurol 98, 449–503, 1953.
903. Wasicky R, Horn AK, Buttner-Ennever JA. Twitch and nontwitch motoneuron subgroups in the oculomotor nucleus of monkeys receive different afferent projections. J Comp Neurol. 479, 117–129, 2004.
904. Weber AL, Dallow RL, Sabates NR. Graves' disease of the orbit. Neuroimag Clin North Am 6, 61–72, 1996.
905. Weber RB, Daroff RB, Mackey EA. Pathology of oculomotor nerve palsy in diabetics. Neurology 20, 835–838, 1970.
906. Weisberg LA. Pituitary apoplexy. Association of degenerative change in pituitary adenoma with radiotherapy and detection by cerebral computed tomography. Am J Med 63, 109–115, 1977.
907. Weizer JS, Lee AG, Coats DK. Myasthenia gravis with ocular involvement in older patients. Can J Ophthalmol 36, 26–33, 2001.
908. Werner DB, Savino PJ, Schatz NJ. Benign recurrent sixth nerve palsies in childhood secondary to immunization or viral illness. Arch Ophthalmol 101, 607–608, 1983.
909. White VA, Cline RA. Pathologic causes of the superior oblique click syndrome. Ophthalmology 106, 1292–1295, 1999.
910. Whitehouse PJ, Wamsley JK, Zarbin MA, Price DL, Kuhar MJ. Neurotransimtter receptors in amyotrophic lateral sclerosis: possible relationship to sparing of eye movements. Ann Neurol 17, 518, 1985.
911. Wilcox LM, Gittinger JW Jr., Breinin GM. Congenital adduction palsy and synergistic divergence. Am J Ophthalmol 91, 1–7, 1981.
912. Wilichowski E, Gruters A, Kruse K, et al. Hypoparathyroidism and deafness associated with pleioplasmic large scale rearrangements of the mitochondrial DNA: a clinical and molecular genetic study of four children with Kearns-Sayre syndrome. Pediatric Res 41, 193–200, 1997.
913. Williams AS, Hoyt CS. Acute comitant esotropia in children with brain tumors. Arch Ophthalmol 107, 376–378, 1989.
914. Wilson WB, Leavengood JM, Ringel SP, Bott AD. Transient ocular motor paresis associated with acute internal carotid artery occlusion. Ann Neurol 25, 286–290, 1989.
915. Wirtschafter JD, Ferrington DA, McLoon LK. Continuous remodeling of adult extraocular muscles as an explanation for selective craniofacial vulnerability in oculopharyngeal muscular dystrophy. J Neuroophthalmol 24, 62–67, 2004.
916. Wist ER, Brandt T, Krafczyk S. Oscillopsia and retinal slip. Evidence supporting a clinical test. Brain 106, 153–168, 1983.
917. Wojno TH. The incidence of extraocular muscle and cranial nerve palsy in orbital floor blow-out fractures. Ophthalmology 94, 682–687, 1987.
918. Wolin MJ, Saunders RA. Aneurysmal oculomotor nerve palsy in an 11-year-old boy. J Clin Neuroophthalmol 12, 178–180, 1992.
919. Wong AM. Listing's law: clinical significance and

implications for neural control. Surv Ophthalmol 49, 563–575, 2004.
920. Wong AM, Sharpe JA, Tweed D. Adaptive neural mechanism for listing's law revealed in patients with fourth nerve palsy. Invest Ophthalmol Vis Sci 43, 1796–1803, 2002.
921. Wong AM, Sharpe JA, Tweed D. The vestibulo-ocular reflex in fourth nerve palsy: deficits and adaptation. Vision Res 42, 2205–2218, 2002.
922. Wong AM, Tweed D, Sharpe JA. Adaptations and deficits in the vestibulo-ocular reflex after sixth nerve palsy. Invest Ophthalmol Vis Sci 43, 99–111, 2002.
923. Wong AM, Tweed D, Sharpe JA. Adaptive neural mechanism for Listing's law revealed in patients with sixth nerve palsy. Invest Ophthalmol Vis Sci 43, 112–119, 2002.
924. Wong AM, Tweed D, Sharpe JA. Vertical misalignment in unilateral sixth nerve palsy. Ophthalmology 109, 1315–1325, 2002.
925. Wong GK, Boet R, Poon WS, Yu S, Lam JM. A review of isolated third nerve palsy without subarachnoid hemorrhage using computed tomographic angiography as the first line of investigation. Clin Neurol Neurosurg 107, 27–31, 2004.
926. Woody RC, Blaw ME. Ophthalmoplegic migraine in infancy. Clin Pediatrics 25, 82–84, 1986.
927. Woody RL, Bradley A, Atchinson DA. Monocular diplopia causes by ocular aberrations and hyperopic defocus. Vision Res 36, 3597–3606, 1996.
928. Worthington JM, Halmagyi GM. Bilateral total ophthalmoplegia due to midbrain hematoma. Neurology 46, 1176–1177, 1996.
929. Wouters RJ, van den Bosch WA, Lemij HG. Saccadic eye movements in Graves' disease. Invest Ophthalmol Vis Sci 198, 39, 1544–1550, 1998.
930. Wray SH, Provenzale JM, John DR, Thulborn KR. MR of the brain in mitochondrial myopathy. Am J Neuroradiol 16, 1167–1173, 1997.
931. Wright RA, Plant GT, Landon DN, Morgan-Hughes JA. Nemaline myopathy: an unusual cause of ophthalmoparesis. J Neuroophthalmol 17, 39–43, 1997.
932. Wutthiphan S, Kowal L, O'Day J, Jones S, Price J. Diplopia folowing subcutaneous injections of botulinum A toxin for facial spasms. J Ped Ophthalmol Strabismus 34, 229–234, 1997.
933. Yamada T, Nishio S, Matsunaga M, Fukui M, Takeshita I. Cavernous haemangioma in the oculomotor nerve. J Neurol 233, 63–64, 1986.
934. Yang MC, Bateman JB, Yee RD, Apt L. Electrooculography and discriminant analysis in Duane's syndrome and sixth-cranial-nerve palsy. Graefe's Arch Clin Exp Ophthalmol 229, 52–56, 1991.
935. Yee RD, Cogan DG, Zee DS. Ophthalmoplegia and dissociated nystagmus in abetalipoproteinemia. Arch Ophthalmol 94, 571–575, 1976.
936. Yee RD, Cogan DG, Zee DS, Baloh RW, Honrubia V. Rapid eye movements in myasthenia gravis. II Electro-oculographic analysis. Arch Ophthalmol 94, 1465–1472, 1976.
937. Yee RD, Duffin RM, Baloh RW, Isenberg SJ. Familial, congenital paralysis of horizontal gaze. Arch Ophthalmol 100, 1449–1452, 1982.
938. Yee RD, Purvin VA, Azzarelli B, Nelson PB. Intermittent diplopia and strabimus caused by ocular neuromyotonia. Trans Am Ophthalmol Soc 94, 223–226, 1996.
939. Yee RD, Whitcup SM, Williams IM, Baloh RW, Honrubia V. Saccadic eye movements in myasthenia gravis. Ophthalmology 94, 219–225, 1987.
940. Yoss RE, Rucker CW, Miller RH. Neurosurgical complications affecting the oculomotor, trochlear, and abducent nerves. Neurology 18, 594–600, 1968.
941. Younge BR, Sutula F. Analysis of trochlear nerve palsies. Diagnosis, etiology, treatment. Mayo Clin Proc 52, 11–18, 1977.
942. Yousem DM, Atlas SW, Grossman RI, et al. MR imaging of Tolosa-Hunt syndrome. AJNR Am J Neuroradiol 10, 1181–1184, 1989.
943. Yousry I, Dieterich M, Naidich TP, Schmid UD, Yousry TA. Superior oblique myokymia: magnetic resonance imaging support for the neurovascular compression hypothesis. Ann Neurol 51, 361–368, 2002.
944. Yu Wai Man CY, Chinnery PF, Griffiths PG. Extraocular muscles have fundamentally distinct properties that make them selectively vulnerable to certain disorders. Neuromuscul Disord 15, 17–23, 2005.
945. Yuki N. Successful plasmaphoresis in Bickerstaff's brain stem encephalitis associated with anti-GQ1b antibody. J Neurol Sci 131, 108–110, 1995.
946. Yuki N, Sato S, Tsuji S, Hozumi I, Miyatake T. An immunological abnormality common to Bickerstaff's brain stem encephalitis and Fisher's syndrome. J Neurol Sci 131, 108–110, 1993.
947. Yuki N, Wakabayashi K, Yamada M, Seki K. Overlap of Guillain-Barré syndrome and Bickerstaff's brainstem encephalitis. J Neurol Sci 145, 119–121, 1997.
948. Yüksel D, Optican LM, Lefèvre P. Properties of saccades in Duane's retraction syndrome. Invest Ophthalmol Vis Sci 46, 3144–3151, 2005.
949. Yumoto E, Kitani S, Okamura H, Yanagihara N Sino-orbital aspergillosis associated with total ophthalmoplegia. Laryngoscope 95, 190–192, 1985.
950. Zackon DH, Sharpe JA. Midbrain paresis of horizontal gaze. Ann Neurol 16, 495–504, 1984.
951. Zasorin NL, Yee RD, Baloh RW. Eye-movement abnormalities in ophthalmoplegia, ataxia, and areflexia (Fisher's Syndrome). Arch Ophthalmol 103, 55–58, 1985.
952. Zee DS, Chu FC, Optican LM, Carl JR, Reingold D. Graphic analysis of paralytic strabismus with the Lancaster red-green test. Am J Ophthalmol 97, 587–592, 1984.
953. Zee DS, Yee RD. Abnormal saccades in paralytic strabismus. Am J Ophthalmol 83, 112–114, 1977.
954. Zhang F. Clinical features of 201 cases with Duane's retraction syndrome. Chin Med J (Engl) 110, 789–791, 1997.
955. Zhou W, King WM. Premotor commands encode monocular eye movements. Nature 393, 692–695, 1998.
956. Zumla A, Lipscomb G, Lewis D. Sixth cranial nerve palsy complicating psittacosis. J Neurol Neurosurg Psychiatry 51, 1462, 1988.
957. Zweifach PH, Walton DS, Brown RH. Isolated congenital horizontal gaze paralysis. Occurrence of the near reflex and ocular retraction on attempted lateral gaze. Arch Ophthalmol 81, 345–350, 1969.

Chapter 10

Diagnosis of Nystagmus and Saccadic Intrusion

THE NATURE AND VISUAL CONSEQUENCES OF ABNORMAL EYE MOVEMENTS THAT PREVENT STEADY FIXATION

Nystagmus and other spontaneous abnormal eye movements that disrupt steady fixation pose a common diagnostic challenge for clinicians. Such eye movements may interfere with vision. Recall the visual requirements for eye movements: to see an object best, its image must be held steadily over the foveal region of the retina.[124] Excessive motion of images on the retina causes vision to decline and may lead to the illusion of motion of the seen world (oscillopsia).[13,74,715] Furthermore, if the image of the object is moved away from the fovea to peripheral retina, it will be seen less clearly.

Abnormal eye movements that prevent steady fixation are of two main types: pathological nystagmus and saccadic intrusions. The essential difference between nystagmus and saccadic intrusions lies in the initial eye movement that takes the line of sight away from the object of regard. Thus, for nystagmus, the initial movement is a slow drift (or "slow-phase"), as opposed to an initial inappropriate saccadic movement that intrudes on steady fixation in saccadic intrusions (Fig. 10–1(A–D)). After the initial movement, corrective or other abnormal eye movements may follow. Thus, a definition of nystagmus is repetitive, to-and-fro movements of the eyes that are initiated by slow phases. Nystagmus may consist mainly of sinusoidal slow-phase oscillations (pendular nystagmus) or, more commonly, of an alternation of slow drift and corrective quick phase (jerk nystagmus). Although nystagmus is often described by the direction of its quick phases (e.g., downbeat nystagmus), it is the slow phase that reflects the underlying disorder. Saccadic intrusions are rapid movements that take the eye away from the target (Fig. 10–14), and comprise a spectrum ranging from single saccades to sustained saccadic oscillations.

Not all nystagmus is pathological. When we move through the environment, and especially when we turn, the slow phases of physiological nystagmus—vestibular and optokinetic—act to preserve clear vision by preventing excessive slip of images on the retina; quick phases reset the eyes into their working range.[245,247,677] Thus, both vestibular and optokinetic nystagmus act to hold retinal images steady, but the

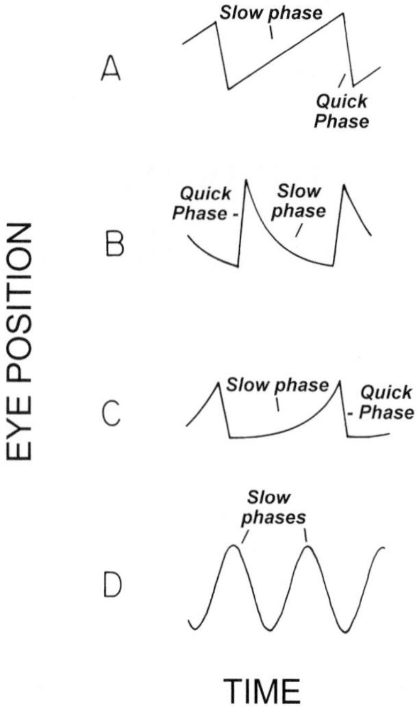

Figure 10–1. Four common slow-phase waveforms of nystagmus. (A) Constant velocity drift of the eyes. This occurs in nystagmus caused by peripheral or central vestibular disease and also with lesions of the cerebral hemisphere. The added quick-phases give a "saw-tooth" appearance. (B) Drift of the eyes back from an eccentric orbital position toward the midline (gaze-evoked nystagmus). The drift shows a negative exponential time course, with decreasing velocity. This waveform reflects an unsustained eye position signal caused by an impaired neural integrator. (C) Drift of the eyes away from the central position with a positive exponential time course (increasing velocity). This waveform suggests an unstable neural integrator and is encountered in the horizontal plane in congenital nystagmus and in the vertical plane in cerebellar disease. (D) Pendular nystagmus, which may be congenital or acquired.

opposite is true of pathologic nystagmus, which causes excessive drift of images of stationary objects on the retina and so degrades vision.

CLINICAL AND LABORATORY METHODS FOR EVALUATING NYSTAGMUS AND SACCADIC INTRUSIONS

History-Taking in Patients with Abnormal Eye Movements that Disrupt Fixation

Accurate diagnosis of nystagmus and saccadic intrusions depends on taking a careful history and performing a systematic examination.[608]

First, ask whether the patient experiences any visual symptoms, such as blurred vision or oscillopsia (illusory motion of the visual world). In general, oscillopsia is a feature of acquired, not congenital, forms of nystagmus. Establish how long the visual symptoms, or ocular oscillations have been present. In children, ask the parents about "jumping eyes," "crossed eyes," "lazy eye," head thrusts or turns, eye patching or eye operations. Determine whether visual symptoms, or ocular oscillations, are worse when viewing far or near objects, when the patient is stationary or in motion, and if they are affected by different gaze angles (e.g., worse on right gaze). If the patient habitually tilts or turns the head, determine whether these findings are evident on old photographs. Establish whether nystagmus is accompanied by other neurologic symptoms. Document the patient's current medications.

Examination of Abnormal Eye Movements that Disrupt Fixation

PRELIMINARY OBSERVATIONS

Before examining eye movements, measure corrected visual acuity at far and near. Test visual fields, color vision and stereopsis. During ophthalmoscopy, note any evidence of optic nerve demyelination or malformation; and look for signs of ocular albinism, such as diffuse transillumination of the iris with a penlight held at the limbus (see Video Display: Congenital Forms of Nystagmus). Test the pupils and note any lid abnormality such as ptosis. During these examinations, note abnormal head posture, such as a tilt or turn, and head tremor.

DIRECTION AND SIZE OF THE ABNORMAL MOVEMENTS

Next, examine the stability of fixation with the eyes close to central position, then viewing far targets at eccentric gaze angles, and during convergence. For each eye, note the planes in which the nystagmus occurs (horizontal, vertical, torsional, mixed). Compare the oscillations of each eye, and note whether the direction or amplitude differs, and whether there is an asynchrony (i.e., a phase shift between the two eyes), which may lead to movements that sometimes are in opposite directions. It is often easiest to appreciate differences in the direction of motion of the two eyes by looking at the bridge of the patient's nose and comparing the nystagmus in the two eyes. When the size of the oscillations differs in each eye, it is referred to as dissociated nystagmus. When the direction of the oscillations in each eye differs, it is called disconjugate nystagmus or disjunctive nystagmus. It is often useful to make a note of the direction and amplitude of nystagmus for each of the cardinal gaze positions. If the patient has a head turn or tilt, the eyes should be observed in various directions of gaze when the head is in that position as well as when the head is held straight. During fixation, occlude each eye in turn to check for latent nystagmus. Some nystagmus is intermittent, or may reverse direction, and requires sustained observation over 2 to 3 minutes. Low-amplitude nystagmus may only be detected while viewing the patient's retina with an ophthalmoscope.[735] (Note that the direction of horizontal or vertical nystagmus is inverted when viewed through the ophthalmoscope, but not the torsional component of nystagmus.) Patients with a head tremor do not show motion of their retina during ophthalmoscopy unless they have also lost their vestibulo-ocular reflex, in which case they have "pseudonystagmus."[101,541,727]

INTERPRETATION OF NYSTAGMUS THAT CHANGES ITS DIRECTION WITH DIFFERENT GAZE DIRECTIONS

At the bedside, a complete description of nystagmus, separating it into horizontal, vertical and torsional components, depends upon the coordinate system in which the observer couches his or her observations. This, in turn, may be influenced by the vantage point of the observer relative to the direction in which the patient is looking (i.e., the patient's line of sight), and also by the position of the patient's eye in the orbit. Describe the direction of motion of the eyes from the patient's viewpoint; for example, clockwise torsional rotations should correspond to rotation of the top poles of the eyes to the patient's right.

Consider a patient with the head still who has a spontaneous jerk nystagmus that appears horizontal in the straight-ahead position of gaze (i.e., the eyes are rotating around the rostral-caudal [yaw] axis relative to the head). If, when the patient looks far up, the eyes continue to rotate around the same (yaw) axis relative to the head (which is typical for a nystagmus of vestibular origin), then the nystagmus would appear to have a developed a torsional component if the line of sight of the observer is moved upward to coincide with that of the eye of the patient. In this case, the observer, by moving the vantage point to match the axis along which the patient is looking, will be describing the nystagmus in an eye-fixed coordinate system. On the other hand, the nystagmus may still be rotating the eye around the same head-fixed (yaw) axis, even though the nystagmus has acquired a "torsional" component. The nystagmus has appeared to change direction when described in an eye-fixed but not when described in a head-fixed coordinate system.

On the other hand, if on upward gaze the nystagmus still appears "horizontal" to the observer, when viewed in an eye-fixed coordinate system (as is typical for congenital forms of nystagmus), then the axis of rotation around which the eye was rotating, relative to the head, must have changed. Note that when the eyes are directed straight ahead, the eye and head frames of reference coincide. Thus, one must examine the eyes in an eccentric position to determine the effect of eye position on the axis of rotation, and hence in what framework a particular nystagmus is organized.

Similar considerations apply to vertical nystagmus in when the eye is close to central position, such as "downbeat" nystagmus, in which the eyes are rotating around the interaural (pitch) axis. If the patient looks far to the right, and if the nystagmus continues to rotate the eyes around the same (pitch) axis relative to head, then the nystagmus would appear to have a developed a torsional component if the nystagmus is described in an eye-fixed coordinate system. Again, the nystagmus may still be rotating the eye around the same head-fixed (pitch) axis, even though the nystagmus has acquired a "torsional" component. The nystagmus has appeared to change direction when described in an eye-fixed but not when described in a head-fixed coordinate system. On the other hand, if on lateral gaze the nystagmus still appears "vertical" to the observer, when viewed in an eye-fixed coordinate system, the axis of rotation around which the eye was rotating, relative to the head, must have changed.

Of course, once cognizant of these frame-of-reference issues, the observer can perform the necessary mental transformation to determine the axis of rotation of nystagmus no matter what the direction of gaze of the patient, or the position of the examiner relative to the patient's line of sight. These distinctions about which axis the eye rotates when the eyes move eccentrically may be important in determining the etiology of nystagmus, since the axis of rotation of nystagmus of vestibular (semicircular canal) origin (peripheral or central) usually remains constant in head-fixed coordinates, no matter what the direction of gaze, whereas other forms of central nystagmus may change their axis of rotation with the position of gaze.

EFFECTS OF VISUAL FIXATION ON NYSTAGMUS

Always examine the effect on nystagmus of removing fixation; nystagmus due to peripheral vestibular imbalance may only be apparent under these circumstances. Removal of fixation can be achieved by eyelid closure; nystagmus is then detected by recording eye movements, by observing movement of the corneal bulge, or by palpating the globes. Because lid closure itself may affect nystagmus, it is better to examine the effects of removing fixation with the eyes open; two clinical methods are available. The first is to observe the nystagmus behind Frenzel goggles, which prevent fixation of objects and also provide the examiner with a magnified, illuminated view of the patient's eyes. The second technique consists of transiently covering the fixating eye during ophthalmoscopy in an otherwise dark room, and noting the effects on retinal motion in the eye being viewed.

OTHER CLINICAL TESTS TO INFLUENCE NYSTAGMUS

Several clinical tests are helpful and should be routinely performed in patients with undiagnosed nystagmus to see if the ocular oscillations are affected. These include positional testing, hyperventilation, the Valsalva maneuver, and head shaking, which are all discussed under the diagnosis of vestibular forms of nystagmus, in the following section. Nystagmus induced by caloric, galvanic, or vibratory stimuli are discussed in Chapters 2 and 11.

EVALUATION OF EACH FUNCTIONAL CLASS OF EYE MOVEMENTS

Evaluation of nystagmus is incomplete without a systematic examination of each functional class of eye movements: vestibular, smooth-pursuit, saccades, and vergence (see Appendix A); selective defects may indicate the nature of the underlying disorder. In patients with spontaneous horizontal nystagmus, it is useful to test the effect of a hand-held optokinetic drum; some individuals with congenital forms of nystagmus show apparent reversal of their oscillations in response to such a stimulus.[294]

Measurement of Abnormal Eye Movements that Disrupt Fixation

It is often helpful to measure abnormal eye movements because analysis of their dynamic properties will usually identify the nature of the oscillation. Thus, recordings will differentiate between nystagmus and saccadic intrusions; this distinction may be difficult on a clinical basis. Moreover, characterization of the nystagmus waveform, especially the slow phase (Fig. 10–1), often provides a pathophysiological "signature" of the underlying disorder; this is especially the case for congenital forms of nystagmus.[5,177,357] Conventionally, nystagmus is measured in terms of its amplitude, frequency, and their product, intensity. However, the visual symptoms due to nystagmus usually correlate best with the speed of images on the retina, and the displacement from the fovea of the image of the object of regard[124,185,437,441]

Although many different methods for recording eye movements are available (Appendix B), the best approach for patients with nystagmus remains the magnetic search coil technique (see Fig. 1–1, Chapter 1). This method is preferable because many patients with ocular oscillations cannot accurately point their eyes at visual targets to allow a reliable calibration; however, the contact lens that the patient wears can be pre-calibrated on a protractor device. Furthermore, this is the only technique to allow precise measurement of horizontal, vertical, and torsional oscillations over an extended range of amplitudes and frequencies. Although originally introduced as a research tool, the technique is now widely used to evaluate clinical disorders of eye movements; in our laboratories, we have studied over 1000 patients with this method without serious adverse effect.

A PATHOPHYSIOLOGICAL APPROACH TO THE DIAGNOSIS OF NYSTAGMUS

Although nystagmus can be classified using descriptive features, our approach will be to identify the pathophysiology of the underlying disorder, and therefore the etiology of the oscillation. In health, three separate mechanisms collaborate to prevent deviation of the line of sight from the object of regard. The first mechanism is the vestibulo-ocular reflex, by which eye movements compensate for head perturbations at short latency, and so maintain clear vision during natural activities, especially locomotion. The second mechanism (referred to as the neural integrator for eye movements) is the brain's ability to hold the eye at an eccentric position in the orbit against the elastic pull of the eyeball's suspensory ligaments and muscles, which tend to return it towards central position. The third mechanism is visual fixation, which has three identifiable components. The first component is visual suppression of unwanted saccades, during such tasks as threading a needle. The second component is the visual system's ability to detect retinal image drift and rapidly program both slow and saccadic corrective eye movements. The third component is a more long-term effect of visual inputs that monitor the visual consequences of eye movements and continuously "recalibrate" them to optimize gaze stability. Such visual inputs are used as error signals and allow the brain to hone the performance of both vestibular and gaze-holding (neural integrator) function.

Disorders of these mechanisms disrupt steady gaze and lead to nystagmus; often the characteristics of the slow-phase drift indicate the ocular motor subsystem that is at fault. First, imbalance of vestibular drives often causes constant velocity drifts (see Fig. 10–1A). Second, if the gaze-holding mechanism is deficient, the eyes cannot be held steadily in an eccentric orbital position, but drift back to the midline with a decreasing-velocity waveform; this is gaze-evoked nystagmus (Fig. 10–1B). Because the gaze-holding mechanism depends, in part, upon the vestibular nuclei, nystagmus due to brainstem lesions often manifests the properties of both vestibular imbalance and disturbed gaze holding. Instability in the gaze-holding mechanism may lead to a slow-phase drift that increases in velocity (Fig. 10–1C). Third, disorders of the visual pathways may interfere with the ability to suppress eye drifts, for example, of vestibular origin, during attempted fixation of a stationary target. Furthermore, visual system disorders may lead to drifts of the eyes, including pendular oscillations (Fig. 10–1D), because adaptive mechanisms cannot null such imbalances if deprived of visual inputs.

Thus, disorders of the vestibular system, the gaze-holding mechanism, and visual stabilization may each lead to nystagmus. First, we will discuss nystagmus due to each of these disorders, in turn. Second, we will then consider other forms of nystagmus that are either due to different causes or for which no satisfactory pathophysiologic basis is known. Third, we will discuss saccadic abnormalities that disrupt steady gaze and are frequently mistaken for nystagmus. Finally, we will discuss current therapies for each of these abnormal eye movements and their visual consequences.

NYSTAGMUS DUE TO VESTIBULAR IMBALANCE

Nystagmus Caused by Peripheral Vestibular Imbalance

Disease affecting the vestibular labyrinth or nerve (including the root entry zone) typically causes nystagmus with linear slow-phase drifts (Box 10–1). The alternation of linear slow phases and corrective quick phases creates a "saw-tooth" pattern of nystagmus (see Fig. 10–1A). Such unidirectional slow-phase drifts reflect an imbalance in the level of tonic neural activity in the vestibular nuclei. If labyrinthine disease leads to reduced activity in, for example, the right vestibular nuclei, then the left vestibular nuclei will drive the eyes, in a slow phase, to the right. In this example, quick phases will be directed to the left, away from the side of the lesion. Such imbalance of vestibular tone also causes vertigo, and a tendency to fall and "past-point" towards the side

Box 10–1. Clinical Features of Peripheral Vestibular Nystagmus

- Mixed horizontal-torsional trajectory; usually beats away from the side of the lesion
- Linear ("constant velocity") slow phases
- Nystagmus increases when eyes are turned in the direction of the quick phases (Alexander's law)
- Suppressed by visual fixation; increased when fixation is removed
- Horizontal component diminished when patient lies with intact ear down; exacerbated with affected ear down
- Increased or precipitated by changes in head position, vigorous head-shaking, hyperventilation, mastoid vibration or Valsalva's maneuver
- Bedside caloric stimulation: unilaterally impaired ability to modulate spontaneous nystagmus
- Saccades and smooth pursuit are relatively preserved

See also: Pathophysiology Of Disorders Of The Vestibular System, in Chapter 2. For a schematic of the nystagmus waveform, see Fig. 10-1A. (Related Video Display: Disorders of the Vestibular System) of the lesion. Paradoxically, some patients will show nystagmus beating towards the side of the lesion; this may be recovery nystagmus, which represents the effects of vestibular adaptation.[470] Two features are helpful in identifying nystagmus as being of peripheral vestibular origin: its trajectory (direction) and whether it is suppressed by visual fixation.

The trajectory of nystagmus can be related to the geometric relationships of the semicircular canals and to the finding that experimental stimulation of an individual canal produces nystagmus in the plane of that canal. Thus, complete unilateral labyrinthine destruction leads to a mixed horizontal-torsional nystagmus (the sum of canal directions from one ear—see Fig. 2–2). In benign paroxysmal positional vertigo, a mixed upbeat-torsional nystagmus reflects posterior semicircular canal stimulation (see Video Display: Positional Nystagmus).[334] Pure vertical or pure torsional nystagmus seldom occurs with peripheral vestibular disease because this would require selective lesions of individual canals from both ears, an unlikely event (Fig. 2–2). However, it has been proposed that downbeat nystagmus induced by positional testing might, in some cases, be due to lithiasis affecting the anterior semicircular canal, perhaps because of the more parasagittal orientation of these canals;[79] this proposition requires confirmation. Rarely, central disease, such as cerebellar infarction may cause mixed horizontal-torsional nystagmus that mimics peripheral vestibular disease.[429] Alcohol produces positional nystagmus that depends on both peripheral and central factors.[228]

Nystagmus due to disease of the vestibular periphery is more prominent, or may only become apparent, when visual fixation is prevented. The reason for this is that visually mediated eye movements are working normally, and will slow or stop the eyes from drifting due to vestibular imbalance. Fixation suppresses the horizontal and vertical components of nystagmus more than the torsional component. The effects of visual fixation on nystagmus can be evaluated at the bedside with Frenzel goggles or during ophthalmoscopy, if the fixating eye is transiently covered.[735]

Another common, but not specific, feature of nystagmus caused by disease of the vestibular periphery is that its intensity increases when the eyes are turned in the direction of the quick phase: Alexander's law.[21,325,567] This phenomenon may be due to an adaptive mechanism developed to counteract the drift of the vestibular nystagmus and so establish an orbital position, in the direction of the slow phases, at which the eyes are quiet and vision is clear. Because the vestibular nuclei contribute to the gaze-holding network (neural integrator), peripheral or central lesions can cause both imbalance of the vestibular nuclei and impairment of gaze holding. Alexander's law provides the basis for a common classification of unidirectional nystagmus. First-degree nystagmus is present only on looking in the direction of the quick phases; second-degree nystagmus is also present in the central position; third-degree nystagmus is present on looking in all directions of gaze. In some patients, a horizontal vestibular nystagmus may become evident in upgaze, with convergence, or during vertical smooth pursuit movements.

Several bedside maneuvers can be employed to bring out nystagmus in patients with peripheral vestibular disease. First, a change of head position may exacerbate nystagmus or induce it in the syndrome of benign positional vertigo; this is discussed further in Chapter 11 (see Video Display: Positional Nystagmus). Second, in patients who have symptomatically recovered from a unilateral, peripheral, vestibular lesion, nystagmus can usually be induced following a period of vigorous head-shaking in the horizontal or the vertical plane for 15 to 20 seconds.[36,291,527,667] After horizontal head shaking, patients may show horizontal nystagmus with quick phases directed away from the side of the lesion (see Video Display: Disorders of the Vestibular System). After vertical head shaking, patients with unilateral peripheral vestibular lesions may show a less prominent nystagmus with horizontal quick phases directed towards the side of the lesion. Development of vertical nystagmus following horizontal head shaking suggests a central, not a peripheral, cause, such as cerebellar disease.[400,481] Third, a Valsalva maneuver may induce nystagmus.[551] Fourth, vibration of the mastoid bone may induce sustained nystagmus with a small torsional component in patients with peripheral vestibular disorders, but much less commonly with central vestibular lesions (see Video Display: Disorders of the Vestibular System).[299] Thus, vibration-induced nystagmus is encountered in patients with perilymph fistula, superior canal dehiscence, unilateral loss of labyrinthine function, and with some central lesions, including cerebellar degeneration.

Fifth, hyperventilation may induce nystagmus in patients with schwannoma of the eighth cranial nerve, and after vestibular neuritis.[58,482] The nystagmus may be directed with slow phases away from the side of the lesion, and a torsional component is often prominent.[583] Measurement of such hyperventilation-induced nystagmus using the 3-D magnetic search coil technique indicates that inputs arising from the horizontal semicircular canal were mainly responsible.[482] An illustrative case is presented in Chapter 11.

Rarely, noises induce peripheral vestibular nystagmus: the Tullio phenomenon (Fig. 11–2) (see Video Display: Disorders of the Vestibular System).[204,483,575] Auditory stimulation of the vestibular organ occurs when there is a breach in the bony labyrinth, especially in the syndrome of superior canal dehiscence, which is discussed in Chapter 11.[483,523]

Whether or not an imbalance of proprioceptive inputs from neck muscles can produce a cervical nystagmus akin to that from peripheral vestibular disease is uncertain. In normal human subjects, cervical proprioception, the cervico-ocular reflex (COR), plays little role in the stabilization of gaze during natural head movements.[103,591] Although the COR does assume more importance in individuals who have lost vestibular function,[104,380] the evidence that cervical disease can induce nystagmus and vertigo is sparse. In human subjects, injection of local anesthetic into the neck has failed to produced nystagmus although slight gait instability or ataxia results.[166,205] However, patients who have undergone radical neck surgery may show reduced vestibular responses.[371] Vibration of the neck may induce nystagmus in patients with labyrinthine disease, an issue that is discussed in Chapter 11. Conversely, a cerebellar lesion has been reported to cause an increase in the COR.[102] Isolated nystagmus and vertigo induced by neck movement are only rarely due to kinking of the vertebral artery,[92,93,664] but may follow chiropractic manipulation of the neck, along with other signs of brainstem compromise.[731]

Nystagmus Caused by Central Vestibular Imbalance

Here we discuss three forms of nystagmus that may be caused by central vestibular pathways: downbeat, upbeat, and torsional nystagmus. We also discuss how central lesions may rarely produce nystagmus with trajectories that are horizontal, or in the plane of a single semicircular canal. After describing the clinical features of each form of nystagmus, we summarize possible pathogenesis. Although periodic alternating nystagmus and seesaw nystagmus may also be viewed as forms of central vestibular nystagmus, they will be discussed separately, below.

CLINICAL FEATURES OF DOWNBEAT NYSTAGMUS

Table 10–1 summarizes some of the clinical disorders with which downbeat nystagmus has been reported. Commonly it occurs with

Table 10–1. **Etiology of Downbeat Nystagmus**[57,105,298,723]

- Cerebellar degeneration,[260,741] including familial episodic ataxia,[54,95] paraneoplastic degeneration,[28,700] and multiple system atrophy[79]
- Craniocervical anomalies, including Arnold–Chiari malformation, Paget's disease, basilar invagination, and syringobulbia[208,525,530]
- Infarction of brainstem or cerebellum[57,518,632]
- Rotational vertebral artery syndrome[129a]
- Dolichoectasia of the vertebrobasilar artery[327,362] or compression of the vertebral artery[572]
- Multiple sclerosis[57,105,464]
- Cerebellar tumor, including hemangioblastoma[595]
- Encephalitis[330]
- Head trauma[57]
- Increased intracranial pressure and hydrocephalus[528,632]
- Toxic-metabolic
  - Anticonvulsant medication[23,24,77,131,347,561]
  - Lithium intoxication[149,296,712]
  - Alcohol intoxication[571] and induced cerebellar degeneration[734]
  - Wernicke's encephalopathy[150,426]
  - Magnesium depletion[211,590]
  - Amiodarone[17]
  - Opioids[576]
  - Deficiency of vitamin B12[468] or thiamine[494]
  - Toluene abuse[460]
- Heat stroke[168a]
- Tetanus[522]
- Congenital[85,97]
- Transient finding in infants[263,342,707]
- Idiopathic form[518]

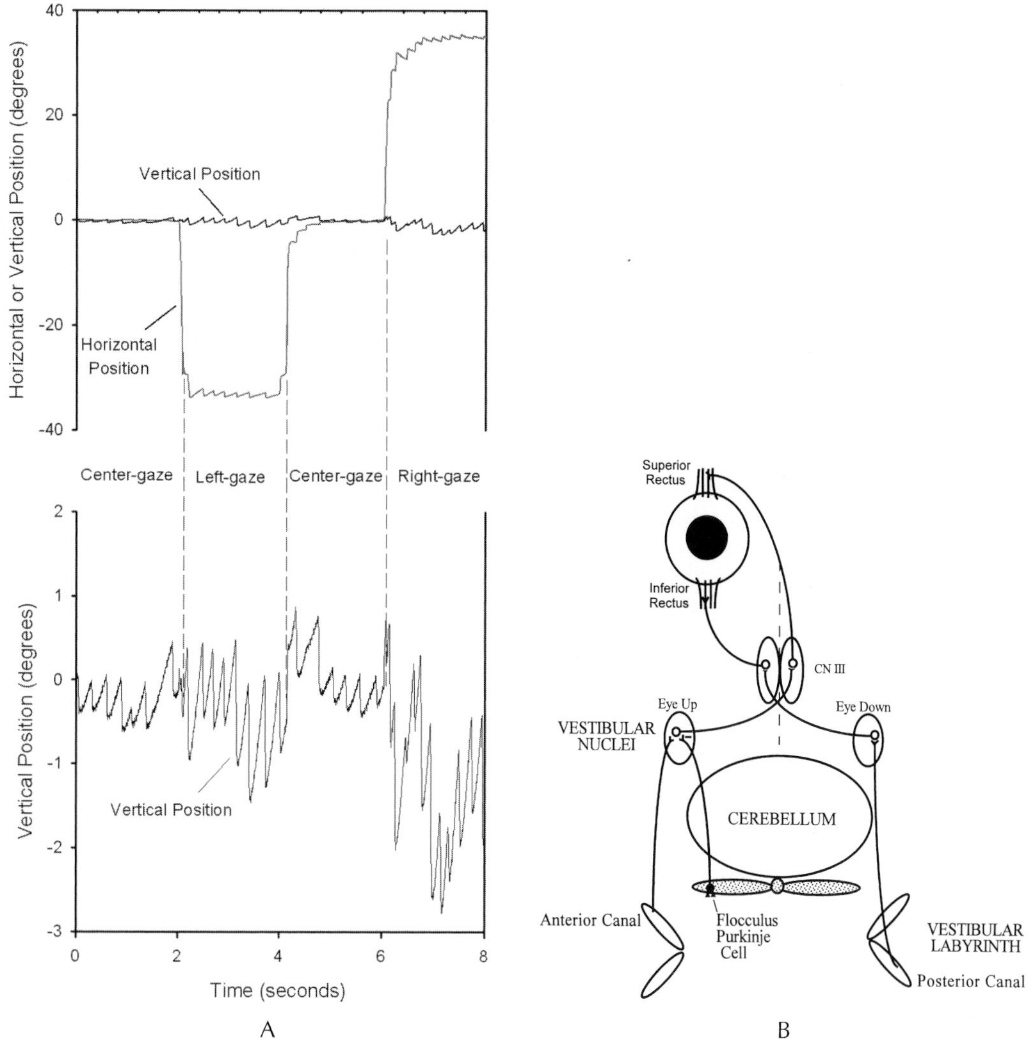

Figure 10–2. Downbeat nystagmus. (A) Example of downbeat nystagmus that was brought out during lateral gaze, when it was accompanied by a horizontal gaze-evoked nystagmus that causes a diagonal (down and lateral) beating nystagmus. The top panel shows horizontal and vertical eye position plotted on the same scale. The bottom panel plots vertical eye position on a more sensitive scale, and it is evident that the nystagmus increases in either left gaze or right gaze compared with center gaze. Positive values indicate rightward or upward rotations from the viewpoint of the patient. The single-position traces are offset to aid clarity of display. (B) Hypothetical scheme for downbeat nystagmus, based on Ito,[354] and Baloh and Spooner.[56] The flocculus preferentially discharges for downward movements; thus lesions will reduce inhibition and cause the eyes to drift up. The flocculus inhibits inputs from anterior semicircular canals of the vestibular labyrinth, which evoke upward eye movements via projections through the superior vestibular nuclei to motoneurons supplying elevator muscles, including the superior rectus (CN III is oculomotor nucleus). Conversely, the flocculus does not govern inputs from the posterior semicircular canals, which evoke downward eye movements via projections through the vestibular nuclei to motoneurons supplying depressor muscles, including the inferior rectus. If inhibition from the flocculus is impaired, the eyes will drift upward causing downbeat nystagmus. Other hypotheses to account for downbeat nystagmus are discussed in the text.

degenerations affecting the vestibulocerebellum, lesions near the craniocervical junction, and with drug intoxications, especially lithium. Vertebral ectasia may also cause downbeat nystagmus. It is less common with multiple sclerosis and stroke.

Patients with downbeat nystagmus often complain of illusory motion of their visual environment (oscillopsia), due to the retinal slip produced by the nystagmus slow phases. This retinal image slip also causes an increased threshold for egocentric detection of object motion.[111] Other complaints are postural instability and clumsiness.[255a] Patients with downbeat nystagmus that report diplopia often have a skew deviation, which alternates in eccentric gaze, the abducting eye usually being the higher one (see Skew Deviation in Chapter 11).

Downbeat nystagmus is usually present with the eyes in central position, although its amplitude may be so small that it is only detected during ophthalmoscopy (Box 10–2). A low-velocity upward drift of the eyes (downward drift of the optic disc) may occasionally be seen during ophthalmoscopy in normal subjects, but it is not present during visual fixation of a stationary target. Often downbeat nystagmus only becomes evident in lateral gaze (see Video Display: Downbeat, Upbeat, Torsional Nystagmus). Since horizontal gaze-evoked nystagmus is also often present, the nystagmus is directed laterally and downward (i.e., diagonally). In most patients with downbeat nystagmus, Alexander's law is obeyed and slow-phase velocity (and nystagmus intensity) is greatest in downgaze, and least in upgaze. Hence, asking patients to look down and laterally is often the best way to bring out downbeat nystagmus. In some patients, however, downbeat nystagmus is greatest on upgaze. In these cases, the slow-phases may not be linear but are, instead, increasing in velocity, see Fig. 10–1C and Fig. 10–7B (see Video Display: Disorders of Gaze Holding);[15,738] this finding indicates an instability of the vertical gaze-holding network. A similar pattern of downbeat nystagmus has also been observed following removal of the vestibulocerebellum (flocculus and paraflocculus) in monkeys.[740] Downbeat nystagmus is occasionally disjunctive, being more vertical in one eye and torsional in the other. In these circumstances, it may be accompanied by internuclear ophthalmoplegia.[244,511]

In most patients, removal of fixation (e.g., by Frenzel goggles) does not substantially affect slow-phase velocity, although quick-phase frequency may diminish. Convergence often accentuates downbeat nystagmus. In some patients, downbeat nystagmus is converted to upbeat nystagmus upon convergence, or vice versa (see Video Display: Downbeat, Upbeat, Torsional Nystagmus).[150,227] Some patients may show combined divergent-downbeat nystagmus.[724]

Downbeat nystagmus is often precipitated or increased when patients are placed in either a "head-hanging" position or prone position for a minute or more.[462] Occasional patients will switch from downbeat to upbeat when they lie supine.[308] However, normal subjects also may show "chin-beating" nystagmus when they are positioned upside-down in darkness.[84,399] These observations imply that otolithic inputs may influence or even cause downbeat nystagmus, an issue that is discussed below, under pathogenesis. The clinical implication of these

Box 10–2. Clinical Features of Downbeat Nystagmus

- Best evoked on looking down and laterally; often in association with horizontal gaze-evoked nystagmus, and so may appear oblique on lateral gaze
- Slow phases may have linear-, increasing-, or decreasing-velocity waveforms
- Poorly suppressed by fixation of a visual target
- May be precipitated or exacerbated or changed in direction, by altering head position, vigorous head-shaking (horizontal or vertical), or hyperventilation
- Convergence may increase, suppress or convert to upbeat nystagmus
- Associated with other signs of vestibulocerebellar involvement

See also: Pathogenesis of Central Vestibular Nystagmus. For a recorded example, see Fig. 10-2. For etiologies, see Table 10-1, (Related Video Display: Downbeat nystagmus, Upbeat, Torsional Nystagmus) findings is that since normal subjects may show chin beating nystagmus behind Frenzel goggles while in dependent or prone positions, further investigations, such as neuroimaging, are only indicated if other abnormalities are present on the ocular motor or neurological examination.[435]

When the vertical vestibulo-ocular reflex is tested in patients with downbeat nystagmus using high-acceleration head thrusts, at least some patients show an asymmetry with greater responses for downward head rotations than could be explained simply by addition of nystagmus slow phases to the vestibular eye movements.[257,701,737] Such findings suggest an asymmetric sensitivity of anterior versus posterior canal influences in some patients with downbeat nystagmus. Furthermore, following horizontal head thrusts, a downward corrective saccade occurs (see Video Display: Downbeat, Upbeat, Torsional Nystagmus).

Vertical smooth pursuit is impaired for downward tracking in patients with downbeat nystagmus;[253] smooth eye-head tracking may be similarly affected. This asymmetry may be greater than can be accounted for by superposition of the upward slow phases of downbeat nystagmus upon the ongoing pursuit movement.[737] Normal subjects may develop downbeat nystagmus after they perform repetitive upward pursuit, suggesting that pursuit asymmetry may contribute to the pathogenesis of downbeat nystagmus, as is discussed below.[461]

CLINICAL FEATURES OF UPBEAT NYSTAGMUS

The more common disorders with which upbeat is associated are summarized in Table 10–2. Upbeat nystagmus is less well localized than downbeat nystagmus, being reported predominantly with paramedian lesions of the medulla,[329,365,424,496,516,671] but also with pontine and midbrain abnormalities. Upbeat nystagmus is a common finding in Wernicke's encephalopathy, in which case its direction may change with convergence.

Upbeat nystagmus with the eyes close to central position (see Video Display: Downbeat, Upbeat, Torsional Nystagmus, and Box 10–3) should be differentiated from upbeat nystagmus evoked exclusively on upgaze. The latter occurs in general gaze-holding failure, with peripheral ocular motor disorders including myasthenia gravis, and in some normal subjects. It should also be differentiated from the transient, mixed upbeat-torsional nystagmus that is induced by positional testing in patients with benign paroxysmal positional vertigo of the posterior canal type (see Video Display: Positional Nystagmus). Unlike downbeat nystagmus, upbeat nystagmus does not usually increase on lateral gaze. Upbeat nystagmus that is present in central position usually follows Alexander's law, becoming greatest in upgaze. Sometimes, however, the nystagmus is accentuated on looking down, and then the slow phase is more likely to be increasing velocity rather than linear (Fig. 10–3C).

Prevention of visual fixation (for example by Frenzel goggles) may alter the frequency of quick phases, but does not influence slow-phase velocity. Convergence enhances the nystagmus in some patients, suppresses it in others, and occasionally converts it to downbeat nystagmus.[150,227] Some patients show a combined upbeat-divergent form of nystagmus (Fig. 10–3B) (see Video Display: Downbeat, Upbeat, Torsional Nystagmus).

Upbeat nystagmus may be influenced by head posture, and downbeat nystagmus may convert to upbeat nystagmus in the supine position.[308] The vestibulo-ocular reflex (VOR) may be abnormal, especially in patients with

Table 10–2. **Etiology of Upbeat Nystagmus[57,229]**

Infarction of medulla[57,114,329,365,390,496,671] or cerebellum and superior cerebellar peduncle[75,742]
Wernicke's encephalopathy[150,229,381,665a,744]
Multiple sclerosis[229,481,516]
Tumors of the medulla,[229,250] cerebellum,[219,675] or midbrain[500,680]
Cerebellar degenerations[241,242] or anomalies[527a]
Brainstem encephalitis[238]
Creutzfeldt–Jacob disease[742a]
Behcet's syndrome[351]
Meningitis[333]
Leber's congenital amaurosis and other congenital disorders of the anterior visual pathways[262]
Thalamic arteriovenous malformation[510]
Congenital[638]
Organophosphate poisoning[366]
Tobacco[627]
Associated with middle ear disease[279]
Transient finding in infants[342]

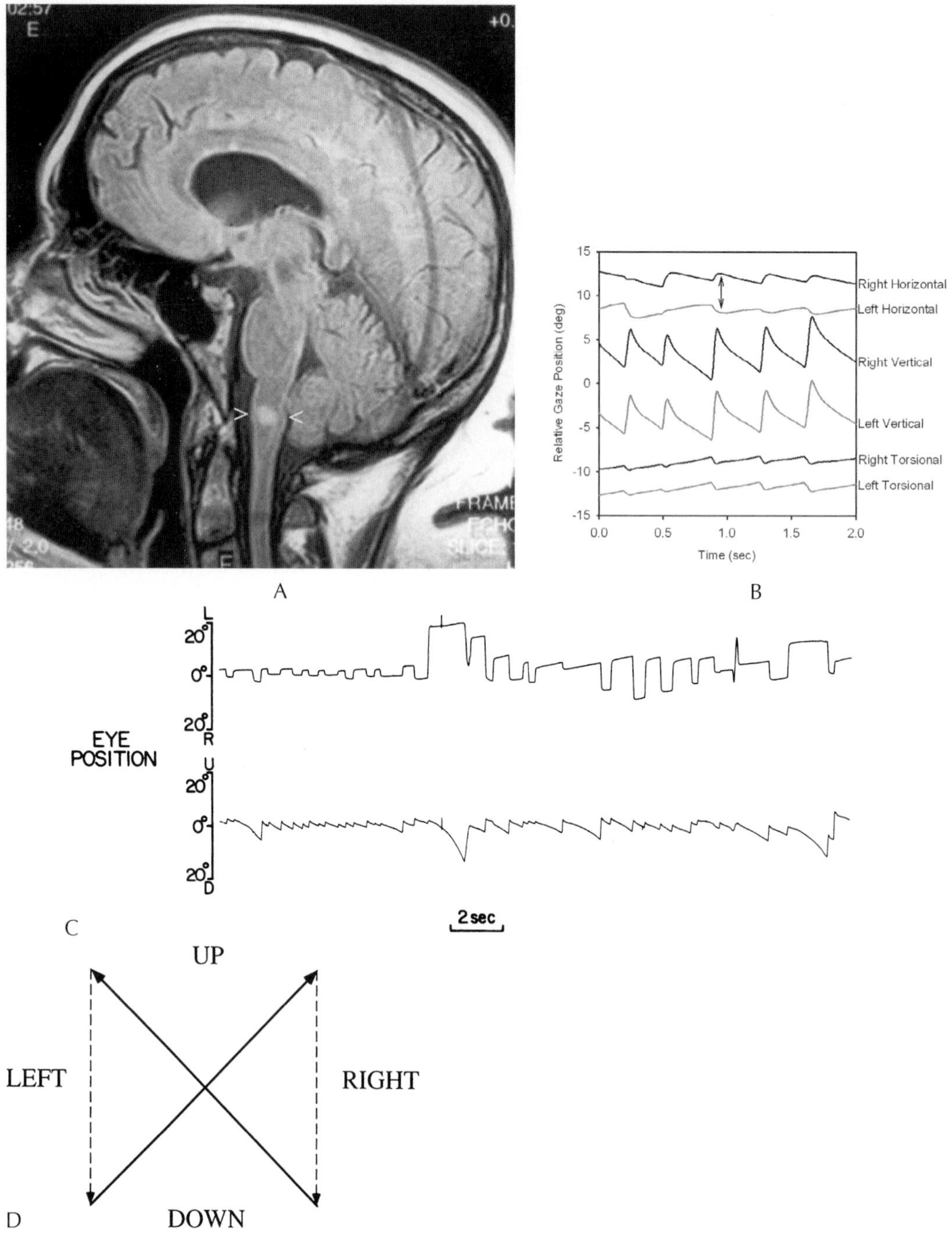

Figure 10–3. Upbeat nystagmus. (A) Magnetic resonance T2-weighted image showing a hyperintense signal in the medulla of a patient with upbeat nystagmus and multiple sclerosis.[481] After horizontal head shaking, she developed downbeating nystagmus (perverted head-shaking nystagmus) and tumbling vertigo. (Reproduced from Minagar et al.,[481] with permission of Lippincott, Williams and Wilkins.) (B) Upbeat nystagmus with an associated divergent component in a 45-year-old woman with multiple sclerosis (see Video Display: Downbeat, Upbeat, Torsional Nystagmus). Not apparent on the video, but evident on this representative record, is that the predominant vertical component and small torsional component are conjugate, but the horizontal movements are disjunctive, having divergent quick phases (double arrowhead). The single-position traces are offset to aid clarity of display; positive deflections indicate rightward (horizontal), upward (vertical) or clockwise (torsional) eye rotations, with respect to the patient. (C) Upbeat nystagmus in a 50-year-old man who had a posterior fossa meningioma removed in 1943 by Dr. Walter Dandy. Note that although each slow phase is directed downward, sometimes with increasing velocity, quick-phases are directed obliquely upward alternately to the right or left, because of the changing direction of each horizontal component. D: down; L: left; R: right; U: up. This creates a trajectory (D) called bow-tie nystagmus;[627,709] quick phases are shown as solid lines and slow phases as dashed lines.

Box 10–3. Clinical Features of Upbeat Nystagmus

- Present in center position; usually increases on looking up
- Slow phases may have linear-, increasing-, or decreasing-velocity waveforms
- Poorly suppressed by visual fixation of a distant target
- Convergence may increase, suppress or convert to downbeat nystagmus
- Associated with abnormal vertical vestibular and smooth-pursuit responses, and saccadic intrusions (square-wave jerks) that produce a bow-tie nystagmus

See also: Pathogenesis of Central Vestibular Nystagmus. For recorded examples, see Fig. 10-3. For etiologies, see Table 10-2. (Related Video Display: Downbeat nystagmus, Upbeat, Torsional Nystagmus)

Wernicke's encephalopathy. Vertical smooth pursuit is abnormal in patients with upbeat nystagmus, but treatment with the potassium channel blocker, 4-aminopyridine lead to improved pursuit and better fixation suppression of the upbeat nystagmus.[255] Some patients may show quick-phases that have small horizontal components (or square wave jerks) that alternate to the right or left; these trajectories create the pattern of a bow-tie nystagmus (Fig. 10–3D).[129,627,709] Upbeat nystagmus may be associated with contrapulsion of saccades (hypermetria away from the side of the lesion, hypometria towards the side of the lesion),[75, 555,671] an issue that may provide clues about its pathogenesis, and which is discussed further below.

CLINICAL FEATURES OF TORSIONAL NYSTAGMUS

Peripheral vestibular, congenital, and seesaw nystagmus all may have torsional components, especially on lateral gaze (when described in an eye-fixed coordinate system). However, nystagmus that is predominantly torsional in central position bespeaks disease affecting central vestibular connections. Often it is difficult to detect, except by careful observation of conjunctival vessels or noting with an ophthalmoscope the opposite direction of retinal movement on either side of the fovea.

Torsional nystagmus is usually associated with medullary lesions, such as syringobulbia and Wallenberg's syndrome (lateral medullary infarction) (Table 10–3).[453] The clinical features of torsional nystagmus (Box 10–4) show similarities to downbeat and upbeat nystagmus, including modulation by head rotations, variable slow-phase waveforms, and suppression by convergence.[509] Torsional nystagmus is probably a common finding in patients with acute ocular tilt reaction,[49] including those with internuclear ophthalmoplegia.[167] It has also been described during vertical smooth pursuit in patients with lesions involving the middle cerebellar peduncle;[232] this phenomenon is discussed further in the section on Ocular Motor Syndromes Caused by Disease of the Cerebellum in Chapter 12. When torsional nystagmus occurs with midbrain disease, the quick phases are usually contralesional (upper poles of the eyes rotate away from the side of the lesion), and both riMLF and inter-

Table 10–3. **Etiology of Torsional Nystagmus*[453]**

Syringobulbia, with or without syringomyelia and Arnold–Chiari malformation[709]
Brainstem stroke (e.g., Wallenberg's syndrome)[491]
Arteriovenous malformation in the brainstem[491,509] or middle cerebellar peduncle[232]
Brainstem tumor[453]
Multiple sclerosis[453]
Oculopalatal tremor ("myoclonus")[53]
Head trauma[453]
Congenital

*Often occurs in association with the ocular tilt reaction[49,658] and unilateral internuclear ophthalmoplegia.[167]

Box 10–4. Clinical Features of Torsional Nystagmus

- Torsional jerk nystagmus (minimal vertical or horizontal components) present with eye close to central position
- Slow phases may have linear-, increasing-, or decreasing-velocity waveforms
- Poorly suppressed by visual fixation of a distant target
- Exacerbated by changes in head position or vigorous head shaking
- May be suppressed by convergence
- Often occurs in association with ocular tilt reaction or unilateral internuclear ophthalmoplegia
- May be precipitated or modulated by vertical smooth pursuit movements

See also: Pathogenesis of Central Vestibular Nystagmus, in Chapter 10. For etiologies, see Table 10-3. (Related Video Display: Downbeat nystagmus, Upbeat, Torsional Nystagmus)

stitial nucleus of Cajal are usually involved.[307] Non-rhythmic but continuous torsional eye movements have been reported as a possible paraneoplastic phenomenon.[573] Finally, patients who have suffered a peripheral vestibular disturbance show a small torsional quick phase with each blink of the eye; the direction of the upper pole of the eye moves away from the side of the lesion. This finding can help with diagnosis if the change in torsional eye position (before and after the blink) is recorded with a video camera.[597]

HORIZONTAL NYSTAGMUS DUE TO CENTRAL VESTIBULAR IMBALANCE

Horizontal nystagmus is most often either congenital or peripheral vestibular in origin, in which case a torsional component is commonly associated. However, central vestibular disturbances occasionally cause nystagmus that is horizontal (when the eyes are close to central position). Sometimes the underlying disorder is a Chiari malformation (Fig. 10–4).[65] The slow-phase waveform may be increasing-velocity, making distinction from congenital forms of nystagmus potentially difficult. However, patients may report recent onset of visual symptoms such as oscillopsia, and measurements usually demonstrate an associated vertical component, which is uncommon in congenital nystagmus. Patients with horizontal nystagmus that is present in the central position should be always be observed for a period of several minutes to exclude the possibility of periodic alternating nystagmus.

PERVERTED NYSTAGMUS

Patients with disease affecting central vestibular connections, including the vestibulocerebellum, sometimes develop nystagmus in a plane other than that being stimulated by either caloric stimulation or head rotation. This is called perverted nystagmus. For example, after horizontal head shaking, downbeat nystagmus may occur—an inappropriate cross-coupling of vestibular nystagmus.[400,699] Following clinical or experimental lesions of the vestibular nuclei, horizontal head rotation or unilateral caloric stimulation may induce responses with vertical components.[481,688] Perverted caloric responses also occur as a manifestation of drug intoxications.[630] However, it is important to note that a small vertical component may also be present in the caloric responses of normal subjects.[60] Brainstem lesions can produce a range of forms of nystagmus, with horizontal, vertical, or torsional components,[702] sometimes as part of the syndrome of oculopalatal tremor.

PATHOGENESIS OF DOWNBEAT, UPBEAT, AND TORSIONAL NYSTAGMUS

Substantial progress has been made in understanding these forms of nystagmus due to the

A

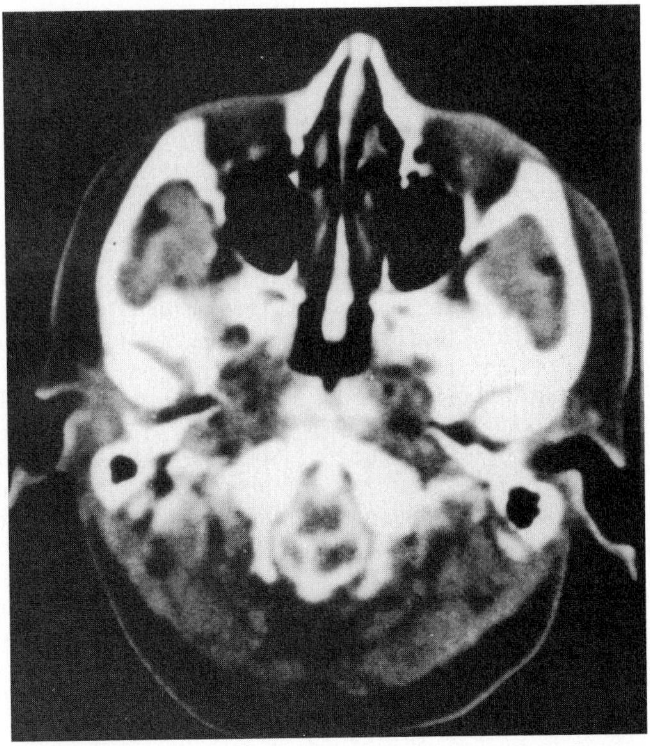

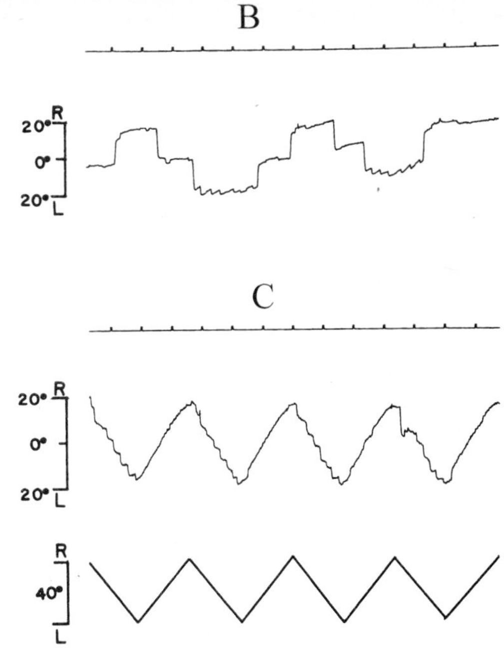

Figure 10–4. Horizontal nystagmus caused by the Arnold–Chiari malformation. The patient was a 40-year-old man who for 12 years had noticed slight imbalance on making turns or negotiating stairs. For the past 3 years, he had experienced episodes of severe vertigo and nausea, which lasted for a few minutes and were precipitated by straining or laughing. (A) CT of his cranio-cervical junction, using metrizamide contrast, showed descent of the cerebellar tonsils behind the medulla, consistent with a diagnosis of Arnold–Chiari malformation. Eye movements were recorded by electro-oculography. The top trace (B) shows a horizontal nystagmus, more marked in left gaze. The lower trace (C) shows asymmetric smooth pursuit, worse during tracking of target motion to the left. The time scale, at top, is in seconds. His vestibulo-ocular reflex was preserved in both directions. Cancellation of the vestibulo-ocular reflex was asymmetrical, consistent with his pursuit deficit (not shown). L: left; R: right.

formulation and testing of hypotheses, which are based on modern neurobiology and clinicopathological correlation.

In the case of downbeat nystagmus, both clinical and experimental studies indicate the importance of lesions of the vestibulocerebellum (especially the flocculus and paraflocculus).[254,462,701,740] Disease that diffusely affects the cerebellum, such as the hereditary calcium channelopathies, also commonly produces downbeat nystagmus.[54,647] Downbeat nystagmus is uncommon with brainstem lesions.[529]

In contrast, upbeat nystagmus is reported most commonly with lesions in the caudal medulla, which variably involve the perihypoglossal group of nuclei, including the nucleus intercalates, the nucleus of Roller, and nucleus pararaphales.[250,329,365,390,496,671] Cases of upbeat nystagmus with more rostral brainstem lesions may interrupt the ventral tegmental tract, which contains projections from the vestibular nuclei that receive inputs from the anterior semicircular canals, and which crosses near the rostral pole of the nucleus reticularis tegmenti pontis (see Fig. 2–3 in Chapter 2).[328,529,556,687] Upbeat nystagmus is also reported with lesions involving the brachium conjunctivum in the rostral pons and midbrain.[75,382,500]

The coexistence of upbeat nystagmus and saccadic contrapulsion, which is discussed in Chapter 3, may provide a clue about the pathogenesis of these two conditions. Lateropulsion of saccades can be attributed to interruption either of climbing fiber pathways running from the inferior olivary nucleus to the cerebellar vermis, or to disruption of outputs from the fastigial nucleus running in the superior cerebellar peduncle (Fig. 3–16, in Chapter 3).[639,697] Contrapulsion (accompanied by upbeat nystagmus) occurs with lesions affecting climbing fibers before they cross the midline (site 1 in Fig. 3–16),[671] or projections from the fastigial nucleus running in the superior cerebellar peduncle (site 5 in Fig. 3–16).[555,742] Note that lesions at sites 2-4 in Fig. 3–16 cause ipsipulsion of saccades but apparently do not produce upbeat nystagmus. Pharmacological inactivation of the fastigial nucleus causes ipsipulsion of saccades but only minor displacement of eye position during fixation, which is towards the side of the injection and variable in the vertical plane;[568] there is no upbeat nystagmus. Thus, unlike downbeat nystagmus, upbeat nystagmus does not seem to occur with cerebellar lesions, but is encountered with lesions throughout the brainstem that may also include cerebellar connections.[529]

Torsional nystagmus is reported with a wider range of lesions throughout the brainstem, including lateral medullary infarction,[491] syringobulbia,[709] pontine tegmental venous angioma,[509] midbrain lesions involving riMLF and interstitial nucleus of Cajal,[307] internuclear ophthalmoplegia,[49] and lesions affecting the middle cerebellar peduncle.[232] Furthermore, many forms of nystagmus have a torsional component and, without reliable 3-D records, it is often difficult to determine what is meant in clinical reports of torsional nystagmus. Thus, our main discussion will address the pathogenesis of vertical forms of nystagmus.

Could any anatomic principles account for the range of sites that are reported with these forms of nystagmus? We suggest that it is possible to account for these findings by considering certain innate asymmetries that characterize the vestibular system and its central connections. First, the anatomical orientation of the labyrinthine semicircular canals may be right-left symmetric, but lacks symmetry in a craniocaudal direction.[88] Second, while the central connections of the horizontal vestibular system are right-left symmetric, those of the vertical vestibular responses are dissimilar for upward or downward eye movements (Fig. 2–3). Third, Purkinje cells of the cerebellar flocculus show an asymmetry of preferred on-directions, most discharging for downward eye movements.[463] These up-down asymmetries are addressed by considering how vertical forms of nystagmus may be due to disorders of: (1) the vertical vestibulo-ocular reflex; (2) the otolith-ocular reflexes; (3) the vestibulocerebellum; (4) the network for eccentric gaze holding (neural integrator); and (5) the smooth pursuit system. In each patient it is possible to identify several different components of the vertical drift: (A) a constant velocity drift (bias); (B) a gaze-dependent drift, which changes when the eye is at eccentric positions, and obeys Alexander's law; (C) a gravity-dependent drift.[254,462,662] The strength of these components differs in individual patients, suggesting that more than one mechanism contributes to downbeat and upbeat nystagmus.

Could an Asymmetry of the Anatomy of the Vertical VOR Account for Vertical Nystagmus?

Excitatory projections for the vertical vestibulo-ocular reflex (see Fig. 2–3) from the *posterior semicircular canals*, which mediate downward eye movements, synapse in the medial and lateral vestibular nuclei and then cross dorsally in the medulla, beneath the nucleus prepositus hypoglossi to reach the contralateral medial longitudinal fasciculus. Experimental lesions that presumably involve this pathway cause upward eye drifts and downbeat nystagmus.[166] Conversely, excitatory connections from the *anterior semicircular canals*, which mediate upward eye movements, take different routes, including the ventral tegmental tract, which crosses in the pons, close to the rostral pole of the nucleus reticularis tegmenti pontis.[471,472,687] Thus, unilateral internuclear ophthalmoplegia mainly impairs the vertical VOR mediated by the posterior canals (which project to ocular motoneurons via the MLF) but has a lesser effect on the VOR mediated by the anterior canals (which project to ocular motoneurons by pathways besides the MLF, including the ventral tegmental tract and brachium conjunctivum.)[152] Thus, it seems possible that brainstem lesions could selectively interrupt either anterior canal excitatory projections, causing upbeat nystagmus, or posterior canal projections, causing downbeat nystagmus. Clinically, the case for anterior canal projections and upbeat nystagmus seems stronger.[529] If downbeat nystagmus were caused by an imbalance of central vestibular connections mediating the rotational VOR, then the 3-D eye rotations should violate Listing's law. Experimental studies show that this prediction is confirmed for some, but not all, patients with downbeat nystagmus.[254,662]

Could Imbalance of Inputs from the Otoliths Cause Vertical Nystagmus?

There is strong experimental evidence that downbeat nystagmus in patients with cerebellar disease is influenced by head position,[462] and may even be converted to upbeat nystagmus in some patients.[308] Furthermore, even normal subjects may develop chin beating nystagmus when they are upside-down in darkness.[84,399] However, not all patients with vertical nystagmus are affected by change of head position or imposed linear accelerations.[278] Indeed, there often appears to be two components of downbeat nystagmus, one dependent on gravity and the other independent of it.[462] Thus, it seems that an otolithic mechanism is the primary mechanisms in some patients,[252] but other mechanisms are more important in other patients. An interesting corroborative line of evidence for the otolithic hypothesis is that convergence often influences vertical nystagmus, and that the viewing distance of a visual target strongly influences the gain of the translational VOR.[704]

How Do Lesions of the Cerebellar Flocculus Account for Vertical Nystagmus?

While there is little argument that lesions of the cerebellar flocculus and paraflocculus (see Box 6–10) in both monkey and humans cause downbeat nystagmus, there is some dispute about the underlying mechanism. One hypothesis rests on the finding that Purkinje cells send inhibitory projections to the central connections of the anterior canal but not of the posterior canal (Fig. 10–2).[56,354] This asymmetry of inhibitory projections would account for the finding that experimental flocculectomy causes downbeat nystagmus;[740] this lesion disinhibits anterior canal (but not posterior canal) projections and so causes the eyes to drift up, producing downbeat nystagmus. An alternative hypothesis concerns the geometric arrangement of the semicircular canals, and the eye movement vectors due to tonic discharge of neurons from each canal; such considerations suggest that the eyes would tend to drift upward.[88] It is postulated that, normally, the vestibulocerebellum would take care of such an imbalance due to the vestibular periphery but, if cerebellar function were compromised, upward eye drifts would lead to downbeat nystagmus. A third hypothesis concerning the flocculus rests on the electrophysiological finding that most Purkinje cells in the vestibulocerebellum preferentially discharge for downward eye movements and that disorders that remove this cerebellar bias would cause the eyes to drift up.[463] The first two of these floccular hypotheses predicts that patients with downbeat nystagmus should show asymmetric responses to vertical head impulses, with greater eye velocities upwards when the head is perturbed down. At least some patients with downbeat nystagmus show such asymmetries.[257,701] Downbeat nystagmus has been reported in patients with autoantibodies to glutamic acid decarboxylase (GAD-ab),[24a,30,670a] raising the possibility that a dysfunction of a specific population of cerebellar neurons could contribute to downbeat nystagmus. However, several diverse clinical disorders have now been described with GAD-ab, making their role in the pathogenesis of neurological disease uncertain.[213a,672,672a]

A new impetus to the floccular hypotheses for vertical nystagmus has been provided by the observation that potassium channel blockers such as 3,4-diaminopyridine and 4-aminopyridine suppress downbeat nystagmus in some subjects, presumably because of increased inhibition of the anterior canal projections by flocculus Purkinje cells.[373,436,665] In some patients, downbeat has been converted to upbeat nystagmus by such treatments.[295,308] However, preliminary evidence suggests different mechanisms for effects on upbeat and downbeat nystagmus, with effects on visually mediated suppression being more important for the former.[255,256]

Could Vertical Nystagmus be Accounted for by Abnormalities of the Neural Integrator for Eye Movements?

A neural network that includes the nucleus prepositus hypoglossi and adjacent medial vestibular nuclei (NPH-MVN region), the interstitial nucleus of Cajal and the vestibulocerebellum is important for the mechanism for holding the eyes steady in eccentric gaze; this neural integrator for eye movements is discussed in Chapter 5. Because patients with downbeat nystagmus also often show gaze-evoked nystagmus, it has been suggested that downbeat nystagmus is due to failure of the neural integrator for eye movements.[254] Several lines of evidence support this hypothesis. First, analysis of 3-D eye movements in patients with downbeat nystagmus indicates failure of the neural integrator for eye movements in either the vertical plane or both vertical and horizontal planes.[254] Second, a patient with lethal lithium intoxication, who developed downbeat nystagmus prior to complete gaze failure, had lesions in the nucleus prepositus hypoglossi.[149] Third, disease of the vestibulocerebellum may rarely cause gaze instability (Fig. 10–7), so that the eyes drift at increasing velocity away from central position in the vertical or horizontal planes, suggesting instability, rather than leakage, of the neural integrator (see Video Display: Disorders of Gaze Holding).[15,65,738]

The cell groups of the paramedian tracts (PMT) (see Box 6–4) also may contribute to neural integrator function by relaying eye movement signals to the vestibulocerebellum.[116,501] One component of the PMT cell groups is the medullary nucleus pararaphales, which receives vertical eye position signals from the interstitial nucleus of Cajal. Thus, medullary lesions that affect this nucleus might lead to upbeat nystagmus.[114,671]

Could Asymmetry of Vertical Smooth Pursuit Account for Vertical Nystagmus?

Based on the observation that the slow-phase velocity of downbeat nystagmus is unaffected by visual fixation, and vertical smooth pursuit is impaired, it was originally proposed that many of the characteristics of downbeat nystagmus could be best explained by a central imbalance in smooth pursuit tone.[737] After normal subjects carry out sustained, asymmetric vertical pursuit, they also may develop downbeat nystagmus.[461] A smooth-pursuit imbalance could contribute to downbeat nystagmus because of compromise of the pursuit pathway either as it passes through the cerebellum or in the vestibular and prepositus nuclei (see Fig. 6–7). Alternatively, the bias of Purkinje cells for discharging for downward movements could account for asymmetric vertical pursuit in patients with downbeat nystagmus.[463] Upbeat or downbeat nystagmus are described as transient findings in otherwise healthy infants,[342,707] and their resolution may reflect "calibration" of the VOR, pursuit or gaze-holding mechanisms as the visual system becomes fully myelinated.

Summary of Current Views about the Pathogenesis of Vertical Forms of Nystagmus

At present there are several hypotheses for upbeat and downbeat nystagmus, each supported by experimental data. Indeed, it seems likely that more that one mechanism accounts for the spectrum of patients with vertical nystagmus encountered in clinical practice.[254] Furthermore, it may prove to be artificial to try and distinguish between some of the different mechanisms in individual patients. For example, vestibular responses require adaptive modification to optimize their performance, and they depend upon visual inputs to achieve this. Thus, asymmetry of smooth pursuit or the VOR may not be mutually exclusive hypotheses. Moreover, the vestibular nuclei and vestibular cerebellum both contribute to the network of neurons that integrates premotor signals, allowing the eyes to be held steadily at eccentric gaze angles. Otolithic inputs may contribute to this gaze-holding network.[251,713] Perhaps the most important hypotheses for clinicians are those that relate to treatment and, in that regard, the role of the vestibulocerebellum, which can be influenced by potassium channel blockers such as 4-aminopyridine, seems most pertinent.[295] Studying the effects of such agents on vertical forms of nystagmus and responses to the vestibulo-ocular reflex seem likely to provide further insights.

PERIODIC ALTERNATING NYSTAGMUS

Acquired periodic alternating nystagmus (PAN) is a spontaneous horizontal nystagmus, present in central gaze, which reverses direction approximately every 2 minutes (Box 10–5) (see Video Display: Periodic Alternating Nystagmus). Because the period of oscillation is about 4 minutes, the diagnosis may be missed unless the examiner observes the nystagmus for several minutes. As the nystagmus finishes one half-cycle (e.g., of right-beating nystagmus), a brief transition period occurs during which there may be upbeating or downbeating nystagmus or square-wave jerks before the next half cycle (e.g., of left-beating nystagmus) starts (Fig. 10–5). Although rare, acquired PAN is perhaps the best understood of all forms of nystagmus and was the first for which an effective treatment was identified.[249,297,440,696]

Several other disorders are characterized by periodic reversals of spontaneous, abnormal eye movements. A congenital form of PAN is usually much less regular in the timing of reversal of direction, and slow-phase waveforms are typical of the infantile nystagmus syndrome (see Video Display: Congenital Forms of Nystagmus).[9,274,609,611] PAN should be differentiated from ping-pong gaze, which is encountered in unconscious patients with large bihemispheric lesions and consists of ocular deviations that reverse direction over

Box 10–5. Clinical Features of Acquired Periodic Alternating Nystagmus

- Horizontal nystagmus, reverses direction approximately every 90–120 seconds
- May be associated with periodic alternating head turns – the head turns in the direction of the quick phase, and the eyes are moved into a position in the orbit that is the same as the direction of the slow phase – so minimizing the nystagmus by Alexander's law
- Nystagmus cycle is usually little affected by visual fixation
- Vestibular stimuli, such as head rotations, can change or transiently stop nystagmus
- Downbeat nystagmus and square wave jerks may become more obvious in the brief null period when the horizontal nystagmus wanes and then reverses

For pathophysiology, see: Effects of Vestibulocerebellar Lesions on the VOR, in Chapter 2. For etiologies, see Table 10-4. (Related Video Display: Periodic Alternating Nystagmus)

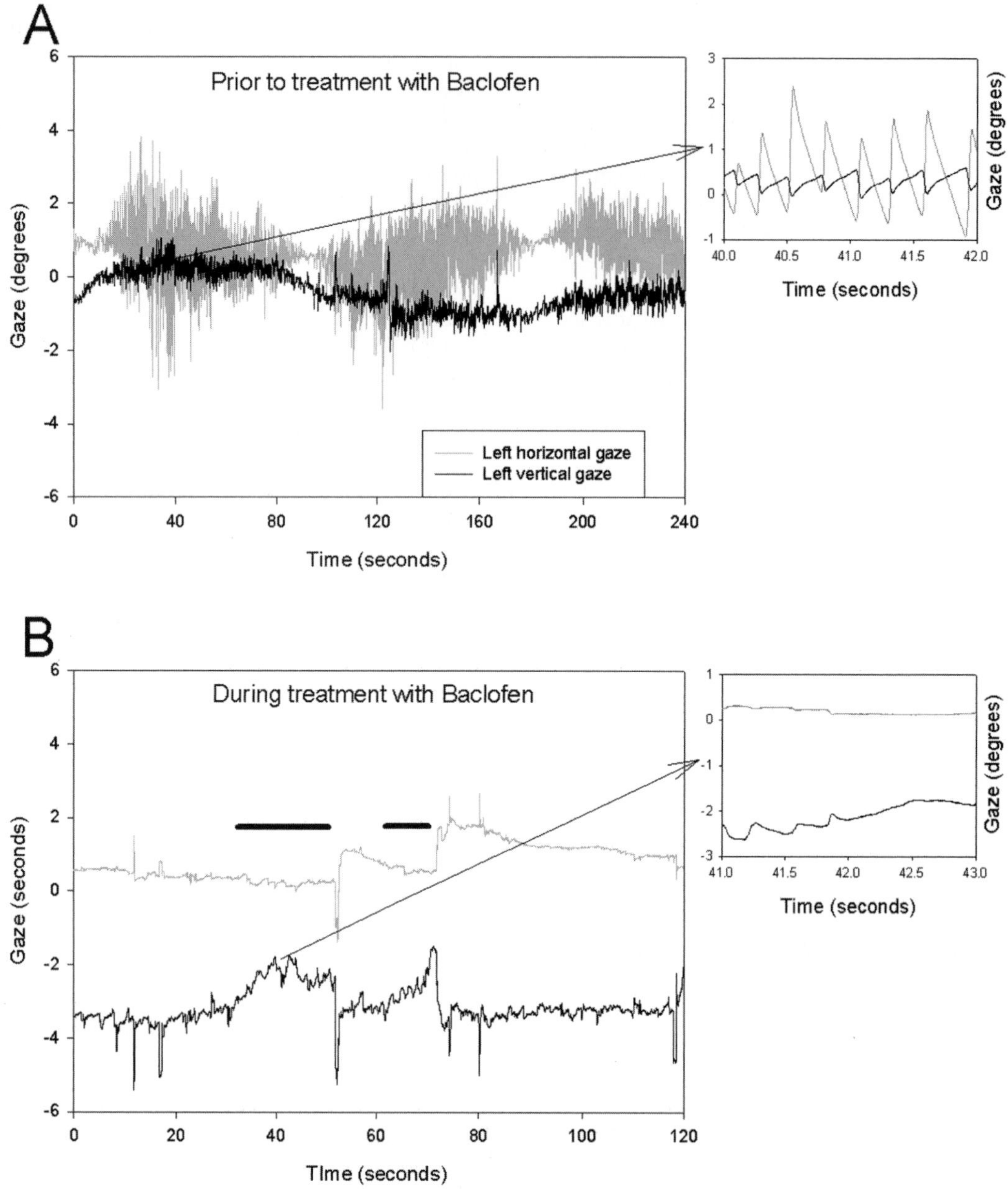

Figure 10–5. Representative records of periodic alternating nystagmus from a 24-year-old woman with multiple sclerosis prior to (A) and during (B) treatment with baclofen. Before treatment, PAN reverses direction approximately every 90 sec; there is an associated downbeat nystagmus (evident in the inset at right, which has a magnified time scale). During treatment with baclofen, PAN is essentially abolished, even when the room was switched to complete darkness (indicated by horizontal bars in B, and shown in more detail in inset at right). Upward deflections indicate rightward or upward eye movements. (Adapted from Garbutt et al.,[249] reproduced by permission of Taylor and Francis Group LLC.)

the course of a few seconds (see Video Display: Eye Movements in Coma).[350] Certain patients with acquired PAN show a "short cycle" of 20 to 40 seconds,[128] and it is uncertain whether their underlying pathophysiology differs from classic acquired PAN.

In most patients with acquired PAN, the nystagmus has the same characteristics in light or in darkness. Some patients, especially children, also show periodic head rotations in the direction of the quick phases, using Alexander's law to partially or completely null the nystagmus.[258,393,653] Smooth pursuit and optokinetic nystagmus are usually impaired,[440] but convergence may be preserved, and can be used to suppress PAN in some patients.[249] Vestibular stimuli are able to "reset" the oscillations, and critically timed rotational stimuli can stop PAN for several minutes.[240,440]

Acquired PAN has been reported in association with a number of conditions (Table 10–4), many of which involve the cerebellum. If the neurologic disorder also involves the brainstem mechanism for generating quick phases, patients may progress to periodic alternating gaze deviation.[46,275] PAN has also been reported to develop following visual loss due to vitreous hemorrhage[154] or cataract,[367] and to be abolished when vision is restored. It may also occur in patients with congenital cerebellar anomalies who later develop vestibular disorders.[128] The $GABA_B$-ergic drug, baclofen, abolishes acquired PAN in most patients,[297] but only helps occasional patients with the congenital form of PAN.[640]

Table 10–4. **Etiology of Periodic Alternating Nystagmus[240,249,415,440]**

Arnold–Chiari malformation and other hindbrain anomalies[128,240,416,440,476]
Multiple sclerosis[249,384,415,465]
Cerebellar degenerations[240,266,301,448]
Cerebellar tumor, abscess, cyst, and other mass lesion[393,440]
Creutzfeldt–Jakob disease[275]
Ataxia telangiectasia[655]
Brainstem infarction[240]
Lithium,[432] anticonvulsant medications[120,601] and seizures[493]
Infections affecting cerebellum, including syphilis[415,440]
Hepatic encephalopathy[46]
Trauma[415]
Following visual loss (due to vitreous hemorrhage or cataract)[154,367]
Aperiodic form as a component of congenital nystagmus, especially in albinos[2,9,609]

Insight into the pathogenesis of PAN has come from experimental studies. Ablation of the cerebellar nodulus and uvula in monkeys causes PAN when they are in darkness; baclofen abolishes this nystagmus.[696] One function of the nodulus and uvula is to control the time course of rotationally induced nystagmus: the velocity-storage mechanism.[144] Thus, following ablation of the nodulus and uvula, the duration of rotationally induced nystagmus is prolonged excessively, and it is postulated that normal vestibular "repair mechanisms" then act to reverse the direction of this nystagmus, so producing the oscillations of PAN.[240,415,440] These oscillations would ordinarily be blocked by visual stabilization mechanisms that tend to suppress nystagmus, but disease of the cerebellum that causes PAN usually also impairs these mechanisms. Finally, pharmacological evidence suggests that the nodulus and uvula maintain inhibitory control on the vestibular rotational responses by using GABA.[144] Thus, the $GABA_B$ agonist baclofen is able to abolish PAN caused by either experimental or clinical lesions of the nodulus and uvula (Fig. 10–5).[144]

Three other unusual disorders, each reported in individual patients, may be related to PAN. The first is a variation of PAN—alternating windmill nystagmus—which consists of oscillations in both the horizontal and vertical planes, 90 degrees out of phase.[587] This phenomenon occurred in a blind patient. The second concerns a patient who developed periodic downbeating nystagmus in the setting of severe hypomagnesemia as a complication of scleroderma.[211] The cycle length was 3.5 minutes, and the period of downbeat lasted 1.5 minutes. The disorder resolved after 84 hours, as the metabolic imbalance was corrected. The third was a patient with paroxysms of mixed torsional-horizontal-vertical nystagmus that occurred every 2 minutes in association with nausea.[427] In this patient, the initial mechanism was probably paroxysmal hyperactivity in one vestibular nucleus complex, unlike PAN, in which prolongation of the vestibular response is the initial mechanism. However, in all three cases, an "adaptive mechanism" appeared to influence the nystagmus about every 2 minutes; taken together, this provides perhaps the most direct evidence that dysfunction of the ocular motor "recalibration mechanism" can modify nystagmus.

SEESAW AND HEMI-SEESAW NYSTAGMUS

In these forms of nystagmus, one half cycle consists of elevation and intorsion of one eye and synchronous depression and extorsion of the other eye; during the next half cycle, the vertical and torsional movements reverse (see Video Display: Nystagmus and Visual Disorders, Figure 10–6, and Box 10–6). The waveform may be pendular,[158,209,210,499] or jerk, in which case the slow phase corresponds to one half-cycle (hemi-seesaw nystagmus).[293] A seesaw component is present in many central forms of nystagmus. Seesaw nystagmus has been reported in association with a variety of disorders (Table 10–5) and may present as a form of infantile nystagmus syndrome (see Video Display: Nystagmus and Visual Disorders).[158,446,594] One patient with congenital seesaw nystagmus was reported to show the opposite pattern of vertical-torsional synchrony seen with acquired cases, so that elevation occurred with extorsion and depression with intorsion,[631] Measurement of horizontal, vertical, and torsional components of these oscillations using the magnetic search coil technique has clarified the characteristics and pathogenesis of hemi-seesaw and seesaw nystagmus occurring with lesions at several sites in the nervous system.

First, jerk seesaw nystagmus (hemi-seesaw nystagmus) is reported in patients with lesions in the region of the interstitial nucleus of Cajal (INC—see Box 6–6).[293] Such patients often have a contralateral ocular tilt reaction; with a left INC lesion, this would cause right head tilt, skew deviation (left hypertropia), tonic intorsion of the left and extorsion of the right eye, and the misperception that earth-vertical is tilted to the right.[94,293] Rarely, the ocular tilt reaction is paroxysmal in form, in which case head tilt is ipsilateral to the INC lesion; some such patients also show corresponding paroxysms of jerk seesaw nystagmus.[293] The ocular tilt reaction represents an imbalance of central otolithic projections from vestibular nuclei to the INC. Stimulation in the region of

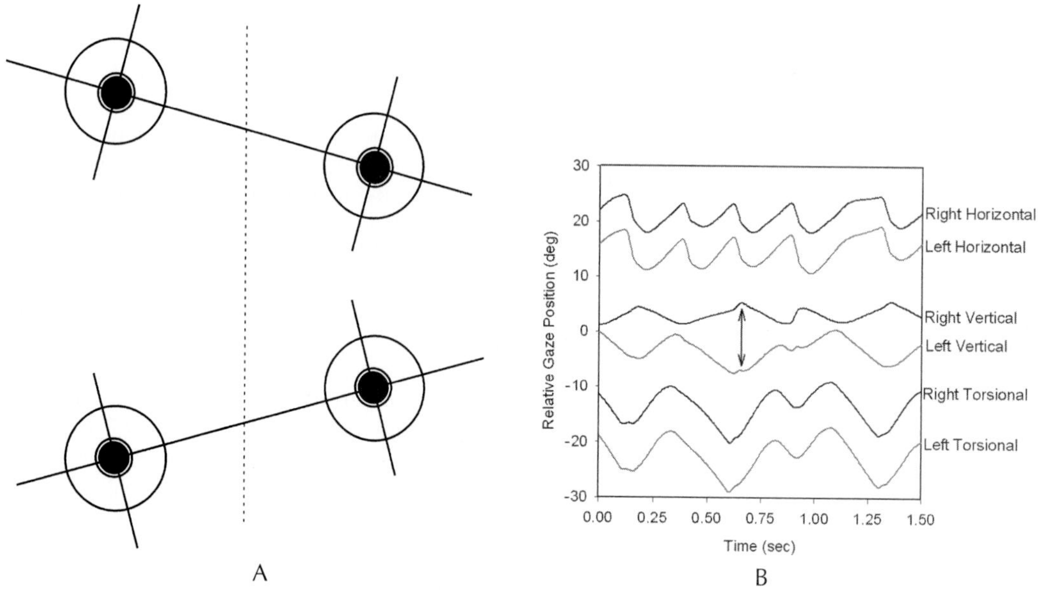

Figure 10–6. Seesaw nystagmus. (A) Schematic of the oscillation showing that during one half-cycle the right eye rises and intorts, and the left falls and extorts (top); during the next half-cycle, the opposite movements occur (bottom). (B) Record of 39-year-old woman with congenital seesaw nystagmus (see Video Display: Nystagmus and Visual Disorders). The horizontal component has a conjugate "pseudocycloid" waveform typical for congenital nystagmus. There is a disconjugate vertical component and a large conjugate torsional component. Note that as either eye goes up, it intorts and as it goes down, it extorts. The single position traces are offset for convenience of display; upward deflections indicate rightward (horizontal), upward (vertical) or clockwise (torsional) eye rotations, with respect to the patient.

Box 10–6. Clinical Features of Seesaw And Hemi-Seesaw Nystagmus

- One half-cycle consists of elevation and intorsion of one eye and synchronous depression and extorsion of the other eye; during the next half-cycle, the vertical and torsional movements reverse
- Waveform may be pendular (seesaw); or jerk (hemi-seesaw), in which the slow phase corresponds to one half-cycle
- Hemi-seesaw form associated with ocular tilt reaction and other manifestations of otolithic imbalance
- Pendular seesaw form associated with bitemporal hemianopia, chiasmal disorders, visual loss
- Reversed congenital form—elevation and extorsion—may be related to dissociated vertical deviation (DVD)

For pathophysiology, see: Disease Affecting the Optic Chiasm and Nystagmus, Skew Deviation And The Ocular Tilt Reaction (OTR). For schematics and a recorded example, see Fig. 10-6. For etiologies, see Table 10-5. (Related Video Display: Nystagmus and Visual Disorders)

INC in monkeys produces an ocular tilt reaction,[710] consisting of extorsion and depression of the eye on the stimulated side and intorsion and elevation of the other eye; somewhat similar results are reported in humans.[457,589] Thus, the various forms of the ocular tilt reaction are similar to the slow phases of jerk seesaw nystagmus. However, experimental inactivation of the interstitial nucleus of Cajal has not induced this form of nystagmus,[552] and in most patients with torsional nystagmus due to midbrain lesions, quick phases are directed contralateral to the side of the lesion (intorsion of ipsilateral eye, extorsion of contralateral eye), which is the opposite that would be expected if they were correcting for an INC lesion.[307]

Hemi-seesaw nystagmus has also been reported in patients with lower brainstem lesions, including the medial medulla,[129] with hindbrain anomalies, such as the Chiari malformation,[742] and as a component of the syndrome of oculopalatal tremor. Pendular seesaw nystagmus has most frequently been described with large parasellar tumors, and so these oscillations have been attributed to either secondary midbrain compression or to the effects of commonly associated visual field defects. Pendular seesaw nystagmus has been reported with visual loss,[78] and has been documented to develop in a patient who progressively lost

Table 10–5. **Etiology of Seesaw and Hemi-Seesaw Nystagmus**[214,293]

Parasellar masses[158,209,210]
Head trauma causing bitemporal visual field defects[214,385]
Lack or loss of crossing fibers in the optic chiasm (e.g., achiasma and septo-optic dysplasia)[32,119,164]
Multiple sclerosis[585]
Arnold–Chiari malformation[742]
Meso-diencephalic disease, such as stroke[293,378]
Medial medullary infarction[129]
Syringobulbia[225]
Progressive visual loss (e.g., due to retinitis pigmentosa)[78,467]
Head trauma[236,385,589]
Whole brain irradiation and intrathecal methotrexate therapy for lymphoma[221]
Congenital[158,171,344,594]

vision due to retinitis pigmentosa.[467] It may also develop and become symptomatic years after head injury causing bitemporal visual field defects,[214] and increase following a blink.[63] Seesaw nystagmus is also reported in patients who have congenital abnormalities of their optic chiasm, such as septoptic dysplasia.[31,32,446] Thus, it is possible that visual loss inactivates the "re-calibration" mechanism for eye movements that compensate for head rotations in roll (ear-to-shoulder). When a normal subject looks at an object located off the midsagittal plane during head roll, a seesaw rotation of the eyes is the geometrically appropriate compensation.[603] It seems that normal calibration of this response, which would require that motion-visual information be sent to the cerebellum, could be impaired with parasellar lesions, which disrupt crossing visual information from the temporal fields, leading to the pendular variant of seesaw nystagmus.[499] Thus, the two variants of seesaw nystagmus probably arise from either imbalance or miscalibration of vestibular responses that normally function to optimize gaze during head rotations in roll. Finally, dissociated vertical deviation (DVD),[691] a form of congenital vertical strabismus in which the covered eye elevates and extorts,[290] is similar to one-half cycle of the variant of congenital seesaw nystagmus,[631] and suggests a relationship between these two disorders.

NYSTAGMUS OCCURRING WHEN THE EYES ARE IN ECCENTRIC GAZE

Gaze-Evoked Nystagmus

Nystagmus induced by moving the eye to an eccentric position in the orbit is called gaze-evoked nystagmus (see Box 10–7 and Video Display: Disorders of Gaze Holding). It is the commonest form of nystagmus encountered in clinical practice. The term gaze-paretic nystagmus is only accurate in those cases with associated paresis of gaze due, for example, to cerebral or brainstem processes, or to weakness of extraocular muscles. Usually gaze-evoked nystagmus occurs on lateral or upward gaze, less often on looking down. If fixation is impaired or prevented (e.g., in darkness or with Frenzel goggles), the slow phases consist of centripetal drifts that may have an exponentially decaying waveform (Fig. 10–1B and Fig. 10–7A). If visual fixation is possible, however, the slow phases have more of a linear profile, and the nystagmus is partially suppressed.

In order to understand how gaze-evoked nystagmus arises, consider the neural command required to hold the eye steadily at an eccentric position in the orbit (see Fig. 1–3, Chapter 1). When the eye is turned towards a

Box 10–7. Clinical Features Of Gaze-Evoked, Centripetal, And Rebound Nystagmus

- Gaze-evoked nystagmus is induced by moving the eye into lateral or upgaze; quick phases are directed away from central position
- With sustained attempts to look eccentrically, gaze-evoked nystagmus declines and may reverse direction—centripetal nystagmus
- After the eyes are then returned to the central position, a short-lived nystagmus with quick phases opposite to the direction of the prior eccentric gaze occurs—rebound nystagmus

For pathophysiology, see: Abnormalities Of The Neural Integrator, in Chapter 5. For a recorded example, see Fig. 10-7. For drug etiologies, see Table 12-11. (Related Video Display: Disorders of Gaze Holding)

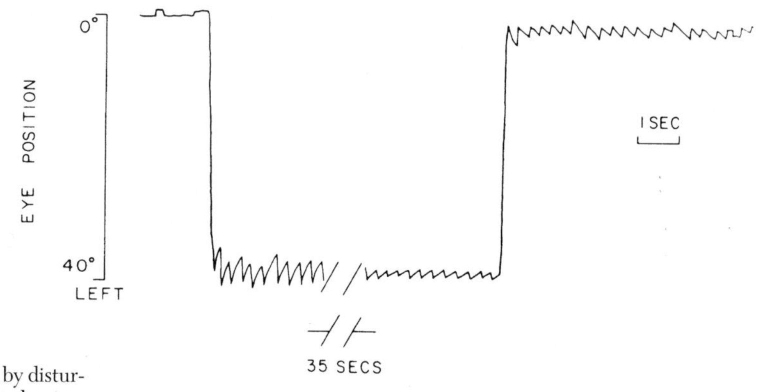

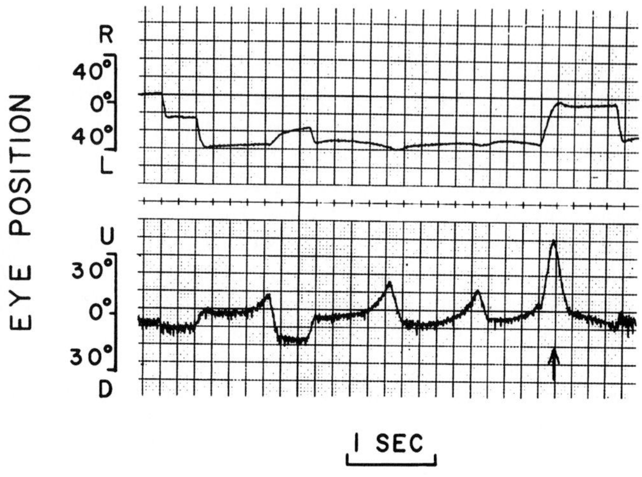

Figure 10–7. Nystagmus caused by disturbance of the gaze-holding mechanism (neural integrator). (A) Gaze-evoked and rebound nystagmus. The electrooculography record is taken from a patient with familial cerebellar degeneration. On looking to the far left, gaze-evoked nystagmus commences, with some individual slow-phases showing declining velocity. After 35 seconds of this sustained effort at maintaining eccentric gaze, the slow-phase drift velocity is reduced. When the eyes are returned to the central position, the nystagmus reverses direction (rebound nystagmus). (From Zee and colleagues,[741] with permission of John Wiley and Sons, Inc.) (B) Downbeat nystagmus with increasing velocity waveforms in a patient with paraneoplastic cerebellar degeneration.[738] The waveform was also evident on clinical examination (see Video Display: Disorders of Gaze Holding) and may represent the consequences of an unstable vertical integrator. Horizontal eye position is shown in the top record and vertical in the lower. The arrow indicates a blink.

corner of the orbit, the tissues that suspend the eye exert an elastic force to return it towards central position. A tonic contraction of the extraocular muscles is required to overcome this elastic, restoring force. This is achieved by a "step" eye position command from the ocular motoneurons, which is generated by a gaze-holding network (the neural integrator for eye movements). Gaze-evoked nystagmus is due to a deficient eye position signal: the eyes cannot be maintained at an eccentric orbital position and they are pulled back towards the central position by the elastic forces of the orbital tissues. Then corrective quick phases move the eyes back toward the desired position in the orbit. Some normal subjects show other waveforms on sustained eccentric gaze such as small pendular oscillations or square-wave jerks (small saccades).[11] The mechanism for gaze holding is discussed further in Chapter 5.

Frequently, lesions that produce gaze-evoked nystagmus also impair visual fixation and smooth pursuit. Crucial structures for horizontal gaze holding are the nucleus prepositus hypoglossi and medial vestibular nucleus (the NPH-MVN region); for vertical gaze holding, the interstitial nucleus of Cajal (see Box 6–6) plays an important role. In addition, the vestibulocerebellum contributes to this gaze-holding function. The cell groups of the paramedian tracts (PMT) are important for relaying the entire range of ocular motor signals back to the vestibular cerebellum,[116] and likely contribute to the process of neural integration, since inactivation of one PMT nucleus impaired gaze-holding.[501]

Most commonly, gaze-evoked nystagmus is a side effect of medications, including sedatives and anticonvulsants,[312,558,641] or is due to intoxications with drugs, especially alcohol.[136,475] Structural lesions involving components of the gaze-holding neural network that contributes to the neural integrator may also cause gaze-evoked nystagmus. Thus, experimental lesions of the NPH-MVN region effectively abolish horizontal gaze-holding function (Fig. 5–5, Chapter 5),[121,376,479] and partially impair vertical gaze-holding as well. Experimental inactivation of the interstitial nucleus of Cajal impairs vertical gaze holding.[151,306] Complete loss of gaze-holding function was described in a patient with lethal lithium intoxication, who showed lesions in the nucleus prepositus hypoglossi.[149] Experimental flocculectomy greatly, but not completely, impairs horizontal gaze holding,[740] and also causes downbeat nystagmus. Disease affecting the vestibulocerebellum commonly causes gaze-evoked nystagmus, often with a downbeating component (see Video Display: Disorders of Gaze Holding). Horizontal gaze-evoked nystagmus due to cerebellar disease may become more prominent during positional testing, if fixation is prevented.[713] Patients with cerebellar atrophy develop gaze-evoked nystagmus with lower serum concentration of anticonvulsants than do patients with a normal cerebellum.[641] Gaze-evoked nystagmus is a feature of familial episodic vertigo and ataxia type 2 (EA-2), which is a calcium channelopathy that is responsive to acetazolamide.[54,95,368] and 4-aminopyridine.[663] Patients with gaze-evoked nystagmus following removal of cerebello-pontine angle tumors often also notice gaze-evoked tinnitus.[452]

Rarely, cerebellar lesions cause the gaze-holding mechanism to become unstable (i.e., hyperactive), so that the eyes drift with increasing velocity *away* from central position either vertically,[738] (see Video Display: Disorders of Gaze Holding) or horizontally.[65] Such gaze-instability nystagmus (Fig. 10–7B) often violates Alexander's law, being greatest in the direction of gaze opposite to that of the quick phases. Horizontal gaze nystagmus in which the quick phases of the adducting eye are slower than those of the abducting eye—a form of dissociated nystagmus — is characteristic of internuclear ophthalmoplegia (see Video Display: Pontine Syndromes).

Differences Between Physiologic "End-Point" Nystagmus and Pathologic Gaze-Evoked Nystagmus

Gaze-evoked nystagmus is commonly encountered in normal subjects, when it is usually called "end-point nystagmus" (Box 10–8).[14,216,]

Box 10–8. Clinical Features that Distinguish "End-Point" Nystagmus from Pathological Gaze-Evoked Nystagmus

- Low-amplitude and frequency
- Horizontal on far lateral gaze; upbeating on far upgaze
- Unsustained
- On lateral gaze, nystagmus is horizontal without vertical component
- Rebound nystagmus is transient or absent
- Ocular motor examination is otherwise normal

For physiological mechanisms, see: Abnormalities Of The Neural Integrator, in Chapter 5. (Related Video Display: Disorders of Gaze Holding)

[612] Typically it occurs on looking far laterally or up, and is poorly sustained. On lateral gaze, the nystagmus is primarily horizontal. It may be asymmetric—for example, more prominent on looking to the right than to the left.[612] Nonetheless, in some normal individuals, the nystagmus is sustained, occurs with less than full deviations of the eye, and may be slightly dissociated or have a small torsional component. A strong downbeating component on lateral gaze, however, implies dysfunction of central vestibular connections (see Video Display: Disorders of Gaze Holding). In normal subjects, physiological gaze-evoked nystagmus can be most reliably identified by the absence of other ocular motor or neurological abnormalities. Thus, pathologic gaze-evoked nystagmus is usually accompanied by other defects such as impaired smooth pursuit.[113]

Another form of gaze-evoked nystagmus in normal subjects is induced by sustained eccentric gaze for a minute or more (fatigue nystagmus).[14] Often the nystagmus is of greater amplitude in the abducting eye, similar to the dissociated nystagmus of internuclear ophthalmoplegia. These findings probably represent the effects of fatigue and may therefore be similar to the gaze-evoked nystagmus seen with myasthenia gravis (see Fig. 9–20A), which also increases with prolonged fixation.[593] Conversely, when subjects are asked to fixate the remembered location of an eccentric target in darkness, gaze-evoked nystagmus decreases with time,[11] suggesting that central mechanisms correct the centripetal eye drift.

Bruns' Nystagmus

Tumors of the cerebellopontine angle (e.g., Schwann cell tumors of the eighth nerve) may produce a combination of low-frequency, large-amplitude nystagmus on looking ipsilaterally, due to defective gaze holding, and high-frequency, small-amplitude nystagmus on looking contralaterally, due to vestibular imbalance.[55,505] This is called Bruns' nystagmus.[109] Even in patients in whom an acoustic schwannoma had been resected years previously, nystagmus in darkness shows a summation of the effects of vestibular imbalance and gaze-evoked nystagmus. It has been proposed that, faced with a vestibular imbalance, the brain deliberately makes the gaze-holding network leaky so that gaze-evoked nystagmus can be used to counteract the vestibular imbalance.[567] In this way there would be at least one position in the orbit in which the eyes would not drift.

Centripetal and Rebound Nystagmus

If patients with gaze-evoked nystagmus sustain their attempt to look eccentrically, the nystagmus may begin to quiet down and, on rare occasion, may even reverse direction, so that the eye begins to drift centrifugally ("centripetal nystagmus").[433] If the eyes are then returned to the central position, a short-lived nystagmus with slow drifts in the direction of the prior eccentric gaze ensues, which is called rebound nystagmus (Box 10–7) (Fig. 10–7A) (see Video Display: Disorders of Gaze Holding).[89,265,335,336] Both centripetal and rebound nystagmus may reflect an attempt by brainstem or cerebellar mechanisms to correct for the centripetal drift of gaze-evoked nystagmus. Rebound nystagmus typically occurs in patients with cerebellar syndromes,[301,450] but has been reported following experimental lesions of the NPH-MVN region,[121] and in normal subjects who show gaze-evoked nystagmus.[612] Torsional rebound nystagmus has been described in association with vestibulocerebellar disease.[661] Extreme gaze deviation away from the side of the lesion in one patient with a lateral medullary infarction was reported to cause paroxysmal nystagmus and vertigo lasting about a minute.[115] Such a phenomenon could be explained by a sustained eye position signal causing an imbalance of central vestibular mechanisms.

The structures that are critical for rebound nystagmus remain undetermined. One patient with a tumor confined to the flocculus was reported to show gaze-evoked nystagmus and rebound nystagmus,[720] but when the tumor spread to involve the vestibular nuclei, the rebound nystagmus disappeared, even though the gaze-evoked nystagmus persisted. Thus, the vestibular nuclei or surrounding medulla may be important for generating rebound nystagmus, and depends upon the ability to internally monitor eye movement signals, such as efference copy, and activate compensatory eye drifts.[89,336,720]

NYSTAGMUS OCCURRING IN ASSOCIATION WITH DISEASE OF THE VISUAL SYSTEM

Pathogenesis of Nystagmus Occurring with Visual System Disorders

Disorders of the visual pathways are often associated with nystagmus (Box 10–9). The most obvious example is the nystagmus that invariably accompanies complete blindness (see Video Display: Nystagmus and Visual Disorders).[445] What is the mechanism? There are at least two separate effects of visual loss: (1) an inability to generate eye movements to correct for drifts of the eyes; and (2) loss of the "error signal" that drives ocular motor adaptation, and tunes eye movements to visual demands.

Visually mediated eye movements such as smooth pursuit and "fixation" stop the eyes from drifting away from a stationary object of regard (see Visual Fixation, in Chapter 4). So, for example, if normal subjects attempt to fixate on the remembered location of a target while in darkness, the eye drifts off target several times faster than if the subject actually views the target (Fig. 4–2).[654] Uncorrected drifts are eventually remedied by a saccade that places the image back on the fovea. The fixation mechanism that generates smooth eye movements to correct for drifts of the eyes depends upon the visual system, which is inherently slow. Thus, a response time of over 70 ms encumbers all visually mediated eye movements, including fixation, smooth pursuit, and optokinetic responses. If the response time is delayed further by disease of the visual system, then the brain's attempts at correcting eye drifts may actually add to the retinal error rather than reducing it, leading to ocular oscillations.[52] This issue is discussed further in the section on Models of Smooth Pursuit in

Box 10–9. Clinical Features Of Nystagmus Associated With Disease Of The Visual Pathways

LESIONS OF THE EYE OR OPTIC NERVE

- Bilateral visual loss causes continuous jerk nystagmus, with horizontal, vertical, and torsional components, and a drifting "null" position
- Monocular visual loss causes slow vertical oscillations and low-amplitude horizontal nystagmus mainly in the blind eye; in children, especially, pendular nystagmus of the blind eye

LESIONS AT THE OPTIC CHIASM

- Seesaw nystagmus with bitemporal visual field loss

LESIONS AFFECTING POSTERIOR CORTICAL AREAS

- Low-amplitude horizontal nystagmus beating towards the side of the lesion

LESIONS AFFECTING CORTICAL-PONTINE-CEREBELLAR OR OLIVOCEREBELLAR PROJECTIONS

- May be responsible for some forms of acquired pendular nystagmus

For pathophysiology, see: Abnormalities of Visual Fixation, in Chapter 4. For recorded examples, see Fig. 10-8. (Related Video Display: Nystagmus and Visual Disorders)

Chapter 4. Another aspect of fixation—the suppression of saccades—is dealt with under saccadic intrusions.

In addition, to minimize drift away from the target, vision is needed for recalibrating and optimizing all types of eye movements. This optimization depends on visual projections to the cerebellum—the "ocular motor repair-shop."[566] Thus, signals from secondary visual areas concerned with moving stimuli project to the cerebellum via the pontine nuclei and middle cerebellar peduncle (Fig. 6–7). Neurons in both the dorsolateral pontine nuclei and Purkinje cells in the cerebellar flocculus respond to moving visual stimuli.[73,519] Visual signals for recalibration may also pass via the inferior olivary nucleus, which sends climbing fibers to the cerebellum.[353,372] If the ocular motor system is to be recalibrated, visual signals need to be compared with eye movement commands. One candidate for this function are the cell groups of the paramedian tracts (PMT) (see Box 6–4), which receive inputs from all premotor structures that project to ocular motoneurons, and which project to the cerebellar flocculus.[116] Alternatively, pathways that coordinate conjugate and vergence movements, involving connections between the nucleus reticularis tegmenti pontis and cerebellar nucleus interpositus (discussed in Chapter 8), might be involved.[243] Thus, lesions at any part of this visual-motor "recalibration" pathway might deprive the brain of signals that are essential to hold each of the eyes on the object of regard; the result would be drifts of the eyes away from the target, leading to nystagmus.

Clinical Features of Nystagmus in Association with Visual System Disease

Disease affecting various parts of the visual system, from retina to cortical visual areas, or that interrupts visual projections to pons and cerebellum, has been associated with nystagmus. First, we review the features of nystagmus reported with disease localized to the different sites in this pathway. Second, we discuss the features of acquired pendular nystagmus, which may sometimes be associated with disease affecting the visual system and its brainstem-cerebellar projections.

NYSTAGMUS ASSOCIATED WITH DISEASE OF THE RETINA AND OCULAR MEDIA

Retinal disorders causing blindness, such as Leber's congenital amaurosis, lead to continuous jerk nystagmus with components in all three planes, which changes in direction over the course of seconds or minutes (Fig. 10–8A) (see Video Display: Nystagmus and Visual Disorders). The drifting null point, the eye position at which nystagmus changes direction, probably reflects an inability to "calibrate" the ocular motor system, and it has also been reported after experimental cerebellectomy.[433,565] Congenital forms of nystagmus have been reported in association with a variety of hereditary retinal disorders (Table 10–7); some, but not all, show the increasing-velocity waveform (Fig. 10–1C) that is characteristic of congenital forms of nystagmus. Animals raised in a strobe illuminated environment, which deprives them of retinal image motion while still providing position cues, develop spontaneous ocular oscillations.[478,585a] Loss of vision later in life also causes nystagmus, which may be pendular (see Video Display: Nystagmus and Visual Disorders) or seesaw nystagmus.[467] Restoration of vision to dogs with retinal disease by gene therapy decreases associated nystagmus.[19,358,502]

DISEASE AFFECTING THE OPTIC NERVES AND NYSTAGMUS

Optic nerve disease is commonly associated with pendular forms of nystagmus. With unilateral disease of the optic nerve, such as tumors or trauma, nystagmus largely affects the abnormal eye ("monocular nystagmus"), with low-frequency, bi-directional drifts that are more prominent vertically and unidirectional drifts with quick phases that occur horizontally (Fig. 10–8B).[57,442,540] Vertical nystagmus that predominantly affects an eye with poor vision is called the Heimann-Bielschowsky phenomenon (see Video Display: Nystagmus and Visual Disorders);[82] it is not confined to primary optic nerve disease, however, and also occurs in patients with amblyopia or longstanding monocular visual loss.[163,442,540,725]

When disease such as demyelination affects both optic nerves, the amplitude of nystagmus is often greater in the eye with poorer vision.[64] Oscillations may also occur after development

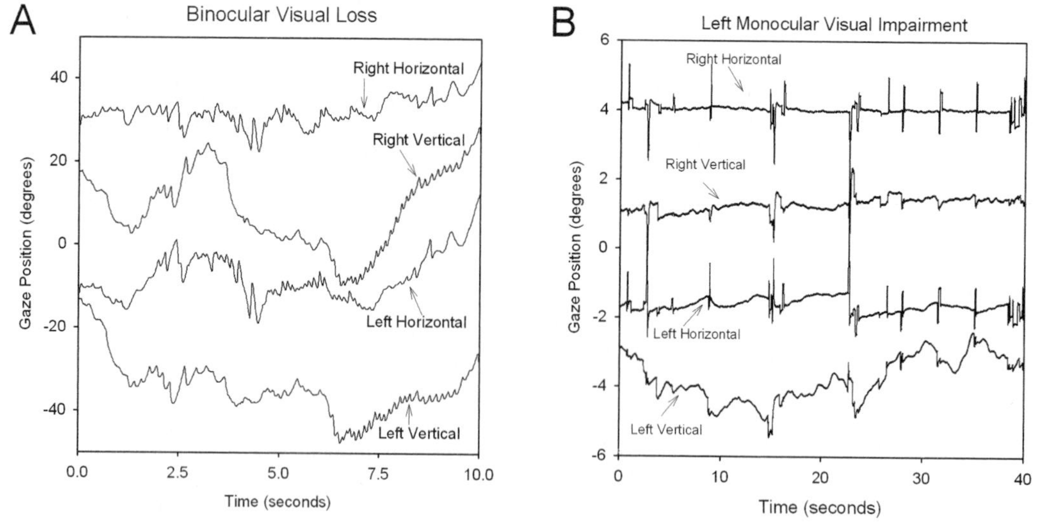

Figure 10–8. Nystagmus associated with visual loss. (A) Horizontal and vertical movements of both eyes of a 25-year-old patient bilaterally blind since birth due to Leber's congenital amaurosis. In the horizontal plane, there is a wandering null point and changes in direction of the quick phases, evident in the velocity channels. Slow-phase waveforms are variably linear, decreasing velocity or, especially in the vertical plane, increasing velocity (see Video Display: Nystagmus and Visual Disorders). (B) Patient who had defocused vision since childhood following eye trauma and removal of his left lens. Following implantation of an artificial lens at age 35 years, his corrected visual acuity was 20/20 OD and 20/25 OS, but he was unable to maintain steady fixation with his left eye and suffered from variable diplopia and abnormal motion of vision in his left eye that he could not control. His left eye shows the Heimann–Bielschowsky phenomenon—vertical instability of fixation with slow drifts. The single-position traces are offset to aid clarity of display; positive deflections indicate rightward (horizontal), upward (vertical) or clockwise (torsional) eye rotations, with respect to the patient.

of a dense cataract or high myopia in childhood; when vision is restored nystagmus may disappear, or persist leading to oscillopsia.[539,718] Those patients in which nystagmus declines after restoration of vision support the contention that these ocular oscillations may be primarily caused by the lack of visual inputs required for "calibration" rather than by any primary disorder of the ocular motor system. The origin of vertical drifts that occur in a blind eye, while the seeing eye holds fixation, is unknown but might be due to disturbance of vertical vergence mechanisms.[442,725] Vertical vergence responses are different from other types of eye movements, including horizontal vergence and visual fixation mechanisms, because they only appear to respond to first-order, luminance-defined stimuli (see Chapter 4 for a discussion of first-order and second-order visual following).[623,657]

In infants, the appearance of monocular, vertical nystagmus raises the possibility of an optic nerve tumor, and imaging studies are indicated.[224,264,425] However, monocular oscillations in children are sometimes spasmus nutans,[706] or other oscillations that spontaneously resolve (see Video Display: Congenital Forms of Nystagmus).[263] Monocular visual impairment, such as amblyopia, also leads to horizontal nystagmus, and if present from birth, the features are those of latent nystagmus, which is discussed in a later section.

DISEASE AFFECTING THE OPTIC CHIASM AND NYSTAGMUS

Parasellar lesions such as pituitary tumors have traditionally been associated with seesaw nystagmus (Box 10–6). As already discussed, seesaw nystagmus is a form of pendular nystagmus in which one half cycle consists of elevation and intorsion of one eye and synchronous depression and extorsion of the other eye, with the vertical and torsional movements reversing during the next half cycle (see Fig. 10–6) (see Video Display: Nystagmus and Visual Disorders). Hemi-seesaw nystagmus has been attributed to disease affecting the interstitial nucleus of Cajal or its connections.[293] Congenital seesaw nystagmus has been reported in a mutant strain of dogs that lack an optic chiasm,[196] and in patients in whom imaging and visual evoked studies suggested a similar developmental defect.[32,413,446] Seesaw nystagmus has also been documented to develop in a patient with progressive visual loss due to retinitis pigmentosa.[467] Thus, it remains possible that visual inputs—especially crossed inputs—are important for optimizing vertical-torsional eye movements. Under natural conditions, seesaw eye movements occur to compensate for ear-to-shoulder head roll, especially when the subject views target located off the midsagittal plane.[603] Crossed visual inputs are presumably necessary to keep this response calibrated and, if removed, might lead to seesaw oscillations.[44,63]

DISEASE AFFECTING THE POST-CHIASMAL VISUAL SYSTEM AND NYSTAGMUS

Horizontal nystagmus occurs in patients with unilateral disease of the cerebral hemispheres, especially when the lesion is large and posterior.[618] Such patients show a constant-velocity drift of the eyes toward the intact hemisphere (i.e., quick phases directed towards the side of the lesion; see Video Display: Nystagmus and Visual Disorders). The nystagmus is low-amplitude, and sometimes is only appreciated during ophthalmoscopy. Such patients usually also show asymmetry of horizontal smooth pursuit (impaired towards the side of the lesion). The asymmetry can be brought out at the bedside using a hand-held optokinetic drum or tape;[143,412] the response is reduced when the stripes move towards the side of the lesion. This asymmetry of visual tracking has led to the suggestion that nystagmus in such patients reflects an imbalance of pursuit "tone" as the cause,[618] but the phenomenon is probably more complex, reflecting imbalances between cortical areas concerned with visual motion, vestibular sense, and directing attention in extrapersonal space.[203,490] As discussed below, one proposed mechanism for congenital latent nystagmus concerns abnormality of such cortical motion-vision processing.

Sometimes, intermittent nystagmus is due to seizure activity affecting cortical areas responsible for generating smooth pursuit movements;[379] this is discussed in Chapter 12 in the section entitled Eye Movements During Epileptic Seizures.

ACQUIRED PENDULAR NYSTAGMUS AND ITS RELATIONSHIP TO DISEASE OF THE VISUAL PATHWAYS

Acquired pendular nystagmus (Fig. 10–9) is one of the more common types of nystagmus and is often associated with disabling visual symptoms – continuous oscillopsia and blurred vision (see Video Display: Acquired Pendular Nystagmus). More than one mechanism appears to be responsible for its pathogenesis, and it is encountered in a variety of conditions (Table 10–6), including several disorders of myelin, the syndrome of oculopalatal tremor, and with Whipple's disease. We will first describe the common features of acquired pendular nystagmus and then discuss characteristics peculiar to the major types separately (Whipple's disease is discussed in the section of convergent-divergent pendular oscillations that follows).

Clinical Characteristics of Acquired Pendular Nystagmus

Acquired pendular nystagmus usually has horizontal, vertical, and torsional components, although one may predominate (Box 10–10).

Table 10–6. **Etiology of Pendular Nystagmus**

Visual loss (including unilateral disease of the optic nerve)[224,442]
Disorders of central myelin:
Multiple sclerosis[52,64,455]
Pelizaeus–Merzbacher disease[678]
Cockayne's syndrome[146,474]
Peroxisomal disorders[414]
Toluene abuse[458]
Syndrome of oculopalatal "myoclonus" or tremor, developing after brainstem stroke[52,498] or as a degenerative[644] or familial disorder[341]
Acute brainstem stroke[388] or with pontine cavernous angioma[702]
Whipple's disease[602]
Spinocerebellar degenerations[51,266]
Hypoxic encephalopathy[51]
Congenital nystagmus[177]

Box 10–10. Clinical Features of Acquired Pendular Nystagmus

COMMON FEATURES

- May have horizontal, vertical, and torsional components; their amplitude and phase relationship determines the trajectory of the nystagmus in each eye
- Phase shift between the eyes is common (horizontally and torsionally; seldom vertically)—may reach 180 degrees, so that the nystagmus becomes convergent-divergent or cyclovergent
- Amplitudes often differ, and nystagmus may appear monocular
- Trajectories may be conjugate, but more often are dissimilar
- Oscillations sometimes suppress momentarily in the wake of a saccade

IN ASSOCIATION WITH DEMYELINATING DISEASES

- Frequency 2–8 Hz (typically 3–4 Hz)
- Generally greater amplitude in the eye with poorer vision
- Internuclear ophthalmoplegia commonly associated
- May have an associated upbeat component

SYNDROME OF OCULOPALATAL TREMOR

- Frequency 1–3 Hz (typically 2 Hz)
- May be vertical (with bilateral lesions) or disconjugate vertical-torsional
- Accentuated by eyelid closure
- Movements of palate and other branchial muscles may be synchronized

WHIPPLE'S DISEASE

- Frequency typically about 1Hz
- Usually convergence-divergence, occasionally vertical; sometimes with associated oscillatory movements of the jaw, face or limbs (oculomasticatory myorhythmia)
- Vertical gaze palsy similar to the clinical picture of progressive supranuclear palsy is usually also present

For pathophysiology, see Models of Smooth Pursuit, in Chapter 4. For recorded examples, see Fig. 10-2, 10-9, 10-10, and 10-17. For etiologies, see Table 10-6. (Related Video Display: Acquired Pendular Nystagmus)

If the horizontal and vertical oscillatory components are in phase, the trajectory of the nystagmus is oblique. If the horizontal and vertical oscillatory components are out of phase, the trajectory will be elliptical (Fig. 10–9B). A special case is when horizontal and vertical components are of equal amplitude but are 90 degrees phase shifted; the trajectory is then circular. When the oscillations of each eye are compared, the nystagmus may be conjugate, but often the trajectories are dissimilar (i.e., disconjugate), and the size of oscillations is dif-

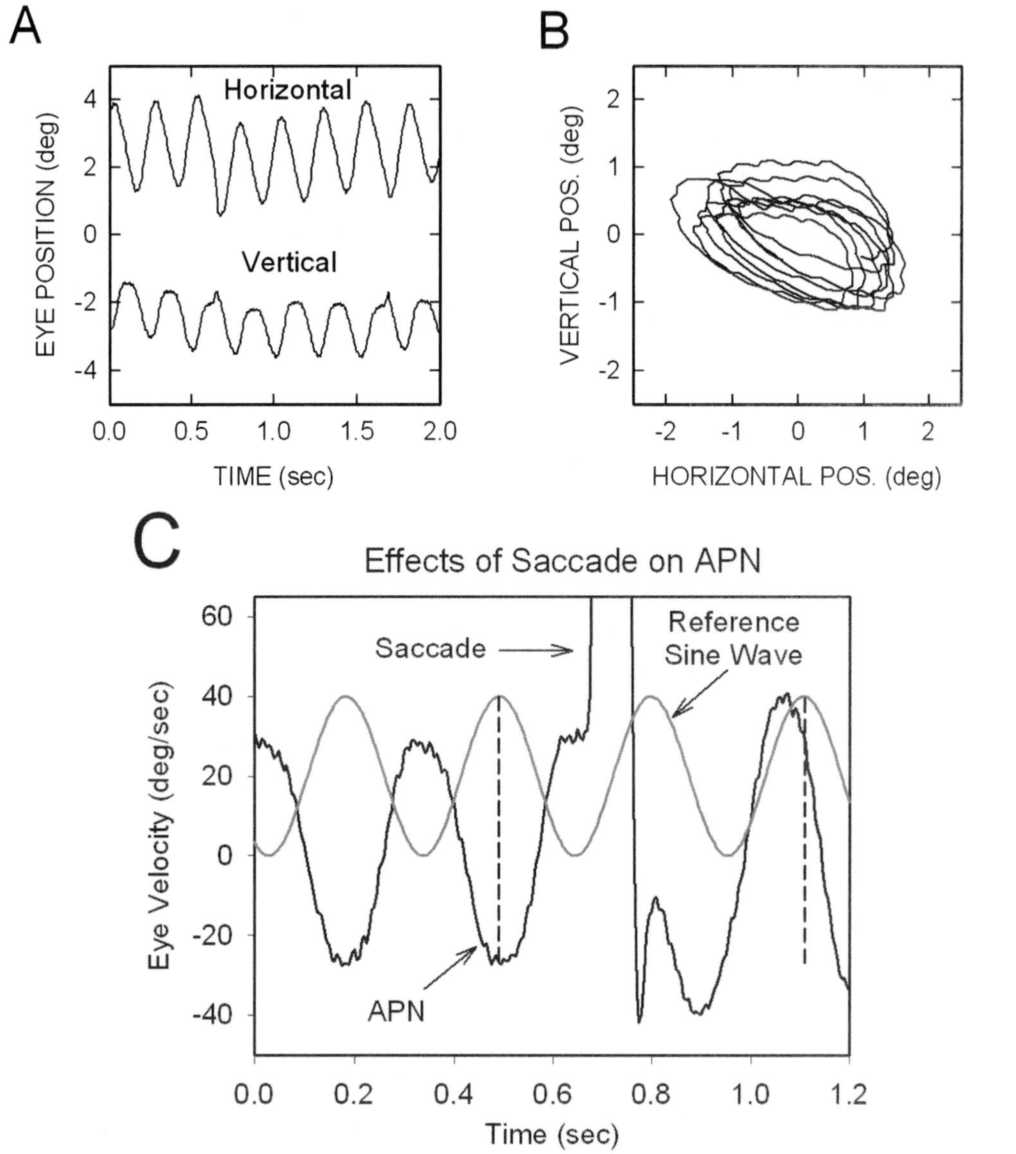

Figure 10–9. Acquired pendular nystagmus. (A) A 2-second record from a patient with multiple sclerosis who showed elliptical nystagmus. (B) Trajectory of nystagmus shown in A, which is quasi-elliptical. In A, upward deflections indicate rightward and upward eye rotations. (C) Example of how a 30 degree rightward horizontal saccade could reset the phase of acquired pendular nystagmus (APN) in a patient with multiple sclerosis. A sine wave at a similar frequency to the oscillations is shown in gray for reference. Note that before the saccade, the horizontal component of APN and sine wave are about 180 degrees out of phase; after the saccade, this phase difference is greatly reduced (compare positions of vertical dashed lines). The single-position traces are offset to aid clarity of display; positive deflections indicate rightward (horizontal) or upward (vertical) eye rotations, with respect to the patient.

ferent (i.e., dissociated). Sometimes the nystagmus appears monocular, and there may be an asynchrony of timing (phase shift), which may reach 180 degrees, in which case the oscillations may be regarded as a form of convergence-divergence nystagmus.[53]

Certain features help to differentiate acquired pendular nystagmus from the congenital form of pendular nystagmus. The latter is predominantly horizontal, with small torsional and negligible vertical components (Fig. 10–11). Foveation periods are often superimposed on congenital pendular nystagmus, but are rare in the acquired form.[651] Oscillopsia is a prominent symptom with acquired pendular nystagmus, but is seldom a complaint with the congenital form.

The waveform of acquired pendular nystagmus may approximate a sine wave, but often is more complex, especially in oculopalatal tremor.[53] The frequency of oscillations of acquired pendular nystagmus ranges from 1 Hz–8 Hz, with a typical value of 3.5 Hz in multiple sclerosis,[282] about 2 Hz in oculopalatal tremor,[199] and about 1 Hz in Whipple's disease, as the convergent-divergent component of oculomasticatory myorhythmia.[602] The horizontal, vertical, and torsional components of each eye's oscillations usually have the same frequency. Rarely one eye may oscillate at a harmonic frequency of the other.[62] For any particular patient, the frequency tends to remain fairly constant, even if partially suppressed by treatment.[51]

Acquired Pendular Nystagmus with Demyelinative Disease

Acquired pendular nystagmus is a common feature of a variety of disorders of central myelin, including multiple sclerosis (MS), congenital disorders such Pelizaeus-Merzbacher disease (see Video Display: Acquired Pendular Nystagmus),[678] peroxisomal assembly disorders,[414] and in toluene abuse.[346,458] Since patients with multiple sclerosis who have pendular nystagmus often also have evidence of optic nerve demyelination, then prolonged response time of the visual processing might be responsible for the ocular oscillations. Support for this hypothesis comes from the observation that oscillations are usually larger in the eye with evidence of more severe optic nerve demyelination.[64] However, the nystagmus often remains unchanged in darkness (when visual inputs have no influence on eye movements). As discussed in the section on Models of Smooth Pursuit, in Chapter 4, spontaneous ocular oscillations can be induced in normal subjects by experimentally delaying the latency of visual feedback during fixation (see Fig. 4–11); however, the frequency of these induced oscillations is less than 2 Hz, which is lower than in most patients with pendular nystagmus due to multiple sclerosis.[52] Furthermore, when this experimental technique was applied to patients with acquired pendular nystagmus, it did not change the characteristics of the nystagmus, but instead superimposed lower-frequency oscillations similar to those induced in normal subjects. Thus, disturbance of visual fixation due to visual delays cannot wholly account for the high-frequency oscillations that often characterize acquired pendular nystagmus. Convergence partially suppresses the oscillations in some patients, and evokes or exacerbates it in others (Fig. 10–16A).[61] Smooth pursuit may be intact so that, despite the oscillations, tracking eye movements occur with nystagmus superimposed.[282] Many affected patients also have internuclear ophthalmoplegia.

An important observation concerning acquired pendular nystagmus in multiple sclerosis is that some patients show transient suppression of their oscillations following a saccade (Fig. 10–9C) (see Video Display: Acquired Pendular Nystagmus).[37] Systematic comparison of the oscillations prior to, and following, a saccade has demonstrated that the oscillations are phase-shifted (reset), and that larger saccades have a greater effect than smaller saccades.[162] This has led to the hypothesis that the oscillations of APN in patients with multiple sclerosis arise in the neural integrator for eye movements, and that large saccades affect the timing of the oscillations by "resetting" the integrator with the large pulse of neural activity.[162] The nucleus prepositus hypoglossi and medial vestibular nucleus are important components of the neural integrator, which is probably affected by feedback of signals via cell groups of the paramedian tracts (PMT) to the cerebellar flocculus (see Box 6–4).[116] Patients with APN show a preponderance of multiple sclerosis plaques in their paramedian pons in the region of the PMT cell groups.[454] Thus, it is postulated that the neural integrator loses normal feedback, becomes unstable, and begins to oscillate, causing acquired pendular nystagmus. Since some information is available about the neurotransmitters used by neurons that contribute to normal neural integration of ocular motor signals,[34,659] this hypothesis for acquired pendular nystagmus in multiple sclerosis suggested drug treatments, and led to therapeutic trials, which are summarized in the section on Treatment of Acquired Pendular Nystagmus.

In patients with multiple sclerosis in whom the oscillations are predominantly convergent-divergent, one possibility is that the instability arises in connections between the nucleus reticularis tegmenti pontis and the cerebellar nucleus interpositus, which both contribute to vergence movements, including the neural integrator for vergence.[53,243]

Oculopalatal Tremor (Myoclonus)

Acquired pendular nystagmus may be one component of the syndrome of oculopalatal (pharyngo-laryngo-diaphragmatic) tremor (see Video Display: Acquired Pendular Nystagmus).[199,288,498] This condition usually develops several weeks or months after brainstem or cerebellar infarction or hemorrhage (Fig. 10–10), though it may not be recognized until years after the stroke. Oculopalatal tremor also occurs with degenerative conditions.[53,644] The term "tremor" is more accurate than "myoclonus," since the movements of affected muscles are to-and-fro, and are approximately synchronized, typically at a rate of about 2 cycles per second. The palate is most often affected, but the eyes, facial muscles, pharynx, tongue, larynx, diaphragm, mouth of the Eustachian tube, neck, trunk, and extremities may also move, in synchrony.

In contrast to symptomatic oculopalatal tremor described above, essential palatal tremor or myoclonus is an idiopathic disorder in which ocular oscillations do not accompany palatal movements. Auditory clicking is a common and annoying symptom in essential palatal tremor.[199] Pendular vertical oscillations of the eyes may sometimes occur acutely with pontine infarctions that cause horizontal gaze palsy,[388] but associated palatal movements usually do not develop for several weeks.

The ocular oscillations of oculopalatal tremor typically have large vertical and torsional components, with a smaller horizontal component (Fig. 10–10B). The waveform of the ocular oscillations is usually irregular and less sinusoidal than that of acquired pendular nystagmus in multiple sclerosis. It has been suggested that, if the palatal tremor is unilateral, the ocular oscillations are vertical-torsional, with the eye on the side of the palatal tremor intorting as it rises and extorting as it falls, whereas the opposite eye extorts as it rises and intorts as it falls (a seesaw pattern).[498] The oscillations are often disconjugate in horizontal, vertical or torsional planes, with some orbital position dependency.[53,282,498] Affected patients often have internuclear ophthalmoplegia or ocular motor palsies as the consequence of their prior strokes.[51,586] Occasionally, following brainstem infarction, patients develop the eye oscillations without movements of the palate. Eyelid closure may sometimes bring out the ocular oscillations.[360] The nystagmus sometimes disappears with sleep, but the palatal movements usually persist. Once established, the condition is usually intractable, and the oscillations only occasionally spontaneously remit.[361]

The main pathologic finding with palatal tremor is hypertrophic degeneration of the inferior olivary nucleus; this may be evident on MRI.[199,272] There may also be destruction of the contralateral dentate nucleus.[288] Histologically, the olivary nucleus has enlarged, vacuolated neurons with enlarged astrocytes. The hypertrophic neurons and their dendrites contain increased acetylcholine esterase reaction products.[405,506] Functional scanning has demonstrated increased glucose metabolism in the medulla, probably due to changes in the inferior olivary nuclei.[212]

Guillain and Mollaret proposed that disruption of connections between the dentate nucleus and the contralateral inferior olivary nucleus, which run via the red nucleus and central tegmental tract, is responsible for the syndrome.[288] However, the red nucleus is not known to have a role in the control of eye movements, and more recent studies have implicated interruption of a pathway from the deep cerebellar nuclei through the superior cerebellar peduncle, which then loops caudally through the central tegmental tract to the inferior olive (Fig. 12–1, Chapter 12).[423,579] How could hypertrophic degeneration of the inferior olive lead to oculopalatal tremor? One hypothesis concerns the peculiar electrotonic coupling of cells in the inferior olivary nucleus, which depend on gap junctions channels, called connexons that permit dendrite-

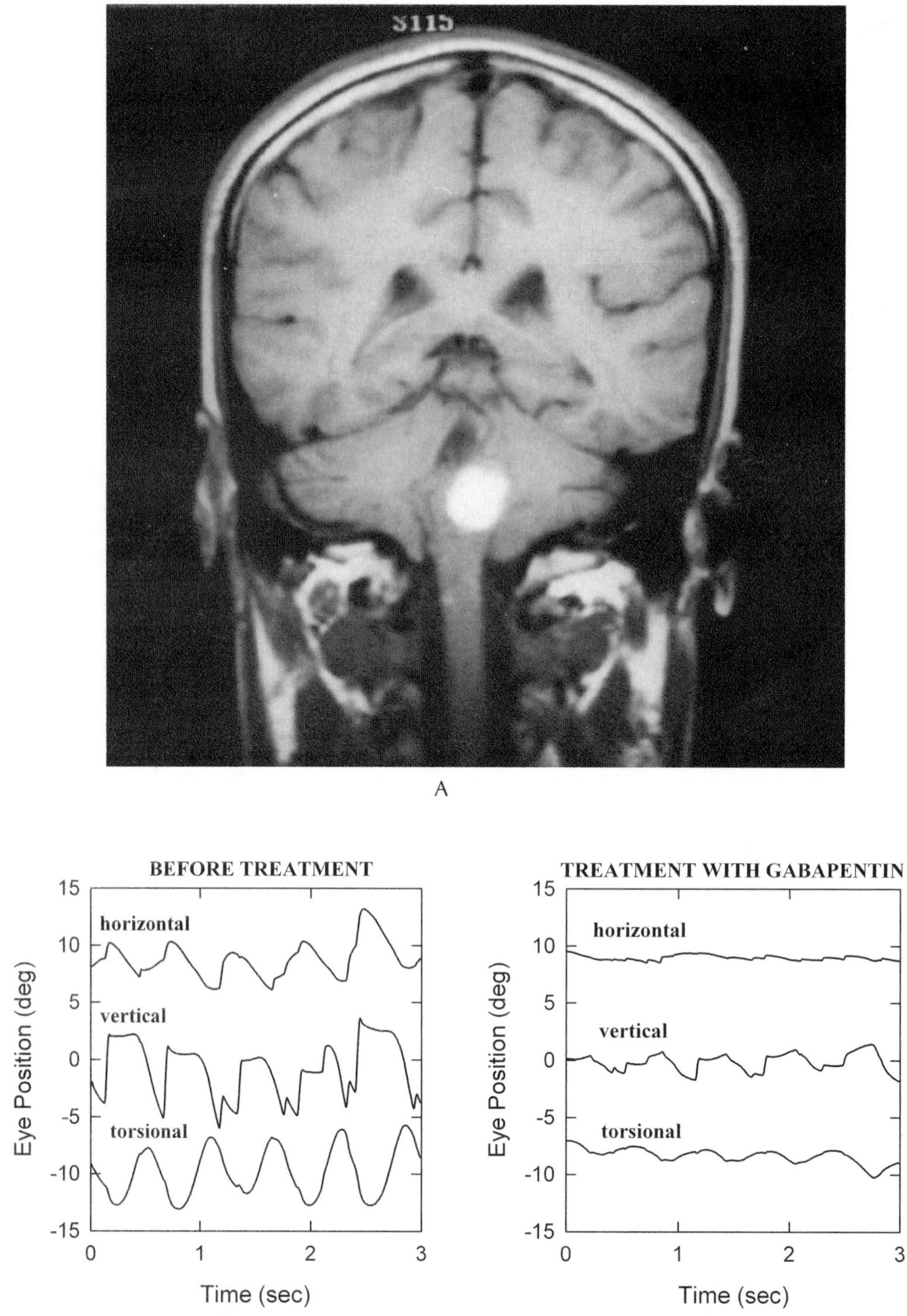

Figure 10–10. Syndrome of oculopalatal tremor following brainstem stroke. The patient was a 25-year-old man who developed this syndrome following brainstem hemorrhage from an arteriovenous malformation. (A) MRI showing brainstem hematoma and a vein draining superiorly from the malformation. (B) The effects of gabapentin on oscillations of his right eye are shown. The horizontal and torsional records have been offset from the vertical records, which are aligned about zero for clarity of display; thus eye positions are relative rather than absolute. Upward deflections indicate rightward, upward, or clockwise eye rotations, with respect to the patient. Gabapentin substantially reduced this patient's nystagmus, as is also evident on the videos (see Video Display: Treatment for Nystagmus).

to-dendrite transmission of ions and small molecules.[147,200] Deafferentation of the inferior olive leads to the development of soma-somatic connexons junctions,[579] and it is postulated that this, in turn, synchronizes the discharge of olivary neurons at about 1Hz–2 Hz. This synchronized signal is then sent to the cerebellar cortex on climbing fibers, and could cause maladaptive learning that produces pendular ocular oscillations with variable waveform.[439] This hypothesis requires testing, but suggests some new treatments for oculopalatal tremor, such as drugs acting on connexons.[147,439]

CONVERGENT-DIVERGENT FORMS OF NYSTAGMUS

Convergent forms of nystagmus are often small in amplitude and may be missed without records to document the phase relationship between each eye. More than one mechanism is likely, and an oscillation that emanates from the vergence mechanism itself is probably rare. Here, we discuss disjunctive forms of pendular nystagmus, vertical jerk nystagmus that has disjunctive horizontal components, and convergence-retraction nystagmus.

Convergence-divergence forms of nystagmus should be differentiated from conjugate nystagmus that is evoked or changed by convergence.[517,617] Thus, in some patients with acquired pendular nystagmus[52,61] or central vestibular forms of nystagmus (downbeat, upbeat, torsional), convergence variably suppresses, increases, or changes the form of the oscillations.[150,227,509] Further, congenital forms of nystagmus are often suppressed by convergence, a factor that also has therapeutic significance (see Video Display: Treatments for Nystagmus).[437]

Convergent-Divergent Pendular Oscillations

Pendular nystagmus with a vergence component occurs in patients with multiple sclerosis,[53] brainstem stroke including oculopalatal tremor,[282] and cerebral Whipple's disease[602] (see Video Display: Acquired Pendular Nystagmus). Disjunctive pendular nystagmus might be due to either a phase difference between the conjugate oscillatory drive reaching each eye (due to a disturbance in the yoking mechanism), or to an oscillation of the vergence system. In cerebral Whipple's disease, the abnormal eye movements have been ascribed to oscillations of the vergence system; hence the term "pendular vergence oscillations."[602] The nystagmus in Whipple's disease typically has a frequency of about 1.0 Hz and is often accompanied by concurrent contractions of the masticatory muscles ("oculomasticatory myorhythmia"). In addition, palsy of vertical saccades occurs, and may mimic the paralysis of progressive supranuclear palsy.[47,456,547]

The issue of whether the vergence system is primarily responsible for pendular nystagmus with a disjunctive component has been addressed in a few studies by measuring 3-D rotations of both eyes. Some patients have been reported with convergent-divergent pendular nystagmus in which the oscillations were about 180 degrees out of phase in the horizontal and torsional planes but had conjugate vertical components.[53] Sometimes, the torsional component of the oscillations had the greatest amplitude ("cyclovergence nystagmus"). In such patients, an oscillation affecting the vergence system itself seems more likely, since there was no phase shift vertically, and the relationship between the horizontal and torsional components was similar to that occurring during normal vergence movements (excyclovergence with horizontal convergence).[53] Under experimental conditions, the vergence system has been made to oscillate at frequencies of up to 2.5 Hz,[566] lower than the frequency reported in patients with conditions other than Whipple's disease. To account for these higher-frequency oscillations, it seems necessary to postulate instability within the brainstem-cerebellar connections of the vergence system, such as between nucleus reticularis tegmenti pontis and the cerebellar posterior interposed nuclei (discussed in Chapter 8).[53]

Vertical Jerk Nystagmus with a Convergent-Divergent Horizontal Component

Like pendular nystagmus, some forms of jerk nystagmus have a convergent or divergent component. For example, the upbeat nystagmus shown in Figure 10–3B in a patient with multiple sclerosis (see Video Display: Downbeat, Upbeat, Torsional Nystagmus) has convergent slow phases. Only occasionally are the horizontal, disjunctive components of the nystagmus large enough to be clinically apparent. Divergence nystagmus has been reported with cerebellar disease such as Arnold–Chiari malformation, when combined divergent and downbeat nystagmus produces slow phases that are directed upward and inward.[141,724] These forms of nystagmus might reflect an otolithic imbalance, since geometric factors require that the normal, translational vestibulo-ocular reflex (see Fig. 1–5) during vertical (bob) or fore-and-aft (surge) head movements combines conjugate vertical and disconjugate horizontal movements, if the subject looks at a near object above or below eye level. Applying translational stimuli to patients with these forms of nystagmus could test such a hypothesis.

Convergence-Retraction Nystagmus

Convergence-retraction nystagmus is elicited either by asking the patient to make an upward saccade, or by using a hand-held optokinetic drum or tape, moving the stripes down (see Video Display: Disorders of Vergence). With the optokinetic stimulus, slow, downward, following eye movements occur, but the upward quick phases are replaced by rapid convergent or retractory movements, or both. Convergence-retraction nystagmus is usually intermittent, being determined by saccadic activity, and so can be differentiated from other, more continuous forms of disjunctive nystagmus such as acquired pendular nystagmus or oculomasticatory myorhythmia. Patients with convergence-retraction nystagmus also often show transient convergence during horizontal saccades, which give the appearance of abduction weakness – pseudoabducens palsy (see Video Display: Disorders of Vergence).[159,543]

Convergence-retraction nystagmus is caused by lesions of the mesencephalon that involve the region of the posterior commissure, classically pineal tumors (see Ocular Motor Syndromes Caused by Lesions of the Mesencephalon, in Chapter 12).[141,513] Convergence nystagmus has also been described in patients with the Arnold–Chiari malformation.[492]

On the basis of measurements in two affected patients, it has been proposed that this is not truly a form of nystagmus, since each cycle of the oscillation is initiated by a disjunctive saccade (or quick phase) that converges and retracts the eyes (see Video Display: Disorders of Vergence).[370,513] However, 3-D measurements of convergence-retraction nystagmus in a third patient indicated that the convergence movements were synchronous, and their dynamic features were more consistent with vergence than saccades [554] Normal subjects typically show small convergence movements with downward movements and small divergence with upward saccades,[736] which is the opposite of the pattern occurring in convergence-retraction nystagmus (see saccade-vergence interactions, in Chapter 8). Thus, further studies are required to better understand normal and abnormal saccade-vergence interactions, and to determine which structures or connections in the dorsal midbrain are responsible. It remains possible that more than one mechanism might lead to the clinical syndrome of convergence-retraction nystagmus.

Pretectal pseudobobbing consists of non-rhythmic, rapid movements which carry the eyes down and medially, and are followed by a slow return to midline; each movement may be preceded by a blink.[387] This disorder is reported in patients with acute obstructive hydrocephalus, and the horizontal component may be a variant of convergence nystagmus.

CONGENITAL FORMS OF NYSTAGMUS

The Nature of Congenital Ocular Oscillations

Progress in understanding the pathogenesis of congenital forms of nystagmus has been advanced by the development of animal models in normal monkeys that are either deprived of binocular vision during early life,[683] or made strabismic,[728] and by the identification of congenital forms of nystagmus in mutant dogs with abnormal anatomy of the visual system.[195,196] However, although some patients with congenital forms of nystagmus show visual abnormalities (Table 10–7), others with similar ocular oscillations do not. Furthermore, the presence of any one type of waveform—such as pendular (see Fig. 10–1D) or jerk (Fig. 10–1A) does not suggest a specific

Table 10–7. **Visual System Disorders Associated With Infantile Nystagmus Syndrome (Congenital Nystagmus)** **2,6a,91,148,165,215,267,270,272a,303,304,391,404,407, 414,480,545,681,690,692,705**

Ocular and oculocutaneous albinism
Hermansky-Pudlak syndrome
Achromatopsia
Cataracts
Corneal opacities
Optic disc atrophy
Cone dystrophy
Optic nerve hypoplasia
Leber's congenital amaurosis
Colobomata
Aniridia
Retinopathy of prematurity
Corectopia
Congenital stationary night-blindness
Chediak–Higashi syndrome
Joubert's syndrome
Peroxisomal disorders

pathogenesis or indicate whether the nystagmus is associated with visual system anomalies.[177] Thus, the underlying mechanisms are not fully understood.

Conventionally, three distinct syndromes have been recognized: congenital nystagmus, latent nystagmus, and spasmus nutans. Recently, the Classification of Eye Movement Abnormalities and Strabismus (CEMAS) Working Group has recommended new names for nystagmus that begins during infancy.[1] Three categories have been defined: (1) infantile nystagmus syndrome (INS), which corresponds to what had previously been called motor or sensory forms of congenital nystagmus; (2) fusional maldevelopment nystagmus syndrome (FMNS), which corresponds to latent nystagmus occurring in association with amblyopia and strabismus; and (3) spasmus nutans syndrome (SNS). Diagnostic features of each of these syndromes are summarized in Boxes 10–11, 10–12, and 10–13. A potential problem posed by the CEMAS classification for some ophthalmologists is that measurement of eye movements, which is necessary to characterize nystagmus waveforms, may not be available. The advantage of the sys-

Box 10–11. Clinical Features Of Infantile Nystagmus Syndrome (Congenital Nystagmus)

- Present since infancy
- Usually conjugate, horizontal; smaller torsional or vertical components
- Pendular or increasing-velocity waveforms punctuated by foveation periods, during which eyes are transiently still and aimed at the object of interest
- Suppresses on convergence or with eyelid closure
- Accentuated by visual attention or arousal
- Often minimal when the eyes are near one particular orbital position (null zone)
- Accompanied by head shaking or head turn

For pathophysiology, see Smooth Pursuit in Patients with Congenital Nystagmus, in Chapter 4. For a recorded example, see Fig. 10-11. (Related Video Display: Congenital Forms of Nystagmus) tem is that it incorporates the broad clinical and laboratory evidence, avoids diagnostic labels based on uncertain pathogenesis, and accepts that overlaps among syndromes sometimes occur.

Infantile Nystagmus Syndrome or Congenital Nystagmus

CLINICAL FEATURES OF INFANTILE NYSTAGMUS SYNDROME

The "congenital" nystagmus of INS may be present at birth but usually develops during infancy.[268,317,321] It occasionally presents during adult life,[235,280] when it may create a diagnostic problem, especially if the patient has other symptoms such as headaches or dizziness. Although variable in form, certain clinical features usually differentiate INS from other ocular oscillations (see Video Display: Congenital Forms of Nystagmus and Box 10–11). In eye-fixed coordinates (i.e., looking along the patient's line of sight), it is almost always conjugate and mainly horizontal, even on up or down gaze. A torsional component to the nystagmus is probably common (Fig. 10–11B), but may be difficult to identify clinically because of the larger horizontal movements.[5,41] Less com-

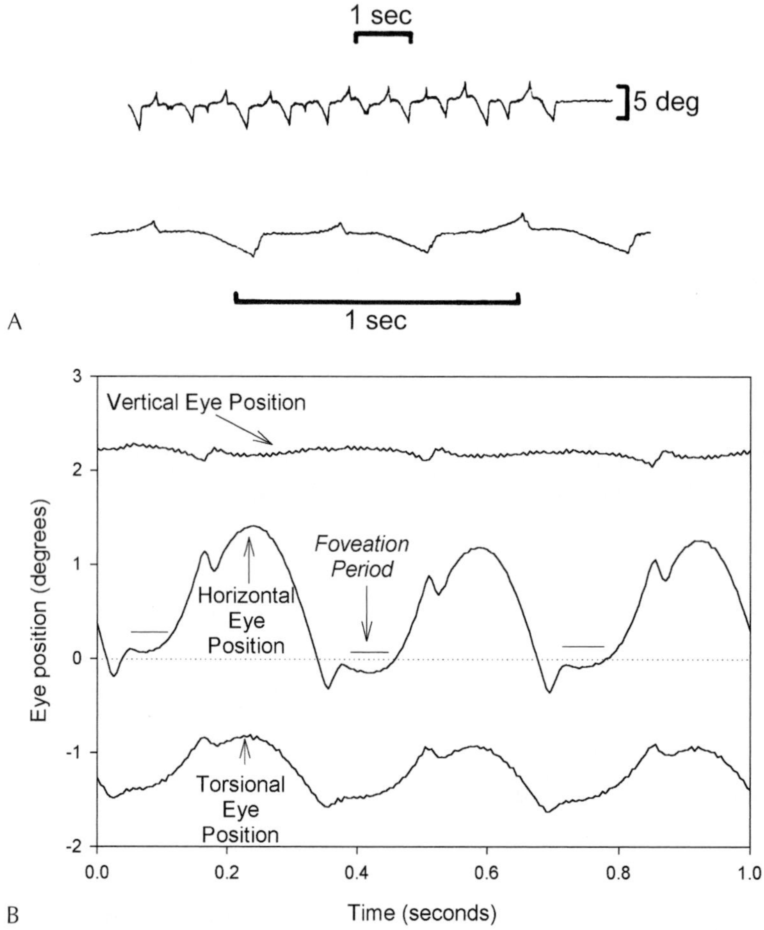

Figure 10–11. Congenital nystagmus. Examples of (A) horizontal jerk waveform, with slow phases that drift away from the fixation position with increasing velocity waveforms (evident on lower, magnified scale) (see Video Display: Congenital Forms of Nystagmus) and (B) A pendular type of congenital nystagmus waveform with superimposed quick phases, showing the large horizontal component, smaller torsional component, and almost absent vertical component. Note that vertical and torsional channels have been offset to aid clarity of display. Foveation periods follow quick phases (when eye position is close to zero), and are indicated by horizontal bars. Upward deflections indicate rightward (horizontal), upward (vertical) or clockwise (torsional) eye rotations, with respect to the patient.

monly, the nystagmus of INS is mainly seesaw (see Video Display: Nystagmus and Visual Disorders), and such patients may have underlying disease of the retina, visual pathways,[32,171] or cerebellum. Lifelong nystagmus that is vertical is not typical of INS,[85,638] and consideration should be given to other diagnoses, such as the calcium channelopathies.

The nystagmus of INS is usually accentuated by the attempt to fixate an object,[673] and by attention or anxiety. Eyelid closure,[626] or convergence, [202] usually suppress it, but occasionally the nystagmus is evoked by viewing a near target.[617,733] Its intensity may also be influenced by viewing the vertical lines of an optokinetic tape.[160] Often, nystagmus decreases when the eyes are moved into a particular position in the orbit; this is called the null point or zone, and corresponds to the range of eye position within which slow-phase eye velocity is at a minimum. In some patients, especially albinos,[2] the nystagmus periodically reverses direction, but this reversal seldom occurs in the regular manner seen in the acquired form of periodic alternating nystagmus.[9,177,274,609] In some patients, the direction of the nystagmus in INS is influenced by which eye is viewing, the nystagmus beating away from the covered eye. This is similar to what happens in the latent nystagmus of fusional maldevelopment nystagmus syndrome, which is discussed below.

Up to 30% of patients with INS have strabismus.[170,317] Stereovision is usually degraded, even in individuals lacking strabismus, partly due to retinal image motion.[689] Individuals with albinism may appear to be exotropic due to a positive angle kappa, which defines the geometric relationship between the pupillary and visual axes.[99] When such patients view a penlight, the examiner notes a medial displacement of the reflected images within the pupils. This finding might be related to the anomalous crossed visual decussation of axons from temporal retina in albinism.[99,332,596]

Head turns are common in INS and are used to bring the eye in the orbit close to the null point or zone, at which nystagmus is minimal.[324,656] The presence of such head turns in childhood photographs is often useful evidence in diagnosing INS. Another strategy used by patients with either INS or the latent nystagmus of FMNS is to purposely induce an esotropia (nystagmus blockage syndrome) in order to suppress the nystagmus; such an esotropia requires a head turn to direct the viewing eye at the object of interest.[180,694]

Some patients with INS also show head oscillations.[123,179,284,553] Such head movements could not act as an adaptive strategy to improve vision unless the vestibulo-ocular reflex was negated. Thus, for most patients with INS, head movements are not compensatory and tend to increase when the individual attends to an object, an effort that also increases the nystagmus. It seems possible, therefore, that in most patients the head tremor and ocular oscillations represent the output of a common neural mechanism.[553]

QUANTITATIVE FEATURES OF INFANTILE NYSTAGMUS SYNDROME

The most distinctive feature of INS is the waveforms of the nystagmus; the commonest are increasing-velocity (see Fig. 10–1C) and pendular (Fig. 10–1D), which may be combined. Frequently superimposed on these waveforms are foveation periods, the "signature" of INS (Fig. 10–11).[3,5,72,177,186] Thus, during each cycle—usually after a quick phase—there is a brief period when the eye is still and is pointed at the object of regard. With jerk waveforms, the quick phases (saccades) may "brake" the oscillation,[178,359] or bring the eye to the target. With pendular waveforms, the oscillation is "flattened" by a foveation period when the eye is closest to the target (Fig. 10–11B).

Foveation periods are probably one reason why many patients with INS have near-normal vision,[133,624] and why most patients do not complain of oscillopsia, in spite of otherwise nearly continuous movement of their eyes.[13,176,259,689] Other factors that contribute to a stable percept of the world despite nystagmus are reduced sensitivity to retinal image motion,[614] and monitoring of internal signals (efference copy) to suppress oscillopsia.[13,70] Oscillopsia may present later in life if, for example, strabismus develops.[320] Based on requirements for clear and stable vision in normal subjects, functions have been described that predict what visual acuity would be expected for any individual with INS from the measured properties of the foveation period.[185] Foveation periods are not an invariable finding in INS, and when they are absent or poorly developed, visual acuity is usually impaired, and visual system disorders are associated.[71,186] Conversely, foveation periods are only rarely reported in acquired forms of nystagmus.[176,651] The waveform also depends upon the child's age; for example, it may be large-amplitude "triangular" in the first few months of life, then pendular and finally jerk as the patient reaches about a year of age.[560] These waveforms are so characteristic of INS that reliable records of eye position and velocity will often secure the diagnosis.

A commonly described associated finding is "inversion" of smooth-pursuit or optokinetic responses.[294] Thus, with a hand-held optokinetic drum or tape, quick phases are directed in the same direction as the drum rotates. The phenomenon can be explained in terms of shifts in the position of the null point of the nystagmus induced by the pursuit or optokinetic stimuli. Measurement of tracking during foveation periods has shown that smooth pursuit and optokinetic eye movements are preserved in at least some individuals.[192,419] Similarly, the higher frequency vestibular responses have generally been found to be normal in patients with INS and, if judged from retinal image stability during the foveation period, performance is normal and allows a similar view of the world while the patient is stationary or in motion.[123,193] However, especially in those patients with associated visual disorders such as albinism, vestibular responses to lower frequencies of head rotations and optokinetic responses (i.e., the velocity-storage mechanism) may be impaired.[198,277] Postural stability shows mild impairment that can be related to the visual "sampling" that occurs during each foveation period.[287] Occasional patients exhibit their nystagmus only during attempted smooth tracking (see Video Display: Disorders of Smooth Pursuit),[392] and others can voluntarily release or inhibit their nystagmus, suggesting that the fixation mechanism plays some role in their oscillations.[684] INS associated with congenital gaze-holding failure (i.e., leaky neural integrator) has been reported in one kindred.[194]

PATHOGENESIS OF INFANTILE NYSTAGMUS SYNDROME

Overall, most individuals with congenital forms of nystagmus have no associated visual system defects. However, about 25% of affected individuals are albinos, and 10% have identifiable visual or ocular anomalies.[2] Some of the visual system disorders associated with nystagmus are listed in Table 10–7, but some such cases may not show the classic features of INS, such as accelerating waveform and foveation periods. Failure to develop a normal optic chiasm may predispose to congenital seesaw nystagmus, both in humans,[31,413] and in mutant dogs who lack any decussation of their visual pathway.[195] Nystagmus that is present at birth, but resolves by 6 months of age, has been associated with delayed visual maturation and uncorrected large hyperopia.[81] Because of the many diagnostic possibilities, a complete ophthalmologic evaluation and an electroretinogram are necessary in patients with nystagmus associated with decreased visual acuity or visual dysfunction.[96,135,261,422,705]

Infantile nystagmus syndrome, either with or without associated visual system abnormalities, may be familial.[2,182,194,395,514] Autosomal dominant,[395] and sex-linked recessive[118,323a,394,477] forms of inheritance have been reported. In X-linked forms,[396] the mothers may show subtle ocular motor abnormalities. INS has been reported in monozygotic twins, but their nystagmus waveforms may vary considerably;[6,8] this is also true of affected members of the same family.[182] These hereditary forms of INS, with the characteristic waveforms (Fig. 10–11) should be differentiated from other genetic disorders that produce forms of nystagmus typical of cerebellar dysfunction.[368,546]

The known anatomical variations of the anterior visual system in individuals with INS, such as excessive crossing at the chiasm in association with albinism,[289,332,469,596] or absent crossing of nasal fibers in achiasmatic subjects with congenital seesaw nystagmus,[31,32,195] have led to development of models for congenital nystagmus based on "miswiring" of visual or proprioceptive pathways.[331a,521,684] Other models have also been proposed that have related the oscillations of congenital nystagmus to chaotic systems,[3] to an underlying instability in visual tracking systems such as smooth pursuit,[357] or to an abnormality of the termination of saccades.[20a,106] These ideas about the pathogenesis of congenital nystagmus are discussed further in Chapter 4, under Smooth Pursuit in Patients with Congenital Nystagmus.

Latent Nystagmus and Fusional Maldevelopment Nystagmus Syndrome (FMNS)

CLINICAL FEATURES OF LATENT NYSTAGMUS

True latent nystagmus is a jerk nystagmus that is absent when both eyes are viewing but appears when one eye is covered: quick phases of both eyes beat away from the covered eye. Usually, the nystagmus reverses direction upon covering of either eye; in some patients, nystagmus is present when one eye is covered but is absent when the other is occluded. True latent nystagmus is rare,[10] and, in most patients, nystagmus (which may be of low amplitude) is present when both eyes are uncovered, then being termed "manifest latent nystagmus" (Box 10–12). An example is shown in Figure 10–12 (see Video Display: Congenital Forms of Nystagmus). However, in such patients, only one eye may be fixating, and vision from the other eye (which is often deviated, e.g., esotropic) is suppressed.[188,285] In some patients, square-wave jerks are prominent during binocular fixation and, in others, torsional nystagmus is evident.[10] A small cyclovertical component may be present, greater in the covered eye, in patients with FMNS that show dissociated vertical deviation (upward deviation of the covered eye).[290,349] Occasional patients with FMNS can control their latent nystagmus at will.[175,411]

Latent nystagmus is one feature of FMNS. Affected patients usually have strabismus, typically esotropia.[189,600] Amblyopia is frequent, whereas binocular vision with normal stereopsis is rare. Like strabismus, latent nystagmus sometimes occurs in individuals who have no other evidence of neurologic dysfunction, but it is also encountered in patients with disorders of cerebral development, such as Down's syndrome.[42] In addition to strabismus, upward deviation of the covered eye (called alternating sursumduction or dissociated vertical deviation) and a torsional component to the nystagmus are frequently associated.[27,691] Individuals with FMNS show asymmetry of monocular smooth pursuit, optokinetic nystagmus,[246] and the cortical visual evoked response (VEP) to motion stimuli; the significance of these findings is discussed in the next section and under Smooth Pursuit, Visual Fixation and Latent Nystagmus, in Chapter 4.[410,600,685]

Fusional maldeveopment nystagmus syndrome with latent nystagmus is quite common,

Box 10–12. Clinical Features of Latent Nystagmus (Fusional Maldevelopment Nystagmus Syndrome)

- Present since infancy; associated with strabismus and lack of binocular vision
- Evoked or enhanced by covering one eye
- Conjugate, horizontal nystagmus beating away from covered eye
- May be have an associated torsional component (pendular or jerk) and vertical upbeating component
- Slow phases may have linear-, or decreasing-velocity waveforms
- Smooth pursuit asymmetry, depending on viewing eye and on-going nystagmus
- Associated with dissociated vertical deviation (eye under cover deviates up)

For pathophysiology, see: Smooth Pursuit, Visual Fixation and Latent Nystagmus, in Chapter 4. For a recorded example, see Fig. 10-12. (Related Video Display: Congenital Forms of Nystagmus)

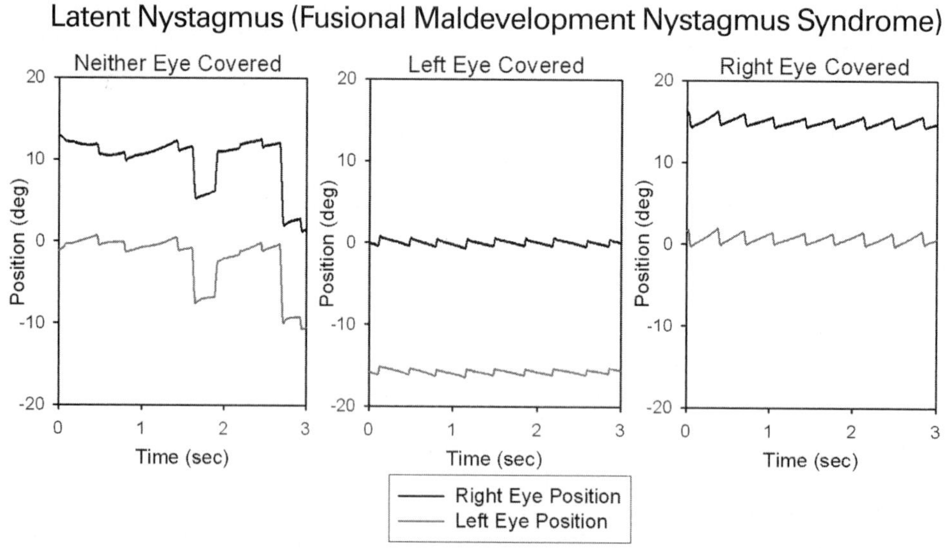

Figure 10–12. The records are from a 56-year-old adult woman with latent nystagmus (fusional maldevelopment nystagmus syndrome), exotropia, and amblyopia (see Video Display: Congenital Forms of Nystagmus). When the patient is asked to view a visual target with both eyes (left panel), she chose to fixate with her left eye and manifests left-beating nystagmus with some saccadic intrusions. When her left eye is covered (center panel), she fixates the target with her right eye and she develops an increased exophoria with right-beating latent nystagmus. When her right eye is covered (right panel), she fixates the target with her left eye and develops an increased exophoria and left-beating latent nystagmus. Upward deflections indicate rightward eye rotations.

and accurate diagnosis is important to avoid inappropriate investigations. Latent nystagmus should be differentiated from gaze-evoked nystagmus in association with strabismus, and especially from abducting nystagmus occurring with internuclear ophthalmoplegia, in which an exotropia may be present but adducting saccades are slow.

QUANTITATIVE FEATURES OF LATENT NYSTAGMUS

The slow phase of latent nystagmus shows a linear or decaying velocity waveform (Fig. 10–1A) (see Video Display: Congenital Forms of Nystagmus), in contrast to the increasing velocity waveform of INS (congenital nystagmus).[10,285] In some patients, a dynamic overshoot of the quick phase effectively produces a small saccade in the direction of the subsequent slow phase.[12] Foveation may occur during the slowest part of the drift if the amplitude of the nystagmus is large, and immediately after the quick phase if the amplitude is small.[187] Latent nystagmus usually follows Alexander's law, the nystagmus being greatest on looking in the direction of the quick phases, away from the covered eye. Some patients take advantage of Alexander's law and turn their head to keep their viewing eye in an adducted position, where nystagmus is minimal;[409] this and other strategies to reduce latent or congenital nystagmus (INS) have been called nystagmus blockage syndrome.[180,273]

Occasionally, congenital nystagmus (INS) and latent nystagmus coexist, and the waveforms may then be more complicated. Rarely, if vision is clearer with the latent nystagmus waveforms than with the congenital nystagmus waveforms, such patients may switch from congenital to latent nystagmus as one eye becomes esotropic and the other takes up fixation.[180]

PATHOGENESIS OF LATENT NYSTAGMUS AND FUSIONAL MALDEVELOPMENT NYSTAGMUS SYNDROME

Latent nystagmus can be induced experimentally in monkeys, either by depriving them of binocular vision early in life,[683] or by surgically creating strabismus.[402] Strabismus also occurs naturally in some monkeys.[729] In strabismic monkeys, the cortical areas that extract motion information from visual stimuli, such as V5 or area MT (see Fig. 6–8, in Chapter 6), have normal responses but are rarely driven binocularly.[402] In humans or monkeys with latent nystagmus, motion-vision cortical evoked potentials are asymmetric, independent of the effects of nystagmus.[29,714] Monocular vertical optokinetic stimulation causes diagonal responses that imply directional abnormalities of motion vision pathways.[246] Normal subjects may develop nystagmus with some similar features to latent nystagmus during monocular viewing of repetitive, stationary flashes of light (flash-induced nystagmus),[524] which is a form of second-order motion (see Chapter 4).[134]

In monkeys with latent nystagmus, the brainstem nucleus of the optic tract (NOT) shows abnormal electrophysiological properties.[497] As summarized in Chapters 2 and 4 (Fig. 4–8), visual motion information from cortical area MT/V5 projects to NOT that, in turn, projects to the velocity-storage mechanism in the vestibular nuclei.[719] In this way, vestibular and optokinetic input can combine to generate appropriate eye movements during and following self-rotation. In normal monkeys, NOT neurons respond to visual stimuli presented to either eye. However, in monkeys with latent nystagmus, NOT neurons are driven mainly by the contralateral eye.[331,497] Thus, for example, during monocular viewing through the right eye, the left NOT will be activated preferentially, producing leftward slow phases of nystagmus. Furthermore, inactivation of NOT with muscimol abolishes latent nystagmus in monkeys who have been deprived of binocular vision.[497,682,683] Taking this evidence together, latent nystagmus may represent the consequences of imbalance of visual inputs to the vestibular system.[100] Thus, in subjects who have failed to develop binocular inputs, occluding one eye causes the contralateral NOT to drive vestibular eye movements as if the subject was being rotated toward the side of the viewing eye.[100]

Latent nystagmus occurs in some, but not all, patients who have congenital uniocular visual loss, suggesting that additional factors beyond visual deprivation are responsible for the development of nystagmus.[420,621] Such factors may include disturbance of directed visual attention or egocentric localization. For example, some patients can change the direction of their nystagmus by "attempting" to view from one eye or the other, without a change of visual inputs.[175,411,620] A model has been proposed to account for the various types of interaction between quick and slow phases of latent nystagmus that have been reported.[184,223]

Spasmus Nutans Syndrome

CLINICAL FEATURES OF SPASMUS NUTANS

This disorder is characterized by the triad of nystagmus, head nodding, and anomalous head positions, such as torticollis (see Video Display: Congenital Forms of Nystagmus and Box 10–13).[508] Its onset is usually during the first

Box 10–13. Clinical Feature of Spasmus Nutans Syndrome

- Characterized by nystagmus, head nodding, and abnormal head positions, developing during first year of life
- Nystagmus is intermittent, small amplitude, high-frequency ("shimmering"), variably disconjugate or disjunctive, greater in the abducting eye, may have vertical component, more evident during convergence
- Head nodding is irregular, with horizontal or vertical components
- Strabismus and amblyopia may coexist
- Normal ophthalmoscopic examination and normal MRI or CT of visual pathways are required to rule out structural lesions
- Spontaneously remits in 2-8 years

See also: Pathogenesis of Spasmus Nutans. For a recorded example, see Fig. 10-13. (Related Video Display: Congenital Forms of Nystagmus) year of life. Neurologic abnormalities are absent, although strabismus or amblyopia may coexist.[730] The syndrome is sometimes familial and has been reported in monozygotic twins.[343] Spasmus nutans spontaneously remits, usually within 1 to 2 years after onset, although it may persist for over 8 years.[271]

The most consistent feature of spasmus nutans is the nystagmus, although head nodding may be the first abnormality to be noticed.[271,276,281,706] The nystagmus is usually intermittent, small amplitude, and with a high-frequency (3 Hz–11 Hz, "shimmering"), pendular waveform; it is easily missed. It may be more evident in the abducting eye during lateral gaze. Characteristically, the nystagmus differs in the two eyes, and sometimes it is uniocular. Another distinguishing feature of these oscillations is the variability of the amplitude in each eye, and the phase relationship between the two eyes. Consequently, even over the course of a few seconds or minutes, the oscillations might variably be conjugate, disconjugate, disjunctive, or purely monocular (Fig. 10–13). The plane of the nystagmus is predominantly horizontal but it may have vertical or torsional components. It may sometimes be brought out by evoking the near response.[130]

The head nodding is irregular, at a frequency of about 3 Hz, with horizontal, vertical, or roll components. It is usually more prominent when the child attempts to inspect something of interest. About two-thirds of the patients have an additional head tilt or turn. In some patients, the head nodding appears to turn off the nystagmus.[276,281] However, it remains unclear whether head nodding, turning, or tilting are always adaptive strategies adopted to reduce the nystagmus, or reflect the underlying abnormality in spasmus nutans.

Two important clinical judgments must be made in children with eye and head oscillations. The first judgment is whether the nys-

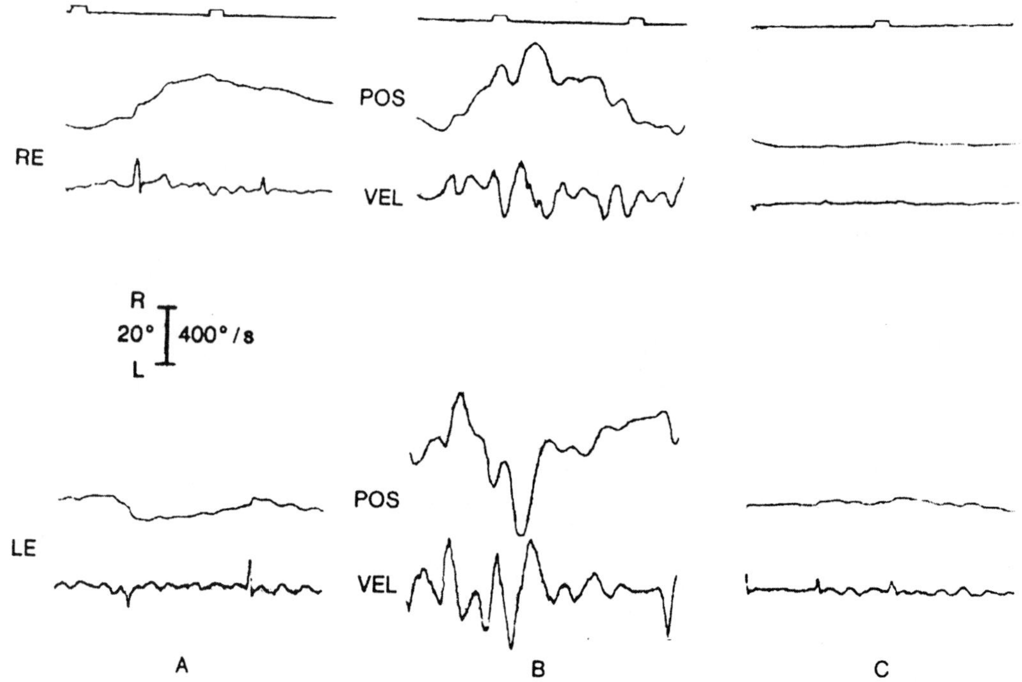

Figure 10–13. Examples of spasmus nutans from one child during one recording session. In A, there are binocular oscillations with no phase difference between the eyes; in B, there are binocular oscillations with approximately 180 degrees phase difference between the eyes; in C, there are uniocular oscillations of the left eye. LE: left eye; RE: right eye; POS: position; VEL: velocity. Timing marks at top are seconds. (Reproduced from Weissman et al.[706] Copyright 1987, American Medical Association. All rights reserved.) See also Video Display: Congenital Forms of Nystagmus.

tagmus reflects a tumor of the optic nerve, chiasm, retina, or more posterior visual pathways,[224,269,270,421,425,619] or a retinal disorder.[269] A careful ophthalmologic evaluation should be performed in all such children; if there is any doubt about the diagnosis, imaging studies and electroretinography should be performed.[633] The second judgment is whether the child has spasmus nutans, which resolves, or congenital nystagmus, which does not. Spasmus nutans can be differentiated from congenital and latent nystagmus by its intermittency, high frequency, vertical component, and dissociated characteristics; if the child will cooperate, eye movement records often help make the distinction.[706]

PATHOGENESIS OF SPASMUS NUTANS

The underlying abnormality in spasmus nutans is unknown; it occurs more commonly in lower socioeconomic groups.[716] Although the ocular oscillations are of high frequency, their disconjugate vertical component makes saccadic oscillations unlikely, since the eyes are tightly yoked during normal vertical saccades. The ability of the active head nodding,[276,281] but not passive rotation in a chair,[706] to stop the ocular oscillations in some patients implies the importance of a voluntary effort. Further, affected children are reported to suppress their nystagmus with a head turn, even though changing eye position in the orbit may have no effect.[132] Thus, voluntary head movements or positions seem essential for returning stability to gaze. Finally, the resolution of spasmus nutans with age might reflect either structural maturation of the nervous system or "full calibration" of eye movements.

LID NYSTAGMUS

Reflecting the anatomic and physiological links between vertical eye and lid movements, upward movements of the eyelids frequently accompany upward movements of vertical nystagmus, especially upbeat nystagmus. An important structure for the normal coordination of vertical saccades is the M-group of neurons, which lie adjacent, medial, and caudal to riMLF (see Fig. 6–3 and Fig. 6–4). The M-group receives inputs from riMLF and project to both the elevator subnuclei of the eye (superior rectus and inferior oblique) and the motoneurons of levator palpebrae superioris in the central caudal subnucleus of CN III.[337] Thus, lid nystagmus unaccompanied by vertical eye nystagmus may reflect midbrain lesions.[98,110,337] Patients with long-standing compression of the central caudal nucleus causing "midbrain ptosis" may develop lid nystagmus.[98]

Twitches of the eyelid may also accompany horizontal nystagmus. This phenomenon has been described in a patient with Wallenberg's syndrome (lateral medullary infarction), in whom lid nystagmus was inhibited by convergence.[161] The opposite—eyelid nystagmus that is evoked by convergence (Pick's sign)—is reported with medullary and cerebellar lesions.[340,581,588] The association of lid nystagmus with convergence may reflect the normal synkinetic lid retraction that occurs during an effort to view a near target. Thus, convergence effort increases innervation to the lids and so may amplify any lid nystagmus.

SACCADIC INTRUSIONS

The Spectrum of Saccadic Intrusions

Several types of inappropriate saccadic movements may intrude upon steady fixation (Box 10–14); these are schematized in Fig. 10–14 and actual recorded examples are shown in Fig. 10–15. Saccadic intrusions should be differentiated from nystagmus, in which a drift of the eyes from the desired position of gaze is the primary abnormality. They should also be differentiated from saccadic dysmetria (see Video Display: Saccadic Oscillations and Intrusions and Fig. 10–14A), in which the eye overshoots or undershoots, sometimes several times, before landing on target.[90,604] Because saccadic intrusions are rapid and brief, it is usually necessary to measure eye and target position and eye velocity in order to identify accurately the saccadic abnormality. We first describe the characteristics of each type of saccadic intrusion and then consider their mechanisms of pathogenesis.

Box 10–14. Clinical Features Of Saccadic Oscillations And Intrusions

SQUARE-WAVE JERKS

- Pairs of small horizontal saccades (typically < 2 deg) that take the eye away from the target and then return it within 200 ms; often occur in a series

MACROSQUARE-WAVE JERKS (MACROSACCADIC PULSES)

- Large (5–15 deg) saccadic intrusions that take the eye away from the target and return it within 70–150 ms

MACROSACCADIC OSCILLATIONS

- Oscillations (hypermetric saccades) around the fixation point that wax and wane, with an intersaccadic interval of about 200 ms

SACCADIC PULSES

- Brief, usually small movements away from the fixation point (saccadic pulse), followed by rapid drift back (due to lack of saccadic step)

OCULAR FLUTTER

- Intermittent bursts of conjugate horizontal saccades without an intersaccadic interval; may be small amplitude and only visible with an ophthalmoscope (microflutter)

OPSOCLONUS

- Combined multidirectional, horizontal, vertical, and torsional saccadic oscillations, without an intersaccadic interval

VOLUNTARY "NYSTAGMUS" OR FLUTTER

- High-frequency (15–25 Hz), conjugate horizontal oscillations
- Unsustained for more than about 30 seconds; often precipitated by convergence

For pathophysiology, see: Inappropriate Saccades (Saccadic Intrusions), in Chapter 3. For schematic and recorded examples, see Fig. 10-15. For etiologies of flutter and opsoclonus, see Table 10-8. (Related Video Display: Saccadic Oscillations and Intrusion)

Square-Wave Jerks

A common finding in healthy subjects, particularly the elderly, is square-wave jerks, also called Gegenrucke.[313,610,613] On eye movement records—see Figure 10–14C and Figure 10–15A—they have a profile that earned them their name. They are small, horizontal, conjugate saccades, typically about 0.5 degree (ranging from 0.1 to 4.0 degrees), which take the

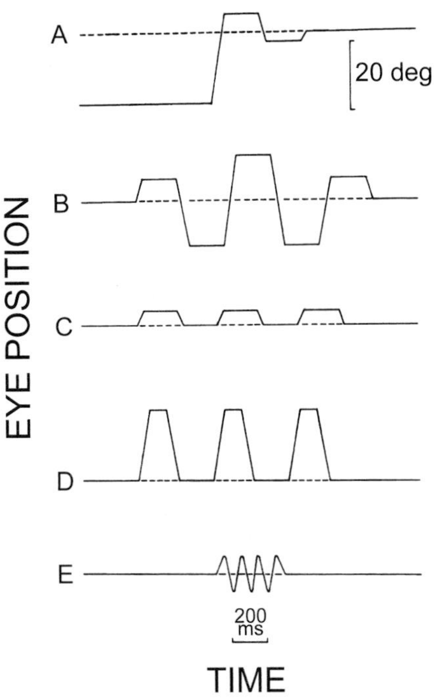

Figure 10–14. Schematic of saccadic intrusions and oscillations. (A) Dysmetria: inaccurate saccades. (B) Macrosaccadic oscillations: hypermetric saccades about the position of the target; (C) Square-wave jerks: small, uncalled-for saccades away from and back to the position of the target; (D) Macrosquare-wave jerks or macrosaccadic pulses: large, uncalled-for saccades away from and back to the position of the target; (E) Ocular flutter: to-and-fro, back-to-back saccades without an intersaccadic interval.

eye away from the fixation position and then return it there after a period of about 200 ms to 400 ms.[7,248] They are most easily detected during ophthalmoscopy. The prevalence of square-wave jerks in healthy subjects depends on the amplitude used to define these movements, but probably most individuals have them, and their frequency may range up to 20 per minute.[7,313] They may be more common,[313] or larger,[7] in normal elderly subjects. Square-wave jerks often show a dynamic overshoot (Fig. 3–4) which is greater in the abducting eye.[12] In certain cerebellar syndromes,[544] progressive supranuclear palsy,[248,557,679] (see Video Display: Saccadic Oscillations and Intrusions) and cerebral hemispheric disease,[616] they may occur almost continuously (but not at more than 2 Hz) and have been called "square-wave oscillations;"[16] these oscillations may be mistaken for nystagmus. Cigarette smoking increases the frequency of square-wave jerks.[629] They are reported to develop following pallidotomy in parkinsonian patients.[50,512] In patients with dementia, fixation is disrupted by larger saccadic intrusions that are usually due to increased distractibility (see section on Alzheimer's disease)

Macrosquare-Wave Jerks (Square-Wave Pulses)

These oscillations are often large (typically greater than 5 degrees) and occur at a frequency of about 2 Hz–3 Hz. After taking the eye off the target, they return it with a latency of about 80 ms (Fig. 10–14D).[191] They occur in light or darkness, but occasionally are suppressed during monocular fixation.[174] Macrosquare-wave jerks occur in bursts and vary in amplitude. They are uncommon, but have been reported in multiple sclerosis and multiple system atrophy.[403]

Macrosaccadic Oscillations

These oscillations usually consist of horizontal saccades that occur in runs, spontaneously building up and then decreasing in amplitude, with intersaccadic intervals of about 200 ms (Fig. 10–14B). Described originally in patients with cerebellar disorders,[606] macrosaccadic oscillations reflect saccadic dysmetria when both primary and corrective saccades are so hypermetric (increased gain) that they overshoot the target continuously in both directions, and so oscillate around the fixation point (Fig. 3–6). They are usually induced by a gaze shift, but may occur during attempted fixation, or even in darkness.[43] They may have vertical or torsional components, and occasionally the vertical may be prominent clinically.[237]

Macrosaccadic oscillations occur most commonly with lesions affecting the fastigial nucleus and its output in the superior cerebellar peduncles. They also occur in some forms of spinocerebellar ataxia.[666] Occasionally, macrosaccadic oscillations occur with pontine lesions, that may compromise either the omni-

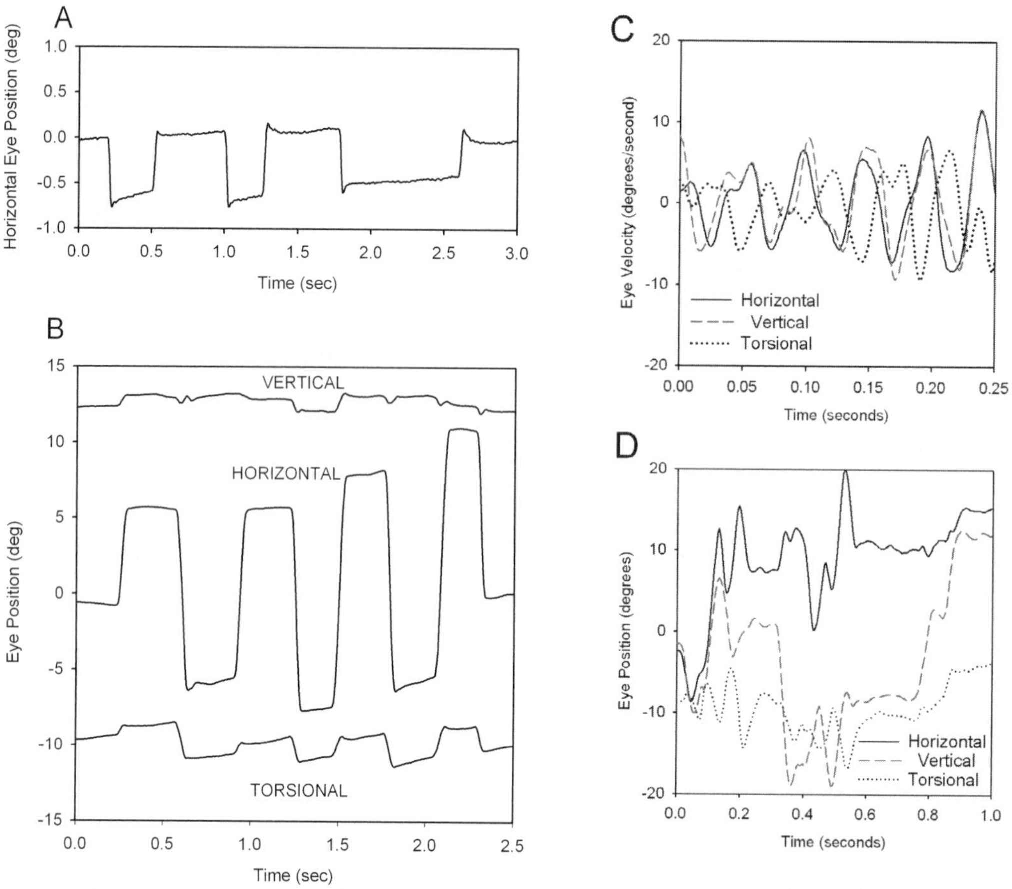

Figure 10–15. Records of saccadic intrusions and oscillations; note different amplitude and times scales. Also see examples on the Video Display: Saccadic Oscillations and Intrusions. (A) Square-wave jerks—small saccades that repeatedly moved the image of regard off the fovea; the patient had progressive supranuclear palsy. (B) Macrosaccadic oscillations from the right eye of a patient with a pontine infarction.[43] Fixation is interrupted by bursts of saccadic intrusions, which are time-locked in the horizontal, vertical, and torsional planes. The return saccade usually overshoots the central fixation point. Torsional and vertical tracings have been offset for convenience of display. Upward deflections correspond to rightward, upward, or clockwise eye rotations, with respect to the patient. (C) Sustained micro-opsoclonus and bursts of opsoclonus in a 40-year-old woman who was asymptomatic. High frequency, small oscillations, with horizontal, vertical, and torsional components, occurred most of the time. She had presumably had these saccadic oscillations all of her life and, like patients with congenital forms of nystagmus, had adapted to their visual consequences. Note that velocity records are shown. (D) Example of a burst of opsoclonus from a 35-year-old woman with the idiopathic variant of this disorder. The single-position traces are offset to aid clarity of display; positive deflections indicate rightward (horizontal), upward (vertical), or clockwise (torsional) eye rotations, from the patient's viewpoint.

pause neurons, or fastigial nucleus input, to premotor burst neurons (Fig. 10–15B) (see Video Display: Saccadic Oscillations and Intrusions).[43] Insights into the pathogenesis of macrosaccadic oscillations come from the observation that they may occur in patients with myasthenia gravis following injection of edrophonium (see Video Display: Diplopia and Strabismus).[408] In this case, they probably reflect cerebellar gain increases to adapt to the ocular motor palsy.

Saccadic Pulses, Ocular Flutter, and Opsoclonus

Saccadic pulses are brief intrusions upon steady fixation. The eye movement is a saccade away from the fixation position with a rapid drift back, since the saccadic pulse has not been integrated to a step. This is unlike square-wave jerks, in which there is a period of 200–400 ms between the saccade taking the eye away from fixation and the returning saccade. Saccadic pulses may occur in series or as double saccadic pulses, which occur in some normal subjects.[7] Frequent saccadic pulses are reported in patients with internuclear ophthalmoplegia.[314]

There is a continuum between saccadic pulses and saccadic oscillations without an intersaccadic interval.[38,76,80,739] The latter may occur in one direction, usually the horizontal plane (called ocular flutter, Fig. 10–14E), or may consist of saccadic oscillations with horizontal, vertical, and torsional components, called opsoclonus or "saccadomania" (Fig. 10–15D). The frequency of oscillations is usually high, typically 10 to 25 cycles per second, being higher with smaller-size movements. Ocular flutter may be intermittent, and is mainly associated with voluntary saccades (flutter dysmetria). Occasionally, the amplitude is very small ("microflutter," see Fig.10–15C) and the oscillations can only be detected with an ophthalmoscope or eye movement recordings, even though visual symptoms such as oscillopsia are produced.[38,233,550] Sometimes such "microflutter" may have components in all three planes.

Sustained opsoclonus is a striking finding, in which multidirectional conjugate saccades, usually of large amplitude, interfere with steady fixation. These oscillations occur during smooth pursuit, convergence,[80] or blinks,[292] and usually persist during eyelid closure or sleep (see Video Display: Saccadic Oscillations and Intrusions). Opsoclonus is often accompanied by myoclonus (brief, jerky involuntary limb movements), hence the term opsoclonus-myoclonus; in children, this syndrome has been called "dancing eyes and dancing feet" (see Video Display: Saccadic Oscillations and Intrusions).[213,622] Ataxia and encephalopathy may also accompany opsoclonus. There are many reported causes of opsoclonus and flutter (Table 10–8), but most patients conform to four clinical settings: parainfectious brainstem encephalitis, paraneoplastic syndromes, metabolic-toxic states, or without evident cause.[48,68,717]

Table 10–8. **Etiology of Ocular Flutter and Opsoclonus***

Parainfectious encephalitis[80,197,207,300,302,418,711]
Paraneoplastic effect of neuroblastoma and other neural crest tumors (in children)†[484,534]
Paraneoplastic effects of other tumors (in adults)[20,417,532,533]
Meningitis[564]
Intracranial tumors[389]
Hydrocephalus[625]
Thalamic hemorrhage[386]
Multiple sclerosis[234,283,599]
Hyperosmolar coma[466,708]
In association with systemic disease: viral hepatitis,[570] sarcoid,[584] AIDS[356,375]
Side effects of drugs: lithium,[145] amitriptyline,[40] cocaine,[217,592] phenytoin with diazepam,[168] phenelzine with imipramine[230]
Toxins: chlordecone,[670] thallium,[459] strychnine,[86] toluene,[428] and organophosphates[542]
As a complication of pregnancy[559]
As a transient phenomenon of normal infants[345,487]

*Not all case reports have documented the abnormality with eye movement recordings.

†As a component of the syndrome of myoclonic encephalopathy of infants ("dancing eyes and dancing feet").[213,401]

OPSOCLONUS AND OCULAR FLUTTER IN BRAINSTEM ENCEPHALITIS

Encephalitis with ocular oscillations and truncal ataxia may follow a prodrome of malaise and mild fever (see Video Display: Saccadic Oscillations and Intrusions).[67,80,140,634] Vertigo may be the presenting neurologic symptom. Such patients develop ocular flutter or opsoclonus and shivering movements of the head and body. Cerebellar and long-tract signs also occur, but the sensorium usually remains clear, apart from emotional liability. Spinal fluid protein and lymphocytic cell count may be elevated. The illness usually resolves in a few weeks or months, although sometimes the course is more protracted with relapses in older individuals.[67] Opsoclonus under closed eyelids is often the last manifestation to resolve. Intravenous immunoglobulin, corticosteroids, ACTH, azathioprine, or monoclonal antibodies directed against B-lymphocytes may hasten recovery.[67,531,537]

OPSOCLONUS AND OCULAR FLUTTER IN PATIENTS WITH CANCER

Opsoclonus occurs in association with cancer in both adults and children (see Video Display: Saccadic Oscillations and Intrusions). In children, about half of the cases are associated with tumors of neural crest origin, such as neuroblastoma.[669] In adults, opsoclonus occurs in association with small-cell lung, breast, or ovarian cancer.[67,69] The electroencephalogram is usually normal, but the cerebrospinal fluid (CSF) may show lymphocytic pleocytosis with or without elevated protein, and oligoclonal bands. Thus, CSF abnormalities may occur in opsoclonus associated with both tumor and encephalitis, and routine tests do not help to distinguish between the infectious and paraneoplastic etiologies. However, children with opsoclonus-myoclonus may show decreased CSF concentrations of 5-hydroxyindolacetic acid (5-HIAA) and homovanillic acid (HVA), and an increased percentage of B-lymphocytes.[535,538]

It is hypothesized that the syndrome is humorally mediated,[32a,532] and antibodies to diverse autoantigens have been reported, but most patients are seronegative.[69] The antineuronal antibodies associated with opsoclonus include anti-Ri, anti-Hu, anti-Yo, anti-Ma1, and anti-amphyphisin antibodies. By probing a complementary DNA library with sera from both paraneoplastic and idiopathic opsoclonus-myoclonus syndrome, it was possible to identify neuronal antigens, including proteins associated with nucleic acid, and post-synaptic density proteins (PSD) that are associated with N-methyl-D-aspartate (NMDA) receptors, and which may eventually provide an insight into the pathogenesis of opsoclonus.[69] However, at the present time, it is probably not worthwhile ordering commercial tests for anti bodies, since even the most consistent marker, anti-Ri is often negative in the serum in paraneoplastic opsoclonus (although it may be present in the CSF), and patients with this antibody may not develop opsoclonus.[69] Instead, body positron emission tomography is more likely to identify an underlying neoplasm. Therapeutic aspects of paraneoplastic opsoclonus in adults and children are discussed in the section Treatments for Nystagmus and Saccadic Oscillations.

OPSOCLONUS AND OCULAR FLUTTER DUE TO METABOLIC-TOXIC PROCESSES

Flutter and opsoclonus are reported secondary to intoxications with drugs (especially combinations of agents) and certain chemicals that are listed in Table 10–8. Agents with a variety of potential effects on neurotransmitters may have produced opsoclonus, including lithium, strychinine,[86] which may have affected the function of glycinergic omnipause neurons, and organophosphate poisoning, which may have had its effect on cholinergic inputs from the pedunculopontine nucleus to the fastigial nucleus.[449] Opsoclonus also occurs in hyperosmolar coma. One problem of many of these reports is that, without records of the ocular oscillations, there is some uncertainty as to whether the disorder was some saccadic oscillations other than flutter or opsoclonus.

OPSOCLONUS AND OCULAR FLUTTER WITHOUT APPARENT CAUSE

Some patients present with saccadic oscillations, especially microsaccadic flutter,[38,233] without apparent cause.[207,534] Their only complaint may be oscillopsia and degraded vision due to the abnormal eye movements. Such patients warrant a careful evaluation for an occult neoplasm, and long-term follow-up. It has been argued that some of the "idiopathic" cases arise as paraneoplastic but that the tumor subsequently undergoes spontaneous regression.[532,533]

Opsoclonus also occurs as a transient phenomenon in otherwise normal infants,[345] and in preterm infants;[487] if persistent diagnostic testing for cancer is warranted.

Voluntary Saccadic Oscillations or "Voluntary Nystagmus"

Some normal subjects possess or can develop the ability to voluntarily induce saccadic oscillations; this has been called voluntary or psychogenic flutter or voluntary nystagmus.[339] When such individuals generate these oscillations as a party trick, they commonly use a vergence effort to initiate them (see Video Display: Saccadic Oscillations and Intrusions). In fact, most normal subjects develop small, high-frequency, conjugate horizontal oscillations when they make a small saccade in combination with a large vergence movement (such as during shifts of fixation between far and near targets aligned on one eye—Fig. 8–3, Chapter 8).[549] Furthermore, recordings of saccades made in association with a blink show that some normal subjects show transient oscillations, such as dynamic overshoots.[292,574] Thus, the phenomenon of conjugate high-frequency oscillations is probably common in normal subjects, but has been overlooked.[548,549] Like ocular flutter, these oscillations have similar dynamic properties to voluntary saccades. Although usually confined to the horizontal plane, voluntary saccadic oscillations nystagmus can sometimes have horizontal, vertical and torsional components.[726] Such oscillations can be superimposed on smooth tracking eye movements,[137] and may be accompanied by a head tremor.[431] The oscillations can cause oscillopsia, due to excessive retinal image motion.

Voluntary nystagmus presents a diagnostic challenge when patients present with visual or ocular complaints due to these oscillations. Distinguishing features of psychogenic flutter are that it is usually not sustained, and is often accompanied by convergence effort, facial grimacing, or eyelid flutter. Pathologic flutter and opsoclonus are more sustained, irrespective of the patient's vergence state.

Pathogenesis of Saccadic Intrusions

PATHOGENESIS OF SACCADIC INTRUSIONS AND OSCILLATIONS WITH INTERSACCADIC INTERVALS

As discussed in Chapter 3, electrophysiological studies in monkey indicate that both the frontal eye field and the rostral pole of the superior colliculus are important for steady visual fixation.[108,495] Pharmacological inactivation at either site leads to disruption of fixation by saccadic intrusions, but does not induce flutter or opsoclonus.[201,495] Similarly, pharmacological inactivation of the inputs to the superior colliculus from the substantial nigra, pars reticulata (SNpr),[326] or of the mesencephalic reticular formation, which has reciprocal connections with the superior colliculus (see Box 6–9),[698] cause irrepressible saccadic intrusions, but not opsoclonus. A discrete infarction in the rostral pole of the superior colliculus of a monkey causes irrepressible saccades.[122] Bilateral inactivation of the caudal fastigial nucleus,[568] cerebellectomy,[520] and cerebellar hemisphere lesions,[703] may cause marked saccadic hypermetria with macrosaccadic oscillations, but flutter and opsoclonus are not reported. Thus, basic studies provide information pertinent to the pathogenesis of large saccadic oscillations, but not for opsoclonus and flutter.

In humans, macrosaccadic oscillations usually occur with cerebellar disease that affects the fastigial nucleus or its outflow; rarely they are reported with focal pontine lesion that could compromise inputs to premotor burst neurons from either omnipause neurons,[43] or the fastigial nucleus.[605] Macrosaccadic oscillations and large saccadic intrusions are not reported with midbrain or basal ganglionic lesions in humans. However, small square-wave jerks are reported to develop or increase following pallidotomy in parkinsonian patients (Fig. 10–15C) (see Video Display: Saccadic Oscillations and Intrusions).[50,512] In such patients, it was postulated that that interruption of the descending nigro-tectal inhibitory projections to the saccade-related cells in the superior colliculus could cause uncontrolled activation of the premotor burst neurons, thereby producing SWJ.[50] Square-wave jerks are also encountered in patients with disease affecting the cerebral hemispheres,[616] and brainstem, especially progressive supranuclear palsy, in which the mesencephalic reticular formation and superior colliculus are both involved.[248] Since square-wave jerks are also encountered in otherwise normal subjects, even at rates of up to 20 per minute, their pathological significance remains to be clarified.[7]

PATHOGENESIS OF OCULAR FLUTTER AND OPSOCLONUS

The pathogenesis of saccadic oscillations without an intersaccadic interval—opsoclonus and flutter—remains controversial since, as noted in the prior section no animal model exists. Traditionally, clinicians have attributed saccadic oscillations, including ocular flutter and opsoclonus, to cerebellar dysfunction.[142,218] However, most reports of flutter and opsoclonus lack reliable measurements of eye movements. Without such records, it is often difficult to determine whether saccadic oscillations are, or are not, separated by an intersaccadic interval. Those that are not probably have a different pathogenesis.

It is also possible that species differences account for the disparate effects of cerebellar inactivation or surgical lesions in monkey, which consist of saccadic hypermetria without flutter or opsoclonus,[520,568] compared with opsoclonus and saccadic dysmetria in humans.[622] Imaging studies have demonstrated activation of the cerebellum, including the fastigial nucleus, in patients with opsoclonus,[305,515] although this may simply reflect increased saccadic activity.

Another proposal to account for opsoclonus and flutter is that these oscillations are due to malfunction of the mechanism by which omnipause neurons control the onset of saccades.[739] However, experimental lesions of the omnipause neurons are reported to cause slowing of both horizontal and vertical saccades,[377,637] rather than saccadic oscillations,[739] although it remains possible that the neurotoxin injected into the pons also affected adjacent burst neurons. Ocular flutter has been reported as a transient phenomenon in a patient with multiple sclerosis and a plaque in the paramedian pons; after recovery from the relapse, the MRI finding had resolved.[599] However, in two patients with saccadic oscillations who came to autopsy, no histopathologic changes were evident in omnipause neurons.[563] Glycine has been identified as the neurotransmitter of omnipause neurons,[338] and poisoning with a glycinergic antagonist, strychnine, is reported to produce opsoclonus and myoclonus.[86] Thus, glycinergic dysfunction (presumably due to autoantibodies) might be responsible for the opsoclonus-myoclonus syndrome.[48]

Although it has been suggested that opsoclonus and flutter are due to delayed feedback control of saccades in patients with cerebellar disease affecting the fastigial nucleus,[717] patients with lesions of the fastigial nucleus lesions can still show conjugate high-frequency oscillations during saccade-vergence responses to the Muller paradigm.[548] Thus, an alternative model (Fig. 3–10) has been proposed in which saccadic oscillations arise because of the synaptic organization of premotor burst neurons, in which positive feedback loops and post-inhibitory rebound properties of burst neurons predispose to saccadic oscillations. Changes in the synaptic weighting of such circuits due to disease could produce oscillations whenever the omnipause neurons were inhibited, and also account for microflutter.[550] This hypothesis is outlined further in Chapter 3.

TREATMENTS FOR NYSTAGMUS AND SACCADIC INTRUSIONS

Rational Basis for Therapy of Abnormal Eye Movements

Before reviewing measures to treat abnormal eye movements that disrupt clear vision, recall the visual requirements of eye movements, which are restated here. Clear vision of an object requires that its image be held fairly steadily on the foveal region of the retina. The image of the object of regard should be within about 0.5 degrees of the center of the fovea, and, for objects with higher spatial frequencies (such as book text and Snellen optotypes), retinal image motion should be held below 5 degrees per second. A "special case" seems to be patients with congenital nystagmus, who may intermittently have images moving across the retina with speeds exceeding 100 degrees per second but seldom complain of oscillopsia.[13] It seems that this is mainly due to foveation periods — a brief epoch during each cycle of the nystagmus when the fovea is pointing at the object of interest and the eye is temporarily still (see Fig. 10–11).

A general point about treatment of abnormal eye movements is that measures that suppress all eye movements (or their effects on vision) may cause problems of their own. Thus, methods that null vergence movements will cause double vision, unless viewing is monocular. And methods that null vestibular eye will compromise vision when the subject is in motion. Therefore, treatments that attempt to quell just the oscillation, without affecting normal eye movements, are to be preferred. Strategies include drug treatments, measures to place the eye in a versional or vergence position in which nystagmus is minimized, optical devices that negate the visual consequences of the oscillations, procedures to weaken the extraocular muscles, and application of somatosensory or auditory stimuli to suppress nystagmus. These approaches are summarized in Table 10–9. Although many therapies have been suggested for abnormal eye movements, few have been properly evaluated with controlled clinical trials.[444,578,660]

Table 10–9. **Treatments for Nystagmus and Its Visual Consequences[444,578]**

Drugs

Gabapentin[51,59]
Memantine[652]
4-aminopyridine,[255,373] and 3,4-diaminopyridine[308,665]
Baclofen[51,206,297]
Clonazepam[157]
Valproate[434]
Trihexyphenidyl[66,311,438]
Benztropine[66]
Scopolamine[66,282]
Isoniazid[676]
Carbamazepine[226,582]
Barbiturates[503]
Alcohol[236]
Acetazolamide[54,286,663]
Cannabis[172,598]
Levetiracetam[157a]

Optical Devices

Prisms (base-in or base-out)[45,169,426]
Retinal image stabilization[580,721]

Special Procedures

Botulinum toxin[443,562,577,674]
Anderson–Kestenbaum procedure to shift null point[26,181,397,743]
Cüppers divergence procedure[155,607]
Recession of horizontal rectus muscles[309,695]
Disinsertion of extraocular muscles[668]
Tenotomy and resuture of the extraocular muscles[318]

Other Measures

Contact lenses[190]
Acupuncture[87,352]
Biofeedback[4,138,615]
Cutaneous head and neck stimulation[624]

(Related Video Display: Treatments for Nystagmus)

Pharmacological Treatments of Abnormal Eye Movements

Knowledge of the pathogenesis of a form of nystagmus may suggest the treatment.[437,444,648,650] The best example is the acquired form of periodic alternating nystagmus (Box 10–5), for which an animal model exists, pharmacological mechanisms have been established, and a drug treatment (baclofen) is usually effective.[249,297,440,696] Such knowledge is still lacking for most forms of nystagmus and saccadic intrusions, although some effective therapies have been established. Caution is required in interpreting reports based on single cases, especially when no reliable measurements have been made of changes in vision or of the ocular oscillations themselves. Most of our summary is derived from evaluations made with reliable measurements and, whenever possible, double-blind controlled trials.[660]

RATIONALE FOR DRUG TREATMENTS OF NYSTAGMUS

Basic pharmacological studies have provided insights concerning the pharmacological substrate for the brainstem elaboration of the VOR and the neural substrate for gaze holding (the neural integrator). Primary vestibular afferents in the eighth cranial nerve, which synapse in the vestibular nuclei, use glutamate as a transmitter.[473] Secondary excitatory projections from the vestibular nuclei to ocular motoneurons employ glutamate and aspartate as transmitters. Secondary inhibitory projections from the vestibular nuclei to the vertical ocular motoneurons employ GABA, whereas those to horizontal motoneurons are glycinergic.[473,643]

The elementary vestibulo-ocular reflex is governed by a number of mechanisms to optimize its performance, including the velocity storage mechanism, which prolongs the peripheral vestibular signal (discussed in Chapter 2). This enhancement of inputs from primary vestibular afferents is achieved by a vestibular commissure, and is controlled by the cerebellar nodulus and uvula.[144] The metabotropic $GABA_B$ receptor, which is a mediator of slow inhibitory postsynaptic potentials, is important in regulating velocity storage. Thus, the velocity-storage phenomenon in normal monkeys is suppressed by the $GABA_B$ agonist baclofen.[144] Furthermore, the cerebellar flocculus seems important in regulating the vertical vestibulo-ocular reflex, probably mediated through GABA. Experimental lesions of the flocculus and paraflocculus cause downbeat nystagmus.[740]

The nucleus prepositus and adjacent medial vestibular nucleus (the NPH-MVN region) play an important role in the gaze-holding network (the neural integrator), which makes it possible to hold the eyes steadily in eccentric gaze.[33] There is evidence that glutamatergic projections from the paramedian pontine reticular formation (PPRF) to NPH, which presumably convey the saccadic pulse signal, which must be integrated into a step, act on AMPA-kainate receptors.[504] Some vestibular inputs to NPH are GABAergic, facilitated by nitric oxide.[488] The projections of NPH (the output of the neural integrator) to the abducens nucleus are cholinergic.[473,642]

Within the NPH-MVN region, several neurotransmitters contribute to the neural integration of eye movements. Thus, pharmacological inactivation of NPH-MVN in monkey by injection of GABA agonist or antagonists, glutamate NMDA antagonist, or kainate antagonist disabled the neural integrator, causing the eyes to drift back to center after a horizontal saccade had taken the eyes to an eccentric position (Fig. 5–5).[34,121,479,659] Occasionally, however, injection of either the $GABA_A$ agonist muscimol or the non-specific GABA antagonist bicuculline into MVN caused the eyes to drift *away* from center position, with increasing velocity, indicating that the neural integrator had become unstable.[34,659] Glycine appears to have no role in the neural integrator.[34] Taken together, these results pose questions: How could agonists and antagonists of GABA and glutamate both cause a leaky integrator? And how could muscimol or bicuculline usually cause the integrator to become leaky, but sometimes cause it to become unstable?

As discussed in Chapter 5, the neural integrator depends on a distributed network of neurons. Pharmacological agents that prevent the constituent neurons of this network from modulating their discharge in response to inputs from other neurons would cause the integrator to become *leaky*. This effect would be predicted both for agents that hyperpolarize cells, thereby silencing their discharge, and agents that depolarize cells, causing their discharge rate to saturate.

To account for how these agents could cause the neural integrator to become *unstable* it is postulated that the constituent neurons remain functional, but that the feedback control of them by the cerebellum is disrupted.[374,738] Thus, injection of GABA agonists or antagonists into that part of the MVN that receives inputs from floccular GABAergic Purkinje cells may block cerebellar control of the neural integrator, leading to instability.[34] Such a suggestion is consistent with reports of patients who show nystagmus with increasing velocity waveforms; such individuals have cerebellar disorders.[65,738] Finally, the interstitial nucleus of Cajal (INC) is an important contributor to eccentric gaze-holding ability in the vertical plane. It is possible to inactivate INC and cause neural integrator failure with muscimol, implying that GABA also contributes to vertical gaze holding.[306]

To this body of basic research must be added the clinical observations that upbeat nystagmus may be induced in darkness in normal subjects by nicotine, and that the 3-D characteristics of this nystagmus imply that it is vestibular in origin.[399,526,628]

Treatment of Peripheral Vestibular Forms of Nystagmus

Most nystagmus due to peripheral vestibular imbalance resolves over the course of a few days, and drug treatments are only helpful during the acute phase of the illness. The management of acute vertigo is summarized in Chapter 11.

Treatment of Downbeat and Upbeat Nystagmus

One hypothesis for downbeat nystagmus is that it arises because of loss of inhibitory control of projections of the anterior semicircular canals by the cerebellar flocculus, thereby leading to upward drifts (Fig. 10–2). Most floccular Purkinje neurons discharge for downward eye movements.[463] Since inhibition of the vestibular nuclei by floccular Purkinje cells is mediated by GABA, then giving a drug with GABAergic effects might be expected to restore normal cerebellar governance and stop the upward drifts.

The $GABA_A$ agonist clonazepam is reported to reduce downbeat nystagmus with a variety of etiologies and the idiopathic variety;[157,732] a single dose of 1 to 2mg of clonazepam may be used to determine whether long-term therapy is feasible. The $GABA_B$ agonist baclofen has been reported to reduce upbeat or downbeat nystagmus velocity and associated oscillopsia.[206,381] However, a double-blind comparison of baclofen and gabapentin (which is discussed below) showed neither drug to produce consistent improvement. In some patients, the nystagmus was made worse.[51]

The effects of cholinergic agents on vertical forms of nystagmus have also been evaluated. On the one hand, the cholinergic drug physostigmine (an acetylcholine-esterase inhibitor), given intravenously, causes worsening of downbeat nystagmus.[206] On the other hand, intravenous scopolamine reduces downbeat nystagmus,[66] but with unacceptable side effects. Oral anticholinergic agents, such as trihexyphenidyl,[438] produce only modest improvement, and are poorly tolerated.

Recently, the potassium channel blockers, 3,4-diaminopyridine and 4-aminopyridine have been shown to suppress downbeat nystagmus in some patients (see Video Display: Treatments for Nystagmus).[373,665] How could they be working? Potassium channels are abundant on cerebellar Purkinje cells, and 4-aminopyridine experimentally increases their discharge by affecting several potassium currents. Then, enhanced Purkinje cell activity could restore normal levels of inhibition of vertical vestibular eye movements (Fig. 10–2). However, 4-aminopyridine also suppresses upbeat nystagmus in some patients,[255] and may occasionally cause downbeat nystagmus to switch to upbeat.[308] It has been proposed that 4-aminopyridine affects upbeat nystagmus mainly through improved visual fixation, whereas the effects on downbeat are mainly vestibular in nature,[256] but more studies are needed to confirm this hypothesis. An alternative hypothesis is that 4-aminopyridine mainly has its effects on otolithic mechanisms that influence vertical nystagmus.[308] Whatever the mechanism, a substantial number of patients are likely to benefit from treatment with 4-aminopyridine, which is generally better tolerated than 3, 4-diaminopyridine, but occasionally causes epileptic seizures.[295,436]

Treatment of Periodic Alternating Nystagmus

This is the best example of a form of nystagmus for which the drug treatment is based on known pathophysiology and pharmacology. Most patients reported respond to the $GABA_B$ agonist baclofen.[240,249,297] Congenital periodic alternating nystagmus, which probably has a different pathogenesis, only occasionally responds to baclofen.[274,640]

Treatment of Acquired Pendular Nystagmus

Acquired pendular nystagmus occurs in association with a variety of disorders affecting central myelin, notably multiple sclerosis; as part of the syndrome of oculopalatal tremor; and in Whipple's disease as a component of oculomasticatory myorhythmia. As discussed in prior sections, each form of acquired pendular nystagmus likely has a separate pathogenesis, requiring different treatment strategies. Acquired pendular nystagmus is one of the most visually disabling forms of nystagmus (see Video Display: Treatments for Nystagmus).

Treatment of Acquired Pendular Nystagmus Associated with Multiple Sclerosis

Drawing on basic research,[33] clinical studies,[52] and neuroimaging data,[454] it was postulated that acquired pendular nystagmus in multiple sclerosis was due to an instability arising in the gaze-holding mechanism (the neural integrator for eye movements—Chapter 5).[162] Evidence implicating both GABA and glutamate in the NPH-MVN,[34,659] which is an important component of the neural integrator, led to clinical trials of drugs thought to have effects on receptors for either of these neurotransmitters.

Early studies that employed drugs with GABAergic properties, such as clonazepam, valproate, and isoniazid, helped some patients.[434,676] After gabapentin, an anticonvulsant with presumed GABAergic action, was introduced, a multicenter double-blind study was conducted comparing it to baclofen, a $GABA_B$

agonist, as therapy for acquired nystagmus.[51] In a group of 15 patients with acquired pendular nystagmus, visual acuity improved significantly with gabapentin, but not with baclofen (see Video Display: Treatments for Nystagmus) (Fig. 10–10). Gabapentin significantly reduced median eye speed in all three planes, but baclofen did so only in the vertical plane. In 10 of the patients with acquired pendular nystagmus, the reduction of nystagmus with gabapentin was substantial, and 8 of these elected to continue taking the drug. However, some patients in that study showed no response to either drug. Furthermore, a significant side effect of gabapentin was increased ataxia in some patients. A subsequent trial compared gabapentin with another anticonvulsant, vigabitrin, and confirmed that gabapentin is an effective treatment for many patients with acquired pendular nystagmus.[59] However, vigabitrin, which is much more purely GABAergic than gabapentin, was ineffective, suggesting that gabapentin suppressed acquired pendular nystagmus by a mechanism other than GABA. Indeed, the mechanism of action of gabapentin is currently not well understood.[107]

An agent with effects on glutamate receptors, memantine, has also been reported to suppress acquired pendular nystagmus in patients with multiple sclerosis.[652] Memantine is a low-to-moderate uncompetitive (open channel) N-methyl-D-aspartate (NMDA) receptor antagonist. It also shows some antagonistic effects at 5HT and nicotinic acetylcholine receptors. It has low-to-negligible affinity for GABA, benzodiazepine, dopamine, adrenergic, histamine, or glycine receptors, and for calcium, sodium, or potassium channels.[569] Memantine has been used for over 20 years in Germany for treatment of a variety of neurological symptoms. More recently, it has received approval from the United States Food and Drug Administration for treatment of advanced Alzheimer's disease. It appears to be generally well tolerated, even at doses of 40 mg per day, which was found to be optimal for suppressing nystagmus, but which is twice the dose recommended for treatment of dementia (see Video Display: Treatments for Nystagmus). Further double-blind evaluations may establish the relative roles of gabapentin and memantine.

In patients who are resistant to both memantine and gabapentin, or cannot tolerate side effects of these drugs, a number of other measures can be tried, although these are based on individual case reports and have not been subjected to controlled trials (see Table 10–9). Optical treatments are another option that is discussed below.

Treatment of the Nystagmus of Oculopalatal Tremor

Some patients with this syndrome following stroke show partial suppression of their nystagmus with gabapentin (see Video Display: Treatments for Nystagmus),[51] and we have observed some improvement with memantine. However, neither drug noticeably suppresses the palatal tremor, although it is usually asymptomatic. In general, the nystagmus of oculopalatal tremor is more refractory to both gabapentin and memantine than the acquired pendular nystagmus with multiple sclerosis.

The hypertrophied inferior olivary nucleus of patients with oculopalatal myoclonus shows increased acetylcholine esterase activity.[405] This finding suggesting cholinergic denervation supersensitivity prompted trials of anticholinergic agents; individual patients may be helped by trihexyphenidyl.[311,355] However, the role of anticholinergic drugs in the treatment of either oculopatal tremor or other forms of acquired pendular nystagmus is not established. Thus, a double-blind crossover trial of trihexyphenidyl and tridihexethyl chloride (a quaternary anticholinergic that does not cross the blood-brain barrier) showed only modest changes that were greater with tridihexethyl chloride.[438] Moreover, no patient in this trial wished to continue with either drug because of anticholinergic side effects. A double-blind comparison of intravenously administered scopolamine, benztropine, and glycopyrrolate (a quaternary agent devoid of central nervous system activity) confirmed an earlier uncontrolled study: a single dose of scopolamine effectively reduces nystagmus and improves vision, whereas benztropine was less effective, and glycopyrrolate had no significant effect.[66] The discrepancy between this study and that of oral trihexyphenidyl might be due to the more selective antagonism of trihexyphenidyl versus scopolamine on muscarinic receptors.[112] Scopolamine by transdermal route is not a reliable therapy for pendular nystagmus and can actually make the nystagmus worse or induce side effects such as confusion in some patients.[398] Future therapies for oculopalatal tremor may capitalize on the unusual electrophysiology of the inferior olive, which depends on electrotonic coupling.[147,200,439] Occasional patients show responses to the other drugs listed in Table 10–9. Optical therapies can also be considered in patients who respond to no drug therapy.

Treatment of Other Forms of Nystagmus

Seesaw nystagmus has been reported to be improved by alcohol,[236,447] and clonazepam.[139] We have observed some improvement in individual patients to gabapentin or memantine.

Familial episodic vertigo and ataxia type 2 (EA-2) with nystagmus usually responds to treatment with acetazolamide,[54,286] The potassium channel blocker, 4-aminopyridine also is effected treatment for EA-2 in some patients.[663] In addition some patients with spinocerebellar atrophy type 6 who suffer episodic attacks of vertigo and nystagmus also benefit from acetazolamide,[369] and 4-aminopyridine is currently being evaluated as treatment for this disorder (M. Strupp, personal communication). Animal models for these disorders, which are channelopathies, are likely to produce a firmer rationale for therapy.[647] Only a few patients with congenital nystagmus have been reported to gain improvement from treatment with drugs.[322,323,640]

Development of gene therapy holds the potential for treatment of forms of nystagmus due to retinal disorders. Thus, in an animal model of Leber's congenital amaurosis, successful gene therapy restored vision, and nystagmus resolved.[19,502]

Treatment of Saccadic Intrusions and Oscillations

RATIONALE FOR DRUG TREATMENTS OF SACCADIC DISORDERS

The excitatory premotor burst neurons that project the pulse of innervation to ocular motoneurons innervating the agonist extraocular muscles utilize glutamate and aspartate. The inhibitory premotor burst neurons that project to motoneurons innervating the antagonist extraocular muscles probably utilize either glycine (for horizontal saccades) or GABA (for vertical saccades). The omnipause neurons that inhibit all premotor burst neurons, except during saccades, utilize glycine. The omnipause neurons receive inhibitory inputs from a number of sites including the rostral pole (fixation zone) of the superior colliculus, the central mesencephalic reticular formation, and cortical eye fields; the transmitters involved in these projections are not yet fully worked out. The excitatory premotor burst neurons receive inputs from long-lead burst neurons that, in turn, are activated by more caudal parts of the superior colliculus. Both inhibitory and excitatory burst neurons receive inputs from the fastigial nucleus. Thus, the further one precedes in a bottom-up process from the ocular motoneurons, the less is known about the influence of each neurotransmitter system, and the more complex interactions become.

Some extra insights can be gained by considering the effects of pharmacological inactivation of the superior colliculus and the fastigial nucleus. As reviewed in Chapter 3, inactivation of more caudal parts of the superior colliculus, using the $GABA_A$ agonist muscimol, resulted in a paucity of saccades.[495] On the other hand, inactivation of the rostral pole of the superior colliculus ("fixation zone") causes an excess of inappropriate saccades.[495] Similar effects are obtained by inactivating the central mesencephalic retinal formation with muscimol.[698] Unilateral inactivation of the fastigial nucleus with muscimol causes hypermetria of ipsilateral saccades and hypometria of contralateral saccades (ipsipulsion).[568] Thus, it has been possible to identify several potential mechanisms that could cause saccadic intrusions, but more research is needed to identify which pharmacological agents could restore normal control.

Drug Treatments of Saccadic Intrusions, Hypermetria, and Macrosaccadic Oscillations

Although saccadic intrusions take the eye away from the visual target, they generally do not cause oscillopsia, with the exception of the nearly continuous oscillations of ocular flutter and opsoclonus. As reviewed in Chapter 3, this is partly due to the phenomena of saccadic suppression and visual masking that occurs with each saccade and maintains a clear, steady percept of the world despite high-speed shifts of the visual fixation point. Thus, in general, saccadic abnormalities cause much less visual distress than does nystagmus. However, patients with saccadic hypermetria and macrosaccadic oscillations often complain of difficulty reading, especially when they make a saccade to the beginning of a new line, and tend to lose their place (Fig. 3–8, Chapter 3). Patients with opsoclonus often complain of vertigo, oscillopsia, and blurring of their visual world, which can be distressing.

Individual saccadic intrusions, such as square-wave jerks are seldom symptomatic and generally do not require treatment, although amphetamines have been reported to reduce them in one preliminary study.[156] When saccadic hypermetria is marked, with macrosaccadic oscillations, as in patients with deep cerebellar lesions, then attempts have been made to reduce saccadic gain. Diazepam, clonazepam, and barbiturates were effective in abolishing high-amplitude square-wave jerks and macrosaccadic oscillations in one patient.[686] Attempts to suppress the macrosaccadic oscillations of a patient with a discrete pontine lesion (Fig. 10–15B) with gabapentin produced only a modest reduction.[45] We have recently noted some decrease in saccadic gain in a patient with a form of spinocerebellar ataxia with saccadic intrusions,[666] in response to memantine. After treatment, he reported less difficulty reading because he no longer lost his place when he looked towards the beginning of a new line (Fig. 3–8B).

Treatments for Ocular Flutter and Opsoclonus

Therapy of these saccadic oscillations falls under two categories: symptomatic and treatment of the underlying disorder. There are no reported trials of symptomatic therapy, but propranolol, verapamil, clonazepam, gabapentin and thiamine have been reported to suppress saccadic oscillations in individual patients.[38,489,532–534] Current models of saccadic oscillations invoke instability of membrane properties of premotor burst neurons,[548] and it seems possible that membrane-stabilizing drugs may find a therapeutic role for flutter and opsoclonus in the future.

For patients with either the syndrome of brainstem encephalitis and opsoclonus, or the idiopathic variety, intravenous immunoglobulin (IVIG), or other immunotherapy may hasten recovery.[67,531] Younger patients are more likely to make a good recovery.

In adults who have opsoclonus associated with cancer, treatment of the tumor itself may cause the neurologic syndrome to improve or resolve, but some patients continue to be neurologically disabled.[67] Thus, the course may or may not improve following tumor therapy, and sometimes waxes and wanes, and occasionally spontaneously resolves in patients with untreated tumor.[239,532] Plasmapheresis and intravenous immunoglobulins (IVIG) have occasionally proved effective.[32a] Immunoadsorption therapy (plasma exchange through a protein A column that binds immune complexes and the Fc portion of IgG molecules) may be effective in abolition of both opsoclonus and myoclonus.[127,220,507] Gabapentin has been reported to suppress opsoclonus in one patient who had an ovarian cancer.[489]

In children with neural crest tumors, opsoclonus often responds to corticosteroids,[406] and sometimes to intravenous immunoglobulin.[231] New therapies with monoclonal antibodies directed against B-lymphocytes may prove effective.[537] Up to 50% of children are left with long-term neurologic disabilities such as ataxia, poor speech, and cognitive problems,[533,534,669] sometimes with recurrent neurological episodes over decades.[536] Similar responses to steroids occur in children with parainfectious or idiopathic opsoclonus.[534] Whether ACTH is superior to corticosteroid has not been systematically studied, although ACTH remains favored and is clearly more effective in some patients.

Optical Treatments of Abnormal Eye Movements

Spectacle correction of refractive errors is worthwhile in most patients with congenital or acquired forms of nystagmus, and may produce appreciable improvement in vision.[25,315] Those patients whose nystagmus decreases during convergence may benefit from wearing spectacle prisms that require convergence for single vision of far targets. An effective arrangement is a pair of 7.00 diopter base-out prisms, with -1.00 diopter spheres added to compensate for the accommodation that accompanies the induced convergence.[169] The spherical correction may not be needed in presbyopic individuals. Especially in some individuals with congenital nystagmus, the improvement of vision due to nystagmus suppression when wearing base-out prisms may be sufficient for them to qualify for a driving license. Some patients with acquired nystagmus may benefit from such prisms.[426] Occasional patients whose nystagmus is worse during near viewing are helped by base-in prisms (Fig. 10–16A).[45]

Theoretically, it should be possible to use prisms to help patients whose nystagmus is quieter when the eyes are moved into a particular position in the orbit (the null point or zone). For patients with congenital nystagmus, there is usually some horizontal eye position in which nystagmus is minimized, and the eyes of patients with downbeat nystagmus may be quieter in upgaze. In practice, however, patients use head-turns to bring their eyes to the quietest position, and only rarely do patients benefit from prisms that produce a conjugate gaze shift.

A different approach has been the development of optical device to negates the visual effects of eye movements. One system consists of a high-plus spectacle lens worn in combina-

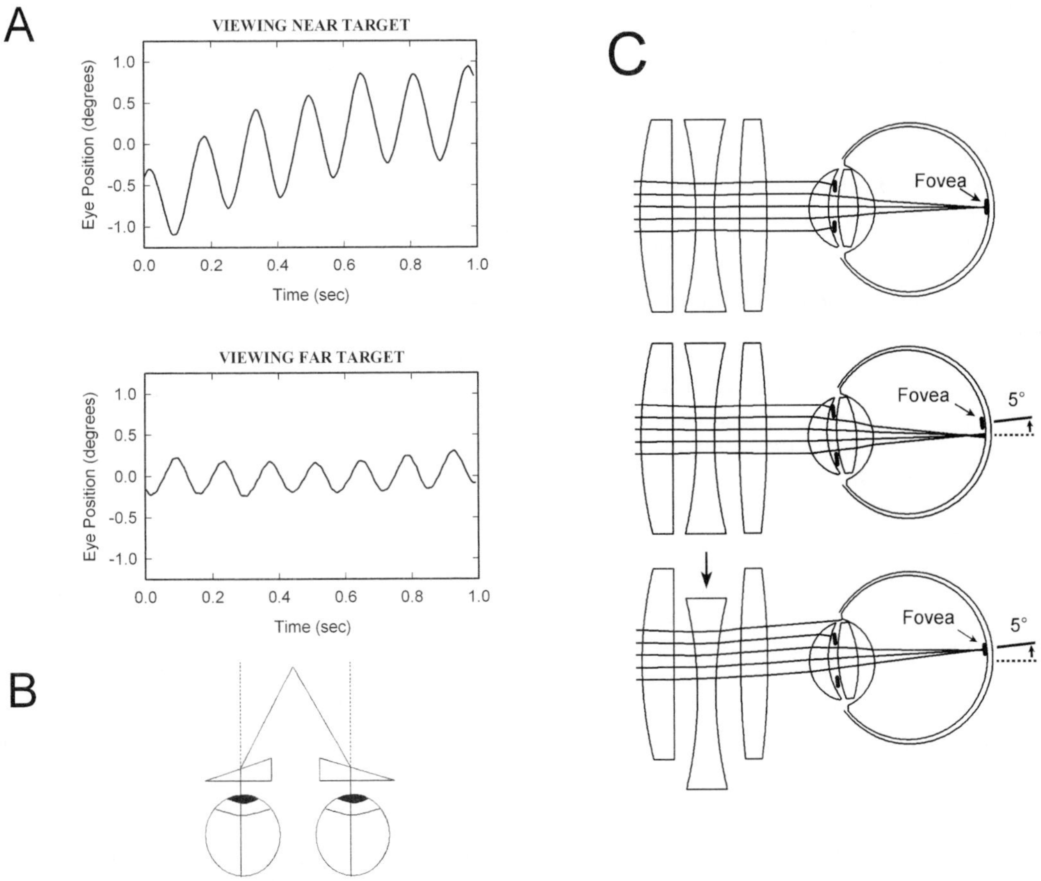

Figure 10–16. Optical treatments for the visual consequences of nystagmus. (A) Acquired pendular nystagmus in a 44-year-old woman with multiple sclerosis that increased during near viewing, making reading difficult. Horizontal records are shown, positive deflections indicating rightward rotations. (B) Vision was improved by wearing base-in prisms, so that the eyes were no longer convergenced during near viewing. (C) Demonstration of how a 3-lens image-shifting device can null the visual effects of ocular oscillations. Starting with the eyes and optics in a neutral position (top), light from a distant target is brought to the fovea of the retina. If the eye is rotated down (middle), the image is displaced from the fovea. However, if the central lens is moved downward by the appropriate amount (bottom), the image is once again brought onto the fovea. (Reproduced, with permission from Smith RM, Oommen BS, Stahl JS. Image-shifting optics for a nystagmus treatment device. J Rehabil Res Dev 41, 325–336, 2004.)

tion with a high-minus contact lens.[580] The system is based on the principle that stabilization of images on the retina could be achieved if the power of the spectacle lens focused the primary image close to the center of rotation of the eye. However, such images are defocused, and a contact lens is required to extend back the focus onto the retina. Since the contact lens moves with the eye, it does not negate the effect of retinal image stabilization produced by the spectacle lens. With such a system it is possible to negate about 90% of the visual effects of eye movements.[441] The system has several limitations, however. One is that it disables all eye movements (including the vestibulo-ocular reflex and vergence), so that it is only useful while the patient is stationary and viewing monocularly. Another is that with the highest-power components (contact lens of -58.00 diopters and spectacle lens of +32 diopters), the field of view is limited. Some patients with ataxia or tremor (such as those with multiple sclerosis) have difficulty inserting the contact lens. However, initial problems posed by rigid polymethyl methacrylate contact lenses have been overcome by development of gas-permeable or even soft contact lenses.[721,722] Most patients do not need the highest power components for oscillopsia to be abolished and vision to be useful. In selected patients, the device may prove useful for limited periods of time, such as the duration of a television program.

A more recent hi-tech approach is an electro-optical device that measures ocular oscillations and moves prism devices to negate the effects of the nystagmus.[649] This approach is best suited for pendular nystagmus, which can be electronically distinguished from normal eye movements, such as voluntary saccades, that are required for clear vision (see Video Display: Treatments for Nystagmus). Figure 10–16B summarizes the image-shifting optics that are being used to develop a portable, battery-driven device.[635,636]

The effects of such optical systems should be differentiated from that of simply wearing contact lenses, which appear to suppress congenital nystagmus in some subjects,[190] but in others may simply be due to better refractive correction.[83] The main therapy for latent nystagmus consists of measures to improve vision, especially patching for amblyopia in children.[693]

Procedures to Weaken the Extraocular Muscles

BOTULINUM TOXIN AS TREATMENT OF NYSTAGMUS

Injection of botulinum toxin into either the extraocular muscles or retrobulbar space has been used to temporarily reduce or abolish acquired nystagmus (Fig. 10–17).[153,310] Several studies have reported that some patients gain improved, more stable vision.[443,562,577,674] Less often, botulinum toxin has been used to treat congenital or latent nystagmus.[125,451] Common side effects are ptosis and diplopia, which may be more troublesome than the visual consequences of the nystagmus. Rarer complications include filamentary keratitis.[674]

A major limitation of botulinum toxin treatment for nystagmus is that it also impairs normal eye movements, static eye position being affected longer than the effect on saccades,[18,348] which become hypometric (Fig. 10–17). Impairment of the vestibulo-ocular reflex causes patients to complain of blurred vision, oscillopsia, or vertigo when they walk. Another effect occurs in patients who habitually view with the injected, paretic eye. After several days, adaptive changes may take place (i.e., increased innervation to compensate for extraocular muscle weakness). Thus, for example, saccadic adaptation is apparent in the non-injected eye as hypermetric saccades (Fig. 10–17). In addition, the nystagmus itself may increase in the non-injected eye.

In summary, botulinum toxin may abolish nystagmus and improve vision in some patients, and may be acceptable to patients who are prepared to view monocularly, but its limited period of action and side effects reduce its therapeutic value.

SURGICAL PROCEDURES FOR NYSTAGMUS

Four surgical procedures on extraocular muscles have been proposed as treatment for selected patients with INF; none have been properly evaluated for acquired nystagmus. One procedure for congenital nystagmus is the Anderson–Kestenbaum operation,[26,397] which aims to move the attachments of the extraocular muscles so that the null point corresponds to the eyes' new central position. It is best

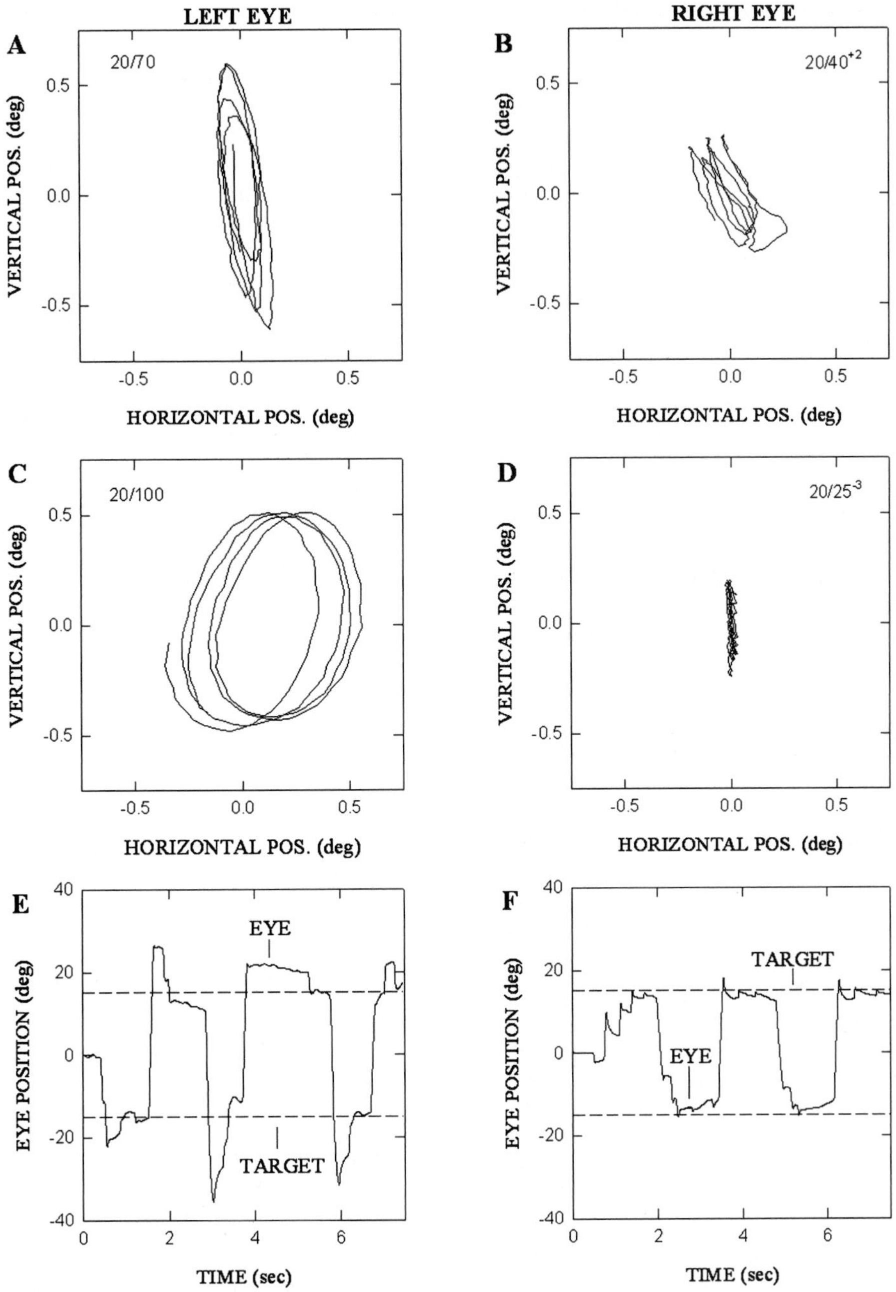

Figure 10–17. Effects of botulinum toxin injected into selected extraocular muscles (A–F) on acquired nystagmus.[443] The records in panels A–F are from a 27-year-old woman with multiple sclerosis. Panels A (left eye) and B (right eye) display representative 1-second records of her nystagmus as "scan paths" prior to injection of botulinum toxin. Panels C and D display characteristics of her nystagmus, 1 week after injection of the right medial rectus and 2 weeks after injection of the right lateral rectus muscle. The horizontal component of nystagmus in the right eye was almost abolished, and visual acuity increased from $20/40^{+2}$ to $20/25^{-3}$ in this eye. The amplitude of the horizontal component of nystagmus in the left, non-injected eye had increased, however, and visual acuity declined from 20/70 to 20/100. Panels E and F show horizontal saccades recorded at the same session as C and D; positive values indicated rightward movements. When the patient viewed with her right eye (F), saccades were generally hypometric with pulse-step mismatches and post-saccadic drifts; some gaze-evoked nystagmus was also present. When she viewed with her left eye (E), there was pronounced saccadic hypermetria, reflecting adaptive changes made in response to viewing habitually with her paretic left eye (which had better vision) over the prior 2 weeks.

planned by measuring visual acuity under different viewing conditions,[645] and the nystagmus at different gaze angles so that the surgeon can calculate what is required to shift the position of the null point.[181,743] In practice, the Anderson-Kestenbaum procedure not only shifts and broadens the null zone, but also decreases nystagmus outside of the null zone, and may improve head posture.[430] However, it is of uncertain value in the treatment of acquired forms of nystagmus.

The second procedure aims to diverge the eyes.[155,607] It may be helpful in patients with congenital nystagmus that suppresses during fixation of near targets, and who have stereopsis. Studies comparing these two methods indicate that either the divergence procedure or combined operations give better visual improvement than the Anderson-Kestenbaum procedure alone.[383,607,743]

A third surgical approach for congenital nystagmus consists of large recession of the horizontal rectus muscles,[22,39,222,274,309,695] sometimes in combination with other procedures.[35] Suppression of nystagmus, improvement of vision and head posture is reported. Nonetheless, a controlled clinical study with evaluation of the changes of nystagmus waveforms by investigators who are unaware of the source of each record is required to establish firmly the role of this procedure. Furthermore, it seems important to determine the frequency with which weakening the extraocular muscles will induce adaptive changes that will cause the nystagmus to increase again. The role of these procedures in the treatment of acquired forms of nystagmus also needs to be established by control trials.[126]

The mechanisms by which any of these operations may damp congenital nystagmus has been re-evaluated by L. F. Dell'Osso, who suggested that simply detaching the muscles, dissecting the perimuscular fascia and then reattaching them at the same site on the globe may suppress congenital nystagmus.[173] Experimental studies in a canine model for congenital nystagmus support this hypothesis,[183] and histological evidence has been presented that the tendo-scleral junction shows certain differences in patients with congenital nystagmus.[316] Preliminary clinical trials indicate that some patients do show improvement on some measures of visual function following horizontal rectus tenotomy,[318,319] but more studies are needed to confirm this effect.[485,486] Recent anatomical studies indicate that insertions of the medial and lateral rectus contain muscle tissue connecting directly with the sclera.[363] Thus, such a procedure might have its effects by altering proprioceptive input from the palisade organs that lie close to the myotendinous junction of the extraocular muscles (see Extraocular Proprioception in Chapter 9).[117] This mechanisms is consistent with the hypothesis that some forms of congenital nystagmus may be due to disturbed proprioceptive control of eye movements.[521]

Extraocular muscle surgery has been tried as treatment of acquired nystagmus, either alone or in combination with drug therapy,[364] and sometimes with success. Formal clinical trials are needed to determine whether orbital surgery has any substantial role in the treatment of acquired nystagmus.

There is a consensus that neurosurgery does have a role in the therapy of the nystagmus associated with the Arnold–Chiari syndrome. Suboccipital decompression has been reported to improve downbeat nystagmus and prevent progression of other neurologic deficits.[208,525,646] Surgical treatment of superior oblique myokymia is discussed in Chapter 9.

Application of Somatosensory or Auditory Stimuli to Suppress Nystagmus

Following up on the finding that wearing contact lenses may suppress congenital nystagmus,[190] it was documented that electrical stimulation or vibration over the forehead may suppress the oscillations in some patients.[624] These effects may be exerted via the trigeminal system, which receives extraocular proprioception (discussed in Chapter 9). Acupuncture administered to the neck muscles may suppress congenital nystagmus in some patients, by a similar mechanism.[87,352] Biofeedback has also been reported to help some patients with this condition,[4,138] but without sustained effects.[615] Indeed, the role of any of these treatments outside the laboratory has yet to be demonstrated, and controlled trials are needed to evaluate these and other measures reported to improve congenital nystagmus.

REFERENCES

1. Classification of Eye Movement Abnormalities and Strabismus (CEMAS) Working Group. http://www.nei.nih.gov/news/statements/cemas 2003.
2. Abadi RV, Bjerre A. Motor and sensory characteristics of infantile nystagmus. Br J Ophthalmol 86, 1152–1160, 2002.
3. Abadi RV, Broomhead DS, Clement RA, Whittle JP, Worfolk R. Dynamical systems analysis: a new method of analysing congenital nystagmus waveforms. Exp Brain Res 117, 355–361, 1997.
4. Abadi RV, Carden D, Simpson J. A new treatment for congenital nystagmus. Br J Ophthalmol 64, 2–6, 1980.
5. Abadi RV, Dickinson CM. Waveform characteristics in congenital nystagmus. Documenta Ophthalmologica 64, 153–167, 1986.
6. Abadi RV, Dickinson CM, Lomas MS, Ackerley R Congenital idiopathic nystagmus in identical twins. Br J Ophthalmol 67, 693–695, 1983.

6a. Abadi RV, Forster JE, Lloyd IC. Ocular motor outcomes after bilateral and unilateral infantile cataracts. Vision Res, in press, 2005.

7. Abadi RV, Gowen E. Characteristics of saccadic intrusions. Vision Res 44, 2675–2690, 2004.
8. Abadi RV, Pascal E. Ocular motor behavior of monozygotic twins with tyrosinase negative oculocutaneous albinism. Br J Ophthalmol 78, 349–352, 1994.
9. Abadi RV, Pascal E. Periodic alternating nystagmus in humans with albinism. Invest Ophthalmol Vis Sci 35, 4080–4086, 1994.
10. Abadi RV, Scallan CJ. Waveform characteristics of manifest latent nystagmus. Invest Ophthalmol Vis Sci 41, 3805–3817, 2000.
11. Abadi RV, Scallan CJ. Ocular oscillations on eccentric gaze. Vision Res 41, 2895–2907, 2001.
12. Abadi RV, Scallan CJ, Clement RA. The characteristics of dynamic overshoots in square-wave jerks and in congenital and manifest latent nystagmus. Vision Res 40, 2813–2829, 2000.
13. Abadi RV, Whittle JP, Worfolk R. Oscillopsia and tolerance to retinal image movement in congenital nystagmus. Invest Ophthalmol Vis Sci 40, 339–345, 1999.
14. Abel LA, Parker L, Daroff RB, Dell'Osso LF. Endpoint nystagmus. Invest Ophthalmol Vis Sci 17, 539–544, 1978.
15. Abel LA, Traccis S, Dell'Osso LF, Ansevin CF. Variable waveforms in downbeat nystagmus imply short-term gain changes. Ann Neurol 13, 616–620, 1983.
16. Abel LA, Traccis S, Dell'Osso LF, Daroff RB, Troost BT. Square wave oscillation: the relationship of saccadic intrusions and oscillations. Neuroophthalmology 4, 21–25, 1984.
17. Abrusow V, Strupp M, Brandt T. Amiodarone-induced severe prolonged head-positional vertigo and vomiting. Neurology 51, 917, 1998.
18. Acheson JF, Bentley CR, Shallo-Hoffmann J, Gresty MA. Dissociated effects of botulinum toxin chemodenervation on ocular deviation and saccade dynamics in chronic lateral rectus palsy. Br J Ophthalmol 82, 67–71, 1998.
19. Acland G, Aguirre GD, Ray J, et al. Gene therapy restores vision in a canine model of childhood blindness. Nature Genet 28, 92–95, 2001.
20. Aggarwal A, Williams D. Opsoclonus as a paraneoplastic manifestation of pancreatic carcinoma. J Neurol Neurosurg Psychiatry 63, 687–688, 1997.

20a. Akman OE, Broomhead DS, Abadi RV, Clement RA. Eye movement instabilities and nystagmus can be predicted by a nonlinear dynamics model of the saccadic system. J Math Biol 51, 661–694, 2005.

21. Alexander G. Die Ohrenkrankheiten im Kindesalter. In Pfaundler M, Schlossman A (eds). Handbuch der Kinderheilkunde. Vogel, Leipzig, 1919, pp 84–96.
22. Alio JL, Chipont E, Mulet E, De La HF. Visual performance after congenital nystagmus surgery using extended hang back recession of the four horizontal rectus muscles. Eur. J Ophthalmol 13, 415–423, 2003.
23. Alkawi A, Kattah JC, Wyman K. Downbeat nystagmus as a result of lamotrigine toxicity. Epilepsy Res 63, 85–88, 2005.
24. Alpert JN. Downbeat nystagmus due to anticonvulsant toxicity. Ann Neurol 4, 471–473, 1978.

24a. Ances BM, Dalmau JO, Tsai J, Hasbani MJ, Galetta SL. Downbeating nystagmus and muscle spasms in a patient with glutamic-acid decarboxylase antibodies. Am J Ophthalmol 140, 142–144, 2005.

25. Anderson J, Lavoie J, Merrill K, King RA, Summers CG. Efficacy of spectacles in persons with albinism. J AAPOS 8, 515–520, 2004.
26. Anderson JR. Causes and treatment of congenital eccentric nystagmus. Br J Ophthalmol 37, 267–281, 1953.
27. Anderson JR. Latent nystagmus and alternating hyperphoria. Br J Ophthalmol 38, 217–231, 1954.
28. Anderson NE, Rosenblum MK, Posner JB. Paraneoplastic cerebellar degeneration: Clinical-immunological correlations. Ann Neurol 24, 559–567, 1988.
29. Anteby I, Zhai HF, Tychsen L. Asymmetric motion visually evoked potentials in infantile strabismus are not an artifact of latent nystagmus. J AAPOS 2, 153–158, 1998.
30. Antonini G, Nemni R, Giubilei F, et al. Autoantibodies to glutamic acid decarboxylase in downbeat nystagmus. J Neurol Neurosurg Psychiatry 74, 998–999, 2003.
31. Apkarian P, Bour LJ. See-saw nystagmus and congenital nystagmus identified in the non-decussating retinal-fugal fiber syndrome. Strabismus 9, 143–163, 2001.
32. Apkarian P, Bour LJ, Barth PG, Wenniger-Prick L, Verbeeten B Jr. Non-decussating retinal-fugal fibre syndrome - An inborn achiasmatic malformation associated with visuotopic misrouting, visual evoked potential ipsilateral asymmetry and nystagmus. Brain 118, 1195–1216, 1995.

32a. Armstrong MB, Robertson PL, Castle VP. Delayed, recurrent opsoclonus-myoclonus syndrome responding to plasmapheresis. Pediatr Neurol 33, 365–367, 2005.

33. Arnold DB, Robinson DA. The oculomotor integrator: testing of a neural network model. Exp Brain Res 113, 57–74, 1997.
34. Arnold DB, Robinson DA, Leigh RJ. Nystagmus induced by pharmacological inactivation of the brainstem ocular motor integrator in monkey. Vision Res 39, 4286–4295, 1999.

35. Arroyo-Yllanes ME, Fonte-Vazquez A, Perez-Perez JF. Modified Anderson procedure for correcting abnormal mixed head position in nystagmus. Br J Ophthalmol 86, 267–269, 2002.
36. Asawavichiangianda S, Fujimoto M, Mai M, Desroches H, Rutka J. Significance of head-shaking nystagmus in the evaluation of the dizzy patient. Acta Otolaryngol Suppl 540, 27–33, 1999.
37. Aschoff JC, Conrad B, Kornhuber HH. Acquired pendular nystagmus with oscillopsia in multiple sclerosis: a sign of cerebellar nuclei disease. J Neurol Neurosurg Psychiatry 37, 570–577, 1974.
38. Ashe J, Hain TC, Zee DS, Schatz NJ. Microsaccadic flutter. Brain 114, 461–472, 1991.
39. Atilla H, Erkam N, Isikcelik Y. Surgical treatment in nystagmus. Eye 13, 11–15, 1999.
40. Au WJ, Keltner JL. Opsoclonus with amitriptyline overdose. Ann Neurol 6, 87, 1979.
41. Averbuch-Heller L, Dell'Osso LF, Leigh RJ, Jacobs JB, Stahl JS. The torsional component of "horizontal" congenital nystagmus. J Neuroophthalmol 22, 22–32, 2002.
42. Averbuch-Heller L, Dell-Osso LF, Jacobs JB, Remler BF. Latent and congenital nystagmus in Down syndrome. J Neuroophthalmol 19, 166–172, 1999.
43. Averbuch-Heller L, Kori AA, Rottach KG, et al. Dysfunction of pontine omnipause neurons causes impaired fixation: macrosaccadic oscillations with a unilateral pontine lesion. Neuroophthalmol 16, 99–106, 1996.
44. Averbuch-Heller L, Leigh RJ. Saccade-induced nystagmus. Neurology 46, 289, 1996.
45. Averbuch-Heller L, Leigh RJ. Medical treatments for abnormal eye movements. Pharmacological and immunological strategies. Austr N Z J Ophthalmol 25, 81–87, 1997.
46. Averbuch-Heller L, Meiner Z. Reversible periodic alternating gaze deviation in hepatic encephalopathy. Neurology 45, 191–192, 1995.
47. Averbuch-Heller L, Paulson GW, Daroff RB, Leigh RJ. Whipple's disease mimicking progressive supranuclear palsy: the diagnostic value of eye movement recording. J Neurol Neurosurg Psychiatry 66, 532–535, 1999.
48. Averbuch-Heller L, Remler BF. Opsoclonus. Semin Neurol 16, 21–26, 1996.
49. Averbuch-Heller L, Rottach AG, Zivotofsky AZ, et al. Torsional eye movements in patients with skew deviation and spasmodic torticollis: responses to static and dynamic head roll. Neurology 48, 506–514, 1997.
50. Averbuch-Heller L, Stahl JS, Hlavin ML, Leigh RJ. Square-wave jerks induced by pallidotomy in parkinsonian patients. Neurology 52, 185–188, 1999.
51. Averbuch-Heller L, Tusa RJ, Fuhry L, et al. A double-blind controlled study of gabapentin and baclofen as treatment for acquired nystagmus. Ann Neurol 41, 818–825, 1997.
52. Averbuch-Heller L, Zivotofsky AZ, Das VE, DiScenna AO, Leigh RJ. Investigations of the pathogenesis of acquired pendular nystagmus. Brain 188, 369–378, 1995.
53. Averbuch-Heller L, Zivotofsky AZ, Remler BF, et al. Convergent-divergent pendular nystagmus: possible role of the vergence system. Neurology 45, 509–515, 1995.
54. Baloh RW, Jen JC. Genetics of familial episodic vertigo and ataxia. Ann N Y Acad Sci 956, 338–345, 2002.
55. Baloh RW, Konrad HR, Dirks D, Honrubia V. Cerebellopontine angle tumors. Arch Neurol 33, 507–512, 1976.
56. Baloh RW, Spooner JW. Downbeat nystagmus: a type of central vestibular nystagmus. Neurology 31, 304–310, 1981.
57. Baloh RW, Yee RD. Spontaneous vertical nystagmus. Rev Neurol (Paris) 145, 527–532, 1989.
58. Bance ML, O'Driscoll M, Patel N, Ramsden RT. Vestibular disease unmasked by hyperventilation. Laryngoscope 108, 610–614, 1998.
59. Bandini F, Castello E, Mazzella L, Mancardi GL, Solaro C. Gabapentin but not vigabatrin is effective in the treatment of acquired nystagmus in multiple sclerosis: How valid is the GABAergic hypothesis? J Neurol Neurosurg Psychiatry 71, 107–110, 2001.
60. Barber HO, Stoyanoff S. Vertical nystagmus in routine caloric testing. Otolaryngol Head Neck Surg 95, 574–580, 1986.
61. Barton JJ, Cox TA, Digre KB. Acquired convergence-evoked pendular nystagmus in multiple sclerosis. J Neuroophthalmol 19, 34–38, 1999.
62. Barton JJS. Is acquired pendular nystagmus always phase locked? J Neurol Neurosurg Psychiatry 57, 1263–1264, 1994.
63. Barton JJS. Blink- and saccade-induced seesaw nystagmus. Neurology 45, 831–833, 1995.
64. Barton JJS, Cox TA. Acquired pendular nystagmus in multiple sclerosis—Clinical observations and the role of optic neuropathy. J Neurol Neurosurg Psychiatry 56, 262–267, 1993.
65. Barton JJS, Sharpe JA. Oscillopsia and horizontal nystagmus with accelerating slow phases following lumbar puncture in the Arnold-Chiari malformation. Ann Neurol 33, 418–421, 1993.
66. Barton JJS, Huaman AG, Sharpe JA. Muscarinic antagonists in the treatment of acquired pendular and downbeat nystagmus—a double-blind randomized trial of three intravenous drugs. Ann Neurol 35, 319–325, 1994.
67. Bataller L, Graus F, Saiz A, Vilchez J. Clinical outcome in adult onset idiopathic or paraneoplastic opsoclonus-myoclonus. Brain 124, 437–443, 2001.
68. Bataller L, Dalmau J. Neuro-ophthalmology and paraneoplastic syndromes. Curr Opin Neurol 17, 3–8, 2004.
69. Bataller L, Rosenfeld MR, Graus F, et al. Autoantigen diversity in the opsoclonus-myoclonus syndrome. Ann Neurol 53, 347–353, 2003.
70. Bedell HE. Perception of a clear and stable visual world with congenital nystagmus. Optom Vis Sci 77, 573–581, 2000.
71. Bedell HE, Bollenbacher MA. Perception of motion smear in normal observers and in persons with congenital nystagmus. Invest Ophthalmol Vis Sci 37, 188–195, 1996.
72. Bedell HE, White JW, Abplanalp PL. Variability of foveations in congenital nystagmus. Clin Vision Sci 4, 247–252, 1989.
73. Belton T, McCrea RA. Role of the cerebellar flocculus region in the coordination of eye and head move-

ments during gaze pursuit. J Neurophysiol 84, 1614–1626, 2000.
74. Bender MB. Oscillopsia. Arch Neurol 13, 204–213, 1965.
75. Benjamin EE, Zimmerman CF, Troost BT. Lateropulsion and upbeat nystagmus are manifestations of central vestibular dysfunction. Arch Neurol 43, 962–964, 1986.
76. Bergenius J. Saccade abnormalities in patients with ocular flutter. Acta Otolaryngol (Stockh) 102, 228–233, 1986.
77. Berger JR, Kovacs AG. Downbeat nystagmus with phenytoin. J Clin Neuroophthalmol 2, 209–211, 1982.
78. Bergin DJ, Halpern J. Congenital see-saw nystagmus associated with retinitis pigmentosa. Ann Ophthalmol 18, 346–349, 1986.
79. Bertholon P, Bronstein AM, Davies RA, Rudge P, Thilo KV. Positional down beating nystagmus in 50 patients: cerebellar disorders and possible anterior semicircular canalithiasis. J Neurol Neurosurg Psychiatry 72, 366–372, 2002.
80. Bhidayasiri R, Somers JT, Kim HI, et al. Ocular oscillations induced by shifts of the direction and depth of visual fixation. Ann Neurol 49, 24–28, 2001.
81. Bianchi PE, Salati R, Cavallini A, Fazzi E. Transient nystagmus in delayed visual maturation. Dev Med Child Neurol 40, 263–265, 1998.
82. Bielschowsky A. Die einseitigen und gegensinnigen ("dissoziierten") vertikal-bewegungen der augen. Albrecht von Graefes Arch Klin Exp Ophthalmol 125, 493–553, 1931.
83. Biousse V, Tusa RJ, Russell B, et al. The use of contact lenses to treat visually symptomatic congenital nystagmus. J Neurol Neurosurg Psychiatry 75, 314–316, 2004.
84. Bisdorff AR, Sancovic S, Debatisse D, et al. Positional nystagmus in the dark in normal subjects. Neuroophthalmology 24, 283–290, 2000.
85. Bixenman WW. Congenital hereditary downbeat nystagmus. Can J Ophthalmol 18, 344–348, 1983.
85a. Blaes F, Fühlhuber V, Korfei M, et al. Surface-binding autoantibodies to cerebellar neurons in opsoclonus syndrome. Ann Neurol 58, 313–317, 2005.
86. Blain PG, Nightingale S, Stoddart JC. Strychnine poisoning: abnormal eye movements. J Toxicol Clin Toxicol 19, 215–217, 1982.
87. Blekher T, Yamada T, Yee RD, Abel LA. Effects of acupunture on foveation charactersitics in congenital nystagmus. Br J Ophthalmol 82, 115–120, 1998.
88. Bohmer A, Straumann D. Pathomechanism of mammalian downbeat nystagmus due to cerebellar lesion: a simple hypothesis. Neurosci Lett 250, 127–130, 1998.
89. Bondar RL, Sharpe JA, Lewis AJ. Rebound nystagmus in olivocerebellar atrophy: a clinicopathological correlation. Ann Neurol 15, 474–477, 1984.
90. Bötzel K, Rottach K, Büttner U. Normal and pathological saccadic dysmetria. Brain 116, 337–353, 1993.
91. Boycott KM, Pearce WG, Bech-Hansen NT. Clinical variability among patients with incomplete X-linked congenital stationary night blindness and a founder mutation in CACNA1F. Can J Ophthalmol 35, 204–213, 2000.
92. Brandt T. Vertigo. Its multisensory syndromes. Springer-Verlag, London, 1999.
93. Brandt T, Bronstein AM. Cervical vertigo. J Neurol Neurosurg Psychiatry 71, 8–12, 2001.
94. Brandt T, Dieterich M. Vestibular syndromes in the roll plane: topographic diagnosis from brain stem to cortex. Ann Neurol 36, 337–347, 1994.
95. Brandt T, Strupp M. Episodic ataxia type 1 and 2 (familial periodic ataxia/vertigo). Audiol Neurootol 2, 373–383, 1997.
96. Brecelj J, Stirn-Kranjc B. Visual electrophysiological screening in diagnosing infants with congenital nystagmus. Clin Neurophysiol 115, 461–470, 2004.
97. Brodsky MC. Congenital downbeat nystagmus. J Pediatr Ophthalmol Strabismus 33, 191–193, 1996.
98. Brodsky MC, Boop FA. Lid nystagmus as a sign of intrinsic midbrain disease. J Neuroophthalmol 15, 236–240, 1995.
99. Brodsky MC, Fray KJ. Positive angle kappa: a sign of albinism in patients with congenital nystagmus. Am J Ophthalmol 137, 625–629, 2004.
100. Brodsky MC, Tusa RJ. Latent nystagmus: vestibular nystagmus with a twist. Arch. Ophthalmol 122, 202–209, 2004.
101. Bronstein AM, Gresty MA, Mossman SS. Pendular pseudonystagmus arising as a combination of head tremor and vestibular failure. Neurology 42, 1527–1531, 1992.
102. Bronstein AM, Hood JD. Cervical nystagmus due to loss of cerebellar inhibition on the cervico-ocular reflex: a case report. J Neurol Neurosurg Psychiatry 48, 128–131, 1985.
103. Bronstein AM, Hood JD. The cervico-ocular reflex in normal subjects and patients with absent vestibular function. Brain Res 373, 399–408, 1986.
104. Bronstein AM, Hood JD. Oscillopsia of peripheral vestibular origin. Central and cervical compensatory mechanisms. Acta Otolaryngol (Stockh) 104, 1987, 307–314.
105. Bronstein AM, Miller DH, Rudge P, Kendall BE. Down beating nystagmus: magnetic resonance imaging and neuro-otological findings. J Neurol Sci 81, 173–184, 1987.
106. Broomhead DS, Clement RA, Muldoon MR, et al. Modelling of congenital nystagmus waveforms produced by saccadic system abnormalities. Biol Cybern 82, 391–399, 2000.
107. Brown JT, Randall A. Gabapentin fails to alter P/Q calcium channel-mediated synaptic transmission in the hippocampus in vitro. Synapse 55, 262–269, 2005.
108. Bruce CJ, Goldberg ME, Bushnell MC, Stanton GB. Primate frontal eye fields. II Physiological and anatomical correlates of electrically evoked eye movements. J Neurophysiol 54, 714–734, 1985.
109. Bruns L. Die Geschwulste des Nervensystems. S Karger Berlin, 1908.
110. Brusa A, Massa S, Piccardo A, Stoehr R, Bronzini E. Le nystagmus palpebral. Rev Neurol (Paris) 140, 288–292, 1984.
111. Büchele W, Brandt T, Degner D. Ataxia and oscillopsia in downbeat-nystagmus vertigo syndrome. Adv Oto-Rhino-Laryngol 30, 291–297, 1983.
112. Buckley NJ, Bonner TI, Buckley CM, Brann MR. Antagonist binding properties of five cloned muscarinic receptors expressed in CHO-K1 cells. Molecular Pharmacol 35, 469–476, 1989.

113. Büttner U, Grundei T. Gaze-evoked nystagmus and smooth pursuit deficits: their relationship studied in 52 patients. J Neurol 242, 384–389, 1995.
114. Büttner U, Helmchen C, Büttner-Ennever JA. The localizing value of nystagmus in brainstem disorders. Neuroophthalmol 15, 283–290, 1995.
115. Büttner U, Straube A, Brandt T. Paroxysmal spontaneous nystagmus and vertigo evoked by lateral eye position. Neurology 37, 1553–1555, 1987.
116. Büttner-Ennever JA, Horn AK. Pathways from cell groups of the paramedian tracts to the floccular region. Ann N Y Acad Sci 781, 532–540, 1996.
117. Büttner-Ennever JA, Horn AK, Graf W, Ugolini G. Modern concepts of brainstem anatomy: from extraocular motoneurons to proprioceptive pathways. Ann N Y Acad Sci 956, 75–84, 2002.
118. Cabot A, Rozet JM, Gerber S, et al. A gene for X-linked idiopathic congenital nystagmus (NYS1) maps to chromosome Xp11.4–p11.3. Am J Hum Genet 64, 1141–1146, 1999.
119. Campbell CL. Septo-optic dysplasia: a literature review. Optometry 74, 417–426, 2003.
120. Campbell WW Jr. Periodic alternating nystagmus in phenytoin intoxication. Arch Neurol 37, 178–180, 1980.
121. Cannon SC, Robinson DA. Loss of the neural integrator of the oculomotor system from brain stem lesions in monkey. J Neurophysiol 57, 1383–1409, 1987.
122. Carasig D, Paul K, Fucito M, Ramcharan E, Gnadt JW. Irrepressible saccades from a tectal lesion in a Rhesus monkey. Vision Res, published online, 2005.
123. Carl JR, Optican LM, Chu FC, Zee DS. Head shaking and vestibulo-ocular reflex in congenital nystagmus. Invest Ophthalmol Vis Sci 26, 1043–1050, 1985.
124. Carpenter RHS. The visual origins of ocular motility. In Carpenter RHS (ed). Eye Movements. Vol 8. MacMillan Press, London, 1991, pp 1–10.
125. Carruthers J. The treatment of congenital nystagmus with Botox. J Pediatr Ophthalmol Strabismus 32, 306–308, 1995.
126. Castillo IG, Reinecke RD, Sergott RC, Wizov S. Surgical treatment of trauma-induced periodic alternating nystagmus. Ophthalmology 111, 180–183, 2004.
127. Cher LM, Hochberg FH, Teruya J, et al. Therapy for paraneoplastic neurologic syndromes in six patients with protein A column immunoadsorption. Cancer 75, 1678–1683, 1995.
128. Chiu B, Hain TC. Periodic alternating nystagmus provoked by an attack of Meniere's disease. J Neuroophthalmol 22, 107–109, 2002.
129. Choi KD, Jung DS, Park KP, Jo JW, Kim JS. Bowtie and upbeat nystagmus evolving into hemi-seesaw nystagmus in medial medullary infarction: possible anatomic mechanisms. Neurology 62, 663–665, 2004.
129a. Choi KD, Shin HY, Kim JS, et al. Rotational vertebral artery syndrome: oculographic analysis of nystagmus. Neurology 65, 1287–1290, 2005.
130. Chrousos GA, Ballen AE, Matsuo V, Cogan DG. Near-evoked nystagmus in spasmus nutans. J Pediatr Ophthalmol Strabismus 23, 141–143, 1986.
131. Chrousos GA, Cowdry R, Schuelein M, et al. Two cases of downbeat nystagmus and oscillopsia associated with carbamazepine. Am J Ophthalmol 103, 221–224, 1987.
132. Chrousos GA, Reingold DR, Chu FC, Cogan DG. Habitual head turning in spasmus nutans: an oculographic study. J Pediatr Ophthalmol Strabismus 22, 113–116, 1985.
133. Chung ST, Bedell HE. Congenital nystagmus image motion: influence on visual acuity at different luminances. Optom Vision Sci 74, 266–272, 1997.
134. Churchland MM, Lisberger SG. Apparent motion produces multiple deficits in visually guided smooth pursuit eye movements of monkeys. J Neurophysiol 84, 216–235, 2000.
135. Cibis GW, Fitzgerald KM. Electroretinography in congenital idiopathic nystagmus. Ped Neurol 9, 369–371, 1993.
136. Citek K, Ball B, Rutledge DA. Nystagmus testing in intoxicated individuals. Optometry. 74, 695–710, 2003.
137. Ciuffreda KJ. Voluntary nystagmus: new findings and clinical implications. Am J Optom Physiol Opt 57, 795–800, 1980.
138. Ciuffreda KJ, Goldrich SG, Neary C. Use of eye movement auditory biofeedback in the control of nystagmus. Am J Optom Physiol Optics 1982, 396–409, 1982.
139. Cochin JP, Hannequin D, Domarcolino C, Didier T, Augustin P. Intermittent see-saw nystagmus abolished by clonazepam. Rev Neurol (Paris) 151, 60–62, 1995.
140. Cogan DG. Ocular dysmetria; flutterlike oscillations of the eyes and opsoclonus. AMA Arch Opthalmol 51, 318–335, 1954.
141. Cogan DG. Convergence nystagmus: with notes on a single case of divergence nystagmus. Arch Ophthalmol 62, 295–299, 1959.
142. Cogan DG. Opsoclonus, body tremulousness and benign encephalitis. Arch Ophthalmol 79, 545–551, 1968.
143. Cogan DG, Loeb DR. Optokinetic response and intracranial lesions. Arch Neurol Psychiatry 61, 183–187, 1949.
144. Cohen B, Helwig D, Raphan T. Baclofen and velocity storage: a model of the effects of the drug on the vestibulo-ocular reflex in the rhesus monkey. J Physiol (Lond) 393, 703–725, 1987.
145. Cohen WJ, Cohen NH. Lithium carbonate, haloperidol and irreversible brain damage. JAMA 230, 1283–1287, 1974.
146. Coker S, Susac J, Sharpe J, Smallridge R. Cockayne's syndrome, neuro-ophthalmic, CAT scan and endocrine observations. In Smith JL (ed). Neuro-ophthalmology Focus. Masson, New York, 1979, pp 379–385.
147. Condorelli DF, Parenti R, Spinella F, et al. Cloning of a new gap junction gene (CX36) highly expressed in mammalian brain neurons. Eur J Neurosci 10, 1202–1208, 1998.
148. Cooke RW, Foulder-Hughes L, Newsham D, Clarke D. Ophthalmic impairment at 7 years of age in children born very preterm. Arch Dis Child Fetal Neonatal Ed 89, F249–F253, 2004.
149. Corbett JJ, Jacobson DM, Thompson HS, Hart MN, Albert DW. Downbeating nystagmus and other ocular motor defects caused by lithium toxicity. Neurology 39, 481–487, 1989.
150. Cox TA, Corbett JJ, Thompson HS, Lennarson L. Upbeat nystagmus changing to downbeat nystagmus with convergence. Neurology 31, 891–892, 1981.

151. Crawford JD, Cadera W, Vilis T. Generation of torsional and vertical eye position signals by the interstitial nucleus of Cajal. Science 252, 1551–1553, 1991.
152. Cremer PD, Migliaccio AA, Halmagyi GM, Curthoys IS. Vestibulo-ocular reflex pathways in internuclear ophthalmoplegia. Ann Neurol 45, 529–533, 1999.
153. Crone RA, de Jong PT, Notermans G. Behandlung des Nystagmus durch Injektion von Botulinustoxin in die Augenmuskeln. Klin Mbl Augenheilk 184, 216–217, 1984.
154. Cross SA, Smith JL, Norton EW. Periodic alternating nystagmus clearing after vitrectomy. J Clin Neuroophthalmol 2, 5–11, 1982.
155. Cüppers C. Probleme der operativen Therapie des okularen Nystagmus. Klin Mbl Augenheilk 159, 145–157, 1971.
156. Currie JN, Goldberg ME, Matsuo V, FitzGibbon EJ. Dyslexia with saccadic intrusions: a treatable reading disorder with a characteristic oculomotor sign. Neurology 36 (Suppl 1), 1986.
157. Currie JN, Matsuo V. The use of clonazepam in the treatment of nystagmus-induced oscillopsia. Ophthalmology 93, 924–932, 1986.
157a. Danchaivijitr C, Nachev P, Rosenthal CR, Bronstein AM, Kennard C. Levetiracetam in acquired pendular nystagmus. Personal communication, 2005.
158. Daroff RB. See-saw nystagmus. Neurology 15, 874–877, 1965.
159. Daroff RB, Hoyt WF. Supranuclear disorders of ocular control systems in man; clinical, anatomical and physiological correlations. In Bach-y-Rita P, Collins CC, Hyde JE (eds). The Control of Eye Movements. Academic Press, New York, 1971, pp 175–235.
160. Daroff RB, Hoyt WF, Bettman JW, Jr., Lessell S. Suppression and facilitation of congenital nystagmus by vertical lines. Neurology 23, 530–533, 1973.
161. Daroff RB, Hoyt WF, Sanders MD, Nelson LR. Gaze-evoked eyelid and ocular nystagmus inhibited by the near reflex: unusual ocular motor phenomena in a lateral medullary syndrome. J Neurol Neurosurg Psychiatry 31, 362–367, 1968.
162. Das VE, Oruganti P, Kramer PD, Leigh RJ. Experimental tests of a neural-network model for ocular oscillations caused by disease of central myelin. Exp Brain Res 133, 189–197, 2000.
163. Davey K, Kowal L, Friling R, Georgievski Z, Sandbach J. The Heimann-Bielschowsky phenomenon: dissociated vertical nystagmus. Aust N Z J Ophthalmol 26, 237–240, 1998.
164. Davis GV, Schock JP. Septo-optic dysplasia associated with see-saw nystagmus. Arch Ophthalmol 93, 137–139, 1975.
165. De Becker I, Walter M, Noel LP. Phenotypic variations in patients with a 1630 A>T point mutation in the PAX6 gene. Can J Ophthalmol 39, 272–278, 2004.
166. de Jong PTVM, De Jong JMBV, Cohen B, Jongkees LB. Ataxia and nystagmus induced by injection of local anesthetics in the neck. Ann Neurol 1, 240–246, 1977.
167. Dehaene I, Casselman JW, Van Zandijcke M. Unilateral internuclear ophthalmoplegia and ipsiversive torsional nystagmus. J Neurology 243, 461–464, 1996.
168. Dehaene I, Van Vleymen B. Opsoclonus induced by phenytoin and diazepam. Ann Neurol 21, 216, 1984.
168a. Deleu D, El Siddig A, Kamran S, Kamha AA, Al Omary, I, Zalabany HA. Downbeat nystagmus following classical heat stroke. Clin Neurol Neurosurg 108, 102–104, 2005.
169. Dell'Osso LF. Improving visual acuity in congenital nystagmus. In Smith JL, Glaser JS (eds). Neuro-Ophthalmology. Volume 7. Mosby, St. Louis, 1973, pp 98–106.
170. Dell'Osso LF. Congenital and latent/manifest latent nystagmus: diagnosis, treatment, foveation, oscillopsia and acuity. Jpn J Ophthalmol 38, 329–336, 1994.
171. Dell'Osso LF. See-saw nystagmus in dogs and humans: an international across-discipline serendipitous collaboration. Neurology 47, 1372–1374, 1996.
172. Dell'Osso LF. Suppression of pendular nystagmus by smoking cannabis in a patient with multiple sclerosis. Neurology 54, 2190–2191, 2000.
173. Dell'Osso LF. Development of new treatments for congenital nystagmus. Ann N Y Acad Sci 956, 361–379, 2002.
174. Dell'Osso LF, Abel LA, Daroff RB. "Inverse latent" macro squarewave jerks and macro saccadic oscillations. Ann Neurol 2, 57–60, 1977.
175. Dell'Osso LF, Abel LA, Daroff RB. Latent/manifest latent nystagmus reversal using an ocular prosthesis. Implications for vision and ocular dominance. Invest Ophthalmol Vis Sci 28, 1873–1876, 1987.
176. Dell'Osso LF, Averbuch-Heller L, Leigh RJ. Oscillopsia suppression and foveation-period variation in congenital latent and acquired nystagmus. Neuroophthalmol 18, 163–183, 1997.
177. Dell'Osso LF, Daroff RB. Congenital nystagmus waveforms and foveation strategy. Documenta Ophthalmologica 39, 155–182, 1975.
178. Dell'Osso LF, Daroff RB. Braking saccade—a new fast eye movement. Aviat Space Environ Med 47, 435–437, 1976.
179. Dell'Osso LF, Daroff RB. Abnormal head positions and head motion associated with nystagmus. In Keller EL, Zee DS (eds). Adaptive Processes in Visual and Oculomotor Systems. Pergamon, Oxford, 1986, pp 473–478.
180. Dell'Osso LF, Ellenberger C, Jr., Abel LA, Flynn JT. The nystagmus blockage syndrome: Congenital nystagmus, manifest latent nystagmus or both? Invest Ophthalmol Vis Sci 24, 1580–1587, 1983.
181. Dell'Osso LF, Flynn JT. Congenital nystagmus surgery: a quantitative evaluation of the effects. Arch Ophthalmol 97, 462–469, 1979.
182. Dell'Osso LF, Flynn JT, Daroff RB. Hereditary congenital nystagmus: an intrafamilial study. Arch Ophthalmol 92, 366–374, 1974.
183. Dell'Osso LF, Hertle RW, Williams RW, Jacobs JB. A new surgery for congenital nystagmus: effects of tenotomy on an achiasmatic canine and the role of extraocular proprioception. J AAPOS 3, 166–182, 1999.
184. Dell'Osso LF, Jacobs JB. A normal ocular motor system model that simulates the dual-mode fast phases of latent/manifest latent nystagmus. Biol Cybern 85, 459–471, 2001.
185. Dell'Osso LF, Jacobs JB. An expanded nystagmus acuity function: intra- and intersubject prediction of

best-corrected visual acuity. Doc Ophthalmol 104, 249–276, 2002.
186. Dell'Osso LF, Leigh RJ. Ocular motor stability of foveation periods. Required conditions for suppression of oscillopsia. Neuroophthalmol 12, 303–326, 1992.
187. Dell'Osso LF, Leigh RJ, Sheth NV, Daroff RB. Two types of foveation strategy in "latent" nystagmus. Visual acuity and stability. Neuroophthalmol 15, 1–20, 1995.
188. Dell'Osso LF, Schmidt D, Daroff RB. Latent, manifest latent and congenital nystagmus. Arch Ophthalmol 97, 1877–1885, 1979.
189. Dell'Osso LF, Traccis S, Abel LA. Strabismus: a necessary condition for latent and manifest latent nystagmus. Neuroophthalmol 3, 247–257, 1983.
190. Dell'Osso LF, Traccis S, Erzurum SI. Contact lenses and congenital nystagmus. Clin Vision Sci 3, 229–232, 1988.
191. Dell'Osso LF, Troost BT, Daroff RB. Macro square wave jerks. Neurology 25, 975–979, 1975.
192. Dell'Osso LF, Van der Steen J, Steinman RM, Collewijn H. Foveation dynamics in congenital nystagmus. II: Smooth pursuit. Documenta Ophthlamologica 79, 25–49, 1992.
193. Dell'Osso LF, Van der Steen J, Steinman RM, Collewijn H. Foveation dynamics in congenital nystagmus. III: Vestibulo-ocular reflex. Documenta Ophthlamologica 79, 51–70, 1992.
194. Dell'Osso LF, Weisman BM, Leigh RJ, Abel RJ, Sheth NV. Hereditary congenital nystagmus and gaze-holding failure: the role of the neural integrator. Neurology 43, 1741–1749, 1993.
195. Dell'Osso LF, Williams RW. Ocular motor abnormalities in achiasmatic mutant Belgian sheepdogs: unyoked eye movements in a mammal. Vision Res 35, 109–116, 1995.
196. Dell'Osso LF, Williams RW, Jacobs JB, Erchul DM. The congenital and see-saw nystagmus in the prototypical achiasma of canines: comparison to the human achiasmatic prototype. Vision Res 38, 1629–1641, 1998.
197. Delreux V, Kevers L, Sindic CJM, Callewaert A. Opsoclonus secondary to Epstein-Barr virus infection. Neuroophthalmol 8, 179–189, 1988.
198. Demer JL, Zee DS. Vestibulo-ocular and optokinetic deficits in albinos with congenital nystagmus. Invest Ophthalmol Vis Sci 25, 74–78, 1984.
199. Deuschl G, Toro C, Valls-Solo J, Zee DS, Hallett M. Symptomatic and essential palatal tremor. 1. Clinical physiological and MRI analysis. Brain 117, 775–788, 1994.
200. Devor A, Yarom Y. Electrotonic coupling in the inferior olivary nucleus revealed by simultaneous double patch recordings. J Neurophysiol 87, 3048–3058, 2002.
201. Dias EC, Segraves MA. Muscimol-induced inactivation of monkey frontal eye field: effects on visually and memory-guided saccades. J Neurophysiol 81, 2191–2214, 1999.
202. Dickinson CM. The elucidation and use of the effect of near fixation in congenital nystagmus. Ophthal Physiol Opt 6, 303–311, 1986.
203. Dieterich M, Bense S, Stephan T, Yousry TA, Brandt T. fMRI signal increases and decreases in cortical areas during small-field optokinetic stimulation and central fixation. Exp Brain Res 148, 117–127, 2003.
204. Dieterich M, Brandt T, Fries W. Otolith function in man: results from a case of otolith Tullio phenomenon. Brain 112, 1377–1392, 1989.
205. Dieterich M, Pollmann W, Pfaffenrath V. Cervicogenic headache: electronystagmography, perception of verticality and posturography in patients before and after C2–blockade. Cephalalgia 13, 285–288, 1993.
206. Dieterich M, Straube A, Brandt T, Paulus W, Büttner U. The effects of baclofen and cholinergic drugs on upbeat and downbeat nystagmus. J Neurol Neurosurg Psychiatry 54, 627–632, 1991.
207. Digre KB. Opsoclonus in adults. Report of three patients and review of the literature. Arch Neurol 43, 1165–1175, 1986.
208. Dones J, De Jesus O, Colen CB, Toledo MM, Delgado M. Clinical outcomes in patients with Chiari I malformation: a review of 27 cases. Surg Neurol 60, 142–147, 2003.
209. Drachman DA. See-saw nystagmus. J Neurol Neurosurg Psychiatry 29, 356–361, 1966.
210. Druckman R, Ellis P, Kleinfeld J, Waldman M. See-saw nystagmus. Arch Ophthalmol 76, 668–675, 1966.
211. Du Pasquier R, Vingerhoets F, Safran AB, Landis T. Periodic downbeat nystagmus. Neurology 51, 1478–1480, 1998.
212. Dubinsky RM, Hallet M, DiChiro G, Fulham M, Schwankhaus J. Increased glucose metabolism in the medulla of patients with palatal myoclonus. Neurology 41, 557–562, 1991.
213. Dyken P, Kolar O. Dancing eye dancing feet: Infantile polymyoclonia. Brain 91, 305–320, 1968.
213a. Economides JR, Horton JC. Eye movement abnormalities in stiff person syndrome. Neurology 65, 1462–1464, 2005.
214. Eggenberger ER. Delayed-onset seesaw nystagmus posttraumatic brain injury with bitemporal hemianopia. Ann N Y Acad Sci 956, 588–591, 2002.
215. Eida H, Ohira A, Amemiya T. Choroidal coloboma in two members of a family. Ophthalmologica 212, 208–211, 1998.
216. Eizenman M, Cheng P, Sharpe JA, Frecker RC. End-point nystagmus and ocular drift: an experimental and theoretical study. Vision Res 30, 863–877, 1990.
217. Elkardoudi-Pijnenburg Y, Van Vliet AG. Opsoclonus a rare complication of cocaine misuse. J Neurol Neurosurg Psychiatry 60, 592, 1996.
218. Ellenberger C, Jr., Campa JF, Netsky MG. Opsoclonus and parenchymatous degeneration of the cerebellum. The cerebellar origin of an abnormal eye movement. Neurology 18, 1041–1046, 1968.
219. Elliott AJ, Simpson EM, Oakhill A, Decock R. Nystagmus after medulloblastoma. Developmental Medicine and Child Neurology 31, 43–46, 1989.
220. Engle EC, Hedley-White T. A 29–month-old girl with worsening ataxia, nystagmus and subsequent opsoclonus and myoclonus. Case records of the Massachusetts General Hospital. New Engl J Med 333, 1995, 1995.
221. Epstein JA, Moster ML, Spiritos M. Seesaw nystagmus following whole brain irradiation and intrathecal methotrexate. J Neuroophthalmol 21, 264–265, 2001.
222. Erbagci I, Gungor K, Bekir NA. Effectiveness of retroequatorial recession surgery in congenital nystagmus. Strabismus 12, 35–40, 2004.

223. Erchul DM, Dell'Osso LF, Jacobs JB. Characteristics of foveating and defoveating fast phases in latent nystagmus. Invest Ophthalmol Vis Sci 39, 1751–1759, 1998.
224. Farmer J, Hoyt CS. Monocular nystagmus in infancy and early childhood. Am J Ophthalmol 98, 504–509, 1984.
225. Fein JM, Williams RDB. See-saw nystagmus. J Neurol Neurosurg Psychiatry 32, 202–207, 1969.
226. Ferro JM, Castro-Caldas A. Palatal myoclonus and carbamazepine. Ann Neurol 10, 402–403, 1981.
227. Fetter M, Dichgans J. Upbeat nystagmus changing to downbeat nystagmus with convergence in a patient with a lower medullary lesion. Neuroophthalmol 10, 89–95, 1990.
228. Fetter M, Haslwanter T, Bork M, Dichgans J. New insights into positional alcohol nystagmus using three-dimensional eye-movement analysis. Ann Neurol 45, 216–223, 1999.
229. Fisher A, Gresty M, Chambers B, Rudge P. Primary position upbeating nystagmus: a variety of central positional nystagmus. Brain 106, 949–964, 1983.
230. Fisher CM. Ocular flutter. J Clin Neuroophthalmol 10, 155–156, 1990.
231. Fisher PG, Wechsler DS, Singer HS. Anit-Hu antibody in a neuroblastoma-associated paraneoplastic syndrome. Ped Neurol 10, 309–312, 1994.
232. FitzGibbon EJ, Calvert PC, Dieterich MD, Brandt T, Zee DS. Torsional nystagmus during vertical pursuit. J Neuroophthalmol 16, 79–90, 1996.
233. Foroozan R, Brodsky MC. Microsaccadic opsoclonus: an idiopathic cause of oscillopsia and episodic blurred vision. Am J Ophthalmol 138, 1053–1054, 2004.
234. Francis DA, Heron JR. Ocular flutter in suspected multiple sclerosis: a presenting paroxysmal manifestation. Postgrad Med J 61, 333–334, 1985.
235. Friedman DI, Dell'Osso LF. "Reappearance" of congenital nystagmus after minor head trauma. Neurology 43, 2414–2416, 1993.
236. Frisén L, Wikkelso C. Posttraumatic seesaw nystagmus abolished by ethanol ingestion. Neurology 136, 841–844, 1986.
237. Fukazawa T, Tashiro K, Hamada T, Kase M. Multisystem degeneration: drugs and square wave jerks. Neurology 36, 1230–1233, 1986.
238. Furman JM, Brownstone PK, Baloh RW. Atypical brainstem encephalitis: magnetic resonance imaging and oculographic features. Neurology 35, 438–440, 1985.
239. Furman JM, Eidelman BH. Spontaneous remission of paraneoplastic ocular flutter and saccadic intrusions. Neurology 38, 499–501, 1988.
240. Furman JM, Wall C, III, Pang D. Vestibular function in periodic alternating nystagmus. Brain 113, 1425–1439, 1990.
241. Furman JMR, Baloh RW, Chugani JH, Waluch V, Bradley WG. Infantile cerebellar atrophy. Ann Neurol 17, 399–402, 1985.
242. Furman JMR, Baloh RW, Yee RD. Eye movement abnormalities in a family with cerebellar vermian atrophy. Acta Otolaryngol (Stockh) 101, 371–377, 1986.
243. Gamlin PD, Clarke RJ. Single-unit activity in the primate nucleus reticularis tegmenti pontis related to vergence and ocular accommodation. J Neurophysiol 73, 2115–2119, 1995.
244. Gamlin PD, Gnadt JW, Mays LE. Lidocaine-induced unilateral internuclear ophthalmoplegia: effects on convergence and conjugate eye movements. J Neurophysiol 62, 82–95, 1989.
245. Garbutt S, Han Y, Kumar AN, et al. Vertical optokinetic nystagmus and saccades in normal human subjects. Invest Ophthalmol Vis Sci 44, 3833–3841, 2003.
246. Garbutt S, Han Y, Kumar AN, et al. Disorders of vertical optokinetic nystagmus in patients with ocular misalignment. Vision Res 43, 347–357, 2003.
247. Garbutt S, Harwood MR, Harris CM. Comparison of the main sequence of reflexive saccades and the quick phases of optokinetic nystagmus. Br J Ophthalmol 85, 1477–1483, 2001.
248. Garbutt S, Riley DE, Kumar AN, et al. Abnormalities of optokinetic nystagmus in progressive supranuclear palsy. J Neurol Neurosurg Psychiatry 75, 1386–1394, 2004.
249. Garbutt S, Thakore N, Rucker JC, et al. Effects of visual fixation and convergence in periodic alternating nystagmus due to MS. Neurophthalmology 28, 221–229, 2004.
250. Gilman N, Baloh RW Primary position upbeat nystagmus. Neurology 27, 294–297, 1977.
251. Glasauer S, Dieterich M, Brandt T. Central positional nystagmus simulated by a mathematical ocular motor model of otolith-dependent modification of Listing's plane. J Neurophysiol 86, 1546–1554, 2001.
252. Glasauer S, Dieterich M, Brandt T. Modeling the role of the interstitial nucleus of Cajal in otolithic control of static eye position. Acta Otolaryngol Suppl 545, 105–107, 2001.
253. Glasauer S, Hoshi M, Büttner U. Smooth pursuit in patients with downbeat nystagmus. Ann N Y Acad Sci 1039, 532–535, 2005.
254. Glasauer S, Hoshi M, Kempermann U, Eggert T, Büttner U. Three-dimensional eye position and slow phase velocity in humans with downbeat nystagmus. J Neurophysiol 89, 338–354, 2003.
255. Glasauer S, Kalla R, Büttner U, Strupp M, Brandt T. 4–aminopyridine restores visual ocular motor function in upbeat nystagmus. J Neurol Neurosurg Psychiatry 76, 451–453, 2005.
255a. Glasauer S, Schneider E, Jahn K, Strupp M, Brandt T. How the eyes move the body. Neurology 65, 1291–1293, 2005.
256. Glasauer S, Strupp M, Kalla R, Büttner U, Brandt T. Effect of 4–aminopyridine on upbeat and downbeat nystagmus elucidates the mechanism of downbeat nystagmus. Ann N Y Acad Sci 1039, 528–531, 2005.
257. Glasauer S, von LH, Siebold C, Büttner U. Vertical vestibular responses to head impulses are symmetric in downbeat nystagmus. Neurology 63, 621–625, 2004.
258. Goldberg RT, Gonzalez C, Breinin GM, Reuben RN. Periodic alternating gaze deviation with dissociation of head movement. Arch Ophthalmol 73, 324–330, 1965.
259. Goldstein HP, Gottlob I, Fendick MG. Visual remapping in infantile nystagmus. Vision Res 32, 1115–1124, 1992.
260. Gomez CM, Thompson RM, Gammack JT, et al. SCA6: Gaze-evoked and vertical nystagmus Purkinje cell degeneration and variable age of onset

despite stable CAG repeat size. Ann Neurol 42, 933–950, 1997.
261. Good PA, Searle AE, Campbell S, Crews SJ. Value of the ERG in congenital nystagmus. Br J Ophthalmol 73, 512–515, 1989.
262. Good WV, Brodsky MC, Hoyt CS, Ahn JC. Upbeating nystagmus in infants: a sign of anterior visual pathway disease. Binocular Vision Quarterly 5, 13–18, 1990.
263. Good WV, Hou C, Carden SM. Transient idiopathic nystagmus in infants. Dev Med Child Neurol 45, 304–307, 2003.
264. Good WV, Jan JE, Hoyt CS, et al. Monocular vision loss can cause bilateral nystagmus in young children. Dev Med Child Neurol 39, 421–424, 1997.
265. Gordon S, Hain T, Zee D, Fetter M. Rebound nystagmus. Soc Neurosci Abstr 12, 1091, 1986.
266. Gorman WF, Brock S. Periodic alternating nystagmus in Friedreich's ataxia. Am J Ophthalmol 33, 860–864, 1950.
267. Gottlob I. Eye movement abnormalities in carriers of blue-cone monochromatism. Invest Ophthalmol Vis Sci 35, 3556–3560, 1994.
268. Gottlob I. Infantile nystagmus. Development documented by eye movement recordings. Invest Ophthalmol Vis Sci 38, 767–773, 1997.
269. Gottlob I, Helbling A. Nystagmus mimicking spasmus nutans as the presenting sign of Bardet-Biedl syndrome. Am J Ophthalmol 128, 770–772, 1999.
270. Gottlob I, Reinecke RD. Eye and head movements in patients with achromatopsia. Graefes Arch Klin Exp Ophthalmol 232, 392–401, 1994.
271. Gottlob I, Wizov SS, Reinecke RD. Spasmus nutans: a long-term follow-up. Invest Ophthalmol Vis Sci 36, 2768–2771, 1995.
272. Goyal M, Versnick E, Tuite P, et al. Hypertrophic olivary degeneration: metaanalysis of the temporal evolution of MR findings. AJNR Am J Neuroradiol 21, 1073–1077, 2000.
272a. Gradstein L, FitzGibbon EJ, Tsilou ET, Rubin BI, Huizing M, Gahl WA. Eye movement abnormalities in hermansky-pudlak syndrome. J AAPOS 9, 369–378, 2005.
273. Gradstein L, Goldstein HP, Wizov SS, Hayashi T, Reinecke RD. Relationships among visual acuity demands, convergence and nystagmus in patients with manifest/latent nystagmus. J AAPOS 2, 218–229, 1998.
274. Gradstein L, Reinecke RD, Wizov SS, Goldstein HP. Congenital periodic alternating nystagmus. Diagnosis and management. Ophthalmology 104, 918–928, 1997.
275. Grant MP, Cohen M, Petersen RB, et al. Abnormal eye movements in Creutzfeldt-Jakob disease. Ann Neurol 34, 192–197, 1993.
276. Gresty M, Leech J, Sanders M, Eggars H. A study of head and eye movement in spasmus nutans. Br J Ophthalmol 60, 652–654, 1976.
277. Gresty MA, Barratt HJ, Page NG, Ell JJ. Assessment of vestibulo-ocular reflexes in congenital nystagmus. Ann Neurol 17, 129–136, 1985.
278. Gresty MA, Barratt HJ, Rudge P, Page N. Analysis of downbeat nystagmus. Otolithic vs semicircular canal influences. Arch Neurol 43, 52–55, 1986.
279. Gresty MA, Bronstein AM, Brookes GB, Rudge P. Primary position upbeating nystagmus associated with middle ear disease. Neuroophthalmol 8, 321–328, 1988.
280. Gresty MA, Bronstein AM, Page NG, Rudge P. Congenital-type nystagmus emerging in later life. Neurology 41, 653–656, 1991.
281. Gresty MA, Ell JJ. Spasmus nutans or congenital nystagmus? Classification according to objective criteria. Br J Ophthalmol 65, 510–511, 1981.
282. Gresty MA, Ell JJ, Findley LJ. Acquired pendular nystagmus: its characteristics localising value and pathophysiology. J Neurol Neurosurg Psychiatry 45, 431–439, 1982.
283. Gresty MA, Findley LJ, Wade P. Mechanism of rotary eye movements in opsoclonus. Br J Ophthalmol 62, 533–535, 1980.
284. Gresty MA, Halmagyi GM. Head nodding associated with idiopathic childhood nystagmus. Ann N Y Acad Sci 374, 614–618, 1981.
285. Gresty MA, Metcalfe T, Timms C, et al. Neurology of latent nystagmus. Brain 115, 1303–1321, 1992.
286. Griggs RC, Moxley R, Lafrance R, McQuillen J. Hereditary paroxysmal ataxia: response to acetazolamide. Neurology 28, 1259–1264, 1978.
287. Guerraz M, Shallo-Hoffmann J, Yarrow K, et al. Visual control of postural orientation and equilibrium in congenital nystagmus. Invest Ophthalmol Vis Sci 41, 3798–3804, 2000.
288. Guillain G, Mollaret P. Deux cas myoclonies synchrones et rhythmées vélo-pharyngo-laryngo-oculodiaphragmatiques: Le problèm anatomique et physiolopathologique de ce syndrome. Rev Neurol (Paris) 2, 545–566, 1931.
289. Guillery RW, Okoro AN, Witkop CJ Jr. Abnormal visual pathways in the brain of a human albino. Brain Res 96, 373–377, 1975.
290. Guyton DL. Dissociated vertical deviation: etiology mechanism and associated phenomena. Costenbader Lecture. J AAPOS 4, 131–144, 2000.
291. Hain TC, Fetter M, Zee DS. Head-shaking nystagmus in patients with unilateral peripheral vestibular lesions. Am J Otolaryngol 8, 36–47, 1987.
292. Hain TC, Zee DS, Mordes M. Blink-induced saccadic oscillations. Ann Neurol 19, 299–301, 1986.
293. Halmagyi GM, Aw ST, Dehaene I, Curthoys IS, Todd MJ. Jerk-waveform see-saw nystagmus due to unilateral meso-diencephalic lesion. Brain 117, 775–788, 1994.
294. Halmagyi GM, Gresty MA, Leech J. Reversed optokinetic nystagmus (OKN): mechanism and clinical significance. Ann Neurol 7, 429–435, 1980.
295. Halmagyi GM, Leigh RJ. Upbeat about downbeat nystagmus. Neurology 63, 606–607, 2004.
296. Halmagyi GM, Lessell I, Curthoys IS, Lessell S, Hoyt WF. Lithium-induced downbeat nystagmus. Am J Ophthalmol 107, 664–670, 1989.
297. Halmagyi GM, Rudge P, Gresty MA, Leigh RJ, Zee DS. Treatment of periodic alternating nystagmus. Ann Neurol 8, 609–611, 1980.
298. Halmagyi GM, Rudge P, Gresty MA, Sanders MD. Downbeating nystagmus: a review of 62 cases. Arch Neurol 40, 777–784, 1983.
299. Hamann KF, Schuster EM. Vibration-induced nystagmus—A sign of unilateral vestibular deficit. ORL J Otorhinolaryngol Relat Spec 61, 74–79, 1999.
300. Hankey GJ, Sadka M. Ocular flutter postural body tremulousness and CSF pleocytosis: a rare postinfec-

tious syndrome. J Neurol Neurosurg Psychiatry 50, 1235–1236, 1987.
301. Hashimoto T, Sasaki O, Yoshida K, Takei Y, Ikeda S. Periodic alternating nystagmus and rebound nystagmus in spinocerebellar ataxia type 6. Mov Disord 18, 1201–1204, 2003.
302. Hattori T, Hirayama K, Imai T, Yamada T, Kojima S. Pontine lesions in opsoclonus-myoclonus syndrome shown by MRI. J Neurol Neurosurg Psychiatry 51, 1572–1575, 1988.
303. Hayashi T, Kozaki K, Kitahara K, et al. Clinical heterogeneity between two Japanese siblings with congenital achromatopsia. Vis Neurosci 21, 413–420, 2004.
304. Hellstrom A, Wiklund LM, Svensson E. The clinical and morphologic spectrum of optic nerve hypoplasia. J AAPOS 3, 212–220, 1999.
305. Helmchen C, Rambold H, Sprenger A, Erdmann C, Binkofski F. Cerebellar activation in opsoclonus: an fMRI study. Neurology 61, 412–415, 2003.
306. Helmchen C, Rambold H, Fuhry L, Büttner U. Deficits in vertical and torsional eye movements after uni- and bilateral muscimol inactivation of the interstitial nucleus of Cajal of the alert monkey. Exp Brain Res 119, 436–452, 1998.
307. Helmchen C, Rambold H, Kempermann U, Büttner-Ennever JA, Büttner U. Localizing value of torsional nystagmus in small midbrain lesions. Neurology 59, 1956–1964, 2002.
308. Helmchen C, Sprenger A, Rambold H, et al. Effect of 3,4–diaminopyridine on the gravity dependence of ocular drift in downbeat nystagmus. Neurology 63, 752–753, 2004.
309. Helveston EM, Ellis FD, Plager DA. Large recession of the horizontal recti for treatment of nystagmus. Ophthalmology 98, 1302–1305, 1991.
310. Helveston EM, Pogrebniak AE. Treatment of acquired nystagmus with botulinum A toxin. Am J Ophthalmol 106, 584–586, 1988.
311. Herishanu Y, Louzoun Z. Trihexyphenidyl treatment of vertical pendular nystagmus. Neurology 36, 82–84, 1986.
312. Herishanu Y, Osimand A, Louzoun Z. Unidirectional gaze-paretic nystagmus induced by phenytoin intoxication. Am J Ophthalmol 94, 122–123, 1982.
313. Herishanu YO, Sharpe JA. Normal square wave jerks. Invest Ophthalmol Vis Sci 20, 268–272, 1981.
314. Herishanu YO, Sharpe JA. Saccadic intrusions in internuclear ophthalmoplegia. Ann Neurol 14, 67–72, 1983.
315. Hertle RW. Examination and refractive management of patients with nystagmus. Surv Ophthalmol 45, 215–222, 2000.
316. Hertle RW, Chan CC, Galita DA, Maybodi M, Crawford MA. Neuroanatomy of the extraocular muscle tendon enthesis in macaque, normal human and patients with congenital nystagmus. J AAPOS 6, 319–327, 2002.
317. Hertle RW, Dell'Osso LF. Clinical and ocular motor analysis of congenital nystagmus in infancy. J AAPOS 3, 70–79, 1999.
318. Hertle RW, Dell'Osso LF, FitzGibbon EJ, et al. Horizontal rectus tenotomy in patients with congenital nystagmus. Ophthalmology 110, 2097–2105, 2003.
319. Hertle RW, Dell'Osso LF, FitzGibbon EJ, Yang D, Mellow SD. Horizontal rectus muscle tenotomy in children with infantile nystagmus syndrome: a pilot study. J AAPOS 8, 539–548, 2004.
320. Hertle RW, FitzGibbon EJ, Avallone JM, Cheeseman E, Tsilou EK. Onset of oscillopsia after visual maturation in patients with congenital nystagmus. Ophthalmology 108, 2301–2307, 2001.
321. Hertle RW, Maldanado VK, Maybodi M, Yang D. Clinical and ocular motor analysis of the infantile nystagmus syndrome in the first 6 months of life. Br J Ophthalmol 86, 670–675, 2002.
322. Hertle RW, Maybodi M, Bauer RM, Walker K. Clinical and oculographic response to Dexedrine in a patient with rod-cone dystrophy exotropia and congenital aperiodic alternating nystagmus. Binocul Vis Strabismus Q 16, 259–264, 2001.
323. Hertle RW, Maybodi M, Mellow SD, Yang D. Clinical and oculographic response to Tenuate Dospan (diethylpropionate) in a patient with congenital nystagmus. Am J Ophthalmol 133, 159–160, 2002.
323a. Hertle RW, Yang D, Kelly K, Hill VM, Atkin J, Seward A. X-linked infantile periodic alternating nystagmus. Ophthalmic Genet 26, 77–84, 2005.
324. Hertle RW, Zhu X. Oculographic and clinical characterization of thirty-seven children with anomalous head postures nystagmus and strabismus: the basis of a clinical algorithm. J AAPOS 4, 25–32, 2000.
325. Hess K, Reisine H, Dursteler M. Normal eye drift and saccadic drift correction in darkness. Neuro-ophthalmol 5, 247–252, 1985.
326. Hikosaka O, Wurtz RH. Modification of saccadic eye movements by GABA-related substances. II Effects of muscimol in monkey substantia nigra pars reticulata. J Neurophysiol 53, 292–308, 1985.
327. Himi T, Kataura A, Tokuda S, et al. Downbeat nystagmus with compression of the medulla oblongata by the dolichoectatic vertebral arteries. Am J Otol 16, 377–381, 1997.
328. Hirose G, Kawada J, Tsukada K, Yoshioka A, Sharpe JA. Upbeat nystagmus: clinicopathological and pathophysiological considerations. J Neurol Sci 105, 159–167, 1991.
329. Hirose G, Ogasawara T, Shirakara T, et al. Primary position upbeat nystagmus due to unilateral medial medullary infarction. Ann Neurol 43, 403–406, 1998.
330. Hirst LW, Clark AW, Wolinsky JS, et al. Downbeat nystagmus. A case report of herpetic brain stem encephalitis. J Clin Neuroophthalmol 3, 245–249, 1983.
331. Hoffmann KP, Distler C, Grusser OJ. Optokinetic reflex in squirrel monkeys after long-term monocular deprivation. Eur J Neurosci 10, 1136–1144, 1998.
331a. Hoffmann MB, Lorenz B, Morland AB, Schmidtborn LC. Misrouting of the optic nerves in albinism: Estimation of the extent with visual evoked potentials. Invest Ophthalmol Vis Sci 46, 3892–3898, 2005.
332. Hoffmann MB, Tolhurst DJ, Moore AT, Morland AB. Organization of the visual cortex in human albinism. J Neurosci 23, 8921–8930, 2003.
333. Holmes GL, Hafford J, Zimmerman AW. Primary position upbeat nystagmus following meningitis. Ann Ophthalmol 13, 935–936, 1981.
334. Honrubia V, Baloh RW, Harris MR, Jacobson KM. Paroxysmal positional vertigo syndrome. Am J Otol 20, 465–470, 1999.
335. Hood JD. Further observations on the phenome-

non of rebound nystagmus. Ann N Y Acad Sci 374, 532–539, 1981.
336. Hood JD, Kayan A, Leech J. Rebound nystagmus. Brain 96, 507–526, 1973.
337. Horn AKE, Büttner-Enever JA, Gayde M, Messoudi A. Neuroanatomical identification of mesencephalic premotor neurons coordinating eyelid with upgaze in the monkey and man. J Comp Neurol 420, 19–34, 2000.
338. Horn AKE, Büttner-Ennever JA, Wahle P, Reichenberger I. Neurotransmitter profile of saccadic omnipause neurons in nucleus raphe interpositus. J Neurosci 14, 2032–2046, 1994.
339. Hotson JR. Convergence-initiated voluntary flutter: a normal intrinsic capability in man. Brain Res 294, 299–304, 1984.
340. Howard RS. A case of convergence evoked eyelid nystagmus. J Clin Neuroophthalmol 6, 169–171, 1986.
341. Howard RS, Greenwood R, Gawler J, et al. A familial disorder associated with palatal myoclonus and other brainstem signs, tetraparesis, ataxia and Rosenthal fibre formation. J Neurol Neurosurg Psychiatry 56, 977–981, 1993.
342. Hoyt CS. Nystagmus and other abnormal ocular movements in children. Ped Clin North Am 34, 1415–1423, 1987.
343. Hoyt CS, Aicardi E. Acquired monocular nystagmus in monozygous twins. J Pediatr Ophthalmol Strabismus 16, 115–118, 1979.
344. Hoyt CS, Gelbart SS. Vertical nystagmus in infants with congenital ocular abnormalities. Ophthalmic Pediatr Genet 4, 155–162, 1984.
345. Hoyt CS, Mousel DK. Transient supranuclear disturbances of gaze in healthy neonates. Am J Ophthalmol 89, 708–713, 1980.
346. Hunnewell J, Miller NR. Bilateral internuclear ophthalmoplegia related to chronic toluene abuse. J Neuroophthalmol 18, 277–280, 1998.
347. Hwang TL, Still CN, Jones JE. Reversible downbeat nystagmus and ataxia in felbamate intoxication. Neurology 45, 846, 1995.
348. Inchingolo P, Optican LM, FitzGibbon EJ, Goldberg ME. Adaptive mechanisms in the monkey saccadic system. In Schmid R, Zambarbieri D (eds). Oculomotor Control and Cognitive Processes. Elsevier, Amsterdam, pp 147–162, 1991.
349. Irving EL, Goltz HC, Steinbach MJ, Kraft SP. Vertical latent nystagmus component and vertical saccadic asymmetries in subjects with dissociated vertical deviation. J AAPOS 2, 344–350, 1998.
350. Ishikawa H, Ishikawa S, Mukuno K. Short-cycle periodic (ping-pong) gaze. Neurology 43, 1067–1070, 1993.
351. Ishikawa S, Nozaki S, Mukuno K. Upbeat and downbeat nystagmus in a single case. Neuroophthalmol 6, 95–99, 1986.
352. Ishikawa S, Ozawa H, Fujiyama Y. Treatment of nystagmus by acupuncture. In Highlights in Neuro-ophthalmology: Proceedings of the Sixth Meeting of the International Neuro-ophthalmology Society (INOS). Aeolus Press, Amsterdam, 1987, pp 227–232.
353. Ito M. Cerebellar flocculus hypothesis. Nature 363, 24–25, 1993.
354. Ito M, Nisimaru N, Yamamoto M. Specific patterns of neuronal connexions involved in the control of the rabbit's vestibulo-ocular reflexes by the cerebellar flocculus. J Physiol (Lond) 265, 833–854, 1977.
355. Jabbari B, Rosenberg M, Scherokman B, et al. Effectiveness of trihexyphenidyl against pendular nystagmus and palatal myoclonus: evidence of cholinergic dysfunction. Mov Disord 2, 93–98, 1987.
356. Jabs DA, Green WR, Fox R, Polk BF, Bartlett JG. Ocular manifestations of acquired immune deficiency syndrome. Am J Ophthalmol 96, 1092–1099, 1989.
357. Jacobs JB, Dell'Osso LF Congenital nystagmus: hypotheses for its genesis and complex waveforms within a behavioral ocular motor system model. J Vis 4, 604–625, 2004.
358. Jacobs JB, Dell'Osso LF, Hertle RW, Bennett J, Acland G. Gene therapy to abolish congenital nystagmus in RPE65–deficient canines. Invest Ophthalmol Vis Sci (ARVO), 4249, 2003.
359. Jacobs JB, Dell'Osso LF, Leigh RJ. Characteristics of braking saccades in congenital nystagmus. Doc Ophthalmol 107, 137–154, 2003.
360. Jacobs L, Bender MB. Palato-ocular synchrony during eyelid closure. Arch Neurol 33, 289–291, 1976.
361. Jacobs L, Newman RP, Bozian D. Disappearing palatal myoclonus. Neurology 31, 748–751, 1981.
362. Jacobson DM, Corbett JJ. Downbeat nystagmus associated with dolichoectasia of the vertebrobasilar artery. Arch Neurol 46, 1005–1008, 1989.
363. Jaggi GP, Laeng HR, Müntener M, Killer HE. The anatomy of the muscle innervation (scleromuscular junction) of the lateral and medial rectus muscle in humans. Invest Ophthalmol Vis Sci 46, 2258–2263, 2005.
364. Jain S, Proudlock F, Constantinescu CS, Gottlob I. Combined pharmacologic and surgical approach to acquired nystagmus due to multiple sclerosis. Am J Ophthalmol 134, 780–782, 2002.
365. Janssen JC, Larner AJ, Morris H, Bronstein AM, Farmer SF. Upbeat nystagmus: clinicoanatomical correlation. J Neurol Neurosurg Psychiatry 65, 380–381, 1998.
366. Jay WM, Marcus RW, Jay MS. Primary position upbeat nystagmus with organophosphate poisoning. J Pediatr Ophthalmol Strabismus 19, 318–319, 1982.
367. Jay WM, Williams BB, De Chicchis A. Periodic alternating nystagmus clearing after cataract surgery. J Clin Neuroophthalmol 5, 149–152, 1985.
368. Jen J, Kim GW, Baloh RW. Clinical spectrum of episodic ataxia type 2. Neurology 62, 17–22, 2004.
369. Jen JC, Yue Q, Karrim J, Nelson SF, Baloh RW. Spinocerebellar ataxia type 6 with positional vertigo and acetazolamide responsive episodic ataxia. J Neurol Neurosurg Psychiatry 65, 565–568, 1998.
370. Johkura K, Komiyama A, Kuroiwa Y. Pathophysiologic mechanism of convergence nystagmus. Eur Neurol 47, 233–238, 2002.
371. Johnson JT, Wall C, Barney SA, Thearle PB. Postoperative vestibular dysfunction following head and neck surgery. Acta Otolaryngol (Stockh) 100, 316–320, 1985.
372. Kahlon M, Lisberger SG. Changes in the responses of Purkinje cells in the floccular complex of monkeys after motor learning in smooth pursuit eye movements. J Neurophysiol 84, 2945–2960, 2000.
373. Kalla R, Glasauer S, Schautzer F, et al. 4–aminopyri-

dine improves downbeat nystagmus, smooth pursuit and VOR gain. Neurology 62, 1228–1229, 2004.
374. Kamath BY, Keller EL. A neurological integrator for the oculomotor control system. Mathematical Biosciences 30, 341–352, 1976.
375. Kaminski HJ, Zee DS, Leigh RJ, Mendez MF. Ocular flutter and ataxia associated with AIDS-related complex. Neuroophthalmol 11, 163–167, 1991.
376. Kaneko CR. Eye movement deficits following ibotenic acid lesions of the nucleus prepositus hypoglossi in monkeys II. Pursuit, vestibular, and optokinetic responses. J Neurophysiol 81, 668–681, 1999.
377. Kaneko CRS. Effect of ibotenic acid lesions of the omnipause neurons on saccadic eye movements in Rhesus macaques. J Neurophysiol 75, 2229–2242, 1996.
378. Kanter DS, Ruff RL, Leigh RJ, Modic M. See-saw nystagmus and brainstem infarction. MRI findings. Neuroophthalmol 7, 279–283, 1987.
379. Kaplan PW, Tusa RJ. Neurophysiologic and clinical correlations of epileptic nystagmus. Neurology 43, 2508–2514, 1993.
380. Kasai T, Zee DS. Eye-head coordination in labyrinthine-defective human beings. Brain Res 144, 123–141, 1978.
381. Kastrup O, Maschke M, Keidel M, Diener HC. Presumed pharmacologically induced change from upbeat- to downbeat nystagmus in a patient with Wernicke's encephalopathy. Clin Neurol Neurosurg 107, 70–72, 2004.
382. Kattah JC, Dagli TF. Compensatory head tilt in upbeating nystagmus. J Clin Neuroophthalmol 10, 27–31, 1990.
383. Kaufmann H, Kolling G. Therapie bei Nystagmuspatienten mit Binokularfunktionen mit und ohne Kopfzwangshaltung. Ber Dtsch Ophthalmol Ges 78, 815–819, 1981.
384. Keane JR. Periodic alternating nystagmus with downward beating nystagmus. Arch Neurol 30, 399–402, 1974.
385. Keane JR. Intermittent see-saw eye movements. Report of a patient in coma after hyperextension head injury. Arch Neurol 32, 119–122, 1978.
386. Keane JR. Transient opsoclonus with thalamic hemorrhage. Arch Neurol 37, 423–424, 1980.
387. Keane JR. Pretectal pseudobobbing. Five patients with 'V'-pattern convergence nystagmus. Arch Neurol 42, 592–594, 1985.
388. Keane JR. Acute vertical ocular myoclonus. Neurology 36, 86–89, 1986.
389. Keane JR, Devereaux MW. Opsoclonus associated with intracranial tumor. Arch Ophthalmol 92, 443–445, 1974.
390. Keane JR, Itabashi HH. Upbeat nystagmus: Clinicopathologic study of two patients. Neurology 37, 491–494, 1987.
391. Kellner U, Wissinger B, Tippmann S, et al. Blue cone monochromatism: clinical findings in patients with mutations in the red/green opsin gene cluster. Graefes Arch Clin Exp Ophthalmol 242, 729–735, 2004.
392. Kelly BJ, Rosenberg ML, Zee DS, Optican LM. Unilateral pursuit-induced congenital nystagmus. Neurology 39, 414–416, 1989.
393. Kennard C, Barger G, Hoyt WF. The association of periodic alternating nystagmus with periodic alternating gaze. J Clin Neuroophthalmol 1, 191–193, 1981.
394. Kerrison JB, Giorda R, Lenart TD, Drack AV, Maumenee IH. Clinical and genetic analysis of a family with X-linked congenital nystagmus (NYS1). Ophthalmic Genet. 22, 241–248, 2001.
395. Kerrison JB, Koenekoop RK, Arnould VJ, Zee DS, Maumenee IH. Clinical features of autosomal dominant congenital nystagmus linked to chromosome 6P12. Am J Ophthalmol 125, 64–70, 1998.
396. Kerrison JB, Vagefi MR, Barmada MM, Maumenee IH. Congenital motor nystagmus linked to Xq26–q27. Am J Hum Genet 64, 600–607, 1999.
397. Kestenbaum A. Nouvelle operation de nystagmus. Bull Soc Ophtalmol Fr 6, 599–602, 1953.
398. Kim JI, Averbuch-Heller L, Leigh RJ. Evaluation of transdermal scopolamine as treatment for acquired nystagmus. J Neuroophthalmol 21, 188–192, 2001.
399. Kim JI, Somers JT, Stahl JS, Bhidayasiri R, Leigh RJ. Vertical nystagmus in normal subjects: effects of head position, nicotine and scopolamine. J Vestib Res 10, 291–300, 2000.
400. Kim JS, Ahn KW, Moon SY, et al. Isolated perverted head-shaking nystagmus in focal cerebellar infarction. Neurology 64, 575–576, 2005.
401. Kinsbourne M. Myoclonic encephalopathy of infants. J Neurol Neurosurg Psychiatry 25, 271–276, 1962.
402. Kiorpes L, Walton PJ, O'Keefe LP, Movshon JA, Lisberger SG. Effects of early-onset artificial strabismus on pursuit eye movements and on neuronal responses in area MT of macaque monkeys. J Neurosci 16, 6537–6553, 1996.
403. Klotz L, Klockgether T. Multiple system atrophy with macrosquare-wave jerks. Mov Disord 20, 253–254, 2005.
404. Koenekoop RK, Loyer M, Dembinska O, Beneish R. Visual improvement in Leber congenital amaurosis and the CRX genotype. Ophthalmic Genet 23, 49–59, 2002.
405. Koeppen AH. Olivary hypertrophy: histochemical demonstration of hydrolytic enzymes. Neurology 30, 471–480, 1980.
406. Koh PS, Raffensperger JG, Berry S, et al. Long-term outcome in children with opsoclonus-myoclonus and ataxia and coincident neuroblastoma. J Pediatrics 125, 712–716, 1994.
407. Kohl S, Varsanyi B, Antunes GA, et al. CNGB3 mutations account for 50% of all cases with autosomal recessive achromatopsia. Eur J Hum Genet 13, 302–308, 2005.
408. Komiyama A, Toda H, Johkura K. Edrophonium-induced macrosaccadic oscillations in myasthenia gravis. Ann Neurol 45, 522–525, 1999.
409. Kommerell G. The relationship between infantile strabismus and latent nystagmus. Eye 10, 274–281, 1996.
410. Kommerell G, Ullrich D, Gilles U, Bach M. Asymmetry of motion VEP in infantile strabismus and in central vestibular nystagmus. Documenta Ophthalmologica 89, 373–381, 1995.
411. Kommerell G, Zee DS. Latent nystagmus. Release and suppression at will. Invest Ophthalmol Vis Sci 34, 1785–1792, 1993.
412. Kömpf D. The significance of optokinetic nystagmus

asymmetry in hemispheric lesions. Neuroophthalmol 6, 61–64, 1986.
413. Korff CM, Apkarian P, Bour LJ, et al. Isolated absence of optic chiasm revealed by congenital nystagmus MRI and VEPs. Neuropediatrics 34, 219–223, 2003.
414. Kori AA, Robin NH, Jacobs JB, et al. Pendular nystagmus in patients with peroxisomal assembly disorder. Arch Neurol 55, 554–558, 1998.
415. Kornhuber HH. Der periodisch alternierende nystagmus (nystagmus alternans) und die Enthemmung des vestibularen Systems. Arch Ohren-Nasen Kehlkopfheilkd 174, 182–209, 1959.
416. Korres S, Balatsouras DG, Zournas C, et al. Periodic alternating nystagmus associated with Arnold-Chiari malformation. J Laryngol Otol 115, 1001–1004, 2001.
417. Koukoulis A, Cimas I, Gomara S. Paraneoplastic opsoclonus associated with papillary renal cell carcinoma. J Neurol Neurosurg Psychiatry 64, 137–138, 1998.
418. Kuban KC, Ephros MA, Freeman RL, Laffell LB, Bresnan MJ. Syndrome of opsoclonus-myoclonus caused by Coxsackie B3 infection. Ann Neurol 13, 69–71, 1983.
419. Kurzan R, Büttner U. Smooth pursuit mechanisms in congenital nystagmus. Neuroophthalmol 9, 313–325, 1989.
420. Kushner BJ. Infantile uniocular blindness with bilateral nystagmus. A syndrome. Arch Ophthalmol 113, 1298–1300, 1995.
421. Lambert SR, Newman NJ. Retinal disease masquerading as spasmus nutans. Neurology 43, 1607–1609, 1993.
422. Lambert SR, Taylor D, Kriss A. The infant with nystagmus normal appearing fundi but an abnormal ERG. Ophthalmology 34, 173–186, 1989.
423. Lapresle J. Rhythmic palatal myoclonus and the dentato-olivary pathway. J Neurol 220, 223–230, 1979.
424. Larner AJ, Bronstein AM, Farmer SF. Role of the nucleus intercalatus in upbeat nystagmus. Ann Neurol 44, 840, 1998.
425. Lavery MA, O'Neill JF, Chu FC, Martyn LJ. Acquired nystagmus in early childhood: a presenting sign of intracranial tumor. Ophthalmology 91, 425–435, 1984.
426. Lavin PJ, Traccis S, Dell'Osso LF, Abel LA, Ellenberger C, Jr. Downbeat nystagmus with a pseudocycloid waveform: improvement with base-out prisms. Ann Neurol 13, 621–624, 1983.
427. Lawden MC, Bronstein AM, Kennard C. Repetitive paroxysmal nystagmus and vertigo. Neurology 45, 276–280, 1995.
428. Lazar RB, Ho SU, Melen O, Daghestani AN. Multifocal central nervous system damage caused by toluene abuse. Neurology 33, 1337–1340, 1983.
429. Lee H, Cho YW. A case of isolated nodulus infarction presenting as a vestibular neuritis. J Neurol Sci 221, 117–119, 2004.
430. Lee IS, Lee JB, Kim HS, Lew H, Han SH. Modified Kestenbaum surgery for correction of abnormal head posture in infantile nystagmus: outcome in 63 patients with graded augmentaton. Binocul Vis Strabismus Q 15, 53–58, 2000.
431. Lee J, Gresty M. A case of voluntary nystagmus and head tremor. J Neurol Neurosurg Psychiatry 56, 1321–1322, 1993.
432. Lee MS, Lessell S. Lithium-induced periodic alternating nystagmus. Neurology 60, 344, 2003.
433. Leech J, Gresty M, Hess K, Rudge P. Gaze failure drifting eye movements and centripetal nystagmus in cerebellar disease. Br J Ophthalmol 61, 774–781, 1977.
434. Lefkowitz D, Harpold G. Treatment of ocular myoclonus with valproic acid. Ann Neurol 17, 103–104, 1985.
435. Leigh RJ. Clinical significance of positionally induced downbeat nystagmus. Ann Neurol 53, 688, 2003.
436. Leigh RJ. Potassium channels, the cerebellum and treatment for downbeat nystagmus. Neurology 61, 158–159, 2003.
437. Leigh RJ, Averbuch-Heller L, Tomsak RL, et al. Treatment of abnormal eye movements that impair vision: strategies based on current concepts of physiology and pharmacology. Ann Neurol 36, 129–141, 1994.
438. Leigh RJ, Burnstine TH, Ruff RL, Kasmer RJ. The effect of anticholinergic agents upon acquired nystagmus. A double-blind study of trihexyphenidyl and tridihexethyl chloride. Neurology 41, 1737–1741, 1991.
439. Leigh RJ, Hong S, Zee DS, Optican LM. Oculopalatal tremor: clinical and computational study of a disorder of the inferior olive. Soc Neurosci Abstr 933.8, 2005.
440. Leigh RJ, Robinson DA, Zee DS. A hypothetical explanation for periodic alternating nystagmus: Instability in the optokinetic-vestibular system. Ann N Y Acad Sci 374, 619–635, 1981.
441. Leigh RJ, Rushton DN, Thurston SE, Hertle RW, Yaniglos SS. Effects of retinal image stabilization in acquired nystagmus due to neurologic disease. Neurology 38, 122–127, 1988.
442. Leigh RJ, Thurston SE, Tomsak RL, Grossman GE, Lanska DJ. Effect of monocular visual loss upon stability of gaze. Invest Ophthalmol Vis Sci 30, 288–292, 1989.
443. Leigh RJ, Tomsak RL, Grant MP, et al. Effectiveness of botulinum toxin administered to abolish acquired nystagmus. Ann Neurol 32, 633–642, 1992.
444. Leigh RJ, Tomsak R. Drug treatments for eye movement disorders. J Neurol Neurosurg Psychiatry 74, 1–4, 2003.
445. Leigh RJ, Zee DS. Eye movements of the blind. Invest Ophthalmol Vis Sci 19, 328–331, 1980.
446. Leitch RJ, Thompson D, Harris CM, et al. Achiasmia in a case of midline craniofacial cleft with seesaw nystagmus. Br J Ophthalmol 80, 1023–1024, 1996.
447. Lepore FE. Ethanol-induced reduction of pathological nystagmus. Neurology 37, 887, 1987.
448. Lewis JM, Kline LB. Periodic alternating nystagmus associated with periodic alternating skew deviation. J Clin Neuroopthalmol 13, 115–117, 1983.
449. Liang TW, Balcer LJ, Solomon D, Messe SR, Galetta SL. Supranuclear gaze palsy and opsoclonus after Diazinon poisoning. J Neurol Neurosurg Psychiatry 74, 677–679, 2003.
450. Lin CY, Young YH. Clinical significance of rebound nystagmus. Laryngoscope 109, 1803–1805, 1999.
451. Liu C, Gresty M, Lee J. Management of symptomatic latent nystagmus. Eye 7, 550–553, 1993.
452. Lockwood AH, Wack DS, Burkard RF, et al. The

functional anatomy of gaze-evoked tinnitus and sustained lateral gaze. Neurology 56, 472–480, 2001.

453. Lopez L, Bronstein AM, Gresty MA, Rudge P, DuBoulay EP. Torsional nystagmus. A neuro-otological and MRI study of thirty-five cases. Brain 115, 1107–1124, 1992.

454. Lopez LI, Bronstein AM, Gresty MA, DuBoulay EP, Rudge P. Clinical and MRI correlates in 27 patients with acquired pendular nystagmus. Brain 119, 465–472, 1996.

455. Lopez LI, Gresty MA, Bronstein AM, DuBoulay EP, Rudge P. Acquired pendular nystagmus: oculomotor and MRI findings. Acta Oto-Laryngologica 285–287, 1995.

456. Louis ED, Lynch T, Kaufmann P, Fahn S, Odel J. Diagnostic guidelines in central nervous system Whipple's disease. Ann Neurol 40, 561–568, 1996.

457. Lueck CJ, Hamlyn P, Crawford TJ, et al. A case of ocular tilt reaction and torsional nystagmus due to direct stimulation of the midbrain in man. Brain 114, 2069–2079, 1991.

458. Maas EF, Ashe J, Spiegel P, Zee DS, Leigh RJ. Acquired pendular nystagmus in toluene addiction. Neurology 41, 282–285, 1991.

459. Maccario M, Seelinger D, Snyder R. Thallotoxicosis with coma and abnormal eye movements. Electroencephalogr Clin Neurophysiol 38, 98–99, 1975.

460. Malm G, Lying-Tunnell U. Cerebellar dysfunction related to toluene sniffing. Acta Neurol Scand 62, 188–190, 1980.

461. Marti S, Bockisch CJ, Straumann D. Prolonged asymmetric smooth-pursuit stimulation leads to downbeat nystagmus in healthy human subjects. Invest Ophthalmol Vis Sci 46, 143–149, 2005.

462. Marti S, Palla A, Straumann D. Gravity dependence of ocular drift in patients with cerebellar downbeat nystagmus. Ann Neurol 52, 712–721, 2002.

463. Marti S, Straumann D, Glasauer S. The origin of downbeat nystagmus: an asymmetry in the distribution of on-directions of vertical gaze-velocity purkinje cells. Ann N Y Acad Sci 1039, 548–553, 2005.

464. Masucci EF, Kurtzke JF. Downbeat nystagmus secondary to multiple sclerosis. Ann Ophthalmol 20, 347–348, 1988.

465. Matsumoto S, Ohyagi Y, Inouye I, et al. Periodic alternating nystagmus in a patient with MS. Neurology 56, 276–277, 2001.

466. Matsumura K, Sonoh M, Tamaoka A, Sakuta M. Syndrome of opsoclonus-myoclonus in hyperosmolar nonketotic coma. Ann Neurol 18, 623–624, 1985.

467. May EF, Truxal AR. Loss of vision alone may result in see-saw nystagmus. J Neuroophthalmol 17, 84–85, 1997.

468. Mayfrank L, Thoden U. Downbeat nystagmus indicates cerebellar or brain-stem lesions in vitamin B_{12} deficiency. J Neurol 233, 145–148, 1986.

469. McCarty JW, Demer JL, Hovis LA, Nuwer MR. Ocular motility anomalies in developmental misdirection of the optic chiasm. Am J Ophthalmol 113, 86–95, 1992.

470. McClure JA, Copp CC, Lycett P. Recovery nystagmus in Meniere's disease. Laryngoscope 91, 1727–1737, 1981.

471. McCrea RA, Strassman A, Highstein SM. Anatomical and physiological characteristics of vestibular neurons mediating the vertical vestibulo-ocular reflexes of the squirrel monkey. J Comp Neurol 264, 571–594, 1987.

472. McCrea RA, Strassman A, May E, Highstein SM. Anatomical and physiological characteristics of vestibular neurons mediating the horizontal vestibulo-ocular reflex of the squirrel monkey. J Comp Neurol 264, 547–570, 1987.

473. McElligott JG, Spencer RF. Neuropharmacological aspects of the vestibulo-ocular reflex. In Anderson JH, Beitz AJ (eds). Neurochemistry of the Vestibular System. CRC Press, Boca Raton, 2000, pp 199–222.

474. McElvanney AM, Wooldridge WJ, Khan AA, Ansons AM. Ophthalmic management of Cockayne's syndrome. Eye 10, 61–64, 1996.

475. McKnight AJ, Langston EA, McKnight AS, Lange JE. Sobriety tests for low blood alcohol concentrations. Accid Anal Prev 34, 305–311, 2002.

476. Meienberg O, Hoyt WF. Ocular motor control disorder during the neutral phase of periodic alternating nystagmus. J Neurol 23, 309–312, 1980.

477. Mellott ML, Brown J Jr., Fingert JH, et al. Clinical characterization and linkage analysis of a family with congenital X-linked nystagmus and deuteranomaly. Arch Ophthalmol 117, 1630–1633, 1999.

478. Melvill JG, Mandl G, Cynader M, Outerbridge JS. Eye oscillations in strobe reared cats. Brain Res 209, 47–60, 1981.

479. Mettens P, Godaux E, Cheron G, Galiana HL. Effect of muscimol microinjections into the prepositus hypoglossi and the medial vestibular nuclei on cat eye movements. J Neurophysiol 72, 785–802, 1994.

480. Michaelides M, Aligianis IA, Ainsworth JR, et al. Progressive cone dystrophy associated with mutation in CNGB3. Invest Ophthalmol Vis Sci 45, 1975–1982, 2004.

481. Minagar A, Sheremata WA, Tusa RJ. Perverted head-shaking nystagmus: a possible mechanism. Neurology 57, 887–889, 2001.

482. Minor LB, Haslwanter T, Straumann D, Zee DS. Hyperventilation-induced nystagmus in patients with vestibular schwannoma. Neurology 53, 2158–2168, 1999.

483. Minor LB, Solomon D, Zinreich JS, Zee DS. Sound- and/or pressure-induced vertigo due to bone dehiscence of the superior semicircular canal. Arch Otolaryngol Head Neck Surg 124, 249–258, 1998.

484. Mitchell WG, Snodgrass SR. Opsoclonus-ataxia due to childhood neural crest tumors: a chronic neurologic syndrome. J Child Neurol 5, 153–158, 1990.

485. Miura K, Hertle RW, FitzGibbon EJ, Optican LM. Effects of tenotomy surgery on congenital nystagmus waveforms in adult patients. Part I Wavelet spectral analysis. Vision Res 43, 2345–2356, 2003.

486. Miura K, Hertle RW, FitzGibbon EJ, Optican LM. Effects of tenotomy surgery on congenital nystagmus waveforms in adult patients. Part II Dynamical systems analysis. Vision Res 43, 2357–2362, 2003.

487. Morad Y, Benyamini OG, Avni I. Benign opsoclonus in preterm infants. Pediatr Neurol 31, 275–278, 2004.

488. Moreno-Lopez B, Escudero M, Estrada C. Nitric oxide facilitates GABAergic neurotransmission in the cat oculomotor system: a physiological mechanism in eye movement control. J Physiol 540, 295–306, 2002.

489. Moretti R, Torre P, Antonello D, Nasuelli D, Cazzato

G. Opsoclonus-myoclonus syndrome: gabapentin as a new therapeutic proposal. Eur J Neurol 7, 455–456, 2000.
490. Morrow MJ. Craniotopic defects of smooth pursuit and saccadic eye movement. Neurology 46, 514–521, 1996.
491. Morrow MJ, Sharpe JA. Torsional nystagmus in the lateral medullary syndrome. Ann Neurol 24, 390–398, 1988.
492. Mossman SS, Bronstein AM, Gresty MA, Kendall B, Rudge P. Convergence nystagmus associated with Arnold-Chiari malformation. Arch Neurol 47, 357–359, 1990.
493. Moster ML, Schnayder E. Epileptic periodic alternating nystagmus. J Neuroophthalmol 18, 292–293, 1998.
494. Mulder AH, Raemaekers JM, Boerman RH, Mattijssen V. Downbeat nystagmus caused by thiamine deficiency: an unusual presentation of CNS localization of large cell anaplastic CD 30–positive non-Hodgkin's lymphoma. Ann Hematol 78, 105–107, 1999.
495. Munoz DP, Wurtz RH. Fixation cells in monkey superior colliculus. II Reversible activation and deactivation. J Neurophysiol 70, 576–589, 1993.
496. Munro NA, Gaymard B, Rivaud S, Majdalani A, Pierrot-Deseilligny C. Upbeat nystagmus in a patient with a small medullary infarct. J Neurol Neurosurg Psychiatry 56, 1126–1128, 1993.
497. Mustari MJ, Tusa RJ, Burrows AF, Fuchs AF, Livingston CA. Gaze-stabilizing deficits and latent nystagmus in monkeys with early-onset visual deprivation: role of the pretectal not. J Neurophysiol 86, 662–675, 2001.
498. Nakada T, Kwee IL. Oculopalatal myoclonus. Brain 109, 431–441, 1986.
499. Nakada T, Kwee IL. Seesaw nystagmus. Role of visuovestibular interaction in its pathogenesis. J Clin Neuroophthalmol 8, 171–177, 1988.
500. Nakada T, Remler MP. Primary position upbeat nystagmus: another central vestibular nystagmus? J Clin Neuroophthalmol 1, 181–185, 1981.
501. Nakamagoe K, Iwamoto Y, Yoshida K. Evidence for brainstem structures participating in oculomotor integration. Science 288, 857–859, 2000.
502. Narfstrom K, Katz ML, Bragadottir R, et al. Functional and structural recovery of the retina after gene therapy in the RPE65 null mutation dog. Invest Ophthalmol Vis Sci 44, 1663–1672, 2003.
503. Nathanson M, Bergman PS. Visual disturbances as the result of nystagmus on direct forward gaze. Arch Neurol Psychiatry 69, 427–435, 1953.
504. Navarro-Lopez JD, Alvarado JC, Marquez-Ruiz J, et al. A cholinergic synaptically triggered event participates in the generation of persistent activity necessary for eye fixation. J Neurosci 24, 5109–5118, 2004.
505. Nedzelski JM. Cerebellopontine angle tumors: bilateral flocculus compression as a cause of associated oculomotor abnormalities. Laryngoscope 93, 1251–1260, 1983.
506. Nishie M, Yoshida Y, Hirata Y, Matsunaga M. Generation of symptomatic palatal tremor is not correlated with inferior olivary hypertrophy. Brain 125, 1348–1357, 2002.
507. Nitschke M, Hochberg F, Dropcho E. Improvement of paraneoplastic opsoclonus-myoclonus after protein A column therapy. N Engl J Med 332, 192, 1995.
508. Norton EW, Cogan DG. Spasmus nutans: a clinical study of twenty cases followed two years or more since onset. Arch Ophthalmol 52, 442–446, 1954.
509. Noseworthy JH, Ebers GC, Leigh RJ, Dell'Osso LF. Torsional nystagmus: quantitative features and possible pathogenesis. Neurology 38, 992–994, 1988.
510. Nowack WJ, Clark GF. Vertical nystagmus and thalamic arteriovenous malformation. Report of a case. Neuro-ophthalmology 6, 169–172, 1986.
511. Nozaki S, Mukuno K, Ishikawa S. Internuclear ophthalmoplegia associated with ipsilateral downbeat and contralateral incyclorotatory nystagmus. Ophthalmologica 187, 210–216, 1983.
512. O'Sullivan JD, Maruff P, Tyler P, et al. Unilateral pallidotomy for Parkinson's disease disrupts ocular fixation. J Clin Neurosci 10, 181–185, 2003.
513. Ochs AL, Stark L, Hoyt WF, D'Amico D. Opposed adducting saccades in convergence-retraction nystagmus. A patient with sylvian aqueduct syndrome. Brain 102, 479–508, 1979.
514. Oetting WS, Armstrong CM, Holleschau AM, DeWan AT, Summers GC. Evidence for genetic heterogeneity in families with congenital motor nystagmus (CN). Ophthalmic Genet 21, 227–233, 2000.
515. Oguro K, Kobayashi J, Aiba H, Hojo H. Opsoclonus-myoclonus syndrome with abnormal single photon emission computed tomography imaging. Pediatric Neurol 16, 334–336, 1997.
516. Ohkoshi N, Komatsu Y, Mizusawa H, Kanazawa I. Primary position upbeat nystagmus increased on downward gaze: clinicopathologic study of a patient with multiple sclerosis. Neurology 50, 551–553, 1998.
517. Oliva A, Rosenberg ML. Convergence-evoked nystagmus. Neurology 40, 161–162, 1990.
518. Olson JL, Jacobson DM. Comparison of clinical associations of patients with vasculopathic and idiopathic downbeat nystagmus. J Neuroophthalmol 21, 39–41, 2001.
519. Ono S, Das VE, Economides JR, Mustari MJ. Modeling of smooth pursuit-related neuronal responses in the DLPN and NRTP of the rhesus macaque. J Neurophysiol 93, 108–116, 2005.
520. Optican LM, Robinson DA. Cerebellar-dependent adaptive control of primate saccadic system. J Neurophysiol 44, 1058–1076, 1980.
521. Optican LM, Zee DS. A hypothetical explanation of congenital nystagmus. Biol Cyber 50, 119–134, 1984.
522. Orwitz JI, Galetta SL, Teener JW. Bilateral trochlear nerve palsy and downbeat nystagmus in a patient with cephalic tetanus. Neurology 49, 894–895, 1997.
523. Ostrowski VB, Byskosh A, Hain TC. Tullio phenomenon with dehiscence of the superior semicircular canal. Otol Neurotol 22, 61–65, 2001.
524. Pasik T, Pasik P, Valciukas A. Nystagmus induced by stationary repetitive light flashes in monkeys. Brain Res 19, 313–317, 1970.
525. Pedersen RA, Troost BT, Abel LA, Zorub D. Intermittent downbeat nystagmus and oscillopsia reversed by suboccipital craniectomy. Neurology 30, 1239–1242, 1980.
526. Pereira CB, Strupp M, Eggert T, Straube A, Brandt

T. Nicotine-induced nystagmus: three-dimensional analysis and dependence on head position. Neurology 55, 1563–1566, 2000.
527. Perez P, Llorente JL, Gomez JR, et al. Functional significance of peripheral head-shaking nystagmus. Laryngoscope 114, 1078–1084, 2004.
527a. Petzold A, Plant GT. Optic flow induced nystagmus. J Neurol Neurosurg Psychiatry 76, 1173–1174, 2005.
528. Phadke JG, Hern JEC, Blaiklock CT. Downbeat nystagmus—a false localizing sign due to communicating hydrocephalus. J Neurol Neurosurg Psychiatry 44, 459, 1981.
529. Pierrot-Deseilligny C, Milea D. Vertical nystagmus: clinical facts and hypotheses. Brain 128, 1237–1246, 2005.
530. Pinel JF, Larmande P, Guegan Y, Iba-Zisen MT. Down-beat nystagmus: case report with magnetic resonance imaging and surgical treatment. Neurosurgery 21, 736–739, 1987.
531. Pless M, Ronthal M. Treatment of opsoclonus-myoclonus with high-dose intravenous immunoglobulin. Neurology 46, 583–584, 1996.
532. Posner JB. Neurological complications of cancer. FA Davis, Philadelphia, 1995.
533. Posner JB, Dalmau JO. Paraneoplastic syndromes affecting the central nervous system. Ann Rev Med 48, 157–166, 1997.
534. Pranzatelli MR. The neurobiology of the opsoclonus-myoclonus syndrome. Clin Neuropharmacol 15, 186–228, 1992.
535. Pranzatelli MR, Huang Y, Tate E, et al. Cerebrospinal fluid 5–hydroxyindoleacetic acid and homovanillic acid in the pediatric opsoclonus-myoclonus syndrome. Ann Neurol 37, 189–197, 1995.
536. Pranzatelli MR, Tate ED, Kinsbourne M, Caviness VC, Mishra B. Forty-one-year follow-up of childhood-onset opsoclonus-myoclonus-ataxia: cerebellar atrophy, multiphasic relapses and response to IVIG. Mov Disord 17, 1387–1390, 2002.
537. Pranzatelli MR, Tate ED, Travelstead AL, Longee D. Immunologic and clinical responses to rituximab in a child with opsoclonus-myoclonus syndrome. Pediatrics 115, e115–e119, 2005.
538. Pranzatelli MR, Travelstead AL, Tate ED, Allison TJ, Verhulst SJ. CSF B-cell expansion in opsoclonus-myoclonus syndrome: a biomarker of disease activity. Mov Disord 19, 770–777, 2004.
539. Pratt-Johnson JA, Tillson G. Intractable diplopia after vision restoration in unilateral cataract. Am J Ophthalmol 107, 23–26, 1989.
540. Pritchard C, Flynn JT, Smith JL. Wave form characteristics of vertical oscillations in longstanding vision loss. J Pediatr Ophthalmol Strabismus 25, 233–236, 1988.
541. Proudlock FA, Gottlob I, Constantinescu CS. Oscillopsia without nystagmus caused by head titubation in a patient with multiple sclerosis. J Neuroophthalmol 22, 88–91, 2002.
542. Pullicino P, Aquilina J. Opsoclonus in organophosphate poisoning. Arch Neurol 46, 704–705, 1989.
543. Pullicino P, Lincoff N, Truax BT. Abnormal vergence with upper brainstem infarcts: pseudoabducens palsy. Neurology 55, 352–358, 2000.
544. Rabiah PK, Bateman JB, Demer JL, Perlman S. Ophthalmologic findings in patients with cerebellar ataxia. Am J Ophthalmol 123, 108–117, 1997.
545. Rabiah PK, Smith SD, Awad AH, et al. Results of surgery for bilateral cataract associated with sensory nystagmus in children. Am J Ophthalmol 134, 586–591, 2002.
546. Ragge NK, Hartley C, Dearlove AM, et al. Familial vestibulocerebellar disorder maps to chromosome 13q31–q33: a new nystagmus locus. J Med Genet 40, 37–41, 2003.
547. Rajput AJ, McHattie JD. Ophthalmoplegia and leg myorhythmia in Whipple's disease. Mov Disord 12, 111–114, 1997.
548. Ramat S, Leigh RJ, Zee DS, Optican LM. Ocular oscillations generated by coupling of brainstem excitatory and inhibitory saccadic burst neurons. Exp Brain Res 160, 89–106, 2005.
549. Ramat S, Somers JT, Das VE, Leigh RJ. Conjugate ocular oscillations during shifts of the direction and depth of visual fixation. Invest Ophthalmol Vis Sci 40, 1681–1686, 1999.
550. Ramat S, Zee DS, Leigh RJ, Optican LM. Familial microsaccadic oscillations may be due to alterations in the inhibitory premotor circuit. Soc Neurosci Abstr 475.15, 2005.
551. Rambold H, Heide W, Sprenger A, Haendler G, Helmchen C. Perilymph fistula associated with pulse-synchronous eye oscillations. Neurology 56, 1769–1771, 2001.
552. Rambold H, Helmchen C, Büttner U. Unilateral muscimol inactivations of the interstitial nucleus of Cajal in the alert rhesus monkey do not elicit seesaw nystagmus. Neurosci Lett 272, 75–78, 1999.
553. Rambold H, Helmchen C, Straube A, Büttner U. Seesaw nystagmus associated with involuntary torsional head oscillations. Neurology 51, 831–837, 1998.
554. Rambold H, Kompf D, Helmchen C. Convergence retraction nystagmus: a disorder of vergence? Ann Neurol 50, 677–681, 2001.
555. Ranalli PJ, Sharpe JA. Contrapulsion of saccades and ipsilateral ataxia: a unilateral disorder of the rostral cerebellum. Ann Neurol 20, 311–316, 1986.
556. Ranalli PJ, Sharpe JA. Upbeat nystagmus and the ventral tegmental pathway of the upward vestibulo-ocular reflex. Neurology 38, 1329–1330, 1988.
557. Rascol O, Sabatini U, Simonetta-Moreau M, et al. Square wave jerks in Parkinsonian syndromes. J Neurol Neurosurg Psychiatry 54, 599–602, 1991.
558. Rashbass C. Barbiturate nystagmus and mechanics of visual fixation. Nature 183, 897–898, 1959.
559. Reiji K, Sakamoto M, Tanaka K, Hayashi H. Opsoclonus-myoclonus syndrome during pregnancy. J Neuroophthalmol 24, 273, 2004.
560. Reinecke RD, Guo S, Goldstein HP. Waveform evolution in infantile nystagmus: an electro-oculo-graphic study of 35 cases. Binocular Vision 31, 191–202, 1988.
561. Remler BF, Leigh RJ, Osorio I, Tomsak RL. The characteristics and mechanisms of visual disturbance associated with anticonvulsant therapy. Neurology 40, 791–796, 1990.
562. Repka MX, Savino PJ, Reinecke RD. Treatment of acquired nystagmus with botulinum neurotoxin A. Arch Ophthalmol 112, 1320–1324, 1994.

563. Ridley A, Kennard C, Scholtz CL, et al. Omnipause neurons in two cases of opsoclonus associated with oat cell carcinoma of the lung. Brain 110, 1699–1709, 1987.
564. Rivner MH, Jay WM, Green JB, Dyken PR. Opsoclonus in hemophilus influenza meningitis. Neurology 32, 661–663, 1982.
565. Robinson DA. The effect of cerebellectomy on the cat's vestibulo-ocular integrator. Brain Res 71, 195–207, 1974.
566. Robinson DA. The control of eye movements. In Brookhart JM, Mountcastle VB (eds). Handbook of Physiology: The Nervous System vol. II part 2. American Physiological Society, Bethesda MD, 1981.
567. Robinson DA, Zee DS, Hain TC, Holmes A, Rosenberg LF. Alexander's law: its behavior and origin in the human vestibulo-ocular reflex. Ann Neurol 16, 714–722, 1984.
568. Robinson FR, Straube A, Fuchs AF. Role of the caudal fastigial nucleus in saccade generation. II Effects of muscimol inactivation. J Neurophysiol 70, 1741–1758, 1993.
569. Rogawski MA, Wenk GL. The neuropharmacological basis for the use of memantine in the treatment of Alzheimer's disease. CNS Drug Reviews 9, 275–308, 2003.
570. Rosa A, Masmoudi K, Barvieux D, Mizon JP, Cartz L. Opsoclonus with virus A hepatitis. Neuroophthalmol 8, 275–279, 1988.
571. Rosenberg ML. Reversible downbeat nystagmus secondary to excessive alcohol intake. J Clin Neuro-ophthalmol 7, 23–25, 1987.
572. Rosengart A, Hedge TR 3rd, Teal PA, et al. Intermittent downbeat nystagmus due to vertebral artery compression. Neurology 43, 216–218, 1993.
573. Rosenthal JG, Selhorst JB. Continuous non-rhythmic cycloversion. A possible paraneoplastic disorder. Neuroophthalmol 7, 291–295, 1987.
574. Rottach KG, Das VE, Wohlgemuth W, Zivotofsky AZ, Leigh RJ. Properties of horizontal saccades accompanied by blinks. J Neurophysiol 79, 2895–2902, 1998.
575. Rottach KG, von Maydell RD, DiScenna NO, et al. Quantitative measurements of eye movements in a patient with Tullio phenomenon. J Vestib Res 6, 255–259, 1996, 1996.
576. Rottach KG, Wohlgemuth WA, Dzaja AE, Eggert T, Straube A. Effects of intravenous opioids on eye movements in humans: possible mechanisms. J Neurol 249, 1200–1205, 2002.
577. Ruben ST, Lee JP, Oneil D, Dunlop I, Elston JS. The use of botulinum toxin for treatment of acquired nystagmus and oscillopsia. Ophthalmology 101, 783–787, 1994.
578. Rucker JC. Current treatment of nystagmus. Curr Treat Options Neurol 7, 69–77, 2005.
579. Ruigrok TJ, de Zeeuw CI, Voogd J. Hypertrophy of inferior olivary neurons: a degenerative regenerative or plasticity phenomenon. Eur J Morphol 28, 224–239, 1990.
580. Rushton D, Cox N. A new optical treatment for oscillopsia. J Neurol Neurosurg Psychiatry 50, 411–415, 1987.
581. Safran AB, Berney J, Safran E. Convergence-evoked eyelid nystagmus. Am J Ophthalmol 93, 48, 1982.
582. Sakai T, Shiraishi S, Murakami S. Palatal myoclonus responding to carbamazepine. Ann Neurol 9, 199–200, 1981.
583. Sakellari V, Bronstein AM, Corna S, et al. The effects of hyperventilation on postural control mechanisms. Brain 120, 1659–1673, 1997.
584. Salonen R, Nikoskelainen E, Aantaa E, Marttila R. Ocular flutter associated with sarcoidosis. Neuroophthalmol 8, 77–79, 1988.
585. Samkoff LM, Smith CR. See-saw nystagmus in a patient with clinically definite MS. Eur Neurol 34, 228–229, 1994.
585a. Sampangi R, Chaudhuri Z, Menon V, Saxena R. Cone-rod dystrophy and acquired dissociated vertical nystagmus. J Pediatr Ophthalmol Strabismus 42, 114–116, 2005.
586. Samuel M, Torun N, Tuite PJ, Sharpe JA, Lang AE. Progressive ataxia and palatal tremor (PAPT): clinical and MRI assessment with review of palatal tremors. Brain 127, 1252–1268, 2004.
587. Sanders MD, Glaser JS. Alternating windmill nystagmus. In Smith JL (ed). Neuro-ophthalmology Vol 7. CV Mosby, St. Louis, 1973, pp 133–136.
588. Sanders MD, Hoyt WF, Daroff RB. Lid nystagmus evoked by ocular convergence: an ocular electromyographic study. J Neurol Neurosurg Psychiatry 31, 368–371, 1968.
589. Sano K, Sekino H, Tsukamoto N, Yoshimasu N, Ishijima B. Stimulation and destruction of the region of the interstitial nucleus in cases of torticollis and see-saw nystagmus. Confin Neurol 34, 331–338, 1972.
590. Saul R, Selhorst JB. Downbeat nystagmus with magnesium depletion. Arch Neurol 38, 650–652, 1981.
591. Sawyer RN, Thurston SE, Becker KR, et al. The cervico-ocular reflex of normal human subjects in response to transient and sinusoidal trunk rotations. J Vestib Res 4, 245–249, 1994.
592. Scharf D. Opsoclonus-myoclonus following the intranasal usage of cocaine. J Neurol Neurosurg Psychiatry 59, 1447–1448, 1989.
593. Schmidt D, Dell'Osso LF, Abel LA, Daroff RB. Myasthenia gravis: saccadic eye movement waveforms. Exp Neurol 68, 346–364, 1980.
594. Schmidt D, Kommerell G. Congenitaler Schaukelnystagmus (seesaw nystagmus): Ein fall mit erhaltenen gesichtsfeldern vertikaler blickparese und kopftremor. Graefes Arch Klin Exp Ophthalmol 191, 265–272, 1974.
595. Schmidt D, Neumann HPH, Eggert HR, Friedburg H. Neuro-Ophthalmologischer Befund bei Hamangioblastom des Kleinhirnsund des Hirnstamms—Downbeat-Nystagmus als Erstsymptom eines Hamangioblastoms beir v. Hippel-Lindau Erkrankung. Fortschr Ophthalmol 85, 427–433, 1988.
596. Schmitz B, Kasmann-Kellner B, Schafer T, et al. Monocular visual activation patterns in albinism as revealed by functional magnetic resonance imaging. Hum Brain Mapp 23, 40–52, 2004.
597. Schneider E, Glasauer S, Dieterich M, Kalla R, Brandt T. Diagnosis of vestibular imbalance in the blink of an eye. Neurology 63, 1209–1216, 2004.
598. Schon F, Hart PE, Hodgson TL, et al. Suppression of pendular nystagmus by smoking cannabis in a patient with multiple sclerosis. Neurology 53, 2209–2210, 1999.

599. Schon F, Hodgson TL, Mort D, Kennard C. Ocular flutter associated with a localized lesion in the paramedian pontine reticular formation. Ann Neurol 50, 413–416, 2001.
600. Schor CM, Fusaro RE, Wilson N, McKee SP. Prediction of early-onset esotropia from components of the infantile squint syndrome. Invest Ophthalmol Vis Sci 38, 719–740, 1997.
601. Schwankhaus JD, Kattah JC, Lux WE, Masucci EF, Kurtzke JF. Primidone/phenobarbital-induced periodic alternating nystagmus. Ann Ophthalmol 21, 230–232, 1989.
602. Schwartz MA, Selhorst JB, Alfred S, et al. Oculomasticatory myorhythmia: s unique movement disorder occurring in Whipple's disease. Ann Neurol 20, 677–683, 1986.
603. Seidman SH, Telford L, Paige GD. Vertical torsional and horizontal eye movement responses to head roll in the squirrel monkey. Exp Brain Res 104, 218–226, 1995.
604. Selhorst JB, Stark L, Ochs AL, Hoyt WF. Disorders in cerebellar ocular motor control. I Saccadic overshoot dysmetria an oculographic control system and clinico-anatomic analysis. Brain 99, 497–508, 1976.
605. Selhorst JB, Stark L, Ochs AL, Hoyt WF. Disorders in cerebellar ocular motor control. II Macrosaccadic oscillation. An oculographic control system and clinico-anatomical analysis. Brain 99, 509–522, 1976.
606. Selhorst JB, Stark L, Ochs AL, Hoyt WF. Disorders in cerebellar ocular motor control. II Macrosaccadic oscillations. An oculographic control system and clinico-anatomic analysis. Brain 99, 509–522, 1976.
607. Sendler S, Shallo-Hoffmann J, Mühlendyck H. Die Artifizielle-Divergenz-Operation beim kongenitale Nystagmus. Fortschr Ophthalmol 87, 85–89, 1990.
608. Serra A, Leigh RJ. Diagnostic value of nystagmus: spontaneous and induced ocular oscillations. J Neurol Neurosurg Psychiatry 73, 615–618, 2002.
609. Shallo-Hoffmann J, Faldon M, Tusa RJ. The incidence and waveform characteristics of periodic alternating nystagmus in congenital nystagmus. Invest Ophthalmol Vis Sci 40, 2546–2553, 1999.
610. Shallo-Hoffmann J, Petersen J, Muhlendyck H. How normal are "normal" square wave jerks? Invest Ophthalmol Vis Sci 30, 1009–1011, 1989.
611. Shallo-Hoffmann J, Riordan-Eva P. Recognizing periodic alternating nystagmus. Strabismus 9, 203–215, 2001.
612. Shallo-Hoffmann J, Schwarze H, Simonsz H, Muhlendyck H. A reexamination of end-point and rebound nystagmus in normals. Invest Ophthalmol Vis Sci 31, 388–392, 1990.
613. Shallo-Hoffmann J, Sendler B, Muhlendyck H. Normal square wave jerks in differing age groups. Invest Ophthalmol Vis Sci 31, 1649–1652, 1990.
614. Shallo-Hoffmann JA, Bronstein AM, Acheson J, Morland AB, Gresty MA. Vertical and horizontal motion perception in congenital nystagmus. Neuroophthalmol 19, 171–183, 1998.
615. Sharma P, Tandon R, Kumar S, Anand S. Reduction of congenital nystagmus amplitude with auditory biofeedback. J AAPOS 4, 287–290, 2000.
616. Sharpe JA, Herishanu YO, White OB. Cerebral square wave jerks. Neurology 32, 57–62, 1982.
617. Sharpe JA, Hoyt WF, Rosenberg MA. Convergence-evoked nystagmus: congenital and acquired forms. Arch Neurol 32, 191–194, 1975.
618. Sharpe JA, Lo AW, Rabinovitch HE. Control of the saccadic and smooth pursuit systems after cerebral hemidecortication. Brain 102, 387–403, 1979.
619. Shaw FS, Kriss A, Russel-Eggitt I, Taylor D, Harris C. Diagnosing children presenting with asymmetric pendular nystagmus. Dev Med Child Neurol 43, 622–627, 2001.
620. Shawkat FS, Harris CM, Taylor DS. Spontaneous reversal of nystagmus in the dark. Br J Ophthalmol 85, 428–431, 2001.
621. Shawkat FS, Harris CM, Taylor DS, et al. The optokinetic response differences between congenital profound and nonprofound unilateral visual deprivation. Ophthalmology 102, 1615–1622, 1995.
622. Shawkat FS, Harris CM, Wilson J, Taylor DS. Eye movements in children with opsoclonus-polymyoclonus. Neuropediatrics 24, 218–223, 1993.
623. Sheliga BM, Chen KJ, FitzGibbon EJ, Miles FA. Short-latency disparity vergence in humans: evidence for early spatial filtering. Ann N Y Acad Sci 1039, 252–259, 2005.
624. Sheth NV, Dell'Osso LF, Leigh RJ, Peckham HP. The effects of afferent stimulation on congenital nystagmus foveation periods. Vision Res 35, 2371–2382, 1995.
625. Shetty L, Rosman NP. Opsoclonus in hydrocephalus. Arch Ophthalmol 88, 585–589, 1972.
626. Shibasaki H, Motomura S. Suppression of congenital nystagmus. J Neurol Neurosurg Psychiatry 41, 1078–1083, 1978.
627. Sibony PA, Evinger C, Manning K. Tobacco-induced primary-position upbeat nystagmus. Ann Neurol 21, 53–58, 1987.
628. Sibony PA, Evinger C, Manning K, Pellegrini JJ. Nicotine and tobacco-induced nystagmus. Ann Neurol 28, 198, 1990.
629. Sibony PA, Evinger C, Manning KA. The effects of tobacco smoking on smooth pursuit eye movements. Ann Neurol 23, 238–241, 1988.
630. Simon RP. Forced downward ocular deviation. Occurrence during oculovestibular testing in sedative drug-induced coma. Arch Neurol 35, 456–458, 1978.
631. Slatt B, Nykiel F. See-saw nystagmus. Am J Ophthalmol 58, 1016–1021, 1964.
632. Slavin ML, Rosenberg ML. Unusual associations of downbeat nystagmus. Neuroophthalmol 5, 265–270, 1985.
633. Smith DE, Fitzgerald K, Stass-Isern M, Cibis GW. Electroretinography is necessary for spasmus nutans diagnosis. Pediatr Neurol 23, 33–36, 2000.
634. Smith JL, Walsh FB. Opsoclonus—ataxic conjugate movements of the eyes. Arch Ophthalmol 64, 244–250, 1960.
635. Smith RM, Oommen BS, Stahl JS. Application of adaptive filters to visual testing and treatment in acquired pendular nystagmus. J Rehabil Res Dev 41, 313–324, 2004.
636. Smith RM, Oommen BS, Stahl JS. Image-shifting optics for a nystagmus treatment device. J Rehabil Res Dev 41, 325–336, 2004.
637. Soetedjo R, Kaneko CR, Fuchs AF. Evidence that the superior colliculus participates in the feedback

control of saccadic eye movements. J Neurophysiol 87, 679–695, 2002.
638. Sogg RL, Hoyt WF. Intermittent vertical nystagmus in a father and son. Arch Ophthalmol 68, 515–517, 1962.
639. Solomon D, Galetta SL, Liu GT. Possible mechanisms for horizontal gaze deviation and lateropulsion in the lateral medullary syndrome. J Neuro-ophthalmol 15, 26–30, 1995.
640. Solomon D, Shepard N, Mishra A. Congenital periodic alternating nystagmus: response to baclofen. Ann N Y Acad Sci 956, 611–615, 2002.
641. Specht U, May TW, Rohde M, et al. Cerebellar atrophy decreases the threshold of carbamazepine toxicity in patients with chronic focal epilepsy. Arch Neurol 54, 427–431, 1997.
642. Spencer RF, Baker R. Histochemical localization of acetycholinesterase in relation to motor neurons and internuclear neurons of the cat abducens nucleus. J Neurocytol 15, 137–154, 1986.
643. Spencer RF, Wenthold RJ, Baker R. Evidence for glycine as an inhibitory neurotransmitter of vestibular reticular and prepositus hypoglossi neurons that project to the cat abducens nucleus. J Neurosci 9, 2718–2736, 1989.
644. Sperling MR, Herrmann J. Syndrome of palatal myoclonus and progressive ataxia: two cases with magnetic resonance imaging. Neurology 35, 1212–1214, 1985.
645. Spielmann A. Clinical rationale for manifest congenital nystagmus surgery. J AAPOS 4, 67–74, 2000.
646. Spooner JW, Baloh RW. Arnold-Chiari malformation. Improvement in eye movements after surgical treatment. Brain 104, 51–60, 1981.
647. Stahl JS. Eye movements of the murine P/Q calcium channel mutant rocker and the impact of aging. J Neurophysiol 91, 2066–2078, 2004.
648. Stahl JS, Averbuch-Heller L, Leigh RJ. Acquired nystagmus. Arch Ophthalmol 118, 544–549, 2000.
649. Stahl JS, Lehmkuhle M, Wu K, et al. Prospects for treating acquired pendular nystagmus with servo-controlled optics. Invest Ophthalmol Vis Sci 41, 1084–1090, 2000.
650. Stahl JS, Plant GT, Leigh RJ. Medical treatment of nystagmus and its visual consequences. J R Soc Med 95, 235–237, 2002.
651. Stahl JS, Rottach KG, Averbuch-Heller L, et al. A pilot study of gabapentin as treatment for acquired nystagmus. Neuroophthalmol 16, 107–113, 1996.
652. Starck M, Albrecht H, Straube A, Dieterich M. Drug therapy for acquired pendular nystagmus in multiple sclerosis. J Neurology 244, 9–16, 1997.
653. Staudenmaier C, Buncic JR. Periodic alternating gaze deviation with dissociated secondary face turn. Arch Ophthalmol 101, 202–205, 1983.
654. Steinman RM, Haddad GM, Skavenski AA, Wyman D. Miniature eye movement. Science 181, 810–819, 1973.
655. Stell R, Bronstein AM, Plant GT, Harding AE. Ataxia telangiectasia: a reappraisal of the ocular motor features and their value in the diagnosis of atypical cases. Mov Disord 4, 320–329, 1989.
656. Stevens DJ, Hertle RW. Relationships between visual acuity and anomalous head posture in patients with congenital nystagmus. J Pediatr Ophthalmol Strabismus 40, 259–264, 2003.
657. Stevenson SB. Visual processing in vertical disparity control. Ann N Y Acad Sci 456, 492–494, 2002.
658. Straube A, Brandt T. Recurrent attacks with skew deviation, torsional nystagmus and contractions of the left frontalis muscle. Neurology 44, 17–18, 1994.
659. Straube A, Kurzan R, Büttner U. Differential effects of bicuculline and muscimol microinjections into the vestibular nuclei on simian eye movements. Exp Brain Res 86, 347–358, 1991.
660. Straube A, Leigh RJ, Bronstein A, et al. EFNS task force—therapy of nystagmus and oscillopsia. Eur J Neurol 11, 83–89, 2004.
661. Straumann D, Müller E. Torsional rebound nystagmus in a patient with type I Chiari malformation. Neuroophthalmol 14, 79–84, 1994.
662. Straumann D, Zee DS, Solomon D. Three-dimensional kinematics of ocular drift in humans with cerebellar atrophy. J Neurophysiol 83, 1125–1140, 2000.
663. Strupp M, Kalla R, Dichgans M, et al. Treatment of episodic ataxia type 2 with the potassium channel blocker 4–aminopyridine. Neurology 62, 1623–1625, 2004.
664. Strupp M, Planck JH, Arbusow V, et al. Rotational vertebral artery occlusion syndrome with vertigo due to "labyrinthine excitation". Neurology 54, 1376–1379, 2000.
665. Strupp M, Schuler O, Krafczyk S, et al. Treatment of downbeat nystagmus with 3,4–diaminopyridine: a placebo-controlled study. Neurology 61, 165–170, 2003.
665a. Suzuki Y, Matsuda T, Washio N, Ohtsuka K. Transition from upbeat to downbeat nystagmus observed in a patient with Wernicke's encephalopathy. Jpn J Ophthalmol 49, 220–222, 2005.
666. Swartz BE, Li S, Bespalova I, et al. Pathogenesis of clinical signs in recessive cerebellar ataxia with saccadic intrusions and sensorimotor neuropathy (SCASI). Ann Neurol 54, 824–828, 2003.
667. Takahashi S, Fetter M, Koenig E, Dichgans J. The clinical significance of head-shaking nystagmus in the dizzy patient. Acta Otolaryngol (Stockh) 109, 8–14, 1990.
668. Talks SJ, Elston JS. Oculopalatal myoclonus: eye movement studies, MRI findings and the difficulty of treatment. Eye 11, 19–24, 1997.
669. Tate ED, Allison TJ, Pranzatelli MR, Verhulst SJ. Neuroepidemiologic trends in 105 US cases of pediatric opsoclonus-myoclonus syndrome. J Pediatr Oncol Nurs 22, 8–19, 2005.
670. Taylor JR, Selhorst JB, Houff SA, Martinez AJ. Chlordecone intoxication in man. I Clinical observations. Neurology 28, 626–630, 1978.
670a. Thakore NJ, Pioro EP, Rucker JC, Leigh RJ. Motor neuronopathy with dropped hands and downbeat nystagmus. A distinctive disorder? BMC Neurology, in press, 2006.
671. Tilikete C, Hermier M, Pelisson D, Vighetto A. Saccadic lateropulsion and upbeat nystagmus: disorders of caudal medulla. Ann Neurol 52, 658–662, 2002.
672. Tilikete C, Vighetto A, Trouillas P, Honnorat J. Potential role of anti-GAD antibodies in abnormal eye movements. Ann N Y Acad Sci 1039, 446–454, 2005.
672a. Tilikete C, Vighetto A, Trouillas P, Honnorat J. Anti-GAD antibodies and periodic alternating nystagmus. Arch Neurol 62, 1300–1303, 2005.

673. Tkalcevic LA, Abel LA. The effects of increased visual task demand on foveation in congenital nystagmus. Vision Res 45, 1139–1146, 2005.
674. Tomsak RL, Remler BF, Averbuch-Heller L, Chandran M, Leigh RJ. Unsatisfactory treatment of acquired nystagmus with retrobulbar botulinum toxin. Am J Ophthalmol 119, 489–496, 1995.
675. Traccis S, Rosati G, Aiello I, et al. Upbeat nystagmus as an early sign of cerebellar astrocytoma. J Neurol 236, 359–360, 1989.
676. Traccis S, Rosati G, Monaco MF, Aiello I, Agnetti V. Successful treatment of acquired pendular elliptical nystagmus in multiple sclerosis with isoniazid and base-out prisms. Neurology 40, 492–494, 1990.
677. Trillenberg P, Zee DS, Shelhamer M. On the distribution of fast-phase intervals in optokinetic and vestibular nystagmus. Biol Cybern 87, 68–78, 2002.
678. Trobe JD, Sharpe JA, Hirsh DK, Gebarski SS. Nystagmus of Pelizaeus-Merzbacher disease. Arch Neurol 48, 87–91, 1991.
679. Troost BT, Daroff RB. The ocular motor defects in progressive supranuclear palsy. Ann Neurol 2, 397–403, 1977.
680. Troost BT, Martinez J, Abel LA, Heros RC. Upbeat nystagmus and internuclear ophthalmoplegia with brain stem glioma. Arch Neurol 37, 453–456, 1980.
681. Tusa RJ, Hove MT. Ocular and oculomotor signs in Joubert syndrome. J Child Neurol 14, 621–627, 1999.
682. Tusa RJ, Mustari MJ, Burrows AF, Fuchs AF. Gaze-stabilizing deficits and latent nystagmus in monkeys with brief early-onset visual deprivation: eye movement recordings. J Neurophysiol 86, 651–661, 2001.
683. Tusa RJ, Mustari MJ, Das VE, Boothe RG. Animal models for visual deprivation-induced strabismus and nystagmus. Ann N Y Acad Sci 956, 346–360, 2002.
684. Tusa RJ, Zee DS, Hain TC, Simonsz HJ. Voluntary control of congenital nystagmus. Clin Vision Sci 7, 195–210, 1992.
685. Tychsen L, Lisberger SG. Maldevelopment of visual motion processing in humans who had strabismus with onset in infancy. J Neurosci 6, 2495–2508, 1986.
686. Tychsen L, Sitaram N. Catecholamine depletion produces irrepressible saccadic eye movements in normal humans. Ann Neurol 25, 444–449, 1989.
687. Uchino Y, Sasaki M, Isu N, et al. Second-order vestibular neuron morphology of the extra-MLF anterior canal pathway in the cat. Exp Brain Res 97, 387–396, 1994.
688. Uemura T, Cohen B. Effects of vestibular nuclei lesions on vestibulo-ocular reflexes and posture in monkeys. Acta Otolaryhgol (Stockh) (Suppl)315, 1–71, 1973.
689. Ukwade MT, Bedell HE. Stereothresholds in persons wtih congenital nystagmus and in normal observers during comparable retinal image motion. Vision Res 39, 2963–2973, 1999.
690. Valenzuela A, Cline RA. Ocular and nonocular findings in patients with aniridia. Can J Ophthalmol 39, 632–638, 2004.
691. Van Rijn LJ, Simonsz HJ, ten Tusscher MPM Dissociated vertical deviation and eye torsion: relation to disparity-induced vertical vergence. Strabismus 5, 13–20, 1997.
692. Vincent MC, Gallai R, Olivier D, et al. Variable phenotype related to a novel PAX 6 mutation (IVS4+5G:C) in a family presenting congenital nystagmus and foveal hypoplasia. Am J Ophthalmol 138, 1016–1021, 2004.
693. von Noorden GK, Campos EC. Binocular Vision and Ocular Motility. Mosby, St. Louis, 2001.
694. von Noorden GK, Munoz M, Wong SY. Compensatory mechanisms in congenital nystagmus. Am J Ophthalmol 104, 387–397, 1987.
695. von Noorden GK, Sprunger DT. Large rectus muscle recession for the treatment of congenital nystagmus. Arch Ophthalmol 109, 221–224, 1991.
696. Waespe W, Cohen B, Raphan T. Dynamic modification of the vestibulo-ocular reflex by the nodulus and uvula. Science 228, 199–202, 1985.
697. Waespe W, Wichmann W. Oculomotor disturbances during visual-vestibular interaction in Wallenberg's lateral medullary syndrome. Brain 113, 821–846, 1990.
698. Waitzman DM, Silakov VL, Palma-Bowles S, Ayers AS. Effects of reversible inactivation of the primate mesencephalic reticular formation. I Hypermetric goal-directed saccades. J Neurophysiol 83, 2260–2284, 2000.
699. Walker MF, Zee DS. Directional abnormalities of vestibular and optokinetic responses in cerebellar disease. Ann N Y Acad Sci 871, 205–220, 1999.
700. Walker MF, Zee DS. The effect of hyperventilation on downbeat nystagmus in cerebellar disorders. Neurology 53, 1576–1579, 1999.
701. Walker MF, Zee DS. Asymmetry of the pitch vestibulo-ocular reflex in patients with cerebellar disease. Ann N Y Acad Sci 1039, 349–358, 2005.
702. Washio N, Suzuki Y, Yamaki T, Kase M, Ohtsuka K. Vertical-torsional oscillations and dissociated bilateral horizontal gaze palsy in a patient with a pontine cavernous angioma. J Neurol Neurosurg Psychiatry 76, 283–285, 2005.
703. Weber H, Fischer B, Rogal L, Spatz WB, Illing RB. Macro square wave jerks in a rhesus monkey: physiological and anatomical findings in a case of selective impairment of attentive fixation. J Hirnforsch 30, 603–611, 1989.
704. Wei M, DeAngelis DC, Angelaki D. Do visual cues contribute to the neural estimate of viewing distance used by the oculomotor system? J Neurosci 23, 8340–8350, 2003.
705. Weiss AH, Biersdorf WR. Visual sensory disorders in congenital nystagmus. Ophthalomology 96, 517–523, 1989.
706. Weissman BM, Dell'Osso LF, Abel LA, Leigh RJ. Spasmus nutans. A quantitative prospective study. Arch Ophthalmol 105, 525–528, 1987.
707. Weissman BM, Dell'Osso LF, DiScenna AO. Downbeat nystagmus in an infant. Spontaneous resolution during infancy. Neuroophthalmol 8, 317–319, 1988.
708. Weissman BM, Devereaux MW, Chandar K. Opsoclonus and hyperosmolar stupor. Neurology 39, 1401–1402, 1989.
709. Weissman JD, Seidman SH, Dell'Osso LF, Naheedy MH, Leigh RJ. Torsional see-saw "bow-tie" nystagmus in association with brain stem anomalies. Neuroophthalmol 10, 315–318, 1990.
710. Westheimer G, Blair SM. The ocular tilt reaction—a brainstem oculomotor routine. Invest Ophthalmol 14, 833–839, 1975.
711. Wiest G, Safoschnik G, Schnaberth G, Mueller C. Ocular flutter and truncal ataxia may be associated

with enterovirus infection. J Neurology 244, 288–292, 1997.
712. Williams DP, Troost BT, Rogers J. Lithium-induced down-beat nystagmus. Arch Neurol 45, 1022–1023, 1988.
713. Wilson E, Sng K, Somers JT, Reschke MF, Leigh RJ. Studies of eccentric gaze stability: effects of pitch head position on horizontal gaze-holding in patients with cerebellar disease. Ann N Y Acad Sci 1039, 593–596, 2005.
714. Wilson JR, Noyd WW, Aiyer AD, et al. Asymmetric responses in cortical visually evoked potentials to motion are not derived from eye movements. Invest Ophthalmol Vis Sci 40, 2435–2439, 1999.
715. Wist ER, Brandt T, Krafczyk S. Oscillopsia and retinal slip: evidence supporting a clinical test. Brain 106, 153–168, 1983.
716. Wizov SS, Reinecke RD, Bocarnea M, Gottlob I, Wizow SS. A comparative demographic and socioeconomic study of spasmus nutans and infantile nystagmus. Am J Ophthalmol 133, 256–262, 2002.
717. Wong AM, Musallam S, Tomlinson RD, Shannon P, Sharpe JA. Opsoclonus in three dimensions: oculographic, neuropathologic and modelling correlates. J Neurol Sci 189, 71–81, 2001.
718. Yagasaki T, Sato M, Awaya S, Nakamura N. Changes in nystagmus after simultaneous surgery for bilateral congenital cataracts. Jpn J Ophthalmol 37, 330–338, 1993.
719. Yakushin SB, Gizzi M, Reisine H, et al. Functions of the nucleus of the optic tract (NOT). II Control of ocular pursuit. Exp Brain Res 131, 433–447, 2000.
720. Yamazaki A, Zee DS. Rebound nystagmus: EOG analysis of a case with a floccular tumor. Br J Ophthalmol 63, 782–786, 1979.
721. Yaniglos SS, Leigh RJ. Refinement of an optical device that stabilizes vision in patients with nystagmus. Optom Vision Sci 69, 447–450, 1992.
722. Yaniglos SS, Stahl JS, Leigh RJ. Evaluation of current optical methods for treating the visual consequences of nystagmus. Ann N Y Acad Sci 956, 598–600, 2002.
723. Yee RD. Downbeat nystagmus: characteristics and localization of lesions. Transactions of the American Ophthalmology Society 87, 984–1032, 1989.
724. Yee RD, Baloh RW, Honrubia V, Lau CG, Jenkins HA. Slow build-up of optokinetic nystagmus associated with downbeat nystagmus. Invest Ophthalmol Vis Sci 18, 622–629, 1979.
725. Yee RD, Jelks GW, Baloh RW, Honrubia V. Uniocular nystagmus in monocular visual loss. Ophthalmology 86, 511–518, 1979.
726. Yee RD, Spiegel PH, Yamada T, Abel LA, Zee DS. Voluntary saccadic oscillations resembling ocular flutter and opsoclonus. J Neuroophthalmol 14, 95–101, 1994.
727. Yen MT, Herdman SJ, Tusa RJ. Oscillopsia and pseudonystagmus in kidney transplant patients. Am J Ophthalmol 128, 768–770, 1999.
728. Yildirim C, Tychsen L. Effect of infantile strabismus on visuomotor development in the squirrel monkey (Saimiri sciureus): optokinetic nystagmus, motion VEP and spatial sweep VEP. Strabismus 7, 211–219, 1999.
729. Yildirim C, Tychsen L. Disjunctive optokinetic nystagmus in a naturally esotropic macaque monkey: interaction between nasotemporal asymmetries of versional eye movement and convergence. Ophthalmic Res 32, 172–180, 2000.
730. Young TL, Weis JR, Summers CG, Egbert JE. The association of strabismus amblyopia and refractive errors in spasmus nutans. Ophthalmology 104, 112–117, 1997.
731. Young YH, Chen CH. Acute vertigo following cervical manipulation. Laryngoscope 113, 659–662, 2003.
732. Young YH, Huang TW. Role of clonazepam in the treatment of idiopathic downbeat nystagmus. Laryngoscope 111, 1490–1493, 2001.
733. Zak TA. Infantile convergence-evoked nystagmus. Ann Ophthalmol 15, 368–369, 1983.
734. Zasorin NL, Baloh RW. Downbeat nystagmus with alcoholic cerebellar degeneration. Arch Neurol 41, 1301–1302, 1984.
735. Zee DS. Ophthalmoscopy in examination of patients with vestibular disorders. Ann Neurol 3, 373–374, 1978.
736. Zee DS, FitzGibbon EJ, Optican LM. Saccade-vergence interactions in humans. J Neurophysiol 68, 1624–1641, 1992.
737. Zee DS, Friendlich AR, Robinson DA. The mechanism of downbeat nystagmus. Arch Neurol 30, 227–237, 1974.
738. Zee DS, Leigh RJ, Mathieu-Millaire F. Cerebellar control of ocular gaze stability. Ann Neurol 7, 37–40, 1980.
739. Zee DS, Robinson DA. A hypothetical explanation of saccadic oscillations. Ann Neurol 5, 405–414, 1979.
740. Zee DS, Yamazaki A, Butler PH, Gücer G. Effects of ablation of flocculus and paraflocculus on eye movements in primate. J Neurophysiol 46, 878–899, 1981.
741. Zee DS, Yee RD, Cogan DG, Robinson DA, Engel WK. Ocular motor abnormalities in hereditary cerebellar ataxia. Brain 99, 207–234, 1976.
742. Zimmerman CF, Roach ES, Troost BT. See-saw nystagmus associated with Chiari malformation. Arch Neurol 43, 299–300, 1986.
742a. Zingler VC, Strupp M, Jahn K, et al. Upbeat nystagmus as the initial clinical sign of Creutzfeldt-Jakob disease. Ann Neurol 57, 607–608, 2005.
743. Zubcov AA, Stark N, Weber A, Wizov SS, Reinecke RD. Improvement of visual acuity after surgery for nystagmus. Ophthalmology 100, 1488–1497, 1993.
744. Zumstein H, Meienberg O. Upbeat nystagmus and visual system disorder in Wernicke's encephalopathy due to starvation. Neuroophthalmol 2, 157–162, 1982.

Chapter 11

Diagnosis and Management of Vestibular Disorders

The diagnosis of the dizzy patient can be challenging for physician and patient alike. But when basic physiological and anatomical principles are applied at the bedside, the exact cause (and often a successful treatment) usually emerges, and even when not, a logical plan for a diagnostic evaluation can be developed. Here we will address patients with the hallmark symptoms of a vestibular disturbance: vertigo and oscillopsia (due to disturbances of the rotational VOR and often associated with nystagmus) and diplopia (due to an imbalance in otolith-ocular reflexes producing a skew deviation). Examples of common and important physical signs of patients with vestibular disorders may be found on the accompanying compact disc in the Video Displays: Disorders of the Vestibular System and Positional Nystagmus. Nystagmus has been discussed in the previous chapter and here we will only highlight the relevant features of vestibular nystagmus. Central disorders that also may produce vestibular disturbances are discussed further in Chapter 12.

VERTIGO AND DIZZINESS

In evaluating the complaint of dizziness, an unhurried history is of paramount importance, especially in the elderly, who often have both general medical and other neurological reasons for dizziness. The side effects of medications must always be considered in evaluating dizzy patients. Whether a patient is complaining of vertigo or some other type of dizziness (such as presyncopal faintness, loss of stable balance, or lightheadedness) can often be determined from a careful history and whether provocative maneuvers at the bedside induce the dizzy feeling (see Table 2–3 and Clinical Examination in Chapter 2). These procedures include testing for orthostatic hypotension, the Valsalva maneuver against pinched nostrils or closed larynx, tragal compression or increasing pressure in the external ear canal with a pneumatic otoscope, presentation of loud tones with an audiometer, mastoid vibration, hyperventilation, looking for head-shaking nystagmus, positional testing, and any other stimulus that the patient has identified as producing the dizziness.

Many patients who present with dizziness have a psychological disorder such as agoraphobia, acrophobia, phobic postural vertigo syndrome, or vestibular symptoms that are a component of panic attacks or depression.[76,196,274,389,490] Some of these patients have had vestibular disorders in the past which have resolved, or have a coexisting vestibular disorder, and may show abnormalities on vestibular function tests.[263,273,285] In other patients the unpredictability of the next attack of severe vertigo, as with benign paroxysmal positional vertigo or Ménière's disease, can be so paralyzing that patients become reclusive and severely depressed. Thus, it is important to evaluate and treat any associated psychological symptoms that dizzy patients have, *in parallel*, with evaluation and treatment of the vestibular disturbance, *per se*.

Vertigo is defined here as an *illusory sensation of motion of self or of the environment.* Rotational vertigo usually indicates disease of the semicircular canals or their central connections. Linear vertiginous sensations such as translation (e.g., lateropulsion and levitation) or body tilt occur with disease of the otoliths or their central connections. The sensation of vertigo is often associated with vegetative symptoms: nausea, weakness, and diaphoresis. Oscillopsia, on the other hand, usually refers to illusory movements of the seen environment that are often to-and-fro; it is absent with the eyes closed.

Not all cases of vertigo are due to disease of the labyrinth or its central connections. Some patients have primarily 'visual vertigo' with extreme sensitivity to visual motion.[96,96a,222] This is often an accompaniment of migraine. Certain individuals are prone to develop vertigo, unsteadiness, or malaise with motion, at height, and when assuming certain postures. Vertigo in these situations and in motion sickness probably occurs because of a mismatch between vestibular and other sensory inputs.[85] For diagnostic purposes, it is helpful to differentiate between acute, recurrent, and position-induced vertigo.

Clinical Features of Acute Peripheral Vestibulopathy

Sudden loss of tonic neural input from one labyrinth or vestibular nerve causes acute vertigo, nystagmus, and postural instability (Box 11–1). Autonomic disturbances also occur.[563a] The nystagmus (Box 10–1) is typically mixed horizontal-torsional, with slow phases directed toward the side of the paretic labyrinth. The nystagmus is more marked on looking in the direction of the quick phases, following Alexander's law (see Chapters 5 and 10). Quantitative three-dimensional recordings of the response to head rotations in different planes in patients with acute loss of labyrinthine function as part of a vestibular neuritis suggest that in most patients the brunt of the pathology is in the superior division of the vestibular nerve.[127,170,205,209,560] The direction of the spontaneous nystagmus alone, however, cannot be used confidently to predict which canals are involved, because some adaptation and rebalancing of tonic levels in the vestibular nuclei usually takes place quickly. Following vestibular neurectomy, the direction of nystagmus may be influenced by whether some canal afferents run in the spared cochlear division of the eighth cranial nerve.[71]

Often the patient cannot decide the direction of perceived rotation. This may be because labyrinthine signals suggest rotation in one direction (toward the side of the intact labyrinth), but the slow phases of spontaneous nystagmus cause motion of the image of the seen world on the retina that, when self-referred, implies turning in the opposite direction (toward the side of the paretic labyrinth). It is helpful, therefore, to inquire about the direction of rotation of the body when the eyes are closed, which is typically away from the side of the lesion.

Usually, the acutely vertiginous patient will lie on one side, with the affected ear uppermost; it has been suggested that this allows otolith influences, which converge centrally with semicircular canal inputs, to reduce the nystagmus caused by imbalance of the semicircular canals.[181] A possible reason for this effect is that the brain may misinterpret the change in the attitude of the head with respect to gravity (which calls for ocular counterroll) as a translation of the head away from the ground (which calls for a horizontal nystagmus with

Box 11–1. Summary of Findings With Acute Unilateral Loss Of Labyrinthine Function

- Spontaneous nystagmus (see Box 10–1)
- Nystagmus induced by head-shaking: after horizontal shaking, nystagmus beats away from affected ear; after vertical shaking, nystagmus beats towards affected ear
- Ocular tilt reaction: skew deviation with ipsilateral hypotropia, head tilt towards side of lesion, ipsilateral cyclodeviation (top poles of eyes rolled ipsilaterally)
- Reduced vestibulo-ocular response to ipsilateral head impulses (r-VOR) and head heaves (t-VOR), requiring corrective saccades
- Absent caloric response on side of lesion; acutely, response from intact side may be diminished
- Past-pointing and turning (Fukuda stepping test) towards the side of the lesion

See also: Pathophysiology Of Disorders of The Vestibular System, in Chapter 2. For etiologies, see Table 11–1. (Related Video: Disorders of the Vestibular System)

slow phases directed toward the intact labyrinth). This could in turn counteract the sustained spontaneous nystagmus from the tone imbalance. Recent behavioral, modeling and physiological studies emphasize the importance of semicircular canal signals in allowing a distinction between utricular activation by linear acceleration during lateral head tilt (which calls for ocular torsion) and by lateral head translation (which calls for horizontal eye motion).[216,570] One can envision that if signals about head translation and head tilt are misinterpreted, as might be the case with a unilateral vestibular imbalance, there could be a diminution or enhancement of any spontaneous nystagmus depending upon the particular pattern of canal-utricular imbalance. In support of this idea is the finding that head-shaking nystagmus in patients with a unilateral peripheral neuritis is modulated by the static attitude of the head, being worse with the affected ear down.[418]

Caloric testing is the traditional method of confirming that the vestibular imbalance is peripheral in location. In patients with spontaneous nystagmus, irrigation with a warm stimulus of the ear toward which the slow phases of nystagmus are directed is especially important; lack of any effect upon the spontaneous nystagmus implies disease affecting the stimulated ear. Central lesions within the brainstem near the root entry zone may lead to a diminution but rarely an absence of the caloric response, and the caloric-induced nystagmus is usually not as well suppressed by visual fixation.[184]

An abnormality with the head impulse maneuver, in which case there is a reduced slow-phase response and a corresponding corrective saccade, with rotation of the head toward the side of the paretic labyrinth, is also a reliable sign of unilateral impairment of labyrinthine function, especially when the loss is marked (see Video Display: Disorders of the Vestibular System).[230] A comparable abnormality with the head heave maneuver, which is a brief, abrupt, high-acceleration, side-to-side translation of the head to elicit the translational VOR mediated by the utricle, also identifies the side of the lesion when the lesion is acute.[401,440] The response is impaired for translation toward the side of the paretic labyrinth (see Video Display: Disorders of the Vestibular System). Rotational testing in patients with acute peripheral lesions shows decreased and asymmetric gain and a decreased time constant of the VOR. Quantitative aspects of the changes in vestibular responses with peripheral lesions are discussed further in Chapter 2.

Acute Vertigo

INFECTIONS CAUSING ACUTE VERTIGO

When acute vertigo occurs without auditory or neurologic disturbances (Table 11–1), particu-

Table 11–1. **Etiology of Vertigo**

Etiology of Vertigo
Acute Vertigo[69,232]
Physiologic vertigo:[80] motion sickness, height vertigo, postural vertigo (on head extension or bending forward at the waist)
Infection of the labyrinth, the vestibular nerve, or both:[29,113,388] by virus,[145,146] including zoster;[17,316,431] acute and chronic bacterial infections; syphilis; Lyme disease.[283,313,432,451]
Ménière's syndrome[13,467]
Trauma: by head injury,[144,179,246,413,477,507,548] complication of ear surgery[235]
Chiropractic manipulation[565]
Vertebral artery compression from neck rotation[79,492]
Perilymph fistula[128a,180,308,433,478,538]
Otosclerosis[457,500]
Congenital anomalies of the inner ear[381,466]
Vestibular atelectasis[358,395]
Vestibular-masseter syndrome[265]
Cogan's syndrome[129,141a,215,244,346,346,469,527]
Occlusive or hemorrhagic vascular disease of the inner ear[14,178,214,441,468]
Brainstem hemorrhage, ischemia and infarction (e.g. Wallenberg's syndrome)[30,174,210, 271, 322,323, 443,501]
Cerebellar hemorrhage[307] or infarction[11,125,126, 324,328,396,547]
Arnold–Chiari malformation (Valsalva-induced vertigo)[9,553]
Multiple sclerosis[10,187,189]
Tumors of the brainstem,[140] cerebellum,[165,219] eighth cranial nerve,[377] and petrous bone, including glomus tumors.[483]
Epilepsy[10a,47,198,295,311,394,462,479,485]
Drugs and toxins[260,275,369,473]
Cerebral hemisphere lesions[73,89,149,461a]
Recurrent Vertigo
Ménière's syndrome[13,39,425,467]
Syphilis[432,554]
Perilymph fistula[179,180,286,433,465,478,538]
Superior canal dehiscence [28,46,92,231,363,364,367,414]
Recurrent Vertigo (cont'd)
Otosclerosis[421,457,500]
Posterior canal dehiscence [314]
Autoimmune conditions[54,240,354,510,534] including Cogan's syndrome,[129,141a,215,244,346,469,527] Susac's syndrome,[26,221,397,494,495] and giant cell arteritis[374,375]
Benign paroxysmal vertigo of childhood[175,320,338, 346a,422,512]
Epilepsy[10a,47,198,295,311,394,462,479,485]
Migraine and its variants including basilar artery migraine[34,60,139,142,197,238,334a,392,409,446,460,499,508,526,531, 536,540]
Familial vertigo, ataxia, and nystagmus[32,41,45,88,111, 192,290,324a,514,515]
Hypothyroidism[59]
Brainstem ischemia[30,174,178,210,214,396,407]
Multiple sclerosis[187]
Posterior fossa tumors[241] or cysts[20]
Microvascular compression[53,82,370]
Vestibular atelectasis[358,395]
Central angioma[321]
Enlarged vestibular aqueduct [408]
Recurrent idiopathic vestibulopathy[455]
Positionally Induced Vertigo
Benign paroxysmal positional vertigo ("cupulolithiasis" and "canalolithiasis")[62,97,98,423,511,530,533]
Alcohol[371]
Head trauma[57,212,379a]
Cochlear implants[337]
Giant cell arteritis[374]
Central causes
Cerebellar infarcts[459]
Cerebellar tumors[219,542]
Cerebellar degenerations[56,559]
Multiple sclerosis[186,187,300]
Brainstem ischemia[214]
Arnold–Chiari malformation and other craniocervical anomalies[42]
Drugs: amiodorone;[19] ototoxicity[66]

larly in young adults, it is usually ascribed to a viral infection affecting the vestibular nerve. The syndrome is often referred to as vestibular neuronitis, vestibular neuritis, or vestibular neurolabyrinthitis.[145,388] In some patients localization within the labyrinth is more likely.[283a, 298,383]Although a definite etiology is not proven in most cases, the histopathology is compatible with a viral or post-viral inflammatory process.[279] Reactivation of latent herpes viruses may be a common mechanism, much as is presumed to be the case for palsies of other cranial nerves.[18,21,493] As noted above, the brunt of the pathology seems to be in the superior division of the vestibular nerve, which may relate to anatomical differences that render the superior division more susceptible to injury.[205,209] High resolution MRI with contrast may show enhancement on the vestibular nerve.[296] Sometimes such attacks of vertigo occur in epidemics, but the responsible agent is usually not identified. Mumps, measles, and infectious mononucleosis are among the infections that may be suspected if acute vertigo is accompanied by deafness. Experimental studies of viral infection of the inner ear have shown a selective vulnerability to specific viruses of the cochlea, labyrinth, or eighth nerve ganglion.[145] One well-recognized cause is herpes zoster, which produces not just vertigo but also a burning pain in the ear followed by a vesicular eruption in the external auditory canal and concha. Deafness, ipsilateral facial pain, and facial paralysis may also occur (Ramsay-Hunt syndrome).[21,205,315,316,431,519] Enhancement of the facial and vestibulocochlear nerves on MRI has been reported.[348] Bacterial infection of the middle ear and serous otitis media also can cause vertigo, especially in children.

TRAUMA CAUSING VERTIGO

Acute vertigo may be associated with head trauma.[144,180,246,413] The injury is often mild; frequently the patient also complains of headache and difficulty with concentration (post-concussion syndrome). Post-traumatic vertigo commonly is caused by whiplash injuries incurred in rear-end automobile accidents. About 50% of such patients show abnormalities on vestibular testing, such as reduced caloric responses, positional nystagmus, and occasionally increased, "hyperactive" vestibular responses.[176,246,305,413] High-impact aerobics have been implicated in patients with otherwise unexplained vestibular symptoms.[544] Temporal bone fractures are often associated with vertigo and vestibular damage.[224,246,548]

Cervical vertigo is commonly invoked as a cause of dizziness after head trauma, presumably due to damage to cervical muscle afferents that do project to the vestibular nuclei.[79,204] In support of this idea, injection of local anesthetic into the neck of volunteer subjects produces a sensation of being drawn toward the side of the cervical injection, with ataxia but not nystagmus. Nystagmus, however, does appear when monkeys are injected with a local anesthetic in their neck muscles.[147,162] Radical neck surgery can lead to abnormal rotational vestibular responses.[292] Vibration of neck muscles can lead to illusions of motion in normal subjects,[299] and to nystagmus in patients with unilateral loss of function.[562] The cervico-ocular reflex may be enhanced in patients with a whiplash injury.[305] Thus, there is a potential substrate for cervical influences on vestibular sensation, but cervical vertigo is still not a clearly defined clinical entity despite efforts to do so. Perhaps the most common mistake is to attribute unexplained dizziness in elderly individuals to cervical osteoarthritis or spondylosis.

Trauma may also cause vertigo by creating a perilymphatic fistula between the inner and middle ear.[461] Perilymph fistula may follow mastoid or stapes surgery, minor head trauma (e.g., from diving into a swimming pool), barotrauma (high altitude or underwater),[277,356,433] strenuous exercise, suppressed sneezing,[471] and air travel.[223,286,308] Symptoms can sometimes be induced by applying manual pressure over the tragus, or better by applying pressure to the tympanic membrane with the pneumatic otoscope. A positive result is production or exacerbation of vertigo or the elicitation of nystagmus (Hennebert's sign). A positive Hennebert's sign is not specific for an oval or round window fistula, however. Other causes include fistulas or dehiscence involving any of the semicircular canals, or abnormal connections between the stapes footplate and the otoliths, including vestibulofibrosis and a hypermobile stapes. Pressure sensitivity may also occur in Ménière's syndrome, when the otolith organs become dilated and abut the stapes footplate. A positive Hennebert's sign has also been associated with bilateral vestibular loss.[4] Pressure-induced signs can sometimes be documented by recording eye movements or measuring body sway as pressure on the tympanic membrane is increased.[415,477] Patients with fistula may show or complain of imbalance, positional vertigo, oscillopsia and nystagmus (sometimes pulsatile) and hearing loss.[223,345,361,442]

TULLIO PHENOMENON

The Tullio phenomenon refers to vestibular symptoms induced by auditory stimuli. These can include vertigo, oscillopsia, nystagmus (Fig. 11–1), the ocular tilt reaction (OTR), and postural imbalance (see Video Display: Disorders of the Vestibular System). The symptoms may be due to abnormal stimulation of the semicircular canals or of the otoliths. Causes include perilymph fistula, superior canal dehiscence (see below), and subluxation of the stapes footplate and other ear pathology.[131,161,415,429,449,452] Normally sounds do not stimulate the semicircular canals or the utricle but when a "third" window is created, as in the case of a perilymphatic fistula, there is a change in compliance such that the labyrinthine motion detectors can become stimulated by fluid flow arising from sound energy.

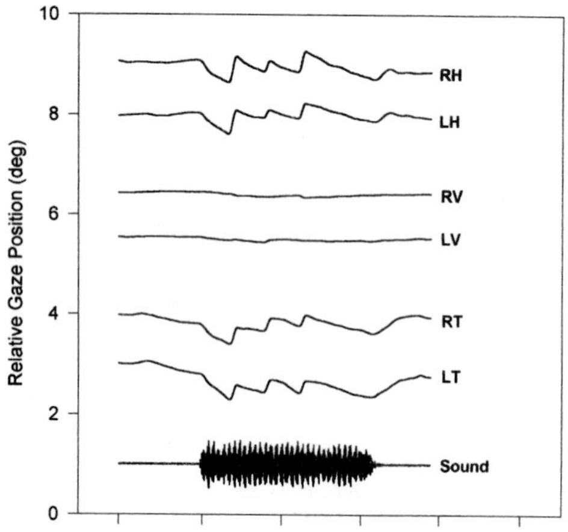

Figure 11–1. Post traumatic Tullio's phenomenon As soon as the acoustic stimulation starts, conjugate horizontal right beating and torsional clockwise beating nystagmus commenced. Note the absence of any spontaneous nystagmus prior to stimulation and also the lack of vertical nystagmus during stimulation. The single position traces are offset for convenience of display; upward deflections indicate rightward (horizontal), upward (vertical), or clockwise (torsional) eye rotations, with respect to the patient. The sound signal is only displayed for timing information. RH: right horizontal; LH: left horizontal; RV: right vertical; LV: left vertical; RT: right torsional; LT: left torsional.[452]

An important cause of the Tullio phenomenon is *dehiscence of the roof of the superior semicircular canal*.[364,367] Many early reports of Tullio phenomenon were probably due to this condition. Other symptoms and signs include vertigo, often induced by Valsalva maneuvers or pressure, positioning and positional nystagmus, drop attacks, pulsatile tinnitus, pulsatile oscillopsia, and conductive hearing loss or hyperacusis (see Video Display: Disorders of the Vestibular System). Vestibular evoked myogenic potentials are commonly abnormal, being more easily elicited on the side of the dehiscent canal. Audiograms may show a lowered threshold for bone conduction hearing with an apparent conductive hearing loss, though stapedius reflexes are spared.[46,92,93,136,153,236,360,361,363,364,414,487,503] A curious manifestation of this syndrome is the malleolus sign; patients may hear rather than feel the vibrating tuning fork applied to their ankle.[543] They also hear their joints crack and their eyes move.[231] The bony abnormality can be identified on coronal and transverse CT scans of the petrous bone with three-dimensional reconstructions in the planes of the vertical canals (Fig. 11–2).[50] MRI scans may also show the anomaly.[313a] The bony abnormality is likely due to a developmental defect, as patients who become symptomatic on one side often have relatively thin bone on the other.[261] Vigorous exercise or a forceful strain may precede the onset of symptoms. One of our patients developed symptoms after pulling a shrub out of her garden. Presumably, the thin bone overlying the superior semicircular canal is broken leading to the frank dehiscence. In particularly bothersome cases, plugging of the superior canal is an effective treatment.[363,364] Recordings of semicircular canal afferent activity in animal models of superior canal dehiscence have suggested that altered activity of irregular vestibular afferents might underlie Tullio's phenomenon.[116] Dehiscence of the *posterior semicircular canal* may also lead to vertigo, hearing loss and tinnitus.[314]

A spontaneous oval or round window fistula has been invoked as a cause of unexplained vertigo and dysequilibrium.[180,538] Unfortunately, there are no reliable diagnostic tests for this syndrome. Many patients in whom no other cause for their vestibular symptoms is uncov-

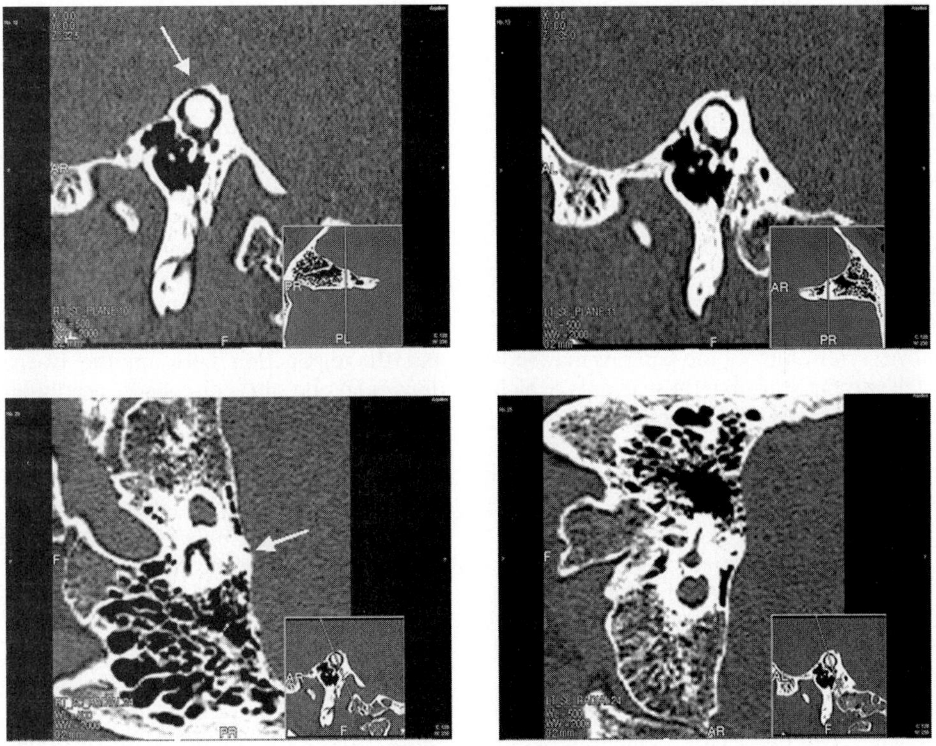

Figure 11–2. Computed tomography with 3D reconstructions in a patient with superior canal dehiscence (left panels) and in a normal subject (right panels). Note the absence of bone at the arrows in the patient over the superior canal. Inset shows the plane of the image; small letters on images indicate the orientation of the reconstruction.

ered have undergone an exploratory tympanotomy with patching of the oval and round windows, even if no fistula is clearly identified. Only a small percentage of patients in this category are permanently helped with this procedure; the problem is how to identify this subgroup that will respond to treatment.[465]

TOXIC CAUSES OF VERTIGO

The most common toxic cause of acute vertigo is ethyl alcohol. It is well known that positional changes exacerbate the vertigo of a hangover. Symptoms are accompanied by a positional nystagmus. The reason may be that alcohol diffuses into the cupula at a faster rate than into the surrounding endolymph and so creates a density gradient, making the cupula gravity-sensitive, the so-called buoyancy hypothesis.[78,371] More recent studies have shown that the nystagmus associated with alcohol has two components: a peripheral component based upon density gradients, and a central vertical component presumably reflecting imbalance within the vestibular nuclei.[171]

The aminoglycoside antibiotics are notorious for causing irreversible failure of vestibular function without vertiginous warning or hearing loss.[234] A number of other causes of acute vertigo are enumerated in Table 11–1, and some are discussed in the following section.

Recurrent Vertigo

MÉNIÈRE'S SYNDROME[366,461]

Ménière's syndrome (endolymphatic hydrops) is a common cause of vertigo that is usually accompanied by aural fullness, fluctuating and usually low-frequency hearing loss, and tinnitus. A failure of resorption of endolymph is presumed to lead to an increase in endolymphatic pressure. Symptoms are probably caused both by direct compression of sensory structures within the cochlea and vestibular labyrinth, and by leakage of potassium-rich endolymph onto the vestibular nerve through breaks in the membrane separating the endolymph and perilymph spaces. The vestibular nerve may first be excited and then depressed in a depolarization block.

A typical attack in Ménière's syndrome is heralded by fullness in the ear, tinnitus, and impaired hearing. The vertigo that ensues is often severe and usually prostrates the patient. After several hours, or sometimes longer, the attack begins to abate. Sometimes the hearing symptoms subside when the vertigo begins (Lermoyez syndrome). Some patients may suddenly fall without warning; these events, which may even occur early in the course of the disease, are referred to as Tumarkin's otolithic crisis,[39] and should be differentiated from other forms of drop attacks.[92,281,282]

Examination during the acute phase commonly shows nystagmus that changes its direction during the attack. At the onset of the attack, an irritative nystagmus with horizontal slow phases directed away from the affected ear (ipsilateral-beating nystagmus) may occur. Slow phases toward the side of the lesion then appear (the "paretic" phase); finally another reversal of the direction of the nystagmus, with slow phases away from the affected ear, can occur a few hours later (recovery nystagmus).[352,425] Postural unsteadiness may persist for several days. Vertigo may be the predominant symptom in some patients with Ménière's syndrome. Commonly, however, audiometric testing shows a characteristic fluctuating low-frequency hearing loss with recruitment. This is usually evident from the history and the clinical examination. Soft sounds are too soft, loud sounds are too loud. Electrocochleography (ECOG) may show an increase in the ratio between the summating and the action potential, a pattern also seen with perilymphatic fistula. MRI scans may show contrast enhancement of labyrinthine structures during attacks, but this finding must be distinguished from enhancement in the labyrinth or nerve due to acute viral infections, autoimmune diseases, and other processes; the enhancement may persist well after the acute episode has subsided.[105,122,188,348,524]

Ménière's syndrome is a disease of adults, often beginning in the third or fourth decade but may start even later; it rarely occurs in children.[27,242] The natural history of Ménière's syndrome is one of progression but often with extended periods of remission.[217] Although the cause of Ménière's syndrome is unknown, endolymphatic hydrops may follow (often after many years) other afflictions of the ear including head trauma and viral infections.[294,318,467] An autoimmune basis has been suggested for some patients with Ménière's syndrome;[240,447,482] patients with arteritis or other vascular disease may present with a Ménière's-like syndrome.[374,375,394] (See also Cogan's syndrome and Susac's syndrome, below.)

The incidence of migraine is probably increased in patients with Ménière's syndrome and the distinction between the two conditions may be difficult, since vestibular and auditory symptoms and signs may occur with classic migraine.[72,107,281,325,327,334a,411,436,445,521,526] A Ménière's like syndrome is described with congenital bony abnormalities of the temporal bone including an enlarged vestibular aqueduct,[408,558] osteogenesis imperfecta,[317] otosclerosis (see below), and occasionally vestibular schwannomas [306]

OTOSCLEROSIS

Otosclerosis, a common cause of dominantly inherited deafness, may also cause attacks of recurrent vertigo that mimic Ménière's syndrome.[421,457,500] Some patients also suffer from positional vertigo. Diagnosis is relatively easy in patients with a conductive hearing loss and an air-bone gap, tinnitus, and a history of affected family members. Superior canal dehiscence may mimic otosclerosis;[231,360] however, with canal dehiscence, there is a *decreased* threshold for bone-conducted hearing, and the stapedius reflex and vestibular-evoked myogenic potentials are intact. CT scanning of the petrous bone may help make the diagnosis.[105,524]

INFLAMMATORY DISORDERS CAUSING RECURRENT VERTIGO

Syphilis is a rare but important cause of recurrent vertigo.[432,554]Inflammation of the membranous labyrinth and osteitis of the surrounding bone occur with both congenital and acquired forms. The clinical picture is episodic vertigo with progressive loss of vestibular and auditory function. Other features of syphilis may be present, especially with the congenital form. The serum fluorescent treponemal antibody absorption test (FTA) is positive, and cerebrospinal fluid abnormalities may be present. Lyme disease, another infectious process, may cause a variety of vestibular syndromes,[283,313,451] though the ocular motor manifestations are more common.[25]

Cogan's syndrome is characterized by interstitial keratitis, hearing loss, and recurrent attacks of vertigo that mimic Ménière's syndrome.[129,141a,215,244,249,469,527] It is often associated with a systemic collagen vascular disease, and some patients develop aortic insufficiency; tests for syphilis are negative. Corticosteroid therapy usually produces improvement, and should be instituted promptly for hearing and vestibular loss.

Susac's syndrome is characterized by a triad of microangiopathy of the brain, retinal vascular disease, and eighth nerve involvement.[221,406,494,495,569] Young women are most commonly affected. Patients have an encephalopathy with characteristic MRI abnormalities in the corpus callosum, visual field loss due to branch retinal artery occlusions, and a Ménière's-like syndrome with spells of vertigo with low-frequency hearing loss. Sarcoid also has a predilection for the eighth cranial nerve and it may cause BPPV, presumably by selectively involving the superior division of the vestibular nerve.[262,534] Other forms of immune mediated inner ear disease leading to progressive vestibular and hearing loss, with or without associated systemic involvement, have also been described.[54,102,188,240,349,354,394,453,472,510]

MIGRAINE AND RECURRENT VERTIGO: VESTIBULAR MIGRAINE

It has become increasingly recognized that recurrent vertigo and other vestibular symptoms may be a common manifestation of migraine.[32,139,155,169,197,326,334a,392,393,436,499,508,528,536,540] Migraine and benign paroxysmal positional vertigo are the most common clinical diagnoses in our dizzy patient clinics. As a component of migraine attacks, vertigo may overshadow the headache and often occurs independently of the headaches. Vertigo in migraine syndromes tends to occurs in three time frames: brief attacks lasting seconds to a minute or two, attacks lasting up to an hour or so, similar to a classic migraine aura, and attacks lasting for days or sometimes weeks in a milder form, producing motion sensitivity and imbalance.[142,540]

Migraine with vestibular symptoms occurs more frequently in women. The vestibular symptoms may begin years after the onset of the migraine headaches.[61] There is often a positional component to vertigo with migraine, and there is also an increased incidence of benign paroxysmal positional vertigo in migraine.[280,334,513,531] Hearing loss may be associated with migraine, further complicating its distinction from Ménière's syndrome.[325,327,436,526] Abnormalities on vestibular testing have been reported in patients with migraine and vertigo, including changes in the phase of the high-frequency vertical VOR[248] and eye movement abnormalities suggestive of vestibulocerebellar dysfunction.[158,239] It is not clear whether these occur with a greater frequency in patients with vestibular symptoms than in patients with migraine without vestibular symptoms.[61] Headache and vertigo associated with other symptoms, such as dysarthria and ataxia, suggest a basilar-artery form of migraine. Such attacks are particularly common in adolescent girls.[60,238]

One distinctive migraine variant is benign paroxysmal vertigo of childhood, which usually begins between the ages of one and four years.[7,166,175,320,346a,422,512] The attacks are typically brief and consist of unsteadiness, pallor, nausea, and vomiting. Older children describe vertigo. Nystagmus or torticollis may be noted; younger children may only show torticollis. Some patients with this syndrome show linkage to the CACNA1A mutation of hemiplegic migraine. The attacks may come every week or month or two, sometimes with a striking periodicity, or in clusters, between which the children feel well. Tests of labyrinthine function sometimes suggest a peripheral abnormality. The attacks usually cease in the course of a few months or years. Migraine and seizure disorders should be considered first in the differential diagnosis of vertigo in childhood.[74,94,140,422,512] Acetazolamide-responsive, familial episodic ataxia type 2 (EA-2) is another cause of episodic vertigo in children and adolescents,[88,192,289,290,514,515,545,566] and like some patients with benign paroxysmal vertigo of childhood,[206] has been linked to a calcium channel defect on chromosome 19.

VASCULAR DISORDERS AND RECURRENT VERTIGO

In older individuals, transient attacks of acute vertigo may be caused by vertebrobasilar insufficiency.[30,43,174,178,210,214,270,322,396,407,475] Usually, associated neurologic symptoms or signs point to a central disorder, but isolated attacks due to ischemia, especially of the caudal cerebellum, can occur;[210,396] they may be the harbinger of brainstem or cerebellar stroke.[535] Isolated attacks of vertigo may also be due to ischemia of the labyrinth, commonly affecting structures within the distribution of the anterior vestibular artery (the anterior and lateral semicircular canals and the utricle). Since the anterior vestibular artery is an end artery with poor collateral supply, isolated attacks of vertigo may occur without hearing loss or tinnitus in patients with hypoperfusion of the labyrinth due to vertebrobasilar insufficiency. Occasionally, such attacks are associated with bilateral hearing loss.[271] Spells of vertigo related to vascular disease are usually short-lived, lasting minutes to an hour or so. In contrast, the spells of vertigo with Ménière's syndrome last longer, hours to a day or so.

Hemorrhage into the vestibular organ is rare, but can cause severe vertigo and deafness.[468] Acute vertigo is often a prominent symptom in brainstem or cerebellar infarction, which are discussed in the next chapter. Vascular lesions in the cerebral hemispheres occasionally give rise to acute vertigo.[73,89,149,461a]

EPILEPSY AND OTHER MISCELLANEOUS CAUSES OF VERTIGO

Seizures—*tornado epilepsy*—may cause vertiginous feelings, but patients with epilepsy more commonly experience vertigo as a side effect of anticonvulsant and other medications (Table 11–1). A posterior fossa tumor rarely causes recurrent vertigo. Tumors of the eighth cranial nerve commonly are associated with progressive hearing loss rather than with vertigo,[55] although nearly half of such patients experience vertigo at some time during the course.[306,377] Hyperventilation, which can provoke seizures, may also provoke vertigo in patients with perilymphatic fistula, compressive lesions on the vestibular nerve, and lesions at the cranio-cervical junction. The following is an illustrative case

A freshman college student developed hemifacial spasms and dizziness precipitated by exercise. On examination the sole findings were a minimal right facial paresis, as reflected in a decreased spontaneous blink, and strong hyperventilation-induced nystagmus with slow phases directed toward the left and clockwise. Laboratory tests initially showed a slightly decreased caloric response on the right side, but hearing was normal. Electroencephalography, temporal bone X-rays and cerebral angiography were normal. The patient's symptoms progressed over several years to a considerable loss of hearing on the right side, absent caloric responses on the right side and moderate right facial paresis with aberrant regeneration. The hyperventilation - induced nystagmus, however, resolved. Computed tomography, repeated with magnification views of the petrous bone, revealed a lytic lesion that proved to be a congenital epidermoid tumor (Fig.11–3).

Comment: The unusual feature of this patient's clinical examination was his hyperventilation-induced nystagmus with slow phases directed away from the side of the lesion (an excitatory nystagmus). We considered four possible explanations. Two of these, seizures and ischemia (due to decreased cerebral blood flow), seemed improbable. More plausible were a perilymph fistula and a "recovery" nystagmus. The former could have occurred because of erosion of the tumor through the bony labyrinth and into the subarachnoid space. Changes in cerebrospinal fluid pressure (as occur with hyperventilation) can be transmitted via the vestibular aqueduct to the perilymph space or directly via the destroyed petrous bone. If this was the mechanism a Valsalva maneuver might have produced nystagmus but this was not attempted.

Alternatively, hyperventilation, by virtue of its effects upon serum pH and free calcium concentration, is known to improve nerve conduction in marginally functional, often demyelinated, fibers, as occurs in multiple sclerosis. In our patient hyperventilation may have improved nerve conduction and thereby increased the level of tonic discharge emanating from the right peripheral labyrinth. Because of a moderate degree of vestibular loss on the right side (which was reflected in the decreased caloric response), central adaptation had occurred beforehand to rebalance the level of activity within the vestibular nuclei. Hence there was no spontaneous nystagmus. Now, with the improved peripheral function due to the hyperventilation, central adaptation became inappropriate (excessive) and a 'recovery' nystagmus ensued with slow phases directed away from the lesioned side. Other mechanisms for hyperventilation nystagmus include the effects

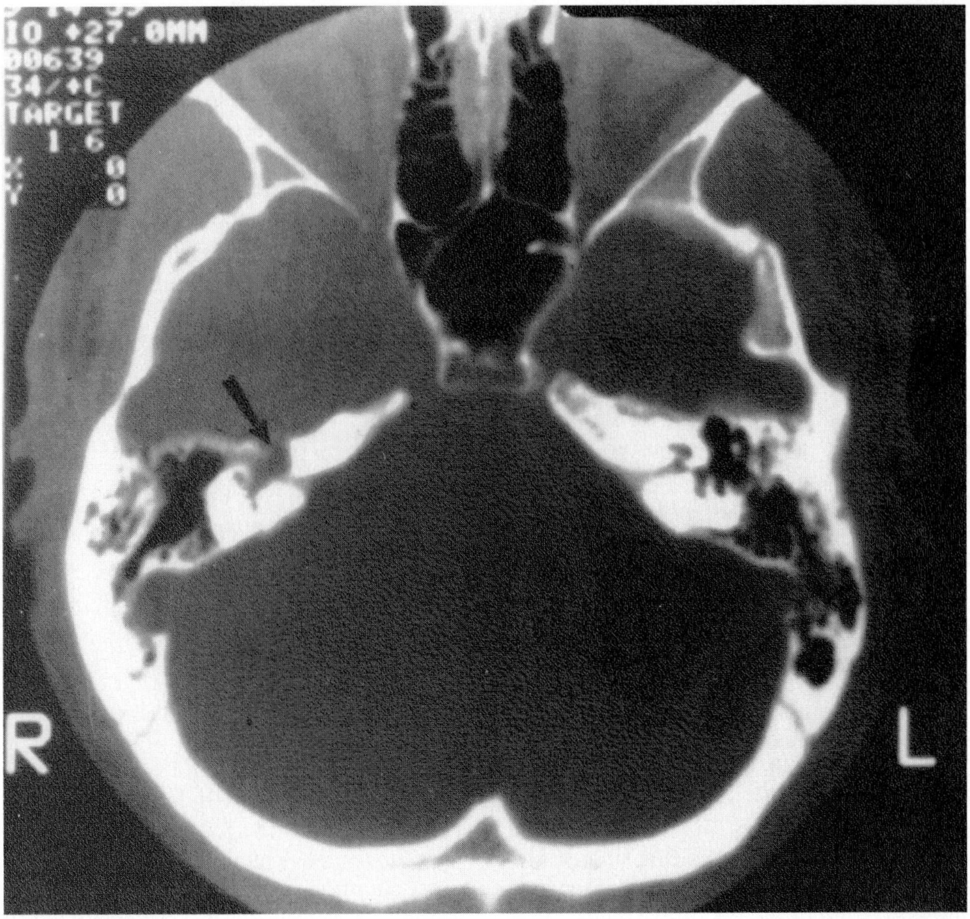

Figure 11–3. Computed tomography showing a lytic lesion (indicated by arrowhead) in the right petrous bone of a patient who presented with hyperventilation-induced vertigo. The lesion was a congenital epidermoid tumor. See Case History: Hyperventilation-induced nystagmus for details, and Video Display: Disorders of the Vestibular System.

of changes of serum pH on central adaptive mechanisms,[458] or on the function of calcium channels.[537] Hyperventilation-induced nystagmus also occurs in patients with acoustic schwannoma and after vestibular neuritis. The nystagmus may be directed with slow phases away from the side of the lesion and a torsional component is often prominent.[365,458]

UNDIAGNOSED RECURRENT VERTIGO

Some patients report episodes of recurrent vertigo for which no cause can be found.[455] Long-term follow-up has shown that about 30% develop into either Ménière's syndrome or benign paroxysmal positional vertigo, while the other 70% remain undiagnosed. Some of these patients almost certainly have vestibular migraine, especially when there is a family history.[169,409] Less commonly, patients may have attacks that affect first one and then the other ear; the bilateral vestibular loss causes oscillopsia with head movements and during walking.[38,285,470] Examination of the temporal bone of three patients who had suffered recurrent episodes of vertigo showed varying degrees of inflammation and destruction within the vestibular system, and mild involvement of the cochlear system.[40]

Some patients with chronic unsteadiness have the syndrome of mal de debarquement.[103,226,384,387] This is an exaggerated form of a normal response that many individuals have when they return to land after sea travel. Patients have a rocking and swaying sensation, usually with no abnormalities on examination or testing. Symptoms typically are absent when the patient is riding in a car or other form of transportation, but often worse afterwards. The pattern of false motion after travel may mimic closely the pattern of motion experienced during travel, suggesting that this is a manifestation of excessive adaptation to sustained, unusual patterns of motion.[336] A possible physiological substrate for this syndrome is in the inferior olive. Rabbits exposed to sustained sinusoidal oscillation will continue to show oscillatory activity in cerebellar climbing fibers even after the rotational stimulus has stopped.[49] The etiology of mal de debarquement in humans is unclear: migraine, fistulas, otolith disturbances, vascular loops and psychiatric disorders have been invoked. Most patients recover spontaneously or respond to antianxiety or antidepressant medications and physical therapy, especially that which invokes slower movements such as Tai Chi exercises.

Recurrent attacks of disabling vertigo have been attributed to vascular loops or tortuous vessels that compress the eighth cranial nerve, analogous to the syndromes of hemifacial spasm and trigeminal neuralgia.[118,148] Microvascular decompression has been reported to produce dramatic cures in some of these patients.[75,370] Clinical features that suggest the diagnosis include short-lived episodes (seconds to minutes) of vertigo or imbalance, often related to a change in head posture; hyperacusis or tinnitus; and a salutary response to carbamazepine or oxycarbazepine.[82] Abnormalities of brainstem auditory evoked potentials and an exacerbation of symptoms or induction of nystagmus with hyperventilation (altering conduction on a compressed and demyelinated nerve) also point to the diagnosis. Unfortunately, reliable laboratory methods to identify such patients have not been established,[53,370] especially since many asymptomatic normal individuals have loops of the anterior inferior cerebellar artery touching the eighth-nerve complex in or near the internal auditory meatus. In patients with unexplained vertigo or disequilibrium, the diagnosis of microvascular compression of the vestibular nerve, or of a spontaneous oval or round window perilymphatic fistula, is raised and exploratory surgery is often considered. There is no convincing evidence; however, that patients will benefit from such procedures unless they meet strict clinical criteria.[75,465] Vestibular migraine, Ménière's syndrome, epilepsy, multiple sclerosis, and even benign paroxysmal positional vertigo may have atypical presentations. Following vestibular nerve section some patients report momentary episodes of vertigo, "quick spins," which are responsive to antiepileptic medications.[372] Unusual conditions such as episodic ataxia type 2 (EA-2) also should be considered and treated empirically before exploratory surgery for a fistula or microvascular compression is performed in patients with unexplained vertigo.

Posturally Induced Vertigo

BENIGN PAROXYSMAL POSITIONAL VERTIGO

Clinical Features of Benign Paroxysmal Positional Vertigo

Benign paroxysmal positional vertigo was first described by Bárány and further characterized by Dix and Hallpike.[31,319] Classic BPPV usually arises when the posterior semicircular canal becomes gravity-sensitive.[194] The syndrome is presumably caused by debris, otoconia, either floating freely within the long arm of the semicircular canal (canalolithiasis, probably the most common occurrence) or adherent to the cupula (cupulolithiasis). Typically, patients complain of brief episodes of vertigo precipitated by changes of head posture such as turning over in bed, looking up to a high shelf, or backing a car out of a garage. Patients can usually identify the offending head position, which they often carefully avoid. Many patients also complain of mild postural instability between attacks, in part due to utricular dysfunction.[532a] The epidemiological features of this syndrome are well described.[120] Women are affected almost twice as often as men. The condition affects all age groups, but is most frequent in the elderly. The average age of onset is 57 years. The annual incidence is about 0.1% though this may be an under representation since many patients with BPPV may never come to medical attention. About 15% of patients have the lateral canal variant. For the posterior canal variant (by far the most common) the right side is more commonly affected,[142a,342,532] though no such side difference exists for the lateral canal variant.[120] Spontaneous remissions are the rule, but symptoms may trouble the patient intermittently for years.[278,398] BPPV may follow head injury, viral neurolabyrinthitis, and labyrinthine ischemia, and occasionally occurs after assumption of unusual head postures (e.g., prolonged reclining in a dentist's chair, at the hairdresser's, or working underneath a car), following prolonged bed rest, or exposure to continuous jarring, such as cycling over rough terrain, or high-impact aerobics.[544] In over half of affected patients, no cause can be identified.[35]

The *clinical examination* may help confirm the diagnosis (Fig. 11–4, A–C). Having reassured the patient (who is often apprehensive of being moved) and emphasized the importance of keeping the eyes open, the patient's head is turned 45° to one shoulder and the head and neck are quickly moved "en bloc" into a head-hanging position (just over the edge of the examining table, about 120° from the upright). This is the Dix-Hallpike maneuver. A variant ('side-lying') in which the patient turns to the side with the nose 45 degrees away from the tested side may be easier for older individuals, especially if they have some limitation of motion of the neck.[132,272] Typically there is a latent period, usually of about 2 to 5 seconds but sometimes as long as 30 seconds, before vertigo, nausea, and a burst of nystagmus appear (see Video Display: Positional Nystagmus). In the typical variant due to involvement of the posterior semicircular canal, the slow phases are directed downward, with intorsion of the dependent eye and extorsion of the upper eye (i.e., top pole of the eyes rotating toward the up, unaffected ear). Hence, the nystagmus is *mixed upbeat and torsional with quick phases beating such that the top pole rotates toward the ground.* The nystagmus appears to change with the direction of gaze: on looking to the dependent ear it seems more torsional, and on looking to the higher ear, more vertical. A small horizontal component, greater in the lower eye, with slow phases toward the dependent ear, may also be evident if eye movements are recorded.

Three-axis search-coil recordings have shown that in most cases the slow phases of BPPV rotate the eye in a plane that is parallel to the posterior semicircular canal.[24,172] This pattern of nystagmus corresponds closely to the results of experimental stimulation of the posterior semicircular canal of the dependent ear (Fig. 2–2).[130] The nystagmus increases for up to 10 seconds, but then begins to fatigue (adaptation), and is usually gone by 40 seconds. In other words, this testing induces positioning nystagmus rather than positional nystagmus. In a small proportion of patients with BPPV, a low-amplitude, secondary nystagmus (in the opposite direction) may occur after the primary nystagmus has resolved, but this reversal is usually most prominent when the patient sits up. Repeating this procedure several times will decrease the symptoms and make the signs more difficult to elicit (habituation); this lessening of the response is of diagnostic value, because positional nystagmus due to central lesions usually does not habituate with repeated testing.

If the classic pattern of nystagmus associated with BPPV is not elicited with the Dix-Hallpike maneuver to either side, the patient should then be brought to the supine position with the head centered on the body. The patient's head (and body, for comfort) should then be turned 90 degrees to one side (right ear down), back to neutral (head supine) and then 90 degrees to the other (left ear down) (Bárány maneuver). This is the best maneuver to elicit a *horizontal positional nystagmus*, as occurs, for example, with the lateral canal variant of BPPV, which is discussed later in this section. When no nystagmus is elicited in a patient with a typical history after both the Dix-Hallpike and the Bárány maneuvers, it is worthwhile repeating the Dix-Hallpike maneuver once again,[525] and also applying a vibrator to the mastoid, in an attempt to bring out the nystagmus.

Nystagmus associated with changes in head posture is sometimes attributed to extension, flexion, or lateral rotation of the head on the body, but with rare exceptions, the nystagmus actually appears because of a change in the position of the head with respect to gravity. To make this distinction, the trunk can be pitched forwards and the head hyperextended at the neck, or the trunk pitched backwards and the head flexed on the neck, in order to keep the attitude of the head with respect to gravity the same as in the normal upright posture. If the vertigo is due to flexion, extension, or rotation at the neck, this maneuver should provoke nystagmus.[128a,450,492]

The *lateral canal variant of BPPV*, while less common than the posterior canal variant, has become increasingly recognized.[24,62,97,98,120,405] There are two variants: geotropic in which the eyes beat toward the lowermost ear and apogeotropic in which the eyes beat toward the uppermost ear. The geotropic variant is about four times more frequent.[120] Lateral canal BPPV may occur as a transient complication following positioning maneuvers used in testing for, or treating, posterior canal BPPV.[258,267] Patients may have both lateral and posterior canal variants simultaneously or sequentially, and treatment of one may lead to the other. Lateral canal BPPV may be associated with a canal paresis on caloric testing that resolves when the BPPV resolves.[529] Lateral canal BPPV produces symptoms in both the right-ear-down and left-ear-down positions. When the nystagmus is geotropic (beating toward the ground) it is usually more intense with the affected ear down; when apogeotropic (beating away from the ground) it is usually more intense with the intact ear down. Thus, in a patient with horizontal positional nystagmus first determine if it beats away or toward the ground, and second to which side it is more intense. If apogeotropic, the affected ear is up when the nystagmus is most intense, if geotropic, the affected ear is down when the nystagmus is most intense. Thus when the nystagmus is most intense it beats toward the side of the affected ear. This difference between the intensity of nystagmus and the affected ear in geotropic and apogeotropic BBPV may represent Ewald's second law (ampulla movement in the excitatory direction elicits a brisker nystagmus than the opposing ampulla movement in the inhibitory direction). In the apogeotropic variant there is often some nystagmus when the patient is in the direct supine position, and a null point with the patient in the supine position and the head turned 10 to 20 degrees toward the side of the affected ear, at which point the lateral canal is aligned with the gravity vector.[62] In other words, in the direct supine position the nystagmus will beat towards the affected ear. In the geotropic variant the nystagmus upon assuming the direct supine position beats toward the intact ear.[404] Likewise, when the head is pitched forward a null can also be identified when the lateral canal reaches an earth-horizontal plane.

The nystagmus of lateral-canal BPPV may reverse its direction if the offending position of the head is maintained.[405] When the head is brought to the supine position from a sustained lateral position, a nystagmus occurs as if the head were being brought from supine to

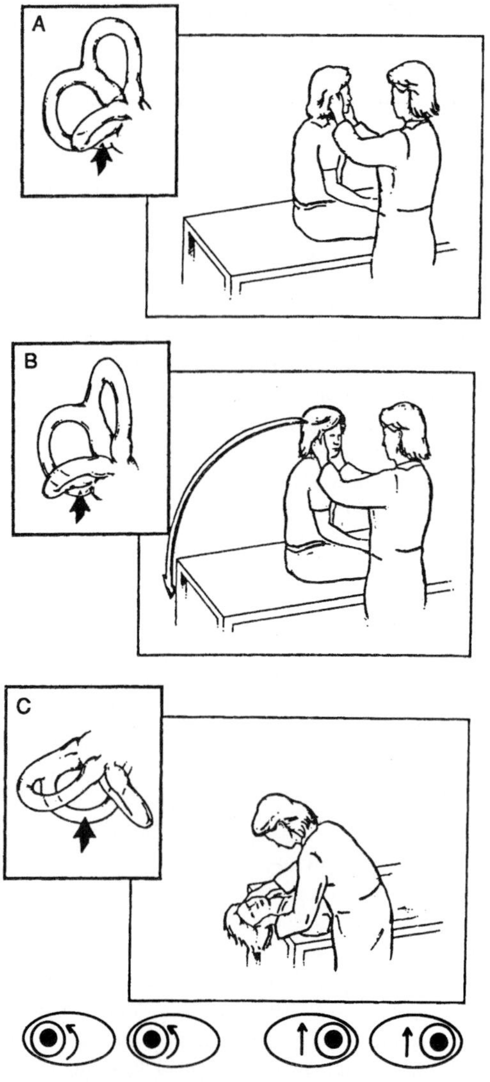

Figure 11–4. Diagnosis (Dix-Hallpike maneuver, A–C) and treatment (Epley maneuver, D–E) of benign paroxysmal positional vertigo due to otolithic debris in the right posterior semicircular canal. For each head position, the corresponding orientation of the right labyrinth is shown, with the arrow pointing to the presumed location of the otolithic debris in the posterior semicircular canal. (A) The patient's head is turned to the right shoulder. (B) The patient is rapidly moved from sitting to head-hanging position, with the head 45 degrees below the horizontal and rotated to the right, as shown in (C). After a brief latency, vertigo is induced and nystagmus commences; the direction of the **quick** phases of nystagmus induced by this maneuver is shown (more upbeat in left gaze and more torsional in right gaze) (see Video Display: Positional Nystagmus). *(continued)*

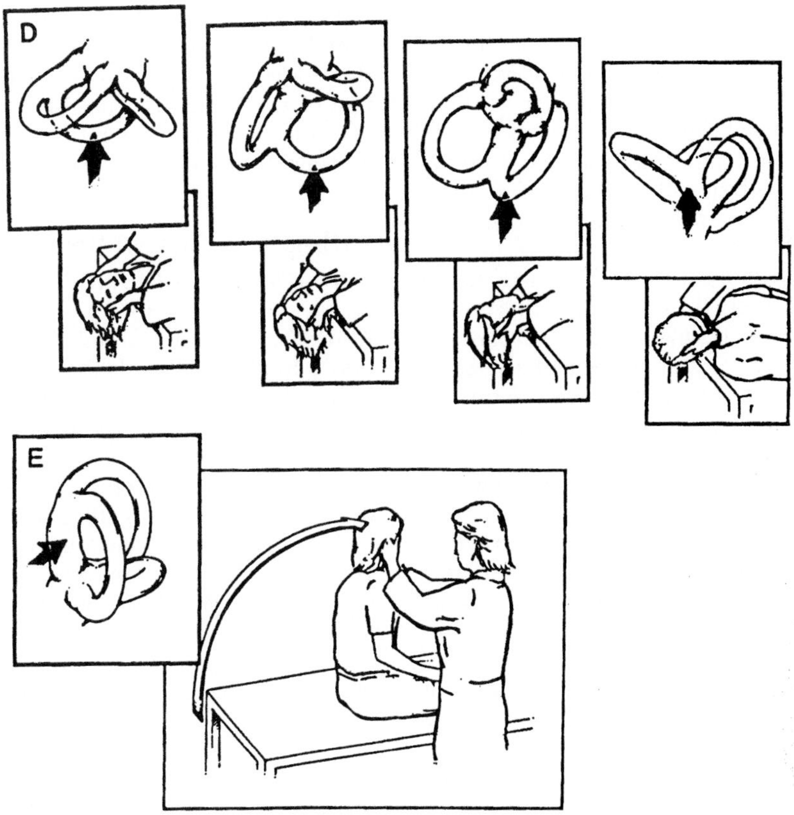

Figure 11–4. *(Continued)* (D) The patient's head is held still for 30 seconds after the nystagmus and vertigo subside. Then the patient's head is extended slightly, and head and body are slowly rotated to the patient's left, so that the head rotates through 180 degrees from the orientation in (C). The patient is held in this position for 30 seconds, to allow time for the otolithic debris to exit from the common crux of the vertical canals (arrow). (E) Finally, the patient sits up, keeping the head turned to the left. The patient is encouraged to sustain a head-erect posture for the rest of the day. (Reproduced from S. J. Herdman,[252] with permission of F.A. Davis, Philadelphia.)

the opposite lateral position (equivalent to the nystagmus reversal that appears with BPPV of the posterior canal when the patient sits upright). With lateral-canal BPPV, the initial horizontal nystagmus may last longer and be less susceptible to habituation with repetitive testing than the vertical-torsional nystagmus of posterior-canal BPPV. The increased duration and the tendency for the nystagmus to increase in intensity as the offending head position is maintained may reflect the action of both the central velocity-storage mechanism (which perseverates peripheral labyrinthine signals, especially from the lateral semicircular canal) and the continuous application of the equivalent of a constant acceleration from gravity causing the nystagmus to grow.

Canalolithiasis and cupulolithiasis both may play a role in lateral-canal BPPV. If the nystagmus is geotropic, the particles probably are in the posterior portion of the long arm of the lateral semicircular canal, relatively far from the cupula. If the nystagmus is apogeotropic, the particles could also be in the long arm, but in its anterior aspect relatively close to the cupula. Finally, if the particles are on the opposite, ampullary side of the cupula the nystagmus will be apogeotropic. Patients may show geotropic nystagmus at some times and apogeotropic at other times, probably reflecting movement of the main body of particles within the canal. There is also the suggestion—in the occasional patient with lateral canal BPPV who also show a vertical component to the nystagmus—that free-floating particles in the utricle could contribute to the pattern of lateral canal BPPV.[561] It remains possible, however, that these patients also have particles floating or adherent in one of the vertical semicircular canals to account for the mixed pattern of positional nystagmus.[342a]

Another variant of BPPV may be due to otolithic debris in the anterior canal. Several authors have suggested that this syndrome can be identified by the direction of the nystagmus during the Dix-Hallpike maneuver (downbeat with a torsional component beating toward the affected ear with the affected ear up) but this syndrome is hard to identify with certainty.[56,309,462a]

Bilateral BPPV occasionally occurs, but if the patient's head is not positioned correctly during positional testing (not moved exactly in the plane of the posterior semicircular canal when testing the unaffected side), debris on the affected side can rest against the cupula and simulate an excitatory nystagmus from the unaffected ear.[484] Rarely, the nystagmus of BPPV may be purely vertical or purely torsional due to debris floating in both vertical canals at the same time (vertical if the debris floats in the same direction, torsional if it floats in opposite directions). This circumstance is an exception to the rule that pure vertical or pure torsional nystagmus always indicates a central problem. There are other patterns of positional nystagmus that do not conform to a specific pattern of involvement of a single canal, yet most are variants of BPPV. Involvement of more than one canal, and the possibility that particles may become adherent to the wall of the canal can lead to diagnostic confusion.[24,342a] The otherwise typical historical features and the lack of additional neurological abnormalities point to the correct diagnosis. On the other hand, BPPV is so common, especially in the elderly, that one must be vigilant for other neurological causes in patients with otherwise typical BPPV who have neurological symptoms that do not fit the typical pattern.

In some patients, no nystagmus will be elicited with postural testing; the diagnosis must then be made based on the history. It is helpful to reexamine the patient if symptoms persist, and especially at a time when they exacerbate. Examination early in the morning may be more fruitful, before the particles disperse as the day progresses, though formal recordings of positional nystagmus have shown no difference depending upon time of day.[312] If the nystagmus is not typical for BPPV, an effort to identify disease of the brainstem or cerebellum is appropriate, although in most cases, no morbid disease process will be found.

Apart from the findings during positional testing, other tests of ocular motility may be normal. In a minority of patients, particularly those with a prior history of viral or ischemic neurolabyrinthitis, the head-impulse maneuver will show a unilateral deficit, or caloric responses are reduced in the affected ear.

Pathophysiology of Benign Paroxysmal Positional Vertigo

A combination of careful clinical observation, pathological correlations, and physiologic experimentation has led to a better understanding of the *pathogenesis* of BPPV.[58,86,168,199,228,268,319,333,416,439,484] Electron microscopic studies have confirmed that the debris consists of otoconia.[546] There is still considerable controversy, however, about exactly what is happening within the semicircular canals to explain the typical characteristics of the nystagmus: latency between assuming the offending head position and the appearance of the positional nystagmus, adaptation (nystagmus decays as the head position is maintained) and diminution on repeat testing (habituation).[228,439] Originally, it was thought that degenerated utricular otoliths became detached and came to rest on the dependent cupula of the posterior semicircular canal, a state called cupulolithiasis.[464] More recent evidence suggests that free-floating debris on the other side of the cupula in the long arm of the posterior semicircular canal is the common cause. This is referred to as canalolithiasis.[376,424] The debris may coalesce and act as a plug so that under the pull of gravity, the moving debris (either with a plunger-like action or simply owing to hydrodynamic drag) causes the cupula to move, inducing nystagmus even when the head is still.[86,168] In other words, the semicircular canal becomes a gravity detector. When the posterior semicircular canal is moved into an earth-vertical position, the net result is to produce false excitatory signals from the affected posterior semicircular canal. These signals cause the eyes to rotate in a plane that is parallel to the stimulated canal, reflecting excitation of the projection targets of the posterior canal VOR, including the primary pathways to the ipsilateral superior oblique and contralateral inferior rectus muscles.

The evidence for involvement of the posterior semicircular canal in BPPV is strengthened by 1) the fact that surgical section of the posterior ampullary nerve, which supplies the posterior semicircular canal, or plugging of the posterior semicircular canal, cures the condition and 2) free-floating particles have been identified within the posterior semicircular canal at the time of surgical plugging.[5,200,202,423,424] There is still some question, though, about other changes in the labyrinth, especially the utricle but also other canals, that contribute to BPPV in some patients.[24,201,243,532a,561] The function of the posterior semicircular canal may also be modestly impaired.[276] Exercises or maneuvers aimed at removing the otolithic debris from the offending semicircular canal promote recovery (see Treatment of Vertigo), although many patients will eventually improve spontaneously.

In patients in whom BPPV follows acute, peripheral vestibulopathy (viral or ischemic in origin), there may be selective damage to the structures innervated by the superior division of the vestibular nerve and perfused by the anterior vestibular artery: the anterior and lateral semicircular canals, and the utricle.[170] By using click-induced EMG potentials in the sternocleidomastoid (a sacculocollic reflex mediated by the inferior vestibular nerve), it was found that this reflex was intact in all patients who developed BPPV after vestibular neurolabyrinthitis, implying sparing of the inferior division of the vestibular nerve.[382] BPPV is not always an isolated phenomenon and may be associated with migraine, Ménière's disease, and other inner disturbances.[280,297,428] Audiograms and sometimes further testing are indicated in any patient with persistent or unusual patterns of positional vertigo and nystagmus.

OTHER CAUSES OF POSITIONAL VERTIGO

Posturally induced vertigo due to *central disorders* (Table 11–1) may be relatively mild, and the nystagmus is usually more impressive than the subjective disturbance (see Video Display: Disorders of the Vestibular System). When the patient is placed in a head-hanging position, usually the nystagmus persists for as long as the head position is maintained; rarely, the findings are similar to BPPV. Multiple sclerosis may cause positional nystagmus, sometimes with accompanying vertigo;[187,300] such symptoms may be the first manifestation of the disease. Occasionally, a cerebellar tumor,[165] infarction, or hematoma[301] may produce postural vertigo or vomiting. Nystagmus typical of BPPV that is present with the patient's head turned to the right and to the left (bilateral BPPV) occasionally may be secondary to head injury or brain stem ischemia,[120,340] but one must watch for improper positioning of the head during positional testing maneuvers before diagnosing bilateral BPPV.[484] Isolated vertigo due to neck movements that lead to kinking of the vertebral artery happens rarely;[128a,450,492] associated neurologic symptoms are usually present.

Some normal subjects may show *sustained positional nystagmus*—nystagmus that persists following a horizontal change in head position (e.g., with the subject supine, head turned to the right or left).[351] It usually is in the same direction as the head. In some patients, the nystagmus changes direction with lateral head turn, either always beating toward the earth (geotropic) or always beating away from the earth (apogeotropic). Such nystagmus most often reflects a lateral canal BPPV syndrome, as discussed above. Alcohol intoxication can produce a horizontal positional nystagmus by making the cupula relatively lighter (during intoxication) or heavier (during sobering up) than the surrounding endolymph, by virtue of differential absorption. During intoxication the nystagmus is geotropic; as the subject sobers up it is apogeotropic.[371]

When due to central causes,[48] horizontal positional nystagmus is relatively unchanging in slow-phase velocity and is almost always associated with other neurological symptoms or signs. The cause of horizontal positional nystagmus in central disorders may relate to abnormalities of the linear (translational) VOR (discussed above and in Chapter 2). Pure vertical positional nystagmus—which is usually downbeating with respect to the head—frequently signals a disturbance in the cerebellum or cranio-cervical junction; it is discussed further in Chapter 10.

Characteristics of horizontal positional nystagmus that suggest a central disturbance and usually demand imaging include: (1) a sustained, large-amplitude nystagmus that is present during visual fixation; (2) nystagmus that occurs in more than one head position; and (3) nystagmus that has an associated vertical (and especially downbeat) component or is pure torsional.

Even with these caveats, most patients with positional vertigo and positional or positioning nystagmus who have no other neurological symptoms or signs will not have a central disturbance as the cause of their vestibular symptoms.[124]

Treatment of Vertigo

Here we summarize some basic principles for the treatment of vertigo.[123,229]In any patient with undiagnosed vestibular symptoms, who have often seen many physicians without a definite diagnosis or treatment, it is helpful to take the time to explain the mechanisms by which disorders of the labyrinth create dizziness, vertigo and imbalance and especially how certain visual environments and types of motion can trigger their symptoms. Much can be accomplished by allaying the patient's fear that their symptoms are 'not real'.

In *acute vertigo* due to a peripheral vestibular lesion such as a viral or ischemic neurolabyrinthitis, recovery is the rule in the ensuing weeks. Prednisone may be helpful in improving the long-term recovery but the case for antiviral medications has not yet been proven.[493] Drugs that have a sedative effect (Table 11–2) should be used sparingly for treatment of vertigo, with the exception of Ménière's syndrome; in this case, the pathophysiology of the attack and the recovery relate to mechanical changes in the labyrinth, not central compensation, so a brief period of moderate sedation need not have any deleterious effects related to retarded central compensation. Patients should be encouraged to get up and increase their activities as soon as possible, since there is evidence that failure to do so might limit the recovery. Much current research is aimed at finding medications that promote vestibular compensation.[143,480,481] A course of specific vestibular exercises may be indicated (see below). Those patients who develop enduring vestibular symptoms may have an underlying central nervous system disorder, typically involving the cerebellum,[193,454] and imaging studies are indicated.

Treatment of *recurrent* vertigo depends upon the nature of the underlying disorder. For example, vertigo due to migraine can usually be successfully treated. Vertigo due to episodic ataxia type 2, may respond to acetazolamide or the diaminopyridines. Vertigo due to Ménière's syndrome may be difficult to manage, although a low-salt diet and diuretics help some patients.[101] Intratympanic gentamicin has been shown to be an effective alternative to surgical ablation for intractable vestibular symptoms in Ménière's syndrome.[114,427] Quantitative recordings of the VOR in response to 'head impulses' often help guide therapy.[115,117]

Benign paroxysmal positional vertigo is treated effectively in most cases by particle repositioning maneuvers. Several effective strategies have been described.[87,133,167,168,211,245,250,258,336a,353,373,399,431a,437,438,474,505,530,557] Patients can often learn to do these maneuvers at home by themselves.[195,264] The use of a cervical collar, daily repetition of Brandt-Daroff exercises, and prolonged periods of sleeping upright seem to be unnecessary in most patients, though there is some disagreement about whether or not mastoid vibration during the maneuver is beneficial.[133,168,227,250,344,373,402] Repeated maneuvers in a single session, however, may be more effective.[211] Even in patients without positional nystagmus it is worthwhile to treat them with a particle repositioning maneuver if the history is otherwise typical.[245]

The *Epley maneuver* is summarized in Figure 11–4 and shown in the Video Display: Positional Nystagmus). We typically repeat the treatment until nystagmus and vertigo are no longer elicited. If the nystagmus remains upbeating through out the treatment maneuver, indicating continued progression of the otolithic debris out of the long arm of the posterior canal, a successful outcome can be predicted confidently. Patients, however, may have successful outcomes even when this pattern is not observed (e.g., there may be some downbeating nystagmus when the patient sits up, which suggests some of the particles have fallen back into the posterior canal). Occasionally a downbeat nystagmus may occur in the dependent position upon repeat testing after the initial mixed upbeat torsional nystagmus can no longer be elicited. This may represent the equivalent of a 'recovery nystagmus' reflecting an adaptive mechanism that would counteract the previously present positional nystagmus. After the treatment patients are advised to sit upright in the clinic for about twenty minutes, and then to be careful when

Table 11–2. **Some Commonly Used Vestibular Sedatives**

Drug	Class	Dosage	Comments	Precautions
Dimenhydrinate (Dramamine)	Antihistamine, increases cAMP	Oral: 50 mg, every 4–6 hr; IM: 50 mg; maximum of 200 mg in 24 hr	Mildly sedative, dryness, moderate antiemetic	Asthma, glaucoma, prostrate enlargement
Promethazine (Phenergan)	Antihistamine Anticholinergic Phenothiazine	Oral: 25 mg, every 6 hr; Supp: 50 mg, every 12 hr; IM: 25 mg; maximum of 75 mg in 24 hr	More sedative, moderate antiemetic	Asthma, glaucoma, prostate enlargement, epilepsy
Meclizine (Antivert, Bonine)	Antihistamine Anticholinergic	Oral: 25 mg or 50 mg, every day or twice daily; maximum of 150 mg in 24 hr	Peak effects 8 hours after ingestion; less sedative	Asthma, glaucoma, prostrate enlargement
Prochlorperazine (Compazine)	Antihistamine, Anticholinergic Phenothiazine	Oral: 5–10 mg every 6 hr; Suppository: 25 mg every 12 hr; IM: 5–10 mg every 6 hr; maximum of 60 mg in 24 hr	Sedative and antiemetic; can cause extrapyramidal reactions	Liver disease; in combination with CNS depressants, propranolol, phenytoin, anticoagulants, levodopa, diuretics
Scopolamine ("Transderm Scop")	Anticholinergic (nonselective muscarinic)	Transdermal patch, every 3 days; Peak effect 4–8 hr after application	Less sedative, more antiemetic, used for prevention of motion sickness Can cause confusion, mydriasis, "dependency"	Asthma, glaucoma, prostrate enlargement, drug dependence.
Ondansetron ("Zofran")	Serotonin 5-HT_3 receptor antagonist	Oral: 4–8 mg, every 8 hr; 4 mg IV	Antiemetic, developed for patients receiving cancer chemotherapy; may be effective for nausea due to CNS disease	Headache; constipation
Lorazepam (Ativan)	Benzodiazepine	0.5 mg every 12 hr; 1 mg IM; maximum of 6 mg in 24 hr	GABA-modulator; may be habit-forming, with habituation	Glaucoma; additive with sedative drugs, scopolamine

first beginning to walk. Some postural instability is common with BPPV and this may be temporarily increased after a successful treatment.

A number of maneuvers have been reported to alleviate the lateral canal variant including log-rolling (270 degrees rotation away from the side of the lesion) and prolonged lying on the side (up to 11 hours) with the affected ear uppermost, and various modified particle repositioning maneuvers.[15,16,121,137,266,506,516] The anterior canal variant has been treated by rapidly sitting up and then rotating the head even further forward; as well as the maneuvers used for the posterior canal variant.[91,138,309] Drugs are not indicated in BPPV except to relieve symptoms during the treatment maneuvers. A small percentage of patients do not improve with exercises and patients with post-traumatic BPPV may be less successfully treated.[212] As previously mentioned, surgical section of the nerve to the posterior semicircular canal has been effective,[200] but occlusion of the posterior semicircular canal is currently the preferred intervention.[5,6,423] We almost never refer a patient with BPPV for surgical intervention though in intractable cases this may be necessary.[5,6,91,266,423]

Physical therapy programs including Tai Chi are often helpful for unilateral and bilateral vestibular loss and motion sensitivity syndromes.[104,207,222,225,251,253–257,355, 488,509,551]

OSCILLOPSIA

Oscillopsia is an illusion of movement of the seen world. It is usually caused by excessive motion of images of stationary objects upon the retina (Table 11–3). Excessive retinal slip not only causes oscillopsia but also impairs vision. The relationship between retinal image velocity and visual acuity is a direct one: for higher spatial frequencies, image motion in excess of about 5 degrees/second impairs vision.[119,151] On the other hand, the relationship between retinal image velocity and the development of oscillopsia is less consistent and varies among subjects. For example, individuals with congenital nystagmus, who often have images moving across the retina with speeds exceeding 100 degrees/second,[2] seldom complain of oscillopsia under normal viewing conditions.[1] Acquired disease affecting eye movements produces oscillopsia in three main ways: an abnormal VOR, paresis of extraocular muscles, and ocular oscillations—such as nystagmus.

Table 11–3. **Etiology of Oscillopsia[99]**

Oscillopsia with Head Movements: Abnormal Vestibulo-Ocular Reflex

- Peripheral vestibular hypofunction[77,260,448]
  - Aminoglycoside toxicity[63,64,234,362,390,541,564]
  - Surgical section of eighth cranial nerve[182]
  - Tumors[350]
  - Meningitis[357]
  - Congenital ear anomalies[347,381]
  - Superior canal dehiscence[153,367,503]
  - Hereditary vestibular areflexia[37,90,517,518]
  - Superficial siderosis[293,522]
  - Cisplatin therapy[108,310,391]
  - Aspirin[491]
  - Idiopathic[38,173,523]
  - Dolichoectatic basilar artery[110,403]
  - Post radiation[128]
  - Trauma[224]
- Central vestibular dysfunction
  - Decreased VOR gain[220,444]
  - Increased VOR gain[502,568]
  - Abnormal VOR phase[220]
  - Abnormal VOR direction[537a]
- Paresis of extraocular muscles (including ocular motor nerve palsies)

Oscillopsia Due to Nystagmus

- Acquired nystagmus (especially pendular nystagmus, upbeat, downbeat, seesaw, dissociated nystagmus)[213,330,331,563]
- Saccadic oscillations (psychogenic flutter/voluntary nystagmus, ocular flutter, microsaccadic flutter and opsoclonus)
- Superior oblique myokymia (monocular oscillopsia—see Chapter 9)
- Congenital nystagmus (uncommon under natural illumination)[259,330]

Central Oscillopsia

- With cerebral disorders: seizures, occipital lobe infarction[51]
- With transcutaneous magnetic stimulation of scalp[299a]
- Extreme motion sensitivity to visual stimulation[96,96a,99,222]

Oscillopsia due to an Abnormal Vestibulo-Ocular Reflex

An abnormal VOR may lead to oscillopsia during head movements via three mechanisms: abnormal gain, abnormal phase shift (timing) between eye and head rotations, and a mismatch between the directions of the vectors of the head rotation and eye rotation (see Quantitative Aspects of the Vestibular-Optokinetic System in Chapter 2). Peripheral or central dysfunction affecting either the angular or the linear VOR can lead to oscillopsia.[152,332,516] Especially in the acute phase of loss of vestibular function due, for example, to bilateral eighth nerve section,[182] or aminoglycoside antibiotic intoxication,[284] head rotations will lead to oscillopsia.

Patients with bilateral vestibular loss may become excessively dependent upon visual inputs for image stabilization and consequently have visual discomfort and inappropriate body sway while standing still and attempting to watch, for example, swaying trees on a windy day. This excessive visual dependence can become a problem in any patient with an active labyrinthine disorder, or even a past history of one. It leads to the common complaint of visual discomfort and unsteadiness when such patients are walking down aisles in a supermarket, seeing action movies on a large screen, looking out of the car through windshield wipers, or walking or riding by a picket fence.[96] On the other hand, patients with vestibular loss often show elevated thresholds for motion detection, a perceptual adaptive mechanism.[476]

Typically, oscillopsia is worse during walking or running, (see Fig. 7–1 in Chapter 7 and Video Display: Disorders of the Vestibular System) but it may be noticed during chewing food and, in the most severe cases, it may occur due to transmitted cardiac pulsation.[284] In addition, dynamic visual acuity declines during head movements; this decline can be easily demonstrated at the bedside.[108,256,257,341,463] Objectively, using the ophthalmoscope, the optic disc will be seen to move with every head rotation. Patients with essential head tremor and vestibular failure may show abnormal oscillations of the optic disc during ophthalmoscopy.[100,564] Because any residual function of the VOR is usually preferentially spared for higher-frequency stimuli,[36] the inadequacy of the vestibulo-ocular reflex may sometimes be more evident during large-amplitude, back-and-forth oscillations of the head at about 1 Hz. During these movements, saccades are necessary to hold gaze steady during attempted fixation. (Video Display: Disorders of the Vestibular System) With time, however, compensation takes place, owing to potentiation of the cervico-ocular reflex, pre-programming of compensatory eye movements, perceptual changes, and other factors (see Table 7–1, Chapter 7 and Chapter 2). Bilateral vestibular loss may be the cause of oscillopsia and gait imbalance in the elderly. Their ability to compensate may be impaired leading to more bothersome symptoms.[173]

Ototoxicity, especially associated with *aminoglycoside* antibiotics, is an important cause of loss of the VOR.[63–65,362,390,539] Intravenous gentamicin is the most common culprit and its toxicity may be insidious. It may occur without hearing symptoms, with therapeutic blood levels, and relatively short periods of administration.[234] Some patients who develop ototoxicity may be genetically predisposed to the toxic side effects of the drug.[177,430] Topical gentamicin may occasionally lead to unwanted labyrinthine loss when used to treat external ear infections.[339] Intratympanic gentamicin is used to purposefully ablate labyrinthine function as part of the treatment of intractable Ménière's syndrome.[114] In contrast, cisplatin is probably not as vestibulotoxic as originally thought.[310,386,391]

The differential diagnosis of bilateral vestibular loss includes toxic, infectious, neoplastic, autoimmune, traumatic and inflammatory processes.[77,224,260,357,400,448] Dolichoectasia of the vertebral or basilar artery also may lead to bilateral loss, usually without involvement of hearing.[403,426] Bilaterally deficient vestibular function may be a feature of congenital ear anomalies.[381] Superficial siderosis leads to hearing and vestibular loss, anosmia, and ataxia.[293,522] Often no cause can be identified for bilateral vestibular deficiency,[37,38,77,517,523] though a nerve location is suggested in some patients.[191]

Idiopathic bilateral vestibular loss is sometimes familial, inherited as a dominant trait, and can be associated with migraine and recurrent attacks of vertigo.[37,90] Hearing is usually intact. There may also be a linkage to chromosome 6.[291] Acetazolamide may help the attacks of vertigo and headaches, but it is not yet clear if the bilateral loss can be arrested or improved. Baloh and colleagues reported autopsy findings in a patient with isolated progressive loss of labyrinthine function who also had ultra-short time constants but preserved amplitude of response on vestibular testing.[40] They found loss of hair cells and altered mitochondria (and presumably abnormal energy metabolism) and suggested that these factors could account for the pattern of vestibular function loss.

Oscillopsia may also occur with disorders of the central nervous system that change the gain direction, or phase of the VOR. Thus, disease of the vestibulocerebellum may cause vestibular hyper-responsiveness, particularly in the vertical plane. This is common in patients with the Arnold–Chiari malformation.[568] Occasionally, patients are reported with increased gain of both the horizontal and vertical VOR.[502] In some patients with vestibulocerebellar dysfunction, the gain of the VOR is normal, but the phase relationship between head and eye movements is abnormal and causes slippage of images on the retina.[220] Lesions of the medial longitudinal fasciculus producing internuclear ophthalmoplegia may cause a low gain of the vertical VOR and produce oscillopsia with vertical head movements.[213,444]

Oscillopsia due to Paresis of Extraocular Muscles

Weakness of extraocular muscles besides causing diplopia may also lead to oscillopsia during head movements.[555] This is because the VOR is prevented from working adequately in the paretic field of gaze. The cause of the muscle weakness may be ocular motor nerve palsy; neuromuscular disease, such as myasthenia gravis; or restrictive diseases in the orbit, such as thyroid ophthalmopathy. Diseases of the extraocular muscles themselves also limit ocular motility, but the slow progression of these disorders seems to allow patients time to make perceptual adaptations, such as raised thresholds for detection of visual motion, to the slip of images on the retina during head movements.[3] These disorders of the extraocular muscles are discussed in Chapter 9. Rarely, subluxation of the lens following head trauma may cause monocular oscillopsia that occurs with each saccade.[385]

Oscillopsia due to Nystagmus and Other Abnormal Eye Movements

Oscillopsia may also be caused by ocular oscillations such as nystagmus (see Chapter 10). In such cases, oscillopsia occurs even when the head is still. Thus, acquired pendular nystagmus, occurring in multiple sclerosis or in association with palatal tremor; downbeat and upbeat nystagmus; and even gaze-evoked nystagmus may lead to oscillopsia (see Video Display: Treatments for Nystagmus). Patients with congenital nystagmus occasionally develop oscillopsia later in life.[259] In addition, certain saccadic disorders such as ocular flutter and opsoclonus (see Video Display: Saccadic Oscillations and Intrusions) may cause oscillopsia.[183] Superior oblique myokymia may cause monocular oscillopsia (see Video Display: Diplopia and Strabismus). One method of bringing out oscillopsia is to ask the patient to fixate on a small light in a dark room and to indicate the direction of the perceived movement of the stationary light. The nystagmus causing oscillopsia is not always obvious on gross examination.[51] A sensitive and convenient way to detect instability of gaze is to view the retina with an ophthalmoscope.

The magnitude of oscillopsia is usually less than the magnitude of nystagmus. For example, in patients with downbeat nystagmus, oscillopsia is equivalent to about one third of what would be predicted from the amplitude of the nystagmus.[106] This finding implies that the brain compensates for the excessive retinal image motion by using an extraretinal signal, such as efference copy, to maintain visual constancy.[150,330] As previously mentioned, oscillopsia is rarely a complaint in individuals with congenital nystagmus, though visual acuity may be impaired due to the oscillation. Motion detection may be impaired in some individuals with congenital nystagmus,[1,157] but this cannot be the entire explanation, since artificial stabilization of images, paradoxically, may cause oscillopsia.[150,330] Methods available for treatment of nystagmus are summarized in Table 10–9 and the Video Display: Treatments for Nystagmus.

Finally, patients occasionally report oscillopsia who do not have excessive retinal image motion (i.e., have no nystagmus or vestibular dysfunction) but, rather, seem to have a disorder of those central mechanisms that normally ensure a sense of visual constancy.[51,498]

SKEW DEVIATION AND THE OCULAR TILT REACTION (OTR)

Clinical Features of Skew Deviation and Ocular Tilt Reaction

Skew Deviation is a vertical misalignment of the visual axes caused by a disturbance of prenuclear inputs (see Video Display: Disorders of the Vestibular System). A torsional and horizontal deviation may be associated. The hypertropia may be nearly the same in all positions of gaze (concomitant) or vary with eye position (nonconcomitant); sometimes it may even alternate with eye position (e.g., right hypertropia on right gaze, left hypertropia on left gaze).[95,303,304,567] When the skew deviation is nonconcomitant, and especially if the pattern of misalignment resembles that of an individual muscle palsy, it may be difficult to differentiate from a vertical extraocular muscle palsy. The direction of any torsion of the elevated eye (intorsion with skew, extorsion with a superior oblique palsy) and coexisting signs of central neurological dysfunction usually clarify the localization.[163,164] Skew deviation has been reported with abnormalities in the vestibular periphery, the brainstem, or the cerebellum.[81,303,380,556a] Skew deviation can also be a transient finding associated with raised intracranial pressure due to supratentorial tumors or pseudotumor.[190] In infants, the presence of a skew deviation may be the harbinger of a subsequent horizontal strabismus.[269]

In some patients, skew deviation is associated with ocular torsion (cyclodeviation and a head tilt (ear to shoulder), the ocular tilt reaction (OTR)—see Figure 11–5. The OTR is commonly tonic (sustained),[84] but may be paroxysmal.[247,434] Rarely, the skew deviation may slowly alternate or vary in magnitude over the course of a few minutes.[135,218,368,435] Usually, any pathological head tilt is toward the lower ear, and the ocular torsion is such that the upper poles of the eyes rotate toward the lower ear. This is in contrast to physiologic counterrolling *in response* to an induced head tilt, when the ocular torsion is such that the upper poles of the eyes rotate toward the higher ear. The ocular torsion may be dissociated between the two eyes, for example in Wallenberg's syndrome with greater extorsion of the lower eye.[83,203] Torsional nystagmus (Box 10–4) can be associated with an acute skew deviation.[22,203] Patients with OTR also show a deviation of the subjective visual vertical.[70,83,84,159] though there may be no perceptual abnormality when the torsion is caused by a semicircular canal lesion alone.[489]

The OTR is usually attributed to an imbalance in otolith-ocular and otolith-collic reflexes; these are part of a phylogenetically old righting response to a lateral tilt of the head. In lateral-eyed animals, tilting the head laterally around the longitudinal (anterior-posterior) axis causes a disjunctive, vertical (skew) deviation (one eye goes up, the other down) that acts to hold the visual axis of each eye close to the horizon. In human subjects, who are frontal-eyed, a static head tilt (ear to shoulder) causes sustained conjugate counter-rolling of the eyes (ocular torsion) equal to about 10% of the head roll;[22,67,134,412,417,420] thus the static ocular response does not compensate for the head tilt and is thought

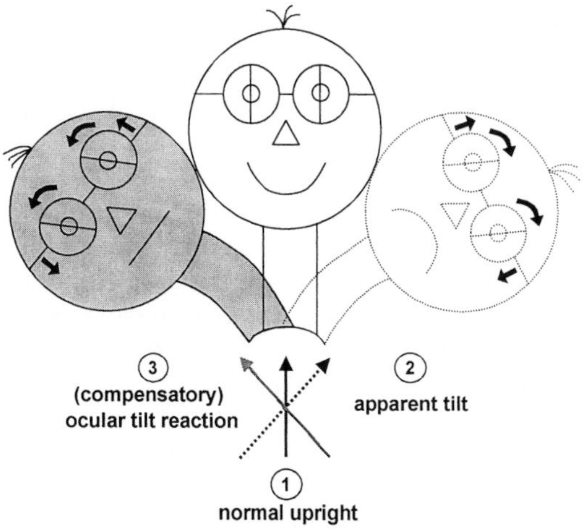

Figure 11–5. The ocular tilt reaction represented as a "motor compensation" of a lesion-induced apparent eye-head tilt (dashed line), and which would be opposite in direction to the apparent tilt. The eyes and head are continuously adjusted to what the lesioned brain computes as being vertical. (From Brandt and Dieterich,[84] with permission.)

to be vestigial. In normal subjects there may be skewing during rotation of the head around its roll (anterior-posterior) axis; the amount depends upon the direction and distance of the point of visual fixation.[52,68,287,288,359,419] In contrast, peripheral or central lesions that disrupt otolithic inputs often cause large amounts of skew deviation (as much as 7 degrees) and ocular torsion (as much as 25 degrees). An imbalance of semicircular canal inputs may also play a role.[84,208] In this case, nystagmus may also be present.[22]

In patients with more rostral lesions in the midbrain, interruption of descending pathways controlling head posture may also contribute to the head tilt of the OTR,[83] and involvement of the oculomotor or trochlear nuclei or nerves may also affect the pattern. Visual factors may also contribute to the head tilt of the OTR. In this case it may be, in part, a compensatory response to the perceived tilt of the subjective visual vertical.[84]

Topologic Diagnosis of Skew Deviation and the Ocular Tilt Reaction

Acute peripheral vestibulopathy—lesions affecting the vestibular organ or its nerve—can cause skew deviation and the complete OTR, based upon an imbalance in inputs from the utricles.[235,324b,449,456,556] The OTR may also occur as a component of the Tullio phenomenon, most often in association with superior canal dehiscence, as discussed above.[367] In one well-studied patient, stimulation of the left ear with a specific auditory tone caused a head tilt to the right, left hypertropia, intorsion of the left eye, and extorsion of the right eye;[161] this effect was ascribed to mechanical stimulation of the left utricle by a hypermobile stapes, though high-resolution CT scanning did not exclude a superior canal dehiscence. These results are consistent with the effects of experimental stimulation of the otoliths[141] and the utricular nerve,[496] which elicits ipsilateral hypertropia and conjugate counter-rolling.

Disease of the *vestibular nuclei* (e.g., as part of Wallenberg's syndrome—lateral medullary infarction) may also cause skew deviation with hypotropia on the side of the lesion.[160] In addition, some patients show an ipsilateral head tilt and disconjugate ocular torsion. The latter is an excyclotropia, with excyclodeviation of the ipsilateral, lower eye, but small or absent incyclodeviation of the contralateral, higher eye.[83,378]

Patients with *cerebellar* lesions may also show a skew deviation.[379,380,435,520,556a,567] Some of these patients show an alternating skew deviation that changes with the direction of horizontal gaze; usually there is a hyperdeviation of the abducting eye. This abnormality, too, is analogous to a phylogenetically old, otolith-mediated, righting reflex present in lateral-eyed animals. In this case, however, the reflex is related to the ocular motor response that compensates for fore and aft pitch of the head when the eyes are directed laterally in the orbit.[95,567] Although involvement of the brainstem is also likely in some of these patients, skew deviation has been reported in patients who appear to have pure cerebellar disease.[379,556a] This suggests that, just as the cerebellum governs the semicircular canal–ocular reflex, it also influences the otolith-ocular reflexes.[44,552] Indeed, downbeat nystagmus (see Video Display: Downbeat, Upbeat, Torsional Nystagmus), which is often attributable to disease of the flocculus, commonly coexists with alternating skew deviation.

Utricular projections from the vestibular nuclei probably cross the midline and ascend in the medial longitudinal fasciculus (see Fig. 2–4, Chapter 2). Therefore, unilateral internuclear ophthalmoplegia is often associated with a skew deviation, usually an *ipsilateral* hypertropia.[504] Patients may also have isolated skew deviation due to brain stem lesions, probably from involvement of the vestibular nuclei or ascending otolith pathways.[497]

In the *midbrain*, otolith projections contact the third and fourth nerve nuclei, and the interstitial nucleus of Cajal (INC) (see Box 6–6). Mesencephalic lesions in or around the INC may cause a skew deviation,[302,303] and the OTR.[84,109,185,233] When the head tilt is sustained (tonic), it is contralateral to the side of the lesion. Usually there is also a hypertropia that is ipsilateral to the lesion and a conjugate torsion, with the ipsilateral eye intorting and the contralateral eye extorting. Associated defects of vertical eye movements and oculomotor or trochlear nerve function, including seesaw nystagmus, are common.[12,237,410] Combined fascicular or nuclear trochlear lesions and prenuclear lesions in the midbrain may cause extorsion of the contralateral eye and a contralateral OTR.[154,156]

Some patients present with a *paroxysmal skew deviation* (with or without a head tilt).[247,434] In one patient with a clearly defined lesion close to the right INC, episodes of contralateral hypertropia and ipsilateral head tilt occurred, suggesting an irritative mechanism.[247] This interpretation of the findings in paroxysmal skew deviation is supported by the results of electrical stimulation near the INC in monkeys, which produces an ocular tilt reaction that consists of depression and extorsion of the ipsilateral eye and elevation and intorsion of the contralateral eye.[550] With the head free to move, an ipsilateral head tilt also occurs.[549] In humans, electrical stimulation in the region of the INC causes an ipsilateral ocular tilt reaction.[343] A microvascular compression syndrome has also been suggested as a cause of paroxysmal skew deviation with torsional nystagmus.[486]

Midbrain lesions may also be associated with a periodic alternating skew deviation that alternates or varies in magnitude over the course of a few minutes.[135,218,368] The periodicity of the phenomenon is reminiscent of periodic alternating nystagmus (Box 10–5), and the two phenomena may coexist.[335] Skew may occasionally be seen as a feature of epilepsy, presumably on the basis of excitation from the cerebral hemispheres to the portions of the vestibular nuclei that mediate otolith-ocular reflexes.[112]

REFERENCES

1. Abadi RV, Whittle JP, Worfolk R. Oscillopsia and tolerance to retinal image movement in congenital nystagmus. Invest Ophthalmol Vis Sci 40, 339–345, 1999.
2. Abadi RV, Worfolk R. Retinal slip velocities in congenital nystagmus. Vision Res 29, 195–205, 1989.
3. Acheson JF, Cassidy L, Grunfeld EA, Shallo-Hoffman JA, Bronstein AM. Elevated visual motion detection thresholds in adults with acquired ophthalmoplegia. Br J Ophthalmol 85, 1447–1449, 2001.
4. Acierno MD, Trobe JD, Shepard NT, Cornblath WT, Disher MJ. Two types of oscillopsia in a patient with idiopathic vestibulopathy. J Neuroophthalmol 17, 92–94, 1997.
5. Agrawal SK, Parnes LS. Human experience with canal plugging. Ann N Y Acad Sci 942, 300–305, 2001.
6. Agrawal SK, Parnes LS. Surgical treatment of benign paroxysmal positional vertigo. Audiological Medicine 3, 63–68, 2005.
7. Al-Twaijri WA, Shevell MI. Pediatric migraine equivalents: occurrence and clinical features in practice. Pediatr Neurol 26, 365–368, 2002.
8. Albano J, Mishkin M, Westbrook L, Wurtz R. Visumotor deficits following ablation of monkey superior colliculus. J Neurophysiol 48, 338–350, 1982.
9. Albers FW, Ingels KJ. Otoneurological manifestations in Chiari-I malformation. J Laryngol Otol 107, 441–443, 1993.
10. Alpini D, Caputo D, Pugnetti L, Giuliano DA, Cesarani A. Vertigo and multiple sclerosis: aspects of differential diagnosis. Neurol Sci 22 Suppl 2, S84–S87, 2001.

10a. Altay EE, Serdaroglu A, Gucuyener K, Bilir E, Karabacak NI, Thio LL. Rotational vestibular epilepsy from the temporo-parieto-occipital junction. Neurology 65, 1675–1676, 2005.

11. Amarenco P, Kase CS, Rosengart A, et al. Very small (border zone) cerebellar infarcts. Distribution, causes, mechanisms and clinical features. Brain 116, 161–186, 1993.
12. Anderson DF, Morris RJ. Parinaud's syndrome and ipsilateral tonic ocular skew deviation from unilateral right paramedian thalamic infarct. Neuro-ophthalmology 19, 13–16, 1998.
13. Andrews JC, Honrubia V. Menier's disease. In Baloh RW, Halmagyi GM (eds). Disorders of the Vestibular System. Oxford, NY, 1996, pp 300–317.
14. Andrews JC, Hoover LA, Lee RS, Honrubia V. Vertigo in the hyperviscosity syndrome. Otolaryngol Head Neck Surg 98, 144–149, 1988.
15. Appiani GC, Catania G, Gagliardi M. A liberatory maneuver for the treatment of horizontal canal paroxysmal positional vertigo. Otol Neurotol 22, 66–69, 2001.
16. Appiani GC, Catania G, Gagliardi M, Cuiuli G. Repositioning maneuver for the treatment of the apogeotropic variant of horizontal canal benign paroxysmal positional vertigo. Otol Neurotol 26, 257–260, 2005.
17. Arbusow V, Dieterich M, Strupp M, et al. Herpes zoster neuritis involving superior and inferior parts of the vestibular nerve causes ocular tilt reaction. Neuro-ophthalmology 19, 17–22, 1998.
18. Arbusow V, Schulz P, Strupp M, et al. Distribution of herpes simplex virus type 1 in human geniculate and vestibular ganglia: implications for vestibular neuritis. Ann Neurol 46, 416–419, 1999.
19. Arbusow V, Strupp M, Brandt T. Amiodarone-induced severe prolonged head-positional vertigo and vomiting. Neurology 51, 917, 1998.
20. Arbusow V, Strupp M, Dieterich M, et al. Alternating episodes of vestibular nerve excitation and failure. Neurology 51, 1480–1483, 1998.
21. Arbusow V, Theil D, Strupp M, Mascolo A, Brandt T. HSV-1 not only in human vestibular ganglia but also in the vestibular labyrinth. Audiol Neurootol 6, 259–262, 2001.
22. Averbuch-Heller L, Rottach KG, Zivotofsky AG, et al. Torsional eye movements in patients with skew deviation and spasmodic torticollis: responses to static and dynamic head roll. Neurology 48, 506–514, 1997.
23. Averbuch-Heller L, Zivotofsky AZ, Das VE, et al. Investigations of the pathogenesis of acquired pendular nystagmus. Brain 188. 368–378, 1995.
24. Aw ST, Todd MJ, Aw GE, McGarvie LA, Halmagyi GM. Benign positional nystagmus: a study of its three-dimensional spatio-temporal characteristics. Neurology 64, 1897–1905, 2005.

25. Balcer LJ, Winterkorn JMS, Galetta SL. Neuroophthalmic manifestations of Lyme disease. J Neuroophthalmol 17, 108–121, 1997.
26. Ballard E, Butzer JF, Doners J. Susac's syndrome: neuropsychological characteristics in a young man. Neurology 47, 266–268, 1996.
27. Ballester M, Liard P, Vibert D, Hausler R. Meniere's disease in the elderly. Otol Neurotol 23, 73–78, 2002.
28. Baloh RW. Superior semicircular canal dehiscence syndrome: leaks and squeaks can make you dizzy. Neurology 62, 684–685, 2004.
29. Baloh RW. Clinical practice. Vestibular neuritis. N Engl J Med 348, 1027–1032, 2003.
30. Baloh RW. Vestibular disorders due to cerebrovascular disease. In Baloh RW, Halmagyi GM (eds). Disorders of the Vestibular System. Oxford, New York, 1996, pp 418–429.
31. Baloh RW. Charles Skinner Hallpike and the beginnings of neurotology. Neurology 54, 2138–2146, 2000.
32. Baloh RW. Episodic vertigo: central nervous system causes. Curr Opin Neurol 15, 17–21, 2002.
33. Baloh RW, DeRossett E, Cloughesy TF, et al. Novel brainstem syndrome associated with prostate cancer. Neurology 43, 2591–2596, 1993.
34. Baloh RW, Foster CA, Yue Q, Nelson SF. Familial migraine with vertigo and essential tremor. Neurology 46, 458–460, 1996.
35. Baloh RW, Honrubia V, Jacobson K. Benign positional vertigo: clinical and oculographic features in 240 cases. Neurology 37, 371–378, 1987.
36. Baloh RW, Honrubia V, Yee RD, Hess K. Changes in the human vestibulo-ocular reflex after loss of peripheral sensitivity. Ann Neurol 16, 222–228, 1984.
37. Baloh RW, Jacobson K, Fife T. Familial vestibulopathy: a new dominantly inherited syndrome. Neurology 44, 20–25, 1994.
38. Baloh RW, Jacobson K, Honrubia V. Idiopathic bilateral vestibulopathy. Neurology 39, 272–275, 1989.
39. Baloh RW, Jacobson K, Winder A. Drop attacks in Meniere's disease. Ann Neurol 28, 384–387, 1990.
40. Baloh RW, Lopez I, Beykirch K, Ishiyama A, Honrubia V. Clinical-pathological correlation in a patient with selective loss of hair cells in the vestibular endorgans. Neurology 49, 1377–1382, 1997.
41. Baloh RW, Winder A. Acetazolamide-responsive vestibulocerebellar syndrome: clinical and oculographic features. Neurology 41, 429–433, 1991.
42. Baloh RW, Yee RD. Spontaneous vertical nystagmus. Rev Neurol (Paris) 145, 527–532, 1989.
43. Baloh RW, Yee RD, Honrubia V. Eye movements in patients with Wallenberg's syndrome. Ann N Y Acad Sci 374, 600–613, 1981.
44. Baloh RW, Yue Q, Demer JL. The linear vestibulo-ocular reflex in normal subjects and patients with vestibular and cerebellar lesions. J Vestib Res 5, 349–361, 1995.
45. Baloh RW, Yue Q, Furman JM, Nelson SF. Familial episodic ataxia: clinical heterogeneity in four families linked to chromosome 19p. Ann Neurol 41, 8–16, 1997.
46. Banerjee A, Whyte A, Atlas MD. Superior canal dehiscence: review of a new condition. Clin Otolaryngol 30, 9–15, 2005.
47. Barac B. Vertiginous epileptic attacks and so-called "vestibulogenic seizures". Epilepsia 9, 137–144, 1968.
48. Barber HO. Positional nystagmus. Otolaryngol Head Neck Surg 92, 649–655, 1984.
49. Barmack NH, Shojaku H. Vestibularly-induced slow phase oscillations in climbing fiber responses of Purkinje cells in the cerebellar nodulus. Neuroscience 50, 1–5, 1992.
50. Belden CJ, Weg N, Minor LB, Zinreich SJ. CT evaluation of bone dehiscence of the superior semicircular canal as a cause of sound- and/or pressure-induced vertigo. Radiology 226, 337–343, 2003.
51. Bender MB. Oscillopsia. Arch Neurol 13, 204–213, 1965.
52. Bergamin O, Straumann D. Three-dimensional binocular kinematics of torsional vestibular nystagmus during convergence on head-fixed targets in humans. J Neurophysiol. 86, 113–122, 2001.
53. Bergsneider M, Becker DP. Vascular compression syndrome of the vestibular nerve: a critical analysis. Otolaryngol Head Neck Surg 112, 118–124, 1995.
54. Berrettini S, Ferri C, La Civita L, et al. Inner ear involvement in mixed cryoglobulinaemia patients. Br J Rheumatol 34, 370–374, 1995.
55. Berrettini S, Ravecca F, Sellari-Franceschini S, et al. Acoustic neuroma: correlations between morphology and otoneurological manifestations. J Neurological Sci 144, 24–33, 1996.
56. Bertholon P, Bronstein AM, Davies RA, Rudge P, Thilo KV. Positional down beating nystagmus in 50 patients: cerebellar disorders and possible anterior semicircular canalithiasis. J Neurol Neurosurg Psychiatry 72, 366–372, 2002.
57. Bertholon P, Chelikh L, Tringali S, Timoshenko A, Martin C. Combined horizontal and posterior canal benign paroxysmal positional vertigo in three patients with head trauma. Ann Otol Rhinol Laryngol 114, 105–110, 2005.
58. Beynon GJ. A review of management of benign paroxysmal positional vertigo by exercise therapy and by repositioning manoeuvers. Br J Audiol 31, 11–26, 1997.
59. Bhatia PL, Gupta OP, Agrawal MK, Mishr SK. Audiological and vestibular function tests in hypothyroidism. Laryngoscope 87, 2082–2089, 1977.
60. Bickerstaff ER. Basilar artery migraine. Lancet 1, 15–17, 1961.
61. Bir LS, Ardic FN, Kara CO, et al. Migraine patients with or without vertigo: comparison of clinical and electronystagmographic findings. J Otolaryngol 32, 234–238, 2003.
62. Bisdorff AR, Debatisse D. Localizing signs in positional vertigo due to lateral canal cupulolithiasis. Neurology 57, 1085–1088, 2001.
63. Black FO, Gianna-Poulin C, Pesznecker SC. Recovery from vestibular ototoxicity. Otol Neurotol 22, 662–671, 2001.
64. Black FO, Pesznecker S, Stallings V. Permanent gentamicin vestibulotoxicity. Otol Neurotol 25, 559–569, 2004.
65. Black FO, Pesznecker SC. Vestibular ototoxicity—clinical considerations. Otolaryngol Clin NA 26, 713–736, 1993.
66. Black FO, Pesznecker SC, Homer L, Stallings V. Benign paroxysmal positional nystagmus in hospitalized subjects receiving ototoxic medications. Otol Neurootol 25, 353–358, 2004.
67. Bockisch CJ, Haslwanter T. Three-dimensional eye position during static roll and pitch in humans. Vision Res 41, 2127–2137, 2001.
68. Bockisch CJ, Straumann D, Haslwanter T. Human

3–DaVOR with and without otolith stimulation. Exp Brain Res 161, 358–367, 2005.
69. Böhmer A. Acute unilateral peripheral vestibulopathy. In Baloh RW, Halmagyi GM (eds). Disorders of the Vestibular System. Oxford, New York, 1996, pp 318–327.
70. Böhmer A, Mast F, Jarchow T. Can a unilateral loss of otolithic function be clinically detected by assessment of the subjective visual vertical. Brain Res Bull 40, 423–429, 1996.
71. Böhmer A, Straumann D, Fetter M. Three-dimensional analysis of spontaneous nystagmus in peripheral vestibular lesions. Ann Otol Rhinol Laryngol 106, 61–68, 1997.
72. Boismier TE, Disher MJ. Spontaneous vertigo and headache: endolymphatic hydrops or migraine? Ear Nose Throat J80, 881–885, 2001.
73. Boiten J, Wilmink J, Kingma H. Acute rotatory vertigo caused by a small haemorrhage of the vestibular cortex. J Neurol Neurosurg Psychiatry 74, 388, 2003.
74. Bower CM, Cotton RT. The spectrum of vertigo in childhood. Arch Otolaryngol Head Neck Surg 121, 911–915, 1995.
75. Brackmann DE, Kesser BW, Day JD. Microvascular decompression of the vestibulocochlear nerve for disabling positional vertigo: the House Ear Clinic experience. Otol Neurotol 22, 882–887, 2001.
76. Brandt T. Phobic postural vertigo. Neurology 46, 1515–1519, 1996.
77. Brandt T. Bilateral vestibulopathy revisited. Eur J Med Res 1, 361–368, 1996.
78. Brandt T. Positional and positioning vertigo and nystagmus. J Neurol Sci 95, 3–28, 1990.
79. Brandt T, Bronstein AM. Cervical vertigo. J Neurol Neurosurg Psychiatry 71, 8–12, 2001.
80. Brandt T, Daroff RB. The multisensory physiological and pathological vertigo syndromes. Ann Neurol 7, 195–203, 1980.
81. Brandt T, Dieterich M. Skew deviation with ocular torsion: a vestibular sign of topographic diagnostic value. Ann Neurol 33, 528–534, 1993.
82. Brandt T, Dieterich M. Vestibular paroxysmia (disabling positional vertigo). Neuro-ophthalmology 14, 359–369, 1994.
83. Brandt T, Dieterich M. Different types of skew deviation. J Neurol Neurosurg Psychiatr 54, 549–550, 1991.
84. Brandt T, Dieterich M. Pathological eye-head coordination in roll: tonic ocular tilt reaction in mesencephalic and medullary lesions. Brain 110, 649–666, 1987.
85. Brandt T, Dieterich M, Strupp M. Vertigo and Dizziness: Common Complaints. Spinger, 2005.
86. Brandt T, Steddin S. Current view of the mechanism of benign paroxysmal positioning vertigo: cupulolithiasis or canalolithiasis. J Vestib Res 3, 373–382, 1993.
87. Brandt T, Steddin S, Daroff RB. Therapy for benign paroxysmal positioning vertigo revisited. Neurology 44, 796–800, 1994.
88. Brandt T, Strupp M. Episodic ataxia type 1 and 2 (familial periodic ataxia/vertigo). Audiol Neurootol 2, 373–383, 1997.
89. Brandt TH, Botzel K, Yousry T, Dieterich M, Schulze S. Rotational vertigo in embolic stroke of the vestibular and auditory cortices. Neurology 45, 42–44, 1995.
90. Brantberg K. Familial early-onset progressive vestibulopathy without hearing impairment. Acta Otolaryngol. 123, 713–717, 2003.
91. Brantberg K, Bergenius J. Treatment of anterior benign paroxysmal positional vertigo by canal plugging: a case report. Acta Otolaryngol 122, 28–30, 2002.
92. Brantberg K, Ishiyama A, Baloh RW. Drop attacks secondary to superior canal dehiscence syndrome. Neurology 64, 2126–2128, 2005.
93. Brantberg K, Lofqvist L, Fransson PA. Large vestibular evoked myogenic potentials in response to bone-conducted sounds in patients with superior canal dehiscence syndrome. Audiol Neurootol 9, 173–182, 2004.
94. Britton BH, Block LD. Vertigo in the pediatric and adolescent age group. Laryngoscope 98, 139–146, 1988.
95. Brodsky MC. Three dimensions of skew deviation. Br J Ophthalmol 87, 1440–1441, 2003.
96. Bronstein AM. Vision and vertigo: some visual aspects of vestibular disorders. J Neurol 251, 381–387, 2004.
96a. Bronstein A. Visual symptoms and vertigo. Neurol Clin 23, 705–713, 2005.
97. Bronstein AM. Benign paroxysmal positional vertigo: some recent advances. Curr Opin Neurol 16, 1–3, 2003.
98. Bronstein AM. Vestibular reflexes and positional manoeuvres. J Neurol Neurosurg Psychiatry 74, 289–293, 2003.
99. Bronstein AM. Oscillopsia: editorial review. Curr Opin Neurol 18, 1–3, 2005.
100. Bronstein AM, Gresty MA, Mossman SS. Pendular pseudonystagmus arising as a combination of head tremor and vestibular failure. Neurology 42, 1527–1531, 1992.
101. Brookes GB. The pharmacological treatment of Menière's disease. Clin Otolaryngol 21, 3–11, 1996.
102. Broughton SS, Meyerhoff WE, Cohen SB. Immune-mediated inner ear disease: 10–year experience. Semin Arthritis Rheum 34, 544–548, 2004.
103. Brown JJ, Baloh RW. Persistent mal de debarquement. Am J Otolaryngol 8, 219–222, 1987.
104. Brown KE, Whitney SL, Wrisley DM, Furman JM. Physical therapy outcomes for persons with bilateral vestibular loss. Laryngoscope 111, 1812–1817, 2001.
105. Bruzzone MG, Grisoli M, De Simone T, Regna-Gladin C. Neuroradiological features of vertigo. Neurol Sci 25 Suppl 1, S20–S23, 2004.
106. Buchele W, Brandt T, Degner D. Ataxia and oscillopsia in downbeat-nystagmus vertigo syndrome. Adv Oto-Rhino-Laryngol 30, 291–297, 1983.
107. Buchholz DW, Reich SG. The menagerie of migraine. Semin Neurol 16, 83–94, 1996.
108. Burgio DL, Blakley BW, Myers SF. The high-frequency oscillopsia test. J Vestib Res 2, 221–226, 1992.
109. Büttner U, Helmchen C. Eye movement deficits after unilateral mesencephalic lesions. Neuro-ophthalmology 24, 469–484, 2000.
110. Büttner U, Ott M, Helmchen C, Yousry T. Bilateral loss of eighth nerve function as the only clinical sign of vertebrobasilar dolichoectasia. J Vestib Res. 5, 47–51, 1995.
111. Calandriello L, Veneziano L, Francia A, et al. Acetazolamide-responsive episodic ataxia in an Italian family refines gene mapping on chromosome 19p13. Brain 120, 805–812, 1997.

112. Galimberti CA, Versino M, Sartori I, et al. Epileptic skew deviation. Neurology 50, 1469–1472, 1998.
113. Canalis RF. Infections of the ear and temporal bone. In Baloh RW, Halmagyi GM (eds). Disorders of the Vestibular System. Oxford, New York, 1996, pp 340–352.
114. Carey J. Intratympanic gentamicin for the treatment of Meniere's disease and other forms of peripheral vertigo. Otolaryngol Clin North Am 37, 1075–1090, 2004.
115. Carey JP, Hirvonen T, Peng GC, et al. Changes in the angular vestibulo-ocular reflex after a single dose of intratympanic gentamicin for Meniere's disease. Ann N Y Acad Sci 956, 581–584, 2002.
116. Carey JP, Hirvonen TP, Hullar TE, Minor LB. Acoustic responses of vestibular afferents in a model of superior canal dehiscence. Otol Neurotol 25, 345–352, 2004.
117. Carey JP, Minor LB, Peng GC, et al. Changes in the three-dimensional angular vestibulo-ocular reflex following intratympanic gentamicin for Meniere's disease. J Assoc Res Otolaryngol 3, 430–443, 2002.
118. Carmona S, Nicenboim L, Castagnino D. Recurrent vertigo in extrinsic compression of the brain stem. Ann N Y Acad Sci 1039, 513–516, 2005.
119. Carpenter RHS. The visual origins of ocular motility. In Carpenter RHS (ed). Eye Movements. Vol 8. MacMillan Press, London, 1991, pp 1–10.
120. Caruso G, Nuti D. Epidemiological data from 2270 PPV patients. Audiological Medicine 3, 7–11, 2005.
121. Casani AP, Vannucci G, Fattori B, Berrettini S. The treatment of horizontal canal positional vertigo: our experience in 66 cases. Laryngoscope 112, 172–178, 2002.
122. Casselman JW. Diagnostic imaging in clinical neuro-otology. Curr Opin Neurol 15, 23–30, 2002.
123. Cesarani A, Alpini D, Monti B, Raponi G. The treatment of acute vertigo. Neurol Sci 25 Suppl 1, S26–S30, 2004.
124. Chang MB, Bath AP, Rutka JA. Are all atypical positional nystagmus patterns reflective of central pathology? J Otolaryngol 30, 280–282, 2001.
125. Chaves CJ, Caplan LR, Chung CS, et al. Cerebellar infarcts in the New England Medical Center Posterior Circulation Stroke Registry. Neurology 44, 1385–1390, 1994.
126. Chaves CJ, Pessin MS, Caplan LR, et al. Cerebellar hemorrhagic infarction. Neurology 46, 346–349, 1996.
127. Chen CW, Young YH, Wu CH. Vestibular neuritis: three-dimensional videonystagmography and vestibular evoked myogenic potential results. Acta Otolaryngol 120, 845–848, 2000.
128. Chen PR, Hsu LP, Tu CE, Young YH. Radiation-induced oscillopsia in nasopharyngeal carcinoma patients. Int J Radiat Oncol Biol Phys 61, 466–470, 2005.
128a. Choi KD, Shin HY, Kim JS, et al. Rotational vertebral artery syndrome: oculographic analysis of nystagmus. Neurology 65, 1287–1290, 2005.
129. Chynn EW, Jakobiec FA. Cogan's syndrome: ophthalmic, audiovestibular and systemic manifestations and therapy. International Ophthalmology Clinics 36, 61–72, 1996.
130. Cohen B, Tokumasu K, Goto K. Semicircular canal nerve eye and head movement: the effect of changes in initial eye and head position on the plane of the induced movement. Arch Ophthalmol 76, 523–531, 1966.
131. Cohen H, Allen JR, Congdon SL, Jenkins HA. Oscillopsia and vertical eye movements in Tullio's phenomenon. Arch Otolaryngol Head Neck Surg 121, 459–462, 1995.
132. Cohen HS. Side-lying as an alternative to the Dix-Hallpike test of the posterior canal. Otol Neurotol 25, 130–134, 2004.
133. Cohen HS, Kimball KT. Treatment variations on the Epley maneuver for benign paroxysmal positional vertigo. Am J Otolaryngol 25, 33–37, 2004.
134. Collewijn H, Van der Steen J, Ferman L, Jansen TC. Human ocular counterroll: assessment of static and dynamic properties from electromagnetic scleral coil recordings. Exp Brain Res 59, 185–196, 1985.
135. Corbett JJ, Schatz NJ, Shults WT, Behrens M, Berry RG. Slowly alternating skew deviation: description of a pretectal syndrome in three patients. Ann Neurol 10, 540–546, 1981.
136. Cremer PD, Minor LB, Carey JP, Della Santina CC. Eye movements in patients with superior canal dehiscence syndrome align with the abnormal canal. Neurology 55, 1833–1841, 2000.
137. Crevits L. A liberatory maneuver for the treatment of horizontal canal paroxysmal positional vertigo. Otol Neurotol 23, 240–241, 2002.
138. Crevits L. Treatment of anterior canal benign paroxysmal positional vertigo by a prolonged forced position procedure. J Neurol Neurosurg Psychiatry 75, 779–781, 2004.
139. Crevits L, Bosman T. Migraine-related vertigo: towards a distinctive entity. Clin Neurol Neurosurg 107, 82–87, 2005.
140. Curless RG. Acute vestibular dysfunction in childhood. Central vs. peripheral. Child's Brain 6, 39–44, 1980.
141. Curthoys IS. Eye movements produced by utricular and saccular stimulation. Aviat Space Environ Med Suppl S8, A192–A197, 1987.
141a. Cundiff J, Kansal S, Kumar A, Goldstein DA, Tessler HH. Cogan's syndrome: a cause of progressive hearing deafness. Am J Otolaryngol 27, 68–70, 2006.
142. Cutrer FM, Baloh RW. Migraine associated dizziness. Headache 32, 300–304, 1992.
142a. Damman W, Kuhweide R, Dehaene I. Benign paroxysmal positional vertigo (BPPV) predominantly affects the right labyrinth. J Neurol Neurosurg Psychiatry 76, 1307–1308, 2005.
143. Darlington CL, Smith PF. Molecular mechanisms of recovery from vestibular damage in mammals: recent advances. Prog Neurobiol 62, 313–325, 2000.
144. Davies RA, Luxon LM. Dizziness following head injury: a neuro-otological study. J Neurol 242, 222–230, 1995.
145. Davis LE. Viruses and vestibular neuritis: review of human and animal studies. Acta Otolaryngol (Stockh) Suppl 503, 70–73, 1993.
146. Davis LE, Johnsson L-G. Viral infections of the inner ear: clinical, virologic and pathologic studies in humans and animals. Am J Otolaryngol 4, 347–362, 1983.
147. de Jong PTVM, de Jong JMBV, Cohen B, Jongkees LB. Ataxia and nystagmus induced by injection of local anesthetics in the neck. Ann Neurol 1, 240–246, 1977.

148. De Ridder D, Moller A, Verlooy J, Cornelissen M, De Ridder L. Is the root entry/exit zone important in microvascular compression syndromes? Neurosurgery 51, 427–433, 2002.
149. Debette S, Michelin E, Henon H, Leys D. Transient rotational vertigo as the initial symptom of a middle cerebral artery territory infarct involving the insula. Cerebrovasc Dis 16, 97–98, 2003.
150. Dell'Osso LF, Averbuch-Heller L, Leigh RJ. Oscillopsia suppression and foveation-period variation in congenital latent and acquired nystagmus. Neuro-ophthalmology 18, 163–183, 1997.
151. Demer JL, Amjadi F. Dynamic visual acuity of normal subjects during vertical optotype and head motion. Invest Ophthalmol Vis Sci 34, 1894–1906, 1993.
152. Demer JL, Honrubia V, Baloh RW. Dynamic visual acuity: a test for oscillopsia and vestibulo-ocular reflex function. Am J Otol 15, 340–347, 1994.
153. Deutschlander A, Strupp M, Jahn K, et al. Vertical oscillopsia in bilateral superior canal dehiscence syndrome. Neurology 62, 784–787, 2004.
154. Dichgans M, Dieterich M. Third nerve palsy with contralateral ocular torsion and binocular tilt of visual vertical indicating a midbrain lesion. Neuro-ophthalmology 15, 315–320, 1995.
155. Dieterich M, Brandt T. Episodic vertigo related to migraine (90 cases): vestibular migraine? J Neurol 246, 883–892, 1999.
156. Dieterich M, Brandt T. Ocular torsion and perceived vertical in oculomotor, trochlear and abducens palsies. Brain 116, 1095–1104, 1993.
157. Dieterich M, Brandt T. Impaired motion perception in congenital nystagmus and acquired ocular motor palsy. Clin Vision Sci 1, 337–345, 1987.
158. Dieterich M, Brandt T. Episodic vertigo related to migraine (90 cases): vestibular migraine? J Neurol 246, 883–892, 1999.
159. Dieterich M, Brandt T. Ocular torsion and tilt of subjective visual vertical are sensitive brainstem signs. Ann Neurol 33, 292–299, 1993.
160. Dieterich M, Brandt T. Wallenberg's syndrome: lateropulsion, cyclorotation and subjective visual vertical in thirty-six patients. Ann Neurol 31, 399–408, 1992.
161. Dieterich M, Brandt T, Fries W. Otolith function in man: results from a case of otolith Tullio phenomenon. Brain 112, 1377–1392, 1989.
162. Dieterich M, Pollmann W, Pfaffenrath V. Cervicogenic headache: electronystagmography, perception of verticality and posturography in patients before and after C2–blockade. Cephalalgia 13, 285–288, 1993.
163. Donahue SP, Lavin PJ, Hamed LM. Tonic ocular tilt reaction simulating a superior oblique palsy: diagnostic confusion with the 3–step test. Arch Ophthalmol 117, 347–352, 1999.
164. Donahue SP, Lavin PJ, Mohney B, Hamed L. Skew deviation and inferior oblique palsy. Am J Ophthalmol 132, 751–756, 2001.
165. Drachman DA, Diamond ER, Hart CW. Postural-evoked vomiting associated with posterior fossa lesions. Ann Otol Rhinol Laryngol 86, 97–101, 1977.
166. Drigo P, Carli G, Laverda AM. Benign paroxysmal vertigo of childhood. Brain Dev 23, 38–41, 2001.
167. Epley JM. Human experience with canalith repositioning maneuvers. Ann N Y Acad Sci 942, 179–191, 2001.
168. Epley JM. Positional vertigo related to semicircular canalithiasis. Otolaryngol Head Neck Surg 112, 154–161, 1995.
169. Evans RW, Baloh RW. Episodic vertigo and migraine. Headache 41, 604–605, 2001.
170. Fetter M, Dichgans J. Vestibular neuritis spares the inferior division of the vestibular nerve. Brain 119, 755–763, 1996.
171. Fetter M, Haslwanter T, Bork M, Dichgans J. New insights into positional alcohol nystagmus using three-dimensional eye-movement analysis. Ann Neurol 45, 216–223, 1999.
172. Fetter M, Sievering M. Three-dimensional eye movement analysis in benign paroxysmal positioning vertigo and nystagmus. Acta Otolaryngol 115, 353–357, 1995.
173. Fife TD, Baloh RW. Disequilibrium of unknown cause in older people. Ann Neurol 34, 674–702, 1993.
174. Fife TD, Baloh RW, Duckwiler GR. Isolated dizziness in vertebrobasilar insufficiency. Clinical features, angiography and follow-up. J Stroke Cerebrovasc Dis 4, 4–12, 1994.
175. Finkelhor BK, Harker LA. Benign paroxysmal vertigo of childhood. Laryngoscope 97, 1161–1163, 1987.
176. Fischer AJEM, Huygen PLM, Folgering HT, Verhagen WIM, Theunissen EJJM. Vestibular hyperreactivity and hyperventilation after whiplash injury. J Neurological Sci 132, 35–43, 1995.
177. Fishel-Ghodsian N, Prezant TR, Bu X, Oztas S. Mitochondrial ribosomal RNA gene mutation in a patient with sporadic aminoglycoside ototoxicity. J Otolaryngol 14, 399–403, 1993.
178. Fisher CM. Vertigo in cerebrovascular disease. Arch Otolaryngol 85, 529–534, 1967.
179. Fitzgerald DC. Head trauma: hearing loss and dizziness. J Trauma 40, 488–496, 1996.
180. Fitzgerald DC. Perilymphatic fistula: a Washington DC, experience. Ann Otol Rhinol Laryngol 106, 830–837, 1997.
181. Fluur E. Interaction between the utricles and the horizontal semicircular canals. IV. Tilting of human patients with acute unilateral vestibular neuritis. Acta Otolaryngol (Stockh) 76, 349–352, 1973.
182. Ford FR, Walsh FB. Clinical observations upon the importance of the vestibular reflexes in ocular movements. Bulletin of the Johns Hopkins Hospital 58, 80–88, 1936.
183. Foroozan R, Brodsky MC. Microsaccadic opsoclonus: an idiopathic cause of oscillopsia and episodic blurred vision. Am J Ophthalmol 138, 1053–1054, 2004.
184. Francis DA, Bronstein AM, Rudge P, du Boulay EP. The site of brainstem lesions causing semicircular canal paresis: an MRI study. J Neurol Neurosurg Psychiatry 55, 446–449, 1992.
185. Frohman EM, Dewey RB, Frohman TC. An unusual variant of the dorsal midbrain syndrome in MS: clinical characteristics and pathophysiologic mechanisms. Mult Scler 10, 322–325, 2004.
186. Frohman EM, Kramer PD, Dewey RB, Kramer L, Frohman TC. Benign paroxysmal positioning vertigo in multiple sclerosis: diagnosis pathophysiology and therapeutic techniques. Mult Scler 9, 250–255, 2003.
187. Frohman EM, Solomon D, Zee DS. Vestibular dysfunction and nystagmus in multiple sclerosis. Int J MS3, 13–26, 1997.
188. Frohman EM, Tusa R, Mark AS, Cornblath DR.

Vestibular dysfunction in chronic inflammatory demyelinating polyneuropathy. Ann Neurol 39, 529–535, 1996.
189. Frohman EM, Zhang H, Dewey RB, et al. Vertigo in MS: utility of positional and particle repositioning maneuvers. Neurology 55, 1566–1569, 2000.
190. Frohman LP, Kupersmith MJ. Reversible vertical ocular deviations associated with raised intracranial pressure. J Clin Neuroophthalmol 5, 158–163, 1985.
191. Fujimoto C, Iwasaki S, Matsuzaki M, Murofushi T. Lesion site in idiopathic bilateral vestibulopathy: a galvanic vestibular-evoked myogenic potential study. Acta Otolaryngol 125, 430–432, 2005.
192. Furman JM. Otolith-ocular responses in familial episodic ataxia linked to chromosome 19p. Ann Neurol 42, 189–193, 1997.
193. Furman JM, Balaban CD, Pollack IF. Vestibular compensation in a patient with a cerebellar infarction. Neurology 48, 916–920, 1997.
194. Furman JM, Cass SP. Benign paroxysmal positional vertigo. N Engl J Med 341, 1590–1596, 1999.
195. Furman JM, Hain TC. "Do try this at home": self-treatment of BPPV. Neurology 63, 8–9, 2004.
196. Furman JM, Jacob RG. Psychiatric dizziness. Neurology 48, 1161–1166, 1997.
197. Furman JM, Marcus DA, Balaban CD. Migrainous vertigo: development of a pathogenetic model and structured diagnostic interview. Curr Opin Neurol 16, 5–13, 2003.
198. Furman JMR, Crumrime PK, Reinmuth OM. Epileptic nystagmus. Ann Neurol 27, 686–688, 1990.
199. Furuya M, Suzuki M, Sato H. Experimental study of speed-dependent positional nystagmus in benign paroxysmal positional vertigo. Acta Otolaryngol 123, 709–712, 2003.
200. Gacek RR. Pathophysiology and management of cupulolithiasis. Am J Otolaryngol 6, 66–74, 1985.
201. Gacek RR. Pathology of benign paroxysmal positional vertigo revisited. Ann Otol Rhinol Laryngol 112, 574–582, 2003.
202. Gacek RR, Gacek MR. Results of singular neurectomy in the posterior ampullary recess. ORLJ Otorhinolaryngol Relat Spec 64, 397–402, 2002.
203. Galetta SL, Liu GT, Raps EC, Solomon D, Volpe NJ. Cyclodeviation in skew deviation. Am J Ophthalmol 118, 509–514, 1994.
204. Gdowski GT, McCrea RA. Neck proprioceptive inputs to primate vestibular nucleus neurons. Exp Brain Res 135, 511–526, 2000.
205. Gianoli G, Goebel J, Mowry S, Poomipannit P. Anatomic differences in the lateral vestibular nerve channels and their implications in vestibular neuritis. Otol Neurotol 26, 489–494, 2005.
206. Giffin NJ, Benton S, Goadsby PJ. Benign paroxysmal torticollis of infancy: four new cases and linkage to CACNA1A mutation. Dev Med Child Neurol 44, 490–493, 2002.
207. Gill-Body KM, Parker SW, Krebs DE, Riley PO. Physical therapy management of peripheral vestibular dysfunction. Physical Therapy 45, 129–142, 1994.
208. Glasauer S, Dieterich M, Brandt T. Simulation of pathological ocular counter-roll and skew-torsion by a 3-D mathematical model. NeuroReport 10, 1843–1848, 1999.
209. Goebel JA, O'Mara W, Gianoli G. Anatomic considerations in vestibular neuritis. Otol Neurotol 22, 512–518, 2001.
210. Gomez CR, Cruz-Flores S, Malkoff MD, Sauer CM, Burch CM. Isolated vertigo as a manifestation of vertebrobasilar ischemia. Neurology 47, 94–97, 1996.
211. Gordon CR, Gadoth N. Repeated vs single physical maneuver in benign paroxysmal positional vertigo. Acta Neurol Scand 110, 166–169, 2004.
212. Gordon CR, Levite R, Joffe V, Gadoth N. Is posttraumatic benign paroxysmal positional vertigo different from the idiopathic form? Arch Neurol 61, 1590–1593, 2004.
213. Gordon RM, Bender MB. Visual phenomenon in lesions of the medial longitudinal fasciculus. Arch Neurol 15, 238–240, 1966.
214. Grad A, Baloh RW. Vertigo of vascular origin. Clinical and electronystagmographic features in 84 cases. Arch Neurol 46, 281–284, 1989.
215. Grasland A, Pouchot J, Hachulla E, et al. Typical and atypical Cogan's syndrome: 32 cases and review of the literature. Rheumatology (Oxford) 43, 1007–1015, 2004.
216. Green AM, Angelaki DE. An integrative neural network for detecting inertial motion and head orientation. J Neurophysiol 92, 905–925, 2004.
217. Green JD, Blum JD, Harner SG. Longitudinal follow-up of patients with Meniere's disease. Otolaryngol Head Neck Surg 104, 783–788, 1991.
218. Greenberg HS, DeWitt LD. Periodic nonalternating ocular skew deviation accompanied by head tilt and pathologic lid retraction. J Clin Neuroophthalmol 3, 181–184, 1983.
219. Gregorius FK, Crandall PH, Baloh RW. Positional vertigo with cerebellar astrocytoma. Surg Neurol 6, 283–286, 1976.
220. Gresty MA, Hess K, Leech J. Disorders of the vestibuloocular reflex producing oscillopsia and mechanisms compensating for loss of labyrinthine function. Brain 100, 693–716, 1977.
221. Gross M, Banin E, Eliashar R, Ben-Hur T. Susac syndrome. Otol Neurotol 25, 470–473, 2004.
222. Guerraz M, Yardley L, Bertholon P, et al. Visual vertigo: symptom assessment, spatial orientation and postural control. Brain 124, 1646–1656, 2001.
223. Gunesh RP, Huber AM. Traumatic perilymphatic fistula. Ann Otol Rhinol Laryngol 112, 221–222, 2003.
224. Guyot JP, Liard P, Thielen K, Kos I. Isolated vestibular areflexia after blunt head trauma. Ann Otol Rhinol Laryngol 110, 562–564, 2001.
225. Hain TC, Fuller L, Weil L, Kotsias J. Effects of T'ai Chi on balance. Arch Otolaryngol Head Neck Surg 125, 1191–1195, 1999.
226. Hain TC, Hanna PA, Rheinberger MA. Mal de debarquement. Arch Otolaryngol Head Neck Surg 125, 615–620, 1999.
227. Hain TC, Helminski JO, Reis IL, Uddin MK. Vibration does not improve results of the canalith repositioning procedure. Arch Otolaryngol Head Neck Surg 126, 617–622, 2000.
228. Hain TC, Squires TM, Stone HA. Clinical implications of a mathematical model of benign paroxysmal positional vertigo. Ann N Y Acad Sci 1039, 384–394, 2005.
229. Hain TC, Yacovino D. Pharmacologic treatment of persons with dizziness. Neurol Clin 23, 831–853, 2005.

230. Halmagyi GM. New clinical tests of unilateral vestibular dysfunction. J Laryngol Otol 118, 589–600, 2004.
231. Halmagyi GM, Aw ST. McGarvie LA, et al. Superior semicircular canal dehiscence simulating otosclerosis. J Laryngol Otol 117, 553–557, 2003.
232. Halmagyi GM, Baloh RW. Overview of the common syndromes of vestibular disease. In Baloh RW, Halmagyi GM (eds). Disorders of the Vestibular System. Oxford, New York, 1996, pp 291–299.
233. Halmagyi GM, Brandt T, Dieterich M, et al. Tonic contraversive ocular tilt reaction due to unilateral meso-diencephalic lesion. Neurology 40, 1503–1509, 1990.
234. Halmagyi GM, Fattore CM, Curthoys IS, Wade S. Gentamicin vestibulotoxicity. Otolaryngol Head Neck Surg 111, 571–574, 1994.
235. Halmagyi GM, Gresty MA, Gibson WPR. Ocular tilt reaction with peripheral vestibular lesion. Ann Neurol 6, 80–83, 1979.
236. Halmagyi GM, McGarvie LA, Aw ST, Yavor RA, Todd MJ. The click-evoked vestibulo-ocular reflex in superior semicircular canal dehiscence. Neurology 60, 1172–1175, 2003.
237. Halmagyi GM, Pamphlett R, Curthoys IS. Seesaw nystagmus and ocular tilt reaction due to adult Leigh's disease. Neuro-ophthalmology 12, 1–9, 1992.
238. Harker LA, Rassekh CH. Episodic vertigo in basilar artery migraine. Otolaryngol Head Neck Surg 96, 239–250, 1987.
239. Harno H, Hirvonen T, Kaunisto MA, et al. Subclinical vestibulocerebellar dysfunction in migraine with and without aura. Neurology 61, 1748–1752, 2003.
240. Harris JP, Ryan AF. Fundamental immune mechanisms of the brain and the inner ear. Otolaryngol Head Neck Surg 112, 639–653, 1995.
241. Harrison MS, Ozsahinoglu C. Positional vertigo. Arch Otolaryngol 101, 675–678, 1975.
242. Hasler R, Toupet M, Guidetti G, Basseres F, Montandon P. Meniere's disease in children. Am J Otolaryngol 8, 187–189, 1987.
243. Hayashi Y, Kanzaki J, Etoh N, et al. Three-dimensional analysis of nystagmus in benign paroxysmal positional vertigo. New insights into its pathophysiology. J Neurol 249, 1683–1688, 2002.
244. Haynes BF, Kaiser-Kupfer MI, Mason P, Fauci AS. Cogan syndrome: studies in thirteen patients long-term follow-up and a review of the literature. Medicine 59, 426–441, 1980.
245. Haynes DS, Resser JA, Labadie RF, et al. Treatment of benign positional vertigo using the Semont maneuver: efficacy in patients presenting without nystagmus. Laryngoscope 112, 796–801, 2002.
246. Healy GB. Hearing loss and vertigo secondary to head injury. N Engl JMed 306, 1029–1031, 1982.
247. Hedges TR, III, Hoyt WF. Ocular tilt reaction due to an upper brainstem lesion: Paroxysmal skew deviation torsion, and oscillation of the eyes with head tilt. Ann Neurol 11, 537–540, 1982.
248. Helm MR. Vestibulo-ocular reflex abnormalities in patients with migraine. Headache 45, 332–336, 2005.
249. Helmchen C, Jäger L, Büttner U, Reiser M, Brandt T. Cogan's syndrome—high resolution MRI indicators of activity. J Vestib Res 8, 155–167, 1998.
250. Helminski JO, Janssen I, Kotaspoiukis D, et al. Strategies to prevent recurrence of benign paroxysmal positional vertigo. Arch Otolaryngol Head Neck Surg 131, 344–348, 2005.
251. Herdman SJ. Assessment and management of bilateral vestibular loss. In Herdman SJ (ed). Vestibular Rehabilitation. FA Davis, Philadelphia, 1994, pp 316–330.
252. Herdman SJ. Vestibular Rehabilitation. FA Davis, Philadelphia, 1994.
253. Herdman SJ, Blatt PJ, Schubert MC. Vestibular rehabilitation of patients with vestibular hypofunction or with benign paroxysmal positional vertigo. Curr Opin Neurol 13, 39–43, 2000.
254. Herdman SJ, Borello-France DF, Whitney SL. Treatment of vestibular hypofunction. In Herdman SJ (ed). Vestibular Rehabilitation. FA Davis, Philadelphia, 1994, pp 287–315.
255. Herdman SJ, Clendaniel RA, Mattox DE, Holliday MJ, Niparko JK. Vestibular adaptation exercises and recovery: acute stage after acoustic neuroma resection. Otolarygol Head Neck Surg 113, 77–87, 1995.
256. Herdman SJ, Schubert MC, Das VE, Tusa RJ. Recovery of dynamic visual acuity in unilateral vestibular hypofunction. Arch Otolaryngol Head Neck Surg 129, 819–824, 2003.
257. Herdman SJ, Schubert MC, Tusa RJ. Role of central preprogramming in dynamic visual acuity with vestibular loss. Arch Otolaryngol Head Neck Surg 127, 1205–1210, 2001.
258. Herdman SJ, Tusa RJ. Complications of the canalith repositioning procedure. Arch Otolaryngol Head Neck Surg 122, 281–286, 1996.
259. Hertle RW, FitzGibbon EJ, Avallone JM, Cheeseman E, Tsilou EK. Onset of oscillopsia after visual maturation in patients with congenital nystagmus. Ophthalmology 108, 2301–2307, 2001.
260. Hess K. Vestibulotoxic drugs and other causes of acquired bilateral peripheral vestibulopathy. In Baloh RW, Halmagyi GM (eds). Disorders of the Vestibular System. Oxford, New York, 1996, pp 360–373.
261. Hirvonen TP, Weg N, Zinreich SJ, Minor LB. High-resolution CT findings suggest a developmental abnormality underlying superior canal dehiscence syndrome. Acta Otolaryngol 123, 477–481, 2003.
262. Hodgson MJ, Furman J, Ryan C, Durrant J, Kern E. Encephalopathy and vestibulopathy following short-term hydrocarbon exposure. J Occup Med 31, 51–54, 1989.
263. Hoffman DL, O'Leary DP, Munjack DJ. Autorotation test abnormalities of the horizontal and vertical vestibulo-ocular reflexes in panic disorder. Otolaryngol Head Neck Surg 110, 259–269, 1994.
264. Honrubia V. Self-treatment of benign paroxysmal positional vertigo: Semont maneuver vs Epley procedure. Neurology 64, 583–584, 2005.
265. Hopf HC. Vertigo and masseter paresis. A new local brainstem syndrome probably of vascular origin. J Neurol 235, 42–45, 1987.
266. Horii A, Imai T, Mishiro Y, et al. Horizontal canal type BPPV: bilaterally affected case treated with canal plugging and Lempert's maneuver. ORLJ Otorhinolaryngol Relat Spec 65, 366–369, 2003.
267. Hornibrook J. Horizontal canal benign positional vertigo. Ann Otol Rhinol Laryngol 113, 721–725, 2004.

268. House MG, Honrubia V. Theoretical models for the mechanisms of benign paroxysmal positional vertigo. Audiol Neurootol 8, 91–99, 2003.
269. Hoyt CS. Nystagmus and other abnormal ocular movements in children. Ped Clin North Am 34, 1415–1423, 1987.
270. Huang CC, Young YH. Vertigo with rebound nystagmus as an initial manifestation in a patient with basilar artery occlusion. Eur Arch Otorhinolaryngol 262, 576–579, 2004.
271. Huang MH, Huang CC, Ryu SJ, Chu NS. Sudden bilateral hearing impairment in vertebrobasilar occlusive disease. Stroke 24, 132–137, 1993.
272. Humphriss RL, Baguley DM, Sparkes V, Peerman SE, Moffat DA. Contraindications to the Dix-Hallpike manoeuvre: a multidisciplinary review. Int J Audiol 42, 166–173, 2003.
273. Huppert D, Kunihiro T, Brandt T. Phobic postural vertigo 154 patients): its association with vestibular disorders. J Audiological Med 4, 97–103, 1995.
274. Huppert D, Strupp M, Rettinger N, Hecht J, Brandt T. Phobic postural vertigo. A long-term follow-up (5 to 15 years) of 106 patients. J Neurol 252, 564–569, 2005.
275. Hybels RL. Drug toxicity of the inner ear. Med Clin North Am 63, 309–319, 1979.
276. Iida M, Hitouji K, Takahashi M. Vertical semicircular canal function: a study in patients with benign paroxysmal positional vertigo. Acta Otolaryngol Suppl 545, 35–37, 2001.
277. Ildiz F, Dündra A. A case of Tullio phenomenon in a subject with oval window fistula due to barotrauma. Aviat Space Environ Med 65, 67–69, 1994.
278. Imai T, Ito M, Takeda N, et al. Natural course of the remission of vertigo in patients with benign paroxysmal positional vertigo. Neurology 64, 920–921, 2005.
279. Ishiyama A, Ishiyama GP, Lopez I, et al. Histopathology of idiopathic chronic recurrent vertigo. Laryngoscope 106, 1340–1346, 1996.
280. Ishiyama A, Jacobson KM, Baloh RW. Migraine and benign positional vertigo. Ann Otol Rhinol Laryngol 109, 377–380, 2000.
281. Ishiyama G, Ishiyama A, Baloh RW. Drop attacks and vertigo secondary to a non-meniere otologic cause. Arch Neurol 60, 71–75, 2003.
282. Ishiyama G, Ishiyama A, Jacobson K, Baloh RW. Drop attacks in older patients secondary to an otologic cause. Neurology 57, 1103–1106, 2001.
283. Ishizaki H, Pyykkö, I, Nozue M. Neuroborreliosis in the etiology of vestibular neuronitis. Acta Otolaryngol (Stockh) Suppl 503, 67–69, 1993.
283a. Iwasaki S, Takai Y, Ozeki H, et al. Extent of lesions in idiopathic sudden hearing loss with vertigo: study using click and galvanic vestibular evoked myogenic potentials. Arch Otolaryngol Head Neck Surg 131, 857–862, 2005.
284. JC. Living without a balancing mechanism. New Engl JMed 246, 458–460, 1952.
285. Jacob RG, Furman JM, Durrant JD, Turner SM. Panic, agoraphobia and vestibular dysfunction. Am J Psychiatr 153, 503–512, 1996.
286. Jaffe BF. Vertigo following air travel. New Engl J Med 301, 1385–1386, 1979.
287. Jáuregui-Renaud K, Faldon M, Clarke A, Bronstein AM, Gresty MA. Skew deviation of the eyes in normal human subjects induced by semicircular canal stimulation. Neurosci Lett 235, 135–137, 1996.
288. Jáuregui-Renaud K, Faldon ME, Gresty MA, Bronstein AM. Horizontal ocular vergence and the three-dimensional response to whole-body roll motion. Exp Brain Res 136, 79–92, 2001.
289. Jen J. Familial episodic ataxias and related ion channel disorders. Curr Treat Options Neurol 2, 429–431, 2000.
290. Jen J, Kim GW, Baloh RW. Clinical spectrum of episodic ataxia type 2. Neurology 62, 17–22, 2004.
291. Jen JC, Wang H, Lee H, et al. Suggestive linkage to chromosome 6q in families with bilateral vestibulopathy. Neurology 63, 2376–2379, 2004.
292. Johnson JT, Wall C, III, Barney SA, Thearle PB. Postoperative vestibular dysfunction following head and neck surgery. Acta Otolaryhgol (Stockh) 100, 316–320, 1985.
293. Kale SU, Donaldson I, West RJ, Shehu A. Superficial siderosis of the meninges and its otolaryngologic connection: a series of five patients. Otol Neurotol 24, 90–95, 2003.
294. Kamei T. Delayed endolymphatic hydrops as a clinical entity. Int Tinnitus J 10, 137–143, 2004.
295. Kaplan PW, Tusa RJ. Neurophysiologic and clinical correlations of epileptic nystagmus. Neurology 43, 2508–2514, 1993.
296. Karlberg M, Annertz M, Magnusson M. Acute vestibular neuritis visualized by 3–T magnetic resonance imaging with high-dose gadolinium. Arch Otolaryngol Head Neck Surg 130, 229–232, 2004.
297. Karlberg M, Hall K, Quickert N, Hinson J, Halmagyi GM. What inner ear diseases cause benign paroxysmal positional vertigo? Acta Otolaryngol 120, 380–385, 2000.
298. Karlberg M, Halmagyi GM, Büttner U, Yavor RA. Sudden unilateral hearing loss with simultaneous ipsilateral posterior semicircular canal benign paroxysmal positional vertigo: a variant of vestibulocochlear neurolabyrinthitis? Arch Otolaryngol Head Neck Surg 126, 1024–1029, 2000.
299. Karnath H-O, Sievering D, Fetter M. The interactive contribution of neck muscle proprioception and vestibular stimulation to subjective "straight ahead" orientation in man. Exp Brain Res 101, 140–146, 1994.
299a. Katims JJ, Long DM, Ng LK. Transcutaneous nerve stimulation. Frequency and waveform specificity in humans. Appl Neurophysiol 49, 86–91, 1986.
300. Katsarkas A. Positional nystagmus of the "central type" as an early sign of multiple sclerosis. J Otolaryngol 11, 91–93, 1982.
301. Kattah JC, Kolsky MP, Luessenhop AJ. Positional vertigo and the cerebellar vermis. Neurology 34, 527–529, 1984.
302. Keane JR. Alternating skew deviation: 47 patients. Neurology 35, 725–728, 1985.
303. Keane JR. Ocular skew deviation. Analysis of 100 cases. Arch Neurol 32, 185–190, 1975.
304. Keane JR. Alternating skew deviation: 47 patients. Neurology 35, 725–728, 1985.
305. Kelders WP, Kleinrensink GJ, van der Geest JN, et al. The cervico-ocular reflex is increased in whiplash injury patients. J Neurotrauma 22, 133–137, 2005.
306. Kentala E, Pyykkö I. Vestibular schwannoma mim-

icking Meniere's disease. Acta Otolaryngol. Suppl 543, 17–19, 2000.
307. Kim JS, Lee JH, Lee MC. Small primary intracerebral hemorrhage. Clinical presentation of 28 cases. Stroke 25, 1500–1506, 1994.
308. Kim SH, Kazahaya K, Handler SD. Traumatic perilymphatic fistulas in children: etiology, diagnosis and management. Int J Pediatr Otorhinolaryngol 60, 147–153, 2001.
309. Kim YK, Shin JE, Chung JW. The effect of canalith repositioning for anterior semicircular canal canalithiasis. ORLJ Otorhinolaryngol Relat Spec 67, 56–60, 2005.
310. Kitsigianis G-A, O'Leary DP, Davis LL. Active head-movement analysis of cisplatin-induced vestibulotoxicity. Otolaryngol Head Neck Surg 98, 82–87, 1988.
311. Kogeorgos J, Scott DF, Swash M. Epileptic dizziness. Br Med J 687–689, 1981.
312. Kramer PD, Kleiman DA. Dix-Hallpike maneuver results are not influenced by the time of day of the test. Acta Oto-Laryngologica 125, 145–147, 2005.
313. Krejcova H, Bojar M, Jerabek J, Tomas J, Jirous J. Otoneurological symptomatology in Lyme disease. Adv Oto-Rhino-Laryngol 42, 210–212, 1988.
313a. Krombach GA, Di Martino E, Martiny S, et al. Dehiscence of the superior and/or posterior semicircular canal: delineation on T2-weighted axial three-dimensional turbo spin-echo images, maximum intensity projections and volume-rendered images. Eur Arch Otorhinolaryngol, published online, 2005.
314. Krombach GA, DiMartino E, Schmitz-Rode T, et al. Posterior semicircular canal dehiscence: a morphologic cause of vertigo similar to superior semicircular canal dehiscence. Eur Radiol 13, 1444–1450, 2003.
315. Kuhweide R, Van de Steene V, Vlaminck S, Casselman JW. Ramsay Hunt syndrome: pathophysiology of cochleovestibular symptoms. J Laryngol Otol 116, 844–848, 2002.
316. Kuo MJ, Drago PC, Proops DW, Chavda SV. Early diagnosis and treatment of Ramsay Hunt syndrome: the role of magnetic resonance imaging. J Laryngol Otol 109, 777–780, 1995.
317. Kuurila K, Kentala E, Karjalainen S, et al. Vestibular dysfunction in adult patients with osteogenesis imperfecta. Am J Med Genet A120, 350–358, 2003.
318. Lambert PR. Delayed vertigo and profound sensorineural hearing loss. Laryngoscope 95, 1541–1544, 1985.
319. Lanska DJ, Remler B. Benign paroxysmal positional vertigo: classic descriptions origins of the provocative positioning technique and conceptual developments. Neurology 48, 1167–1177, 1997.
320. Lanzi G, Balottin U, Fazzi E. Benign paroxysmal vertigo of childhood. Cephalgia 14, 458–460, 1994.
321. Lawden MC, Bronstein AM, Kennard C. Repetitive paroxysmal nystagmus and vertigo. Neurology 45, 276–280, 1995.
322. Lee H, Ahn BH, Baloh RW. Sudden deafness with vertigo as a sole manifestation of anterior inferior cerebellar artery infarction. J Neurol Sci 222, 105–107, 2004.
323. Lee H, Baloh RW. Sudden deafness in vertebrobasilar ischemia: clinical features, vascular topographical patterns and long-term outcome. J Neurol Sci 228, 99–104, 2005.
324. Lee H, Cho YW. A case of isolated nodulus infarction presenting as a vestibular neuritis. J Neurol Sci 221, 117–119, 2004.
324a. Lee H, Jen JC, Wang H, et al. A genome-wide linkage scan of familial benign recurrent vertigo: Linkage to 22q12 with evidence of heterogeneity. Hum Mol Genet, published online, 2005.
324b. Lee H, Lee SY, Lee SR, Park BR, Baloh RW. Ocular tilt reaction and anterior inferior cerebellar artery syndrome. J Neurol Neurosurg Psychiatry 76, 1742–1743, 2005.
325. Lee H, Lopez I, Ishiyama A, Baloh RW. Can migraine damage the inner ear? Arch Neurol 57, 1631–1634, 2000.
326. Lee H, Sohn SI, Jung DK, et al. Migraine and isolated recurrent vertigo of unknown cause. Neurol Res 24, 663–665, 2002.
327. Lee H, Whitman GT, Lim JG, et al. Hearing symptoms in migrainous infarction. Arch Neurol 60, 113–116, 2003.
328. Lee H, Yi HA, Cho YW, et al. Nodulus infarction mimicking acute peripheral vestibulopathy. Neurology 60, 1700–1702, 2003.
329. Lee MY, Kim MS, Park BR. Adaptation of the horizontal vestibuloocular reflex in pilots. Laryngoscope 114, 897–902, 2004.
330. Leigh RJ, Dell'Osso LF, Yaniglos SS, Thurston SE. Oscillopsia retinal image stabilization and congenital nystagmus. Invest Ophthalmol Vis Sci 29, 279–282, 1988.
331. Leigh RJ, Rushton DN, Thurston SE, Hertle RW, Yaniglos SS. Effects of retinal image stabilization in acquired nystagmus due to neurologic disease. Neurology 38, 122–127, 1988.
332. Lempert T, Gianna CC, Gresty MA, Bronstein AM. Effect of otolith dysfunction. Impairment of visual acuity during linear head motion in labyrinthine defective subjects. Brain 120, 1005–1113, 1997.
333. Lempert T, Gresty MA, Bronstein AM. Benign positional vertigo: recognition and treatment. Br Med J 311, 489–491, 1995.
334. Lempert T, Leopold M, von Brevern M, Neuhauser H. Migraine and benign positional vertigo. Ann Otol Rhinol Laryngol 109, 1176, 2000.
334a. Lempert T, Neuhauser H. Migrainous vertigo. Neurol Clin 23, 715–730, 2005.
335. Lewis JM, Kline LB. Periodic alternating nystagmus associated with periodic alternating skew deviation. J Clin Neuroophthalmol 13, 115–117, 1983.
336. Lewis RF. Frequency-specific mal de debarquement. Neurology 63, 1983–1984, 2004.
336a. Li JC, Epley J. The 360-degree maneuver for treatment of benign positional vertigo. Otol Neurotol 27, 71–77, 2006.
337. Limb CJ, Francis HF, Lustig LR, Niparko JK, Jammal H. Benign positional vertigo after cochlear implantation. Otolaryngol Head Neck Surg 132, 741–745, 2005.
338. Lindskog U, Odkvist L, Noaksson L, Wallquist J. Benign paroxysmal vertigo in childhood: a long-term follow-up. Headache 39, 33–37, 1999.

339. Longridge NS. Topical gentamicin vestibular toxicity. J Otolaryngol 23, 444–446, 1994.
340. Longridge NS, Barber HO. Bilateral paroxysmal positioning nystagmus. J Otolaryngol 7, 395–400, 1978.
341. Longridge NS, Mallinson AL. The dynamic illegible Etest. A technique for assessing the vestibuloocular reflex. Acta Otolaryngol (Stockh) 103, 273–279, 1987.
342. Lopez-Escamez JA, Gamiz MJ, Finana MG, Perez AF, Canet IS. Position in bed is associated with left or right location in benign paroxysmal positional vertigo of the posterior semicircular canal. Am J Otolaryngol 23, 263–266, 2002.
342a. Lopez-Escamez JA, Molina MI, Gamiz M, et al. Multiple positional nystagmus suggests multiple canal involvement in benign paroxysmal vertigo. Acta Otolaryngol 125, 954–961, 2005.
343. Lueck CJ, Hamlyn P, Crawford TJ, et al. A case of ocular tilt reaction and torsional nystagmus due to direct stimulation of the midbrain in man. Brain 114, 2069–2079, 1991.
344. Macias JD, Ellensohn A, Massingale S, Gerkin R. Vibration with the canalith repositioning maneuver: a prospective randomized study to determine efficacy. Laryngoscope 114, 1011–1014, 2004.
345. Maitland CG. Perilymphatic fistula. Curr Neurol Neurosci Rep 1, 486–491, 2001.
346. Manto MU, Jacquy J. Cerebellar ataxia in Cogan syndrome. J Neurological Sci 136, 189–191, 1996.
346a. Marcelli V, Piazza F, Pisani F, Marciano E. Neuro-otological features of benign paroxysmal vertigo and benign paroxysmal positioning vertigo in children: A follow-up study. Brain Dev, published online, 2005.
347. Marietta J, Walters KS, Burgess R, et al. Usher's syndrome type IC: clinical studies and fine-mapping the disease locus. Ann Otol Rhinol Laryngol 106, 123–128, 1997.
348. Mark AS. Vestibulocochlear system. Neuroimag Clin North Am 3, 153–170, 1993.
349. Mathews J, Kumar BN. Autoimmune sensorineural hearing loss. Clin Otolaryngol 28, 479–488, 2003.
350. Mautner V-F, Lindenau M, Baser ME, et al. The neuroimaging and clinical spectrum of neurofibromatosis 2. Neurosurgery 38, 880–886, 1996.
351. McAuley JR, Dickman JD, Mustain W, Anand VK. Positional nystagmus in asymptomatic human subjects. Otolarygnol Head Neck Surg 114, 545–553, 1996.
352. McClure JA, Copp CC, Lycett P. Recovery nystagmus in Meniere's disease. Laryngoscope 91, 1727–1737, 1981.
353. McClure JA, Parnes LS. A cure for benign positional vertigo. Baillière's Clinical Neurology 3, 535–545, 1994.
354. McCombe PA, Sheean GI, McLaughlin DB, Pender MP. Vestibular and ventilatory dysfunction in sensory and autonomic neuropathy associated with primary Sjögren's syndrome. J Neurol Neurosurg Psychiatry 55, 1211–1212, 1992.
355. McGibbon CA, Krebs DE, Parker SW, et al. Tai Chi and vestibular rehabilitation improve vestibulopathic gait via different neuromuscular mechanisms: preliminary report. BMC Neurol 5, 3, 2005.
356. Melamed Y, Shupak A, Bitterman H. Medical problems associated with underwater diving. N Engl J Med 326, 30–35, 1992.
357. Merchant SN, Gopen Q. A human temporal bone study of acute bacterial meningogenic labyrinthitis. Am J Otol 17, 375–385, 1996.
358. Merchant SN, Schuknecht HF. Vestibular atelectasis. Ann Otol Rhinol Laryngol 97, 565–576, 1988.
359. Migliaccio AA, Della Santina CC, Carey JP, Minor LP, Zee DS. The effect of binocular eye position and head rotation plane on the human torsional vestibuloocular reflex. Vision Res 2006.
360. Mikulec AA, McKenna MJ, Ramsey MJ, et al. Superior semicircular canal dehiscence presenting as conductive hearing loss without vertigo. Otol Neurotol 25, 121–129, 2004.
361. Minor LB. Labyrinthine fistulae: pathobiology and management. Curr Opin Otolaryngol Head Neck Surg 11, 340–346, 2003.
362. Minor LB. Gentamicin-induced bilateral vestibular hypofunction. J Am Med Assoc 279, 541–544, 1998.
363. Minor LB, Carey JP, Cremer PD, et al. Dehiscence of bone overlying the superior canal as a cause of apparent conductive hearing loss. Otol Neurotol 24, 270–278, 2003.
364. Minor LB. Clinical manifestations of superior canal dehiscence. Larynogoscope 115, 1717–1727, 2005.
365. Minor LB, Haslwanter T, Straumann D, Zee DS. Hyperventilation-induced nystagmus in patients with vestibular schwannoma. Acta Otolaryngol (Stockh), 1998.
366. Minor LB, Schessel DA, Carey JP. Meniere's disease. Curr Opin Neurol 17, 9–16, 2004.
367. Minor LB, Solomon D, Zee DS, Zinreich JS. Sound- and/or pressure-induced vertigo due to bone dehiscence of the superior semicircular canal. Arch Otolaryngol Head Neck Surg 124, 249–258, 1998.
368. Mitchell JM, Smith CL, Quencer RB. Periodic alternating skew deviation. J Clin Neuroophthalmol 1, 5–8, 1981.
369. Moller C, Odkvist LM, Thell J, et al. Otoneurological findings in psycho-organic syndrome caused by industrial solvent exposure. Acta Otolaryngol (Stockh) 107, 5–12, 1989.
370. Møller MB, Møller AR, Jannetta PJ, Jho HD, Sekhar LN. Microvascular decompression of the eighth nerve in patients with disabling positional vertigo: selection criteria and operative results. Acta Neurochir (Wien) 125, 75–82, 1993.
371. Money KE, Scott JW. Heavy water nystagmus and effects of alcohol. Nature 247, 404–406, 1974.
372. Moon IS, Hain TC. Delayed quick spins after vestibular nerve section respond to anticonvulsant therapy. Otol Neurotol 26, 82–85, 2005.
373. Moon SJ, Bae SH, Kim HD, Kim JH, Cho YB. The effect of postural restrictions in the treatment of benign paroxysmal positional vertigo. Eur Arch Otorhinolaryngol 2004.
374. mor-Dorado JC, Llorca J, Costa-Ribas C, Garcia-Porrua C, Gonzalez-Gay MA. Giant cell arteritis: a new association with benign paroxysmal positional vertigo. Laryngoscope 114, 1420–1425, 2004.
375. mor-Dorado JC, Llorca J, Garcia-Porrua C, et al. Audiovestibular manifestations in giant cell arteritis: a prospective study. Medicine (Baltimore) 82, 13–26, 2003.
376. Moriarty B, Rutka J, Hawke M. The incidence and

distribution of cupular deposits in the labyrinth. Laryngoscope 102, 56–59, 1992.
377. Morrison GAJ, Sterkers JM. Unusual presentations of acoustic tumours. Clin Otolaryngol 21, 80–83, 1996.
378. Morrow MJ, Sharpe JA. Torsional nystagmus in the lateral medullary syndrome. Ann Neurol 24, 390–398, 1988.
379. Mossman S, Halmagyi GM. Partial ocular tilt reaction due to unilateral cerebellar lesion. Neurology 49, 491–493, 1997.
379a. Motin M, Keren O, Groswasser Z, Gordon CR. Benign paroxysmal positional vertigo as the cause of dizziness in patients after severe traumatic brain injury: diagnosis and treatment. Brain Inj 19, 693–697, 2005.
380. Moster ML, Schatz NJ, Savino PJ, et al. Alternating skew on lateral gaze (bilateral abducting hypertropia). Annals of Neurology 23, 190–192, 1988.
381. Murofushi T, Ouvrier RA, Parker GD, et al. Vestibular abnormalities in CHARGE association. Ann Otol Rhinol Laryngol 106, 129–134, 1997.
382. Murofushi T, Halmagyi GM, Yavor RA, Colebatch JG. Absent vestibular evoked myogenic potentials in vestibular neurolabyrinthitis. An indicator of inferior vestibular nerve involvement? Arch Otolaryngol Head Neck Surg 122, 845–848, 1996.
383. Murofushi T, Monobe H, Ochiai A, Ozeki H. The site of lesion in "vestibular neuritis": study by galvanic VEMP. Neurology 61, 417–418, 2003.
384. Murphy TP. Mal de Debarquement: a forgotten entity. Otolaryngol Head Neck Surg 109, 10–13, 1993.
385. Murray RS, Ajax ET. Monocular oscillopsia secondary to lens subluxation. Ann Neurol 20, 544–545, 1986.
386. Myers SF, Blakely BW, Schwan S. Is cis-platin vestibulotoxic? Otolaryngol Head Neck Surg 108, 322–328, 1993.
387. Nachum Z, Shupak A, Letichevsky V, et al. Mal de debarquement and posture: reduced reliance on vestibular and visual cues. Laryngoscope 114, 581–586, 2004.
388. Nadol JB. Vestibular neuritis. Otolaryngol Head Neck Surg 112, 162–172, 1995.
389. Nagarkar AN, Gupta AK, Mann SB. Psychological findings in benign paroxysmal positional vertigo and psychogenic vertigo. J Otolaryngol. 29, 154–158, 2000.
390. Nakashima T, Teranishi M, Hibi T, Kobayashi M, Umemura M. Vestibular and cochlear toxicity of aminoglycosides—a review. Acta Otolaryngol. 120, 904–911, 2000.
391. Nakayama M, Riggs LC, Matz GJ. Quantitative study of vestibulotoxicity induced by gentamicin or cisplatin in the guinea pig. Laryngoscope 106, 162–167, 1996.
392. Neuhauser H, Lempert T. Vertigo and dizziness related to migraine: a diagnostic challenge. Cephalalgia 24, 83–91, 2004.
393. Neuhauser H, Leopold M, von Brevern M, Arnold G, Lempert T. The interrelations of migraine, vertigo and migrainous vertigo. Neurology 56, 436–441, 2001.
394. Nielsen JM. Tornado epilepsy simulating Ménière's syndrome. Neurology 9, 794–796, 1959.
395. Nomura Y, Okuno T, Hara M, Young Y. 'Floating' labyrinth. Acta Otolaryngol (Stockh) 112, 186–191, 1992.
396. Norrving B, Magnusson M, Holtas S. Isolated acute vertigo in the elderly; vestibular or vascular disease? Acta Neurol Scand 91, 43–48, 1995.
397. Notis CM, Kitei RA, Cafferty MS, Odel JG, Mitchell JP. Microangioathy of brain retina and inner ear. J Neuroopthalmol 15, 1–8, 1995.
398. Nunez RA, Cass SP, Furman JM. Short- and long-term outcomes of canalith repositioning for benign paroxysmal positional vertigo. Otolaryngol Head Neck Surg 122, 647–652, 2000.
399. Nuti D, Agus G, Barbieri M-T, Passali D. The management of horizontal-canal paroxysmal positional vertigo. Acta Otolaryngol (Stockh) 118, 455–460, 1998.
400. Nuti D, Biagini C, Salerni L, Gaudini E, Passali GC. Use of mammalian inner ear antigens for the diagnosis of autoimmune sudden loss of vestibular function. Acta Otolaryngol. Suppl 34–37, 2002.
401. Nuti D, Mandala M, Broman AT, Zee DS. Acute vestibular neuritis: prognosis based upon bedside clinical tests (thrusts and heaves). Ann N Y Acad Sci 1039, 359–367, 2005.
402. Nuti D, Nati C, Passali D. Treatment of benign paroxysmal positional vertigo: no need for postmaneuver restrictions. Otolaryngol Head Neck Surg 122, 440–444, 2000.
403. Nuti D, Passero S, Di Girolamo S. Bilateral vestibular loss in vertebrobasilar dolichoectasia. J Vestib Res 6, 85–91, 1996.
404. Nuti D, Vannucchi P, Pagnini P. Lateral canal BPPV: which is the affected side? Audiological Medicine 3, 16–20, 2005.
405. Nuti D, Vannucchi P, Pagnini P. Benign paroxysmal positional vertigo of the horizontal canal: a form of canalolithiasis with variable clinical features. J Vestib Res 6, 173–184, 1996.
406. O'Halloran HS, Pearson PA, Lee WB, Susac JO, Berger JR. Microangiopathy of the brain retina and cochlea (Susac syndrome). A report of five cases and a review of the literature. Ophthalmology 105, 1038–1044, 1998.
407. Oas J, Baloh RW. Vertigo and the anterior inferior cerebellar artery syndrome. Neurology 42, 2274–2279, 1992.
408. Oh AK, Ishiyama A, Baloh RW. Vertigo and the enlarged vestibular aqueduct syndrome. J Neurol 248, 971–974, 2001.
409. Oh AK, Lee H, Jen JC, et al. Familial benign recurrent vertigo. Am J Med Genet 100, 287–291, 2001.
410. Ohashi N, Nakagawa H, Kanda K, Mizukoshi K. Otoneurological manifestations of the Shy-Drager syndrome. Eur Arch Otorhinolaryngol 248, 150–152, 1991.
411. Olsson JE. Neurotologic findings in basilar migraine. Laryngoscope 101, 1–41, 1991.
412. Ooi D, Cornell ED, Curthoys IS, Burgess AM, MacDougall HG. Convergence reduces ocular counterroll (OCR) during static roll-tilt. Vision Res 44, 2825–2833, 2004.
413. Oosterveld WJ, Kortschot HW, Kingma GG, de John HAA, Saatci MR. Electronystagmographic findings following cervical whiplash injuries. Acta Otolaryngol (Stockh) 111, 201–205, 1993.
414. Ostrowski VB, Byskosh A, Hain TC. Tullio phenomenon with dehiscence of the superior semicircular canal. Otol Neurotol 22, 61–65, 2001.

415. Ostrowski VB, Hain TC, Wiet RJ. Pressure-induced ocular torsion. Arch Otolaryngol Head Neck Surg 123, 646–649, 1997.
416. Otsuka K, Suzuki M, Furuya M. Model experiment of benign paroxysmal positional vertigo mechanism using the whole membranous labyrinth. Acta Otolaryngol 123, 515–518, 2003.
417. Palla A, Bockisch CJ, Bergamin O, Straumann D. Residual torsion following ocular counterroll. Ann N Y Acad Sci 1039, 81–87, 2005.
418. Palla A, Marti S, Straumann D. Head-shaking nystagmus depends on gravity. J Assoc Res Otolaryngol 6, 1–8, 2005.
419. Pansell T, Schworm HD, Ygge J. Torsional and vertical eye movements during head tilt dynamic characteristics. Invest Ophthalmol Vis Sci 44, 2986–2990, 2003.
420. Pansell T, Tribukait A, Bolzani R, Schworm HD, Ygge J. Drift in ocular counterrolling during static head tilt. Ann N YAcad Sci 1039, 554–557, 2005.
421. Paparella MM, Mancini F, Liston SL. Otosclerosis and Meniere's syndrome: diagnosis and treatment. Laryngoscope 94, 1414–1417, 1984.
422. Parker W. Migraine and the vestibular system in childhood and adolescence. Am J Otol 10, 364–371, 1989.
423. Parnes LS, Agrawal SK, Atlas J. Diagnosis and management of benign paroxysmal positional vertigo (BPPV). CMAJ 169, 681–693, 2003.
424. Parnes LS, McClure JA. Free floating endolymph particles: a new operative finding during posterior semicircular canal occlusion. Laryngoscope 102, 988–992, 1992.
425. Parnes LS, McClure JA. Rotatory recovery nystagmus: an important localizing sign in endolymphatic hydrops. J Otolaryngol 19, 96–99, 1990.
426. Passero S, Nuti D. Auditory and vestibular findings in patients with vertebrobasilar dolichoectasia. Acta Neurologica Scandinavia 93, 50–55, 1996.
427. Perez N, Martin E, Garcia-Tapia R. Intratympanic gentamicin for intractable Meniere's disease. Laryngoscope 113, 456–464, 2003.
428. Perez N, Martin E, Zubieta JL, Romero MD, Garcia-Tapia R. Benign paroxysmal positional vertigo in patients with Meniere's disease treated with intratympanic gentamycin. Laryngoscope 112, 1104–1109, 2002.
429. Pillsbury NC, Postma DS. The Tullio phenomenon, fistula test, and Hennebert's sign: Clinical significance. Otolaryngol Clin North Am 16, 205–207, 1983.
430. Prezant TR, Agapian JV, Bohlman MC, et al. Mitochondrial ribosomal RNA mutation associated with both antibiotic-induced and nonsyndromic deafness. Nat Genet 4, 289–294, 1993.
431. Proctor L, Perlman H, Lindsay J, Matz G. Acute vestibular paralysis in herpes zoster oticus. Ann Otol Rhinol Laryngol 88, 303–310, 1979.
431a. Prokopakis EP, Chimona T, Tsagournisakis M, et al. Benign paroxysmal positional vertigo: 10-year experience in treating 592 patients with canalith repositioning procedure. Laryngoscope 115, 1667–1671, 2005.
432. Pulec JL. Meniere's disease of syphilitic etiology. Ear Nose Throat J 76, 508–10, 512, 1997.
433. Pullen FW. Perilymphatic fistula induced by barotrauma. Am J Otol 13, 270–272, 1992.
434. Rabinovitch HE, Sharpe JA, Sylvester TO. The ocular tilt reaction. A paroxysmal dyskinesia associated with elliptical nystagmus. Arch Ophthalmol 95, 1395–1398, 1977.
435. Radtke A, Bronstein AM, Gresty MA, et al. Paroxysmal alternating skew deviation and nystagmus after partial destruction of the uvula. J Neurol Neurosurg Psychiatry 70, 790–793, 2001.
436. Radtke A, Lempert T, Gresty MA, et al. Migraine and Meniere's disease: is there a link? Neurology 59, 1700–1704, 2002.
437. Radtke A, Neuhauser H, von Brevern M, Lempert T. A modified Epley's procedure for self-treatment of benign paroxysmal positional vertigo. Neurology 53, 1358–1360, 1999.
438. Radtke A, von Brevern M, Tiel-Wilck K, et al. Self-treatment of benign paroxysmal positional vertigo: Semont maneuver vs Epley procedure. Neurology 63, 150–152, 2004.
439. Rajguru SM, Ifediba MA, Rabbitt RD. Three-dimensional biomechanical model of benign paroxysmal positional vertigo. Ann Biomed Eng 32, 831–846, 2004.
440. Ramat S, Zee DS, Minor LB. Translational vestibulo-ocular reflex evoked by a "head heave" stimulus. Ann N Y Acad Sci 942, 95–113, 2001.
441. Rambold H, Boenki J, Stritzke G, et al. Differential vestibular dysfunction in sudden unilateral hearing loss. Neurology 64, 148–151, 2005.
442. Rambold H, Heide W, Sprenger A, Haendler G, Helmchen C. Perilymph fistula associated with pulse-synchronous eye oscillations. Neurology 56, 1769–1771, 2001.
443. Rambold H, Helmchen C. Spontaneous nystagmus in dorsolateral medullary infarction indicates vestibular semicircular canal imbalance. J Neurol Neurosurg Psychiatry 76, 88–94, 2005.
444. Ranalli PJ, Sharpe JA. Vertical vestibulo-ocular reflex, smooth pursuit and eye-head tracking dysfunction in internuclear ophthalmoplegia. Brain 111, 1299–1317, 1988.
445. Rassekh CH, Harker, LA. The prevalence of migraine in Meniere's disease. Laryngoscope 102, 135–138, 1992.
446. Reploeg MD, Goebel JA. Migraine-associated dizziness: patient characteristics and management options. Otol Neurotol 23, 364–371, 2002.
447. Riente L, Bongiorni F, Nacci A, et al. Antibodies to inner ear antigens in Meniere's disease. Clin Exp Immunol 135, 159–163, 2004.
448. Rinne T, Bronstein AM, Rudge P, Gresty MA, Luxon LM. Bilateral loss of vestibular function: clinical findings in 53 patients. J Neurol 245, 314–321, 1998.
449. Riordan-Eva P, Harcourt JP, Faldon M, Brookes GB, Gresty MA. Skew deviation following vestibular nerve surgery. Ann Neurol 41, 94–99, 1997.
450. Rosengart A, Hedges TR, III, Teal PA, et al. Intermittent downbeat nystagmus due to vertebral artery compression. Neurology 43, 216–218, 1993.
451. Rosenhall U, Hanner P, Kaijser B. Borrelia infection and vertigo. Acta Otolaryngol (Stockh) 106, 111–116, 1988.
452. Rottach KG, von Maydell RE, DiScenna AO, et al. Quantitative measurements of eye movements in a

patient with Tullio phenomenon. J Vestib Res 6, 255–259, 1996, 1996.
453. Ruckenstein MJ. Autoimmune inner ear disease. Curr Opin Otolaryngol Head Neck Surg 12, 426–430, 2004.
454. Rudge P, Chambers BR. Physiological basis for enduring vestibular symptoms. J Neurol Neurosurg Psychiatry 45, 126–130, 1982.
455. Rutka JA, Barber HO. Recurrent vestibulopathy: third review. J Otolaryngol 15, 105–107, 1986.
456. Safran AB, Vibert D, Issoua D. Skew deviation after vestibular neuritis. Am J Ophthalmol 118, 238–245, 1994.
457. Saim L, Nadol JB. Vestibular symptoms in otosclerosis—Correlations of otosclerotic involvement of vestibular apparatus and Scarpa's ganglion cell count. Am J Otol 17, 263–270, 1996.
458. Sakellari V, Bronstein AM, Corna S, et al. The effects of hyperventilation on postural control mechanisms. Brain 120, 1659–1673, 1997.
459. Samson M, Mihout B, Thiebot J, et al. Forme benigne des infarctus cerebelleux. Rev Neurol (Paris) 137, 373–382, 1981.
460. Savundra PA, Carroll JD, Davies RA, Luxon LM. Migraine-associated vertigo. Cephalgia 17, 505–510, 1997.
461. Schessel DA, Minor LB, Nedzelski J. Meniere's disease and other peripheral vestibular disorders. In Cummings CW (ed). Otolaryngology Head, Neck Surgery. Elsevier Mosby, Philadelphia, 2005, pp 3209–3253.
461a. Schneider JP, Reinohs M, Prothmann S, et al. Subcortical right parietal AVM rotational vertigo and caloric stimulation fMRI support a parietal representation of vestibular input. J Neurol, published online, 2005.
462. Schneider RC, Calhoun HD, Crosby EC. Vertigo and rotational movement in cortical and subcortical lesions. J Neurol Sci 6, 493–516, 1968.
462a. Schratzenstaller B, Wagner-Manslau C, Strasser G, Arnold W. Canalolithiasis of the superior semicircular canal: an anomaly in benign paroxysmal vertigo. Acta Otolaryngol 125, 1055–1062, 2005.
463. Schubert MC, Herdman SJ, Tusa RJ. Vertical dynamic visual acuity in normal subjects and patients with vestibular hypofunction. Otol Neurotol 23, 372–377, 2002.
464. Schuknecht HF. Cupulolithiasis. Arch Otolaryngol 90, 765–768, 1969.
465. Schuknecht HF. Myths in neurotology. Am J Otol 13, 124–126, 1992.
466. Schuknecht HF. Pathology of the Ear. Lea, Febiger, Philadelphia, 1993.
467. Schuknecht HF, Gulya AJ. Endolymphatic hydrops. An overview and classification. Ann Otology 92 (suppl 106), 1–20, 1983.
468. Schuknecht HF, Igarashi M, Chasin WE. Inner ear hemorrhage in leukemia. Laryngoscope 75, 662–668, 1965.
469. Schuknecht HF, Nadol JB. Temporal bone pathology in a case of Cogan's syndrome. Laryngoscope 104, 1135–1142, 1994.
470. Schuknecht HF, Witt RL. Acute bilateral sequential vestibular neuritis. Am J Otolaryngol 6, 255–257, 1985.
471. Schuknecht HF, Witt RL. Suppressed sneezing as a cause of hearing loss and vertigo. Am J Otolaryngol 6, 468–470, 1985.
472. Schuler O, Strupp M, Arbusow V, Brandt T. A case of possible autoimmune bilateral vestibulopathy treated with steroids. J Neurol Neurosurg Psychiatr 74, 825, 2003.
473. Scott PM, Griffiths MV. A clinical review of ototoxicity. Clin Otolaryngol 19, 3–8, 1994.
474. Semont A, Freyss G, Vitte E. Curing the BPPV with a liberatory maneuver. Adv Otorhinolaryngol 42, 290–293, 1988.
475. Seo SW, Shin HY, Kim SH, et al. Vestibular imbalance associated with a lesion in the nucleus prepositus hypoglossi area. Arch Neurol 61, 1440–1443, 2004.
476. Shallo-Hoffmann J, Bronstein AM. Visual motion detection in patients with absent vestibular function. Vision Res 43, 1589–1594, 2003.
477. Shepard NT, Telian SA, Niparko JK, Kemink JL, Fujita S. Platform pressure test in identification of perilymph fistula. Am J Otol 13, 49–54, 1992.
478. Singleton CT. Diagnosis and treatment of perilymph fistulas without hearing loss. Otolaryngol Head Neck Surg 94, 426–429, 1984.
479. Smith BH. Vestibular disturbances in epilepsy. Neurology 10, 465–469, 1960.
480. Smith PF. Pharmacology of the vestibular system. Curr Opin Neurol 13, 31–37, 2000.
481. Smith PF, Darlington CL. Can vestibular compensation be enhanced by drug treatment? A review of recent evidence. J Vestib Res 4, 169–180, 1994.
482. Soliman AM. A subpopulation of Meniere's patients produce antibodies that bind to endolymphatic sac antigens. Am J Otol 17, 76–80, 1996.
483. Spector GJ, Druck NS, Gado M. Neurological manifestations of glomus tumors in the head and neck. Arch Neurol 33, 270–274, 1976.
484. Steddin S, Brandt T. Unilateral mimicking bilateral benign paroxysmal positional vertigo. Arch Otolaryngol Head Neck Surg 120, 1341, 1994.
485. Stodieck SRG, Brandt T, Büttner U. Visual and vestibular epileptic seizures. Electroencephalogr Clin Neurophysiol 75, 65–66, 1990.
486. Straube A, Brandt T. Recurrent attacks with skew deviation torsional nystagmus and contractions of the left frontalis muscle. Neurology 44, 17–18, 1994.
487. Streubel SO, Cremer PD, Carey JP, Weg N, Minor LB. Vestibular-evoked myogenic potentials in the diagnosis of superior canal dehiscence syndrome. Acta Otolaryngol Suppl 545, 41–49, 2001.
488. Strupp M, Arbusow V, Brandt T. Exercise and drug therapy alter recovery from labyrinth lesion in humans. Ann N Y Acad Sci 942, 79–94, 2001.
489. Strupp M, Glasauer S, Schneider E, et al. Anterior canal failure: ocular torsion without perceptual tilt due to preserved otolith function. J Neurol Neurosurg Psychiatr 74, 1336–1338, 2003.
490. Strupp M, Glaser M, Karch C, et al. The most common form of dizziness in middle age: phobic postural vertigo. Nervenarzt 74, 911–914, 2003.
491. Strupp M, Jahn K, Brandt T. Another adverse effect of aspirin: bilateral vestibulopathy. J Neurol Neurosurg Psychiatr 74, 691, 2003.
492. Strupp M, Planck JH, Arbusow V, et al. Rotational

vertebral artery occlusion syndrome with vertigo due to "labyrinthine excitation". Neurology 54, 1376–1379, 2000.
493. Strupp M, Zingler VC, Arbusow V, et al. Methylprednisolone, valacyclovir or the combination for vestibular neuritis. N Engl J Med 351, 354–361, 2004.
494. Susac JO. Susac's syndrome: the triad of microangiopathy of the brain and retina with hearing loss in young women. Neurology 44, 591–593, 1994.
495. Susac JO, Murtagh FR, Egan RA, et al. MRI findings in Susac's syndrome. Neurology 61, 1783–1787, 2003.
496. Suzuki JI, Tokumasu K, Goto K. Eye movements from single utricular nerve stimulation in the cat. Acta Otolaryngol (Stockh) 68, 350–362, 1969.
497. Suzuki T, Nishio M, Chikuda M, Takayanagi K. Skew deviation as a complication of cardiac catheterization. Am J Ophthalmol 132, 282–283, 2001.
498. Suzuki Y, Kiyosawa M, Mochizuki M, et al. Oscillopsia associated with dysfunction of visual cortex. Jpn J Ophthalmol 48, 128–132, 2004.
499. Thakar A, Anjaneyulu C, Deka RC. Vertigo syndromes and mechanisms in migraine. J Laryngol Otol 115, 782–787, 2001.
500. Thomas JE, Cody DTR. Neurologic perspectives of otosclerosis. Mayo Clin Proc 56, 17–21, 1981.
501. Thömke F, Hopf HC. Pontine lesions mimicking acute peripheral vestibulopathy. J Neurol Neurosurg Psychiatr 66, 340–349, 1999.
502. Thurston SE, Leigh RJ, Abel LA, Dell'Osso LF. Hyperactive vestibuloocular reflex in cerebellar degeneration: pathogenesis and treatment. Neurology 37, 53–57, 1987.
503. Tilikete C, Krolak-Salmon P, Truy E, Vighetto A. Pulse-synchronous eye oscillations revealing bone superior canal dehiscence. Ann Neurol 56, 556–560, 2004.
504. Tilikete C, Vighetto A. Internuclear ophthalmoplegia with skew deviation. Two cases with an isolated circumscribed lesion of the medial longitudinal fasciculus. Eur Neurol 44, 258–259, 2000.
505. Tirelli G, D'Orlando E, Giacomarra V, Russolo M. Benign positional vertigo without detectable nystagmus. Laryngoscope 111, 1053–1056, 2001.
506. Tirelli G, Russolo M. 360–Degree canalith repositioning procedure for the horizontal canal. Otolaryngol Head Neck Surg 131, 740–746, 2004.
507. Toglia JU. Acute flexion-extension injury of the neck. Electronystagmographic study of 309 patients. Neurology 26, 808–814, 1976.
508. Troost BT. Vestibular migraine. Curr Pain Headache Rep 8, 310–314, 2004.
509. Tsang WW, Wong VS, Fu SN, Hui-Chan CW. Tai Chi improves standing balance control under reduced or conflicting sensory conditions. Arch Phys Med Rehabil 85, 129–137, 2004.
510. Tsunoda I, Awano H, Kayama H, et al. Idiopathic AA amyloidosis manifested by autonomic neuropathy, vestibulocochleopathy and lattice corneal dystrophy. J Neurol Neurosurg Psychiatry 57, 635–637, 1994.
511. Tusa RJ. Benign paroxysmal positional vertigo. Curr Neurol Neurosci Rep 1, 478–485, 2001.
512. Tusa RJ, Saada AA, Niparko JK. Dizziness in childhood. J Child Neurol 9, 261–274, 1994.
513. Uneri A. Migraine and benign paroxysmal positional vertigo: an outcome study of 476 patients. Ear Nose Throat J 83, 814–815, 2004.
514. Vahedi K, van Bogaert P, et al. A gene for hereditary paroxysmal cerebellar ataxia maps to chromosome 19p. Ann Neurol 37, 289–293, 1995.
515. van Bogaert P, Van Nechel C, Goldman S, Szliwowski HB. Acetazolamide-responsive hereditary paroxysmal ataxia: report of a new family. Acta Neurologica Belgica 93, 268–275, 1993.
516. Vannucchi P, Giannoni B, Pagnini P. Treatment of horizontal semicircular canal benign paroxysmal positional vertigo. J Vestib Res 7, 1–6, 1997.
517. Verhagen W, Huygen PLM, Horstink MWIM. Familial congenital vestibular areflexia. J Neurol Neurosurg Psychiatr 50, 933–935, 1987.
518. Verhagen WIM, Huygen PLM, Joosten EMG. Familial progressive vestibulocochlear dysfunction. Arch Neurol 45, 766–768, 1988.
519. Verhulst E, Van Lammeren M, Dralands L. Diplopia from skew deviation in Ramsey-Hunt syndrome. A case report. Bull Soc Belge Ophtalmol 27–32, 2000.
520. Versino M, Hurko O, Zee DS. Disorders of binocular control of eye movements in patients with cerebellar dysfunction. Brain 119, 1933–1950, 1996.
521. Versino M, Sances G, Anghileri E, et al. Dizziness and migraine: a causal relationship? Funct Neurol 18, 97–101, 2003.
522. Vibert D, Hausler R, Lovblad KO, Schroth G. Hearing loss and vertigo in superficial siderosis of the central nervous system. Am J Otolaryngol 25, 142–149, 2004.
523. Vibert D, Liard P. Bilateral idiopathic loss of peripheral vestibular function with normal hearing. Acta Otolaryngol 115, 611–615, 1995.
524. Vignaud J, Marsot-Dupitch K, Pharaboz C, Derosier C, Cordoliani Y-S. Imaging of the vestibule. Otolaryngol Head Neck Surg 112, 36–49, 1995.
525. Viirre E, Purcell I, Baloh RW. The Dix-Hallpike test and the canalith repositioning maneuver. Laryngoscope 115, 184–187, 2005.
526. Viirre ES, Baloh RW. Migraine as a cause of sudden hearing loss. Headache 36, 24–28, 1996.
527. Vollersten RS, MacDonald TJ, Banks PM, Stanson AW, Ilstrup DM. Cogan's syndrome: 18 cases and a review of the literature. Mayo Clin Proc 61, 344–361, 1986.
528. von Brevern M, Arnold G, Lempert T. Migrainous vertigo. Schmerz. 18, 411–414, 2004.
529. von Brevern M, Clarke AH, Lempert T. Continuous vertigo and spontaneous nystagmus due to canalolithiasis of the horizontal canal. Neurology 56, 684–686, 2001.
530. von Brevern M, Lezius F, Tiel-Wilck K, Radtke A, Lempert T. Benign paroxysmal positional vertigo: current status of medical management. Otolaryngol Head Neck Surg 130, 381–382, 2004.
531. von Brevern M, Radtke A, Clarke AH, Lempert T. Migrainous vertigo presenting as episodic positional vertigo. Neurology 62, 469–472, 2004.
532. von Brevern M, Seelig T, Neuhauser H, Lempert T. Benign paroxysmal positional vertigo predominantly affects the right labyrinth. J Neurol Neurosurg Psychiatry 75, 1487–1488, 2004.
532a. von Brevern M, Schmidt T, Schonfeld U, Lempert T, Clarke AH. Utricular dysfunction in patients with benign paroxysmal positional vertigo. Otol Neurotol 27, 92–96, 2006.

533. von Brevern M, Lempert T. Benign paroxysmal positional vertigo. Arch Neurol 58, 1491–1493, 2001.
534. von Brevern M, Lempert T, Bronstein AM, Kocen R. Selective vestibular damage in neurosarcoidosis. Ann Neurol 42, 117–120, 1997.
535. von Campe G, Regli F, Bogousslavsky J. Heralding manifestations of basilar artery occlusion with lethal or severe stroke. J Neurol Neurosurg Psychiatry 74, 1621–1626, 2003.
536. von Brevern M, Zeise D, Neuhauser H, Clarke AH, Lempert T. Acute migrainous vertigo: clinical and oculographic findings. Brain 128, 365–374, 2005.
537. Walker MF, Zee DS. The effect of hyperventilation on downbeat nystagmus in cerebellar disorders. Neurology 53, 1576–1579, 1999.
537a. Walker MF, Zee DS. Cerebellar disease alters the axis of the high-acceleration vestibuloocular reflex. J Neurophysiol 94, 3417–3429, 2005.
538. Wall C, III, Rauch SD. Perilymphatic fistula. In Baloh RW, Halmagyi GM (eds). Disorders of the Vestibular System. Oxford, New York, 1996, pp 396–406.
539. Waterson JA, Halmagyi GM. Unilateral vestibulotoxicity due to systemic gentamicin therapy. Acta Otolaryngol (Stockh) 118, 474–478, 1998.
540. Waterston J. Chronic migrainous vertigo. J Clin Neurosci 11, 384–388, 2004.
541. Waterston JA, Halmagyi GM. Unilateral vestibulotoxicity due to systemic gentamicin therapy. Acta Otolaryngol 118, 474–478, 1998.
542. Watson P, Barber HO, Deck J, Terbrugge K. Positional vertigo and nystagmus of central origin. Can J Neurol Sci 8, 133–137, 1981.
543. Watson SR, Halmagyi GM, Colebatch JG. Vestibular hypersensitivity to sound (Tullio phenomenon): structural and functional assessment. Neurology 54, 722–728, 2000.
544. Weintraub MI. Vestibulopathy induced by high impact aerobics. A new syndrome: discussion of 30 cases. J Sports Med Phys Fitness 34, 56–63, 1994.
545. Weisleder P, Fife TD. Dizziness and headache: a common association in children and adolescents. J Child Neurol 16, 727–730, 2001.
546. Welling DB, Parnes LS, Bakaletz LO, Brackmann DE, Hinojosa R. Particulate matter in the posterior semicircular canal. Laryngoscope 107, 90–94, 1997.
547. Welsh LW, Welsh JJ, Jaffe SC, Healy MP. Syndromal vertigo identified by magnetic resonance imaging and angiography. Laryngoscope 106, 1144–1151, 1996.
548. Wennmo C, Svensson C. Fractures of the temporal bone-chain incongruencies. Am J Otolaryngol 141, 38–42, 1993.
549. Westheimer G, Blair SM. Synkinesis of head and eye movements evoked by brainstem stimulation in the alert monkey. Exp Brain Res 24, 89–95, 1975.
550. Westheimer G, Blair SM. The ocular tilt reaction—a brainstem oculomotor routine. Invest Ophthalmol 14, 833–839, 1975.
551. Whitney SL, Rossi MM. Efficacy of vestibular rehabilitation. Otolaryngol Clin North Am 33, 659–672, 2000.
552. Wiest G, Tian JR, Baloh RW, Crane BT, Demer JL. Otolith function in cerebellar ataxia due to mutations in the calcium channel gene CACNA1A. Brain 124, 2407–2416, 2001.
553. Williams B. Cough headache due to craniospinal pressure dissociation. Arch Neurol 37, 226–230, 1980.
554. Wilson WR, Zoller M. Electronystagmography in congenital and acquired syphilitic otitis. Ann Otol Rhinol Laryngol 90, 21–24, 1981.
555. Wist ER, Brandt T, Krafczyk S. Oscillopsia and retinal slip: Evidence supporting a clinical test. Brain 106, 153–168, 1983.
556. Wolfe GI, Taylor CL, Flamm ES, et al. Ocular tilt reaction resulting from vestibuloacoustic nerve surgery. Surg Neurol 32, 417–420, 1993.
556a. Wong AM, Sharpe JA, Cerebellar skew deviation and the torsional vestibuloocular reflex. Neurology 65, 412–419, 2005.
557. Woodworth BA, Gillespie MB, Lambert PR. The canalith repositioning procedure for benign positional vertigo: a meta-analysis. Laryngoscope 114, 1143–1146, 2004.
558. Wu CC, Chen YS, Chen PJ, Hsu CJ. Common clinical features of children with enlarged vestibular aqueduct and Mondini dysplasia. Laryngoscope 115, 132–137, 2005.
559. Yabe I, Sasaki H, Takeichi N, et al. Positional vertigo and macroscopic downbeat positioning nystagmus in spinocerebellar ataxia type 6 (SCA6). J Neurol 250, 440–443, 2003.
560. Yagi T, Ohyama Y, Suzuki K, Kamura E, Kokawa T. 3D analysis of nystagmus in peripheral vertigo. Acta Otolaryngol (Stockh) 117, 135–138, 1997.
561. Yagi T, Morishita M, Koizumi Y, et al. Is the pathology of horizontal canal benign paroxysmal positional vertigo really localized in the horizontal semicircular canal? Acta Otolaryngol. 121, 930–934, 2001.
562. Yagi T, Ohyama Y. Three-dimensional analysis of nystagmus induced by neck vibration. Acta Otolaryngol (Stockh) 116, 167–169, 1996.
563. Yaniglos SS, Leigh RJ. Refinement of an optical device that stabilizes vision in patients with nystagmus. Optometry and Vision Science 69, 447–450, 1992.
563a. Yates BJ, Bronstein AM. The effects of vestibular system lesions on autonomic regulation: observations, mechanisms, and clinical implications. J Vestib Res 15, 119–129, 2005.
564. Yen MT, Herdman SJ, Tusa RJ. Oscillopsia and pseudonystagmus in kidney transplant patients. Am J Ophthalmol 128, 768–770, 1999.
565. Young YH, Chen CH. Acute vertigo following cervical manipulation. Laryngoscope 113, 659–662, 2003.
566. Yue Q, Jen JC, Thwe MM, Nelson SF, Baloh RW. De novo mutation in CACNA1A caused acetazolamide-responsive episodic ataxia. Am J Med Gen 77, 298–301, 1998.
567. Zee DS. Considerations on the mechanisms of alternating skew deviation in patients with cerebellar lesions. J Vestib Res 6, 395–401, 1996.
568. Zee DS, Friendlich AR, Robinson DA. The mechanism of downbeat nystagmus. Arch Neurol 30, 227–237, 1974.
569. Zeidman LA, Melen O, Gottardi-Littell N, et al. Susac syndrome with transient inverted vision. Neurology 63, 591, 2004.
570. Zupan LH, Merfeld DM, Darlot C. Using sensory weighting to model the influence of canal, otolith and visual cues on spatial orientation and eye movements. Biol Cybern 86, 209–230, 2002.

Chapter 12

Diagnosis of Central Disorders of Ocular Motility

USING EYE MOVEMENTS FOR TOPOLOGICAL DIAGNOSIS

In this chapter we review the effects of focal disease in the nervous system, starting in the medulla, and proceeding rostrally. Especially at the level of the brainstem, abnormal eye movements can aid the clinician in topological diagnosis. We also discuss certain other disorders affecting distributed systems of neurons and use our knowledge of the neurobiology of eye movements to provide insights into genetic, degenerative, metabolic, and toxic disorders, whenever possible. Throughout the text, we provide links to the Video Displays that are available on the accompanying compact disc.

OCULAR MOTOR SYNDROMES CAUSED BY LESIONS IN THE MEDULLA

Medullary Lesions Impairing Gaze Holding

Examples of the effects of medullary lesions on eye movements are shown in the Video Display: Medullary Syndromes. The medulla contains nuclei and tracts that are important in the control of eye movements, including the vestibular nuclei, perihypoglossal nuclei, medullary reticular formation, inferior olivary nuclei, and restiform body (inferior cerebellar peduncle).

The perihypoglossal nuclei consist of the nucleus prepositus hypoglossi (NPH), which lies in the floor of the fourth ventricle, the nucleus of Roller, and the nucleus intercalatus. These nuclei have connections with other brainstem structures controlling eye movements and the cerebellum (see Table 5–1, Chapter 5). The NPH and the adjacent medial vestibular nuclei (MVN)— the NPH-MVN region—are critical for holding horizontal positions of gaze (the neural integrator), and experimental lesions abolish the ability to hold the eye in an eccentric lateral position.[169] The NPH-MVN region also participates in vertical gaze holding, along with contributions from rostral structures, especially the interstitial nucleus of Cajal (see Box 6–6). Another group of paramedian neurons in the medulla that probably contributes to gaze holding is the nucleus pararaphales, which lies about halfway between the abducens and hypoglossal nucleus, receives inputs from the interstitial nucleus of Cajal, and sends axons laterally, running close to the ventral surface of the brainstem, before entering the inferior cerebellar peduncle. The nucleus paraphales is one component of cell groups of the paramedian tracts (PMT), which receive inputs from premotor nuclei concerned with eye movements and relay information to the vestibulocerebellum (Box 6–4).[161]

Strokes that affect the NPH may cause gaze-evoked nystagmus as well as postural imbalance and vertigo.[980] Wernicke's encephalopathy commonly involves the NPH-MVN region, which may account for the gaze-evoked nystagmus and other ocular motor features of this disease (see Video Display: Disorders of Gaze Holding). A patient who developed complete gaze failure following a lethal dose of lithium intoxication showed selective loss of neurons and gliosis in the NPH-MVN region.[219]

Upbeat nystagmus is a common finding in patients with lesions in the paramedian medulla, sometimes with a horizontal component (see Fig. 10–3 and Video Display: Downbeat, Upbeat, Torsional Nystagmus).[840,1107] Upbeat nystagmus has been attributed to involvement, by tumor or infarction, of the perihypoglossal nuclei, including the nucleus intercalatus,[466,510,753] and the nucleus of Roller.[562] It also seems possible that such reported medullary lesions, which are often neither discrete nor confirmed by postmortem examination, might affect nucleus paraphales and its long axons, thereby causing failure of vertical gaze holding.[155,760,1100] More rostral lesions might cause upbeat nystagmus by affecting projections from the superior vestibular nucleus that run in the crossing ventral tegmental pathway for the upward vestibulo-ocular reflex (Fig. 2–3, Chapter 2).[881] The pathogenesis of upbeat nystagmus is discussed further in Chapter 10.

Effects of Disease Involving the Inferior Olivary Nucleus

Lesions of the inferior olivary nucleus or its connections may produce the syndrome of oculopalatal tremor (or myoclonus) (Fig. 10–10) (see Video Display: Medullary Syndromes). This condition, which usually develops weeks to months after infarction or hemorrhage affecting the brainstem, cerebellum, or superior cerebellar peduncle,[953,1190] is discussed in the section on acquired pendular nystagmus in Chapter 10. Oculopalatal tremor may also occur with degenerative conditions.[275,1025] In some patients, a progressive ataxia accompanies development of the syndrome,[304,953] and they may show impairment of motor learning.[274] Essential palatal tremor, without ocular oscillations, is distinct from the symptomatic form that follows brainstem stroke;[275] the idiopathic form affects different palatal muscles, and causes auditory clicking.[273]

The main pathologic finding with palatal tremor is hypertrophy of the inferior olivary nucleus, which may be seen using MRI.[96,275,404,1025] When the syndrome is due to unilateral infarction of the dentate nucleus and superior cerebellar peduncle, changes in the olive appear on the contralateral side.[1190] Histologically, the olivary nucleus is enlarged, due to hypertrophy of neurons that contain increased acetylcholinesterase reaction product.[582,780] Such changes begin within a month of the stroke and maximize in about six months, and are accompanied by astrocytosis, and synaptic and axonal remodelling. At the same time, the number of olivary neurons progressively declines, so that after about six years, they are less than 10% of control brains. Furthermore, efferent axons from olivary neurons are severely degenerated in patients who survive several years.[780] Despite the anatomic demonstration of atrophy, functional imaging studies suggest increased metabolism of the inferior olive.[293]

Guillain and Mollaret postulated that disruption of connections between the dentate and the contralateral olivary nucleus, which run via the red nucleus and central tegmental tract, is responsible for the syndrome.[416] Since the red nucleus has no known role in eye movements,[158] an alternative hypothesis concerns the peculiar electrotonic coupling of cells in the inferior olivary nucleus, which depend on gap junctions channels, called connexons. Connexons permit dendrite-to-dendrite transmission of ions and small molecules.[211, 278] The syndrome of oculopalatal tremor may arise because of interruption of inhibitory projections from the deep cerebellar nuclei, which may project out of the superior cerebellar peduncle before looping back to the inferior olive in the central tegmental tract (Fig. 12–1).[602] Loss of this cerebellar inhibition is followed by degenerative changes in the inferior olivary nucleus.[257,278,945] It is postulated that this hypertrophic degeneration includes development of connexons and electrotonic coupling between cell bodies of inferior olivary neurons, causing large groups of olivary neurons to synchronize, creating a 1 Hz to 2 Hz oscillator.[476] This synchronized signal is sent to the cerebellar cortex on climbing fibers, stimulating the cerebellar motor learning network to produce a maladaptive response consisting of pendular ocular oscillations with variable waveform.[622]

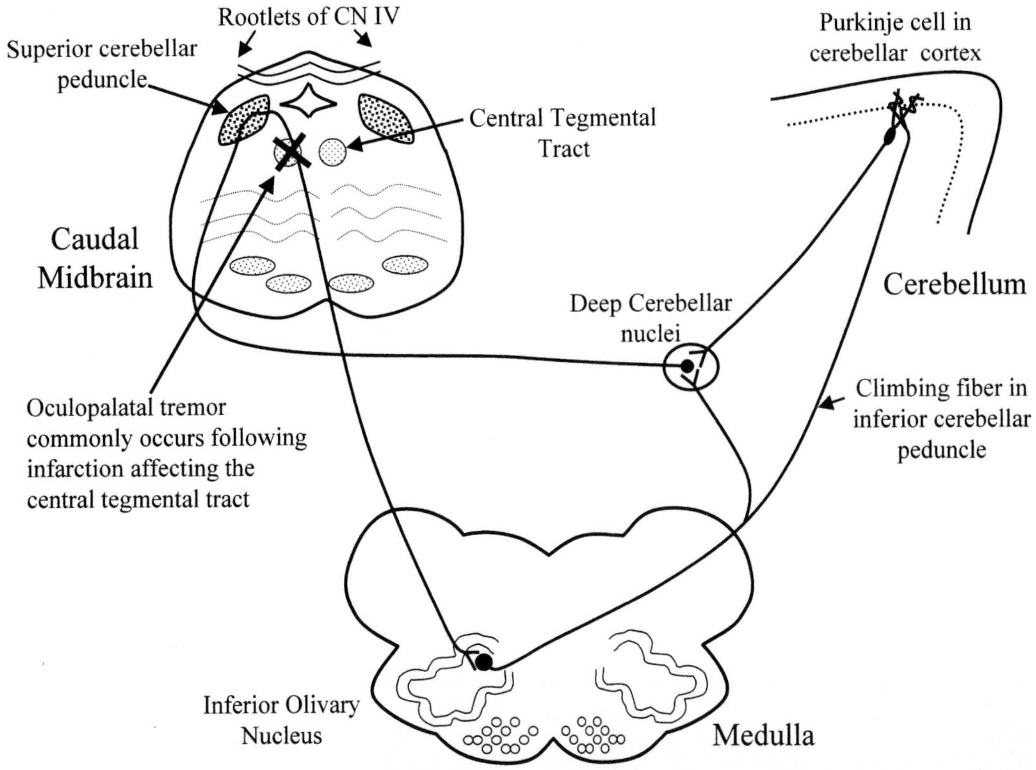

Figure 12–1. Hypothetical scheme to account for the syndrome of oculopalatal tremor with degenerative hypertrophy of the inferior olivary nucleus (IO). Normally, the deep cerebellar nuclei inhibit the IO via a pathway that runs through superior cerebellar peduncle and the central tegmental tract. Disruption by a stroke (indicated by X) leads to hypertrophic degeneration of the IO, with formation of abnormal electrotonic coupling between cell bodies of neurons and development of synchronous discharge at about 2 Hz. This IO activity passes on climbing fibers to cerebellar Purkinje cells, and causes maladaptive learning expressed as ocular oscillations, which may be in the planes of the vestibular semicircular canals, as well as tremor of other branchial muscles, including the palate.[476,622]

Only rarely does oculopalatal tremor resolve spontaneously. Gabapentin, ceruletide, memantine, and anticholinergic agents may help some patients (see Table 10–9).[47,501] Drugs that block connexin channels,[231] and thereby reduce synchronized discharge of electrontonically coupled olivary neurons might provide a new therapeutic approach.[622]

Effects of Disease Restricted to the Vestibular Nuclei

Occasionally, the acute manifestation of a generalized disease process may be restricted to the vestibular nuclei. For example, vertigo may be the sole symptom of an exacerbation of multiple sclerosis[543] or of brainstem ischemia.[297,395,405] Nystagmus caused by disease of the vestibular nuclei may be purely horizontal, vertical, or torsional, or mixed patterns may occur. Moreover, nystagmus from a central vestibular lesion can mimic that caused by peripheral vestibular disease.[711] Paroxysmal vertigo and nystagmus has been reported with an arteriovenous malformation near the vestibular nucleus, and close to the middle cerebellar peduncle.[611] The attacks were successfully treated with carbamazepine. Dolichoectasia of the basilar artery may produce a variety of combinations of central and peripheral vestibular syndromes.[155,785] Central causes of vertigo are discussed further in Chapter 11.

Wallenberg's Syndrome (Dorsolateral Medullary Infarction)

Most commonly, lesions of the vestibular nuclei also affect neighboring structures, in particular the cerebellar peduncles and the perihypoglossal nuclei. The best recognized syndrome involving the vestibular nuclei is that due to dorsolateral medullary infarction—Wallenberg's syndrome (Fig. 12–2; Box 12–1).[528, 567] The typical findings of Wallenberg's syndrome are *ipsilateral* impairment of pain and temperature sensation over the face, Horner's syndrome, limb ataxia, and bulbar disturbance causing dysarthria and dysphagia and, commonly, hiccups.[948] *Contralaterally*, pain and temperature sensation is impaired over the trunk and limbs. Dysphagia, facial paresis and dysarthria are more common with rostral lesions.[567] The stroke is caused most commonly by occlusion of the ipsilateral vertebral artery; occasionally the posterior inferior cerebellar artery is selectively involved.[330, 528,567] Dissection of the vertebral artery (either spontaneous or traumatic, sometimes following chiropractic manipulation) is occasionally the cause.[460] Rarely, demyelinating disease may produce this syndrome.[1013]

The symptoms of Wallenberg's syndrome include vertigo and a variety of unusual sensations of body and environmental tilt, often so bizarre as to be thought to be a psychiatric symptom.[1099] Patients may report the whole room tilted on its side or even upside down; such misperceptions tend to be transient, but sometimes recur. Smaller tilts of the subjective visual vertical tend to be more persistent.[122] Similar symptoms are occasionally reported in patients without signs of dorsolateral medullary infarction and may be due to transient brainstem or cerebellar ischemia.[181,659] Such symptoms may also occur with lesions in the cerebral hemispheres.[1018]

Lateropulsion, a compelling sensation of being pulled toward the side of the lesion, is

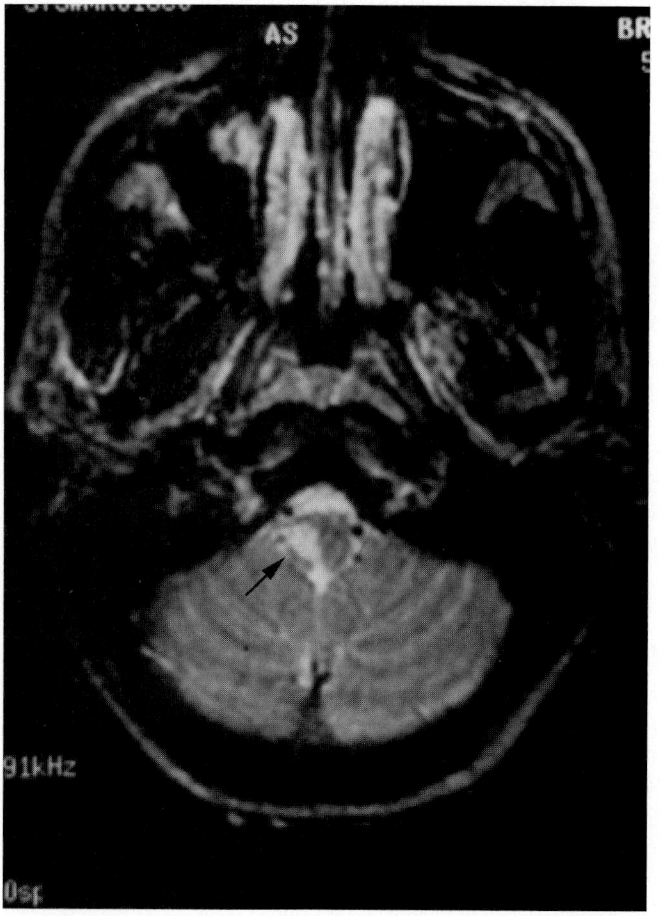

Figure 12–2. T2-weighted MRI scan of a patient with Wallenberg's syndrome, showing an area of infarction (hyperintense signal indicated by arrow) that involved the left side of the medulla.

Box 12–1. Ocular Motor Findings In Wallenberg's Syndrome Of Dorsolateral Medullary Infarction

- Lateropulsion (deviation) of the eyes towards the side of the lesion occurs in darkness, behind closed lids, or with a blink
- Lateropulsion (ipsipulsion) of horizontal saccades: Ipsilateral (to the lesion side) saccades are hypermetric, contralateral are hypometric
- Lateropulsion of vertical saccades causing an oblique trajectory, with an inappropriate horizontal component towards the side of the lesion
- Torsipulsion—inappropriate torsional "blips"— may occur during horizontal saccades
- Smooth pursuit is impaired for targets moving away from the side of the lesion
- Spontaneous nystagmus (often mixed horizontal-torsional) occurs with the eyes in central position; slow phases may be directed towards or away from the side of the lesion
- Ocular tilt reaction (OTR): Skew deviation with ipsilateral hypotropia, head tilt towards side of lesion, ipsilateral cyclodeviation (top poles of eyes rolled ipsilaterally); ipsilateral deviation of subjective visual vertical

For pathophysiology, see: Disorders of Saccadic Accuracy in Chapter 3, and Skew Deviation And The Ocular Tilt Reaction (OTR) and Fig. 11-4 in Chapter 11. (Related Video Display: Medullary Syndromes)

often a prominent complaint and is also evident in the ocular motor findings.[57,482,589] If the patient is asked to fixate straight ahead and then gently close the lids, the eyes deviate conjugately toward the side of the lesion (see Video Display: Medullary Syndromes). This is reflected by the corrective saccades that the patient must make on eye opening to reacquire the target. Lateropulsion may appear with a blink.

Saccadic eye movements are also affected by lateropulsion.[57,129,156,1019,1146,1148,1150] Horizontal saccades directed toward the side of the lesion usually overshoot the target, whereas saccades directed away from the side of the lesion undershoot the target (see Video Display: Medullary Syndromes); this is referred to as *ipsipulsion* of saccades and should be differentiated from *contrapulsion* of saccades that occurs with infarcts due to occlusion of the superior cerebellar artery. Contrapulsion is also reported with demyelinative lesions affecting the superior cerebellar penducle.[350] Quick phases of nystagmus are similarly affected, so that in Wallenberg's syndrome those directed away from the side of the lesion are smaller than those toward the lesion. On attempting a purely vertical refixation, an oblique saccade directed toward the side of the lesion is produced (see Video Display: Medullary Syndromes). Corrective saccades then bring the eyes back to the target.[571] Saccades made in total darkness also show lateropulsion, although in one report the patient was still able to make corrective saccades to the remembered location of a previously seen target, implying that the central nervous system had a knowledge of actual eye position.[796] With time, vertical saccades may become more perverse; S-shaped saccadic trajectories can appear a week or more after the onset of the illness and may reflect an adaptive strategy to correct the saccadic abnormality. Torsipulsion (inappropriate torsional saccades during attempted horizontal or vertical saccades) may also occur in association with torsional nystagmus.[447,734,1046]

When present, *spontaneous nystagmus* in Wallenberg's syndrome is usually horizontal or mixed horizontal-torsional with a small vertical component.[734] The waveform of the nystagmus is usually linear and analysis of its rotational vectors suggests disruption of central pathways from horizontal and anterior semicircular canals, rather than the otoliths.[874] In central position, the slow phase is usually directed toward the side of the lesion, although it may reverse direction in eccentric positions, suggesting coexistent involvement of the gaze-holding mechanism. Lid nystagmus (synkinetic lid twitches with horizontal quick phases) can also occur.[242]

The *ocular tilt reaction* commonly occurs in Wallenberg's syndrome.[283] The skew deviation manifests as an ipsilateral hypotropia (see Video Display: Medullary Syndromes).[125] The eyes are cyclodeviated toward the side of the lesion, but unequally so that the lower eye is more extorted. The head tilt is ipsilateral.[124] The skew deviation and head tilt arise from imbalance in pathways mediating otolith responses. The subjective sensations of tilt or inversion of the world probably also reflect involvement of central projections from the gravireceptors, the utricle, and the saccule.

Smooth pursuit is usually impaired, particularly for tracking targets moving away from the side of the lesion.[57,1150] Caloric testing usually shows intact horizontal canal function. During both rotational and caloric testing, there is a directional preponderance of slow phases, usually toward the side of the lesion.[57,310] Head nystagmus also occurs in some patients with Wallenberg's syndrome.[589]

Some of the findings in Wallenberg's syndrome, including the bizarre visual disturbances and the skew deviation, may reflect imbalance of otolith influences due to direct involvement of the caudal aspects of the vestibular nuclei. The nystagmus appears to represent an ipsilesional lesion of central projections from horizontal and anterior semicircular canals.[874] Involvement of the inferior cerebellar peduncle, which carries olivocerebellar projections, may also account for some of the ocular motor findings, especially the steady-state deviation of the eyes toward the side of the lesion and the ipsipulsion of saccades (Fig. 3–16, Chapter 3).[156,1019,1146,1148,1150] Ipsipulsion of saccades, with deviation of the eyes to the side of the lesion, can be produced experimentally by fastigial nucleus lesions.[912] This finding supports the hypothesis that in Wallenberg's syndrome the interruption of climbing fiber input to the dorsal cerebellar vermis releases Purkinje cell inhibition upon the underlying fastigial nucleus, leading to the equivalent of a lesion in the fastigial nucleus.[1150] Also consistent with this scheme, contrapulsion has also been reported with a medial medullary lesion that affected olivary climbing-fiber projections before they crossed the midline.[569a,1100] An analogous increase in Purkinje cell inhibition from the flocculus to the vestibular nucleus may also play a role in the nystagmus that these patients may develop (with the slow phase toward the side of the lesion).

The vestibular nuclei and adjacent dorsolateral brainstem are also supplied by the anterior inferior cerebellar artery (AICA). In addition, the AICA supplies the inferior lateral cerebellum and is the origin of the labyrinthine artery in most individuals. Consequently, ischemia in the distribution of the AICA (Fig. 12–3) may cause vertigo, vomiting, hearing loss, facial palsy, and ipsilateral limb ataxia, along with

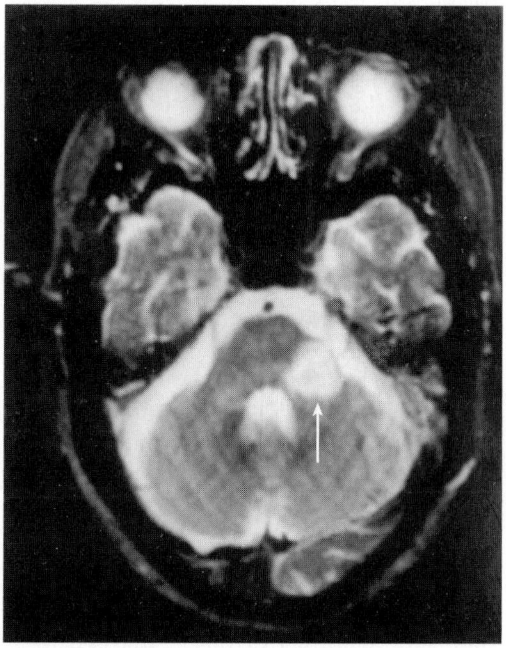

Figure 12–3. MRI scan showing infarction in the distribution of the anterior inferior cerebellar artery (AICA), with the characteristic finding of bright signal on a T2-weighted image in the left middle cerebellar peduncle (arrowhead). The patient also suffered loss of left vestibular function due to occlusion of the labyrinthine artery (see Video Display: Cerebellar Syndromes).

gaze-holding and pursuit deficits, and vestibular imbalance (see Video Display: Cerebellar Syndromes).[405,787] The AICA syndrome is discussed further under Cerebellar Infarction.

OCULAR MOTOR SYNDROMES CAUSED BY DISEASE OF THE CEREBELLUM

Examples of the effects of cerebellar lesions on eye movements are shown in the Video Display: Cerebellar Syndromes. Clinicians have been somewhat reluctant to embrace disorders of eye movements as diagnostic aids when evaluating patients with cerebellar syndromes. For example, in the bourgeoning field of genetically identified spinocerebellar ataxia (SCA), careful description of eye movement abnormalities is often lacking. This is unfortunate, since abnormal properties of eye movements provide insights into which cerebellar circuits are involved. Gordon Holmes[472] and David G. Cogan[193] were among the first to recognize specific cerebellar eye signs that could be distinguished from the effects of coexistent brainstem involvement. Most of their observations have been confirmed by modern clinical and experimental studies, which have also clarified the functional deficits that are caused by specific cerebellar lesions.[77,78,652,805,890,912,913,1046,1062–1064,1137,1149,1215]

Three Principal Cerebellar Syndromes

A substantial body of research concerning the effects of discrete lesions and pharmacological inactivation in monkeys have made it possible to define three principal cerebellar syndromes: (1) The syndrome of the flocculus and paraflocculus (see Box 6–10 and Box 12–2); (2) The syndrome of the nodulus and ventral uvula (see Box 6–11 and Box 12–3); (3) The syndrome of the dorsal vermis (lobules VI and VII) and underlying caudal fastigial nuclei (see Box 6–12, Box 6–13, Box 12–4). These are discussed in turn below, and examples are provided on the Video Display: Cerebellar Syndromes.

In addition, there is evidence that the cerebellar hemispheres contribute to the control of eye movements. Thus, during voluntary saccades made between either two visual targets, or remembered target locations in darkness, fMRI demonstrates increased activation in the hemispheres as well as in the midline (vermis and fastigial nuclei), as is shown in Figure 3–14

Box 12–2. Clinical Findings With Lesions Affecting The Cerebellar Flocculus And Paraflocculus

- Impaired smooth pursuit and combined eye-head tracking ("VOR suppression")
- Impaired ability to suppress caloric nystagmus by fixating a stationary target
- Impaired gaze-holding function, leading to gaze-evoked nystagmus; centripetal and rebound nystagmus
- Downbeat nystagmus, often greatest on looking laterally and downward and with convergence
- Impaired ability to adapt the VOR to changing visual needs (*e.g.*, new spectacle correction)
- Post-saccadic drift (pulse-step mismatch)

For related anatomy, see Box 6-10 and Fig. 6-6 in Chapter 6. For related etiologies, see Table 12-1 and Table 12-2. (Related Video Display: Cerebellar Syndromes)

Box 12–3. Clinical Findings With Lesions Affecting The Cerebellar Nodulus And Ventral Uvula

- Prolongation of vestibular responses (increased velocity storage)
- Loss of ability to suppress post-rotational nystagmus by tilting the head when the rotation stops
- Positional nystagmus; downbeat nystagmus
- Periodic alternating nystagmus in darkness (present in light if floccular and paraflocculus are also lesioned, which impairs visual fixation)

For related anatomy, see Box 6-11 and Fig. 6-6 in Chapter 6. For some related etiologies, see Table 10-4. (Related Video Displays: Periodic Alternating Nystagmus and Cerebellar Syndromes)

Box 12–4. Deficits Caused By Lesions Of Dorsal Vermis, Fastigial Nucleus, And Uncinate Fasciculus*

Dorsal Vermis Lesion

- Ipsilateral hypometria and mild contralateral hypermetria of saccades
- Gaze is tonically deviated away from the side of the lesion
- Smooth pursuit is impaired for targets moving towards the side of the lesion

Unilateral Fastigial Nucleus Lesion†

- Ipsilateral hypermetria and contralateral hypometria of saccades – "ipsipulsion"
- Gaze is tonically deviated towards the side of the lesion
- Smooth pursuit is impaired for targets moving away from the side of the lesion
- Similar defects are features of Wallenberg's syndrome

Uncinate Fasciculus (Which Runs In Superior Cerebellar Peduncle)

- Ipsilateral hypometria and contralateral hypermetria of saccades – "contrapulsion"

*Based on experimental pharmacological inactivation.
† Corresponds to saccadic lateropulsion in Wallenberg's lateral medullary infarction (see Box 12-1)
For related anatomy, see Box 6-12 and Box 6-13 in Chapter 6, and Fig. 3-16 in Chapter 3. (Related Video Display: Cerebellar Syndromes)

of Chapter 3. Furthermore, lesions restricted to one cerebellar hemisphere impair ipsilateral smooth pursuit.[1044]

LESIONS OF THE FLOCCULUS AND PARAFLOCCULUS

Experimental lesions of the flocculus and paraflocculus in animals cause gaze-evoked nystagmus, rebound nystagmus, and downbeat nystagmus,[1215] clinical features of which are discussed in Chapter 10. Inactivation of the flocculus with muscimol severely impairs smooth tracking with the eyes alone, but active eye-head tracking is spared.[78] Saccades are generally accurate, but show postsaccadic drift. There is loss of the ability to adaptively adjust the gain and direction of the vestibulo-ocular reflex (VOR),[654] or the pulse-step match for saccades. Unilateral lesions produce ipsilateral deficits in pursuit and gaze holding.[1044]

In patients with cerebellar disease, defects of smooth pursuit with the head still, combined eye-head tracking, and gaze-holding frequently occur together, reflecting their common substrate in the flocculus and vestibular nuclei;[154] quantitatively, though, pursuit with the head still tends to be relatively more impaired.[409,1161] During tracking of a smoothly moving target, patients with cerebellar disease often show temporal differences between eye and target motion (phase errors),[1161] but there is some preservation of predictive capability.[633] The ability to generate anticipatory smooth eye movements is also impaired in some cerebellar patients.[738]

LESIONS OF THE NODULUS AND VENTRAL UVULA

Experimental or clinical lesions of the nodulus and ventral uvula lead to an increase in the duration of vestibular responses that predisposes the individual to the development of periodic alternating nystagmus, which is discussed in Chapter 10 (see Video Display: Periodic Alternating Nystagmus).[368,1149] Other abnormalities of the velocity-storage mechanism are present, including a failure of tilt-suppression of postrotatory nystagmus,[420,1174a] and loss of habituation to repetitive vestibular stimulation. Positional nystagmus, especially downbeat, may occur in patients with cerebellar disorders that involve the nodulus and ventral uvula (see Video Display: Positional Nystagmus).[692] A patient with a tumor involving the uvula showed horizontal nystagmus with increasing velocity waveforms, implying an unstable neural integrator;[869] following tumor biopsy she developed paroxysmal alternating skew deviation, a condition which is described further in Chapter 11.

LESIONS OF THE DORSAL VERMIS AND FASTIGIAL NUCLEI

Experimental lesions of the dorsal vermis and fastigial nuclei (fastigial oculomotor region—FOR) cause saccadic dysmetria, typically hypometria if the vermis alone is involved, and hypermetria if the deep nuclei are involved (Fig. 12–4).[912,1062] Similarly, clinical lesions predominantly affecting vermal cerebellar cortex cause hypometria, whereas those affecting the fastigial nuclei cause marked saccadic hypermetria (see Fig. 12–4 and Video Display: Cerebellar Syndromes).[978] The pattern of saccadic dysmetria that occurs in cerebellar disease, as well as whether or not corrective saccades occur, is influenced by the type of visual stimulus.[140,374,530] Thus, memory-guided saccades are dysmetric, especially if the target moves during the memory period.[374,530, 593] In some patients with cerebellar disease, corrective saccades are dysmetric.[120] Saccadic dysmetria may be present for externally triggered movements to a visual target but not for internally triggered saccades during scanning of a visual scene.[156] Large torsional "blips" that occur during voluntary saccades constitute violations of Listing's law (see Chapter 9) and have been reported in patients with lesions involving the vermis and fastigial nuclei.[447]

Experimental lesions of the dorsal vermis also produce deficits of smooth pursuit, especially its onset.[1064] Dorsal vermis lesions also impair the ability to adapt smooth pursuit to novel visual demands.[1064] Patients with dorsal vermis lesions show moderate, ipsilateral deficits of sustained pursuit,[1124] as well as defects in motion perception.[766] Similarly, inactivation of one fastigial nucleus impairs the onset of contralateral pursuit onset but increases the acceleration of ipsilateral pursuit onset; sustained pursuit is impaired in all directions, but more so contralaterally. In humans, fastigial nucleus lesions are invariably bilateral because their axons cross in the opposite nucleus; such lesions

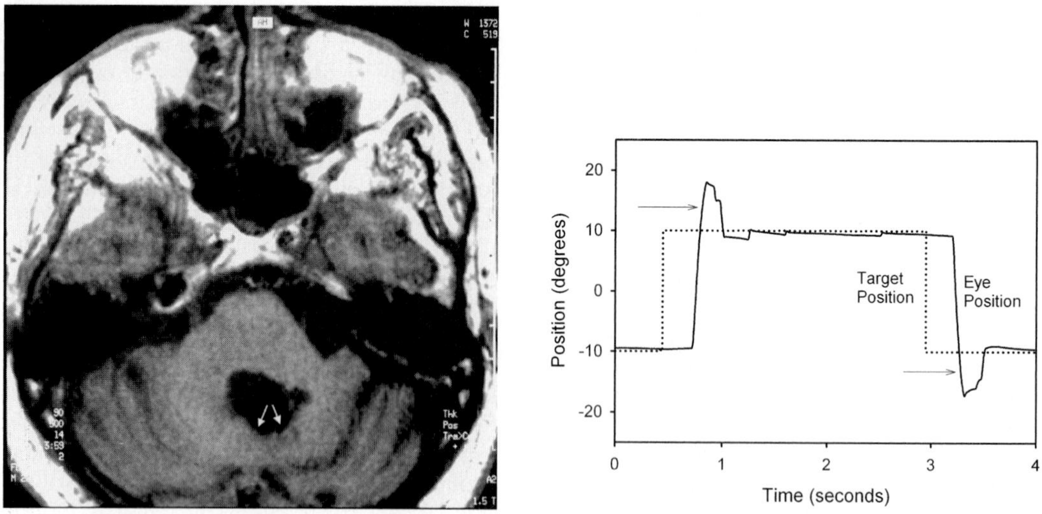

A B

Figure 12–4. Cerebellar disease causing saccadic dysmetria. (A) MRI of a 50-year-old man who had undergone resection of a cystic astrocytoma, with a surgical lesion involving the fastigial nuclei (arrow). (B) The patient's main ocular motor deficit was saccadic hypermetria, indicated by arrows. Rightward eye rotations correspond to upward deflections (see Video Display: Disorders of Saccades).

are reported to cause marked saccadic hypermetria but to have little effect on sustained pursuit,[156] since the main deficit is probably one of eye acceleration at pursuit onset.

Other Disorders of Eye Movements Attributed to Cerebellar Disease

Disorders of *ocular alignment* encountered in association with cerebellar disease include esotropia, especially for distance viewing (divergence paralysis); loss of comitancy (ocular alignment varying with orbital position); defects in prism adaptation; alternating skew deviations;[1137,1182a,1205] disconjugate (poorly yoked) saccades; and disconjugate gaze-evoked nystagmus.[1063,1137]

Fixation is commonly disrupted in patients with cerebellar disease, either by nystagmus or saccadic intrusions. In addition to the forms of nystagmus that are part of the three principal cerebellar syndromes, nystagmus with a divergent component (Fig. 10–3B),[1192] centripetal nystagmus (Box 10–7),[616] central position upbeating nystagmus (see Video Display: Positional Nystagmus),[243] seesaw nystagmus (see Fig. 10–6 and Video Display: Nystagmus and Visual Disorders),[1223] and acquired pendular nystagmus (see Fig. 10–9 and Video Display: Acquired Pendular Nystagmus),[47] have all been reported in patients with cerebellar disease. Hyperventilation-induced downbeat nystagmus may occur in some patients with cerebellar disease, perhaps reflecting abnormalities of calcium channels that are known to occur in some forms of cerebellar degeneration.[1155] A variety of saccadic intrusions occur with cerebellar disease, but may not be specific for it. One example is square-wave jerks (see Fig. 10–15A and Video Display: Saccadic Oscillations and Intrusions), which are a common finding in patients with Friedreich's ataxia,[867,1026] but occur in many of other neurological disorders, and in some normal subjects.[1] However, in cerebellar disorders that affect the deep nuclei,[979] and in certain spinocerebellar ataxias,[1055] macrosaccadic oscillations prominently disrupt steady fixation (see Fig. 10–15B and Video Display: Saccadic Oscillations and Intrusions).

A singular disturbance of *smooth pursuit* is the presence of torsional nystagmus during vertical tracking.[334] This has been described in patients with cavernous angiomas in the middle cerebellar peduncle. The direction of such torsional nystagmus changes with the direction of the pursuit, with the eye velocity of the slow phase of the torsional nystagmus being directly proportional to the eye velocity of the slow phase of pursuit (see Video Display: Disorder of Smooth Pursuit). This sign may occur because smooth pursuit is programmed in, or superimposed upon, a phylogenetically old, vertical "labyrinthine-optokinetic" coordinate system, so that for a pure vertical pursuit movement to occur, opposite torsional components must cancel (as is the case for a pure vertical vestibular nystagmus). The middle cerebellar peduncle carries information to the cerebellum from the pontine nuclei, including the nucleus reticularis tegmenti pontis (NRTP), which may contain vertical pursuit signals encoded with a torsional component.

Other *vestibular* abnormalities are reported in patients with cerebellar disease, including vestibular hyper-responsiveness (increased VOR gain),[1088] and increased responsiveness of the cervico-ocular reflex.[137] In addition, abnormalities of the response to off-vertical axis rotation (OVAR), such as barbecue-spit rotation, occur with an increase in the component that modulates according to head position with respect to gravity, and a decrease in the steady-state bias component of nystagmus.[22] There are also impaired responses to linear translation (L-VOR)[58,1176] and static and dynamic counter-roll.[1182a]

The cerebellum is also important in long-term *adaptive functions* that keep eye movements appropriate to the visual stimulus. For example, adaptive properties of the VOR,[1189] and of smooth pursuit,[1064] are impaired in patients with cerebellar lesions. This adaptive or "repair shop" function of the cerebellum probably accounts for both the enduring nature of the ocular motor deficits that accompany diffuse cerebellar lesions and, perhaps, the somewhat variable effects of cerebellar lesions. Thus, inherent, idiosyncratic abnormalities in brainstem or peripheral ocular motor mechanisms that are normally "repaired" by the cerebellum may reappear after cerebellar lesions. For example, some patients with cerebellar disease may not be able to adapt to a phoria induced by wearing prisms.[419,592a,715]

Some children with congenital cerebellar disorders, such as the Dandy-Walker syndrome, are less affected than adults with lesions at similar locations.[623,1158] If cerebellar ablation is performed in neonatal monkeys, almost complete recovery occurs, provided that the deep cerebellar nuclei are left intact; if they are not, gaze holding and smooth pursuit never fully recover.[300]

Developmental Anomalies of the Hindbrain and Cerebellum

The Arnold–Chiari malformation is an anomaly of the hindbrain involving the caudal cerebellum, including the vestibulocerebellar flocculus, paraflocculus (tonsils), uvula, and nodulus, and the caudal medulla. In the Chiari type I malformation, the cerebellar tonsils are displaced caudally into the foramen magnum, the medulla is elongated, and a meningomyelocele is only rarely present. Such patients often present with symptoms in adult life, occasionally as late as the ninth decade. In the Chiari type II malformation, both the fourth ventricle and inferior vermis extend below the foramen magnum, the brainstem and spinal cord are thin, and a lumbar meningomyelocele is usually present. Patients with type II malformation usually present in childhood, but, in milder cases, onset of symptoms is delayed until adulthood.

Presenting symptoms include oscillopsia (brought on or exacerbated by head movements), postural disequilibrium, and Valsalva-induced dizziness, vertigo, cervical pain, and headaches.[1177] A variety of ocular motor abnormalities, especially downbeat nystagmus (both spontaneous and positional), have been reported in patients with the Arnold-Chiari malformation (Table 12–1). Many of these signs are reproduced by vestibulocerebellar lesions in monkeys.[1215] The positional nystagmus of posterior fossa lesions usually differs from the transient mixed upbeat-torsional nystagmus typical of posterior-canal, benign paroxysmal positional nystagmus.[88,413,545,1163] Diagnosis is by MRI, with sagittal views of the cranio-cervical junction (Fig. 12–5).[119,861] Patients often improve after suboccipital decompression, although it may take months for the eye movement abnormalities to diminish.[286,826,1027]

The Dandy-Walker syndrome consists of malformation of the cerebellar vermis, a membranous cyst of the fourth ventricle, and malformations of the cerebellar cortex and deep cerebellar nuclei. Despite the large cerebellar defect, patients may show only mild saccadic dysmetria, and eye movements may be normal.[623] The preservation of eye movements

Table 12–1. **Disturbances in Eye Movements in the Arnold–Chiari Malformation**

Downbeat nystagmus (occasionally with a torsional component), worse on lateral gaze and with convergence[196,424,545,1027,1192,1209]
Divergence nystagmus[1192]
Convergence nystagmus[747]
Horizontal nystagmus (unidirectional, present with eyes in central position—see Fig. 10–7)
Periodic alternating nystagmus[360]
Gaze-evoked nystagmus[16]
Rebound nystagmus including torsional rebound[1045]
Seesaw nystagmus[1223]
Impaired pursuit (and VOR cancellation)[1209]
Impaired OKN with slow build-up of eye velocity in response to a constant velocity stimulus[1191]
Strabismus, esotropia[11,649]
Divergence paralysis[649]
Skew deviation accentuated or alternating on lateral gaze,[1205] with dissociated vertical nystagmus[832]
Saccadic may be dysmetria[34] or accurate[951]
Internuclear ophthalmoplegia[34]
Increased VOR gain[1209]
Shortened VOR time constant and impaired tilt-suppression[420]
Positional nystagmus[55]

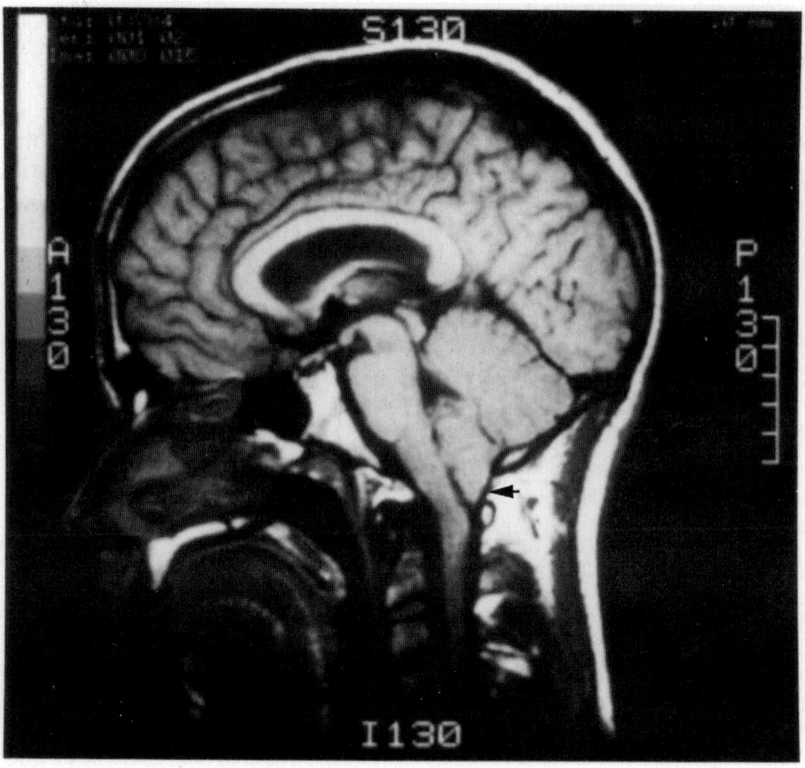

Figure 12–5. MRI scan showing caudal displacement of the cerebellar tonsils below the foramen magnum (arrow), with flattening of the brainstem, typical of the Arnold–Chiari malformation.

in Dandy-Walker syndrome may reflect the preservation of the pontomesencephalic junction in these patients;[689] experimental evidence suggests some compensation is possible for some cerebellar defects that are present since birth.[300] However, ocular motor abnormalities, including nystagmus and strabismus, have also been reported in patients with agenesis of the vermis[166] or hypoplasia of the entire cerebellum.[957]

Other rare syndromes associated with anomalous cerebellar development include Coffin–Siris syndrome (developmental delay, hypotonia, cutaneous changes, and abnormalities of the roof of the fourth ventricle),[259] and Joubert's syndrome, which manifests with a variable combination of episodic tachypnea, psychomotor retardation, retinal dystrophy, torsional nystagmus, skew deviation, ocular motor apraxia, agenesis of the cerebellar vermis, and fibrosis of the extraocular muscles (see Video Display: Congenital Ocular Motor Apraxia).[380,601,690,956]

Ocular Motor Findings in the Hereditary Ataxias

Substantial advances have been made in defining and understanding the molecular biology of the hereditary ataxias.[687,1070] On the one hand, the recessive ataxias are often associated with loss of protein function in pathways normally concerned with prevention of damage due to oxidative stress, and DNA repair and maintenance. Consequently, patients with some recessive ataxias have manifestations outside of the nervous system, such as cardiomyopathy, and increased risk of developing cancer. On the other hand, most autosomal dominant ataxias are associated with an expanded CAG-repeat in the coding region of abnormal genes, which translates into an abnormal protein with an excessively long polyglutamine segment. The expanded polyglutamine stretches have a "toxic gain-of-function" effect that interferes with normal protein folding, responses to stress, and regulation of transcription. Longer polyglutamine segments are associated with earlier disease onset and more severe disease in later generations (the phenomenon of anticipation).

With the identification of genes responsible for the hereditary ataxias has come an attempt to link phenotype with genotype. Substantial efforts have been made to achieve this goal by identifying distinctive syndromes of abnormal eye movements.[566a,695a] Some results of these studies are summarized in Table 12–2. While it appears that certain findings are quite distinctive for some gene mutations, there is substantial phenotypic variation in others due to several factors. For example, some patients with genetically confirmed SCA1 have been reported to show clinical and neuropathologic findings indistinguishable from multiple system atrophy.[387] Even monozygotic twins with SCA2 and episodic ataxia type 2 show some differences of their eye movements.[25] Furthermore, the clinical picture may change as the disease develops.[576] Neuropathological studies have shown widespread involvement of nuclei important for eye movement control in three types of spinocerebellar ataxia (SCA 1-3).[386,937,939] Thus, caution is necessary in trying to assign an individual to one group on the basis of eye movement findings alone. Nonetheless, some reported families show very stereotyped findings, and eye movement studies may provide insights into the pathogenesis of certain components of the clinical picture.[1055]

With these caveats, the presence of very slow saccades is suggestive of SCA2, (see Video Display: Disorders of Saccades) formerly called olivopontocerebellar degeneration of Wadia and Swami, in which pontine saccadic burst cells are also involved.[480,673,1009,1144,1195a,1212] The degree of saccadic slowing in SCA2 has been related to the size of the polyglutamine expansion.[1129] However, saccades may also be slow in patients with SCA1,[147] SCA7,[795] and SCA28.[162a]

Impairment of the vestibulo-ocular reflex is a common feature in SCA3 (Machado-Joseph disease),[152,398] consistent with neuropathological findings.[935] The presence of prominent downbeat, gaze-evoked, and rebound nystagmus, with normal saccade speed is typical of SCA6,[394,1216] which may also correspond to the late-onset, Holmes type of cerebellar degeneration and to the autosomal dominant "pure" cerebellar ataxia (autosomal dominant cerebellar ataxia– ADCA—type 3 of Harding) (see Video Display: Disorders of Gaze Holding).[430] There is some overlap between SCA6 and familial episodic vertigo and ataxia type 2 (EA-2), both of which affect the calcium channel (CACNL1A4) gene.[59,127,381,511] A corollary of

Table 12–2. **Ocular Motor Findings in Hereditary Ataxias***

Current Name (Possible Former Name)	Chromosome	Ocular Motor Findings†	Other Distinguishing Features
Dominant Forms			
SCA1/ATXN1[147]	6p23	Saccades mildly slow and hypermetric; GEN; RBN; VOR gain decreased	Pyramidal tract signs; dysphagia; optic nerve pallor
SCA2/ATXN2 (Olivopontocerebellar atrophy)[939,1129,1143]	12q23-q24.1	Very slow saccades, especially horizontally	Cerebellar dysarthria; hypoactive tendon reflexes
SCA3/ATXN3 (Machado-Joseph disease)[398,936,939]	14q21	Saccadic hypometria and hypermetria; GEN; RBN; SWJ; VOR gain decreased	Faciolingual myokymia; dystonia; parkinsonism
SCA6 (Holmes type; ADCA3 of Harding)[394,1066,1216]	19p13	Normal velocity, dysmetric saccades; DBN; GEN; RBN; PAN; SWJ; VOR gain increased or decreased or normal; eye-head tracking superior to ocular pursuit	Late onset; "pure" cerebellar atrophy with loss of Purkinje cells
SCA7/ATXN10 (ADCA2 of Harding)[737,795]	3p21.1-p12	Slow saccades; supranuclear ophthalmoplegia	Pigmentary maculopathy and visual loss; hearing loss; extrapyramidal signs
SCA8[249]	13q21 (CTG repeats)	Gaze-evoked nystagmus; saccadic hypermetria	Athetosis and myoclonus in some; maternal inheritance common
SCA20[577]	11	Saccadic hypermetria; impaired smooth pursuit; square-wave jerks	Present with dysarthria; palatal tremor; dentate nucleus calcification
Dentatorubral-pallidoluysian atrophy (Haw River syndrome)[127,149,776]	12p	Slow saccades	Epilepsy, myoclonus, choreoathetosis, dementia
Episodic ataxia (EA)1[127]	12p13 (potassium channel)	No vertigo	Brief attacks of ataxia; interictal myokymia
Episodic ataxia (EA)2[511,1176]	19p (calcium channel)	Vertigo; interictal GEN, DBN, INO, impaired translational VOR	Prolonged attacks; may show progressive ataxia; possible overlap with SCA6
Recessive Forms			
Friedreich's ataxia (classic and atypical forms)	9q13	SWJ; ocular flutter in some patients; variable saccadic dysmetria; VOR gain decreased	Onset usually before 20 years; sensory loss; areflexia; Babinski responses; cardiomyopathy; diabetes
Hereditary Vitamin E deficiency (alpha-tocopherol transfer protein gene); also abetalipoproteinemia[1193]	8q13	Progressive gaze restriction; slow saccades; dissociated nystagmus, in which adduction is faster than abduction	Friedreich-like picture; retinitis pigmentosa may be associated

Ataxia telangiectasia (Louis-Bar syndrome)[317,651,1038]	11q22	Saccade initiation defects; hypometria, increased latency, substitution of smooth pursuit; head thrusts; GEN; PAN; SWJ; esodeviation	Oculocutaneous telangiectasia; radiosensitivity; immunological disorders; cancer; elevated alpha-fetoprotein
SCASI (Spinocerebellar ataxia with saccadic intrusions)[1055]	1p36	Saccadic hypermetria, macrosaccadic oscillations, frequent saccades intrusions; large saccades faster than normal	Axonal neuropathy, fasciculations, corticospinal tracts
Ataxia with oculomotor apraxia 1 (AOA1)[613]	9p13	Onset 2–10 years; gaze shifts achieved with a series of small saccades	Severe axonal motor neuropathy; chorea early in course; hypoalbuminaemia, hypercholesterolemia
Ataxia with oculomotor apraxia 2 (AOA2)[612]	9q34	Onset 11–20 years	Sensorimotor neuropathy; elevated alpha-fetoprotein

* Includes only those diseases for which eye movements have been clearly delineated. General references.[147,152,249,298,317,436,566a,651,695a]

† Impaired smooth pursuit eye movements are a common finding in most forms of cerebellar degeneration.

ADCA: autosomal dominant cerebellar ataxia (Harding's classification)[431]: ADCA2: ataxia with macular retinopathy; ACDA3: pure cerebellar ataxia); ATXN, ataxin gene symbol (www.gene.ucl.ac.uk); DBN: downbeat nystagmus; GEN: gaze-evoked nystagmus; INO: internuclear ophthalmoplegia; PAN: periodic alternating nystagmus; RBN: rebound nystagmus; SCA: spinocerebellar ataxia; SWJ: square-wave jerks; VOR: vestibulo-ocular reflex.

this overlap is that not only EA-2, but also some patients with SCA6 who have episodic worsening show improvement of symptoms with acetazolamide (see Treatments for Nystagmus and Saccadic Intrusions, in Chapter 10).[511] The syndrome of cerebellar ataxia with bilateral vestibulopathy is usually sporadic; affected patients show corrective saccades during head rotation while they view a stationary target since both smooth pursuit and the vestibulo-ocular reflex are impaired.[714]

Friedreich's ataxia, the commonest recessive ataxia, usually presents before age 20 years with ataxia, hyporeflexia, extensor plantar responses, neuropathy, cardiomyopathy and diabetes. Affected patients show disruption of steady fixation by saccadic intrusions, which are usually square-wave jerks but occasionally ocular flutter.[1026] There is variable saccadic dysmetria, but vestibular responses tend to be reduced. Some patients with gluten sensitivity develop an illness with features similar to Friedreich's ataxia, but more striking eye movement abnormalities. They show gaze-evoked nystagmus, slow saccades and upward gaze difficulties may be present.[148] Such patients often also have the human leukocyte antigen (HLA) DQB1*0201 haplotype, an axonal peripheral neuropathy, and may have memory difficulties. Since patients with this cerebellar syndrome may not have evidence of gluten enteropathy on mucosal biopsy, the pathophysiology of this syndrome remains unclear, although patients are advised to maintain a gluten-free diet.[148] A later-onset recessive disorder is spinocerebellar ataxia with saccadic intrusions (SCASI); there is an associated axonal neuropathy and saccadic hypermetria with macrosaccadic oscillations.[1055] Other recessive ataxias, including ataxia telangiectasia, and ataxia with oculomotor apraxia types 1 and 2 are discussed in a later section of this chapter that deals with ocular motor apraxia.

In this rapidly growing field, clinicians must keep in mind the broadening spectrum of differential diagnoses when confronted by a patient with progressive ataxia and abnormal eye movements. Progress in understanding the underlying molecular genetics of these disorders may clarify why certain populations of neurons that contribute to specific eye movements, such as saccades, are predominantly affected.

Paraneoplastic Cerebellar Degeneration

This rare "remote effect" of cancer usually occurs in post-menopausal women with ovarian or breast cancer, but also in both men and women with small-cell lung cancer and Hodgkin's lymphoma.[71,87,697,829,856] Patients usually present with subacute vertigo, diplopia, or oscillopsia (due to downbeat nystagmus), and subsequently develop midline and appendicular ataxia, and dysarthria, all of which may become severe. Downbeat nystagmus is a common finding, sometimes with increasing velocity waveforms, which imply an unstable neural integrator for eye movements.[1211] Other reported findings are horizontal gaze-evoked nystagmus, impaired smooth pursuit, and saccadic intrusions and dysmetria. Paraneoplastic cerebellar degeneration should be differentiated from a cerebellar syndrome that may complicate treatment of cancer or leukemia with cytosine arabinoside.[104]

About half of all patients with paraneoplastic cerebellar degeneration have antineuronal antibodies, more commonly in their cerebrospinal fluid than serum, usually anti-Yo or anti-Tr.[71] Rarely, autoantibodies against zinc-finger proteins may also cause a cerebellar syndrome.[70] There is evidence that the findings in paraneoplastic cerebellar degeneration, which may coexist with Lambert-Eaton myasthenic syndrome, are caused by antibodies against P/Q voltage-gated calcium channels,[410] which are common in the cerebellum.[1028] In addition, antibodies to metabotropic glutamate receptors have been demonstrated,[190] which are present on Purkinje cells. Thus, although current treatment is unsatisfactory,[697,856] the identification of possible mechanisms for this syndromes suggest new therapeutic approaches. When this disorder is suspected, body proton emission tomography (PET) is the best means to detect an undiagnosed primary cancer.

Cerebellar Stroke

Three arteries of the posterior circulation supply the cerebellum: the posterior-inferior cerebellar artery, the anterior-inferior cerebellar artery, and the superior cerebellar artery.[1071] Occlusion in these vessels often produces concurrent brainstem infarction, making precise clinicopathological correlation difficult.

The *posterior-inferior cerebellar artery* (PICA) arises from the vertebral artery and supplies the lateral medulla, the inferior cerebellar peduncle, and the nodulus and uvula. Thus, occlusion of the PICA may cause Wallenberg's syndrome.[567] Infarction in the distribution of the distal PICA may cause acute vertigo and nystagmus that often simulates an acute peripheral vestibular lesion.[297,680,941] These symptoms and signs are probably due to a central vestibular imbalance created by asymmetric infarction in the vestibulocerebellum, which normally has a tonic inhibitory effect upon the vestibular nuclei. Such patients may have prominent gaze-evoked nystagmus, which helps differentiate this cerebellar lesion from an acute peripheral vestibulopathy.

The *anterior-inferior cerebellar artery* (AICA) is usually the most caudal large vessel arising from the basilar artery. It supplies portions of the vestibular nuclei, adjacent dorsolateral brainstem, and inferior lateral cerebellum. In addition, the AICA is the origin of the labyrinthine artery in most individuals and also sends small branches to the cerebellar flocculus and facial nerve in the cerebellopontine angle. Consequently, ischemia in the AICA distribution (Fig. 12–3) may cause vertigo, vomiting, hearing loss,[614] facial palsy, and ipsilateral limb ataxia. Unilateral loss of vestibular function may cause asymmetric responses with rapid head turns (see Video Display: Cerebellar Syndromes). In addition, there may be gaze-evoked nystagmus, impaired smooth pursuit, and vestibular nystagmus.[19,405,787]

The *superior cerebellar artery* (SCA) arises from the rostral basilar artery and supplies the superior surface of the cerebellar hemisphere and vermis, and the superior cerebellar peduncle. Infarction in the territory of the superior cerebellar artery causes ataxia of gait and limbs, and vertigo.[81,880,1122] A characteristic abnormality is saccadic contrapulsion. This consists of an overshooting of contralateral saccades and an undershooting of ipsilateral saccades; attempted vertical saccades are oblique, with a horizontal component away from the side of the lesion. Thus, the disorder is the opposite of the saccadic ipsipulsion seen in Wallenberg's syndrome (see Video Display: Medullary Syndromes), and probably reflects interruption of outputs from the fastigial nucleus running in the uncinate fasciculus next to the superior cerebellar peduncle (Fig. 3–16, Chapter 3).[1041,1147] Infarction restricted to the posterior-inferior vermis has been reported to selectively impair pursuit and optokinetic eye movements.[834]

Cerebellar Mass Lesions

Cerebellar hemorrhage, tumors, infarction, abscesses, cysts, and extra-axial hematomas may all cause cerebellar eye signs by direct involvement of cerebellar parenchyma. However, acutely expanding or large cerebellar mass lesions, such as hemorrhage, often also compress the brainstem and produce additional signs. Either horizontal or vertical gaze disorders can occur depending upon whether the direction of compression is forward or rostral, respectively. Acute cerebellar hemorrhage frequently causes nystagmus, horizontal gaze palsy (usually toward the side of the lesion), and skew deviation; it can even cause ocular bobbing (see Video Display: Eye Movements in Coma). The third, fourth, and sixth cranial nerves may also be affected. Ocular motor dysfunction may also be caused by secondary obstructive hydrocephalus and increased intracranial pressure.

Medulloblastoma arising in the posterior medullary velum frequently causes positional nystagmus, presumably due to involvement of the nodulus and uvula.[407] Such involvement may also account for the inability to suppress post-rotational nystagmus by tilting the head.[420] Tumors within the fourth ventricle may affect the cerebellar nuclei, vestibulocerebellum, and dorsal medulla, sometimes producing upbeat or downbeat nystagmus, the pathogenesis of which is discussed in Chapter 10.

Schwannoma of the eighth cranial nerve may compress the cerebellar flocculus and paraflocculus, which lie in the cerebellopontine angle, and so produce this vestibulocerebellar syndrome (Box 12–2). In addition, patients may show Bruns' nystagmus, in which there is a "coarse" gaze-evoked nystagmus beating towards the side of the lesion and a "fine" vestibular nystagmus beating away from the side of the lesion.[53,143,768] Hyperventilation-induced nystagmus may be an early sign of a vestibular schwannoma (see Video Display: Disorders of the Vestibular System).[721] Asymmetry of the caloric responses and of rotational testing may be observed,[84] but the most sensitive and specific method used to detect small tumors of the eighth cranial nerve is MRI with gadolinium.[858]

OCULAR MOTOR SYNDROMES CAUSED BY DISEASE OF THE PONS

Disease affecting the pons causes classic disorders of gaze. Examples of the effects of pontine lesions on eye movements are shown in the Video Display: Pontine Syndromes.

Lesions of the Abducens Nucleus

Lesions of the abducens nucleus (see Box 6–1) cause an ipsilateral palsy of horizontal conjugate gaze (see Box 12–5 and Video Display: Pontine Syndromes). Movements of both eyes are affected because the abducens nucleus contains two main groups of neurons: abducens motoneurons, which innervate the ipsilateral lateral rectus muscle, and abducens internuclear neurons, which cross the midline and ascend in the medial longitudinal fasciculus to innervate the contralateral medial rectus motor neurons (see Fig. 6–1, Chapter 6). Vergence movements of the eyes are spared, so that some adduction of the contralateral eye may be possible with a near stimulus. Recall that vergence depends mainly on inputs passing directly to medial rectus motoneurons in the oculomotor nucleus (Fig. 6–1). Vergence may substitute for gaze shifting movements during recovery.[584] Saccadic, pursuit, optokinetic, and vestibular movements are still present in the contralateral hemifield, but are impaired when directed towards the side of the lesion. Thus, in the case of a left abducens nucleus lesion, saccades from center to right gaze are preserved, because they depend on projections to the intact abducens nucleus from the excitatory burst neurons of the right paramedian pontine reticular formation (PPRF). Saccades from right gaze to center are slow, because they are generated solely due to projections to the intact, right abducens nucleus from the inhibitory burst neurons of the left medullary reticular formation; thus eye velocity is a function of antagonist muscle relaxation rather than agonist contraction. Another factor in asymmetry of residual movements may be horizontal gaze-evoked nystagmus on looking contralaterally (to the right, in the above example). Such nystagmus may be due to interruption either of fibers of passage from the medial vestibular nucleus, which provide an eye position signal to the contralateral abducens

Box 12–5. Clinical Findings With Lesions Of The Abducens Nucleus

- Loss of all conjugate movements towards the side of the lesion – "ipsilateral, horizontal gaze palsy"
- Contralateral gaze deviation, in acute phase
- Vergence and vertical movements are spared
- In the intact hemifield of gaze, horizontal movements may be preserved, but ipsilaterally directed saccades are slow
- Horizontal gaze-evoked nystagmus on looking contralaterally
- Ipsilateral facial palsy often associated

For related anatomy, see Box 6-1 and Fig. 6-1 in Chapter 6. (Related Video Display: Pontine Syndromes) nucleus,[21] or of fibers from cell groups of the paramedian tracts (PMT), which lie at the rostral end of the abducens nucleus (see Box 6–4).[754] Clinical lesions restricted to the abducens nucleus are rare.[82,465,708,754,754] More commonly, the abducens nucleus is affected in association with adjacent tegmental structures, especially the medial longitudinal fasciculus and the paramedian reticular formation. An ipsilateral facial palsy usually occurs with abducens nucleus lesions, owing to involvement of the adjacent genu of the seventh cranial nerve, but may be absent.[719] Complete horizontal gaze palsy occurs with bilateral pontine lesions such as infarction and demyelination.[717] Other causes to be considered in patients with horizontal gaze palsy include myasthenia gravis, botulism, Miller Fisher syndrome, Wernicke's encephalopathy, drug intoxications (see Table 12–11) and, rarely, as a remote effect of occult neoplasm.[50,752] Congenital forms of horizontal gaze palsy are discussed in Chapter 9.

Lesions of the Paramedian Pontine Reticular Formation (PPRF)

Although the predominant effect of destructive lesions of the paramedian pontine reticular formation (PPRF) falls on ipsilateral horizontal saccades (Box 12–6), other horizontal and vertical eye movements may be affected because the PPRF contains several different populations of neurons that are important for generating saccades (see Box 6-3), as well as fibers of passage. Excitatory burst neurons, which are important in the generation of horizontal saccades, lie in the dorsomedial portions of the nucleus pontis centralis caudalis (see Fig. 6–2, Chapter 6 and Fig. 3–10, Chapter 3), rostral to the abducens nucleus.[480] Excitatory burst neurons project to the ipsilateral abducens nucleus. At the level of the abducens nucleus lies the nucleus raphe interpositus, which contains omnipause neurons that inhibit all burst neurons (horizontal and vertical) except during saccades. Caudal to the abducens nucleus, in the dorsomedial tegmentum of the rostral medulla, lie the inhibitory burst neurons, which receive inputs from the ipsilateral excitatory burst neurons, but project to the contralateral abducens nucleus (Fig. 3–10). Another group of neurons involved in the control of eye movements that lies close to the PPRF is the cell groups of the paramedian tracts (PMT) (see Box 6–4), which project to the cerebellar flocculus.[161] Finally, the PPRF and adjacent pons contain axons of passage that carry vestibular, pursuit, and gaze-holding signals to the abducens nucleus.

Unilateral lesions of the PPRF, such as infarction, cause an ipsilateral, conjugate, horizontal gaze palsy that may involve all classes of

Box 12–6. Clinical Findings With Lesions Of The Paramedian Pontine Reticular Formation (PPRF)

- Loss of horizontal saccades directed towards the side of the lesion, in all fields of gaze
- Contralateral gaze deviation, in acute phase
- Gaze-evoked nystagmus on looking contralateral to the lesion
- Ipsilateral smooth pursuit and vestibular eye movements may be preserved or impaired
- Bilateral lesions cause total horizontal gaze palsy and slowing of vertical saccades

For related anatomy, see Box 6-3 and Fig. 6-2 in Chapter 6. (Related Video Display: Pontine Syndromes) eye movements, but vestibular and even pursuit eye movements are sometimes spared.[518,588,838] Acutely, the eyes may be deviated contralaterally. Nystagmus occurs when gaze is directed into the intact contralateral field of movement, with quick phases directed away from the lesioned side; this is usually accentuated in darkness. Ipsilaterally directed saccades and quick phases are small and slow and do not carry the eye past the midline.

The degree of slowing of saccades directed toward the lesioned side, when made in the intact field of gaze, may depend upon whether or not inhibitory burst neurons, which project to the *contralateral* abducens nucleus, are involved. Recall that excitatory saccadic inputs reach the abducens nucleus from the ipsilateral population of excitatory burst cells in the PPRF, whereas inhibitory saccadic inputs originate from contralateral inhibitory burst cells in the medulla (Fig. 6–1, Chapter 6 and Fig. 3–10). Thus, if the lesion is restricted to the ipsilateral abducens nucleus, then saccades from the opposite field of gaze to the midline may be present but slow, since inhibition of the antagonists (i.e., the ipsilateral medial rectus and contralateral lateral rectus) are intact. However, if the PPRF is extensively involved, particularly in its more caudal part, inhibition is also affected, so that saccades directed towards the lesioned side are absent.[754] Rapid eye movements directed to the side opposite the lesion appear normal. Vertical saccades may be slightly slow and misdirected obliquely away from the side of the lesion, owing to an inappropriate horizontal component.[521]

Smooth pursuit movements and slow phases of optokinetic nystagmus may be preserved, in both directions, within the intact field of movement, but usually they cannot bring the eyes across the midline. Sometimes, horizontal pursuit or optokinetic responses are asymmetrically impaired. It has been suggested that more rostral brainstem lesions tend to cause ipsilateral smooth pursuit deficits, whereas caudal brainstem lesions lead to contralateral deficits.[519] On the other hand, more basal lesions in the pons tend to impair ipsilateral or bilateral pursuit.[373,1084,1145] Because of the confluence of pursuit pathways in the brainstem and its cerebellar connections, the direction of a pursuit deficit with a brainstem lesion is not reliable for determining the side of the lesion.[359]

In some patients, vestibular stimuli drive the eyes past the midline.[241] Presumably, either the PPRF lesion is more rostral in such individuals, or the ipsilateral abducens nucleus and its direct vestibular input are intact.[266,518] In an occasional patient, vestibular stimuli can only drive the contralateral adducting eye into the ipsilateral field. This finding implies a lesion of one PPRF and the ipsilateral abducens nerve but sparing the abducens nucleus. The following case illustrates the range of abnormalities that can occur with pontine lesions.

CASE HISTORY: Horizontal Gaze Palsy due to Pontine Metastasis (see Video Display: Pontine Syndromes)

A 52-year-old woman presented with a history of left-sided paresthesia and unsteadiness for 6 weeks and the recent onset of horizontal diplopia. She was alert and her cranial nerves were intact apart from a right Horner's syndrome and her abnormal eye movements. She had a mild left hemiparesis with a left extensor plantar response. Joint position and vibration senses were impaired on the left side of the body. Her gait was markedly ataxic. CT (Fig. 12–6A) and vertebral arteriography demonstrated a right brainstem mass, suggestive of tumor.

She was unable to move her eyes to the right past the midline, using either saccadic or pursuit eye movements. Head rotation to the left, however, drove the eyes past the midline, but the right eye abducted incompletely. Vergence movements also induced the left eye to cross the midline. Vertical eye movements appeared normal. Figure 12–6B shows that her saccades to the right were slow, whereas saccades to the left were of normal velocity. Gaze-evoked nystagmus was present on looking to the left, with slow phases toward the midline. When she was rotated to the right in darkness (Fig.12–6C), there was a good vestibular response with the eyes moving to the left. However, quick phases directed to the right were small, slow, and infrequent. When she was rotated to the left (Fig.12–6D), slow phases to the right occurred, with good quick phases directed to the left.

The patient was treated with radiation and steroids but her disease progressed. She subsequently lost all abduction of the right eye (sixth nerve palsy) but she could still adduct the left eye during head rotation. The patient died a few months later; no autopsy was performed.

Comment. A figure presenting a hypothetical explanation for her gaze disorder is provided in the Video Display: Pontine Syndromes. This patient initially showed a right horizontal gaze palsy that selectively impaired saccades and smooth pursuit. In addition, she had partial involvement of the fascicles of the right abducens nerve. Thus, preservation of rightward movements of her left eye for the vestibulo-ocular reflex indicated that her right abducens nucleus was intact, but its saccadic and smooth pursuit inputs were selectively interrupted. (She also lacked a facial palsy, which is often associated with abducens nucleus lesions.) In the intact hemifield of gaze, saccades and quick phases to the right were very slow. This finding probably reflects loss of not only the excitatory connections from the right PPRF to the right abducens nucleus, but also the projections from the right PPRF, via the inhibitory burst neurons, to the contralateral abducens nucleus. Impaired gaze-holding function to the left may have reflected involvement of fibers of passage providing an eye position signal to the contralateral abducens nucleus,[21] or interruption of projections from cell groups of the paramedian tracts to the flocculus.[161,754] As the disease progressed, she lost all abduction of her right eye, consistent with

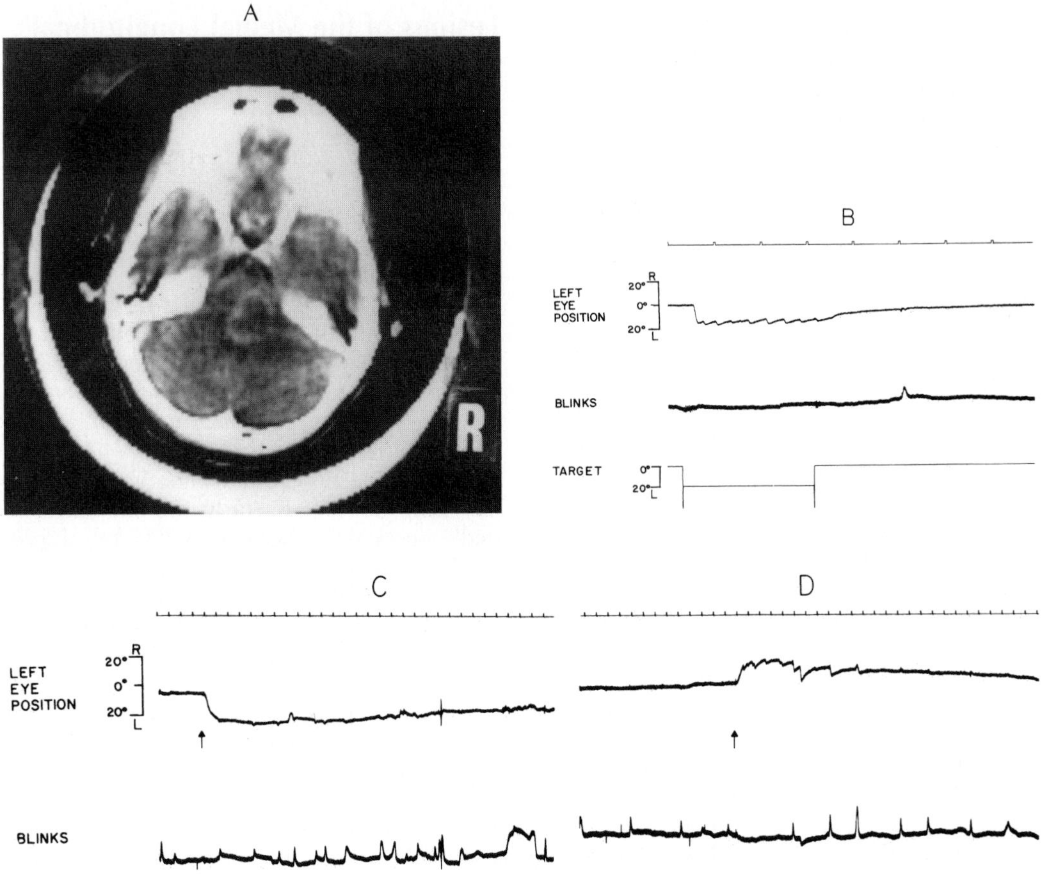

Figure 12–6. Horizontal gaze palsy (see Case History: Horizontal gaze palsy due to pontine metastasis for clinical details) (see Video Display: Pontine Syndromes). (A) CT demonstrates a right-sided brainstem mass with a ring of contrast enhancement. (B, C, and D) Movements of the left eye, recorded by electro-oculography. The time scale, at top, is in seconds. (B) The patient is able to make normal saccades to the left but saccades to the right are slow. Gaze-evoked nystagmus is present on gaze to the left. The patient is unable to make saccades into the right field of gaze. (C) The patient is rotated clockwise in a vestibular chair, in darkness, at 60 degrees per second, starting at the arrow time mark. The vestibulo-ocular reflex drives her eyes to the left, but quick phases of nystagmus are small, infrequent, and slow. (D) She is rotated counterclockwise, in darkness, at 60 degrees per second, starting at the arrow time mark. The vestibulo-ocular reflex drives her eyes over into the right field of gaze, which saccades and pursuit could not do. Normal slow and quick phases of nystagmus occur.

the right fascicular sixth nerve palsy. She could still adduct the left eye with a vestibular stimulus, however, suggesting that the right abducens nucleus and its internuclear pathway to the left oculomotor nucleus (via the medial longitudinal fasciculus) were intact. Alternatively, preserved adduction could be attributed to the ascending tract of Dieters (Fig. 6–1, Chapter 6). Convergence was preserved because these inputs mainly reach the medial rectus motoneurons directly in the midbrain.

Bilateral lesions restricted to the PPRF are uncommon. Discrete infarction,[429] or tumor,[779] can cause a selective loss of saccades, leaving smooth pursuit and the vestibulo-ocular reflex relatively preserved. Such a selective deficit implies loss or dysfunction of saccadic burst neurons but sparing of fibers of passage conveying smooth pursuit and the vestibulo-ocular reflex.

Inactivation of the PPRF with lidocaine in monkeys causes slow saccades that generally get on target.[66] Experimental lesions of the PPRF in monkeys, using neurotoxins that spare fibers of passage, may cause a similar deficit.[451] During the recovery phase from horizontal gaze palsies, patients may substitute convergence for impaired conjugate adduction and then cross-fixate to extend their range of view.[74] Furthermore, during recovery from bilateral gaze palsies due to vascular lesions, involuntary synkinetic divergence and convergence movements may appear with horizontal or vertical gaze.[108,145] Although bilateral pontine lesions can abolish all horizontal eye movements, with chronic lesions such as tumors, vestibular eye movements may be spared.[52,838]

Bilateral pontine lesions may also impair vertical eye movements, especially saccades.[285,429,1106] Thus, slow vertical saccades are reported in patients with discrete, bilateral pontine lesions,[429,452,1010] and in monkeys following bilateral lesions of the PPRF using neurotoxins.[451,532] Since omnipause cells project to both horizontal burst neurons in the pons and to vertical burst neurons located in the midbrain, pontine lesions could lead to desynchronization of the discharge of both sets of burst neurons and, consequently, to slow vertical as well as horizontal saccades. It is postulated that the large acceleration that characterizes saccadic eye movements is partly due to normal function of omnipause neurons;[724] this issue is discussed in Chapter 3. When vertical vestibular and smooth pursuit eye movements are also affected, involvement of the medial longitudinal fasciculus (MLF) and other pathways ascending through the pons may be the explanation.

Pontine lesions that affect the dorsolateral pontine nuclei may disrupt ipsilateral pursuit.[1084] Lesions affecting the nucleus reticularis tegmenti pontis (NRTP) may cause disturbances of vergence eye movements,[876,877] and these are discussed in Chapter 8.

Lesions of the Medial Longitudinal Fasciculus: Internuclear Ophthalmoplegia (INO)

Lesions affecting the medial longitudinal fasciculus (MLF) (see Box 6–2) cause internuclear ophthalmoplegia (INO); examples are provided on the Video Display: Pontine Syndromes. Both horizontal and vertical eye movements are affected (Box 12–7). This is because some of the axons in the MLF carry a command for conjugate horizontal movements from abducens internuclear neurons to the medial rectus subdivision of the contralateral oculomotor nucleus (Fig. 6–1, in Chapter 6), while other axons carry vestibular and smooth pursuit signals from neurons in the vestibular nuclei to midbrain nuclei concerned with vertical gaze (Fig. 6–5, in Chapter 6). We first summarize the clinical findings of INO, then review the etiologies, and finally discuss the pathophysiology of each component of the syndrome.

CLINICAL MANIFESTATIONS OF INTERNUCLEAR OPHTHALMOPLEGIA

The cardinal sign of INO is paresis of adduction by the eye on the side of the MLF lesion during conjugate movements (see Video Display: Pontine Syndromes). The same eye may be able to adduct during convergence movements. In INO, impaired adduction can range from total paralysis to a paresis that is only apparent as slowing of adducting saccades. Thus, making the clinical diagnosis of INO often rests on judging the conjugacy of large horizontal saccades, looking for relative slowing

Box 12–7. Clinical Features Of Internuclear Ophthalmoplegia (INO)

- Weakness of the ipsilateral medial rectus muscle for conjugate eye movements—especially saccades, leading to "adduction lag"
- Adduction may be preserved during convergence
- Nystagmus or postsaccadic drift on abduction of the eye contralateral to the lesion—"dissociated nystagmus"
- Skew deviation—hypertropia on the side of the lesion
- Dissociated vertical nystagmus—downbeat with greater torsional component in the contralateral eye
- Bilateral INO also causes gaze-evoked vertical nystagmus, impaired vertical pursuit, and decreased vertical vestibular responses
- Small-amplitude saccadic intrusions may interrupt fixation

For related anatomy, see Box 6-2, Fig. 6-1 and Fig. 6-5 in Chapter 6. For records of eye movements, see: Fig. 12-8 and Fig. 12-9 of Chapter 12. For related etiologies, see Table 12-3. (Related Video Display: Pontine Syndromes)

of the adducting movement, called adduction lag. A commonly associated feature is nystagmus on abduction of the eye contralateral to the lesion. Disconjugacy of the quick phases of this nystagmus, with slowing of the adducting eye (a form of dissociated nystagmus) is suggestive of INO. Convergence eye movements may be preserved or impaired; acutely, an esophoria may be present, suggesting increased vergence tone.[44] INO is also often accompanied by skew deviation, with hypertropia on the side of the lesion (see Video Display: Disorders of the Vestibular System). Dissociated vertical nystagmus—downbeat, with a greater torsional component in the contralateral eye—may be present. Asymmetry of vertical vestibulo-ocular responses may be evident with rapid head rotations; thus, in a patient with right INO, the vertical vestibulo-ocular reflex (VOR) induced by stimulating the left posterior semicircular canal was deficient, whereas stimulation of the left anterior semicircular canal was preserved.[227] Bilateral INO often causes additional findings: gaze-evoked vertical nystagmus, impaired vertical pursuit, and decreased vertical vestibular responses. Small-amplitude saccadic intrusions may interrupt fixation. INO may cause diplopia or oscillopsia.

ETIOLOGY OF INTERNUCLEAR OPHTHALMOPLEGIA

Many disorders have been reported to cause INO (Table 12–3).[561] As a generalization, unilateral INO is most commonly related to ischemia, although even in these cases the other side is often subtly involved. Disease throughout the posterior circulation, including both small and large vessel occlusion, may cause INO, often accompanied by other brainstem signs.[568] In some patients, one, rather than two, paramedian perforating pontine arteries supplies both MLF, accounting for the rarer cases of bilateral INO due to stroke.[329] Bilateral INO is most commonly due to demyelination associated with multiple sclerosis, but even in multiple sclerosis the INO may be asymmetric.[354] In some patients, it may be possible to demonstrate a lesion in the MLF

Table 12–3. **Etiology of Internuclear Ophthalmoplegia**[561]

Multiple sclerosis (commonly bilateral);[755,1048] post-irradiation demyelination.[112,638]
Brainstem infarction (commonly unilateral),[112,117,587,726,1110] including vasculitis,[5,8,12] complication of arteriography[306,596,894] and hemorrhage[171]
Brainstem and fourth ventricular tumors[33,203,970,1115] and mesencephalic clefts[598]
Arnold–Chiari malformation and associated hydrocephalus and syringobulbia[34,197,253,781,952,1183]
Infection: bacterial, viral, and other forms of meningoencephalitis;[139,234,695] in association with AIDS[425,831,1048]
Hydrocephalus,[781] subdural hematoma,[277] supratentorial arteriovenous malformation[216]
Nutritional disorders: Wernicke's encephalopathy,[201] pernicious anemia[531]
Metabolic disorders: hepatic encephalopathy,[172] maple syrup urine disease,[1208] abetalipoproteinemia,[1193] Fabry's disease[467]
Drug intoxications: phenothiazines,[215] tricyclic antidepressants,[287,485] narcotics,[307,910] propranolol,[233] lithium,[265] barbiturates[64]
Cancer: carcinomatous infiltration[343] or remote effect[849]
Head trauma,[116,180,214,411,557,748,756,1047] and cervical hyperextension,[507] or manipulation[1203]
Degenerative conditions: progressive supranuclear palsy[698]
Syphilis[197]
Episodic ataxia type 2 (channelopathy)[942]
Pseudo-internuclear ophthalmoplegia of myasthenia gravis,[389] and Miller Fisher syndrome[1061]

with MRI (Fig. 12–7);[757] thin cuts, sagittal and axial views, and proton density images may be required.[355] A large number of unusual causes of INO have been reported.[561,942]

Overall, INO persists in about half of all patients who develop this disorder, chances for recovery being better for demyelinative than vascular etiologies,[112,305] and recovery being

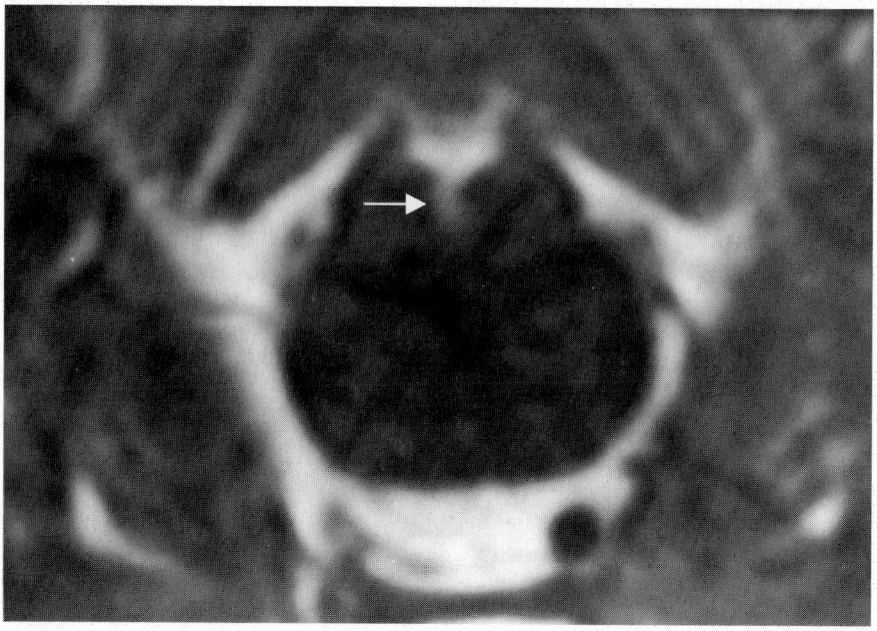

Figure 12–7. T2-weighted MRI scan showing an infarct involving the left medial longitudinal fasciculus (hyperintense signal indicated by arrow), in a patient with internuclear ophthalmoplegia, skew deviation (left hyperdeviation), and ocular tilt reaction (see Video Display: Disorders of the Vestibular System).

slower if there is other clinical evidence of brainstem infarction.[568]

PATHOGENESIS OF FINDINGS IN INTERNUCLEAR OPHTHALMOPLEGIA

Paresis of Adduction in Internuclear Ophthalmoplegia

Adduction weakness for conjugate movements is due to involvement of axons of abducens internuclear neurons, so that conjugate commands coming into the abducens nucleus are not properly relayed to the medial rectus motoneurons in the contralateral oculomotor nucleus (Fig. 6–1, Chapter 6). Although the weakness of the medial rectus affects all types of conjugate eye movements, it is most evident during saccades, the speed of which depends on a strong agonist contraction. When INO is due to demyelinating diseases, there may be a discrepancy between the involvement of saccades and other movements because demyelinated fibers cannot carry the high-frequency discharges required during the saccadic pulse, but can sustain lower-frequency discharges that occur with other movements. This dissociation is reflected in a pulse-step mismatch (see Fig. 3–19, Chapter 3) since saccade speed (determined by the high-frequency "pulse" of innervation) is diminished out of proportion to the limitation in range of adduction (determined by the low-frequency "step" of innervation). These findings are evident in the records shown in Figure 12–8 (top right panel) (see Video Display: Pontine Syndromes), which are taken from a patient with a right-sided INO.

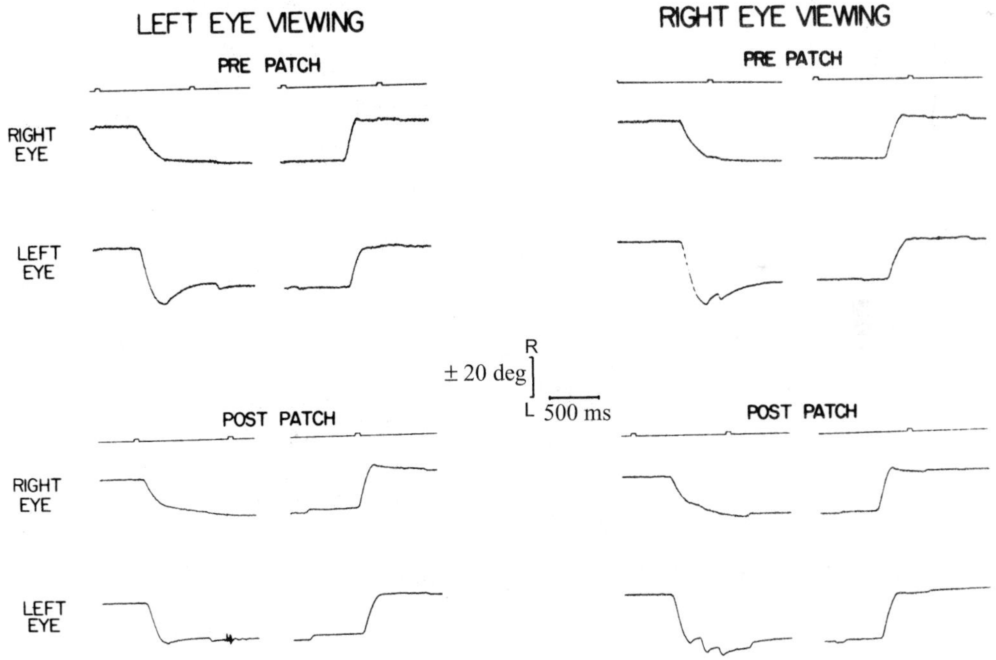

Figure 12–8. Effects of habitual monocular viewing on the eye movements of a patient with unilateral, right internuclear ophthalmoplegia. "Pre-patch" data were obtained after habitual binocular viewing, but the patient preferred to fixate with the right eye. "Post-patch" data were obtained after 5 days of patching of the right eye to ensure habitual left-eye viewing. "Left Eye Viewing" and "Right Eye Viewing" refer to the viewing conditions at the time the eye movements were recorded. Note the post-patch decrease in the abduction nystagmus of the left eye (decrease in the size of the abduction saccadic pulse and of the backward post-saccadic drift), with a commensurate decrease in the size of the saccadic pulse and increase of the onward post-saccadic drift for the adduction saccades made by the right eye. These changes were independent of which eye was viewing during the recording session. Patching led to little change in the adducting saccades made by the left eye or abducting saccades made by the right eye (vertical bar indicates ± 20 degrees; horizontal bar, 500 ms). (From Zee, Hain, and Carl,[1210] reprinted with permission of John Wiley and Sons, Inc.)

When she attempted to look to the left, the adducting saccades of the right eye were slow and hypometric; each consisted of a hypometric pulse followed by a glissadic drift of the eye towards the target. In the left eye, abducting saccades were hypermetric—overshooting the target—and were followed by a glissadic backward drift of the eye. A series of such small saccades and drifts would give the appearance of dissociated nystagmus.

As noted above, adduction lag is brought out clinically by asking the patient to make large horizontal saccades back and forth across the midline or by using a hand-held optokinetic drum or tape to produce nystagmus that allows easy comparison of the movements of the two eyes.[267] Measurement of saccades to compare the peak velocity of abduction and adduction allows identification of subtle degrees of INO (Fig. 12–9), but these results should be interpreted with caution because normal subjects show greater peak velocities in the abducting eye.[207,872] A solution to this problem is to compare the ratio of measurements from the two eyes. Thus, normal subjects show little variation in the ratio either of peak eye velocity,[1130] or of peak acceleration,[342] of the adducting saccades to abducting saccades. Patients with INO show adduction/abduction ratios of peak velocity or peak acceleration that consistently fall outside the ranges for normal subjects.[351] If it is not possible to differentiate eye movement records, then comparison of the size of the movement of each eye during the time it takes the abducting eye to get on target may determine whether a patient has INO.[353] To be reliable, any of these analytic methods require that confidence intervals for a group of control subjects first be established using the same method for recording eye movements.

Internuclear ophthalmoplegia may also be characterized by mild abnormalities of saccadic abduction in the affected eye: hypometria with centripetal drifts[364] and slowing.[1086] These changes in abducting saccades might be due to impaired ability to inhibit the affected medial rectus, although Komerell was unable to find any evidence of impaired medial rectus inhibition in one patient with a unilateral INO in whom he performed electromyography.[587]

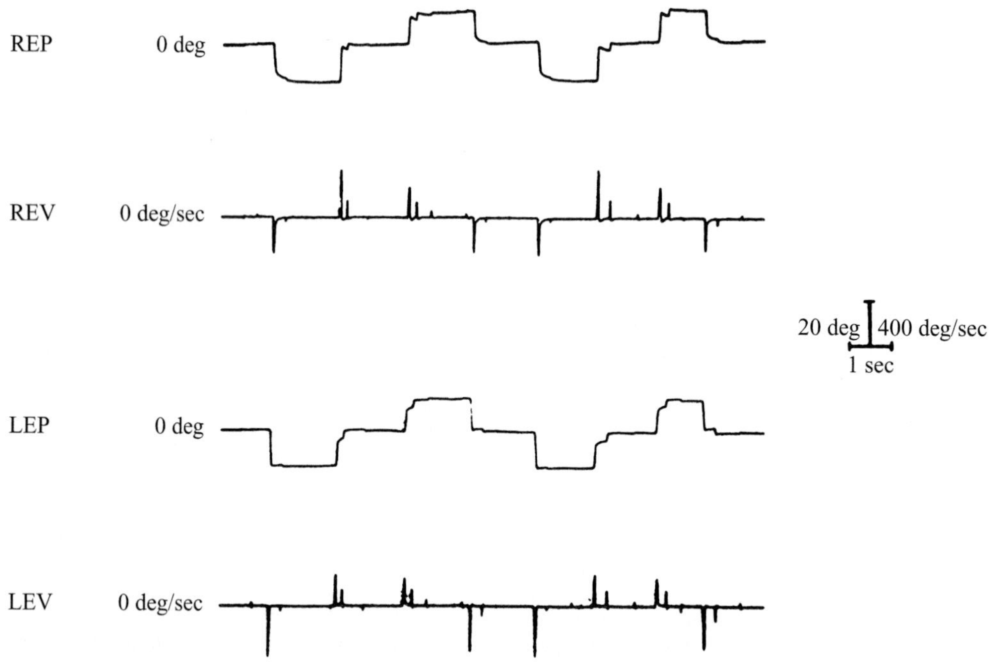

Figure 12–9. Subtle adduction lag due to bilateral internuclear ophthalmoplegia (infrared reflection technique). The patient makes saccades to targets located at 0 degrees, and at 15 degrees right and left. The velocity of adducting saccades of either eye is lower than that of corresponding abducting saccades. For rightward movements, the initial saccade of the right eye is hypometric and the right eye drifts back toward primary position, causing abduction or dissociated nystagmus. LEP: left eye position; LEV: left eye velocity; REP: right eye position; REV: right eye velocity.

Dissociated Horizontal Nystagmus in Internuclear Ophthalmoplegia

Several explanations have been offered to account for the dissociated nystagmus of INO, which are not necessarily mutually exclusive. The hypothesis that has received the most experimental support is that the nystagmus reflects the brain's attempts to compensate for the adduction weakness. Such compensation entails an adaptive increase in innervation to the adducting eye, which, because of Hering's law of equal innervation, must be accompanied by a commensurate change in the innervation to the strong, abducting eye. Although this adaptive change may help get the paretic eye on target, it leads to overshooting saccades and postsaccadic drift of the abducting eye—a pulse-step mismatch that has the appearance of an abducting nystagmus. If this is the case, the oscillation is initiated by a saccade and, thus, is not truly nystagmus.

One line of support for this proposal comes from the observation that abduction nystagmus is not observed in acute experimental INO induced by injecting lidocaine into the MLF.[364] This result implies that the cause of abduction nystagmus must be due to processes outside the MLF, or to an adaptive response to the initial adduction weakness. Second, in patients with unilateral INO, patching the eye with the adduction weakness for several days almost abolished the overshoot and pulse-step mismatch of the abducting eye (Fig. 12–8B).[1210] A third line of support for the proposition that the abduction nystagmus is a compensatory response to a "peripheral" weakness comes from the observation that surgically-caused medial rectus weakness leads to a similar nystagmus, and that this nystagmus resolves if the eye with the weak medial rectus is patched for several days.[1142]

Another probable mechanism for an abduction nystagmus is a dissociated gaze-evoked nystagmus that appears more prominent in the abducting eye because of the adduction weakness. In contrast to the abducting nystagmus produced by adaptation, such gaze-evoked abduction nystagmus is usually relatively sustained, and the postsaccadic drift would bring the eye to the central position if it were not interrupted by corrective eccentric saccades. Interruption of paramedian tracts that run near the MLF and carry fibers to and from the flocculus might be responsible for the finding.[161]

Centripetal drift of the eye in abduction nystagmus does not seem to be due to loss of inhibition of the medial rectus of the eye contralateral to the lesion, since both electrophysiological studies in animals[462] and an electromyographic study in one patient showed no evidence for such loss of inhibition.[587] Furthermore, as noted above, experimental INO produced by local anesthetic blockade of the MLF does not acutely produce abducting nystagmus in the contralateral eye.[364] The possibility of increased convergence tone has some experimental support,[364,1049] and is discussed further in the following section. However, of these hypotheses, the only one that accounts for the observed hypermetria of the abducting eye is the one that proposes that the abduction nystagmus is a compensatory response.

Abnormalities of Vergence in Internuclear Ophthalmoplegia

Changes in vergence in patients with INO are variable, and preclude a single explanation. When patients are able to converge despite absence of voluntary adduction, a caudal lesion with preservation of the medial rectus motoneurons has been assumed.[596] However, some caution is required in applying this "rule," since medial rectus motoneurons lie in three subgroups (Fig. 9–9B, Chapter 9) and recent evidence suggests that the smaller motoneurons that are located on the perimeter of the oculomotor nucleus receive a larger vergence input than do the larger motoneurons that lie ventrally.[160] Furthermore, even when experimental INO is induced by injecting lidocaine into the MLF between the levels of the trochlear and abducens nuclei, vergence is affected; the reported *increase* in accommodative vergence led to the suggestion that the MLF normally carries an inappropriate vergence signal.[364] We have encountered occasional patients with acute INO and esophoria.[44] A more common finding, however, especially with bilateral INO, is exotropia ("wall-eyed bilateral INO"—WEBINO).[586] Such exotropia does not necessarily imply loss of vergence (see Video Display: Pontine Syndromes). In one patient with bilateral INO, clinicopathologic correlation failed to find a cause for the loss of convergence.[1048] Although the presence of intact convergence is important, its absence does not necessarily imply a rostral lesion involving the medial rectus nuclear subdivision. This may be because some patients simply cannot produce a strong convergence effort, and the vertical disparity that occurs when a unilateral INO is associated with a skew deviation (see following section) may interfere with convergence effort. In this regard, convergence can often be best elicited in patients with a vertical stimulus, such as a pencil. Thus, caution is required in trying to localize INO on the basis of whether convergence is "preserved" or "absent" (corresponding to the posterior INO and anterior INO of Cogan,[193] respectively). More systematic studies are required to better understand the changes in vergence that occur with INO.

Skew Deviation in Internuclear Ophthalmoplegia

Skew deviation commonly occurs with unilateral INO; the higher eye is usually on the side of the adduction weakness (see Video Display: Disorders of the Vestibular System). Skew deviation is probably due to interruption of central projections from otolithic inputs that ascend in the MLF (see Skew Deviation and the Ocular Tilt Reaction, in Chapter 11). The associated adduction defect, as well as incyclorotation of the hypertropic eye, makes it possible to distinguish this vertical deviation from trochlear nerve palsy. Oculomotor nerve palsy can also cause a vertical deviation along with weakness of adduction; however, in this case, the eye is down on the affected side, and ptosis or pupillary changes may also be present.

Vertical Nystagmus in Internuclear Ophthalmoplegia

Downbeat nystagmus with a greater torsional component in the eye contralateral to a unilateral INO,[784] can be related to interruption of the pathways mediating the vertical VOR (Fig. 2–3, Chapter 2). Thus, posterior semicircular canal pathways mediating excitation pass through the MLF, but some anterior semicircular canal pathways do not. Experimental INO, produced by lidocaine blockade, causes ipsilateral hypertropia and unilateral downbeating nystagmus.[364] Patients with a unilateral INO may also have an ipsiversive torsional nystagmus (top poles of the eyes cyclorotate so as to beat toward the side of the lesion).[261] The torsional nystagmus is sometimes dissociated, and is usually but not always associated with a skew deviation. It may relate to interruption of pathways between the vestibular nuclei and the interstitial nucleus of Cajal (INC) (see Box 6–6, Chapter 6).

Bilateral Internuclear Ophthalmoplegia

Bilateral lesions of the MLF cause bilateral adduction weakness, bilateral abduction nystagmus, and impaired vertical vestibular and pursuit eye movements (see Fig. 6–5). Studies of the effects of experimental[313] and clinical[882] bilateral lesions of the MLF have clarified the deficits in vertical gaze that occur with INO. These deficits follow both unilateral and bilateral lesions, though they are more enduring with bilateral ones.[882] Both the upward and downward vestibulo-ocular reflex have reduced gain, and eye velocity may lag head velocity; the consequence is appreciable drift of images upon the retina and oscillopsia during vertical head rotations. In one patient with a right unilateral INO, asymmetry of the vertical vestibulo-ocular responses was evident with rapid head rotations applied in the planes of the canals.[227] Thus, the vertical VOR induced by stimulating the left posterior semicircular canal was deficient binocularly, whereas stimulation of the left anterior semicircular canal was preserved. This result suggests that while posterior canal projections travel up the MLF to contact ocular motoneurons, anterior canal projections also take other routes, including possibly the brachium conjunctivum and the crossing ventral tegmental tract (see Fig. 2–3,Chapter 2). Vertical optokinetic nystagmus is impaired and vertical optokinetic after-nystagmus is abolished. Vertical smooth pursuit is moderately impaired. The vestibulo-ocular reflex is not canceled during combined eye-head tracking. Vertical gaze-holding is also impaired. However, the partial preservation of vertical gaze-holding in INO—or after lesions of the prepositus and medial vestibular nuclei—confirms that the interstitial nucleus of Cajal plays a major role as the vertical neural integrator.[221]

Some patients with bilateral INO have been noted to have impaired fixation. In such patients, sporadic bursts of monocular abducting saccades may occur in each eye. The presence of saccadic intrusions in patients with bilateral INO suggests involvement of the brainstem adjacent to the MLF.[456]

Visual Symptoms Due to Internuclear Ophthalmoplegia

Patients with INO may have no visual symptoms, particularly when there is no limitation of adduction. In other cases, the presence of either limitation of adduction or skew deviation may cause diplopia that is horizontal, vertical, or oblique. Some patients with INO complain of oscillopsia.[400] In the horizontal plane, this usually occurs from either the adduction lag or the abduction nystagmus. In the vertical plane, however, it occurs during head movements and is caused by a deficient vertical vestibulo-ocular reflex.[414] In many patients, visual symptoms become less bothersome or resolve completely, either because of recovery of function of MLF axons,[290] or because of more central adaptive mechanisms.

Variants of Internuclear Ophthalmoplegia

Lesions that damage the MLF may also damage adjacent structures such as the abducens nucleus; these syndromes are discussed in the following section on the "one-and-a-half syndrome." The so-called posterior INO of Lutz, [670] in which abduction (but not adduction) is impaired during saccades and pursuit but not during vestibular stimuli, is rare. Three explanations may account for these findings. First, patients with an abducens palsy may show nystagmus in the contralateral adducting eye, if the weak abducting eye is used preferentially for fixation.[800] This nystagmus could reflect the same type of mechanisms (an adaptive response or a dissociated nystagmus) that accounts for the abducting nystagmus that develops in patients with typical INO. Second, it has been suggested that interruption of an extra-MLF pathway from the PPRF, which inhibits medial rectus motoneurons, causes increased tone in the medial rectus and the appearance of abduction paresis.[1085,1086] However, anatomical verification of this pathway is lacking; in fact, the major projection from the PPRF to the midbrain is from pontine omnipause neurons to the riMLF, which is concerned with vertical, not horizontal, saccades (see Fig. 6–5).[158] Third, it has been shown that experimental inactivation of the oculomotor internuclear neurons, which project to the contralateral abducens nucleus via the MLF, causes hypometria and slowing of abducting saccades.[189] Thus, midbrain lesions might lead to contralateral abduction weakness (see Video Display: Midbrain Syndromes).

Combined Unilateral Conjugate Gaze Palsy and Internuclear Ophthalmoplegia: "One-and-a-half Syndrome" and Other Variants

Combined lesions of the abducens nucleus or PPRF and adjacent MLF on one side of the brainstem cause an ipsilateral horizontal gaze palsy and INO, so that the only preserved horizontal eye movement is abduction of the contralateral eye (see Box 12–8 and Video Display: Pontine Syndromes) —hence the name "one-

Box 12–8. Clinical Features Of "One-And-A-Half" Syndrome

- Ipsilateral horizontal gaze palsy and internuclear ophthalmoplegia
- Only surviving horizontal conjugate movement is abduction of the contralateral eye
- Paralytic pontine exotropia on looking straight ahead (one eye is deviated laterally)
- Vergence and vertical movements may be spared

For related anatomy, see Box 6-2, Box 6-3 and Fig. 6-1 in Chapter 6. (Related Video Display: Pontine Syndromes) and-a-half syndrome."[105,105,139,266,327,1157] Such patients may show an exotropia when attempting to look straight ahead: the eye opposite the side of the lesion is deviated outward. This strabismus may be more evident when fixation is prevented by Frenzel goggles.[514] It has been attributed to the unopposed drives of the intact pontine gaze center (paralytic pontine exotropia).[586,993] The spared abduction saccades of the contralateral eye are followed by centripetal drift so that a nystagmus similar to that of the abducting eye in INO is present. Occasionally, the ipsilateral horizontal vestibular responses may be preserved when voluntary gaze is abolished,[105,266] suggesting that the pontine lesion is more rostral in the PPRF, or more discrete in the caudal PPRF,[518] sparing the vestibular projections to the abducens nucleus. Although attempts at conjugate (versional) movements elicit no adduction, vergence movements may be preserved. Ocular bobbing (see Eye Movements in Stupor and Coma) may accompany the one-and-a-half syndrome.[538] The presence of a peripheral facial weakness on the same side as the gaze palsy in one-and-a-half syndrome suggests involvement of the abducens nucleus, genu of CN VII, and the adjacent MLF.[24,258,303] Involvement of the central tegmental tract, may predispose to development of the syndrome of oculopalatal tremor.[1182]

The one-and-a-half syndrome may be due to brainstem ischemia,[105,539,993,1195] multiple sclerosis,[1157] tumor,[503,773] hemorrhage,[804] trauma,[1014] or infection.[720] Occasionally focal hemorrhage producing the one-and-a-half syndrome can be treated surgically.[884]

The conventional explanation for one-and-a-half syndrome is that the pontine lesion affects both one abducens nucleus (causing the gaze palsy) and the crossing internuclear axons from the contralateral abducens nucleus (causing the INO). C. Miller Fisher has recently pointed out that an alternative explanation is possible in cases in which one (rather than two) paramedian tegmental pontine artery bifurcates into terminal branches at the level of the abducens nucleus, thereby supply the MLF on both sides;[329] the abducens nucleus would presumably be infarcted on the side of the penetrator, causing a bilateral INO and unilateral gaze palsy.

A case of "one-and-a-half syndrome" has been described in which only adduction in one eye was spared.[174] The patient had mucormycosis that caused a sixth-nerve palsy due to cavernous sinus involvement on one side, and on the other side had horizontal gaze palsy due to carotid artery occlusion. Lesions that damage the MLF and ipsilateral abducens fascicle produce horizontal ophthalmoplegia in the ipsilateral eye from the combination of an INO and a sixth-nerve palsy. Lesions that damage the MLF on one side and the PPRF or abducens nucleus on the opposite side produce horizontal gaze palsy toward the same side as the involved PPRF or abducens nucleus. In such cases, the INO cannot be diagnosed because of the overriding horizontal gaze palsy. Damage to the MLF on one side and to the contralateral abducens nerve fascicle will produce abduction weakness of the contralateral eye combined with adduction weakness of the ipsilateral eye. In this setting, there will be a "pseudo–horizontal gaze palsy" on attempted horizontal gaze away from the side of the MLF lesion. This diagnosis may be suspected in a patient who appears to have a horizontal gaze palsy that is asymmetric, with one eye (usually the adducting eye) being more limited than the other.

Selective Cell Vulnerability in the Pons

Many metabolic, toxic, and degenerative conditions may cause selective deficits of ocular motility that suggest a predominant loss of one population of brainstem neurons concerned with eye movements. By applying hypotheses based on current concepts of the neurobiology of saccades (Chapter 3), it is possible to propose explanations for slow saccades and saccadic oscillations (see Video Display: Disorders of Saccades).

SLOW SACCADES WITH PONTINE DISEASE

Disorders that are reported to cause slow saccades are listed in Table 12–4. Predominant slowing of horizontal saccades generally occurs in hereditary degenerative disorders that involve the pons, especially spinocerebellar ataxia type 2 (SCA2 or olivopontocerebellar atrophy of Wadia and Swami) (see Video Display: Disorders of Saccades).[673,1129,1144,1212] Slow horizontal saccades also occur after pon-

Table 12–4. **Etiology of Slow Saccades**

Spinocerebellar ataxias (SCA), especially SCA2 (olivopontocerebellar atrophy)[147,477,673,798,906,958,1129,1144,1175,1212]
Huntington's disease[103,208,607,624]
Progressive supranuclear palsy[92,367,933,1139]
Parkinson's (advanced cases)[1171] and related diseases;[251,1185] Lytico-Bodig[639]
Whipple's disease[43,580]
Lipid storage diseases[365,934,1020]
Wilson's disease[572]
Drug intoxications: anticonvulsants,[1075,1087] benzodiazepines[928]
Tetanus[707]
In dementia: Alzheimer's disease (stimulus-dependent),[338] and in association with AIDS[775]
Lesions of the paramedian pontine reticular formation[429,1105]
Internuclear ophthalmoplegia[1210]
Paraneoplastic syndromes[50,230]
Amyotrophic lateral sclerosis (some cases)[40]
Peripheral nerve palsy, diseases affecting the neuromuscular junction and extraocular muscle, restrictive ophthalmopathy

tine infarction but, even in cases with neuropathological confirmation of neuronal loss and gliosis confined to the paramedian pons, vertical saccades may also show some slowing.[429] Genetic storage disorders, notably Gaucher's disease, may be characterized by horizontal saccadic slowing, along with ocular motor apraxia.[435] However early in the course of Gaucher's disease,[6] and especially in late-onset Tay-Sachs disease,[943] saccades may be of normal velocity but stall in mid-flight (Fig. 3–20, Chapter 3); these transient decelerations have been ascribed to a defect of the hypothetical latch circuit, which inhibits omnipause neurons until the saccade is complete (see Fig. 3–9, Chapter 3). In diseases that principally affect the midbrain, such as progressive supranuclear palsy (PSP), vertical saccades become slow before horizontal ones.[92]

Selective slowing of horizontal saccades in association with facial spasms has been described as a probable paraneoplastic phenomenon in association with prostatic cancer.[50] Other forms of paraneoplastic brainstem encephalitis, especially with anti-Ma2 antineuronal antibodies and testicular carcinoma, may produce saccadic slowing, but vertical gaze is usually also affected.[239]

Some patients with slow horizontal saccades use blinks of the eyelids to speed up their eye movements,[1206] perhaps because blinks inhibit omnipause neurons. In patients with very slow saccades, there may be some doubt as to whether the residual movements are really saccades or rather pursuit or non-saccadic drifts of the eyes. One strategy is to induce optokinetic or vestibular nystagmus and determine whether the quick phases are similarly slowed to saccades. Another strategy is to ask the patient to make diagonal saccades, when a curved trajectory will demonstrate that the vertical component is faster than the horizontal (see Video Display: Disorders of Saccades). Some patients with slow saccades are able to generate smooth-pursuit movements of up to about 20 degrees per second. It is difficult to distinguish a considerably slowed saccade from pursuit, however, so that whether or not pursuit function is truly intact in such patients is not established. In those patients in whom smooth pursuit is relatively preserved, if the saccades are so slow that they cannot catch up with the moving target, then pursuit may appear very deficient, as the eyes appear to lag behind the target. Patients with SCA2 usually make normal-amplitude saccades despite their low velocity, and are able to respond to targets flashed during these prolonged movements by turning the eye around in midflight.[673,1212] Nonetheless, patients who make slow saccades seldom complain of motion of their environment and appear to suppress vision during the movements even though they are able to respond to intrasaccadic visual stimuli.[673] Patients with slow saccades may use a variety of strategies of eye-head coordination to move their eyes more quickly to the target (see Eye-Head Movements in Patients with Slow or Inaccurate Saccades, Chapter 7).

The simplest explanation for slow horizontal saccades in disorders such as SCA2 is that excitatory burst neurons in the PPRF are involved.[480] However, experimental lesions of the omnipause neurons using excitotoxins are also reported to cause slow horizontal and vertical saccades.[532] In some patients with selective slowing of horizontal saccades, both burst and omnipause cell populations may be affected,[429] and involvement of omnipause neurons in nucleus raphe interpositus is confirmed in patients with SCA3.[936] Thus, an alternative explanation for saccadic slowing is that the premotor burst neurons need the omnipause neurons to abruptly discontinue inhibition in order to generate a high-acceleration movement.[724] It is also possible that disturbance of other inputs to the premotor burst neurons could lead to slow saccades. For example, acute inactivation of the superior colliculus causes slow saccades in monkey.[464] These issues are discussed further in Chapter 3 (Pathophysiology of Saccadic Abnormalities).

SACCADIC OSCILLATIONS WITH PONTINE LESIONS

Saccadic oscillations that lack any intersaccadic interval (ocular flutter and opsoclonus—Fig. 10–14E) (see Video Display: Saccadic Oscillations and Intrusions) are discussed in Chapter 10. They have been attributed to disease that selectively affects the omnipause neurons,[1213] which are located in the nucleus raphe interpositus in the midline of the pons at the level of the abducens nucleus (Fig. 6–2, Chapter 6). However, experimental lesions of the omnipause region with excitotoxin cause slow saccades rather than oscillations.[532] Furthermore, neuropathologic examination of the brain of two patients who had manifest opsoclonus as the remote effect of lung cancer did not disclose changes in the omnipause population.[898] Nonetheless, transient ocular flutter was reported in one patient during an exacerbation of multiple sclerosis with a plaque in the parmedian pons; the oscillations resolved as the MRI became normal.[968] Thus, it remains possible that omnipause neuron dysfunction may contribute to saccadic oscillations. Another possibility is that the brainstem network of premotor burst neurons is inherently unstable,[873] a proposal that is developed further in Chapter 3.

OCULAR MOTOR SYNDROMES CAUSED BY LESIONS OF THE MIDBRAIN

Modern Concepts of Vertical Gaze Palsies

The midbrain is important in the control of vertical eye movements, especially saccades and gaze holding. Examples of the effects of midbrain lesions on eye movements are shown in the Video Display: Midbrain Syndromes. Patients with acute palsies of vertical gaze usually have lesions localized to structures lying in the high midbrain (Box 12–9).[91] In evaluating the patient with a disturbance of vertical gaze, it is crucial to test not just range of movement, but also to determine whether there are selective defects of saccades, smooth pursuit, vestibular, or vergence eye movements. Although certain lesions may cause paralysis of all upward or downward movements, or both, selective defects of ocular motility are more common. Second, it is also important to test the torsional vestibulo-ocular reflex, noting whether quick phases of nystagmus occur in both directions as the patient's head rolls from side to side. Third, exam ocular alignment, looking for signs of oculomotor or trochlear palsy, and for evidence for skew deviation and the ocular tilt reaction. Fourth, look for abnormalities of eyelid movements and the pupils, which are common features of vertical gaze disorders.

Although human studies have made important contributions to understanding the control of vertical gaze, the value of many older reports is limited either by lack of information concerning the effects of lesions on each class of eye movements, or uncertainty as to the degree of involvement of the critical structures for vertical gaze. Over the past 25 years, the pathways critical for vertical gaze have been defined using modern anatomical and physiological techniques, and the measurement of behavioral deficits when such pathways are selectively lesioned or pharmacologically inactivated. These experimental studies, which are summarized in Chapter 6, have defined the roles of three key structures in the control of vertical gaze: the rostral interstitial nucleus of the medial longitudinal fasciculus (riMLF), the interstitial nucleus of Cajal (INC), and the posterior commissure.

Lesions of the riMLF and Vertical Saccadic Palsy

In interpreting vertical saccadic palsies, it is helpful to bear in mind several key facts. The first is the anatomic location of the riMLF (see Box 6–5), which contains the burst neurons that generate vertical and torsional saccades. The riMLF lies dorsomedial to the rostral pole

Box 12–9. Commonly Reported Localization Of Acute Vertical Gaze Palsies

Paralysis of downgaze:

- Selective saccadic loss: bilateral riMLF lesions
- Involvement of all types of eye movement: INC or PC affected

Paralysis of upgaze:

- All types of eye movements are involved: PC and INC

Combined upgaze and downgaze:

- Selective saccadic loss: bilateral riMLF lesion
- Involvement of all eye movements: INC or PC also affected

riMLF: Rostral interstitial nucleus of MLF; INC: Interstitial nucleus of Cajal; PC: Posterior commissure. For related anatomy, see: Brainstem Connections for Vertical and Torsional Movements, Fig. 6-4 and Fig. 6-5 in Chapter 6. For related etiologies, see Table 12-6. (Related Video Display: Midbrain Syndromes)

of the red nucleus, medial to the fields of Forel, lateral to the periaqueductal gray and the nucleus of Darkschewitsch, and immediately rostral to the interstitial nucleus of Cajal (see Figs. 6–3 to 6–5, Chapter 6). Second, the riMLF receives its blood supply from a small perforating vessel (the posterior thalamo- subthalamic paramedian artery) that arises between the bifurcation of the basilar artery and the origin of the posterior communicating artery, with a single vessel often supplying both riMLFs.[175,827] Third, each riMLF projects bilaterally to motoneurons for the elevator muscles (superior rectus and inferior oblique) but ipsilaterally to motoneurons for the depressor muscles (inferior rectus and superior oblique).[741,742] Note that these bilateral projections probably are not via the posterior commissure, but occur at the level of the oculomotor and trochlear nuclei. What this means is that unilateral riMLF lesions are more likely to affect downward than upward saccades. Furthermore, each burst neuron in the riMLF sends axon collaterals to motoneurons supplying yoke muscle pairs; this appears to be part of the neural substrate for Hering's law in the vertical plane.[740] Thus, riMLF lesions (unilateral or bilateral) would be expected to cause vertical saccadic defects that are mainly conjugate. Fourth, although each riMLF contains burst neurons to drive upward or downward saccades, the right riMLF is responsible for torsional quick phases that are clockwise from the point of view of the patient (extorsion of the right eye and intorsion of the left eye), and the left riMLF is responsible for counter-clockwise quick phases. Thus, although the effects of a unilateral riMLF lesion on vertical saccades may be minor, it will abolish ipsitorsional quick phases and produce a cyclodeviation. A final anatomical point is that the riMLF shows no neuronal loss or atrophy, or gliosis with increasing age,[453] so that slow vertical saccades cannot be attribute simply to aging.

Lesions of the riMLF are usually infarcts in the distribution of the posterior thalamo-subthalamic paramedian artery, which may be paired or single, and which may also supply the rostromedial red nucleus, adjacent subthalamus, the posterior-inferior portion of the dorsomedial nucleus and the parafascicular nucleus of the thalamus. Older reports of vertical gaze disorders have been reviewed in a modern context,[159,835] and here we focus on recent reports.

Based on experimental studies,[1054] a *unilateral lesion of the riMLF* would be expected to cause a minimal defect in vertical saccades (mainly downward), but a defect in generating ipsitorsional quick phases (with top poles of eyes towards the side of the lesion) (Box 12–10). Patients have been reported with such findings,[628,903] as well as a static, contralesional torsional deviation with torsional nystagmus beating contralesionally.[153,449,450]

Other patients with a unilateral riMLF lesion have been described as having greater defects of vertical saccades or other eye movements. In the case of Ranalli and colleagues,[883] the infarct had spread partly into the adjacent interstitial nucleus of Cajal; saccades were absent above the central position, and slow and limited below. Smooth pursuit and the vestibulo-ocular reflex were also affected in the vertical plane, being restricted in range, and of reduced gain. These additional defects might be attributed to involvement of the interstitial nucleus of Cajal. In a second patient who had a vertical saccadic palsy (up and down) in association with a discrete, unilateral riMLF lesion, there was also bilateral infarction in the base of the pons.[107] In a third patient with a left thalamic lesion on MRI, upward saccades in her left eye were impaired, but with sparing of upward pursuit and other eye movements.[803] This patient's monocular vertical saccadic defect is difficult to explain, since excitatory burst neurons in the riMLF project to superior rectus motoneuron bilaterally, with axons crossing within the oculomotor nucleus.[741] Lacking autopsy verification, it remains possible that bilateral lesions were present. However, this third case raises the issue of the role played by inhibitory burst neurons in vertical saccades. The anatomical connections of vertical burst neurons are only recently being elucidated, but it seems that those projecting to the inferior rectus and superior oblique lie not in riMLF, but in the interstitial nucleus of Cajal.[481]

Bilateral lesions of the riMLF are more common, and have been reported to cause loss either of downward saccades (Fig. 12–10) (see Video Display: Midbrain Syndromes), or of all

Box 12–10. Clinical Findings with Lesions of the Rostral Interstitial Nucleus of the MLF (riMLF)

Unilateral Lesion:

- A mild and variable defect of downward saccades
- Loss of ipsitorsional quick phases (e.g., clockwise* quick phases are lost with right riMLF lesions)
- Static, contralesional torsional deviation with torsional nystagmus beating contralesionally

Bilateral lesion:

- More profound defect of vertical saccades that may be more pronounced for downward than upward eye movements
- Vertical gaze-holding, VOR and pursuit, and horizontal saccades are preserved

* Torsional rotations are defined from the viewpoint of the patient, not the observer, so that clockwise means that the upper pole of the right eye would rotate temporally (extorsion) and the upper pole of the left eye, nasally (intorsion)

For related anatomy, see Box 6-5, Fig. 6-4, and Fig. 6-5 in Chapter 6. For related etiologies, see Table 12-6. (Related Video Display: Midbrain Syndromes)

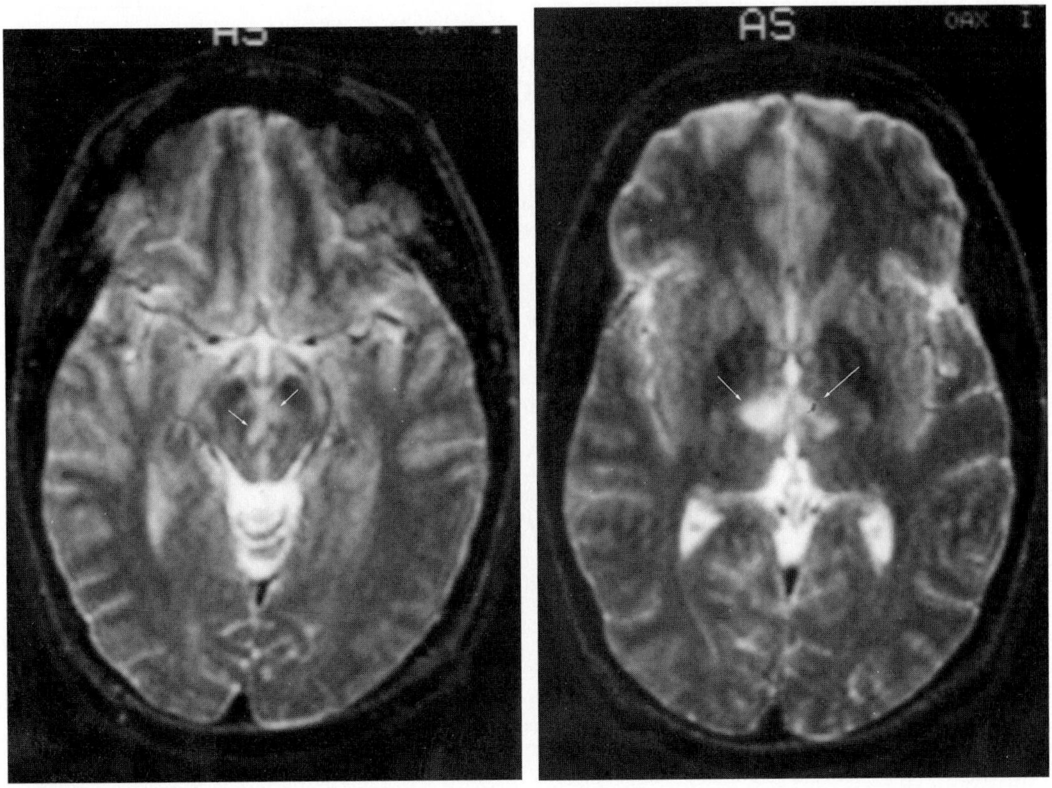

A B

Figure 12–10. MRI findings in a patient with acute vertical saccadic palsy and disturbance of consciousness (see Video Display: Midbrain Syndromes). T2-weighted MRI scans showing small, hyperintense bilateral lesions (arrowheads) within the rostral midbrain (A) and caudal thalamus (B), which presumably involved the rostral interstitial nucleus of the MLF. This stroke was in the distribution of the thalamic and subthalamic perforating vessels coming off of the proximal portion of the posterior cerebral artery.

vertical saccades. The explanation for selective paralysis of downward saccades had centered on which part of the riMLF is affected, and how this partial lesion might affect emerging axons from burst neurons for upward or downward saccades.[835] However, a more cogent explanation is that motoneurons innervating upward acting extraocular muscles receive bilateral innervation from the riMLF, whereas motoneurons innervating downward acting muscles receive only a unilateral innervation.[741,742] Impairment of vertical smooth pursuit and the vestibulo-ocular reflex probably reflects involvement of adjacent structures such as the MLF and interstitial nucleus of Cajal.[990] Somnolence or memory impairment may imply coexistent involvement of medial thalamic nuclei.

A *vertical one-and-a-half syndrome* has been reported, with either loss of all downward movements and selective loss of upward movements in one eye,[264] or impairment of all upward eye movements and a selective deficit of downward saccades in the eye on the side of the lesion.[109] Since each burst neuron in the riMLF sends axon collaterals to yoke muscle pairs, such deficits imply a lesion close to the motoneurons of the muscle responsible for the disconjugate deficit.

Lesions of the Interstitial Nucleus of Cajal (INC)

Recent experimental work has demonstrated that the INC (see Box 6–6) plays a key role in

Box 12–11. Findings with Lesions of the Interstitial Nucleus of Cajal (INC)*

Unilateral Lesions or Inactivation

- Impaired gaze-holding in the vertical and torsional planes following saccades to tertiary positions; VOR less affected
- Ocular tilt reaction: skew deviation (ipsilateral hypertropia), extorsion of the contralateral eye and intorsion of the ipsilateral eye, and contralateral head tilt
- Torsional nystagmus that has ipsilesional quick phases—top pole rotates to the side of the lesion; downbeat component may also be present

Bilateral Lesions or Inactivation

- Reduced range of all vertical eye movements but saccades not slowed
- Impaired gaze-holding after all vertical and torsional movements; upbeat nystagmus
- Neck retroflexion

*Based mainly on experimental pharmacological inactivation.
For related anatomy, see Display 6-6, Fig. 6-4, and Fig. 6-5 in Chapter 6. For schematic of OTR, see Fig. 11-4 of Chapter 11. For related etiologies, see Table 12-6. (Related Video Display: Midbrain Syndromes)

holding eccentric vertical gaze (Box 12–11).[221,449] Furthermore, the INC appears to project exclusively to the ocular motoneurons via the posterior commissure (see next section). However, it seems that the defect of vertical gaze associated with INC lesions is not just one of vertical gaze-evoked nystagmus.[818] Bilateral pharmacological inactivation of INC in monkeys greatly restricts the vertical range of all classes of conjugate eye movements, although saccades do not become slow.[449] The INC is frequently involved in cases of vertical gaze disturbance.[159,835,883]

While bilateral lesions of INC mainly affect vertical gaze, unilateral lesions produce the ocular tilt reaction and ipsilesional torsional nystagmus with quick phases moving the top poles of the eyes towards the side of the lesion (which helps differentiate it from torsional nystagmus due to riMLF lesions, in which torsional quick phases moving the top poles of the eyes towards the side of the lesion are abolished).[153,446,450]

Effects of Lesions of the Posterior Commissure and Nucleus of the Posterior Commissure

Lesions of the posterior commissure are traditionally equated with a syndrome of loss of upward gaze and associated findings (Table 12–5) generally known by a variety of names: dorsal midbrain syndrome, Parinaud's syndrome, Koeber-Salus-Elschig syndrome, pretectal syndrome, and Sylvian aqueduct syndrome.[241,819,821] In the past, selective paralysis of upward gaze was ascribed to destruction of the superior colliculi, but this is not the case.[13,820] Unilateral midbrain lesions can create the same ocular motor syndrome by interrupting both projections through the posterior commissure.[38,159,883,1015] Experimental inactivation of the posterior commissure with lidocaine causes vertical gaze-evoked nystagmus,[818] but electrolytic lesions cause greater deficits (Box 12–12).[819,821] Thus, it seems that the clinical syndrome associated with posterior commissure lesions is due

Table 12–5. Features of the Dorsal Midbrain Syndrome[159,241,559,835,862,1095]

Limitation of upward eye movements
Saccades
Smooth pursuit
Vestibulo-ocular reflex
Bell's phenomenon
Dissociation of lid and eye movements: Lid retraction (Collier's sign), occasionally ptosis
Disturbances of downward eye movements:
Downward gaze preference ("setting sun" sign)
Downbeating nystagmus
Downward saccades and smooth pursuit may be impaired, but vestibular movements are relatively preserved
Disturbances of vergence eye movements:
Convergence-retraction nystagmus
Paralysis of convergence
Spasm of convergence
Paralysis of divergence
"A" or "V"-pattern exotropia
Pseudo-abducens palsy
Fixation instability (square-wave jerks)
Skew deviation
Pupillary abnormalities (light-near dissociation)

to more than axon projections of the INC (see Box 6–7), but also represents lesioning the nucleus of the posterior commissure (nPC), which may be important for the control of vertical gaze and eyelid movements. Cells in the nPC project through the posterior commissure and may contact the riMLF, INC, and the M-group of neurons, which relays to the central caudal subdivision of the oculomotor nucleus (Fig. 9–9), and may coordinate vertical eye and lid movements.[965]

The vertical gaze defect observed with clinical lesions affecting the posterior commissure usually affects all types of eye movements, though the vestibulo-ocular reflex (VOR) and Bell's phenomenon (upward eye deviation during forceful lid closure) may sometimes be spared. Eyelid abnormalities occur: Collier's "tucked lid" sign (or lid retraction),[209] or less commonly, ptosis. Some patients show transient eyelid lag with downward gaze shifts, but without sustained eyelid retaction;[362] this defect could be attributed to involvement of the midbrain M-group that normally coordinates vertical saccades and lid movements.[479] Below the horizontal meridian, vertical saccades can be made but are usually slow. Acutely, the eyes may be tonically deviated downward ("setting sun sign"); this finding is prominent in premature infants who have suffered intraventricular hemorrhage.[1067] Transient downward deviation of the eyes occasionally occurs in normal infants, but, in such cases, the eyes can be easily driven above the horizontal meridian by the vertical doll's-head maneuver.[489] Tonic upward gaze deviation of the eyes has been reported in some patients with midbrain lesions,[63] and following

Box 12–12. Findings With Lesions Of The Posterior Commissure

- Impairment of all classes of vertical eye movements, especially upward, with loss of vertical gaze-holding (neural integrator) function
- Attempted upward or horizontal saccades evoke "convergence-retraction nystagmus"—asynchronous convergent saccades
- Pathologic lid retraction while looking straight ahead (Collier's sign)
- Pupils are mid-dilated and show a smaller reaction to light than to a near stimulus

For related anatomy, see Box 6-7, Fig. 6-4, and Fig. 6-5 in Chapter 6. For related etiologies, see Table 12-6. (Related Video Display: Midbrain Syndromes) hypoxic-ischemic insults.[552] Oculogyric crises are discussed under the section on Parkinson's disease. Episodic tonic upgaze may also occur in otherwise normal infants,[9] although some may later show horizontal strabismus and intellectual or language disability.[439,809]

The dorsal midbrain syndrome also includes disturbance of horizontal eye movements, especially vergence. In some patients, convergence is paralyzed, while in others it is excessive and causes convergence spasm. During horizontal saccades, the abducting eye may move more slowly than its adducting fellow. This finding has been called *pseudo-abducens palsy*,[241,862] and may reflect excess of convergence tone (see Video Display: Midbrain Syndromes). Alternatively, abduction weakness with midbrain lesions that cause sustained esotropia could be due to effects on oculomotor internuclear neurons that project to the pons, since experimental inactivation of these cells causes paresis of abduction.[189] Pseudoabducens palsy may lead to an early symptom of posterior commissure lesions: reading difficulty caused by a transient inability to find, and to focus both eyes on, the beginning of the next line when a horizontal saccade is made.

Convergence-retraction nystagmus may also occur following experimental lesions of the posterior commissure,[819,821] and in patients with disease of the midbrain.[789] Convergence-retraction nystagmus had been regarded as a saccadic disorder, consisting of asynchronous, opposed saccades whenever upward quick phases are stimulated. However, other studies indicate that, at least in some patients, convergence-retraction nystagmus is a primary disorder of the vergence system.[875] Convergence is often evident during attempted large upward movements, and contrasts with the transient divergence that occurs in normal subjects.[1207] Pupillary reactions are also commonly affected. Usually, the pupils are large and react better with a near stimulus than to light—"light-near dissociation."

A variety of disease processes may affect the region of the posterior commissure and disrupt vertical gaze (Table 12–6). Pineal tumors produce the dorsal midbrain syndrome either by direct pressure on the posterior commissure or by causing obstructive hydrocephalus.[51] Hydrocephalus may produce this syndrome by enlarging the aqueduct and third ventricle or the suprapineal recess, and so stretching or compressing the posterior commissure.[218] The following case history illustrates certain features of the dorsal midbrain syndrome.

Table 12–6. **Etiology of Disorders of Vertical Gaze**

TUMOR. Classically, pineal germinoma or teratoma in an adolescent male; also pineocytoma, pineoblastoma, glioma, metastasis,[17,38,52,157,855] or as a remote effect of cancer in anti MA2 encephalitis.[239]

HYDROCEPHALUS. Usually aqueductal stenosis leading to dilatation of the third ventricle and aqueduct or enlargement of the suprapineal recess with pressure on the posterior commissure.[356,807]

VASCULAR. Midbrain or thalamic hemorrhage,[324,325,954,1083] infarction,[93,106,110,159,591,705,835] or subdural hematoma.[862,904]

METABOLIC. Niemann-Pick variants,[198,322,934] Gaucher's disease,[1141,1164] Tay-Sachs disease,[509] Maple syrup urine disease,[677,1208] Wilson's disease,[572] kernicterus.[488]

DRUG-INDUCED. Barbiturates,[301] carbamazepine,[83] neuroleptic agents.[151,620]

DEGENERATIVE. Progressive supranuclear palsy,[933,1033,1139] Huntington's disease,[208,607,624] cortical basal degeneration,[383,901,902] diffuse Lewy body disease,[648] others[958,1185]

MISCELLANEOUS. Multiple sclerosis,[349,1011] Whipple's disease,[7,580,973] hypoxia,[563] encephalitis,[51] syphilis,[815,1029] aneurysm,[217] trauma,[548] neurosurgical procedure,[974] mesencephalic clefts,[598] tuberculoma, trauma, benign transient form of childhood,[9,167,489,809,810] variant of hereditary spastic ataxia[415]

CASE HISTORY: Vertical Gaze Palsy with Midbrain Hemorrhage

A 38-year-old woman presented with a 10-day history of fever, sores in her mouth, bruises, and profound tiredness. Hematological findings were consistent with monocytic leukemia in blastic crisis. One day after admission she became stuporous and developed a right hemiparesis.

On examination the left pupil was oval, approximately 5 mm in diameter, and fixed. The right pupil was 3 mm and fully reactive. There was a full range of horizontal eye movements, but with continuous square-wave jerks during attempted fixation. She had complete paralysis of vertical eye movements above the midline. Below the horizontal meridian, downward pursuit was abnormal and saccades, both up and down, appeared slow. There was a downward beating nystagmus on attempting to look down. Horizontal saccades appeared to be of normal velocity but horizontal pursuit was bilaterally impaired. There was some horizontal gaze-evoked nystagmus. Vergence could not be elicited.

Computed tomography (Fig. 12–11A) demonstrated a hemorrhage in the left midbrain. The patient died a few days later. Examination of the brain confirmed the presence of the midbrain hemorrhage with compression and displacement of the aqueduct and the posterior commissure (Fig. 12–11B).

Comment: This patient showed evidence of left oculomotor nerve dysfunction and dorsal midbrain syndrome. Although CT indicated a unilateral midbrain lesion, autopsy showed that the posterior commissure was compressed. Moreover, the hemorrhage was located so as to affect fibers coursing into and out of the posterior commissure. Involvement of the left cerebral peduncle accounted for the right hemiparesis.

Clinical Manifestations of Other Midbrain Lesions

The effects of lesions affecting other midbrain structures are less certain. The periaqueductal gray matter of the midbrain is known to contain burst-tonic neurons that cease discharge during saccades. Selective loss of downgaze with tonic upward deviation of the eyes has been reported with lesions affecting the periaqueductal gray matter of the midbrain.[504,1083]

Rarely, both elevator muscles of one eye may be selectively impaired with midbrain lesions. This *double elevator palsy* may be a supranuclear paresis of monocular elevation, because in the central position, the eyes are nearly straight and only on looking upward does a vertical disconjugacy become evident.[474,508] This disorder has been described with midbrain infarction and tumor, and the lesion may be located ipsilaterally or contralaterally to the palsy.[474] Rarely, it is congenital.[75,1220] Monocular elevator palsy may be associated with a contralateral depressor paresis.[1174]

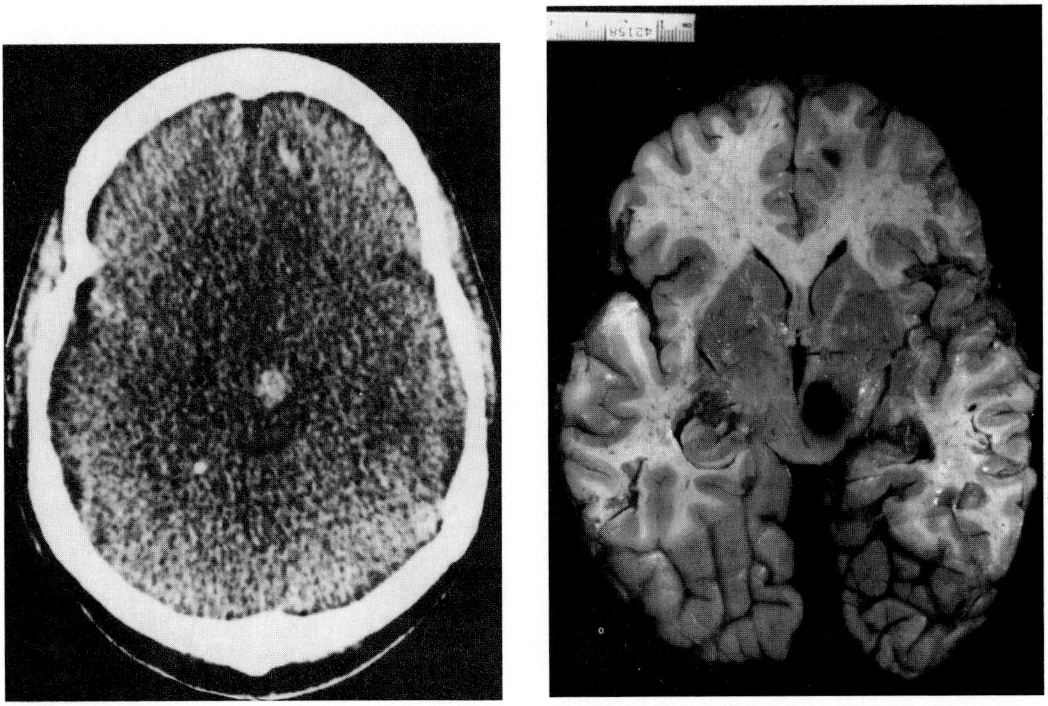

A B

Figure 12–11. Upgaze paralysis due to midbrain hemorrhage (see Case History: Vertical gaze palsy with midbrain hemorrhage; see text for details). (A) This CT scan shows the appearance of a left midbrain hemorrhage (right side of scan shows left side of brain). (B) At autopsy, the hemorrhage was shown to compress the aqueduct and posterior commissure (basal view).

If both the superior rectus and inferior oblique muscles are weak, then a nuclear lesion is unlikely, because the inferior oblique is supplied by the ipsilateral oculomotor nucleus and the superior rectus is supplied by the contralateral nucleus. It is possible, therefore, that the site of the lesion for monocular elevator palsy is prenuclear. However, if this is the case, the lesion must lie close to the ocular motoneurons because the saccadic signals from each riMLF project bilaterally to the elevator subnuclei (see Fig. 6–5, Chapter 6). A more plausible explanation for monocular elevator palsy is that it is due to a lesion selectively involving the oculomotor fascicles supplying the inferior oblique and superior rectus muscles, as the third nerve exits the brainstem.[370] Orbital MRI in some affected patients shows atrophy of the superior rectus muscle.[162] In most instances, however, patients with restricted elevation of one eye will have more common processes such as thyroid ophthalmopathy, blowout fracture of the orbit, myasthenia gravis, and restrictive ophthalmopathies (see Table 9–4 in Chapter 9).

Unilateral, paramedian midbrain lesions may cause midbrain paresis of horizontal gaze, with impairment of ipsilateral, horizontal smooth pursuit by affecting the descending smooth-pursuit pathway.[1200] Contralateral saccades may also be affected,[115,696,1200] but the horizontal VOR tends to be spared (Roth-Bielschowsky phenomenon).[241] Paramedian midbrain lesions often involve the oculomotor nerve nucleus, producing a combination of nuclear and prenuclear deficits. Nuclear oculomotor nerve palsies are often characterized by bilateral elevator and lid weakness, and pupillary abnormalities are common (discussed in Chapter 9). Occasionally, large midbrain lesions may lead to complete ophthalmoplegia.[918,1184]

As discussed in Chapter 3, the central midbrain reticular formation (cMRF) has extensive connections with structures concerned with saccadic eye movements, such as the superior colliculus, supplementary eye fields, and PPRF (see Box 6–9). The effects of lesions in this area are summarized in Box 12–13 and discussed in the following section on progressive supranuclear palsy.

Selective Cell Vulnerability in the Midbrain

PROGRESSIVE SUPRANUCLEAR PALSY

General Features of Progressive Supranuclear Palsy

Progressive supranuclear palsy is a degenerative disease of later life (mean age of onset about 65 years), which is characterized by abnormal eye movements (Box 12–14), difficulties with swallowing and speech, mental slowing, and disturbance of tone and posture that leads to falls within a year of onset.[656,764] Patients have a characteristic look of astonishment and may also show retrocollis with their eyes also being somewhat elevated in the

Box 12–13. Findings With Unilateral Lesions Of The Central Mesencephalic Reticular Formation (cMRF)*

- Ipsilateral gaze shift
- Hypermetria of contralateral and upward saccades; hypometria of ipsilateral and downward saccades
- Fixation disrupted by saccadic intrusions directed away from the side of inactivation

* Based on experimental pharmacological inactivation
For related anatomy and pathophysiology, see Box 6-9, and Fig. 6-3 in Chapter 6. For related clinical etiologies, see Table 12-6.

Box 12–14. Clinical Features Of Progressive Supranuclear Palsy (PSP)

- Slow vertical saccades, especially down, with a preserved range of movement, may be the first sign of the disorder; later, loss of vertical saccades and quick phases
- Horizontal saccades become slow and hypometric
- Disruption of steady gaze by horizontal saccadic intrusions (square-wave jerks)
- Impaired smooth pursuit, vertically (reduced range) and horizontally (with catch-up saccades)
- Smooth eye-head tracking may be relatively preserved, especially vertically
- Preservation of vestibulo-ocular reflex
- Horizontal disconjugacy suggesting INO
- Loss of convergence
- Ultimately, all eye movements may be lost, but vestibular movements are the last to go
- Eyelid disorders: apraxia of lid opening, lid lag, repetitive blinking in response to flashlight stimulus (failure to habituate), blepharospasm
- Tonic head deviation opposite to direction of body rotation (vestibulocollic reflex)
- Inability to clap *just* three times (applause sign)

For related anatomy, see: Brainstem Connections for Vertical and Torsional Movements, Fig. 6-4, and Fig. 6-5 in Chapter 6. For recorded examples, see Fig. 7-9B in Chapter 7, and Fig. 12-12. (Related Video Display: Parkinsonian Syndromes)

orbits. Median survival time is about six years after onset;[392,682] death is commonly due to aspiration pneumonia or the consequence of falls. The disease is uncommon and most cases are sporadic.[256,1076]

Patients with PSP may present with visual complaints such as blurred vision or photophobia,[764] and have often had several different spectacle refractions. By talking with the patient, it is usually possible to determine that these visual symptoms are a consequence of vertical saccadic palsy, so that they have difficulty looking down to eat from a plate of food or to tie their shoe laces. Falls are also a common early complaint.

Eye Movement Examination in Progressive Supranuclear Palsy

The disturbance of eye movements is often present early in the course, but occasionally is noted late or not at all.[248,900,933] The initial ocular motor deficit consists of slowing of *vertical saccades,* either down or up or both, evident as the patient voluntarily redirects gaze between two stationary targets that are separated in the vertical plane (see Figure 12–12 and see Video Display: Parkinsonian Syndromes). Quick phases of optokinetic nystagmus may be reduced or absent, so that the direction of gaze moves up or down with the optokinetic stimulus into the extremes of gaze.[92,367] Early on, vertical saccades may take a curved or oblique trajectory to the target ("round the houses" sign).[865,933] Vertical smooth pursuit may appear impaired but this is partly due to inability to make catch-up saccades. Thus, tracking is improved when patients attempt to track larger visual displays.[976] Combined eye-head tracking may also be relatively spared, although neck stiffness may limit its range (see Fig. 7–9B, Chapter 7). Eventually, smooth pursuit and saccades are both lost, and this combined deficit constitutes voluntary gaze palsy.

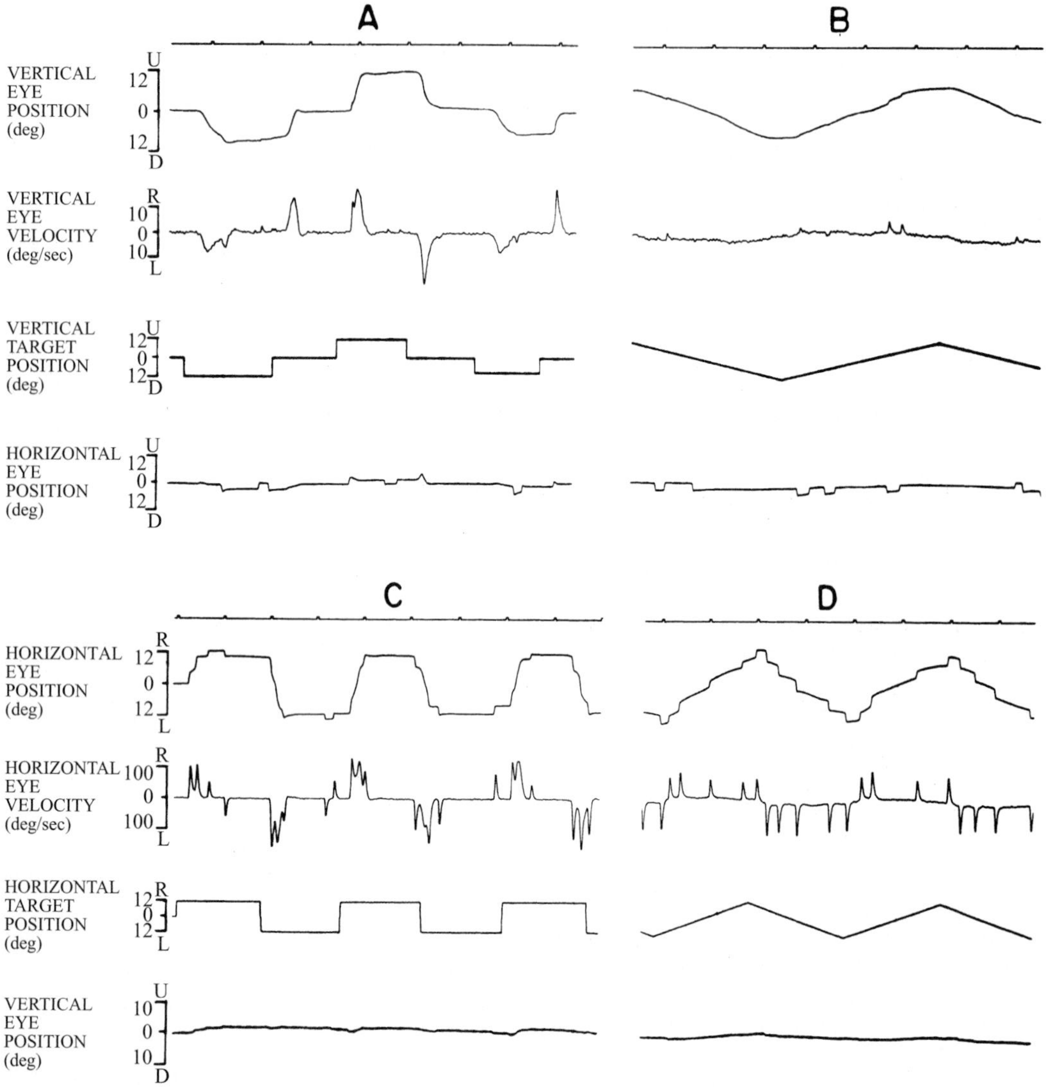

Figure 12–12. Ocular motor findings in progressive supranuclear palsy. Horizontal and vertical eye movements were recorded by the magnetic search coil technique; the time scale at the top of each record is in seconds. (A) Vertical saccades, particularly downward, are slow but generally orthometric. (B) Vertical smooth pursuit is relatively preserved, with occasional, small catch-up saccades best seen on the velocity trace. In both A and B, the horizontal fixation abnormality, square-wave jerks, is evident. (C) Horizontal saccades are hypometric; a "staircase" of small saccades is necessary to acquire the target. (D) Horizontal smooth pursuit shows decreased gain (eye velocity/target velocity) and the superimposed, corrective saccades.

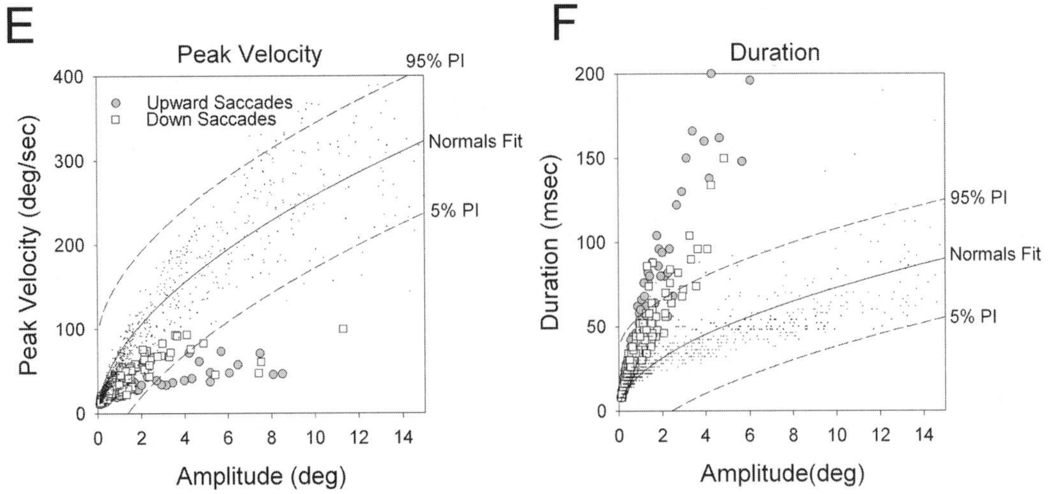

Figure 12–12. *(Continued)* (E and F) Representative plots of amplitude versus peak-velocity (E) or duration (F) for upward and downward saccades of a patient with SPS. Prediction intervals (PI) for a group of normal subjects are also shown.

However, the vestibulo-ocular reflex is preserved until late in the disease (although a characteristic nuchal rigidity may make the vertical doll's head maneuver difficult).

Horizontal eye movements show several characteristic changes, notably disruption of steady fixation by square-wave jerks (see Video Display: Parkinsonian Syndromes).[367,888,933] Horizontal saccades tend to be hypometric, but they only become slow later in the disease.[92] Both horizontal smooth pursuit and eye-head tracking appear impaired, partly by superimposed saccadic intrusions.[246,887,1113] The horizontal vestibulo-ocular reflex is preserved. In some patients, the involvement of voluntary horizontal eye movements resembles internuclear ophthalmoplegia, although vestibular stimulation may overcome the limitation of adduction.[340,698] Convergence eye movements are also commonly impaired. The horizontal vestibulo-ocular reflex is preserved so that patients with absent quick phases but intact vestibular responses may show sustained gaze and head deviations in the opposite direction to body rotation (see Video Display: Parkinsonian Syndromes).[97,595] Late in the disease, the ocular motor deficit may progress to a complete ophthalmoplegia.

Patients with PSP may show several disorders of eyelid movements, including blepharospasm, lid-opening apraxia (see Video Display: Parkinsonian Syndromes), eye-closing apraxia, lid retraction, and lid lag.[260,347] Quite consistently, PSP patients show an inability to inhibit a blink when a penlight is shone in their eyes, a "visual glabellar" or Myerson's sign (see Video Display: Parkinsonian Syndromes).[595] Bell's phenomenon is usually absent.

Measurement of Eye Movements

Saccades: Reliable measurements of saccades in PSP usually requires the scleral search coil technique (Appendix B) because patients often cannot reliably look at target lights during calibration, and are prone to blepharospasm, which disrupts video or reflection techniques. Such studies have demonstrated that vertical saccades are slower than horizontal saccades of similar size.[92] When vertical saccades become small, it is still possible to show that they remain slower than similar sized movements made by controls.[366] The saccadic reaction time (latency) of horizontal saccades in PSP is prolonged in some patients, but others retain the ability to make short-latency express saccades.[847] Patients with PSP make errors on the antisaccade task, when they are required to look in the opposite direction to a suddenly appearing target (Fig. 3–2D). Taken together, the presence of express saccades and errors on the antisaccade task indicate defects in frontal lobe function, and this idea is supported by evidence for frontal hypometabolism on positron emission tomography,[391] as well as other signs of frontal lobe dysfunction.[295]

Smooth-pursuit is usually impaired in both horizontal and vertical planes, although this is more evident in the vertical plane, where no corrective "catch-up" saccades can be made. Tracking of larger moving visual displays is superior to small targets,[976] so that during vertical optokinetic stimulation, PSP patients often show tonic deviation of the eyes in the direction of stripe motion, with small or absent resetting quick phases. When PSP patients make vergence movements combined with saccades to shift their fixation point between distant and near targets, the vergence movement is slowed compared to control subjects.[575]

Vestibular Eye Movements: Measurement of eye movements during horizontal rotation, either in darkness, or during fixation of a stationary target, confirms that the vestibulo-ocular is preserved in PSP patients,[246] but quick phases are often impaired leading to tonic deviation of the eyes opposite to the direction of rotation.

Structural Abnormalities in Progressive Supranuclear Palsy

Progressive supranuclear palsy is a disorder of tau-protein (along with cortical-basal ganglionic degeneration and frontotemporal dementia with chromosome 17).[150,723,1017,1030] There is also evidence for other mechanisms, such as impaired mitochondrial function.[15] Pathologically, there are widespread neurofibrillary tangles, with neuronal loss and gliosis in many subcortical and brainstem areas, partially sparing the neocortex and hippocampus.[210,525,1033,1135] Affected structures include the globus pallidus, substantia nigra (pars compacta and reticulata), periaqueductal gray, brainstem reticular formation, and superior colliculi.[210,432] Decrease of neurons in substantia nigra, pars reticulata is reported to be correlated with the presence of gaze palsy.[421] Some brains show hypertrophy of the inferior olivary nucleus,[428,544] although oculopalatal tremor in PSP is rare.[1053] Recently two phenotypic forms of PSP have been differentiated, one typical for this disorder and the other looking more like Parkinson's disease.[1179] The two forms show differences in the isoform composition of tangle-tau protein in the basal pons (discussed further below).

The atrophy of the midbrain and dilatation of the quadrigeminal cisterns, aqueduct, and third and fourth ventricles, as well as frontal atrophy is often evident on MRI scans.[825,969] The midbrain atrophy leads to the characteristic "humming bird" sign on MRI images (see Video Display: Parkinsonian Disorders).[541] Measurement of the area of the midbrain tegmentum on a midsagittal MRI section appears to provide a reliable way of differentiating PSP from other parkinsonian disorders, especially when the ratio of midbrain to pontine area is calculated.[788]

Pathogenesis of Ocular Motor Findings in Progressive Supranuclear Palsy

The clinical feature that is most distinctive early in the course of PSP is the selective slowing of vertical saccades. This finding probably reflects involvement of the riMLF and adjacent midbrain brainstem reticular formation.[1033] In addition, the nucleus raphe interpositus in the pons is involved, in which are located omnipause neurons (see Fig. 6–2).[897] However, selective involvement of vertical saccades early in the course of the disease indicates that burst neurons in riMLF, rather than omnipause neurons in the pons, are mainly responsible for the clinical finding of slow vertical saccades.[92] If involvement of omnipause neurons were the primary cause of slow saccades in PSP, then both horizontal and vertical saccades should show commensurate slowing early in the course, and this is not the case.[92]

Another common finding is saccadic intrusions (square-wave jerks), which might be related to involvement of the superior colliculus and the adjacent central midbrain reticular formation (cMRF) (see Box 6–9), which have reciprocal connections. Experimental lesions or inactivation of either the cMRF or the rostral pole of the superior colliculus causes fixation to become disrupted by saccadic intrusions (see Box 12–13).[1152,1154] Furthermore, involvement of the substantia nigra, pars reticulata (SNpr) in PSP might interfere with the normal initiation and suppression of saccades via its projections to the superior colliculus (discussed in Chapter 3). Thus, antisaccade responses are abnormal in some PSP patients.[847] Abnormalities of smooth pursuit in PSP might be related to extensive involvement of the dorsolateral pontine nuclei,[684] which are known to be an important relay in the pursuit pathway between visual cortical areas and the cerebellum (see Fig. 6–7, in Chapter 6).

Differential Diagnosis of Progressive Supranuclear Palsy

Recently, it has been suggested that pathologically proven PSP comprises two distinct phenotypes.[1179] One is characterized by early falls, cognitive disturbances and vertical gaze abnormalities, and has been dubbed Richardson's syndrome. The second more closely resemble Parkinson's disease with asymmetric findings, tremor, and some response to levodopa. The two forms also show neuropathological differences that are described below. Unfortunately, eye movements were not carefully examined in half of the patients studied, and more research is required to validate this phenotypic dichotomy.

A number of other conditions can mimic PSP, although patients who show slow vertical saccades, horizontal square-wave jerks, and normal vestibular eye movements, and report dysphagia and frequent falls usually have this disorder. Similar syndromes may be caused by multiple infarcts affecting the basal ganglia, internal capsule, and midbrain.[294,745] Whipple's disease, discussed in the following section, can also closely mimic PSP, and oculomasticatory myorhythmia, so characteristic of Whipple's disease, may be absent. Frontotemporal lobar degeneration can produce a progressive frontal type of dementia with a PSP-like picture,[824] as can Creutzfeldt–Jakob disease.[524] Disorders causing the dorsal midbrain syndrome (Table 12–6), such as hydrocephalus,[235] can produce a clinical picture that has some similarities to PSP. A syndrome resembling PSP that occurs following cardiac surgery is discussed below under Ocular Motor Apraxia.[727,1105]

Of the parkinsonian degenerative disorders, few produce slow vertical saccades early in the course, although the vertical range of movement may be limited.[933,1139,1171] Thus, idiopathic Parkinson's disease may cause slow saccades late in the course,[933,1139,1171] but, unlike PSP, shows responsiveness to levodopa.

Pure akinesia is characterized by profound disturbances of slowing of gait, speech, and handwriting.[900] For example, affected patients may suffer episodes during which they stand "frozen" for hours on end when they get up during the night to go to the bathroom. Tremor, limb rigidity, akinesia, dementia, or responsiveness to levodopa are absent. Such patients may show some slowing and hypometric vertical saccades. The disorder may be a restricted form of PSP with a longer, more benign course.[900]

Cortical-basal ganglionic degeneration usually does not cause slow saccades, but is associated with increased saccadic latency.[908,933,998] Other features of this degeneration are focal dystonia, ideomotor apraxia, alien hand syndrome, myoclonus, and an asymmetric akinetic-rigid syndrome with late onset of gait or balance disturbances.[86,383,657,901]

Multiple system atrophy (MSA) may also present with features similar to PSP.[887] Measurements of vertical saccadic velocity in MSA have been normal,[933] or showed some mild slowing,[92] whereas positionally induced downbeat nystagmus may be a feature.[88] Diffuse Lewy body disease is reported to mimic PSP,[251,319,648,762] and Parkinson's disease,[662] but descriptions or measurements of vertical saccade dynamics are not yet available. Other basal ganglia disorders that have been reported to show features similar to PSP include familial Lewy body disease,[132] idiopathic striopallidodentate calcification,[958] autosomal dominant parkinsonism and dementia with pallido-ponto-nigral degeneration,[1185] and the amyotrophic lateral sclerosis – parkinsonism dementia complex of Guam (Lytico-Bodig disease).[639]

A group of patients unresponsive to levodopa with a neurological disorder similar to PSP has been described in Guadeloupe;[170,1104] it is possible that this disorder might be attributable to herbal tea containing mitochondrial complex 1 inhibitors, such as quinolines, but more studies are needed to confirm this interesting finding.

Although patients are reported with autopsy-proven PSP in whom abnormal eye movements were not documented, our experience is that careful clinical examination of vertical saccades usually shows slowing;[626] measurements of eye movements often help in difficult cases. In such patients, a history of falls, and the presence of certain associated findings, including lack of habituation of blink to a flashlight stimulus, persistence of a vestibulocollic reflex, and impaired ability to clap the hand just three times, makes the diagnosis of PSP likely.[295,595]

Presently, there are no effective treatments for PSP, although individual patients may benefit from tricyclic antidepressants, serotonergic or adrenergic agents, or dopamine agonists such as bromocriptine.[382,772] Studies of the pharmacological imbalance in PSP may suggest novel approaches for drug therapy.[1159]

WHIPPLE'S DISEASE

This is a rare systemic disorder, caused by *Tropheryma Whippelii* (Whipple-associated bacillus), and characterized by weight loss, diarrhea, arthralgia, lymphadenopathy, and fever.[722] It may involve, and even be confined to, the nervous system.[580,663] *Tropheryma whippelii* shows a predilection for specific areas of the gray matter, in particular, the basal ganglia, which can result in movement disorders, parkinsonism and a clinical picture resembling PSP. Thus, involvement of the rostral mesencephalon, with abnormal vertical gaze, is not uncommon in patients with Whipple's disease of the central nervous system. Initially, vertical saccades may be slow and curved whereas horizontal saccades may be relatively preserved.[43] Eventually, all eye movements may be lost. Oculomasticatory or oculofacioskeletal myorhythmia is virtually pathognomonic of this disease, and consists of rhythmic movements of the masticatory and occasionally other skeletal muscles, synchronized with pendular vergence oscillations of the eyes (see Video Display: Parkinsonian Syndromes).[973,1007] It is almost always accompanied by a supranuclear vertical gaze palsy. However, many patients with Whipple's disease have no ocular oscillations and, in them, study of the dynamic properties of eye movements, including vertical saccades, may help diagnosis[43] Ophthalmoplegia with myorhythmia of the leg, but not of the eyes or jaw, is reported.[871]

Whipple's disease can be diagnosed using polymerase chain reaction (PCR) analysis of involved tissue.[664] PCR analysis of small-bowel biopsy material can be positive in the absence of clinical signs of gastrointestinal involvement, and even when the intestinal tissue is microscopically negative. Positive PCR of the cerebrospinal fluid may also clinch the diagnosis.[617] However, while positive PCR confirms the diagnosis, negative PCR does not exclude it, and sometimes repeat biopsies are indicated. Whipple's disease can be treated with antibiotics,[336] although bacteria may persist in the cerebrospinal fluid even after treatment.[683]

AMYOTROPHIC LATERAL SCLEROSIS AND EYE MOVEMENTS

Clinically, amyotrophic lateral sclerosis (ALS) spares eye movements until very late in the course of the disease, despite severe weakness of the skeletal and bulbar muscles. Neuropathologic studies have indicated that the ocular motoneurons themselves are spared except in very advanced cases.[725,797] The sparing of ocular motoneurons has been related to lower concentrations of glycinergic and muscarinic receptors, or differences in glutamate transporter molecules, compared with motoneurons in other nuclei affected by ALS.[703,1173]

Studies using reliable methods for measuring eye movements and modern test paradigms have defined the spectrum of disturbances of eye movements that may be encountered in ALS. In most patients, the velocities and latencies of visually guided saccades are normal. However, memory-guided saccades are inaccurate, and there are increased errors on the antisaccade task.[995] These findings are consistent with frontal lobe involvement in ALS. Square-wave jerks are more frequent than in control subjects.[995] Impaired or asymmetric smooth pursuit has also been reported.[2,4]

Standing apart from this general picture is a subset of patients in whom disordered eye movements are more prominent early in the course. Such patients usually show slowing of vertical saccades, impairment of smooth pursuit, and gaze-evoked nystagmus.[388,597,691] In two well-studied patients, slow vertical saccades correlated with loss of neurons in the riMLF at autopsy.[40] Another patient with slow saccades and ballismus was reported to show neuronal loss in the interstitial nucleus of Cajal as well as the lower motoneurons in the spinal cord.[578]

We have also studied three patients with abnormal eye movements who had clinical and electrodiagnostic evidence of progressive loss of anterior horn cells.[1077] They showed disproportionately severe involvement of finger and wrist extensors, and relative sparing of facial, pharyngeal, tongue and respiratory musculature. All three had a long course and lack of a family history of similar disorder. Their eye movement abnormalities included downbeat nystagmus with alternating skew deviation, and saccadic oscillations, that suggested cerebellar dysfunction. One patient had modest levels of anti-glutamic acid decarboxylase (GAD) antibodies, which have been reported with idiopathic downbeat nystagmus and also in a patient with spinocerebellar degeneration showing periodic alternating nystagmus. However, these antibodies have also been associated with insulin-dependent diabetes and stiff-person syndrome, raising the possibility that they are an epiphenomenona caused by neuronal damage rather than a factor in pathogenesis.[1101] Thus, the biological significance of slow saccades, downbeat nystagmus and other ocular motor abnormalities in variants of ALS has yet to be determined.

OCULAR MOTOR SYNDROMES CAUSED BY LESIONS IN THE SUPERIOR COLLICULUS

Lesions confined to the superior colliculi are rare in humans. One patient who had undergone removal of an angioma from the right superior colliculus showed persistent limitation of upward gaze, implying pretectal damage, but a full range of horizontal eye movements.[459] Systematic testing of horizontal saccades demonstrated a paucity of spontaneous refixations contralateral to the side of the lesion. Saccades to the left occurred after a normal latency but were hypometric. A second patient who had a hematoma largely restricted to the right superior colliculus showed defects in latency and accuracy for contralateral saccades and increased numbers of inappropriate saccades in the antisaccade task.[848] These findings show similarities to results of surgical ablation of the superior colliculi in monkeys.[13] More discrete lesions of the superior colliculus in monkey cause increased latency of saccades, with some slowing, deficits which endure; however, the accuracy of saccades recovers to normal.[426] Thus, enduring effects on saccadic accuracy probably reflect involvement of adjacent reticular formation beyond the superior colliculus.

A number of more diffuse disorders, such as progressive supranuclear palsy, involve the superior colliculus and adjacent mesencephalic reticular formation at autopsy.[210] For reasons similar to those given above for the effects of vascular disease, it is difficult to draw conclusions about the role of the superior colliculus in such disorders. For example, express saccades, which are considered to be the most sensitive index of superior colliculus function, are preserved in some patients with PSP.[847] At present, it seems that the ability to view the human superior colliculus by fMRI is the most promising way to confirm whether the superior colliculus plays the same pivotal role in the control of saccades that has been shown in the monkey; preliminary studies indicate that it does.[769]

OCULAR MOTOR SYNDROMES CAUSED BY LESIONS IN THE DIENCEPHALON

Effects of Thalamic Lesions on Eye Movements

Lesions affecting the thalamus (see Box 6–22) are characterized by disturbances of both horizontal and vertical gaze (Box 12–15).[324] Conjugate deviation of the eyes *contralateral* to the side of the lesion—wrong-way deviation—may occur with hemorrhage affecting the medial thalamus.[327,549] The reason for this contraversive deviation is unclear. The descending pathways from the frontal eye fields to the pons have not yet crossed at this level, although the notion of a discrete ocular motor decussation lacks confirmation. Involvement of the descending pathway for smooth pursuit might lead to a paretic, contraversive deviation of the eyes,[986] but a patient with a defect of smooth pursuit directed toward the side of a small hemorrhage in the posterior thalamus and adjacent internal capsule still showed an ipsiversive gaze preference.[133a] Another possibility is that wrong-way deviation may be an irritative phenomenon; electrical stimulation in the region of the thalamic intramedullary lamina (IML) elicits contralaterally directed saccades (discussed in Chapter 3).

Tonic downward gaze deviation of the eyes, with convergence and miosis, is another common feature of thalamic hemorrhage; affected patients appear to peer at their noses.[325] However, in autopsied cases, the hemorrhage usually has extended into or compressed the midbrain.[182] Hence, forced downward deviation of the eyes probably represents a compressive effect of the hemorrhage on structures

Box 12–15. Clinical Effects Of Diencephalic Lesions

Thalamic Lesions (Central Nuclei)

- Conjugate gaze deviation away from the side of the lesion ("wrong-way deviation")
- Sustained downward deviation of the eyes, (due to compression of the dorsal midbrain), sometimes with convergence—"thalamic esotropia"
- Inaccuracy of memory-guided saccades if gaze changes during the memory period

Lesions Of The Pulvinar

- Difficulties in shifting gaze into the contralateral hemifield
- Decrease in spontaneous scanning
- No reduction of the saccadic reaction time if fixation point is turned off when the visual target is presented

For related anatomy, see Box 6-18, and Box 6-22 in Chapter 6. For pathophysiology of saccadic defects see: The role of the internal medullary lamina (IML) in saccade generation and the role of the pulvinar in saccade generation in Chapter 3.

responsible for upgaze. Resolution of the downward deviation has followed treatment of raised intracranial pressure,[1151] suggesting that traction on midbrain structures or hydrocephalus may be responsible in some patients.

Thalamic esotropia occurring with caudal thalamic lesions may be marked and sometimes is unassociated with downward deviation;[396,458] it may reflect a disturbance of vergence inputs to the oculomotor nuclei (organic convergence spasm, see Chapter 8). Patients with posterolateral thalamic infarctions may have disturbances of the subjective visual vertical (either ipsilateral or contralateral),[284] and show reduced activation of multisensory vestibular temporo-parietal cortex ipsilateral to the lesion on fMRI.[282] However, the ocular tilt reaction is not present unless the rostral midbrain is also involved. Saccades made to sounds may be hypometric contralateral to the side of central thalamic lesions.[1136]

Infarction of the caudal thalamus, caused by occlusion of the proximal portion of the posterior cerebral artery or its perforator branch, the posterior thalamosubthalamic paramedian artery, is reported to produce paralysis of downgaze. In fact, this deficit is probably due to involvement of the adjacent riMLF or its immediate premotor inputs (see Box 12–9).[186,1000] Some patients also show impairment of horizontal gaze, perhaps due to interruption of descending pathways,[93,637] or of the mesencephalic reticular formation.[1153] Associated disturbances of arousal and short-term memory have been ascribed to involvement of adjacent thalamic nuclei.[90,1167] Experimentally, combined lesions of the superior colliculus and caudal thalamus in monkeys lead to an enduring saccadic hypometria without corrective saccades;[14] similar results in humans would confirm the importance of the caudal thalamus and superior colliculus in the generation of saccades.

Patients with lesions affecting the central thalamic nuclei show a specific defect: memory-guided saccades become inaccurate only if the eyes move to a new position during the memory period (e.g., a smooth-pursuit movement or saccade).[76,377] We have observed similar effects in a patient with a large central thalamic lesion (Fig. 12–13): memory-guided saccades were only inaccurate if gaze shifted during the memory period in a smooth-pursuit movement. Visually guided saccades were similar to

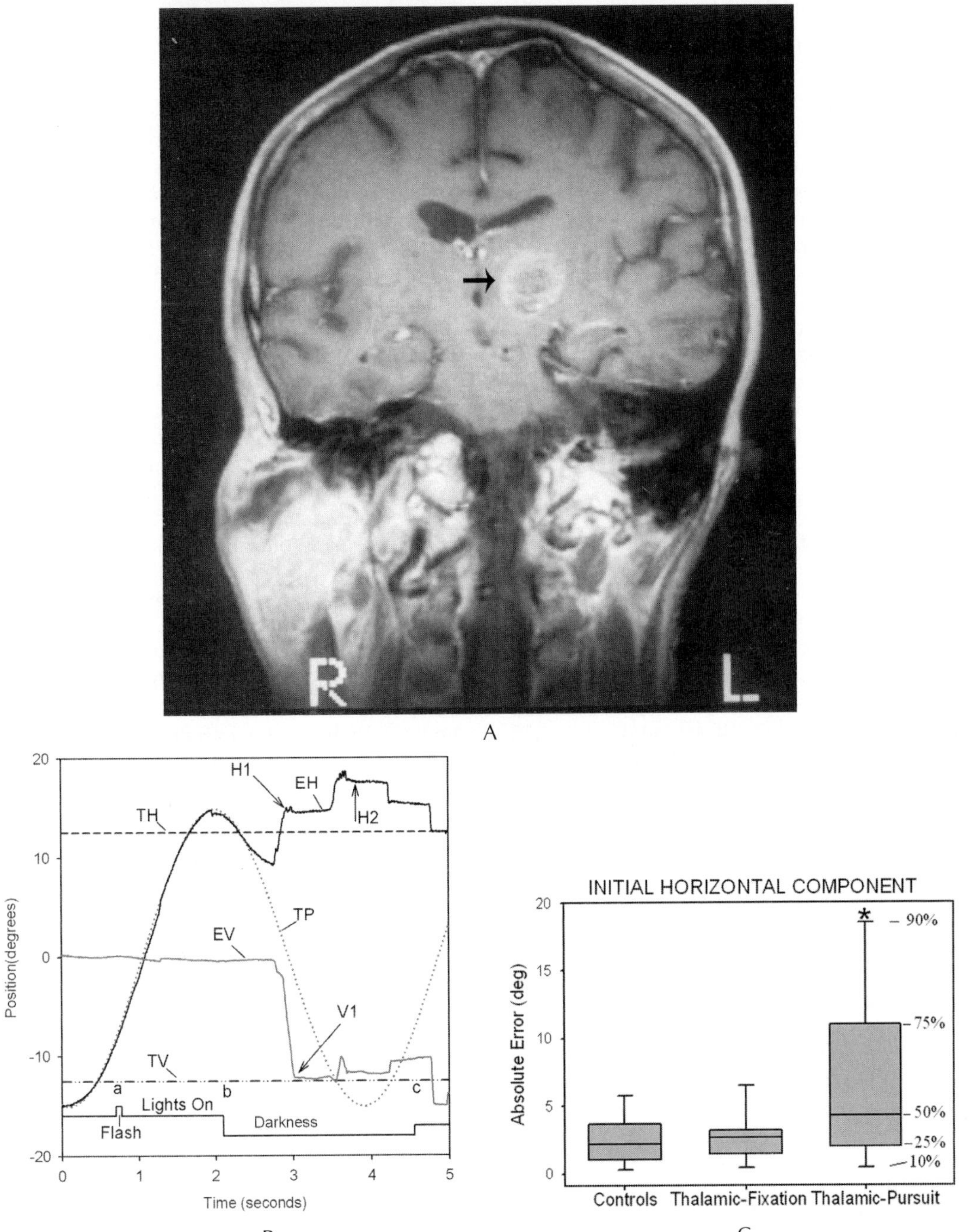

Figure 12–13. Patient with a metastasis in his left central thalamus (A) showed inaccurate memory-guided saccades only when his eyes moved (in horizontal smooth pursuit) during the memory period (B). At the beginning, he smoothly pursues a white spot of light (TP) moving sinusoidally in the horizontal plane; EH is horizontal eye position; EV is vertical eye position. At 0.6 s, a red visual target is flashed for 75 ms (a); it is located 12 degrees to the right and below center (TH and TV indicate its horizontal and vertical coordinates). The patient continues to horizontally track the primary target until 2 seconds (b), when the room is switched to complete darkness; this is the cue to make a memory-guided saccade. After the visual target is switched on again (c), the patient starts to make corrective movements towards the target. The initial horizontal saccade (H1) is in the correct direction but overshoots the target location, and the second saccade (H2) increases this error, whereas the vertical saccade (V1) is accurate. Thus, the patient has not fully taken into account the horizontal pursuit eye movement that occurred during the memory period of 1.4s (from a until b). (C) Comparison of absolute error of horizontal components of first memory-guided saccade (corresponding to H1 in panel B) made by a group of 11 control subjects and the thalamic patient. Controls showed no difference whether gaze was stationary in fixation, or moved in pursuit, during the memory period, and data are pooled. The patient only showed an increase in error if his gaze moved during the memory period (*indicates $p < 0.05$ with rank-sum test). The patient's visually guided saccades were similar to controls.

controls.[593] This finding suggests that the central thalamus normally relays an efference copy (in this case a smooth-pursuit shift of gaze during the memory period) to cortical areas that program memory-guided saccades, and is consistent with experimental inactivation of the medial dorsal or ventrolateral thalamus in monkey.[1022,1069] Lesions in the posterior parietal cortex and the supplementary eye field of the frontal lobes create similar deficits.[296,442] Lesions affecting the ventrolateral (cerebellar) thalamus show impaired ability to adapt saccades to novel visual stimuli.[378]

Effects of Pulvinar Lesions on Eye Movements

Studies of patients with lesions of the posterior thalamus, the pulvinar (see Box 6–18), have shown difficulties in shifting attention and gaze into the contralateral hemifield, manifest by a paucity and prolonged latency for visually guided saccades (Box 12–15), and, with right-sided lesions, hemispatial neglect.[537] Thus, such patients show no reduction of the saccadic reaction time if the fixation point is turned off when the visual target is presented, whereas normal subjects do.[870] This result, which was obtained in patients without visual neglect, replicates older studies showing that pulvinar lesions in humans cause a prolongation of fixation and difficulties in shifting gaze into the contralateral hemifield.[793,1222] Taken along with studies in monkey, which are summarized in Chapter 6, current evidence indicates that the pulvinar is important for disengaging visual fixation when a shift of attention (and gaze) is to be made.[793,1222]

OCULAR MOTOR ABNORMALITIES AND DISEASE OF THE BASAL GANGLIA

Parkinson's Disease and Conditions Causing Parkinsonism

PARKINSON'S DISEASE

Clinical Findings in Parkinson's Disease

Routine bedside examination of the eye movements of most patients with Parkinson's disease (PD) shows only minor findings, and most of these also occur in age-matched control subjects. Thus, steady fixation may be disrupted by saccadic intrusions (square-wave jerks),[888,1171] but these are also seen in some normal subjects.[1,455] Many clinicians look for restriction of the range of upward gaze, but this is similarly limited in normal, elderly individuals as well as in patients with PD,[178,187,794] possibly due to age-related changes in orbital tissues.[268] Moreover, both smooth pursuit and convergence are impaired in both parkinsonian patients and otherwise healthy elderly subjects,[933] although convergence insufficiency is more likely to be symptomatic in PD.[95,868,895] Thus, unlike progressive supranuclear palsy, PD calls for special testing to bring out abnormalities that generally require laboratory testing, (Box 12–16 and Fig. 3–2, Chapter 3). One exception is the difficulty that most PD patients have in making self-paced saccades between two continuously visible targets. This is brought out by asking the patient to look between to widely spaced targets, such as the examiners fingers positioned to elicit horizontal saccades through about three-quarters of the patient's ocular motor range. Under these circumstances, PD patients typically make near-accurate saccades when verbally instructed ("right, left, right" etc.). However, when they are instructed to maintain this activity on their own, their saccades invariably become hypometric (see Video Display: Parkinsonian Syndromes). PD patients also show a variety of disorders of eyelid movements, including lid retraction on looking straight ahead and lid lag on downgaze.[39] Unlike patients with PSP, they habituate their blink response when a flashlight is repetitively shone into one eye.[595]

Saccadic Abnormalities in Parkinson's Disease

Saccades in PD are typically *hypometric*, especially vertically.[751,885,933,1171] The characteristic finding noted above–hypometria that becomes more marked when patients are asked to perform self-paced refixations between two continuously visible targets (see Video Display: Parkinsonian Syndromes)— is not, however, due simply to the persistence of the target light. Thus, saccades made in anticipation of the appearance of a target light, or to a remembered target location (Fig. 3–2C), are also

Box 12–16. Clinical Findings In Parkinson's Disease

- Fixation may be disrupted by square-wave jerks
- Hypometria of horizontal and vertical saccades, especially when patients are asked to perform rapid, self-paced refixations between two continuously visible targets
- Normal saccadic velocity except in some advanced cases
- Impaired smooth pursuit, horizontally and vertically, due partly to inadequate catch-up saccades
- Vestibular eye movements normal for natural head movements
- Impaired convergence
- Oculogyric crises
- Lid lag

For pathophysiology, see: The Role of the Basal Ganglia in Saccade Generation, in Chapter 3. (Related Video Display: Parkinsonian Syndromes)

hypometric.[222,666,668] In fact, patients with PD have difficulty in generating memory-guided saccades to a range of stimuli,[761,994,1133,1138] with "fragmented" multistep responses.[570] Paradoxically, if the memory period is prolonged from 3 to 30 seconds, performance is actually improved.[618] Taken with other studies,[841] the inference is that intermediate spatial memory, which depends on dorsolateral prefrontal cortex, is impaired in Parkinson's disease, whereas longer-term memory, which depends on parahippocampal cortex and medial temporal lobe, is preserved. Patients with PD may also make large errors when they make saccades to remembered target locations,[228] including to a sequence of remembered targets.[179] These deficits suggest both impaired ability to inhibit saccades and deficits in spatial working memory.[179]

In contrast, saccades made reflexively to novel visual stimuli are of normal amplitude and usually are promptly initiated.[933,1139] Thus, it appears that parkinsonian patients are unable to generate saccades internally that accurately shift gaze.[138,1131,1162] Despite this tendency to hypometria, PD patients can still shift their gaze, using a series of saccades, to the location of a target that is briefly flashed; this indicates a retained ability to encode the location of objects in extrapersonal space.[222,1171] Adaptation of saccades to novel visual stimuli is impaired in Parkinsonian patients, who are able to decrease, but not increase, the saccade gain.[674] The saccadic initiation defect to command or to continuously visible targets appears to be more marked in the vertical plane; upward saccades especially may be hypometric. In contrast, vertical saccades to randomly appearing visual targets are normal.[667] If downward saccades are abnormal or the velocity of vertical saccades in either direction is decreased, a diagnosis of progressive supranuclear palsy (PSP) is more likely.

Saccadic reaction time (latency) during non-predictable tracking may be normal, mildly increased or even decreased compared with controls.[138,179,1171] During self-paced refixations between two visible targets, intersaccadic intervals increase above values during non-predictable tracking.[222,1131] Application of the "gap" paradigm (turning out the fixation light before the target light is turned on—Fig. 3–2B) has demonstrated that PD patients are able to make short-latency express saccades.[179,1139] Saccadic velocity is usually normal, except in some advanced cases.[933,1139,1171]

Patients with advanced PD may show greater defects on certain tests than patients with mild or moderate disease. Thus, on the one hand, some patients with mild PD perform normally on the antisaccade task.[574,667] On the other hand, other patients show more directional errors,[133,179] and this increases with advancing disease,[228] especially when patients are also taking anticholinergic drugs.[574]

Rapid eye-head movements (gaze saccades) may also be abnormal in PD; affected patients tend not to move their heads unless instructed to do so.[1172] During rapid eye-head gaze shifts, in response to either predictable or nonpredictable step displacements of the target, patients show increased latency and slowing of head movements.

Smooth Pursuit in Parkinson's Disease

Smooth-pursuit movements are usually impaired in PD, though mildly affected patients differ little from age-matched control subjects.[933,1162] During tracking of a target moving in a predictable, sinusoidal pattern, pursuit gain (eye velocity/target velocity) is decreased leading to catch-up saccades.[885,1171] It appears that at least part of the defect during tracking of a smoothly moving target is that the catch-up saccades are hypometric; thus, the cumulative tracking eye movement (pursuit plus saccades) is less than that of the target.[1162] Despite the impairment of smooth-pursuit gain, the phase relationship between eye and target movement during tracking of a periodic target is normal;[138] which implies a normal predictive smooth tracking strategy in PD. This is in contrast to predictive tracking of saccades, which is impaired in PD.

Visuo-Vestibular Interactions in Parkinson's Disease

Low-frequency rotational and caloric vestibular responses, in darkness, may be reduced in patients with PD.[891,1170] However, at higher frequencies of head rotation corresponding to those during natural activities such as locomotion, and particularly during visual fixation, the gain of the vestibulo-ocular reflex (VOR) is close to 1.0, which accounts for the lack of complaint of oscillopsia in patients with PD.[1170]

Combined eye-head tracking (VOR cancellation or suppression) is abnormal to a similar degree as smooth pursuit with the head stationary in most patients with PD (see Disorders Of Smooth Eye-Head Tracking in Chapter 7).[409,1162,1172]

Effects of Treatment on Eye Movements in Parkinson's Disease

In general, levodopa treatment of PD has little effect on the ocular motor deficits except for some improvement of saccadic accuracy (i.e., saccades become larger),[385,885] and improvement of convergence insufficiency in occasional patients.[868] Despite general improvement with add-on therapy such as pergolide, errors on the antisaccade task may increase.[229] Some newly diagnosed patients with idiopathic PD may show improved smooth pursuit after the institution of dopaminergic therapy.[385] In one patient with advanced PD, electrical stimulation of the pallidum was reported to improve performance on memory-guided and antisaccade tasks.[1042] Bilateral, high-frequency stimulation of the subthalamic nucleus improved the accuracy of memory-guided saccades, but had no effect on visually guided saccades or on responses to the antisaccade test.[907] Conversely, pallidotomy is reported to induce square-wave jerks in parkinsonian patients,[45,786] and reduce the velocity of internally generated saccades.[102]

In patients with parkinsonism due to methyl-4-phenyl-1,2,3,6-tetrahydropyridine (MPTP) toxicity, saccadic reaction time was shortened and accuracy was improved by dopaminergic agents; additionally, reflex blepharospasm in these patients was improved.[483] Similarly, in monkeys who received MPTP, saccadic abnormalities, including increased latency, increased duration, decreased rate of spontaneous saccades, and inappropriate saccades, were all reversed by dopaminergic therapy.[141,971]

In those patients with idiopathic PD who show pronounced drug-related fluctuations, there is disagreement as to whether smooth pursuit shows an increase in gain during "on" periods.[384,885,987] The dopaminergic pars compacta of the substantia nigra does not appear to contain neurons related to eye movement, whereas the pars reticulata does.[463] (The influence of the substantia nigra pars reticulata (SNpr) and the nigro-collicular pathway in the control of saccades is discussed in Chapters 3 and 6.) In monkeys with MPTP-induced parkinsonism, cerebral metabolic rate was reduced in the frontal eye fields and paralamellar mediodorsal thalamus;[468] it is possible that these metabolic changes are secondary to loss of projections from the dopamine-depleted substantia nigra.

OTHER CONDITIONS CAUSING PARKINSONISM

A common diagnostic challenge is to differentiate patients with other parkinsonian states from those with PD; although general neurologic findings and response to levodopa are important factors, a careful observation or measurement of eye movements can often help. Thus, as discussed above, slow vertical saccades usually indicate progressive supranuclear palsy and pure akinesia, which may be a precursor of PSP.[900] Slow saccades are also characteristic of Creutzfeldt–Jakob disease, but in both horizontal and vertical planes.[408] Cortical-basal ganglionic degeneration does not cause slow saccades, but the latency of visually guided saccades is increased beyond that typical of PD.[933,1139] In some patients with multiple system atrophy (MSA), saccades may show mild slowing and are hypometric.[92,933] An additional finding in MSA is positionally induced downbeat nystagmus.[88] At present there are no published quantitative data on the velocity of vertical saccades in diffuse Lewy-body disease, which is reported to cause a vertical gaze palsy.[251,648] However, patients with diffuse Lewy body dementia as well as patients with Parkinson's disease dementia or Alzheimer's disease show more errors on complex tasks such as the antisaccade test (Fig. 3–2D) than patients with idiopathic Parkinson's disease.[746] Furthermore, patients with diffuse Lewy body dementia or Parkinson's disease dementia show increased reaction time in response to the gap paradigm (Fig. 3–2B). Patients with the syndrome of amyotrophic lateral sclerosis, parkinsonism, and dementia (Lytico-Bodig), which is encountered in the inhabitants of the islands of the South Pacific Ocean, including Guam, may show more severe deficits than those with idiopathic PD, including limitation of vertical gaze.[639,811]

OCULOGYRIC CRISIS

This unusual state was a common feature of postencephalitic parkinsonism but is now usually a side effect of drugs, especially neuroleptic agents.[83,151,302,345,401,512,620,879,955] A typical attack of oculogyric crisis is ushered in by feelings of fear or depression, which give rise to an obsessive fixation on a thought. The eyes typically deviate upward, and sometimes laterally; they rarely deviate downward (see Video Display: Parkinsonian Syndromes). During the period of upward deviation, the movements of the eyes in the upper field of gaze appear nearly normal. Affected patients have great difficulty in looking down, except when they combine a blink and downward saccade. Thus, the ocular disorder may reflect an imbalance of the vertical gaze-holding mechanism (neural integrator). Anticholinergic drugs promptly terminate the thought disorder and ocular deviation, a finding that has led to the suggestion that the disorders of thought and eye movements are linked by a pharmacological imbalance common to both.[620] Delayed oculogyric crises have been described after striatocapsular infarction,[658] and due to bilateral putaminal hemorrhage.[997]

Oculogyric crises can usually be distinguished from the brief upward ocular deviations that occur in Tourette's syndrome, Rett's syndrome,[333] Lesch-Nyhan disease,[513] in many patients with tardive dyskinesia,[332] and rarely as a dopa-induced dyskinesia in Parkinson's disease.[653] Occasional patients with tardive dyskinesias show more sustained eye deviations, and also have the characteristic neuropsychological syndrome of oculogyric crises.[949] Episodic brief spells of tonic upgaze have been noted after bilateral lentiform lesions.[569] Some infants show paroxysmal tonic upgaze, accompanied by neck flexion, and an otherwise normal neurological examination;[489,809] about half of all children make a good recovery whereas ataxia, mild cognitive or ocular motor abnormalities persist in the remander.[809] A genetic defect may be present in some affected children.[523]

Huntington's Disease (HD)

CLINICAL FINDINGS IN HUNTINGTON'S DISEASE

Huntington's Disease (HD) is due to a defect of the IT15 gene on chromosome 4 causing increased CAG triplet repeat length and the protein "huntingtin." HD produces

Box 12–17. Ocular Motor Findings In Huntington's Disease

- Difficulties initiating saccades—facilitated by an associated head thrust or blink
- Difficulties suppressing reflexive saccades to novel visual stimuli (especially during the antisaccade task)
- Slow saccades, especially vertically, and in patients with early age of onset
- Impairment of smooth pursuit
- Preservation of VOR and gaze-holding

For pathophysiology, see: The Role of the Basal Ganglia in Saccade Generation, in Chapter 3. For a recorded example, see Fig. 12-14 of Chapter 12. (Related Video Display: Parkinsonian Syndromes)

disturbances of voluntary gaze, especially saccades (Box 12–17).[208,607,607,608,1091] Often there is impaired initiation of saccades with prolonged latencies, especially when the saccade is made to command or in anticipation of a target that is moving in a predictable fashion. Patients use an obligatory blink or head turn to start the eye movement component of the gaze shift (see Video Display: Parkinsonian Syndromes).[1202] Paradoxically, there are often difficulties in suppressing saccades during fixation, with increased visual distractibility. In some patients, saccades may be slow in the horizontal or vertical plane. Although this is more evident later in the course of the disease,[624] saccadic slowing can be detected at an earlier stage in the disease if eye movements are measured.[208] Saccades tend to be slower in patients who become symptomatic at an earlier age; it has been suggested that such individuals are more likely to have inherited the disease from their father.[609] Smooth pursuit may also be impaired but gaze holding and the vestibulo-ocular reflex (VOR) are well preserved, although the ability to adapt the VOR to new visual demands is impaired.[321] Late in the disease, rotational stimulation causes the eyes to tonically deviate with few or no quick phases. Fixation is abnormal in some patients with Huntington's disease because of saccadic intrusions.[624] This defect of steady fixation is particularly evident when patients view a textured background.[208]

LABORATORY STUDIES AND THE PATHOGENESIS OF OCULAR MOTOR FINDINGS IN HUNTINGTON'S DISEASE

The paradoxical finding of difficulty in initiating voluntary saccades, but with an excess of extraneous saccades during attempted fixation, has been clarified using novel test stimuli (Fig. 3–2). For example, HD patients make increased errors during the antisaccade task (Fig. 12–14), consistent with the excessive distractibility during clinical testing.[608] A second finding is that saccades to visual stimuli are made at normal latency, while those made to command are delayed. Longitudinal studies of saccades have documented progressive slowing and prolongation of reaction time.[940] These findings can be related to the parallel pathways that control the various types of saccadic responses (Fig. 3–12). Thus, on the one hand, disease affecting either the frontal lobes or the caudate nucleus, which inhibits the substantia nigra, pars reticulata (SNpr), may lead to difficulties in initiating voluntary saccades in tasks that require learned or predictive behavior.[463] On the other hand, Huntington's disease also affects the SNpr.[812] Since this structure inhibits the superior colliculus (nigro-collicular projection), and so suppresses reflexive saccades to visual stimuli, one might expect excessive distractibility during attempted fixation. The slowing of saccades might reflect involve-

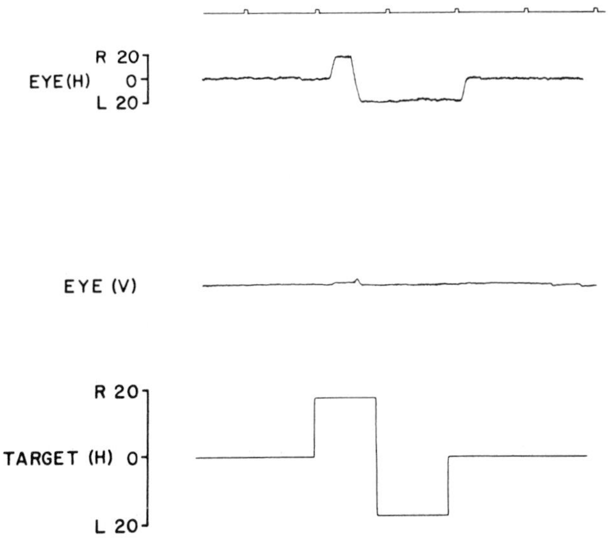

Figure 12–14. The antisaccade task. A patient, who had Huntington's disease, was instructed to look in the opposite "mirror" location of the target light as soon as it was turned on. She was unable to do this and, instead, first made a saccade towards the target light and then corrected her mistake and looked in the opposite (correct) direction. The target reappeared in the mirror location, at which time the patient held fixation and then, when the target returned to primary position, made a saccade to it to await the onset of the next trial. H: horizontal; V: vertical; time marks at top indicate one-second intervals. Similarly abnormalities are encountered on the antisaccade task in a range of disorders affecting the cerebral hemispheres and basal ganglia.(From Lasker and colleagues,[608] with permission of Lippincott, Williams and Wilkins.)

ment of saccadic burst neurons,[581] but at least some pathologic evidence suggests that disturbance of prenuclear inputs, such as the superior colliculus or frontal eye fields, is responsible.[625] The ability of blinks to initiate or speed-up saccades is reviewed in Saccades and Movements of the Eyelids, in Chapter 3).

EYE MOVEMENTS AND THE DIAGNOSIS OF HUNTINGTON'S DISEASE

Even though most patients with HD show some abnormalities of eye movements, individuals who have been studied at a presymptomatic point in their disease have shown normal eye movements.[208,932] Thus, despite the report of increased clinical abnormalities of eye movements, including slow saccades, in presymptomatic Huntington gene carriers,[573] eye movements cannot be regarded as a reliable method for determining which offspring of affected patients will go on to develop the disease. Newer testing that incorporates more natural eye tasks, such as visual scanning, may prove to be more revealing of an underlying disorder.[16a,103]

Disorders to be considered in the differential diagnosis of HD include neuroacanthocytosis and dentatorubropallidoluysian atrophy. One form of neuroacanthocytosis, chorea-acanthanocytosis is an autosomal recessive disorder that may be mistaken for Huntington's disease.[406] Affected patients have dystonia, chorea, parkinsonism, dysarthria, dysphagia, seizures and cognitive impairment. Their eye movement abnormalities consist of frequent square-wave jerks, and multistep hypometric saccades that may be slow, especially vertically.[406] Dentatorubropallidoluysian atrophy,[776] also called the Haw River syndrome,[149] is another CAG triplet repeat disease (B37, chromosome 12) and is characterized by slow saccades but more myoclonus and ataxia than in HD. Slowing of vertical saccades is probably not a feature of chorea due to non-degenerative conditions or tardive dyskinesia.[484]

Other Diseases of Basal Ganglia

A number of other conditions that involve the basal ganglia may cause abnormal eye movements. Wilson's disease and Niemann-Pick variants are discussed under Ocular Motor Manifestations of Metabolic and Deficiency Diseases.

Caudate nucleus hemorrhage may cause ipsilateral gaze preference,[1034] consistent with the effects of experimental dopamine depletion of this nucleus.[540] Patients with bilateral *lentiform nucleus* lesions show abnormalities of internally generated predictive and memory-guided saccades, but saccades and antisaccades triggered by visual stimuli are reported to be normal.[1134] Defects in the control of predictive smooth-pursuit eye movements are a feature of striatal damage,[632] consistent with pursuit projections from the frontal eye fields to the caudate nucleus.[232]

Patients with *Gilles de la Tourette's syndrome* may show abnormalities such as blepharospasm and eye tics with involuntary gaze deviations.[309, 344] Saccades, fixation, and pursuit to visual targets are normal.[114] However, Tourette patients show increased latency and decreased peak velocity of antisaccades, and impaired sequencing of memory-guided saccades.[763,1043] The lid abnormalities of Tourette's syndrome should be distinguished from benign eye-movement tics that are unaccompanied by vocal utterances, and which children often outgrow.[94,996]

Most patients with *essential blepharospasm* have normal eye movements,[269] although saccadic reaction time may be increased to visually guided and memory-guided tests.[30,113] Some patients with *spasmodic torticollis* show abnormalities of vestibular function, including the torsional vestibulo-ocular reflex (VOR).[44, 1037] Whether such vestibular abnormalities are the cause, or the effect, of spasmodic torticollis is not settled. Affected patients show changes in their perceptions of the visual vertical and straight ahead.[23,23,701]

Patients with *tardive dyskinesia* may show increased saccade distractibility.[1079] Patients with active *Sydenham's chorea* may show saccadic hypometria.[173] In *Lesch-Nyhan disease*, an hereditary disorder characterized by hyperuricemia, recurrent self-injurious behavior and extrapyramidal features, patients show impaired ability to make voluntary saccades, errors on the antisaccade task, blepharospasm, and intermittent gaze deviations similar to Tourette's syndrome.[513] Patients with essential tremor show reduced gain of pursuit initiation, and impaired suppression of post-rotational nystagmus with head tilt, suggestive of underlying cerebellar dysfunction.[448]

OCULAR MOTOR SYNDROMES CAUSED BY LESIONS IN THE CEREBRAL HEMISPHERES

In reviewing the effects of cerebral hemisphere lesions on eye movements, first we describe the effects of acute lesions; second, we identify the enduring effects of large, unilateral lesions; and then we will discuss the effects of lesions limited to specific lobes, referring to the scheme laid out in Chapter 6. Ocular motor apraxia, the manifestations of epileptic seizures, and the effects of diffuse processes, such as those causing dementia, are dealt with subsequently.

Disturbances of Gaze with Acute Hemispheric Lesions

Following an acute lesion of one cerebral hemisphere, the eyes often deviate conjugately towards the side of the lesion, Prevost's or Vulpian's sign (Box 12–18).[397,1004,1098] The head is also often turned in the same direction (see Chapter 7). Sustained horizontal gaze deviation is more common after large, right-sided strokes that predominantly involve post-Rolandic cortex or the subcortical fronto-parietal region and the internal capsule.[255, 1093,1098] Left hemispheric lesions that produce gaze deviations are usually large, covering the entire fronto-temporal-parietal area. With right-sided lesions, visual hemineglect is also often present, and may contribute to the "gaze preference".[590] In general, the larger the lesion, the more persistent is the conjugate deviation. However, most horizontal gaze deviations that occur following a hemispheric stroke resolve within a week. When gaze deviations are more persistent, there is often a prior lesion in the contralateral hemisphere.[1035]

Most patients show a conjugate gaze deviation that is ipsilateral to the side of the hemispheric lesion; they appear to "look away from their hemiparesis." Rarely, hemispheric lesions (usually hemorrhages) may cause a contralateral gaze deviation, so that the patient appears to "look towards the hemiparesis";[828,986] such *wrong-way deviations* are more common with thalamic lesions.[327,549] Another cause of a wrong-way deviation is epilepsy; when the patient is first examined, it should be confirmed that the gaze deviation is sustained, and not a transient phenomenon that would suggest seizures.

Although the gaze deviation due to a hemispheric lesion may be quite marked during the acute phase, it is usually possible to drive the eyes across the middle of the orbits with a head rotation or caloric stimulation. This preservation of the range of reflexive eye movements is

Box 12–18. Topological Diagnosis Of Acute Conjugate Deviations Of The Eyes

Sustained Horizontal Conjugate Gaze Deviation

- Ipsilateral ("looks away from the hemiparesis"): destructive hemispheric lesions (e.g., infarcts), especially with large, posterior, and right-sided location
- Contralateral ("looks towards the hemiparesis"): pontine lesions; thalamic lesions, and rarely with other supratentorial disease ("wrong-way deviation")

Intermittent Horizontal Conjugate Gaze Deviation

- Usually a manifestation of epileptic seizures

Sustained Upward Gaze Deviation

- Following hypoxic-ischemic insult
- Drug effects and oculogyric crisis

Sustained Downward Gaze

- Thalamic hemorrhage
- Lesions compressing the dorsal midbrain, such as hemorrhage, tumor, hydrocephalus

For related anatomy, see: Descending, Parallel Pathways that Control Voluntary Gaze, Brainstem Connections for Vertical and Torsional Movements, Fig. 6-4, and Fig. 6-5 in Chapter 6.

helpful in distinguishing the gaze deviation from a pontine lesion, in which vestibular stimuli often fail to drive the eyes across the midline.[241] When quick phases of caloric nystagmus are absent, consciousness is usually, but not always, impaired owing to increased intracranial pressure and shift of intracranial contents.[194,854]

The defect of eye movements after a large hemispheric lesion often corresponds to craniotopic coordinates (i.e., head-centered rather than eye-centered): there is difficulty moving the eyes in the contralateral hemifield. Even within the remaining field of movement, however, other abnormalities are evident. For example, some patients show a small-amplitude nystagmus with ipsilateral quick phases; a similar finding is reported acutely after hemidecortication in the monkey.[1119] The slow phases of this nystagmus may reflect unopposed pursuit, or perhaps vestibular, drives directed away from the side of the lesion. Recall that unilateral hemispheric lesions produce predominant deficits for contralateral saccades, but ipsilateral smooth-pursuit and optokinetic responses (see Fig. 4–12, Chapter 4 and Video Display: Disorders of Smooth Pursuit). Support for this interpretation comes from measurement of optokinetic visual tracking in patients with ipsiversive gaze deviation; responses to stimulus motion towards the intact hemisphere are much greater.[733] Within the preserved field of movement, contralateral saccades are hypometric.[733,1097] Vertical saccades may have an inappropriate horizontal component, similar to the effects of acute inactivation of one frontal eye field in monkey.[279] In general, for comparably sized lesions, ocular motor defects—both pursuit and saccades—are more profound when the lesion is in the nondominant hemisphere.[631] Whether this is a true hemispheric motor asymmetry, or is related to the greater effects of the non-dominant hemisphere lesions on attention, which leads to neglect, is not yet settled.

Some further insights into the effects of acute inactivation of one hemisphere come from observations of gaze control following *intracarotid injection of barbiturate* (the Wada test to determine cerebral dominance).[641,702] At the onset of hemiparesis, a transient horizontal gaze deviation may occur, which is more common with right-sided injections, providing further evidence for the dominance of the right hemisphere in directing attention. During the period of hemiparesis of the Wada test, contralateral and ipsilateral saccades are still possible, with relatively minor slowing of the contralateral ones. This persistence of voluntary saccades is probably due to the influence of posterior cerebral areas, which receive blood supply from the vertebrobasilar system and which project, independently of the frontal eye fields, to the superior colliculus.[641]

Enduring Disturbances of Gaze Caused by Unilateral Hemispheric Lesions

Persisting ocular motor deficits caused by large lesions (such as hemidecortication for intractable seizures) are summarized in Table 12–7. Although there may be no resting deviation of the eyes, Cogan pointed out that forced closure of the eyelids may cause a *contralateral "spastic" conjugate eye deviation*, the mechanism of which is not understood,[191] but which occurs most frequently with parietotemporal lesions.[1051] Conjugate deviation during attempted lid closure in patients with hemispheric lesions differs from the deviation

Table 12–7. **Enduring Effects of Large Unilateral Lesions of the Cerebral Hemispheres upon Ocular Motor Function**

Fixation

In darkness, eyes usually drift away from the side of the lesion. This may also be evident during fixation (on ophthalmoscopic examination*) as nystagmus with quick phases towards the side of the lesion.[992] Square-wave jerks.[989]

Saccades

Slower horizontal saccades to both sides, especially contralaterally; latency longer for small saccades directed contralateral to the side of the lesion;[1116] inaccurate (hypometric and hypermetric) saccades into the "blind" hemifield.[992,1116] Vertical saccades may have inappropriate horizontal component.[337]

Smooth Pursuit

Reduced pursuit gain towards the side of the lesion; smooth pursuit gain away from the side of the lesion may be increased for low-velocity targets.[992,1114]

Optokinetic

Reduced gain for stimuli directed toward the side of the lesion; may be relatively preserved compared with pursuit, with prolonged build-up of slow-phase velocity; impaired optokinetic after-nystagmus.[56,443]

Vestibular

During sinusoidal head rotation, VOR gain in darkness may be slightly asymmetric (greater for eye movements away from the side of the lesion); with attempted fixation of an imagined or real stationary target, the asymmetry is increased.[311,311,490] No asymmetry of response with rapid head turns[490]

Forced Eyelid Closure

Eyes usually deviate conjugately away from the side of the lesion (Cogan's "spasticity of conjugate gaze")[1051]

*Remember that the direction of eye movements appears inverted during ophthalmoscopy.

(lateropulsion) that occurs in Wallenberg's syndrome (dorsolateral medullary infarction) (see Video Display: Medullary Syndromes). With hemispheric lesions, the eyes deviate only with forceful eyelid closure or attempted lid closure, but in Wallenberg's syndrome, the deviation occurs even with the eyes open in darkness.

In central position, a small-amplitude nystagmus may be present (best seen during ophthalmoscopy), with slow phases directed toward the side of the intact hemisphere; as discussed in the prior section, it may represent an *asymmetry of smooth pursuit* (imbalance of pursuit tone).[992] Horizontal pursuit gain (eye velocity/target velocity) is low for tracking of targets moving toward the side of the lesion for all stimulus velocities (see Video Display: Disorders of Smooth Pursuit). For targets moving slowly toward the intact hemisphere, the eye movements may be too fast (pursuit gain greater than 1.0), requiring back-up saccades (see Fig. 4–12B); for higher target velocities, pursuit gain toward the intact side is normal.[992,1114] This disturbance of smooth pursuit probably reflects loss of both posterior (occipital-parietal-temporal) and frontal influences; possible pathogenic mechanisms are discussed in the following sections, in which the effects of lobar lesions are separately considered.

A convenient way to demonstrate this asymmetry of smooth pursuit is with a hand-held optokinetic drum or tape.[200] The response is decreased when the stripes are moved toward the side of the lesion. This bedside optokinetic response is usually judged according to the frequency and amplitude of quick phases. Since these quick-phase variables also depend on slow-phase velocity, a decreased response (reduced gain) may reflect impaired slow-phase generation, impaired quick-phase generation, or a combination of the two.

Hemidecortication causes abnormalities of both contralateral and ipsilateral *horizontal saccades*.[992,1116] Saccades are usually slower than normal for refixations into the hemianopic field, and sometimes into the intact hemifield. Saccadic latency is also prolonged in both directions.[992] For small refixations, contralaterally directed saccades have greater latencies than ipsilateral saccades. Prolonged saccadic reaction time may reflect (1) defects in visual detection due to the hemianopia, (2) defects in directing visual attention, and (3) abnormal motor programming. Saccadic accuracy is impaired asymmetrically: most contralaterally directed saccades do not put the eye on target (see Video Display: Disorders of Smooth Pursuit).[1116]

The horizontal *vestibulo-ocular reflex* may be mildly asymmetric in hemidecorticate patients at lower test frequencies; the gain (eye velocity/head velocity) is greater for compensatory eye movements directed away from the side of the lesion.[311] More asymmetry appears when visual fixation and vestibular stimulation are combined (during rotation while fixating a stationary object), probably reflecting the ipsilateral smooth pursuit deficit. The asymmetry is still present during head rotation if the patient imagines a stationary object.[991] However, if the head is suddenly and rapidly rotated during fixation of a stationary target, gaze is perturbed no more than in normal subjects,[490] consistent with the absence of oscillopsia in patients with hemispheric lesions as they make head movements during natural activities.

Effects of Focal Hemispheric Lesions on Gaze

EFFECTS OF LESIONS OF POSTERIOR OCCIPITO-TEMPORAL CORTICAL AREAS ON GAZE

Unilateral lesions of the occipital lobes cause a contralateral visual field defect and an ocular motor deficit (saccadic dysmetria) that reflects the patient's *homonymous hemianopia* (Box 12–19). Saccades into the hemianopic visual field are dysmetric (usually hypometric), and similar patterns of saccades are reported with acoustic targets, implying some degree of common motor programming, perhaps influenced by associated defects in directing spatial attention.[1108]

Patients with hemianopia may show compensatory strategies to increase saccadic accuracy,[712] unless hemineglect is also present. These strategies include a staircase of search saccades with backward, glissadic drifts; a deliberate overshooting saccade to bring the target into the intact hemifield of vision; and, with predictable targets, saccades using memory of previous attempts. Such findings have been used to develop simple clinical tests for distinguishing hemianopia with and without neg-

Box 12–19. Effects of Lesions of Posterior Cortical Areas

Primary Visual Cortex

- Acutely: Unable to make saccades or generate smooth pursuit in response to visual stimuli presented into the blind field
- Chronically: Strategies develop to scan the environment and place the image of an object of interest in the intact visual field

Middle Temporal Visual Area (MT, V5)

- Retinotopic defect of motion vision causing saccades and smooth pursuit to be impaired when visual stimuli fall in the affected visual field

Medial Superior Temporal Visual Area (MST)

- Directional defect of smooth pursuit, with decreased gain for ipsilateral target motion
- Superimposed retinotopic defect, similar to MT lesions

Posterior Insula ("Vestibular Cortex")

- Contralateral tilts of subjective visual vertical
- Circularvection abolished during optokinetic stimulation

For related anatomy, see Box 6-14, Box 6-15, Fig. 6-7, and Fig. 6-8, in Chapter 6. For review of vestibular cortex, see Chapter 2. For recorded examples of the effects of clinical lesions, see Fig.4-9 and Fig.4-12 in Chapter 4. (Related Video Display: Disorders of Smooth Pursuit)

lect.[706] Rapid gaze shifts achieved by combined movements of eye and head also show increased latency of head movements and development of compensatory strategies when looking to the hemianopic side.[1201] There is some evidence that patients with hemianopia can be trained to improve their visual search.[816] Smooth pursuit remains intact with unilateral lesions of the striate cortex, provided the moving stimulus is presented to the intact hemifield,[977] and optokinetic nystagmus elicited at the bedside is usually symmetric. Within the affected visual field, motion detection is usually abolished.[68] However, functional imaging suggests that secondary visual areas at the occipitoparietal region, lying anterior to an occipital lesion, may still respond to moving stimuli either due to extrastriate or interhemispheric callosal inputs.[123]

Bilateral occipital lesions cause *cortical blindness*. A patient with bilateral, congenital occipital lesions and little residual vision was reported to be able to make voluntary saccades but not smooth pursuit.[911] Optokinetic responses are present in monkeys following bilateral occipital lobectomy, and pursuit of small targets shows some degree of recovery;[1214] but this is probably not the case in humans.[136,1132]

Patients with more anterior lesions that involve cortex at the junction of areas 19, 37, and 39 (see Box 6–14), close to the intersection of the ascending limb of the inferior temporal sulcus and the lateral occipital sulcus (see Fig. 6–8, Chapter 6), are reported to show defects of motion perception (akinetopsia),[999,1125] and impaired smooth pursuit,[619,1089] similar to those described in monkeys with lesions in the middle temporal visual area (MT or V5) (see Fig. 4–9). Similar lesions may also involve the adjacent homologue of the medial superior temporal visual area (MST) and produce a tracking deficit similar to that in monkeys, with impairment of ipsilateral pursuit and a defect of motion processing affecting the contralateral visual hemifield (Fig.4–11).[67,69,444,619,735,1089] These tracking defects with lesions affecting posterior cortical lesions are most evident when the responses to step-ramp stimuli are measured (see Abnormalities of pursuit initiation in Chapter 4). A patient with bilateral MST lesions experienced illusory motion of the stationary world during smooth pursuit, presumably because he could not use an internal (efference) copy of eye movements to determine whether retinal slip was due to the smooth pursuit eye movement or motion of the visual stimulus.[418]

Lesions affecting vestibular cortex, a component of which lies in the posterior aspect of the superior temporal gyrus (parieto-insular-vestibular cortex (PIVC)) (see Box 6–15 and Fig. 6–8) cause contralateral tilts of the subjective visual vertical.[126] In addition, such lesions may abolish the sense of self-rotation (circularvection) that normally occurs with optokinetic stimulation,[1040] and may impair memory-guided saccades if patients are rotated to a new position during the memory period.[500]

Recent studies of memory-guided saccades have indicated that lesions involving the parahippocampal cortex impair "medium-term" spatial memory of up to 30 seconds,[851] whereas the hippocampal formation contributes to "long-term" spatial memory, which ranges up to minutes.[843]

Seizures emanating in the temporal lobes may cause a range of vestibular sensations. Though a mild feeling of dizziness is common with a variety of seizure types, a true sensation of rotation, vestibular or tornado epilepsy, is a rare but well-described epileptic phenomenon.[61,361,583,777,967,1012]

EFFECTS OF PARIETAL LOBE LESIONS ON GAZE

Acute unilateral lesions involving the parietal lobe (see Box 6–16, Box 6–17 and Fig. 6–8) often cause an ipsilateral horizontal gaze deviation or preference. Especially when the lesion is right-sided, there is also contralateral inattention. Bilateral ptosis may also occur with acute right parietal lesions,[41,46] although it more commonly occurs with disease located in midbrain (especially involving the oculomotor nucleus), with Miller Fisher syndrome, disorders of the neuromuscular junction, or the extraocular muscles (see Chapter 9). The defect of ocular motility with lesions of the parietal lobe often corresponds to craniotopic (head-centered) coordinates, reflecting the normal role of parietal areas in directing visual attention in head-centered spatial coordinates, as is discussed further under Disturbances of Gaze with Acute Hemispheric Lesions. Although ocular motor defects associated with parietal lesions may be partly due to difficulties in shifting attention from one position to another in extrapersonal space,[857] there are also distinct and specific effects on saccadic and pursuit eye movements (Box 12–20).[371a,833,1156]

The latency of visually guided saccades to targets presented in either visual hemifield is increased with right-sided lesions; with left-sided lesions, only saccades to contralateral targets are delayed.[844] These increases in saccadic latency are more marked when the fixation light remains on during testing (overlap paradigm, Fig. 3–2A, Chapter 3) than when it is turned off just before the target light appears (gap paradigm, Fig. 3–2B);[845] this may reflect difficulties in disengaging attention prior to initiating the saccade. The accuracy of saccades to contralateral targets may also be impaired, but the most impressive dysmetria occurs when patients are required to respond to a *double-step stimulus*, in which the target jumps twice before a response can be initiated.[296,442] If the target jumps first into the contralateral hemifield and then into the ipsilateral field, patients cannot make accurate saccades to the final target position, even though it lies in the "intact" hemifield. This finding has been taken as evidence that the parietal lobe plays a pivotal role in computing target position from both visual stimuli and an efference copy of eye movements (in this case, the change in eye position due to the first saccade).[296,442]

Patients suffering from hemispatial neglect show an inability to attend to the contralateral half of space, which biases their attention towards the ipsilesional side and impairs ability to search the contralesional space.[564] Furthermore, search behaviour in hemispatial neglect appears to combine a spatial bias with a loss of working memory for locations previously

Box 12–20. Effects Of Parietal Lobe Lesions

Unilateral Lesions (Especially Right-Sided)

- Contralateral inattention
- Ipsilateral gaze deviation or preference
- Increased latency for visually guided saccades
- Errors on responses to double-step stimulus
- Impaired smooth pursuit of target moving across textured background

Bilateral Parietal Lesions

- Balint's syndrome: peripheral visual inattention (simultanagnosia), inaccurate arm pointing ("optic ataxia"), difficulty in making visually guided saccades (If all voluntary eye movements are affected, involvement of frontal lobes is likely, and the term "ocular motor apraxia" has been used.)

For related anatomy, see Box 6-16, Box 6-17 and Fig. 6-8 in Chapter 6. (Related Video Display: Acquired Ocular Motor Apraxia)

searched.[492] During visual scanning, patients return too frequently to fixation locations that they have previously visited. In patients with hemispatial neglect, saccadic reaction time is influenced by the position of the eyes in the head,[72] being greater when the eyes are in the orbital positions away from the side of the lesion.

Asymmetry of smooth pursuit and optokinetic tracking has traditionally been ascribed to parietal lobe lesions. Thus, decreased nystagmus elicited when a hand-held optokinetic drum or tape moves towards the side of the lesion has been taken as indicating involvement of the inferior parietal lobule and underlying deep white matter.[200,444] Functional imaging studies suggest that secondary visual areas at the temporo-occipito-parietal junction are probably responsible for these defects in smooth tracking (see Fig. 6–7). More specific to parietal lobe lesions is the loss of ability to attend to the image of a moving target and to "ignore" the smeared images of the stationary background consequent to the eye movement. Thus, patients with lesions affecting Brodmann area 40 show impaired smooth pursuit when the target moves across a structured background, compared with pursuit across a dark background.[610] Impairment of the same mechanism may explain why, in patients with parietal lesions, responses to full-field optokinetic stimuli are relatively spared; such stimuli demand less selective visual attention.[56] Bilateral posterior parietal lesions cause Balint's syndrome,[839] which is discussed below, under Ocular Motor Apraxia.

EFFECTS OF FRONTAL LOBE LESIONS ON GAZE

Experimental and clinical studies, reviewed in Chapter 6, have made it possible to identify three distinct regions in the frontal lobes that contribute to the control of eye movements (see Fig. 6–8): the frontal eye field (FEF) (see Box 6–19), the supplementary eye field (SEF) (see Box 6-20) in the supplementary motor area, and the dorsolateral prefrontal cortex (DLPC) (see Box 6–21). Although there is some overlap of function, lesions affecting each of these three areas produce certain behavioral deficits that are distinctive (Box 12–21).[837] We also discuss the effects of lesions of cingulate cortex.

Box 12–21. Effects Of Frontal Lobe Lesions

Effects Of Lesions Of The Frontal Eye Field (FEF)
In monkeys, acute unilateral pharmacological inactivation of FEF with muscimol produces:

- An "ocular motor scotoma," so that all voluntary contralateral saccades with sizes and directions corresponding to the injection site are abolished
- Gaze preference toward the side of the lesion
- Impaired smooth pursuit, especially toward side of the lesion

In humans, chronic unilateral lesions affecting the FEF cause:

- Bilateral increase in reaction time of saccades made to visual targets in "overlap" task, to remembered target locations, and imagined targets during the "antisaccade" task
- Hypometria of saccades made to visual or remembered targets located contralateral to the side of the lesion
- Reduced ability to make saccades in anticipation of predictable stepping movement of a target, when the target moves away from the side of the lesion
- Impaired ability to inhibit inappropriate saccades to a novel visual stimulus
- Impairment of smooth pursuit and optokinetic following of targets moving towards the side of the lesion

Effects Of Lesions Of The Supplementary Eye Field (SEF)

- Memory-guided saccades become inaccurate if gaze shifts during the memory period
- Impaired ability to make a remembered sequence of saccades to an array of visible targets (especially with left-sided lesions)
- Impaired ability to reverse saccade direction from an established pattern of response

Effects Of Lesions Of Dorsolateral Prefrontal Cortex (DLPC)

- Pharmacological blockade of D1 dopamine receptors causes inaccuracy of saccades made to remembered target locations lying contralateral to the side of injection
- Patients with lesions affecting this area show defects of predictive saccades, memory-guided saccades and antisaccades

For related anatomy, see Box 6-19, Box 6-20, Box 6-21 and Fig. 6-8, in Chapter 6. For pathophysiology of saccadic disorders, see: The Role of the Frontal Lobe in Saccade Generation.

Effects of Frontal Eye Field Lesions on Gaze

Acute lesions restricted to the FEF in humans are uncommon, but may produce an ipsilateral horizontal gaze deviation and head rotation that resolves with time.[241,1068] Experimental inactivation of the FEF in monkey with muscimol does cause ipsilateral gaze deviation and an "ocular motor scotoma" so that the horizontal component of contralateral saccades is impaired or abolished; additionally, visual fixation is frequently broken by spontaneous ipsilateral saccades.[279,1021] Rarely, contralateral deviation has been observed in patients with acute, hemorrhagic frontal lesions[986] or frontoparietal lesions.[828]

The enduring deficits of saccades and smooth pursuit with FEF lesions are often not obvious at the bedside, and require laboratory testing to identify. Thus, saccades made in response to the overlap paradigm (Fig. 3–2A), during which the fixation light remains on when the target light is presented, show increased reaction time, both ipsilaterally and contralaterally.[678,905] This finding suggests a role for the FEF in disengaging fixation. Memory-guided saccades are also mildly impaired, especially to contralateral targets.[853] Errors during the antisaccade task (Fig. 12–14) may be due to difficulties in initiating the correct antisaccade, whereas suppression of inappropriate saccades towards the visual stimulus appears to depend more on the dorsolateral prefrontal cortex, which is discussed below.[842] Another deficit is in the ability to make saccades in anticipation of target jumps that occur predictably, when the target moves away from the side of the lesion.[271,845,985] Mild slowing of contralateral saccades occurs in some patients.[985] Deep, unilateral frontal lobe lesions cause increased latency for contralateral saccades.[846] This deficit is probably due to damage of efferent and afferent connections of the frontal eye fields.

Frontal eye field lesions also impair smooth pursuit.[128,444,631,632,736,905] With unilateral FEF lesions, horizontal pursuit is impaired bilaterally, but more so for tracking of targets moving towards the side of the lesion. Both the initiation and maintenance of pursuit are affected, more so at higher target speeds and frequencies. Since neurons in the FEF also discharge for vergence movements (reviewed in Chapter 8), it is likely that lesions in this area will impair vergence, possibly more so when vergence is made with pursuit to a target moving smoothly in depth, or with a saccade to change the depth and direction of the point of fixation.

Effects of Supplementary Eye Field Lesions on Gaze

The supplementary eye field (SEF), which is part of a network that includes the presupplementary cortex, cingulate cortex, and hippocampus, seems important for programming sequences of eye movements as part of learned forms of behavior. Thus, the most characteristic defect of SEF lesions is a loss of the ability to make a sequence of saccades to an array of visible targets in the order that they were turned on (Fig. 3–2E, Chapter 3).[372,376] This is especially true with left-sided SEF lesions. Memory-guided saccades are impaired if patients with SEF lesions are rotated in a vestibular chair during the memory period. Another effect of SEF lesions is difficulty in changing the direction of saccades as part of a reversal of a previously established pattern of response.[493] SEF lesions may also impair predictive, ipsilateral smooth-pursuit response.[444,631]

Effects of Lesions of Dorsolateral Prefrontal Cortex on Gaze

Goldman-Rakic and colleagues established the importance of DPLC for making saccades to remembered target locations. Thus, pharmacological inactivation of the DLPC with D1-dopamine antagonists specifically impairs the ability of monkeys to make accurate memory-guided saccades toward contralateral targets.[959] Similarly, patients with lesions affecting the DLPC show impaired ability to make saccades to remembered target locations, if the memory period is less than about 30 seconds (after this period, other cortical areas, including the parahippocampal gyrus, assume more importance).[842,843] Lesions of the DLPC also impair responses on the antisaccade task (Fig. 12–14), with an increased percentage of errors.[842] Errors on antisaccades also occur with lesions involving the anterior limb, genu, and anterior half of the posterior limb of the internal capsule, through which pass projections from DLPC to brainstem.[212,852] Pursuit defects with unilateral DLPC lesions may be bilateral.[631]

Effects of Lesions of Cingulate Cortex on Gaze

As discussed in Chapter 6, the anterior cingulate cortex contributes to programming of more complex aspects of saccades. It has been proposed that there is a "cingulate eye field," located in the posterior part of the anterior cingulate cortex, at the junction of Brodmann areas 23 and 24,[375] which makes oligosynaptic connections with brainstem ocular motor structures.[739] Thus, the anterior cingulate cortex is reported to show changes in regional cerebral blood flow during self-paced saccades, memory-guided saccades, memorized triple saccades, and antisaccades.[26,289,441,830]

In two patients with small infarcts in the cingulate eye field of the right hemisphere, saccadic reaction time was increased and the gain decreased for saccades made during the overlap task, and also for memory-guided saccades.[375] Both patients also made errors on the antisaccade task in both directions, and during sequences of saccades to remembered target locations. In a second study, patients who had undergone resection of a tumor involving the anterior cingulate cortex also showed deficits on the antisaccade task.[716] The function of the posterior cingulate is less well worked out, although electrophysiological studies suggest that it assign spatial coordinates to retinal images following gaze shifts.[802] Taken together, it seems likely that the cingulate lobe will assume greater importance as its functions are better worked out.

Ocular Motor Apraxia

ACQUIRED OCULAR MOTOR APRAXIA

Acute bilateral frontal or frontoparietal lesions may produce a striking disturbance of ocular motility that has been called acquired ocular motor apraxia.[262,379,836] It is usually due to bihemispheric infarcts. It is characterized by loss of voluntary control of saccades and pursuit, with preservation of reflex movements, especially slow and quick phases of the vestibulo-ocular reflex. Patients have difficulties making horizontal and vertical saccades to command, and following a pointer moved by the examiner (see Video Display: Acquired Ocular Motor Apraxia). Gaze shifts are achieved more easily with combined eye-head movements, often in association with a blink. Vestibular eye movements (both slow and quick phases) are preserved. In addition, some patients are able to initiate saccades reflexively to novel visual targets. The defect of voluntary eye movements probably reflects disruption of descending pathways both from the frontal eye fields and the parietal cortex (see Fig. 6–8 and Fig. 3–12), so that the superior colliculus and brainstem reticular formation are bereft of their cortical inputs. The behavioral deficit is similar to that produced by bilateral, combined, experimental lesions of the frontal eye fields and superior colliculus,[963] or frontal and parietal eye fields.[671]

When a similar disorder of ocular motility, called psychic paralysis of gaze, is associated with inaccurate arm pointing (optic ataxia) and disturbance of visual attention (simultagnosia), the eponym *Balint's syndrome* has been used.[194,471,473,494,836,909,1123] The lesions are more parietal or occipital, and voluntary saccades may be made more easily than in response to visual stimuli.[839] Thus, the main abnormality appears to be a defect in the visual guidance of saccades, manifest by increased latency and decreased accuracy, and impaired ability to conduct visual search.[73,669,1221] Smooth pursuit is also impaired.[630] Spontaneous blinking may be absent.[1164] In one patient, the visual scene was reported to fade during fixation and be restored by intentional blinks.[402] The effects of blinks on eye movements are reviewed in Saccades and Movements of the Eyelids, in Chapter 3.

Some patients with ocular motor apraxia may show spasm of fixation, the inability to generate a voluntary eye movement to shift gaze when a fixation target is continuously present; only when the fixation target is removed can a gaze shift be made.[473] Holmes,[473] assisted by Denny-Brown, noted that if affected patients viewed a homogenous white screen, then voluntary eye movements became possible. The anatomic basis for this disturbance is uncertain, although defects in the inhibitory control of the superior colliculus by the substantia nigra pars reticulata (SNpr) have been proposed.[520]

The following case history illustrates some features of the syndrome of acquired ocular motor apraxia.

CASE HISTORY: Acquired Ocular Motor Apraxia in Multiple Sclerosis (see Video Display: Acquired Ocular Motor Apraxia)

A 28-year-old woman was in good health until 8 months prior to admission, when she suffered a "whiplash" neck injury in an automobile accident. Subsequently, she developed transient mild weakness of the left side of the body, which resolved in a few weeks. She suffered several further transient neurologic deficits, including loss of vision in first the right and then the left eye. Just prior to admission, she developed right-sided weakness, difficulty with speech and emotional behavior that her husband characterized as "child-like."

On examination, she had striking immobility of gaze. She was emotionally labile and had difficulties with calculations and short-term memory, but was cooperative and could follow instructions. Both optic discs were pale. Her visual acuity was 20/200 OS and 20/100 OD. She had no difficulty in recognizing or naming objects. There were bilateral pyramidal tract signs.

With the head still, she had great difficulty initiating saccades to command or to visual targets. When saccades did occur, they were often associated with a blink. With her head free to move, she could change gaze more easily. Her saccades were of small amplitude, but appeared to be of normal velocity. On occasion, she would change gaze by moving first the trunk, then her head, and finally making a small saccade. With an optokinetic tape, quick phases of nystagmus were easily elicited, though they seemed to be reduced in frequency. Smooth tracking was also impaired. Rotational testing elicited normal quick and slow phases of vestibular nystagmus.

Computed tomography (Fig. 12–15) showed bilateral lucencies in the centrum semiovale and deep portions of the posterior frontal and parietal lobes. Spinal fluid findings supported a diagnosis of multiple sclerosis. She improved while in the hospital, and 1 year later was reported to have no ocular motor deficit.

Comment: This patient's ocular motor deficit was restricted to voluntary eye movements: saccades and pursuit. Her "reflex" eye movements, slow and quick phases of vestibular nystagmus, and eye-head gaze shifts were relatively spared. Use of eye-head movements to shift gaze is similar to normal behavior in afoveate animals, such as the rabbit, and probably reflects use of a phylogenetically old linkage between head and saccadic eye movements (see Rapid Gaze Shifts Achieved by Combined Eye-Head Movements, in Chapter 7). Since brainstem generation of reflexive eye movements was intact, the term "ocular motor apraxia" might be correctly applied to this deficit, which reflects disease involving both cerebral hemispheres.

One clinical presentation deserving special mention is the syndrome of *loss of voluntary gaze following cardiac surgery*, especially of the aortic valve, and requiring cardiopulmonary bypass and hypothermia. Affected patients may report difficulties in seeing their environment clearly as they recover from their surgery, but often their symptoms are either not appreciated or ignored. Two distinct syndromes can be recognized.

The first syndrome is a form of ocular motor apraxia in which voluntary saccades, pursuit, and vergence are lost, whereas reflexive eye movements, including slow and quick phases of vestibular nystagmus are preserved. Such patients may be able to make normal velocity gaze shifts using a combined eye-head movement. In such cases, bihemispheric lesions are likely, but are only rarely demonstrated on imaging.[276] Since the frontal and parietal eye fields lie close to the watershed zone between the major cerebral arteries, they are at particular risk of infarction. Sometimes, other cortical deficits are present, such as Balint's syndrome. Affected patients show slow and incomplete recovery.

The second syndrome is a selective palsy of all rapid eye movements, including all saccades and quick phases, but with sparing of voluntary smooth pursuit or vergence (see Video Display: Acquired Ocular Motor Apraxia).[429,629,727,1105] Saccades may be very hypometric, requiring a "staircase" of small movements to shift gaze to a visual targets. Other patients show slow saccades with mild hypometria. The saccadic deficit may be prominent horizontally or vertical, but often saccades in all directions are involved, making visual search and reading difficult. Other symptoms, such as labile affect, dysarthria, and ataxia or dystonia, are sometimes associated. In one such patient who came to autopsy, neuronal loss and gliosis were confined to the paramedian pons, involving the omnipause and premotor burst neurons areas;

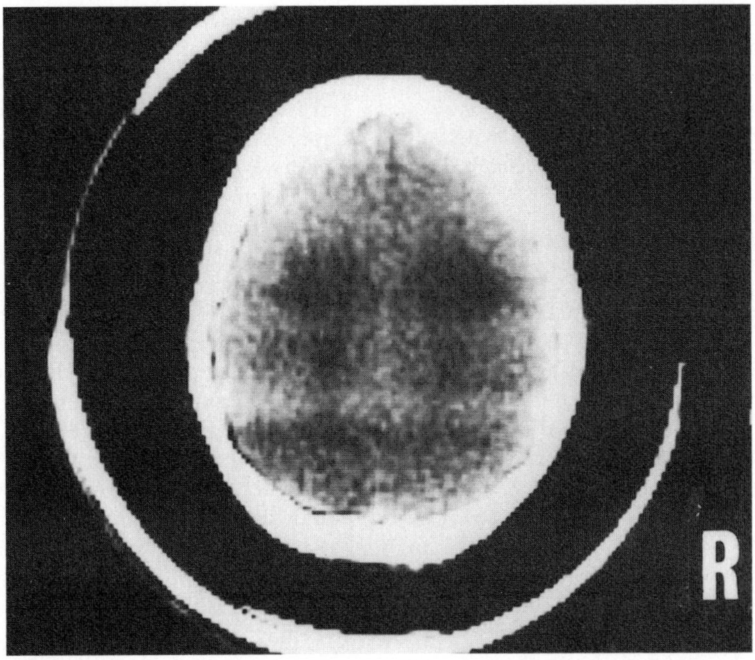

A

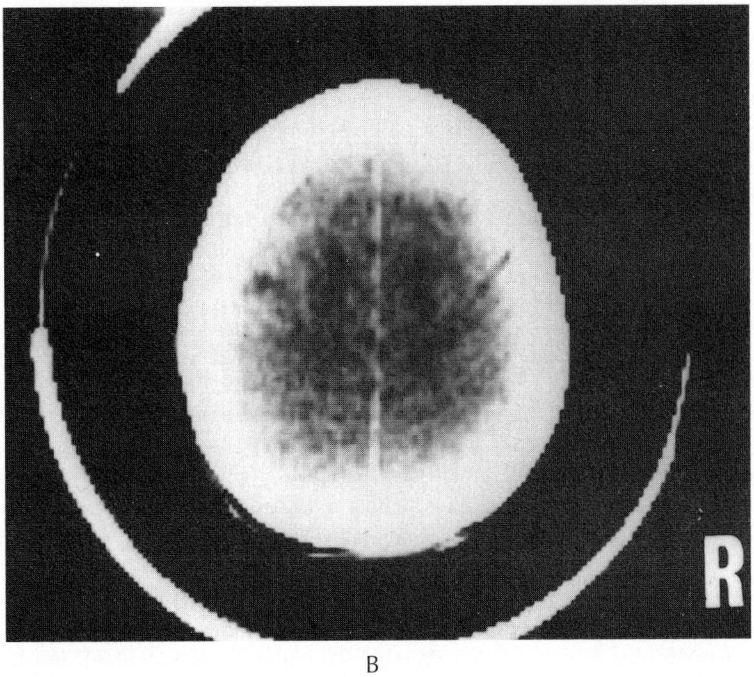

B

Figure 12–15. CT scans of the cerebral hemispheres of a patient with multiple sclerosis, who presented with "apraxia of gaze" (see Case history: Acquired ocular motor apraxia in multiple sclerosis and Video Display: Acquired Ocular Motor Apraxia). The scans show bilateral lucencies located in the centrum semiovale (A) and in the deep portions of the posterior frontal and adjacent parietal lobes (B).

other parts of the neuraxis, including the cerebral hemispheres, were normal (see Video Display: Disorders of Saccades).[429] The prognosis for recovery from this saccadic palsy syndrome is slow, and some patients may actually show progression of certain symptoms.[727]

CONGENITAL OCULAR MOTOR APRAXIA

Congenital ocular motor apraxia was first clearly defined by David G. Cogan.[192] Since his description, ocular motor apraxia has been recognized as a component of a number of hereditary disorders, often associated with ataxia, several of which have now been genetically defined. Here we first summarize the features of Cogan's form of the disorder and then review genetic disorders of which ocular motor apraxia is a common feature; Table 12–8 summarizes key features of each condition.

Cogan's Congenital Ocular Motor Apraxia

An abnormality may be recognized at several months of age, when the child does not appear to fixate upon objects normally and may be thought to be blind.[192,195,199] Some children with congenital ocular motor apraxia have also been reported to have a transient head and limb tremor in the first few days of life. Between the ages of 4 and 6 months, characteristic, thrusting horizontal head movements develop (see Video Display: Congenital Ocular Motor Apraxia), sometimes with prominent blinking or even rubbing the eyelids, when the child attempts to change fixation. In children with poor head control, development of head thrusting may be delayed or absent. Almost all patients also show a defect in generating quick phases of nystagmus,[434] which can usually be appreciated at the bedside by manual spinning of the patient, either when holding the child out at arm's length or by rotating the child on a swivel chair, if necessary sitting in an adult's lap (see Video Display: Congenital Ocular Motor Apraxia). A large-field optokinetic stimulus may also prove useful in identifying those children who lack normal responses.[365] Despite difficulties in shifting horizontal gaze, vertical voluntary eye movements are normal.

Measurements of eye and head movements have documented the characteristics of this disorder.[320,434,1217] With the head immobilized, patients show both impaired initiation (increased latency) and decreased amplitude (hypometria) of voluntary saccades in response to either a simple verbal command to look left or right or, less so, to track a step displacement

Table 12–8. **Disorders Associated with Congenital Ocular Motor Apraxia**[6,607,612,613,943,1020,1070,1112,1117,1193]

Disorder	Distinguishing Features
Ataxia telangiectasia (Louis-Bar syndrome)	Oculocutaneous telangiectasia; radiosensitivity; immunological disorders; cancer; elevated alpha-fetoprotein
Ataxia with oculomotor apraxia 1 (AOA1)	Hypercholesterolemia, hypoalbumineua, deficient coenzyme Q10
Ataxia with oculomotor apraxia 2 (AOA2)	Elevated alpha-fetoprotein
Pelizaeus-Merzbacher disease	Pendular nystagmus, upbeat nystagmus, saccadic dysmetria
Niemann-Pick type C	Predominant vertical deficit with slow vertical saccades and other eye movements preserved
Gaucher's disease	Horizontal and vertical gaze palsy
Tay-Sachs (infantile form)	Vertical gaze defect precedes horizontal
Late-onset Tay-Sachs	Vertical and horizontal saccades both affected
Joubert's syndrome	Alternating skew deviations, pigmentary retinal degeneration, breathing disorder
Abetaliproteinemia (vitamin E deficiency)	Slowing of abduction compared with adduction during horizontal saccades
Huntington's disease	Slow saccades and skeletal rigidity

of a target (Fig. 12–16). Saccades are also delayed during attempted refixations between auditory targets in complete darkness, so that the saccadic initiation abnormality cannot be ascribed to a defect of disengaging visual fixation. Saccadic velocities are normal and saccades or quick phases of nystagmus of large amplitude can occasionally be generated. These findings indicate that, in these patients, the premotor brainstem burst neurons that generate saccadic eye movements are intact. Especially in younger patients, however, the timing and amplitude (but not velocity) of quick phases of vestibular and optokinetic nystagmus may be impaired; the eyes intermittently deviate tonically in the direction of the slow phase because of a defect in the initiation of the quick phase of nystagmus. Sometimes the saccade defect (and head thrusts) is asymmetric.[176] Pursuit eye movements may also be of low gain, but the corrective saccades are usually promptly generated. The defects in congenital ocular motor apraxia are usually restricted to the horizontal plane, an important differential diagnostic point, because most acquired cases also have defects in the vertical plane.

The head thrusts made by affected patients probably reflect one of several adaptive strategies to facilitate changes in gaze.[74,1217] Younger patients appear to use their intact vestibulo-ocular reflex (VOR), which drives their eyes into an extreme contraversive position in the orbit. As the head continues to move past the target, the eyes are dragged along in space until they become aligned with the target. Then the head rotates backward and the eyes maintain fixation as they are brought back to the central position in the orbit by the VOR. In contrast, older patients appear to use the head movement per se to trigger the generation of a saccadic eye movement that cannot normally be made with the head still (Fig. 12–16). This strategy may reflect the use of a phylogenetically old linkage between head and saccadic eye movements that occurs reflexively in afoveate animals, when they desire to redirect their center of visual attention (see Rapid Gaze Shifts Achieved by Combined Eye-Head Movements, in Chapter 7).

The pathogenesis of this disorder remains unknown. Cogan suggested that it may reflect a delay in the normal development of the mechanisms by which we assume voluntary control over eye movements.[199] Delay in learning to speak and read, infantile hypotonia, strabismus, torsional nystagmus, and clumsiness may be associated.[946] Genetic testing may ultimately provide more specific diagnoses in some patients with ataxia (as discussed in the following sections). Affected patients usually improve with age: the head movements

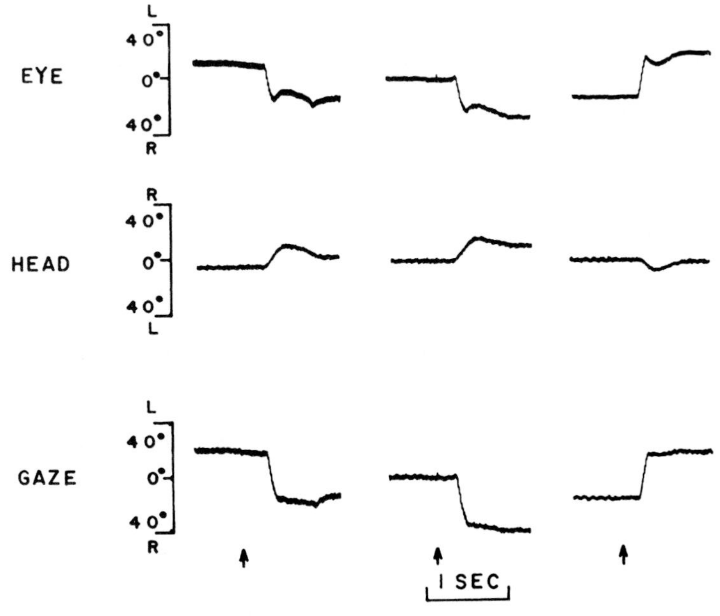

Figure 12–16. Eye-head coordination in congenital ocular motor apraxia. Responses to non-predictable 40-degree changes in target position (arrow indicate target steps). Eye: eye position in the head; Head: head position in space; Gaze: eye position in space (sum of head in space and eye in head). Note that the head positions axis is inverted. Left panel: Initial saccade and head movement begin nearly synchronously; Head movement overshoots its final position. Center panel: Head moves first and causes a brief, backward eye movement before the initial saccade; Right panel: Net change of head movement is negligible, but it facilitates an accurate gaze shift (see Video Display: Congenital Ocular Motor Apraxia).

become less prominent as the patients are better able to direct their eyes voluntarily. The presence of normal-velocity saccades suggests an intact brainstem mechanism for generating eye movements. The propensity of these children to blink in order to initiate a saccade suggests a problem with gating of brainstem burst neurons.[1206] The effects of blinks on eye movements is reviewed in Saccades and Movements of the Eyelids, in Chapter 3).

Ataxia Telangiectasia (Louis-Bar syndrome)

Ataxia Telangiectasia is an autosomal recessive disorder characterized by ocular motor apraxia in childhood, progressive ataxia, dysarthria, chorea, and oculocutaneous telangiectasia, which may develop later in the course (see Video Display: Congenital Ocular Motor Apraxia).[184,317,1038] The responsible ATM gene maps to chromosome 11q22–23. Affected individual often show head thrusts when they shift gaze. When their heads are fixed, patients shift gaze using a combination of hypometric saccades made at increased latency, and very slow eye movements.[651] They may also show gaze-evoked nystagmus, alternating skew deviation, vertical nystagmus, prolonged post-rotational nystagmus, periodic alternating nystagmus, square-wave jerks, and esotropia. Affected individuals show a number of immunological disorders leading to recurrent pulmonary infections, elevated alpha-fetoprotein, and radiosensitivity with a propensity to develop cancer, especially lymphoma. Ataxia telangiectasia-like disease is due to a genetic disorder on chromosome 11q21, and has a similar but milder course than the classic form.[1070]

Ataxia with Ocular Motor Apraxia (AOA)

This term is applied to two forms of congenital ocular motor apraxia associated with ataxia that have been identified genetically. AOA1 is an autosomal recessive disorder caused by mutations in the aprataxin gene (APTX) on chromosome 9p13.[247,369,613,729,771] Aprataxin is a nuclear protein with a role in DNA repair. Onset is usually between ages 2 and 10 years (mean 6.8), with ataxia, cerebellar atrophy, and severe axonal motor neuropathy.[613] There is some phenotypic variability, but oculomotor apraxia is present in more than 80% of affected children, who use a series of small saccades to shift gaze, giving the appearance of slow saccades (see Video Display: Congenital Ocular Motor Apraxia). Chorea is present early in the course, but may resolve.[20] Metabolic abnormalities such as hypercholesterolemia, hypoalbuminaemia, and deficiency of muscle coenzyme Q10 may be present.[866] The main diagnostic challenge posed by AOA1 is to differentiate it from Friedreich's ataxia (which does not cause ocular motor apraxia), ataxia-telangiectasia (characterized by cutaneous and conjunctival telangiectasia), and Huntington's disease (which may cause chorea and ocular motor apraxia).

Ataxia with ocular motor apraxia type 2 (AOA2) is also autosomal recessive, with mutations in the senataxin gene on chromosome 9q34.[730] The age of onset is later (11–20 years) with sensory motor neuropathy, chorea, and ocular motor apraxia in about half of affected patients.[612,730] A consistent laboratory finding is elevation of alpha-fetoprotein.

Joubert's Syndrome

Children with Joubert's syndrome present with developmental delay, breathing disorders in infancy, and ocular motor apraxia in both the horizontal and vertical planes (see Video Display: Congenital Ocular Motor Apraxia).[1117] On MRI scans, they show the "molar tooth sign," reflecting cerebellar vermian dysplasia or hypoplasia, a deep posterior interpeduncular fossa, and thick, elongated superior cerebellar peduncles.[1188] Other features include alternating skew deviation, seesaw and pendular nystagmus, impaired ocular and eye-head tracking, and pigmentary degeneration of the retina.[690]

Other Childhood Disorder that Manifest Ocular Motor Apraxia

Apart from the idiopathic type of congenital ocular motor apraxia, a variety of hereditary disorders that directly involve the brainstem mechanisms for generating saccades are characterized by the development of a strategy of head thrusting or blinking to shift gaze, and hence superficially appear as congenital ocular motor apraxia (Table 12–8). Some of these conditions are discussed in the section on Ocular Motor Manifestations Of Metabolic And Deficiency Disorders. Other disorders reported in association with horizontal saccadic failure include GM1 gangliosidosis,

Krabbe's leukodystrophy, peroxisomal assembly disorders, Lesch-Nyhan disease,[513] proprionic acidemia, Bardet-Biedl syndrome, Cornelia de Lange syndrome, and a variety of developmental abnormalities of the midline cerebellum.[434] These disorders can be distinguished from Cogan's form of congenital ocular motor apraxia when vertical saccades are affected, and when saccades are slow. In early stages of these diseases, however, distinguishing the ocular motor apraxia from Cogan's type may be difficult.[198] Purely vertical ocular motor apraxia is rare and usually acquired, reflecting direct involvement of saccade-generating pathways in the midbrain or pons.[299]

Eye Movements During Epileptic Seizures

Abnormal eye and head movements are common manifestations of epileptic seizures. Abnormalities include various forms of nystagmus, horizontal or vertical conjugate gaze deviation, and skew deviation.[363] Horizontal gaze deviations are usually contralateral, but occasionally ipsilateral, to the side of the seizure focus.[533,1039,1094] Epileptic gaze deviation can usually be distinguished from a paretic deviation due to a large cerebral infarction (Box 12–18) by observing the patient's eye for a few minutes: epileptic deviations are seldom sustained.

Epileptic seizures also cause a variety of forms of nystagmus: conjugate, retraction, convergence, or monocular (see Video Display: Disorders of Gaze Holding).[433,506,534,535,920,1006,1090,1118] Convergence nystagmus has been reported with either periodic lateralizing epileptiform discharges[1198] or burst-suppression patterns.[131,770] Epileptic nystagmus has also been reported with typical absence seizures[1160] and with infantile spasms.[478] Eyelid flutter may be the only clinical manifestation of seizures.[718] Some patients may show both intermittent gaze deviations and nystagmus.[1090] How can these diverse manifestations be related to the known mechanisms that control gaze, which we summarized in Chapter 6?

Although eye movements may be a manifestation of a seizure focus in any lobe,[732] the most commonly reported site in patients with epileptic nystagmus is the temporo-occipital-parietal region.[534–536] In most such cases, *the eyes initially deviate contralateral to the seizure focus*. This initial deviation may be due to activation of the parietal eye fields, which, in the monkey homologue (the lateral intraparietal area, LIP), have a low electrical threshold for eliciting *saccades*. In one such patient, who had a right temporo-occipital focus, the seizure began with a contraversive (leftward) gaze deviation due to a staircase of small saccades.[1090] After a few seconds, left-beating nystagmus commenced, with slow phases that showed a decreasing-velocity waveform. The nystagmus was accompanied by high-voltage 11Hz to 14 Hz spike activity that did not spread to frontal cortex. At the end of the seizure, the eyes returned to central position. It seems possible that the centripetal slow phases of such nystagmus, drifting towards center position, are similar to those of gaze-evoked nystagmus (Fig. 10–1B, Chapter 10). The reason for the unsustained gaze deviation, centripetal drifts, and nystagmus may be either effects of anticonvulsants,[1090] impaired consciousness,[621] or a deficient eye position signal due to seizure activity emanating from cortical areas.[732] Contraversive gaze deviation is also reported during periodic lateralized epileptiform discharges (PLEDS) over the right fronto-central region.[533]

Rarely, the patient's eyes *initially deviate ipsilateral to the seizure focus*, being followed by quick phases, which generate nystagmus.[535,536, 1118] In such cases, activation of *pursuit mechanisms* at the occipito-temporo-parietal junction (Fig. 6–8, Chapter 6) may be responsible. Experimental studies in awake monkeys indicate that the threshold for stimulating pursuit eye movements in this region is lower than that for stimulating saccades.[585] Support of this hypothesis comes from the observation that the slow phases of subsequent nystagmus are linear (see Fig. 10–1A, Chapter 10) and move the eyes across the midline. A further point is that such patients are usually awake, and the quick phases are then generated in response to the pursuit-mediated eye deviation. Finally, a patient with a temporoparietal seizure focus has been described who showed *no gaze deviation* prior to onset of nystagmus.[361] Her attacks were accompanied by vertigo, and slow phases were linear, suggesting involvement of the cortical areas involved in vestibular and optokinetic or pursuit mechanisms (Fig. 6–7, Chapter 6).

Thus, contraversive quick phases in epileptic patients may be due to two different mechanisms: (1) primary, contraversive saccades due to epileptic activity in the saccadic regions, followed by centripetal drift due to impaired gaze-holding; and (2) secondary, reflexive contraversive saccades, which correct for slow ipsiversive deviation across the midline, due to epileptic activation of either the smooth-pursuit or optokinetic regions. In patients with coexistent brainstem lesions, the only manifestation of epileptic activity may be rapid, small-amplitude, vertical eye movements.[1006] The absence of horizontal movements suggests dysfunction of the paramedian pontine reticular formation (PPRF—see Box 12–6).

Frontal lobe foci may cause contraversive deviations but, if bilateral, will lead to *vertical deviations of gaze*.[533,534] These results are consistent with stimulation studies in monkeys: unilateral stimulation of the frontal eye field typically causes oblique saccades with a contralateral horizontal component; the direction of the vertical saccade depends upon a cortical map.[142] Purely vertical movements require bilateral stimulation of the frontal eye fields. Because there are also neurons in the frontal eye fields that contribute to smooth pursuit, it is theoretically possible that frontal lobe foci could lead to an ipsiversive deviation.

Head turning common accompanies epileptic gaze deviation (see Head Turning in Epilepsy, in Chapter 7). In patients who are conscious during the seizure, a frontal focus is likely, and the initial direction of head turning is usually contralateral to the seizure focus.[1186,1187] A contralateral focus is also likely in a patient who shows forced and sustained lateral positioning of the head and eyes. In patients who are unconscious during the seizure, the focus may arise from any lobe and head turning may be toward or away from the side of the lesion.[390,790]

As discussed above, seizures emanating in the superior temporal lobes may cause a variety of vestibular sensations, and occipital lobe seizures may produce oscillopsia.[79] Rarely, seizures may be precipitated by movements of the eyes such as convergence[1140] or sustained lateral deviation.[983] We have observed a patient in whom left horizontal gaze deviation consistently precipitated adversive seizures, with head turning to the left and tonic flexion of the left elbow. He had recently undergone partial resection of a right frontotemporal glioblastoma.

Finally, gaze deviations during disturbance of consciousness need not imply epilepsy. Experimentally induced syncope is reported to cause tonic upward gaze deviation and downbeat nystagmus.[634]

ABNORMALITIES OF EYE MOVEMENTS IN PATIENTS WITH DEMENTIA

A variety of disease processes that cause global impairment of cognitive function may also impair the control of eye movements. Often the clinical ocular motor examination may be normal, and when findings such as vertical gaze palsy or slowed saccades are present, disorders such as progressive supranuclear palsy (PSP), frontotemporal lobar degeneration, which presents as a frontal type of dementia with a PSP-like picture,[661,713a,824] diffuse Lewy-body disease,[762] Huntington's disease, and Whipple's disease should be considered.

Application of experimental paradigms (Fig. 3–2) that are known to test specific cortical and subcortical areas has proved useful in better defining the extent of involvement in these diseases. For example, patients with diffuse Lewy body dementia as well as patients with Parkinson's disease dementia or Alzheimer's disease show more errors on complex tasks such as the antisaccade test (Fig. 3–2D) than patients with idiopathic Parkinson's' disease.[746] Although no test is diagnostically specific, serial testing provides one index of progression of the disease, and so may be useful in evaluating new therapies.

Alzheimer's Disease

Most disorders of eye movements in Alzheimer's disease reflect an underlying loss of the ability to direct or shift visual attention. Thus, the ability to sustain steady fixation of a visual target may be disrupted by large saccadic intrusions, which are distinct from the small, to-and-fro square-wave jerks (Fig. 10–15A) that are also common in the elderly.[1,455,522,744,962,982,989] These larger, inappropriate saccades are often due to a distracting stimulus, or occur because patients cannot suppress eye movements made in anticipation of the expected appearance of a stimulus.[486] They have been studied using the antisaccade test stimulus, in which the subject is required to suppress a reflexive saccade towards a visual stimulus and, instead, look in the opposite direction (Fig. 12–14),[3,237,338,982] Patients affected by Alzheimer's disease are unable to suppress such reflexive saccades; this has been called a visual grasp reflex.[338] The frequency of errors on the antisaccade task correlates with impairment on cognitive testing.[224]

When patients with Alzheimer's disease make visually guided saccades, the reaction time is prolonged if the appearance of the target is unpredictable.[338,457,850] Saccades are hypometric,[338,982] and may be mildly slowed if the target stimulus is unpredictable,[338] more so vertically.[486] Slowing of vertical saccades is consistent with neuropathological studies, which have demonstrated cytoskeletal changes in the riMLF.[938] When patients with Alzheimer's disease are asked to study a complex visual scene, their ability to scan it with saccades is diminished.[238,744] This impaired ability to direct visual attention may mimic Balint's syndrome.[470]

Smooth pursuit in patients with Alzheimer's disease often shows reduced gain, with catch-up saccades, for all frequencies and velocities of target motion, with a further decline for higher target accelerations.[339,1199] Similar to what occurs during fixation, smooth pursuit may be disrupted by large saccadic intrusions as the patient looks towards the anticipated target position. Predictive aspects of smooth pursuit are relatively preserved in Alzheimer's disease. The vestibulo-ocular reflex is normal.[600]

In summary, in Alzheimer's disease, the impaired ability to suppress saccades to novel visual stimuli on the antisaccade task suggests frontal lobe involvement, whereas patients who show impaired ability to shift visual attention probably have parietal lobe involvement.

Creutzfeldt–Jakob Disease

Patients with Creutzfeldt–Jakob disease may show limitation of vertical gaze and slow vertical saccades, and two rare forms of nystagmus, periodic alternating nystagmus (see Box 10–5) and centripetal nystagmus (see Box 10–7).[408,445] Eventually, patients may lose saccades and quick phases, but continue to show periodic alternating gaze deviation.[408] Other affected patients show sustained gaze or skew deviations with head turns.[1197] This spectrum of disturbance of eye movements attests to prominent involvement of the cerebellum and brainstem in some patients with Creutzfeldt-Jakob disease. Overdoses of lithium or bismuth may lead to syndromes that mimic Creutzfeldt-Jakob disease.[399,1016] Cerebellar eye signs are typically found in another prion disorder, Gerstmann-Sträussler-Scheinker disease.[316,1194]

AIDS and Dementia

HIV encephalopathy may cause several disturbances of ocular motility reflecting frontal lobe involvement, including increased errors on the antisaccade task (Fig. 12–14), increased fixation instability, and increased latencies of saccades, especially vertically.[517,713,758] Some patients may develop acquired ocular motor apraxia.[130] Others show signs suggesting cerebellar and brainstem involvement, including gaze-evoked and dissociated nystagmus,[831] slow saccades,[775] and ocular flutter.[529] Decreased or asymmetric pursuit gain is a common finding.[517,1057] In addition, patients with AIDS may show a number of ocular motor abnormalities reflecting the effects of opportunistic infection or coexistent neoplasia.[236,425,440,560]

EYE MOVEMENT DISORDERS IN PSYCHIATRIC ILLNESSES

Although abnormalities of voluntary gaze have long been associated with insanity, it was Diefendorf and Dodge who, in 1908, first suggested that eye tracking is abnormal in dementia praecox (schizophrenia).[280] A sustained research effort has gone into trying to delineate the eye movement abnormalities encountered in psychosis, with the goal of identifying behavioral markers for major genes that could contribute to this disorder.[646,700,947]

Smooth Pursuit in Schizophrenia

Initial studies were thwarted by poor recording techniques and methods of analysis that bear no relevance to the physiologic properties of eye movements.[495] More recent reports agree that smooth pursuit is abnormal in most schizophrenics: eye acceleration at onset of pursuit is decreased, the gain of sustained pursuit is reduced, and the number of catch-up saccades is increased.[315,348,496,643,743,1058,1060,1081] Predictive aspects of smooth pursuit show some abnormalities in schizophrenics.[47a,1111]

Another abnormality that interferes with smooth pursuit in schizophrenics is saccadic intrusions.[642,655] These consist of small, to-and-fro square-wave jerks (Fig 10–15A, Chapter 10), which also occur in normal subjects,[1] but also larger anticipatory or "leading" saccades in the direction of target motion that are followed, after about 0.5 to 1.5 seconds, by a corrective saccade that brings the eyes back to the target.[48] Large studies have confirmed that both pursuit and saccadic abnormalities are shown by both schizophrenics and their unaffected relatives.[927]

How specific for schizophrenia are the abnormalities of eye movements that occur during tests of smooth pursuit? Low-gain pursuit eye movements may occur in patients with affective disorders, and it is debated whether the disruption of pursuit by saccades is more specific for schizophrenia.[315,348,1060] Furthermore, square-wave jerks occur in a variety of conditions, and anticipatory saccades are not peculiar to schizophrenics; they also occur in Alzheimer's disease,[339] and in normal subjects as they track a target moving across a textured background.[547] Another potentially confounding factor is that cigarette smoking—a habit common among schizophrenics—is known to induce square-wave jerks,[1003] and may influence smooth pursuit performance. The converse view is that nicotine normalizes smooth pursuit in schizophrenics,[799] reducing the number of leading saccade,[48] possibly by improving function in regions of cerebral cortex that are important for motion vision.[1109]

The possible contribution of neuroleptic medications to the saccadic intrusions is not completely settled, although unmedicated schizophrenics do show lower smooth-pursuit gain than controls and patients who have been receiving neuroleptic medicines for years tend to show poorer tracking.[348,495,496,1059] It has been suggested that the drug ketamine, a non-competitive N-methyl-D-aspartate (NMDA) receptor antagonist is a pharmacological model for schizophrenia and, some changes in eye movements similar to those encountered in schizophrenia, such as reduced pursuit gain, increased leading saccades, and increased distractibility during the antisaccade task have been reported.[49,213,1166]

There is some evidence that impaired smooth pursuit may be due to a deficit in motion perception.[1050] However, the disorder of smooth pursuit in schizophrenia resembles the disorder occurring in monkeys after frontal lobe lesions.[675] Functional imaging has supported this hypothesis, linking impaired smooth tracking with hypometabolism in the frontal eye fields, supplementary eye fields, medial superior temporal visual area (MST) and anterior cingulate.[475,926]

Saccades in Schizophrenia

The most consistent abnormalities in schizophrenia have concerned the voluntary control of saccades, and especially those functions that depend on the frontal lobes.[497] Simple tests of saccades demonstrate increased saccadic reaction times, decreasing velocity as reaction time increases, and hypometria compared with control subjects or patients with affective disorders.[679,743,878,964] However, the most impressive findings are with tests requiring imagination, memory, or prediction. Thus, schizophrenics show saccade abnormalities similar to those in patients with frontal lobe or basal ganglia disease, including increased errors on the antisaccade task (Fig. 12–14).[165,223,225,778,1080] Errors on the antisaccade task correlate with other measures of working memory in schizophrenics.[497] First-degree relatives of schizophrenics also show increased errors on the antisaccade task compared with controls.[225,1082] Nicotine reduces errors on the antisaccade task in schizophrenics, but not control subjects.[606] Schizophrenics also show defects in memory-guided saccades, suggesting dysfunction of dorsolateral prefrontal cortex.[817] On the other hand, schizophrenics are able to generate express saccades, depending on the length of the gap between the disappearance of the fixation light and the appearance of the target.[188] Prior to starting therapy, schizophrenics may show smaller reaction times than controls during visually guided saccades.[892] Taken together with results from basic studies of frontal lobe function,[358] the disorder of saccades in schizophrenics implicates an abnormal neural substrate in the dorsolateral prefrontal cortex.[497] However, other evidence suggests involvement of other basal ganglia and cerebellar circuits.[312,592]

Eye Movements in Other Psychiatric Disorders

Evidence has also been presented from tests of saccadic eye movements showing disturbed frontal lobe function in patients with obsessive-compulsive disorder.[921,1092] Individuals with attention-deficit hyperactivity disorder (ADHD) are less able to hold steady gaze during attentional tasks,[31] and to countermand saccades than controls, perhaps reflecting parallel difficulties with impulse control.[32] Eye movement studies have been used to investigate the gaze-avoidance behavior shown in autism.[240] Patients with Asperger's syndrome show increased errors and latencies on the antisaccade task (Fig. 3-2D), implicating dysfunction of prefrontal cortex,[686] as well as impairment of pursuit especially for targets presented into the right visual hemifield, suggesting disturbance in left extrastriate cortex.[1065]

EYE MOVEMENTS IN STUPOR AND COMA

The ocular motor examination is especially useful for evaluating the unconscious patient because both arousal and eye movement are controlled by neurons in the brainstem reticular formation. Comatose patients do not make eye movements that depend upon cortical visual processing; voluntary saccades and smooth pursuit are in abeyance. Quick phases of nystagmus, too, may be absent. The ocular motor examination of the unconscious patient, therefore, consists of observing the resting position of the eyes, looking for any spontaneous movements, and reflexively inducing eye movements (see Video Display: Eye Movements in Coma).[146,328,621,854]

Resting Position of the Eyes in Unconscious Patients

Conjugate, horizontal deviation of the eyes is common in coma (Box 12–18). If this is due to lesions above the presumed brainstem ocular motor decussation (between the midbrain and pons), then the eyes are usually directed toward the side of the lesion and away from the hemiparesis. A vestibular stimulus, though, can usually drive the eyes across the midline. If the conjugate deviation is due to a lesion below the ocular motor decussation, then the eyes will be directed away from the side of the lesion and toward the hemiparesis. This situation is typically seen with pontine lesions, but also in some patients with thalamic lesions,[327] and rarely with hemispheric disease above the thalamus (so-called *wrong-way deviation*).[828,986]

Intermittent deviation of the eyes and head turning are usually due to seizure activity. At the onset of each attack, gaze is usually deviated contralateral to the side of the seizure focus; it may be followed by nystagmus with contralaterally directed quick phases. Toward the end of the seizure, gaze drifts to an ipsilateral (paretic) position (see Eye Movements during Epileptic Seizures).

Tonic downward gaze deviation of the eyes, often accompanied by convergence, occurs in thalamic hemorrhage,[182,324,325] and with lesions affecting the *dorsal midbrain*. It may be induced by unilateral caloric stimulation, after the initial horizontal deviation subsides, in patients with coma due to sedative drugs, usually barbiturates.[1005] Forced downward deviation of the eyes (always looking towards the ground) has also been reported in patients feigning coma or seizures.[923]

Tonic upward gaze deviation of the eyes occurs following a hypoxic-ischemic insult, even when no pathologic lesions are found in the midbrain.[552] Some patients go on to develop downward gaze deviation associated with a vegetative state.[515] In those patients that survive, downbeating nystagmus may develop,[552] and it has been suggested that upward drift is due to loss of inhibition on the upward vertical vestibulo-ocular reflex.[759] Upward deviation also occurs as a component of oculogyric crises, which usually occur as a side effect of certain drugs, especially neuroleptic agents.[620] Tonic uninhibited elevation of the lids (eyes-open coma) rarely occurs in unconscious patients and may be related to pontomesencephalic dysfunction.[550]

Deviations of the visual axes in coma may be due to palsied oculomotor, trochlear, or abducens nerves (see Clinical Features of

Ocular Nerve Palsies, in Chapter 9) skew deviation, or a phoria that is normally compensated for by fusional mechanisms. Thalamic and brainstem hemorrhages also cause ocular deviations, including eyes that are turned in and down.[182,863] Restrictive ophthalmopathy, particularly blow-out fracture of the orbit, may be a mechanism in patients who have suffered head trauma. Diagnosis of the cause of the deviation depends upon determining whether the range of movement of the eyes, induced by head rotation or caloric stimulation (see Reflex Eye Movements in Unconscious Patients, below), is reduced in a pattern corresponding to specific muscle weakness. In addition, involvement of the pupils and other brainstem reflexes may help with the diagnosis. Complete oculomotor nerve palsy causes pupillary dilatation, ptosis, and deviation of the eye "down and out." Pupillary involvement is an early sign of uncal herniation,[854] and disturbance of eye movements usually follows.[556] Vertical tropias are usually due to skew deviation or to trochlear nerve palsy, which is common following head trauma. Bilateral abducens palsy occurs when increased intracranial pressure compromises the nerves as they bend over the petroclinoid ligament. Occasionally, skew deviation and internuclear ophthalmoplegia are encountered in metabolic encephalopathy,[172,331] or with drug intoxication.[215,287,307,485,910]

Spontaneous Eye Movements in Unconscious Patients

Always consider epileptic seizures in the unconscious patient who shows spontaneous eye movements (see discussion in preceding section). Slow conjugate or disconjugate roving eye movements are similar to the eye movements of light sleep (but slower than the rapid movements of paradoxical or REM sleep). They imply that brainstem gaze mechanisms are intact.[328] A spectrum of abnormal eye movements are encountered almost exclusively in unconscious patients, and are summarized in Table 12–9.

Ocular bobbing consists of intermittent, usually conjugate, rapid downward movement of the eyes followed by a slower return to the central position (see Video Display: Eye Movements in Coma).[80,326,704] Reflex horizontal eye movements are usually absent. Ocular

Table 12–9. **Spontaneous Eye Movements Occurring in Unconscious Patients**

Term	Description	Significance
Ocular bobbing	Rapid, conjugate, downward movement; slow return to primary position	Pontine strokes;[80,245,326,546,605, 919,1052, 1096,1218] other structural,[118,806,944] metabolic,[292] or toxic disorders[437]
Ocular dipping or inverse ocular bobbing	Slow downward movement; rapid return to primary position	Unreliable for localization; follows hypoxic-ischemic insult or metabolic disorder[579,665,916,917,950,1032,1128]
Reverse ocular bobbing	Rapid upward movement; slow return to primary position	Unreliable for localization; may occur with metabolic disorders[244,1102]
Reverse ocular dipping or converse bobbing	Slow upward movement; rapid return to primary position	Unreliable for localization; pontine infarction and with AIDS[393,704]
Ping-pong gaze	Horizontal conjugate deviation of the eyes, alternating every few seconds	Bilateral cerebral hemispheric dysfunction[499]
Periodic alternating gaze deviation	Horizontal conjugate deviation of the eyes, alternating every 2 minutes	Hepatic encephalopathy;[42] disorders causing periodic alternating nystagmus and unconsciousness or vegetative state[408]
Vertical "myoclonus"	Vertical pendular oscillations (2–3 Hz)	Pontine strokes[555]
Monocular movements	Small, intermittent, rapid monocular horizontal, vertical, or torsional movements	Pontine or midbrain destructive lesions, perhaps with coexistent seizures[1006]

bobbing is a classic sign of intrinsic pontine lesions, usually hemorrhage, but it has also been reported with cerebellar lesions that secondarily compress the pons (Fig. 12–17), as well as in metabolic or toxic encephalopathy. A variant, inverse bobbing has an initial downward movement that is slow and the return to midposition is rapid; this has also been called ocular dipping. Reverse ocular bobbing consists of rapid deviation of the eyes upward and a slow return to the horizontal. Finally, the term reverse ocular dipping or converse bobbing has been used to describe a slow upward drift of the eyes followed by a rapid return to central position. Sometimes, the bobbing is variably disconjugate.[371] These variants of ocular bobbing are less reliable for localization. Nevertheless, the report that some patients have shown several types of bobbing suggests a common underlying pathophysiology.[144,393,924,1102] Since the pathways that mediate upward and downward eye movements differ anatomically, and probably pharmacologically, it seems likely that these movements represent a varying imbalance of mechanisms for vertical gaze. Rarely, large-amplitude vertical pendular oscillations ("myoclonus"), in association with horizontal gaze palsy, occur in the acute phase of a brainstem stroke;[555] some patients survive to develop oculopalatal tremor. Repetitive vertical eye movements, including variants of ocular bobbing, that contain convergent-divergent components usually indicate disease affecting the dorsal midbrain.[553,782,925]

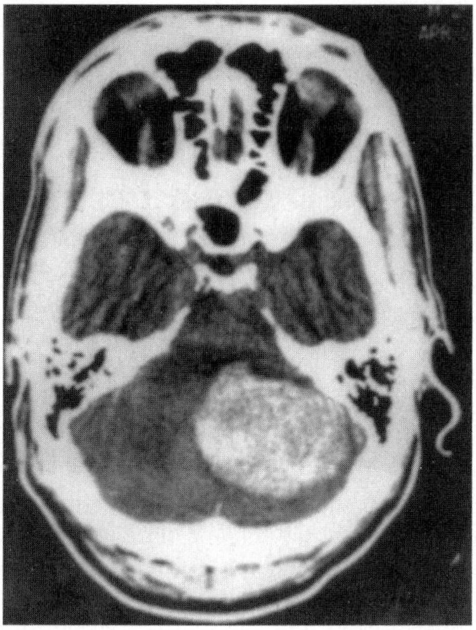

A

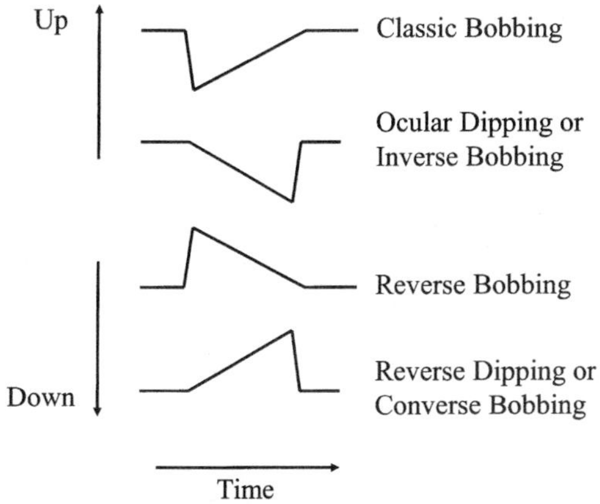

B

Figure 12–17. (A) MRI of a patient who developed ocular bobbing (see Video Display: Eye Movements in Coma), showing acute hemorrhagic infarction of the cerebellum with swelling that compressed the pons. (B) Schematic summary of nomenclature of reported variants of ocular bobbing.

Ping-pong gaze consists of slow, horizontal, conjugate deviations of the eyes alternating every few seconds (see Video Display: Eye Movements in Coma);[499] affected patients are usually obtunded. Ping-pong gaze usually occurs with bilateral infarction of the cerebral hemispheres or of the cerebral peduncles,[603] but also has been ascribed to diffuse ischemia following cardiac surgery.[281] Sometimes a rapid horizontal head rotation will induce transient oscillations with a similar periodicity to ping-pong gaze in patients with bilateral hemispheric disease.[621] A saccadic form of ping-pong gaze has been reported as a transient finding in patients who are more awake or who survive in a persistent vegetative state.[516] Ping-pong gaze has been reported as a manifestation of drug intoxication with tranylcypromine, thioridazine, and clomipramine.[860] Periodic alternating gaze deviation, in which conjugate gaze deviations change direction every 2 minutes, has been reported in hepatic encephalopathy.[42] This phenomenon is related to periodic alternating nystagmus (without the quick phases), which is discussed in Chapter 10.

Rapid, small-amplitude, vertical eye movements may be the only manifestation of epileptic seizures in patients with coexistent brainstem injury.[1006] Rapid, monocular eye movements with horizontal, vertical, or torsional components, can occur in coma, and may also indicate brainstem dysfunction.

Identification of patients who are conscious but quadriplegic, the *locked-in or de-efferented state*, depends upon identifying preserved voluntary vertical eye movements.[604,636,854] The syndrome is typically caused by pontine infarction with a variable loss of voluntary and reflex horizontal movements, so that eyelid or vertical eye movements may be the only means of communication in the acute illness. The locked-in syndrome also occurs with midbrain lesions, in which case ptosis and ophthalmoplegia may be associated.[709]

Reflex Eye Movements in Unconscious Patients

The examination of the unconscious patient is incomplete without attempting to elicit reflex eye movements, either by head rotation (the doll's-head or oculocephalic maneuver) or by caloric stimulation (see Video Display: Eye Movements in Coma).[146,765,854] Always check that there has been no neck injury or abnormality before rotating the head, and inspect the tympanic membranes before carrying out caloric testing.

What do these time-honored clinical methods test? Head rotation, with the patient supine, potentially stimulates the labyrinthine semicircular canals, the otoliths, and neck muscle proprioceptors. Unless there has been prior loss of vestibular function (e.g., from aminoglycoside antibiotic toxicity, for example), the contribution made by neck muscle proprioceptors in generating reflex eye movements (the cervico-ocular reflex (COR)) is insignificant.[621] Furthermore, the otolithic contribution is probably small compared with that of the labyrinthine semicircular canals. Finally, although visually mediated eye movements, such as fixation and smooth pursuit, can influence the eye movements produced by head rotation in normal, awake subjects, this is unlikely to be the case in unconscious patients. Therefore, eye rotations induced by head rotation in unconscious individuals are principally due to the effects of the semicircular canals and their central connections: the vestibulo-ocular reflex (VOR). Conventionally, high-frequency (1 Hz to 2 Hz) quasi-sinusoidal rotations are applied, or position-step stimuli, which consist of a sudden head turn to a new steady position. Both horizontal and vertical rotations should be performed. If small-amplitude head rotations are performed, the adequacy of the VOR can be estimated by observing the optic disc of one eye with an ophthalmoscope.[1204] If reflex eye movements are intact in an unconscious patient, then when the head is rapidly rotated horizontally to a new position (position-step stimulus), the eyes are carried into a corner of the orbit (Fig. 12–18). If the head is held stationary in its new position, the eyes may drift back to the midline. This implies that the gaze-holding mechanism (neural integrator) is not functioning normally. Patients with more rapid centripetal drift may have more severe brain injury.[621]

Caloric irrigation of the external auditory meatus causes convection currents of the vestibular endolymph that displace the cupula of a semicircular canal; thus, this procedure tests the VOR (see Video Display: Eye Movements in Coma). The canal stimulated depends upon the orientation of the head; with the head elevated 30 degrees from supine position, the horizontal canals are principally stimulated. Large quantities (100 ml or more) of ice water may be necessary. Caloric stimulation with ice water may sometimes be a more effective stimulus than head rotation, perhaps owing to the sustained nature of the stimulus as well as the arousing effect of the cold water. Combined cold caloric stimulation and head rotation may be the most effective stimulus in the deeply unconscious patient,[328] producing tonic deviation of the eyes toward the irrigated ear.

In testing reflex eye movements in unresponsive patients, it is important to note the magnitude of the response and whether or not the ocular deviation is conjugate; the dynamic response to position-step head rotations; and the occurrence of any quick phases of nystagmus, particularly during caloric stimulation. When reflex eye movements are present in an unresponsive patient, the brainstem is likely to be structurally intact. When reflex eye movements are abnormal or absent, the cause may be structural disease (especially brainstem strokes), metabolic and deficiency states (including Wernicke's encephalopathy), or drug intoxication (Table 12–11).[427,922] Complete ophthalmoplegia in an unresponsive patient should also prompt consideration of acute neu-

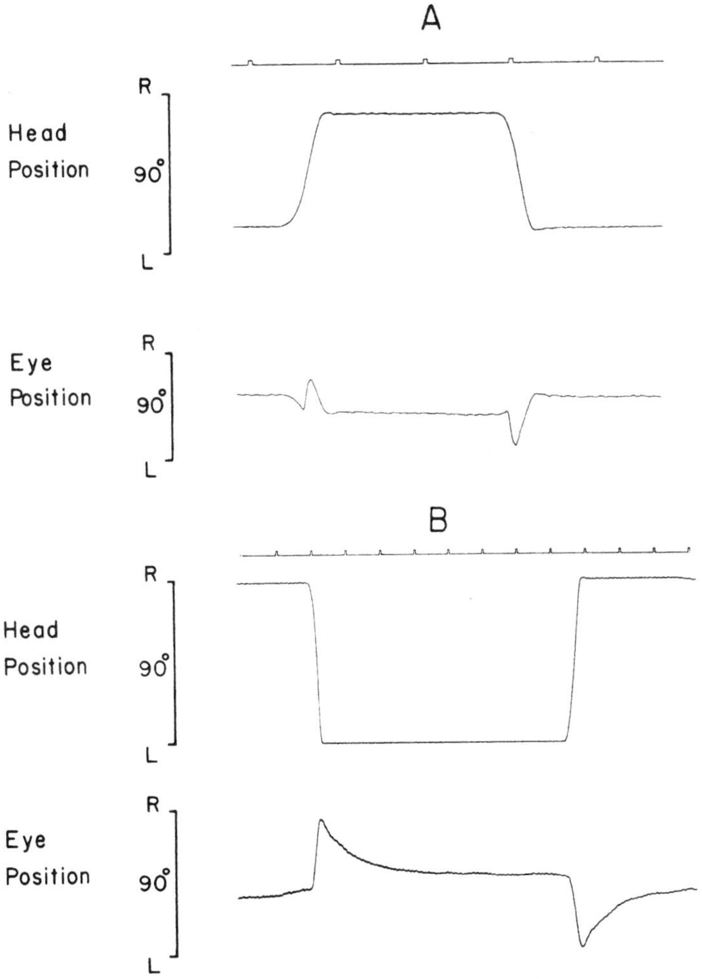

Figure 12–18. The vestibulo-ocular reflex in coma. (A) The response of a normal subject, in darkness, to a sudden, rapid or "step" head turn. An initial vestibular slow phase is interrupted by a quick phase. The new eye position is held steadily. (B) Eye movements of an unconscious patient. The patient had suffered bilateral infarction of the cerebral hemispheres and also had hepatic dysfunction. Pupils were 3 mm, equal, and reactive to light. Noxious stimuli produced no eye opening or verbal response but caused extensor posturing in the right upper extremity and abnormal flexor posturing in the left upper extremity. A step rotation of the head to the left produced a vestibular eye movement to the right, without any quick phase. Subsequently, the eyes drifted back to the midline with a negative exponential waveform. This reflects the "leaky" nature of the neural integrator, which depends upon brainstem reticular structures. Eye movements were recorded by electro-oculography. Calibration is approximate for the unconscious patient. Time scale, at top, is in seconds (see also Video Display: Eye Movements in Coma).

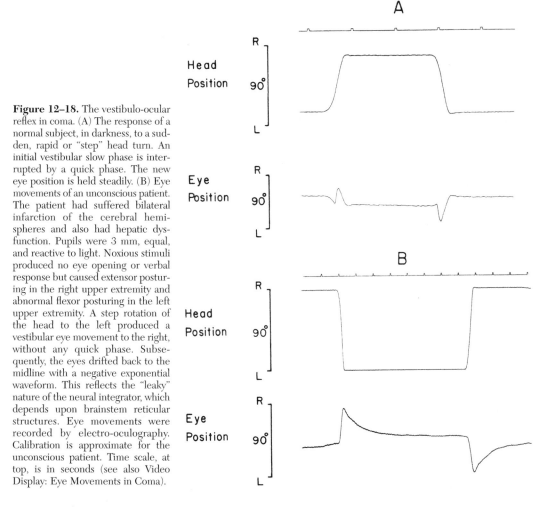

ropathy (such as Guillain-Barre syndrome) and neuromuscular block, due to drugs or botulism.[554] Vertical reflex eye movements may be impaired with disease of the midbrain[1120] or bilateral lesions of the MLF. Pontine lesions may abolish the reflex eye movements in the horizontal plane but relatively spare the vertical responses. Impaired abduction suggests sixth nerve palsy; impaired adduction implies either internuclear ophthalmoplegia or third nerve palsy. Occasionally, impaired adduction to vestibular stimulation may be observed in patients with metabolic coma[172] or drug intoxication.[215,287,307,485,910] Patients in barbiturate coma may show downward deviation of their eyes with caloric stimuli,[1005] or no response. When used in combination with other clinical signs, reflex eye movements have been useful in predicting the outcome of coma.[644,749]

Quick phases of nystagmus are usually absent in acutely unconscious patients, so their presence, without a tonic deviation of the eyes, should raise the possibility of feigned coma. In patients who are stuporous but uncooperative, caloric nystagmus may be a useful way of inducing eye movements that cannot be initiated voluntarily. For example, in a patient with a pineal tumor, retraction nystagmus was induced with caloric stimulation.[1008] Patients who survive coma but who are left in a persistent vegetative state, with severe damage of the cerebral hemispheres but preservation of the brainstem,[854] regain nystagmus with caloric or rotational stimulation.[621] Recovery of eye tracking of the examiner or family members is an indication of those patients who may show some recovery from this state.[27] Caloric induced nystagmus has been reported in patients with neocortical death and an isoelectric electroencephalogram.[767]

OCULAR MOTOR DYSFUNCTION AND MULTIPLE SCLEROSIS (MS)

Value of Examining Eye Movements in Multiple Sclerosis Patients

No evaluation of a patient either suspected or diagnosed with MS is complete without a systematic examination of their eye movements. A hundred-and-fifty years of clinical experience, and numerous published studies, attest to the value of eye movements in making a diagnosis of MS, tracking its progress, and even estimating prognosis.[272] It is unfortunate, therefore, that current standard evaluations of MS lack a systematic approach for testing each of the functional classes of eye movements. Here we aim to describe the common findings in MS, and interpret their significance using our pathophysiologic approach.

Clinical Evaluation

Multiple sclerosis causes a variety of ocular motor deficits (Box 12–22), of which bilateral internuclear ophthalmoplegia (INO) (see Video Display: Pontine Syndromes), cerebellar eye signs (including gaze-evoked nystagmus), and acquired pendular nystagmus (Fig.10–9, Chapter 10) are most commonly recognized.[352,354,1036] The pendular nystagmus is frequently visually disabling (see Video Display: Acquired Pendular Nystagmus).[35,660] Acute vertigo with nystagmus may occur during an exacerbation, and sometimes is recurrent and troublesome.

Systematic examination of eye movements in patients with MS commonly reveals other abnormalities, especially saccadic dysmetria.[291,981] Some patients also show deviation of the subjective visual vertical, assessed with a

Box 12–22. Common Ocular Motor Manifestations of Multiple Sclerosis

- Internuclear ophthalmoplegia (INO), usually bilateral
- Gaze-evoked nystagmus
- Acquired pendular nystagmus
- Upbeat, downbeat, or torsional nystagmus
- Positionally induced nystagmus
- Saccadic dysmetria
- Saccadic oscillations, such as flutter
- Impaired smooth pursuit and combined eye-head tracking (VOR suppression)
- Impaired optokinetic responses

For recorded examples, see Fig. 10-10 of Chapter 10 and Fig. 12-7, Fig. 12-8, and Fig. 12-9 of Chapter 12. (Related Video Displays: Pontine Syndromes; Disorders of Saccades; Acquired Pendular Nystagmus) simple laser pointer fitted with inexpensive line-generating optics.[981] Such clinical studies have established that patients who have abnormal eye movements are more disabled than those with normal motility, and that this difference is sustained after two years. The reason for the increased disability in MS patients with abnormal eye movements is less due to their impaired vision than to their disturbance of gait. Both are caused by prominent involvement of the brainstem and cerebellar pathways.[981]

Measuring Eye Movements in Multiple Sclerosis

Clinical detection of INO may be challenging,[357] and measurement of eye movements may help confirm the diagnosis during early stages of the disease (Fig. 12–9). Detection of a saccadic abnormality may be better when targets are presented randomly, so that neither their time of onset nor their location can be predicted. Large saccades (20 degrees or greater) are more likely to show changes in velocity than are small saccades.[710] Paired comparison of the peak velocity of abducting and adducting saccades can be misleading since normal subjects show somewhat greater peak velocities in the abducting eye,[207] depending on the methodology being used. A more reliable approach is to measure the ratio of abducting/adducting movements during horizontal saccades, and compare the patient's value with that of group of normal subjects. Thus, normal subjects show little variation in the abducting/adducting ratio of either peak eye velocity[1130] or peak acceleration.[341,342] Patients with INO have abduction/adduction ratios for peak velocity or peak acceleration that exceed the 95% prediction intervals for normal subjects.[351]

Other saccadic abnormalities in multiple sclerosis include prolonged reaction time (latency), inaccuracy, and decreased velocity.[134,710,896] Some patients with multiple sclerosis show saccadic oscillations and intrusions.[36,456]

Smooth-pursuit gain may be decreased,[896,988] and there may be impaired cancellation of the horizontal vestibulo-ocular reflex (VOR) during eye-head rotation.[988] Unilateral internuclear ophthalmoplegia may impair the vertical vestibulo-ocular reflex during stimulation of the contralateral posterior semicircular canal, which depends on the medial longitudinal fasciculus for normal responses.[227] Bilateral internuclear ophthalmoplegia impairs the vertical vestibulo-ocular reflex, gaze holding, smooth pursuit, and eye-head tracking, functions which also depend on the medial longitudinal fasciculus (Box 6–2).[882] Patients with severe head tremor and an impaired vestibulo-ocular reflex may report oscillopsia.[859]

Other reported abnormalities include horizontal and vertical gaze palsies,[694,1157] gaze-evoked blepharoclonus,[551] upbeat and downbeat nystagmus,[55,323,699] various vestibular and optokinetic abnormalities,[498,543,1103] superior oblique myokymia (Chapter 9) and convergence spasm (Chapter 8). Patients may also develop oculomotor, trochlear or abducens palsies (see Chapter 9). An MRI is often helpful in identifying brainstem or cerebellar lesions responsible for such abnormalities; thin cuts and proton density images may be required.[355]

The Role of Eye Movements in Diagnosis and Management of Multiple Sclerosis

Diagnosis of early multiple sclerosis depends on demonstration of lesions disseminated throughout the nervous system. Early diagnosis has become more important because prompt initiation of immunotherapy appears to provide the best opportunity to arrest the disease. Although detection of subtle deficits of ocular motility, such as INO, may be useful in making a diagnosis, some caution is required since these tests are not specific for multiple sclerosis. Thus, the clinician must weigh the results of ocular motor studies with other clinical or laboratory findings before making a diagnosis. Routine examination of eye movements during follow-up visits to the MS clinic (along with careful evaluation of vision) may provide a useful method of evaluating progress and prognosis. Patients who are more generally disabled are more likely to develop abnormalities of eye movements, probably because the brunt of the disease is affecting brainstem and cerebellar connections.[272,291,981]

As discussed in Chapter 10, clinical trials have demonstrated that gabapentin,[47,60] and memantine,[1031] may ameliorate the visually disabling acquired pendular nystagmus that occurs in multiple sclerosis (see Video Display: Treatments for Nystagmus).

OCULAR MOTOR MANIFESTATIONS OF METABOLIC AND DEFICIENCY DISORDERS

The genetic revolution has identified the biochemical basis for many disorders and so redefined the spectrum of diseases considered "metabolic" and "degenerative". With this progress in mind, we review selected metabolic and deficiency disorders. Some of the main ocular motor findings of selected hereditary disorders are listed in Table 12–10. First, we address the issue of whether abnormal eye movements in infants imply a genetic disorder or a syndrome that will spontaneously resolve.

Eye Movement Disorders in Infants who Eventually Develop Normally

It is important to note that some normal infants who ultimately develop normally may show transient ocular motor "abnormalities". These include upward or downward deviation of the eyes (but with a full range of reflex vertical movement), intermittent saccadic oscillations (flutter or opsoclonus), and skew deviation.[9,439,487,489,809,810] However, skew deviation and transient tonic upgaze may be associated with later appearance of horizontal strabismus and intellectual or language disability.[439] Premature babies may show reduced excursion of the adducting eye with caloric stimulation, suggest-

Table 12–10. **Ocular Motor Manifestations of Certain Neurogenetic, Metabolic, and Deficiency Disorders**

Disorder	Disturbance of Eye Movement
Tay-Sachs disease	Impairment of vertical and horizontal gaze[509]
Adult-onset hexosaminidase A deficiency (late-onset Tay-Sachs disease)	Horizontal and vertical saccades show transient decelerations, especially for large saccades[943]
Gaucher's disease (non-infantile, neuronopathic form)	Initially, horizontal saccadic palsy; later, loss of voluntary gaze[6,822,1141,1180]
Niemann-Pick type C	Initially, selective vertical saccadic palsy;[934] later, loss of voluntary gaze[198,322,461,1020]
Branch-chain aminoacid disorders (e.g., Maple syrup urine disease)	Adduction and upgaze impairment[677,1208]
Glutaric aciduria, type 1	Gaze palsy[527]
Wernicke's encephalopathy	Spectrum ranging from gaze-evoked and upbeat nystagmus to complete ophthalmoplegia (see text)[201,254,566,984]
Leigh's syndrome	Similar to that in Wernicke's encephalopathy[288,423,731,975,1073]
Vitamin E deficiency: hereditary (e.g., abetalipoproteinemia) or acquired	Progressive restriction of horizontal and vertical gaze; dissociated nystagmus, in which adduction is faster than abduction[226,1193]
Pelizaeus-Merzbacher disease	Pendular nystagmus; upbeat nystagmus; ocular motor apraxia; saccade dysmetria and other cerebellar signs including truncal titubation[774,1112]
Wilson's disease	Slow vertical saccades;[572] gaze distractibility;[635] oculogyric crisis[615]
Kernicterus	Vertical gaze palsy[488]
Joubert's syndrome	Alternating skew deviation; ocular motor apraxia; seesaw and pendular nystagmus; pigmentary degeneration of the retina[690,690]
Ataxia telangiectasia (Louis-Bar syndrome, 11q22–23) and variants	Saccade initiation defects with head thrusts; gaze-evoked and periodic alternating nystagmus[10,369,650,1038]

ing internuclear ophthalmoparesis, but a full deviation of both eyes usually occurs with rotational stimuli, although quick phases of nystagmus may be absent.[1168] The time constant (as a reflection of duration) of the vestibulo-ocular reflex in newborns is low (typically 6 seconds) and does not reach adult values until the infant is about 2 months old.[1168]

Lipid Storage Diseases

These disorders are often characterized by disturbances of gaze. Thus, infantile Tay-Sachs disease impairs vertical and, subsequently, horizontal eye movements. Late-onset Tay-Sachs disease is due to a partial defect of hexosaminidase A, and is characterized by a progressive course and variable clinical picture that includes, ataxia, signs suggestive of motoneuron disease, and psychiatric symptoms. Horizontal and vertical saccades may appear slow of multistep; measurements have demonstrated that large saccades stall in mid-flight, evident as transient decelerations (Fig. 3–20).[943]

Variants of Niemann-Pick disease that begin after the first year of life (previously called the sea-blue histiocyte syndrome or juvenile dystonic lipidosis) are characterized by deficits of voluntary vertical eye movements.[198] Early in the course of Niemann-Pick type C (2S) disease, which presents during adolescence with intellectual impairment, ataxia, and dysarthria, there may be selective slowing of vertical saccades; other eye movements (including horizontal saccades) are normal (see Video Display: Disorders of Saccades).[198,627,934,1020] Diagonal saccades may show a curved trajectory (Fig. 3–5B), evident during the clinical examination. Histopathological examination of the brain of a patient with Niemann-Pick type C disease showed glial fibrillary lesions affecting the posterior commissure and neuronal loss in the riMLF, but with preservation of the interstitial nucleus of Cajal and of ocular motoneurons.[1020]

Gaucher's disease is an autosomal recessive lysosomal glycolipid storage disease due to deficient glucocerebrosidase enzyme, which is located in chromosome 1q21. Gaucher's disease comprises three phenotypic variants.[6] Type 1 is the most common and lacks neurological features. Type 2 is the infantile neuronopathic form, which is characterized by trismus, strabismus, ocular motor apraxia, opisthotonus and death by about 2 years. Type 3 is a juvenile neuronopathic form with a milder course. Neuronopathic Gaucher's disease causes a prominent deficit of horizontal gaze, with impaired saccadic initiation and loss of optokinetic quick phases;[111,435] in adult patients, slow saccades may be a prominent finding,[822,1141] and may provide a therapeutic index during enzyme therapy for this disorder.[18] Interestingly, even adults with Type 1 Gaucher's disease may show some saccadic abnormalities, such as abnormal velocity profiles, which may be evidence for subclinical neurological involvement.[6]

Wernicke's Encephalopathy

Wernicke's encephalopathy is characterized by the triad of ophthalmoplegia, mental confusion, and gait ataxia,[163] though there are probably many *formes fruste* with lesser manifestations. It is caused by thiamine deficiency and is commonly encountered in alcoholics, but other causes to be considered include malnutrition related to gastric bypass, eating disorders, bulimia, fad diets, deficient soy-based infant formula,[318] and nausea and vomiting due to pregnancy or chemotherapy.

The ocular motor findings in Wernicke's encephalopathy include weakness of abduction, gaze-evoked nystagmus (see Video Display: Disorders of Gaze Holding), internuclear ophthalmoplegia, central vertical nystagmus (usually upbeat, see Video Display: Downbeat, Upbeat, Torsional Nystagmus), impaired vestibular responses to caloric and rotational stimulation (see Video Display: Disorders of the Vestibular System), and horizontal and vertical gaze palsies that may progress to total ophthalmoplegia.[201,220,254,566] The ophthalmoplegia is bilateral but may be asymmetric. Saccades may show transient decelerations of their velocity profiles,[502] somewhat similar to that seem in late-onset Tay-Sachs disease (Fig. 3–20, Chapter 3).

Experimental thiamine deficiency in monkeys causes an orderly progression of ophthalmoplegia associated with well-circumscribed histopathologic changes.[202] These changes consist of neuronal loss and gliosis in the oculomotor, trochlear, abducens, and vestibular nuclei. In humans, demyelination, vascular changes, and hemorrhage may occur; in addition to the sites listed above, the lesions are found in the periventricular regions of the thalamus, the hypothalamus, periaqueductal gray matter, superior vermis of the cerebellum, and dorsal motor nucleus of the vagus (Fig. 12–19). Thus, gaze-evoked nystagmus and the impaired caloric responses can be attributed to vestibular nucleus involvement (NPH-MVN region). The abduction weakness may reflect involvement of the abducens nerve, and the internuclear ophthalmoplegia (INO) may reflect involvement of the medial longitudinal fasciculus. Paralysis of horizontal gaze may be due to involvement of the abducens nucleus, and total ophthalmoplegia may indicate involvement of all the ocular motor nerve nuclei. Affected areas of the brain most likely contain neurons that use high amounts of glucose and are therefore particularly dependent upon thiamine, an important coenzyme in glucose metabolism.[1181] Administration of thiamine usually causes rapid improvement of the ocular motor signs, although complete recovery may take several weeks. Coexistent magnesium deficiency should also be treated.

In those patients with Wernicke's disease who go on to develop Korsakoff's syndrome, which is primarily characterized by a severe and enduring memory loss, ocular motor abnormalities may persist, consisting of slow and inaccurate saccades, impaired smooth pursuit, vertical and gaze-evoked nystagmus.[565,566]

Leigh's Syndrome

Leigh's syndrome is a subacute necrotizing encephalopathy of infancy or childhood characterized by psychomotor retardation, seizures, and brainstem abnormalities that involve eye movements.[1219] It may be caused by either abnormalities of mitochondrial DNA,[1073] or be

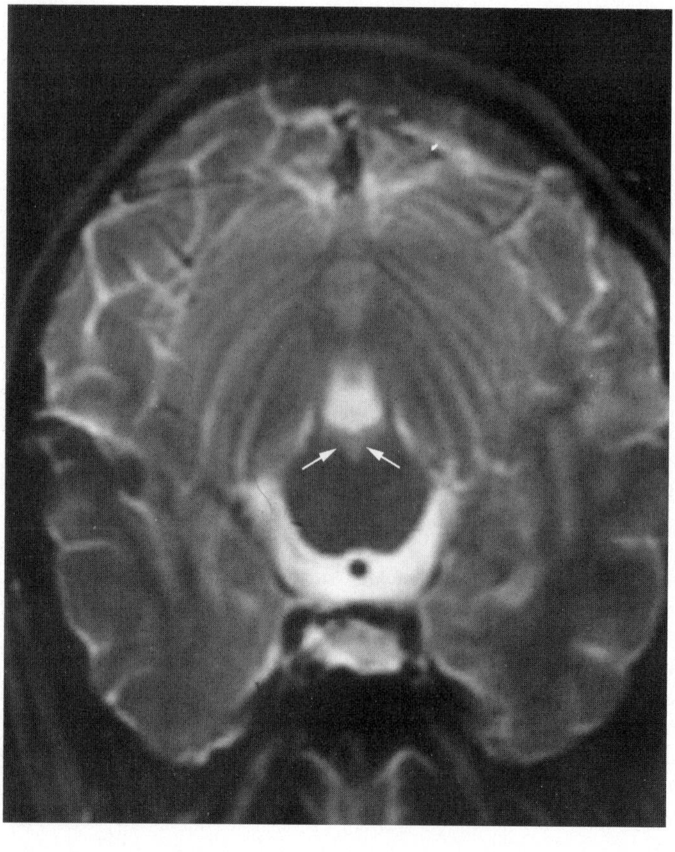

Figure 12–19. MRI scan of a patient with Wernicke's encephalopathy showing signal changes under the floor of the fourth ventricle (arrowheads) that indicate involvement of the medial vestibular nucleus–nucleus prepositus hypoglossi complex at the ponto-medullary junction (see Video Display: Disorders of Gaze Holding).

inherited as an autosomal recessive disorder. Deficiency of respiratory chain complexes I and IV has been identified.[731] Patients with onset early in life show disturbances of ocular motility similar to that caused by experimental thiamine deficiency or Wernicke's encephalopathy. In addition, seesaw nystagmus (Box 10–6) and the ocular tilt reaction (OTR) are reported in Leigh's syndrome.[423] Later-onset cases share clinical features with other disorders of mitochondrial DNA (discussed in Chapter 9).

Genetic Disorders of Central Myelin

Pelizaeus-Merzbacher disease is an X-linked recessive dysmyelinating disease.[403] Affected children may have ocular motor apraxia, cerebellar signs, including saccadic dysmetria and pendular nystagmus (see Video Display: Acquired Pendular Nystagmus).[774,1112] The peroxisomal assembly disorders, such as the neonatal form of adrenoleukodystrophy, also may be associated with pendular nystagmus.[594] Patients with another congenital disorder affecting myelin, Cockayne's syndrome, show similar findings.[206] Alexander's disease is a leukoencephalopathy due to mutation of the gene that encodes the glial fibrillary acid protein. It usually presents in infancy with macrocephaly, spasticity, dementia and seizures. Juvenile and adult-onset cases have been reported that show gaze-evoked and rebound nystagmus, impaired pursuit and oculopalatal myoclonus.[693,972] Diagnosis is made either by histological demonstration of Rosenthal fibers or by DNA analysis.

Hereditary Disorders Causing Vitamin E Deficiency

Vitamin E deficiency due to a range of disorders may cause a progressive neurologic condition characterized by areflexia, cerebellar ataxia, and loss of joint position sense.[177] Ocular motor involvement includes progressive gaze restriction, sometimes with strabismus. Typically, there is a dissociated ophthalmoplegia, and nystagmus in which adduction is fast but with a limited range and abduction is slow but with a full range.[1193] These findings presumably reflect a mixture of central and peripheral pathology.

Vitamin E deficiency occurs in childhood, when it may be due to abetalipoproteinemia (Bassen-Kornzweig disease), which is inherited on chromosome 4q24.[1070,1193] It is also reported in adults, with bowel disease that interferes with fat absorption,[135] or as an inherited ataxia on chromosome 8q13, the site of the alpha-tocopherol transfer protein gene.[808,1196]

Wilson's Disease

Hepatolenticular degeneration is an autosomal recessive, inherited disorder of copper metabolism. The defect is in a copper-transporting ATPase with the gene at q14.3 on chromosome 13. CT scans typically show hypodense areas, and PET scanning indicates a decreased rate of glucose metabolism in the globus pallidum and putamen.[438] The classic clinical picture is a movement disorder with prominent dysarthria, psychiatric symptoms and associated liver disease. Detection of Kayser-Fleischer rings during the neuro-ophthalmologic examination is diagnostic. Ocular motor disorders in Wilson's disease include a distractibility of gaze, with inability to fix voluntarily upon an object unless other, competing, visual stimuli are removed (e.g., fixation of a solitary light in an otherwise dark room).[635] Slow vertical saccades have also been reported in one patient with Wilson's disease.[572] A lid-opening apraxia has also been noted.[558] We have measured the eye movements of a 19-year-old man, who showed marked distractibility of gaze but whose saccades were of normal velocity. The eye movements of Wilson's disease, therefore, show some similarities to those described in Huntington's disease and Alzheimer's disease. The distractibility in both conditions may be due to involvement of the inhibitory pathways from the basal ganglia to the superior colliculus, as discussed in Chapter 3.

EFFECTS OF DRUGS ON EYE MOVEMENTS

Many drugs affect eye movements; Table 12–11 summarizes reports of effects of certain individual agents. Drugs taken in combination (e.g., anticonvulsants) can cause defects in ocular motility with relatively nontoxic blood

Table 12–11. **Effects of Drugs on Eye Movements**

Drug	Reported Effect
Benzodiazepines	Reduced velocity and increased duration of saccades;[99,314,526,813,928,1126,1127] increase errors on antisaccade task[412]
	Impaired smooth pursuit[100,929,960]
	Decreased gain and change of time constant of VOR[101,813]
	Divergence paralysis[29]
Tricyclic antidepressants	Internuclear ophthalmoplegia[287,485]
	Partial or total gaze palsy[864,1024]
	Opsoclonus[37]
Phenytoin	Impaired smooth pursuit and VOR suppression[98]
	Gaze-evoked nystagmus[454,899]
	Downbeat nystagmus[85]
	Periodic alternating nystagmus[168]
	Partial or total gaze palsy[346]
	Convergence spasm[417]
Carbamazepine	Decreased velocity of saccades[1075]
	Impaired smooth pursuit[252]
	Gaze-evoked nystagmus[893,1023,1121]
	Oculogyric crisis[83]
	Downbeat nystagmus[183]
	Partial or total gaze palsy[750,783]
Phenobarbital and other barbiturates	Reduced peak saccadic velocity[960,1075]
	Gaze-evoked nystagmus[889]
	Impaired smooth pursuit[960]
	Impaired vergence[1169]
	Decreased VOR gain[250]
	Internuclear ophthalmoplegia[64]
	Perverted caloric responses[1005]
	Vertical nystagmus[640]
	Partial or total gaze palsy[64,301]
Phenothiazines	Oculogyric crisis[620]
	Internuclear ophthalmoplegia[215]
	Slow saccades (haloperidol)
Lithium carbonate	Saccadic dysmetria[28]
	Impaired smooth pursuit[645]
	Gaze-evoked nystagmus[28]
	Downbeat nystagmus[219,335,422,1178]
	Opsoclonus[205]
	Oculogyric crisis[955]
	Internuclear ophthalmoplegia[265]
	Partial or total gaze palsy[219]
Amphetamines	Reduced saccadic latency[1074]
	Increased accommodative convergence/accommodation ratio[1169]
Alcohol (ethanol)	Reduced peak velocity, increased latency, and hypometria of saccades[54,542]
	Impaired smooth pursuit[54] and VOR suppression[62]
	Gaze-evoked nystagmus[54,185]
	Positionally induced nystagmus[121,185]
	Reversal of compensation of vestibular lesions[89]

Table 12–11. *(continued)*

Drug	Reported Effect
Tobacco and nicotine	Decreased saccadic latency[914]
	Upbeat nystagmus in darkness[1001,1002]
	Square-wave jerks[1001,1078]
	Impaired horizontal and vertical smooth pursuit[1002]
Methadone and other narcotics	Saccadic hypometria[930]
	Impaired smooth pursuit[931]
	Internuclear ophthalmoplegia[307]
Baclofen	Reduced VOR time constant[204]
	Partial or total gaze palsy[823]
	For therapeutic effects see Table 10–9
Betablockers	Diplopia[1165]
	Internuclear ophthalmoplegia[233]
Choral hydrate	Impaired smooth pursuit[647]
Nitrous oxide	Reduced saccadic peak velocity[681]
	Impaired smooth pursuit[681]
Risperidone	Reduced peak velocity and increased latency of saccades[1056]
Cocaine	Opsoclonus[308,961]
Phencyclidine (PCP)	Nystagmus[65]

levels.[1087] For example, patients taking a combination of phenytoin and carbamazepine may complain of oscillopsia, which is due to spontaneous nystagmus, an inappropriate vestibulo-ocular reflex (VOR), or diplopia.[893] Many drugs affect central vestibular and cerebellar connections and cause ataxia and gaze-evoked nystagmus.[886]

Although all classes of eye movements may be affected by *therapeutic doses* of various drugs, smooth pursuit, eccentric gaze holding and convergence are particularly susceptible. So, for example, diazepam, methadone, phenytoin, barbiturates, chloral hydrate, and alcohol all impair smooth-pursuit tracking. However, some drugs have specific effects on ocular motility and thus have provided insights into both the function of the ocular motor system and the mode of drug action. For example, diazepam (a benzodiazepine) reduces saccadic peak velocity but does not impair accuracy, whereas methadone shows the converse effect. Diazepam reduces the gain of the VOR; in experimental animals the time constant is prolonged, but in humans it is reduced.[814] Ketamine, given in non-anesthetic doses causes defects of smooth-pursuit tracking,[49] and errors on the antisaccade task.[213] These findings are similar to those reported in schizophrenia, and have been interpreted as evidence that N-methyl-D-aspartate (NMDA) mechanisms are involved in this disorder; however, some caution is necessary because of the widespread effect of the drug in the nervous system. The immunosuppressive drug, tacrolimus (FK506) is reported to cause reversible brainstem findings, including internuclear ophthalmoplegia.[599,801] Cyclosporin-A has been associated with opsoclonus.[688]

In *toxic doses*, all eye movements may be impaired by neuroactive drugs, particularly when consciousness is impaired. Phenytoin may cause a complete ophthalmoplegia in an awake patient, and therapeutic levels may cause ophthalmoplegia in patients in stupor.[922] Phenytoin and diazepam can lead to opsoclonus.[263] The tricyclic antidepressants may cause complete, or internuclear, ophthalmoplegia in stuporous patients. Lithium intoxication causes a variety of abnormalities, including fixation instability and downbeat nystagmus.[335] In one patient, a lethal dose of lithium caused marked impairment of all types of horizontal eye movements and downbeat nystagmus, neuronal loss was mainly confined to the nucleus prepositus hypoglossi and adjacent medial vestibular nuclei.[219] Thus, the pathophysiology was similar to that produced by experimental lesions of these nuclei in monkeys:[169] the neural integrator (gaze-holding network) was disrupted. The propensity of lithium to damage this area of the medulla has been attributed to the proximity to the choroid plexus of the fourth ventricle (and hence high local levels of lithium).[505] Cerebellar damage may also occur after lithium intoxication.[966]

In addition to drugs, certain *toxins* are reported to affect eye movements. Some, such as chlordecone,[1072] and thallium,[676] cause saccadic oscillations. Intoxication with hydrocarbons is reported to cause vestibulopathy.[469,792] and exposure to trichloroethylene and other solvents may affect pursuit, visual suppression of the VOR, and saccades.[791] Prolonged toluene abuse, due to solvent-inhalation, affects central myelin causing a clinical picture similar to multiple sclerosis, and may lead to downbeat and acquired pendular nystagmus (see Video Display: Acquired Pendular Nystagmus),[672,685] internuclear ophthalmoplegia, [491] and saccadic oscillations.[728] Chronic sniffing of gasoline (petroleum) with high lead levels may cause lead encephalopathy; affected individuals show increased saccadic reaction times and increased errors on the antisaccade task.[164]

Tobacco and nicotine have a number of ocular motor effects. They cause upbeat nystagmus,[1001,1002] impaired pursuit,[1003] decrease in saccade latency,[914] and increased square-wave jerks during pursuit,[1078] but with normal performance on the antisaccade test.[915] Cocaine also can affect eye movements. The most dramatic abnormality is opsoclonus.[270,308,961] A variety of drugs are ototoxic, notably the aminoglycoside antibiotics. These are discussed in Chapter 11.

Finally, novel clinical observations and systematic study of the effects of new drugs on eye movements is likely to provide insights into the pharmacological substrate of the ocular motor system, and lead to the development of novel treatments for abnormal eye movements that prevent clear vision.

REFERENCES

1. Abadi RV, Gowen E. Characteristics of saccadic intrusions. Vision Res 44, 2675–2690 2004.
2. Abel LA, Gibson K, Williams IA, Chengwei L. Asymmetric smooth pursuit impairment and nystagmus in motor neurone disease. Neuro-ophthalmology 12, 197–206, 1992.
3. Abel LA, Unverzagt F, Yee RD. Effects of stimulus predictability and interstimulus gap on saccades in Alzheimer's disease. Dement Geriatr Cogn Disord 13, 235–243, 2002.
4. Abel LA, Williams IM, Gibson KL, Levi L. Effects of stimulus velocity and acceleration on smooth pursuit in motor neuron disease. J Neurol 242, 419–424, 1995.
5. Abel MP, Murphy FT, Enzenauer RJ, Enzenauer RW. Internuclear ophthalmoplegia (INO): an unusual presentation of neuropsychiatric lupus erythematosus. Binocul Vis Strabismus Q 18, 29–30, 2003.
6. Accardo AP, Pensiero S, Perissutti P. Saccadic analysis for early identification of neurological involvement in Gaucher disease. Ann N Y Acad Sci 1039, 503–507, 2005.
7. Adams M, Rhyner PA, Day J, DeArmond S, Smuckler EA. Whipple's disease confined to the central nervous system. Ann Neurol 21, 104–108, 1987.
8. Ahmad I, Zaman M. Bilateral internuclear ophthalmoplegia: an initial presenting sign of giant cell arteritis. J Am Geriatr Soc 47, 734–736, 1999.
9. Ahn JC, Hoyt WF, Hoyt CS. Tonic upgaze in infancy. A report of three cases. Arch Ophthalmol 107, 57–58, 1989.
10. Aicardi J, Barbosa C, Andermann E, et al. Ataxia-ocular motor apraxia: a syndrome mimicking ataxia-telangiectasia. Ann Neurol 24, 497–502, 1988.
11. Akman S, Dayanir V, Sanac AS, Kansu T. Acquired esotropia as presenting sign of craniocervical junction anomalies. Neuro-ophthalmology 15, 311–314, 1995.
12. Al-Abdulla NA, Rismondo V, Minkowski JS, Miller NR. Herpes zoster vasculitis presenting as giant cell arteritis with bilateral internuclear ophthalmoplegia. Am J Ophthalmol 134, 912–914, 2002.
13. Albano JE, Mishkin M, Westbrook LE, Wurtz RH. Visuomotor deficits following ablation of monkey superior colliculus. J Neurophysiol 48, 338–350, 1982.
14. Albano JE, Wurtz RH. Deficits in eye position following ablation of monkey superior colliculus pretectum and posterior-medial thalamus. J Neurophysiol 48, 318–337, 1982.
15. Albers DS, Beal MF. Mitochondrial dysfunction in progressive supranuclear palsy. Neurochem Int 40, 559–564, 2002.
16. Albers FW, Ingels KJ. Otoneurological manifestations in Chiari-I malformation. J Laryngol Otol 107, 441–443, 1993.

16a. Ali FR, Michell AW, Barker RA, Carpenter RH. The use of quantitative oculometry in the assessment of Huntington's disease. Exp Brain Res, e-publication 2005.

17. Allmer DM, Golis TA. Dorsal midbrain syndrome secondary to a pineocytoma. Optometry 72, 234–238, 2001.
18. Altarescu G, Hill S, Wiggs E, et al. The efficacy of enzyme replacement therapy in patients with chronic neuronopathic Gaucher's disease. J Pediatr 138, 539–547, 2001.
19. Amarenco P, Hauw J-J. Cerebellar infarction in the territory of the anterior and inferior cerebellar artery. Brain 113, 139–155, 1999.
20. Amouri R, Moreira MC, Zouari M, et al. Aprataxin gene mutations in Tunisian families. Neurology 63, 928–929, 2004.
21. Anastasio TJ, Robinson DA. Failure of the oculomotor neural integrator from a discrete midline lesion

between the abducens nuclei in the monkey. Neurosci Lett 127, 82–86, 1991.
22. Anastasopoulos D, Haslwanter T, Fetter M, Dichgans J. Smooth pursuit eye movements and otolith-ocular responses are differently impaired in cerebellar ataxia. Brain 121, 1497–1505, 1998.
23. Anastasopoulos D, Nasios G, Psilas K, et al. What is straight ahead to a patient with torticollis? Brain 121, 91–101, 1998.
24. Anderson CA, Sandberg E, Filley CM, Harris SL, Tyler KL. One and one-half syndrome with supranuclear facial weakness: magnetic resonance imaging localization. Arch Neurol 56, 1509–1511, 1999.
25. Anderson JH, Christova PS, Xie TD, et al. Spinocerebellar ataxia in monozygotic twins. Arch. Neurol. 59, 1945–1951, 2002.
26. Anderson TJ, Jenkins IH, Brooks DJ, et al. Cortical control of saccades and fixation in man. A PET study. Brain 117, 1073–1084, 1994.
27. Andrews K. Recovery of patients after four months or more in the persistent vegetative state. Br Med J 306, 1597–1600, 1993.
28. Apte SN, Langston JW. Permanent neurological deficits due to lithium toxicity. Ann Neurol 13, 453–455, 1983.
29. Arai M, Fujii S. Divergence paralysis associated with ingestion of diazepam. J Neurol 237, 45–46, 1990.
30. Aramideh M, Bour LJ, Koelman JH, Speelman JD, Ongerboer de Visser BW. Abnormal eye movements in blepharospasm and involuntary levator palpebrae inhibition. Brain 117, 1457–1474, 1994.
31. Armstrong IT, Munoz DP. Attentional blink in adults with attention-deficit hyperactivity disorder. Influence of eye movements. Exp Brain Res 152, 243–250, 2003.
32. Armstrong IT, Munoz DP. Inhibitory control of eye movements during oculomotor countermanding in adults with attention-deficit hyperactivity disorder. Exp Brain Res 152, 444–452, 2003.
33. Arnold AC. Internuclear ophthalmoplegia from intracranial tumor. J Clin Neuro-ophthalmol 10, 278–286, 1990.
34. Arnold AC, Baloh RW, Yee RD, Helper RS. Internuclear ophthalmoplegia in the Chiari type II malformation. Neurology 40, 1850–1854, 1990.
35. Aschoff JC, Conrad B, Kornhuber HH. Acquired pendular nystagmus with oscillopsia in multiple sclerosis: a sign of cerebellar nuclei disease. J Neurol Neurosurg Psychiatry 37, 570–577, 1974.
36. Ashe J, Hain TC, Zee DS, Schatz NJ. Microsaccadic flutter. Brain 114, 461–472, 1991.
37. Au WJ, Keltner JL. Opsoclonus with amitriptyline overdose. Ann Neurol 6, 87, 1979.
38. Auerbach SH, DePiero TJ, Romanul F. Sylvian aqueduct syndrome caused by unilateral midbrain lesion. Ann Neurol 11, 91–94, 1982.
39. Averbuch-Heller L. Neurology of the eyelids. Curr Opin Ophthalmol 8, 27–34, 1997.
40. Averbuch-Heller L, Helmchen C, Horn AKE, Leigh RJ, Büttner-Ennever JA. Slow vertical saccades in motor neuron disease: correlation of structure and function. Ann Neurol 44, 641–648, 1998.
41. Averbuch-Heller L, Leigh R J, Mermelstein V, Zagalsky L, Streifler JY. Ptosis in patients with hemispheric strokes. Neurology 58, 620–624, 2002.
42. Averbuch-Heller L, Meiner Z. Reversible periodic alternating gaze deviation in hepatic encephalopathy. Neurology 45, 191–192, 1995.
43. Averbuch-Heller L, Paulson GW, Daroff RB, Leigh RJ. Whipple's disease mimicking progressive supranuclear palsy: the diagnostic value of eye movement recording. J Neurol Neurosurg Psychiatry 66, 532–535, 1999.
44. Averbuch-Heller L, Rottach KG, Zivotofsky AZ, et al. Torsional eye movements in patients with skew deviation and spasmodic torticollis: responses to static and dynamic head roll. Neurology 48, 506–514, 1997.
45. Averbuch-Heller L, Stahl JS, Hlavin ML, Leigh RJ. Square-wave jerks induced by pallidotomy in parkinsonian patients. Neurology 52, 185–188, 1999.
46. Averbuch-Heller L, Stahl JS, Remler BF, Leigh RJ. Bilateral ptosis and upgaze palsy with right hemispheric lesions. Ann Neurol 40, 465–468, 1996.
47. Averbuch-Heller L, Tusa RJ, Fuhry L, et al. A double-blind controlled study of gabapentin and baclofen as treatment for acquired nystagmus. Ann Neurol 41, 818–825, 1997.
47a. Avila MT, Hong LE, Moates A, Turano KA, Thaker GK. The role of anticipation in schizophrenia-related pursuit initiation deficits. J Neurophysiol, e-publication, 2005.
48. Avila MT, Sherr JD, Hong E, Myers CS, Thaker GK. Effects of nicotine on leading saccades during smooth pursuit eye movements in smokers and nonsmokers with schizophrenia. Neuropsychopharmacology 28, 2184–2191, 2003.
49. Avila MT, Weiler MA, Lahti AC, Tamminga CA, Thaker GK. Effects of ketamine on leading saccades during smooth-pursuit eye movements may implicate cerebellar dysfunction in schizophrenia. Am J Psychiatry 159, 1490–1496, 2002.
50. Baloh RW, DeRossett SE, Cloughesy TF, et al. Novel brainstem syndrome associated with prostate carcinoma. Neurology 43, 2591–2596, 1993.
51. Baloh RW, Furman JM, Yee RD. Dorsal midbrain syndrome: clinical and oculographic findings. Neurology 35, 54–60, 1985.
52. Baloh RW, Furman JM, Yee RD. Eye movements in patients with absent voluntary horizontal gaze. Ann Neurol 17, 283–286, 1985.
53. Baloh RW, Konrad H R, Dirks D, Honrubia V. Cerebellopontine angle tumors. Arch Neurol 33, 507–512, 1976.
54. Baloh RW, Sharma S, Moskowitz H, Griffith R. Effect of alcohol and marijuana on eye movements. Aviat Space Environ Med 50, 18–23, 1979.
55. Baloh RW, Yee RD. Spontaneous vertical nystagmus. Rev Neurol (Paris) 145, 527–532, 1989.
56. Baloh RW, Yee RD, Honrubia V. Optokinetic nystagmus and parietal lobe lesions. Ann Neurol 7, 269–276, 1980.
57. Baloh RW, Yee RD, Honrubia V. Eye movements in patients with Wallenberg's syndrome. Ann N Y Acad Sci 374, 600–613, 1981.
58. Baloh RW, Yue Q, Demer JL. The linear vestibulo-ocular reflex in normal subjects and patients with vestibular and cerebellar lesions. J Vestib Res 5, 349–361, 1995.
59. Baloh RW, Yue Q, Furman JM, Nelson SF. Familial episodic ataxia: clinical heterogeneity in four families linked to chromosome 19p. Ann Neurol 41, 8–16, 1997.

60. Bandini F, Castello E, Mazzella L, Mancardi GL, Solaro C. Gabapentin but not vigabatrin is effective in the treatment of acquired nystagmus in multiple sclerosis: How valid is the GABAergic hypothesis? J Neurol Neurosurg Psychiatry 71, 107–110, 2001.
61. Barac B. Vertiginous epileptic attacks and so-called "vestibulogenic seizures". Epilepsia 9, 137–144, 1968.
62. Barnes GR, Crombie JW, Edge A. The effects of ethanol on visual-vestibular interaction during active and passive head movements. Aviat Space Environ Med 56, 695–701, 1985.
63. Barontini F, Simonetti C, Ferranini F, Sita D. Persistent upward eye deviation. Report of two cases. Neuro-ophthalmology 3, 217–224, 1983.
64. Barret LG, Vincent FM, Arsac PL, Debru J-L, Faure JR. Internuclear ophthalmoplegia in patients with toxic coma. Frequency prognostic value diagnostic significance. J Toxicol Clin Toxicol 20, 373–379, 1983.
65. Barton CH, Sterling ML, Vaziri ND. Phencyclidine intoxication: clinical experience in 27 cases confirmed by urine assay. Ann Emergency Med 10, 243–246, 1981.
66. Barton EJ, Nelson JS, Gandhi NJ, Sparks DL. Effects of partial lidocaine inactivation of the paramedian pontine reticular formation on saccades of macaques. J Neurophysiol. 90, 372–386, 2003.
67. Barton JJS, Sharpe JA, Raymond JE. Directional defects in pursuit and motion perception in humans with unilateral cerebral lesions. Brain 119, 1535–1550, 1996.
68. Barton JJS, Sharpe JA. Motion direction discrimination in blind hemifields. Ann Neurol 41, 255–264, 1997.
69. Barton JJS, Sharpe JA, Raymond JE. Retinotopic and directional defects in motion discrimination in humans with cerebral lesions. Ann Neurol 37, 665–675, 1995.
70. Bataller L, Wade DF, Fuller GN, Rosenfeld MR, Dalmau J. Cerebellar degeneration and autoimmunity to zinc-finger proteins of the cerebellum. Neurology 59, 1985–1987, 2002.
71. Bataller L, Dalmau J. Neuro-ophthalmology and paraneoplastic syndromes. Curr Opin Neurol 17, 3–8, 2004.
72. Behrmann M, Ghiselli-Crippa T, Sweeney JA, Di MI, Kass R. Mechanisms underlying spatial representation revealed through studies of hemispatial neglect. J Cogn Neurosci. 14, 272–290, 2002.
73. Behrmann M, Watts S, Black SE, Barton JJ. Impaired visual search in patients with unilateral neglect: an oculographic analysis. Neuropsychologia 35, 1445–1458, 1997.
74. Beigi B, Logan P, Eustace P. Convergence substitution for paralysed horizontal gaze. Br J Ophthalmol 79, 229–232, 1995.
75. Bell JA, Fielder AR, Viney S. Congenital double elevator palsy in identical twins. J Clin Neuro-ophthalmol 10, 32–34, 1990.
76. Bellebaum C, Daum I, Koch B, Schwarz M, Hoffmann KP. The role of the human thalamus in processing corollary discharge. Brain 128, 1139–1154, 2005.
77. Belton T, McCrea RA. Role of the cerebellar flocculus region in cancellation of the VOR during passive whole body rotation. J Neurophysiol 84, 1599–1613, 2000.
78. Belton T, McCrea RA. Role of the cerebellar flocculus region in the coordination of eye and head movements during gaze pursuit. J Neurophysiol 84, 1614–1626, 2000.
79. Bender MB. Oscillopsia. Arch Neurol 13, 204–213, 1965.
80. Benitez JT, Ernstoff RM, Wang AM, Arsenault MD. BAER, EOG, MRI and 3–D MR angiography correlates in a case of locked-in syndrome. Ear Nose Throat J 73, 23–24, 1994.
81. Benjamin EE, Zimmerman CF, Troost BT. Lateropulsion and upbeat nystagmus are manifestations of central vestibular dysfunction. Arch Neurol 43, 962–964, 1986.
82. Bennett A, Savill T. A case of permanent conjugate deviation of the eyes and head the result of a lesion limited to the sixth nucleus; with remarks on associated lateral movements of the eyeballs and rotation of the head and neck. Brain 12, 102–116, 1889.
83. Berchou RC. Carbamazepine-induced oculogyric crisis. Arch Neurol 36, 522–523, 1979.
84. Bergenius J, Magnusson M. The relationship between caloric response oculomotor dysfunction and size of cerebello-pontine angle tumours. Acta Otolaryngol (Stockh) 106, 361–367, 1998.
85. Berger JR, Kovacs AG. Downbeat nystagmus with phenytoin. J Clin Neuro-ophthalmol 2, 209–211, 1982.
86. Bergeron C, Pollanen MS, Weyer L, Black SE, Lang AE. Unusual clinical presentations of cortical-basal ganglionic degeneration. Ann Neurology 40, 893–900, 1996.
87. Bernal F, Shams'ili S, Rojas I. Anti-Tr antibodies as markers of paraneoplastic cerebellar degeneration and Hodgkin's disease. Neurology 60, 230–234, 2003.
88. Bertholon P, Bronstein AM, Davies RA, Rudge P, Thilo KV. Positional down beating nystagmus in 50 patients: cerebellar disorders and possible anterior semicircular canalithiasis. J Neurol Neurosurg Psychiatry 72, 366–372, 2002.
89. Berthoz A, Young L, Oliveras F. Action of alcohol on vestibular compensation and habituation in the cat. Acta Otolaryngol (Stockh) 84, 317–327, 1977.
90. Beversdorf DQ, Jenkyn LR, Petrowski IJ, Cromwell LD, Nordgren RE. Vertical gaze paralysis and intermittent unresponsiveness in a patient with a thalamo-mesencephalic stroke. J Neuro-ophthalmology 15, 230–235, 1995.
91. Bhidayasiri R, Plant GT, Leigh RJ. A hypothetical scheme for the brainstem control of vertical gaze. Neurology 54, 1985–1993, 2000.
92. Bhidayasiri R, Riley DE, Somers JT, et al. Pathophysiology of slow vertical saccades in progressive supranuclear palsy. Neurology 57, 2070–2077, 2001.
93. Biller J, Sand JJ, Corbett JJ, Adams HP Jr., Dunn V. Syndrome of the paramedian thalamic arteries: clinical and neuroimaging correlation. J Clin Neuro-ophthalmol 5, 217–223, 1985.
94. Binyon S, Prendergast M. Eye-movement tics in children. Dev Med Child Neurol 33, 343–355, 1991.
95. Biousse V, Skibell BC, Watts RL, et al. Ophthalmologic features of Parkinson's disease. Neurology 62, 177–180, 2004.
96. Birbamer G, Gerstenbrand F, Aichner F, et al. MR-imaging of post-traumatic olivary hypertrophy. Funct Neurol 9, 183–187, 1994.
97. Bisdorff AR, Bronstein AM, Wolsley C, Lees AJ. Torticollis due to disinhibition of the vestibulo-collic reflex in a patient with Steele-Richardson-Olszewski syndrome. Mov Disord 12, 328–336, 1997.

98. Bittencourt PRM, Gresty MA, Richens A. Quantitative assessment of smooth-pursuit eye movements in healthy and epileptic subjects. J Neurol Neurosurg Psychiatry 43, 1119–1124, 1980.
99. Bittencourt PRM, Wade P, Smith AT, Richens A. The relationship between peak velocity of saccadic eye movements and serum benzodiazepine concentration. Br J Clinical Pharmacol 12, 523–533, 1981.
100. Bittencourt PRM, Wade P, Smith AT, Richens A. Benzodiazepines impair smooth pursuit eye movements. Br J Clin Pharmacol 15, 259–262, 1983.
101. Blair SM, Gavin M. Modifications of vestibulo-ocular reflex induced by diazepam. Arch Otolaryngol 105, 698–701, 1979.
102. Blekher T, Siemers E, Abel LA, Yee RD. Eye movements in Parkinson's disease: before and after pallidotomy. Invest Ophthalmol Vis Sci 41, 2177–2183, 2000.
103. Blekher TM, Yee RD, Kirkwood SC, et al. Oculomotor control in asymptomatic and recently diagnosed individuals with the genetic marker for Huntington's disease. Vision Res 44, 2729–2736, 2004.
104. Boesen P, Fallingboro J, Spaun E. Severe persistent cerebellar dysfunction complicating cytosine arabinoside therapy. Acta Med Scand 224, 189–191, 1988.
105. Bogousslavsky J, Miklossy J, Regli F, Deruaz JP, Despland PA. One-and-a-half syndrome in ischemic locked-in state. J Neurol Neurosurg Psychiatry 47, 927–935, 1984.
106. Bogousslavsky J, Miklossy J, Regli F, Deruaz JP, Despland PA. Unilateral left paramedian infarction of thalamus and midbrain: a clinico-pathological study. J Neurol Neurosurg Psychiatry 49, 686–694, 1986.
107. Bogousslavsky J, Miklossy J, Regli F, Janzer R. Vertical gaze palsy and selective unilateral infarction of the rostral interstitial nucleus of the medial longitudinal fasciculus (riMLF). J Neurol Neurosurg Psychiatry 53, 67–71, 1990.
108. Bogousslavsky J, Regli F. Convergence and divergence synkinesis. A recovery pattern in benign pontine hematoma. Neuro-ophthalmology 4, 219–225, 1984.
109. Bogousslavsky J, Regli F. Upgaze palsy and monocular paresis of downgaze from ipsilateral thalamo-mesencephalic infarction. A vertical "one-and-a-half syndrome". J Neurol 231, 43–45, 1984.
110. Bogousslavsky J, Regli F, Uske A. Thalamic syndromes: clinical syndromes etiology and prognosis. Neurology 38, 837–848, 1988.
111. Bohlega S, Kambouris M, Shahid M, Al Homsi M, Al Sous W. Gaucher disease with oculomotor apraxia and cardiovascular calcification (Gaucher type IIIC). Neurology 54, 261–263, 2000.
112. Bolanos I, Lozano D, Cantu C. Internuclear ophthalmoplegia: causes and long-term follow-up in 65 patients. Acta Neurol Scand 110, 161–165, 2004.
113. Bollen E, Van Exel E, van der Velde EA, et al. Saccadic eye movements in idiopathic blepharospasm. Mov Disord 11, 678–682, 1996.
114. Bollen EL, Roos RA, Cohen AP, et al. Oculomotor control in Gilles de la Tourette syndrome. J Neurol Neurosurg Psychiatry 51, 1081–1083, 1988.
115. Bolling J, Lavin PJM. Combined gaze palsy of horizontal saccades and pursuit contralateral to a midbrain haemorrhage. J Neurol Neurosurg Psychiatry 50, 789–791, 1987.
116. Bonilha L, Fernandes YB, Mattos JP, Borges WA, Borges G. Bilateral internuclear ophthalmoplegia and clivus fracture following head injury: case report. Arq Neuropsiquiatr 60, 636–638, 2002.
117. Borsini W, Giuliacci G, Torricelli F, et al. Anderson-Fabry disease with cerebrovascular complications in two Italian families. Neurol Sci 23, 49–53, 2002.
118. Bosch EP, Kennedy SS, Aschenbrener CA. Ocular bobbing: the myth of its localizing value. Neurology 25, 949–953, 1975.
119. Bosley TM, Cohen DA, Schatz NJ, et al. Comparison of metrizamide computed tomography and magnetic resonance imaging in the evaluation of lesions at the cervicomedullary junction. Neurology 35, 485–492, 1985.
120. Bötzel K, Rottach K, Büttner U. Normal and pathological saccadic dysmetria. Brain 116, 337–353, 1993.
121. Brandt T. Positional and positioning vertigo and nystagmus. J Neurol Sci 95, 3–28, 1990.
122. Brandt T. Cortical matching of visual and vestibular 3–D coordinate maps. Ann Neurol 42, 983–984, 1997.
123. Brandt T, Bucher SF, Seelos KC, Dieterich M. Bilateral functional MRI activation of the basal ganglia and middle temporal/medial superior temporal motion-sensitive areas. Optokinetic stimulation in homonymous hemianopia. Arch Neurol 55, 1126–1131, 1998.
124. Brandt T, Dieterich M. Pathological eye-head coordination in roll: tonic ocular tilt reaction in mesencephalic and medullary lesions. Brain 110, 649–666, 1987.
125. Brandt T, Dieterich M. Different types of skew deviation. J Neurol Neurosurg Psychiatry 54, 549–550, 1991.
126. Brandt T, Dieterich M. Vestibular syndromes in the roll plane: topographic diagnosis from brain stem to cortex. Ann Neurol 36, 337–347, 1994.
127. Brandt T, Strupp M. Episodic ataxia type 1 and 2 (familial periodic ataxia/vertigo). Audiology Neurootology 2, 373–383, 1997.
128. Braun DI, Boman DK, Hotson JR. Anticipatory smooth eye movements and predictive pursuit after unilateral lesions in human brain. Exp Brain Res 110, 111–116, 1996.
129. Brazis P. Ocular motor abnormalities in Wallenberg's lateral medullary syndrome. Mayo Clin Proc 67, 365–368, 1992.
130. Brekelmans GJF, Tijssen CC. Acquired ocular motor apraxia in an AIDS patient with bilateral frontoparietal lesions. Neuro-ophthalmology 10, 53–56, 1990.
131. Brenner RP, Carlow TJP. PLEDs and nystagmus retractorius. Ann Neurol 5, 403, 1979.
132. Brett FM, Henson C, Staunton H. Familial diffuse Lewy body disease eye movement abnormalities and distribution of pathology. Arch Neurol 59, 464–467, 2002.
133. Briand KA, Strallow D, Hening W, Poizner H, Sereno AB. Control of voluntary and reflexive saccades in Parkinson's disease. Exp Brain Res 129, 38–48, 1999.
133a. Brigell M, Babikian V, Goodwin JA. Hypometric saccades and low-gain pursuit resulting from a thalamic hemorrhage. Ann Neurol 15, 374–378, 1984.

134. Brigell MG, Goodwin JA, Lorance R. Saccadic latency as a measure of afferent visual conduction. Invest Ophthalmol Vis Sci 29, 1331–1338, 1988.
135. Brin MF, Fetell MR, Green PH, et al. Blind loop syndrome, vitamin E malabsorption and spinocerebellar degeneration. Neurology 35, 338–342, 1985.
136. Brindley GS, Gautier-Smith PC, Lewin W. Cortical blindness and the functions of the non-geniculate fibers of the optic tracts. J Neurol Neurosurg Psychiatry 32, 259–264, 1969.
137. Bronstein AM, Hood JD. Cervical nystagmus due to loss of cerebellar inhibition on the cervico-ocular reflex: a case report. J Neurol Neurosurg Psychiatry 48, 128–131, 1985.
138. Bronstein AM, Kennard C. Predictive ocular motor control in Parkinson's disease. Brain 108, 925–940, 1985.
139. Bronstein AM, Rudge P, Gresty MA, du Boulay EPGH, Morris J. Abnormalities of horizontal gaze. Clinical oculographic and magnetic resonance imaging findings. II Gaze palsy and internuclear ophthalmoplegia. J Neurol Neurosurg Psychiatr 53, 200–207, 1990.
140. Bronstein AM, Shallo-Hoffmann J, Kanayama R, Rudge P. Corrective saccades in cerebellar dysmetria. Ann Neurol 37, 413–414, 1995.
141. Brooks BA, Fuchs AF, Finochio D. Saccadic eye movement deficits in the MTPT monkey model of Parkinson's disease. Brain Res 383, 402–407, 1986.
142. Bruce CJ, Goldberg ME, Bushnell MC, Stanton GB. Primate frontal eye fields. II Physiological and anatomical correlates of electrically evoked eye movements. J Neurophysiol 54, 714–734, 1985.
143. Bruns L. Die Geschwulste des Nervensystems. S Karger Berlin, 1908.
144. Brusa A, Firpo MP, Massa S, Piccardo A, Bronzini E. Typical and reverse bobbing: a case with localizing value. European Neurol 23, 151–155, 1984.
145. Brusa G, Meneghini S, Piccardo A, Pizio N. Regressive pattern of horizontal gaze palsy. case report. Neuro-ophthalmology 7, 301–306, 1987.
146. Buettner UW, Zee DS. Vestibular testing in comatose patients. Arch Neurol 46, 561–563, 1989.
147. Bürk K, Abele M, Fetter M, et al. Autosomal dominant cerebellar ataxia type I Clinical features and MRI in families with SCA1, SCA2 and SCA3. Brain 119, 1497–1505, 1996.
148. Bürk K, Bosch S, Muller CA, et al. Sporadic cerebellar ataxia associated with gluten sensitivity. Brain 124, 1013–1019, 2001.
149. Burke JR, Wingfield MS, Lewis KE, et al. The haw river syndrome:dentatorubropallidoluysian atrophy (DRPLA) in an African-American family. Nat Genet 7, 521–524, 1994.
150. Burn DJ, Lees AJ. Progressive supranuclear palsy: where are we now? Lancet Neurol. 1, 359–369, 2002.
151. Burstein AH, Fullerton T. Oculogyric crisis possibly related to pentazocine. Ann Pharmacother 27, 874–876, 1993.
152. Büttner N, Geschwind D, Jen JC, et al. Oculomotor phenotypes in autosomal dominant ataxias. Arch Neurol 55, 1353–1357, 1998.
153. Büttner U, Büttner-Ennever JA, Rambold H, Helmchen C. The contribution of midbrain circuits in the control of gaze. Ann N Y Acad Sci 956, 99–110, 2002.
154. Büttner U, Grundei T. Gaze-evoked nystagmus and smooth pursuit deficits: their relationship studied in 52 patients. J Neurol 242, 384–389, 1995.
155. Büttner U, Helmchen C, Büttner-Ennever JA. The localizing value of nystagmus in brainstem disorders. Neuro-ophthalmology 15, 283–290, 1995.
156. Büttner U, Straube A. The effect of cerebellar midline lesions on eye movements. Neuro-ophthalmology 15, 75–82, 1995.
157. Büttner-Ennever JA, Acheson JF, Buttner U, et al. Ptosis and supranuclear downgaze palsy. Neurology 39, 385–389, 1989.
158. Büttner-Ennever JA, Büttner U. The reticular formation. In Büttner-Ennever JA (ed). Neuroanatomy of the Oculomotor System. Elsevier, New York, 1988, pp 119–176.
159. Büttner-Ennever JA, Büttner U, Cohen B, Baumgartner G. Vertical gaze paralysis and the rostral interstitial nucleus of the medial longitudinal fasciculus. Brain 105, 125–149, 1982.
160. Büttner-Ennever JA, Cohen B, Horn AKE, Reisine H. Pretectal projections to the oculomotor complex of the monkey and their role in eye movements. J Comp Neurol 366, 348–359, 1996.
161. Büttner-Ennever JA, Horn AK. Pathways from cell groups of the paramedian tracts to the floccular region. Ann N Y Acad Sci 781, 532–540, 1996.
162. Cadera W, Bloom JN, Karlik S, Viirre E. A magnetic resonance imaging study of double elevator palsy. Can J Ophthalmol 32, 250–253, 1997.
162a. Cagnoli C, Mariotti C, Taroni F, et al. SCA28, a novel form of autosomal dominant cerebellar ataxia on chromosome 18p11.22–q11.2. Brain, e-publication, 2005.
163. Caine D, Halliday GM, Kril JJ, Harper CG. Operational criteria for the classification of chronic acoholics: identification of Wernicke's encephalopathy. J Neurol Neurosurg Psychiatry 62, 51–60, 1997.
164. Cairney S, Maruff P, Burns CB, Currie J, Currie BJ. Saccade dysfunction associated with chronic petrol sniffing and lead encephalopathy. J Neurol Neurosurg Psychiatry 75, 472–476, 2004.
165. Calkins ME, Iacono WG, Curtis CE. Smooth pursuit and antisaccade performance evidence trait stability in schizophrenia patients and their relatives. Int J Psychophysiol 49, 139–146, 2003.
166. Calogero JA. Vermian agenesis and unsegmented midbrain tectum. Case report. J Neurosurg 47, 605–608, 1977.
167. Camarata PJ, McGeachie RE, Haines SJ. Dorsal midbrain encephalitis caused by Propionibacterium acnes. Report of two cases. J Neurosurg 72, 654–659, 1990.
168. Campbell WW Jr. Periodic alternating nystagmus in phenytoin intoxication. Arch Neurol 37, 178–180, 1980.
169. Cannon SC, Robinson DA. Loss of the neural integrator of the oculomotor system from brain stem lesions in monkey. J Neurophysiol 57, 1383–1409, 1987.
170. Caparros-Lefebvre D, Sergeant N, Lees A, et al. Guadeloupean parkinsonism: a cluster of progressive supranuclear palsy-like tauopathy. Brain 125, 801–811, 2002.
171. Caplan LR, Goodwin JA. Lateral tegmental brainstem hemorrhages. Neurology 32, 252–260, 1982.

172. Caplan LR, Scheiner D. Dysconjugate gaze in hepatic coma. Ann Neurol 8, 328–329, 1980.
173. Cardosa F, Eduardo C, Silva AP, Mota CCC. Chorea in fifty consecutive patients with rheumatic fever. Mov Disord 12, 701–703, 1997.
174. Carter JE, Rauch RA. One-and-a-half syndrome type II. Arch Neurol 51, 87–89, 1994.
175. Castaigne P, Lhermitte F, Buge A, et al. Paramedian thalamic and midbrain infarcts: clinical and neuropathological study. Ann Neurol 10, 127–148, 1981.
176. Catalano RA, Calhoun JH, Reinecke RD, Cogan DG. Asymmetry in congenital ocular motor apraxia. Can J Ophthalmol 23, 318–321, 1988.
177. Cavalier L, Ouahchi K, Kayden HJ, et al. Ataxia with isolated vitamin E defiency: heterogeneity of mutations and phenotypic variability in a large number of families. Am J Hum Genet 62, 301–310, 1998.
178. Chamberlain W. Restriction of upward gaze with advancing age. Am J Ophthalmol 71, 341–346, 1971.
179. Chan F, Armstrong IT, Pari G, Riopelle RJ, Munoz DP. Deficits in saccadic eye-movement control in Parkinson's disease. Neuropsychologia 43, 784–796, 2005.
180. Chan JW. Isolated unilateral post-traumatic internuclear ophthalmoplegia. J Neuroophthalmol 21, 212–213, 2001.
181. Charles N, Froment C, Rode G, et al. Vertigo and upside down vision due to an infarct in the territory of the medial branch of the posterior inferior cerebellar artery caused by dissection of a vertebral artery. J Neurol Neurosurg Psychiatry 55, 188–189, 1992.
182. Choi KD, Jung DS, Kim JS. Specificity of "peering at the tip of the nose" for a diagnosis of thalamic hemorrhage. Arch Neurol 61, 417–422, 2004.
183. Chrousos GA, Cowdry R, Schuelein M, et al. Two cases of downbeat nystagmus and oscillopsia associated with carbamazepine. Am J Ophthalmol 103, 221–224, 1987.
184. Chun HH, Gatti RA. Ataxia-telangiectasia an evolving phenotype. DNARepair (Amst) 3, 1187–1196, 2004.
185. Citek K, Ball B, Rutledge DA. Nystagmus testing in intoxicated individuals. Optometry 74, 695–710, 2003.
186. Clark JM, Albers GW. Vertical gaze palsy from paramedian thalamic stroke without midbrain involvement. Stroke 26, 1467–1470, 1996.
187. Clark RA, Isenberg SJ. The range of ocular movements decreases with aging. J AAPOS 5, 26–30, 2001.
188. Clementz BA. The ability to produce express saccades as a function of gap interval among schizophrenic patients. Exp Brain Res 111, 121–130, 1996.
189. Clendaniel RA, Mays LE. Characteristics of antidromically identified oculomotor internuclear neurons during vergence and versional eye movements. J Neurophysiol 71, 1111–1127, 1994.
190. Coesmans M, Sillevis-Smitt P, Linden DJ. Mechanisms underlying cerebellar motor deficits due to mGluR1-autoantibodies. Ann Neurol 53, 325–336, 2003.
191. Cogan DG. Neurologic significance of conjugate lateral deviation of the eyes on forced closure of the lids. Arch Ophthalmol 39, 37–42, 1948.
192. Cogan DG. A type of congenital ocular motor apraxia presenting jerky head movements. Trans Am Acad Ophthalmol 56, 853–862, 1952.
193. Cogan DG. Neurology of the Ocular Muscles. Charles C Thomas, Springfield Ilinois, 1956.
194. Cogan DG. Ophthalmic manifestations of bilateral non-occipital cerebral lesions. Br J Ophthalmol 49, 281–297, 1965.
195. Cogan G. Congenital ocular motor apraxia. Can J Ophthalmol 1, 253–260, 1966.
196. Cogan DG. Downbeat nystagmus. Arch Ophthalmol 80, 757–768, 1968.
197. Cogan DG. Internuclear ophthalmoplegia typical and atypical. Arch Ophthalmol 84, 583–589, 1970.
198. Cogan DG, Chu FC, Reingold DR, Barranger J. Ocular motor signs in some metabolic diseases. Arch Ophthalmol 99, 1802–1808, 1981.
199. Cogan DG, Chu FC, Reingold DR, Tychsen L. A long-term follow-up of congenital ocular motor apraxia. Neuro-ophthalmology 1, 145–147, 1980.
200. Cogan DG, Loeb DR. Optokinetic response and intracranial lesions. Arch Neurol Psychiatry 61, 183–187, 1949.
201. Cogan DG, Victor M. Ocular signs of Wernicke's disease. Arch Ophthalmol 103, 1212–1220, 1954.
202. Cogan DG, Witt ED, Goldman-Rakic PS. Ocular signs in thiamine-deficient monkeys and in Wernicke's disease in humans. Arch Ophthalmol 103, 1212–1220, 1985.
203. Cogan DG, Wray SH. Internuclear ophthalmoplegia as an early sign of brainstem tumors. Neurology 20, 629–633, 1970.
204. Cohen B, Helwig D, Raphan T. Baclofen and velocity storage: A model of the effects of the drug on the vestibulo-ocular reflex in the rhesus monkey. J Physiol (Lond) 393, 703–725, 1987.
205. Cohen WJ, Cohen NH. Lithium carbonate, haloperidol and irreversible brain damage. JAMA 230, 1283–1287, 1974.
206. Coker S, Susac J, Sharpe J, Smallridge R. Cockayne's syndrome. Neuro-ophthalmic, CAT scan and endocrine observations. In Smith JL (ed). Neuro-ophthalmology Focus. Masson, New York, 1979, pp 379–385.
207. Collewijn H, Erkelens CJ, Steinman RM. Binocular co-ordination of human horizontal saccadic eye movements. J Physiol (Lond) 40, 157–182, 1988.
208. Collewijn H, Went LN, Tamminga EP, Vegter-Van der Vlis M. Oculomotor defects in patients with Huntington's disease and their offspring. J Neurol Sci 86, 307–320, 1988.
209. Collier J. Nuclear ophthalmoplegia with especial reference to retraction of the lids and ptosis and to lesions of the posterior commissure. Brain 50, 488–498, 1927.
210. Collins SJ, Ahlskog JE, Parsi JE, Maragnore DM. Progressive supranuclear palsy: neuropathologically based diagnostic clinical criteria. J Neurol Neurosurg Psychiatry 58, 167–173, 1995.
211. Condorelli DF, Parenti R, Spinella F, et al. Cloning of a new gap junction gene (CX36) highly expressed in mammalian brain neurons. Eur J Neurosci 10, 1202–1208, 1998.
212. Condy C, Rivaud-Pechoux S, Ostendorf F, Ploner CJ, Gaymard B. Neural substrate of antisaccades: role of subcortical structures. Neurology 63, 1571–1578, 2004.
213. Condy C, Wattiez N, Rivaud-Pechoux S, Gaymard B.

Ketamine-induced distractibility: An oculomotor study in monkeys. Biol Psychiatry 57, 366–372, 2005.
214. Constantoyannis C, Tzortzidis F, Papadakis N. Internuclear ophthalmoplegia following minor head injury: a case report. Br J Neurosurg 12, 377–379, 1998.
215. Cook FF, Davis RG, Russo LS Jr. Internuclear ophthalmoplegia caused by phenothiazine intoxication. Arch Neurol 38, 465–466, 1981.
216. Coppeto JR, Greco P. Unilateral internuclear ophthalmoplegia migraine and supratentorial arteriovenous malformation. Am J Ophthalmol 104, 191–192, 1987.
217. Coppeto JR, Lessell S. Dorsal midbrain syndrome from giant aneurysm of the posterior fossa: report of two cases. Am J Ophthalmol 104, 191–192, 1987.
218. Corbett JJ. Neuro-ophthalmological complications of hydrocephalus and shunting procedures. Semin Neurol 6, 111–123, 1986.
219. Corbett JJ, Jacobson DM, Thompson HS, Hart MN, Albert DW. Downbeating nystagmus and other ocular motor defects caused by lithium toxicity. Neurology 39, 481–487, 1989.
220. Cox TA, Corbett JJ, Thompson HS, Lennarson L. Upbeat nystagmus changing to downbeat nystagmus with convergence. Neurology 31, 891–892, 1981.
221. Crawford JD, Cadera W, Vilis T. Generation of torsional and vertical eye position signals by the interstitial nucleus of Cajal. Science 252, 1551–1553, 1991.
222. Crawford T, Goodrich S, Henderson L, Kennard C. Predictive responses in Parkinson's disease: manual key presses and saccadic eye movements to regular stimulus events. J Neurol Neurosurg Psychiatry 52, 1033–1042, 1989.
223. Crawford TJ, Haeger B, Kennard C, Reveley MA, Henderson L. Saccadic abnormalities in psychotic patients. I Neuroleptic free psychotic patients. Psychological Medicine 25, 461–471, 1995.
224. Crawford TJ, Higham S, Renvoize T, et al. Inhibitory control of saccadic eye movements and cognitive impairment in Alzheimer's disease. Biol Psychiatry 57, 1052–1060, 2005.
225. Crawford TJ, Sharma T, Puri BK, et al. Saccadic eye movements in families multiply affected with schizophrenia: the Maudsley Family Study. Am J Psychiatry 155, 1703–1710, 1998.
226. Cremer PD, Halmagyi GM. Eye movement disorders in a patient with liver disease. Neuro-ophthalmology 16 (Suppl), 276, 1996.
227. Cremer PD, Migliaccio AA, Halmagyi GM, Curthoys IS. Vestibulo-ocular reflex pathways in internuclear ophthalmoplegia. Ann Neurol 45, 529–533, 1999.
228. Crevits L, De Ridder K. Disturbed striatoprefrontal mediated visual behavior in moderate to severe parkinsonism patients. J Neurol Neurosurg Psychiatry 63, 296–299, 1997.
229. Crevits L, Versijpt J, Hanse M, De Ridder K. Antisaccadic effects of a dopamine agonist as add-on therapy in advanced Parkinson's patients. Neuropsychobiology 42, 202–206, 2000.
230. Crino PB, et al. Clinicopathological study of paraneoplastic brainstem encephalitis and ophthalmoparesis. J Neuro-ophthalmology 16, 44–48, 1996.
231. Cruikshank SJ, Hopperstad M, Younger M, Connors BW, Spray DC. Potent block of Cx36 and Cx50 gap junction channels by mefloquine. Proc Natl Acad Sci U S A 33, 12365–12369, 2004.
232. Cui DM, Yan YJ, Lynch JC. Pursuit subregion of the frontal eye field projects to the caudate nucleus in monkeys. J Neurophysiol 89, 2678–2684, 2003.
233. Cunningham GM. Drug-induced internuclear ophthalmoplegia. Can Med Assoc J 128, 892–893, 1983.
234. Curless RG. Acute vestibular dysfunction in childhood. Central vs. peripheral. Child's Brain 6, 39–44, 1980.
235. Curran T, Lang AE. Parkinsonian syndromes associated with hydrocephalus: case reports, a review of the literature and pathophysiological hypotheses. Mov Disord 9, 508–520, 1994.
236. Currie J, Benson E, Ramsden B, Perdices M, Cooper D. Eye movement abnormalities as a predictor of the acquired immunodeficiency syndrome dementia complex. Arch Neurol 45, 949–953, 1988.
237. Currie JN, Ramsden B, McArthur C, Maruff P. Validation of a clinical antisaccade eye movement test in the assessment of dementia. Arch Neurol 48, 644–648, 1991.
238. Daffner KR, Scinto LF, Weintraub S, Guinessey JE, Mesulam MM. Diminished curiosity in patients with probable Alzheimer's disease as measured by exploratory eye movements. Neurology 42, 320–328, 1992.
239. Dalmau J, Graus F, Villarejo A, et al. Clinical analysis of anti-Ma2–associated encephalitis. Brain 127, 1831–1844, 2004.
240. Dalton KM, Nacewicz BM, Johnstone T, et al. Gaze fixation and the neural circuitry of face processing in autism. Nat Neurosci, 2005.
241. Daroff RB, Hoyt WF. Supranuclear disorders of ocular control systems in man: Clinical, anatomical and physiological correlations—1969. In Bach-y-Rita P, Collins CC, Hyde JE (eds). The Control of Eye Movements. Academic Press, New York, 1971, pp 175–235.
242. Daroff RB, Hoyt WF, Sanders MD, Nelson LR. Gaze-evoked eyelid and ocular nystagmus inhibited by the near reflex: unusual ocular motor phenomena in a lateral medullary syndrome. J Neurol Neurosurg Psychiatry 31, 362–367, 1968.
243. Daroff RB, Troost BT. Upbeat nystagmus. JAMA 225, 312, 1973.
244. Daroff RB, Troost BT, Dell'Osso LF. Nystagmus and saccadic intrusions and oscillations. In Glaser JS (ed). Neuro-Ophthalmology. JB Lippincott, Philadelphia, 1990, pp 325–356.
245. Daroff RB, Waldman AL. Ocular bobbing. J Neurol Neurosurg Psychiatry 28, 375–377, 1965.
246. Das VE, Leigh RJ. Visual-vestibular interaction in progressive supranuclear palsy. Vision Res 40, 2077–2081, 2000.
247. Date H, Onodera O, Tanaka H, et al. Early-onset ataxia with ocular motor apraxia and hypoalbuminemia is caused by mutations in a new HIT superfamily gene. Nat Genet 29, 184–188, 2001.
248. Davis PH, Bergeron C, McLachlan DR. Atypical presentation of progressive supranuclear palsy. Ann Neurol 17, 337–343, 1985.
249. Day JW, Schut LJ, Moseley ML, Durand AC, Ranum LP. Spinocerebellar ataxia type 8: clinical features in a large family. Neurology 55, 649–657, 2000.

250. Dayal VS, Mai M, Tomlinison RD, Farkashidy J. Effects of barbituate on the vestibular and oculomotor systems: a sequential study. In Graham RD, Kemink JL (eds). The Vestibular System: Neurophysiologic and Clinical Research. Raven Press, New York, 1987, pp 169–175.
251. de Bruin VM, Lees AJ, Daniel SE. Diffuse Lewy body disease presenting with supranuclear gaze palsy, parkinsonism and dementia: a case report. Mov Disord 7, 355–358, 1992.
252. De Kort PLM, Gielen G, Tijssen CC, Declerck AC. The influence of antiepileptic drugs on eye movements. Neuro-ophthalmology 10, 59–68, 1990.
253. De La Monte SM, Horowitz SA, Larocque AA, Richardson EP Jr. Keyhole aqueduct syndrome. Arch Neurol 43, 926–929, 1986.
254. De La Paz MA, Chung SM, McCrary JA. Bilateral internuclear ophthalmoplegia in a patient with Wernicke's encephalopathy. J Clin Neuro-ophthalmol 12, 116–120, 1992.
255. De Renzi E, Colombo A, Faglioni P, Gibertoni M. Conjugate gaze paresis in stroke patients with unilateral damage. An unexpected instance of hemispheric asymmetry. Arch Neurol 39, 482–486, 1982.
256. de Yébenes JG, Sarasa JL, Daniel SE, Lees AJ. Familial progressive supranuclear palsy-description of a pedigree and review of the literature. Brain 118, 1095–1103, 1995.
257. De Zeeuw CI, Simpson JI, Hoogenraad CC, et al. Microcircuitry and function of the inferior olive. Trends Neurosci 21, 391–400, 1998.
258. de Seze J, Lucas C, Leclerc X, et al. One-and-a-half syndrome in pontine infarcts: MRI correlates. Neuroradiology 41, 666–669, 1999.
259. DeBassio WA, Kemper TL, Knoefel JE. Coffin-Siris syndrome. Neuropathological findings. Arch Neurol 42, 350–353, 1985.
260. Dehaene I. Apraxia of eyelid opening in progressive supranuclear palsy. Ann Neurol 15, 115–116, 1985.
261. Dehaene I, Casselman JW, Van Zandijcke M. Unilateral internuclear ophthalmoplegia and ipsiversive torsional nystagmus. J Neurol 243, 461–464, 1996.
262. Dehaene I, Lammens M. Paralysis of saccades and pursuit: clinicopathologic study. Neurology 41, 414–415, 1991.
263. Dehaene I, Van Vleymen B. Opsoclonus induced by phenytoin and diazepam. Ann Neurol 21, 216, 1984.
264. Deleu D, Buisseret T, Ebinger G. Vertical one-and-a-half syndrome. Supranuclear downgaze paralysis with monocular elevation palsy. Arch Neurol 46, 1361–1363, 1989.
265. Deleu D, Ebinger G. Lithium-induced internuclear ophthalmoplegia. Clin Neuropharmacol 12, 244–226, 1989.
266. Deleu D, Solheid C, Michotte A, Ebinger G. Dissociated ipsilateral horizontal gaze palsy in one-and-a-half syndrome: clinicopathological study. Neurology 38, 1278–1280, 1988.
267. Dell'Osso LF, Robinson DA, Daroff RB. Optokinetic asymmetry in internuclear ophthalmoplegia. Arch Neurol 31, 138–139, 1974.
268. Demer JL. Pivotal role of orbital connective tissues in binocular alignment and strabismus: the Friedenwald lecture. Invest Ophthalmol Vis Sci 45, 729–738, 2004.
269. Demer JL, Holds JB, Hovis LA. Ocular movements in essential blepharospasm. Am J Ophthalmol 110, 674–682, 1990.
270. Demer JL, Volkow ND, Ulrich I, et al. Eye movements in cocaine abusers. Psychiat Res 29, 123–136, 1989.
271. Deng S-Y, Goldberg ME, Segraves MA, Ungerleider LG, Mishkin M. The effect of unilateral ablation of the frontal eye fields on saccadic performance in the monkey. In Keller EL, Zee DS (eds). Adaptive Processes in Visual and Oculomotor Systems. Pergamon, Oxford, 1986, pp 201–208.
272. Derwenskus J, Rucker JC, Serra A, et al. Abnormal eye movements predict disability in MS: two-year follow-up. Ann N Y Acad Sci 1039, 521–523, 2005.
273. Deuschl G, Toro C, Hallett M. Symptomatic and essential palatal tremor. 2. Differences of palatal movements. Mov Disord 9, 676–678, 1994.
274. Deuschl G, Toro C, Valls-Sole J, Hallett M. Symptomatic and essential palatal tremor. 3. Abnormal motor learning. J Neurol Neurosurg Psychiatry 60, 520–525, 1996.
275. Deuschl G, Toro C, Valls-Sole J, et al. Symptomatic and essential palatal tremor. 1. Clinical physiological and MRI analysis. Brain 117, 775–788, 1994.
276. Devere TR, Lee AG, Hamill MB, et al. Acquired supranuclear ocular motor paresis following cardiovascular surgery. J Neuro-ophthalmol 17, 189–193, 1997.
277. Devereaux MW, Brust JCM, Keane JR. Internuclear ophthalmoplegia caused by subdural hematoma. Neurology 29, 251–255, 1979.
278. Devor A, Yarom Y. Electrotonic coupling in the inferior olivary nucleus revealed by simultaneous double patch recordings. J Neurophysiol 87, 3048–3058, 2002.
279. Dias EC, Segraves MA. Muscimol-induced inactivation of monkey frontal eye field: effects on visually and memory-guided saccades. J Neurophysiol 81, 2191–2214, 1999.
280. Diefendorf AR, Dodge R. An experimental study of the ocular reactions of the insane from photographic records. Brain 31, 451–489, 1908.
281. Diesing TS, Wijdicks EF. Ping-pong gaze in coma may not indicate persistent hemispheric damage. Neurology 63, 1537–1538, 2004.
282. Dieterich M, Bartenstein P, Spiegel S, et al. Thalamic infarctions cause side-specific suppression of vestibular cortex activations. Brain 128, 2052–2067, 2005.
283. Dieterich M, Brandt T. Wallenberg's syndrome: lateropulsion cyclorotation and subjective visual vertical in thirty-six patients. Ann Neurol 31, 399–408, 1992.
284. Dieterich M, Brandt T. Thalamic infarctions: differential effects on vestibular function in the roll plane (35 patients). Neurology 43, 1732–1740, 1993.
285. Dominguez RO, Bronstein AM. Complete gaze palsy in pontine haemorrhage. J Neurol Neurosurg Psychiatry 51, 150–151, 1988.
286. Dones J, De Jesus O, Colen CB, Toledo MM, Delgado M. Clinical outcomes in patients with Chiari I malformation: a review of 27 cases. Surg Neurol 60, 142–147, 2003.
287. Donhowe SP. Bilateral internuclear ophthalmoplegia from doxepin overdose. Neurology 34, 259, 1984.
288. Dooling EC, Richardson EP, Jr. Ophthalmoplegia

and Ondine's curse. Arch Ophthalmol 95, 1790–1793, 1977.
289. Doricchi F, Perani D, Incoccia C, et al. Neural control of fast-regular saccades and antisaccades: an investigation using positron emission tomography. Exp Brain Res 116, 50–62, 1997.
290. Doslak MJ, Kline LB, Dell'Osso LF, Daroff RB. Internuclear ophthalmoplegia: Recovery and plasticity. Invest Ophthalmol Vis Sci 19, 1506–1511, 1980.
291. Downey DL, Stahl JS, Bhidayasiri R, et al. Saccadic and vestibular abnormalities in multiple sclerosis: sensitive clinical signs of brainstem and cerebellar involvement. Ann N Y Acad Sci 956, 438–440, 2002.
292. Drake ME Jr., Erwin CW, Massey EW. Ocular bobbing in metabolic encephalopathy: Clinical pathologic and electrophysiologic study. Neurology 32, 1029–1031, 1982.
293. Dubinsky RM, Hallett M, Di Chiro G, Fulham M, Schwankhaus J. Increased glucose metabolism in the medulla of patients with palatal myoclonus. Neurology 41, 557–562, 1991.
294. Dubinsky RM, Jankovic J. Progressive supranuclear palsy and a multi-infarct state. Neurology 37, 570–576, 1987.
295. Dubois B, Slachevsky A, Pillon B, et al. "Applause sign" helps to discriminate PSP from FTD and PD Neurology 64, 2132–2133, 2005.
296. Duhamel J, Goldberg ME, FitzGibbon EJ, Sirigu A, Grafman J. Saccadic dysmetria in a patient with a right frontoparietal lesion: the importance of corollary discharge for accurate spatial-behavior. Brain 115, 1387–1402, 1992.
297. Duncan GW, Parker SW, Fisher CM. Acute cerebellar infarction in the PICA territory. Arch Neurol 32, 364–368, 1975.
298. Durig JS, Jen JC, Demer JL. Ocular motility in genetically defined autosomal dominant cerebellar ataxia. Am J Ophthalmol 133, 718–721, 2002.
299. Ebner R, Lopez L, Ochoa S, Crovetto L. Vertical ocular motor apraxia. Neurology 40, 712–713, 1990.
300. Eckmiller R, Westheimer G. Compensation of oculomotor deficits in monkeys with neonatal cerebellar ablations. Exp Brain Res 49, 315–326, 1983.
301. Edis RH, Mastaglia FL. Vertical gaze palsy in barbiturate intoxication. Br Med J 1, 144, 1977.
302. Edwards M, Koo MW, Tse RK. Oculogyric crisis after metoclopramide therapy. Optom Vis Sci 66, 179–180, 1989.
303. Eggenberger E. Eight-and-a-half syndrome: one-and-a-half syndrome plus cranial nerve VII palsy. J Neuroophthalmol 18, 114–116, 1998.
304. Eggenberger E, Cornblath W, Stewart DH. Oculopalatal tremor with tardive ataxia. J Neuro-ophthalmol 21, 83–86, 2001.
305. Eggenberger E, Golnik K, Lee A, et al. Prognosis of ischemic internuclear ophthalmoplegia. Ophthalmology 109, 1676–1678, 2002.
306. Eggenberger ER, Desai NP, Kaufman DI, Pless M. Internuclear ophthalmoplegia after coronary artery catheterization and percutaneous transluminal coronary balloon angioplasty. J Neuroophthalmol 20, 123–126, 2000.
307. El-Mallakh RS. Internuclear ophthalmoplegia with narcotic overdosage. Ann Neurol 20, 107, 1986.
308. Elkardoudi-Pijnenburg Y, Van Vliet AG. Opsoclonus a rare complication of cocaine misuse. J Neurol Neurosurg Psychiatry 60, 592, 1996.
309. Elston JS, Casgranje F, Lees AJ. The relationship between eye-winking tics, frequent eye-blinking and blepharospasm. J Neurol Neurosurg Psychiatry 52, 477–480, 1989.
310. Estanol B, Lopez-Rios G. Neurotology of the lateral medullary infarct syndrome. Arch Neurol 39, 176–179, 1982.
311. Estanol B, Romero R, de Viteri MS, Mateos JH, Corvera J. Oculomotor and oculovestibular functions in a hemispherectomy patient. Arch Neurol 37, 365–368, 1980.
312. Ettinger U, Kumari V, Chitnis XA, et al. Volumetric neural correlates of antisaccade eye movements in first-episode psychosis. Am J Psychiatry 161, 1918–1921, 2004.
313. Evinger LC, Fuchs AF, Baker R. Bilateral lesions of the medial longitudinal fasciculus in monkeys: effects on the horizontal and vertical components of voluntary and vestibular induced eye movements. Exp Brain Res 28, 1–20, 1977.
314. Fafrowicz M, Unrug A, Marek T, et al. Effects of diazepam and buspirone on reaction time of saccadic eye movements. Neuropsychobiology 32, 156–160, 1995.
315. Farber RH, Clementz BA, Swerdlow NR. Characteristics of open- and closed-loop smooth pursuit responses among obsessive-compulsive disorder schizophrenia and nonpsychiatric individuals. Psychophysiology 34, 157–162, 1997.
316. Farlow MR, Yee RD, Dloughy SR, et al. Gerstmann-Sträussler-Scheinker disease. I Extending the clinical spectrum. Neurology 39, 1446–1452, 1989.
317. Farr AK, Shalev B, Crawford TO, et al. Ocular manifestations of ataxia-telangiectasia. Am J Ophthalmol 134, 891–896, 2002.
318. Fattal-Valevski A, Kesler A, Sela BA, et al. Outbreak of life-threating thiamine deificiency in infants in Israel caused by a defective soy-based formula. Pediatrics 115, 233–238, 2005.
319. Fearnley JM, Revesz T, Brooks DJ, Frackowiak RS, Lees AJ. Diffuse Lewy body disease presenting with a supranuclear gaze palsy. J Neurol Neurosurg Psychiatry 54, 159–161, 1991.
320. Fielder AR, Gresty MA, Dodd KL, Mellor DH, Levene MI. Congenital ocular motor apraxia. Trans Ophthalmol Soc UK 105, 589–598, 1986.
321. Fielding J, Gerogiou-Karistianis N, Bradshaw J, et al. Impaired modulation of the vestibulo-ocular reflex in Huntington's disease. Mov Disord 19, 68–75, 2004.
322. Fink JK, Filling-Katz MR, Sokol J, et al. Clinical spectrum of Niemann-Pick type C disease. Neurology 39, 1040–1049, 1989.
323. Fisher A, Gresty M, Chambers B, Rudge P. Primary position upbeating nystagmus: a variety of central positional nystagmus. Brain 106, 949–964, 1983.
324. Fisher A, Knezevic W. Ocular and ocular motor aspects of primary thalamic haemorrhage. Clin Exp Neurol 21, 129–139, 1985.
325. Fisher CM. The pathologic and clinical aspects of thalamic hemorrhage. Trans Am Neurological Assoc 84, 56–59, 1959.

326. Fisher CM. Ocular bobbing. Arch Neurol 11, 543–546, 1964.
327. Fisher CM. Some neuro-ophthalmological observations. J Neurol Neurosurg Psychiatry 30, 383–392, 1967.
328. Fisher CM. Neurological examination of the comatose patient. Acta Neurol Scand 45 (Suppl 36), 1–56, 1969.
329. Fisher CM. Neuroanatomic evidence to explain why bilateral internuclear ophthalmoplegia may result from occlusion of a unilateral pontine branch artery. J Neuroophthalmol 24, 39–41, 2004.
330. Fisher CM, Tapia J. Lateral medullary infarction extending to the lower pons. J Neurol Neurosurg Psychiatry 50, 620–624, 1987.
331. Fisher M. Ocular skew deviation in hepatic coma. J Neurol Neurosurg Psychiatry 44, 458, 1981.
332. FitzGerald PM, Jankovic J. Tardive oculogyric crisis. Neurology 39, 1434–1437, 1989.
333. FitzGerald PM, Jankovic J, Glaze DG, Schultz R, Percy AK. Extrapyramidal involvement in Rett's syndrome. Neurology 40, 293–295, 1990.
334. FitzGibbon E J, Calvert PC, Dieterich MD, Brandt T, Zee DS. Torsional nystagmus during vertical pursuit. J Neuroophthalmol 16, 79–90, 1996.
335. Flechtner K-M, Mackert A, Thies K, Frick K, Muller-Oerlinghausen B. Lithium effect on smooth pursuit eye movements of healthy volunteers. Biol Psychiatr 32, 932–938, 1992.
336. Fleming JL, Wiesner RH, Shorter RG. Whipple's disease: clinical, biochemical and histopathological features and assessment of treatment in 29 patients. Mayo Clin Proc 63, 539–551, 1988.
337. Fletcher WA, Gellman RS. Saccades in humans with lesions of frontal eye fields (FEF). Soc Neuro Sci 15, 1203, 1989.
338. Fletcher WA, Sharpe JA. Saccadic eye movement dysfunction in Alzheimer's disease. Ann Neurol 20, 464–471, 1986.
339. Fletcher WA, Sharpe JA. Smooth pursuit dysfunction in Alzheimer's disease. Neurology 38, 272–277, 1988.
340. Flint AC, Williams O. Bilateral internuclear ophthalmoplegia in progressive supranuclear palsy with an overriding oculocephalic maneuver. Mov Disord 20, 1069–1071, 2005.
341. Flipse JP, Straathof CS, Van der Steen J, et al. Binocular saccadic acceleration in multiple sclerosis. Neuroophthalmol 16, 43–46, 1996.
342. Flipse JP, Straathof CS, Van der Steen J, et al. Binocular saccadic eye movements in multiple sclerosis. J Neurol Sci 148, 53–65, 1997.
343. Ford CS, Cruz J, Biller J, Laster W, White DR. Bilateral internuclear ophthalmoplegia in carcinomatous meningitis. J Clin Neuroophthalmol 3, 127–130, 1983.
344. Frankel M, Cummings JL. Neuro-ophthalmic abnormalities in Tourette's syndrome. Functional and anatomical implications. Neurology 34, 359–361, 1984.
345. Fraunfelder FW, Fraunfelder FT. Oculogyric crisis in patients taking cetirizine. Am J Ophthalmol 137, 355–357, 2004.
346. Fredericks CA, Gianotta SL, Sadun AA. Dilantin-induced long-term bilateral total external ophthalmoplegia. J Clin Neuro-ophthalmol 6, 22–26, 1986.
347. Friedman DI, Jankovic J, McCrary JA. Neuro-ophthalmic findings in progressive supranuclear palsy. J Clin Neuro-ophthalmol 12, 104–109, 1992.
348. Friedman L, Jesberger JA, Siever LJ, et al. Smooth pursuit performance in patients with affective disorders or schizophrenia and normal controls: analysis with specific oculomotor measures RMS error and qualitative ratings. Psychological Medicine 25, 387–403, 1995.
349. Frohman EM, Dewey RB, Frohman TC. An unusual variant of the dorsal midbrain syndrome in MS: clinical characteristics and pathophysiologic mechanisms. Mult Scler 10, 322–325, 2004.
350. Frohman EM, Frohman TC, Fleckenstein J, et al. Ocular contrapulsion in multiple sclerosis: clinical features and pathophysiological mechanisms. J Neurol Neurosurg Psychiatry 70, 688–692, 2001.
351. Frohman EM, Frohman TC, O'Suilleabhain P, et al. Quantitative oculographic characterisation of internuclear ophthalmoparesis in multiple sclerosis: the versional dysconjugacy index Z score. J Neurol Neurosurg Psychiatry 73, 51–55, 2002.
352. Frohman EM, Frohman TC, Zee DS, McColl R, Galetta S. The neuro-ophthalmology of multiple sclerosis. Lancet Neurol 4, 111–121, 2005.
353. Frohman EM, O'Suilleabhain P, Dewey RB, Jr., Frohman TC, Kramer PD. A new measure of dysconjugacy in INO: the first-pass amplitude. J Neurol Sci 210, 65–71, 2003.
354. Frohman EM, Solomon D, Zee DS. Vestibular dysfunction and nystagmus in multiple sclerosis. Intl J MS 3, 13–26, 1997.
355. Frohman EM, Zhang H, Kramer PD, et al. MRI characteristics of the MLF in MS patients with chronic internuclear ophthalmoparesis. Neurology 57, 762–768, 2001.
356. Frohman LP, Kupersmith MJ. Reversible vertical ocular deviations associated with raised intracranial pressure. J Clin Neuro-opthalmol 5, 158–163, 1985.
357. Frohman TC, Frohman EM, O'Suilleabhain P, et al. Accuracy of clinical detection of INO in MS: corroboration with quantitative infrared oculography. Neurology 61, 848–850, 2003.
358. Fukushima J, Fukushima K, Miyasaka K, Yamashita I. Voluntary control of saccadic eye movement in patients with frontal cortical lesions and parkinsonian patients in comparison with that in schizophrenics. Biol Psychiatry 36, 21–30, 1994.
359. Furman JM, Hurtt M R, Hirsch WL. Asymmetrical ocular pursuit with posterior fossa tumors. Ann Neurol 30, 208–211, 1991.
360. Furman JM, Wall C, III, Pang D. Vestibular function in periodic alternating nystagmus. Brain 113, 1425–1439, 1990.
361. Furman JMR, Crumrime PK, Reinmuth OM. Epileptic nystagmus. Ann Neurol 27, 686–688, 1990.
362. Galetta SL, Raps EC, Liu GT, Saito NG, Kline LB. Eyelid lag without eyelid retraction in pretectal disease. J Neuro-ophthalmol 16, 96–98, 1996.
363. Galimberti CA, Versino M, Sartori I, et al. Epileptic skew deviation. Neurology, 1998.
364. Gamlin PD, Gnadt JW, Mays LE. Lidocaine-induced unilateral internuclear ophthalmoplegia: effects on convergence and conjugate eye movements. J Neurophysiol 62, 82–95, 1989.

365. Garbutt S, Harris CM. Abnormal vertical optokinetic nystagmus in infants and children. Br J Ophthalmol 84, 451–455, 2000.
366. Garbutt S, Harwood MR, Kumar AN, Han YH, Leigh RJ. Evaluating small eye movements in patients with saccadic palsies. Ann N Y Acad Sci 1004, 337–346, 2003.
367. Garbutt S, Riley DE, Kumar AN, et al. Abnormalities of optokinetic nystagmus in progressive supranuclear palsy. J Neurol Neurosurg Psychiatry 75, 1386–1394, 2004.
368. Garbutt S, Thakore N, Rucker J, et al. Effects of visual fixation and convergence in periodic alternating nystagmus due to MS. Neuro-ophthalmology 28, 221–229, 2004.
369. Gascon GG, Abdo N, Sigut D, Hemidan A, Hannan MA. Ataxia-oculomotor apraxia syndrome. J Child Neurol 10, 118–122, 1995.
370. Gauntt CD, Kashii S, Nagata I. Monocular elevation paresis caused by an oculomotor fascicular impairment. J Neuroophthalmol 15, 11–14, 1995.
371. Gaymard B. Disconjugate ocular bobbing. Neurology 43, 2151, 1993.
371a. Gaymard B, Lynch J, Ploner CJ, Condy C, Rivaud-Pechoux R. The parieto-collicular pathway: an anatomical location and contribution to saccade generation. Eur J Neurosci 17, 1518–1526, 2003.
372. Gaymard B, Pierrot-Deseilligny C, Rivaud S. Impairment of sequences of memory-guided saccades after supplementary motor area lesions. Ann Neurol 28, 622–626, 1990.
373. Gaymard B, Pierrot-Deseilligny C, Rivaud S, Velut S. Smooth pursuit eye movement deficits after pontine nuclei lesions in humans. J Neurol Neurosurg Psychiatry 56, 799–807, 1993.
374. Gaymard B, Rivaud S, Amarenco P, Pierrot-Deseilligny C. Influence of visual information on cerebellar saccadic dysmetria. Ann Neurol 35, 108–112, 1994.
375. Gaymard B, Rivaud S, Cassarini JF. Effects of anterior cingulate cortex lesions on ocular saccades in humans. Exp Brain Res 120, 173–183, 1998.
376. Gaymard B, Rivaud S, Pierrot-Deseilligny C. Role of the left and right supplementary motor areas in memory-guided saccade sequences. Ann Neurol 34, 404–406, 1993.
377. Gaymard B, Rivaud S, Pierrot-Deseilligny C. Impairment of extraretinal eye position signals after central thalamic lesions. Exp Brain Res 102, 1–9, 1994.
378. Gaymard B, Rivaud-Pechoux S, Yelnik J, Pidoux B, Ploner CJ. Involvement of the cerebellar thalamus in human saccade adaptation. Eur J Neurosci 14, 554–560, 2001.
379. Genc BO, Genc E, Acik L, Ilhan S, Paksoy Y. Acquired ocular motor apraxia from bilateral frontoparietal infarcts associated with Takayasu arteritis. J Neurol Neurosurg Psychiatry 75, 1651–1652, 2004.
380. Gentile M, Di Carlo A, Susca F, et al. COACH syndrome: report of two brothers with congenital hepatic fibrosis, cerebellar vermis hypoplasia, oligophrenia, ataxia and mental retardation. Am J Med Genet 64, 514–520, 1996.
381. Geschwind DH, Perlman S, Figueroa KP, et al. Spinocerebellar ataxia type 6. Frequency of the mutation and genotype-phenotype correlations. Neurology 49, 1247–1251, 1997.
382. Ghika J, Tennis M, Hoffman E, Schoenfeld D, Growdon J. Idazoxan treatment in progressive supranuclear palsy. Neurology 41, 986–991, 1991.
383. Gibb WRG, Luthert PJ, Marsden CD. Corticobasal degeneration. Brain 112, 1171–1192, 1989.
384. Gibson JM, Kennard C. Quantitative study of "on-off" fluctuations in the ocular motor system in Parkinson's disease. Adv Neurol 45, 329–333, 1986.
385. Gibson JM, Pimlott R, Kennard C. Ocular motor and manual tracking in Parkinson's disease and the effect of treatment. J Neurol Neurosurg Psychiatry 50, 853–860, 1987.
386. Gierga K, Burk K, Bauer M, et al. Involvement of the cranial nerves and their nuclei in spinocerebellar ataxia type 2 (SCA2). Acta Neuropathol (Berl), 2005.
387. Gilman S, Sima AA, Junck L, et al. Spinocerebellar ataxia type 1 with multiple system degeneration and glial cytoplasmic inclusions. Ann Neurol 39, 241–255, 1996.
388. Gizzi M, DiRocco A, Sivak M, Cohen B. Ocular motor function in motor neuron disease. Neurology 42, 1037–1046, 1992.
389. Glaser JS. Myasthenic pseudo-internuclear ophthalmoplegia. Arch Ophthalmol 75, 363–366, 1966.
390. Gloor P, Quesney F, Ives J, Ochs R, Olivier A. Significance of direction of head turning during seizures. Neurology 37, 1092, 1987.
391. Goffinet AM, De Volder AG, Gillain C, et al. Positron tomography demonstrates frontal lobe hypometabolism in progressive supranuclear palsy. Ann Neurol 25, 131–139, 1989.
392. Golbe LI, Davis PH, Schoenberg BS, Duvoisin RC. Prevalence and natural history of progressive supranuclear palsy. Neurology 38, 1031–1034, 1988.
393. Goldschmidt TJ, Wall M. Slow-upward ocular bobbing. J Clin Neuro-ophthalmol 7, 241–243, 1987.
394. Gomez CM, Thompson RM, Gammack JT, et al. Spinocerebellar ataxia type 6: gaze-evoked and vertical nystagmus Purkinje cell degeneration and variable age of onset. Ann Neurol 42, 933–950, 1997.
395. Gomez CR, Cruz-Flores S, Malkoff MD, Sauer CM, Burch CM. Isolated vertigo as a manifestation of vertebrobasilar ischemia. Neurology 47, 94–97, 1996.
396. Gomez CR, Gomez SM, Selhorst JB. Acute thalamic esotropia. Neurology 38, 1759–1762, 1988.
397. Goodwin JA, Kansu T. Vulpian's sign: conjugate eye deviation in acute cerebral hemisphere lesions. Neurology 36, 711–712, 1986.
398. Gordon CR, Joffe V, Vainstein G, Gadoth N. Vestibulo-ocular arreflexia in families with spinocerebellar ataxia type 3 (Machado-Joseph disease). J Neurol Neurosurg Psychiatry 74, 1403–1406, 2003.
399. Gordon MF, Abrams RI, Rubin DB, Barr WB, Correa DD. Bismuth subsalicylate toxicity as a cause of prolonged encephalopathy with myoclonus. Mov Disord 10, 220–222, 1995.
400. Gordon RM, Bender MB. Visual phenomenon in lesions of the medial longitudinal fasciculus. Arch Neurol 15, 238–240, 1966.
401. Gorman M, Barkley GL. Oculogyric crisis induced by carbamazepine. Epilepsia 36, 1158–1160, 1995.
402. Gottlieb D, Calvanio R, Levine DN. Reappearance of the visual percept after intentional blinking in a patient with Balint's syndrome. J Clin Neuro-ophthalmol 11, 62–65, 1991.

403. Gow A, Southwood CM, Lazzarini RA. Disrupted proteolipid protein trafficking results in oligodendrocyte apoptosis in an animal model for Pelizaeus-Merzbacher disease. J Cell Biol 140, 925–934, 1998.
404. Goyal M, Versnick E, Tuite P, et al. Hypertrophic olivary degeneration: metaanalysis of the temporal evolution of MR findings. AJNR Am J Neuroradiol 21, 1073–1077, 2000.
405. Grad A, Baloh RW. Vertigo of vascular origin. Clinical and electronystagmographic features in 84 cases. Arch Neurol 46, 281–284, 1989.
406. Gradstein L, Danek A, Grafman J, FitzGibbon E. Eye movements in chorea-acanthocytosis. Invest Ophthalmol Vis Sci 46, 1979–1987, 2005.
407. Grand W. Positional nystagmus: an early sign in medulloblastoma. Neurology 21, 1157–1159, 1971.
408. Grant MP, Cohen M, Petersen RB, et al. Abnormal eye movements in Creutzfeldt-Jakob disease. Ann Neurology 34, 192–197, 1993.
409. Grant MP, Leigh RJ, Seidman SH, Riley DE, Hanna JP. Comparison of predictable smooth ocular and combined eye-head tracking behaviour in patients with lesions affecting the brainstem and cerebellum. Brain 115, 1323–1342, 1992.
410. Graus F, Lang B, Pozo-Rosich P. P/Q type calcium channel antibodies in paraneoplastic cerebellar degeneration with lung cancer. Neurology 59, 764–766, 2002.
411. Gray M, Forbes RB, Morrow JI. Primary isolated brainstem injury producing internuclear ophthalmoplegia. Br J Neurosurg 15, 432–434, 2001.
412. Green JF, King DJ, Trimble KM. Antisaccade and smooth pursuit eye movements in healthy subjects receiving sertraline and lorazepam. J Psychopharmacol 14, 30–36, 2000.
413. Gregorius FK, Crandall PH, Baloh RW. Positional vertigo with cerebellar astrocytoma. Surg Neurol 6, 283–286, 1976.
414. Gresty MA, Hess K, Leech J. Disorders of the vestibuloocular reflex producing oscillopsia and mechanisms compensating for loss of labyrinthine function. Brain 100, 693–716, 1977.
415. Grewal KK, Stefanelli MG, Meijer IA, et al. A founder effect in three large Newfoundland families with a novel clinically variable spastic ataxia and supranuclear gaze palsy. Am J Med Genet 131A, 249–254, 2004.
416. Guillain G, Mollaret P. Deux cas myoclonies synchrones et rhythmées vélo-pharyngo-laryngo-oculodiaphragmatiques: Le problèm anatomique et physiolopathologique de ce syndrome. Rev Neurol (Paris) 2, 545–566, 1931.
417. Guiloff RJ, Whiteley A, Kelly RE. Organic convergence spasm. Acta Neurol Scand 61, 252–259, 1980.
418. Haarmeier T, Thier P, Repnow M, Petersen D. False perception of motion in a patient who cannot compensate for eye movements. Nature 389, 849–852, 1997.
419. Hain TC, Luebke A. Phoria adaptation in patients with cerebellar lesions. Invest Ophthalmol Vis Sci 31, 1394–1397, 1990.
420. Hain TC, Zee DS, Maria B. Tilt-suppression of the vestibulo-ocular reflex in patients with cerebellar lesions. Acta Otolaryngol (Stockh) 105, 13–20, 1988.
421. Halliday GM, Hardman CD, Cordato NJ, Hely MA, Morris JG. A role for the substantia nigra pars reticulata in the gaze palsy of progressive supranuclear palsy. Brain 123, 724–732, 2000.
422. Halmagyi GM, Lessell I, Curthoys IS, Lessell S, Hoyt WF. Lithium-induced downbeat nystagmus. Am J Ophthalmol 107, 664–670, 1989.
423. Halmagyi GM, Pamphlett R, Curthoys IS. Seesaw nystagmus and ocular tilt reaction due to adult Leigh's disease. Neuro-ophthalmology 12, 1–9, 1992.
424. Halmagyi GM, Rudge P, Gresty MA, Sanders MD. Downbeating nystagmus: a review of 62 cases. Arch Neurol 40, 777–784, 1983.
425. Hamed LM, Schatz NJ, Galetta SL. Brainstem ocular motility defects and AIDS. Am J Ophthalmol 106, 437–442, 1988.
426. Hanes DP, Smith MK, Optican LM, Wurtz RH. Recovery of saccadic dysmetria following localized lesions in monkey superior colliculus. Exp Brain Res 160, 325, 2005.
427. Hanid MA, Silk DBA, Williams R. Prognostic value of the oculovestibular reflex in fulminant hepatic coma. Br Med J 1, 1029, 1978.
428. Hanihara T, Amano N, Takahashi T, Itoh Y, Yagishita S. Hypertrophy of the inferior olivary nucleus in patients with progressive supranuclear palsy. Eur Neurol 39, 97–102, 1998.
429. Hanson MR, Hamid MA, Tomsak RL, Chou SS, Leigh RJ. Selective saccadic palsy caused by pontine lesions: clinical, physiological and pathological correlations. Ann Neurol 20, 209–217, 1986.
430. Harding AE. Classification of the hereditary ataxias and paraplegia. Lancet 1, 1151–1155, 1983.
431. Harding AE, Young EP, Schon F. Adult onset supranuclear ophthalmoplegia cerebellar ataxia and neurogenic proximal muscle weakness in a brother and sister: another hexosaminidase A deficiency syndrome. J Neurol Neurosurg Psychiatry 50, 687–690, 1987.
432. Hardman CD, Halliday GM, McRitchie DA, Cartwright HR, Morris JG. Progressive supranuclear palsy affects both the substantia nigra pars compact and reticulata. Exp Neurol 144, 183–192, 1997.
433. Harris CM, Boyd S, Chong K, Harkness W, Neville BG. Epileptic nystagmus in infancy. J Neurol Sci 151, 111–114, 1997.
434. Harris CM, Shawkat F, Russell-Eggitt I, Wilson J, Taylor D. Intermittent horizontal saccade failure ('ocular motor apraxia') in children. Br J Ophthalmol 80, 151–158, 1996.
435. Harris CM, Taylor DS, Vellodi A. Ocular motor abnormalities in Gaucher disease. Neuropediatrics 30, 289–293, 1999.
436. Hashimoto T, Sasaki O, Yoshida K, Takei Y, Ikeda S. Periodic alternating nystagmus and rebound nystagmus in spinocerebellar ataxia type 6. Mov Disord 18, 1201–1204, 2003.
437. Hata S, Bernstein E, Davis LE. Atypical ocular bobbing in acute organophosphate poisoning. Arch Neurol 43, 185–186, 1986.
438. Hawkins RA, Mazziotta JC, Phelps ME. Wilson's disease with FDG and positron emission tomography. Neurology 37, 1707–1711, 1987.
439. Hayman M, Harvey AS, Hopkins IJ, Kornberg AJ, Coleman LT. Paroxysmal tonic upgaze—a reappraisal of outcome. Ann Neurol 43, 514–520, 1998.
440. Hedges TR. Ophthalmoplegia associated with AIDS. Surv Ophthalmol 39, 43–51, 1994.

441. Heide W, Binkofski F, Seitz RJ, et al. Activation of frontoparietal cortices during memorized triple-step sequences of saccadic eye movements: an fMRI study. Eur J Neurosci 13, 1177–1189, 2001.
442. Heide W, Blankenburg M, Zimmermann E, Kömpf D. Cortical control of double-step saccades: implications for spatial orientation. Ann Neurol 38, 739–748, 1995.
443. Heide W, Koenig E, Dichgans J. Optokinetic nystagmus, selfmotion sensation and their aftereffects in patients with occipitoparietal lesions. Clin Vision Sci 5, 145–156, 1990.
444. Heide W, Kurzidim K. Deficits of smooth pursuit eye movements after frontal and parietal lesions. Brain 119, 1951–1969, 1996.
445. Helmchen C, Büttner U. Centripetal nystagmus in a case of Creutzfeldt-Jakob disease. Neuroophthalmol 15, 187–192, 1995.
446. Helmchen C, Glasauer S, Bartl K. Contralesionally beating torsional nystagmus in a unilateral rostral midbrain lesion. Neurology 47, 482–486, 1996.
447. Helmchen C, Glasauer S, Buttner U. Pathological torsional eye deviation during voluntary saccades: a violation of Listing's law. J Neurol Neurosurg Psychiatry 62, 253–260, 1997.
448. Helmchen C, Hagenow A, Miesner J, et al. Eye movement abnormalities in essential tremor may indicate cerebellar dysfunction. Brain 126, 1319–1332, 2003.
449. Helmchen C, Rambold H, Fuhry L, Büttner U. Deficits in vertical and torsional eye movements after uni- and bilateral muscimol inactivation of the interstitial nucleus of Cajal of the alert monkey. Exp Brain Res 119, 436–452, 1998.
450. Helmchen C, Rambold H, Kempermann U, Büttner-Ennever JA, Büttner U. Localizing value of torsional nystagmus in small midbrain lesions. Neurology 59, 1956–1964, 2002.
451. Henn V, Lang W, Hepp K, Reisine H. Experimental gaze palsies in monkeys and their relation to human pathology. Brain 107, 619–636, 1984.
452. Hennerici M, Fromm C. Isolated complete gaze palsy: An unusual ocular movement deficit probably due to bilateral parapontine reticular formation (PPRF) lesion. Neuro-ophthalmology 1, 165–173, 1981.
453. Henson C, Staunton H, Brett FM. Does ageing have an effect on midbrain premotor nuclei for vertical eye movements? Mov Disord 18, 688–694, 2003.
454. Herishanu Y, Osimand A, Louzoun Z. Unidirectional gaze-paretic nystagmus induced by phenytoin intoxication. Am J Ophthalmol 94, 122–123, 1982.
455. Herishanu YO, Sharpe JA. Normal square wave jerks. Invest Ophthalmol Vis Sci 20, 268–272, 1981.
456. Herishanu YO, Sharpe JA. Saccadic intrusions in internuclear ophthalmoplegia. Ann Neurol 14, 67–72, 1983.
457. Hershey LA, Whicker L Jr, Abel LA, et al. Saccadic latency measurements in dementia. Arch Neurol 40, 592–593, 1983.
458. Hertle RW, Bienfang DC. Oculographic analysis of acute esotropia secondary to a thalamic hemorrhage. J Clin Neuro-ophthalmol 10, 21–26, 1990.
459. Heywood S, Ratcliff G. Long-term consequences of unilateral colliculectomy in man. In Lennerstrand G, Bach-y-Rita P (eds). Basic Mechanisms of Ocular Motility and Their Clinical Implications.1975, pp 561–564.
460. Hicks PA, Leavitt J, Mokri B. Ophthalmic manifestations of vertebral artery dissection. Ophthalmology 101, 1786–1792, 1994.
461. Higgins JJ, Patterson MC, Dambrosia JM, et al. A clinical staging classification for type C Niemann-Pick disease. Neurology 42, 2286–2290, 1992.
462. Highstein SM, Baker R. Excitatory termination of abducens internuclear neurons on medial rectus motoneurons: relationship to syndrome of internuclear ophthalmoplegia. J Neurophysiol 41, 1647–1661, 1978.
463. Hikosaka O. Role of basal ganglia in saccades. Rev Neurol (Paris) 145, 580–586, 1989.
464. Hikosaka O, Wurtz RH. Modification of saccadic eye movements by GABA-related substances. I Effect of muscimol and bicuculline in monkey superior colliculus. J Neurophysiol 53, 266–291, 1985.
465. Hirose G, Furui K, Yoshioka A, Sakai K. Unilateral conjugate gaze palsy due to a lesion of the abducens nucleus. J Clin Neuro-ophthalmol 13, 54–58, 1993.
466. Hirose G, Ogasawara T, Shirakawa T, et al. Primary position upbeat nystagmus due to unilateral medial medullary infarction. Ann Neurol 43, 403–406, 1998.
467. Ho PC, Feman SS. Internuclear ophthalmoplegia in Fabry's disease. Ann Ophthalmol 13, 951, 1981.
468. Ho VW, Porrino LJ, Crane AM, et al. Metabolic mapping of the oculomotor system in MPTP-induced parkinsonian monkeys. Ann Neurol 23, 86–89, 1988.
469. Hodgson MJ, Furman J, Ryan C, Durrant J, Kern E. Encephalopathy and vestibulopathy following short-term hydrocarbon exposure. J Occup Med 31, 51–54, 1989.
470. Hof PR, Bouras C, Constantinidis J, Morrison JH. Balint's syndrome in Alzheimer disease. Specific disruption of the occipito-parietal visual pathways. Brain Res 493, 368–375, 1989.
471. Holmes G. Disturbances of visual orientation. Br J Ophthalmol 2, 449–468, 1918.
472. Holmes G. Clinical symptoms of cerebellar disease and their interpretation (Croonian lectures III). Lancet ii, 59–65, 1922.
473. Holmes G. Spasm of fixation. Trans Ophthalmol Soc UK 50, 253–262, 1930.
474. Hommel M, Bogousslavsky J. The spectrum of vertical gaze palsy following unilateral brainstem stroke. Neurology 41, 1229–1234, 1991.
475. Hong LE, Tagamets M, Avila M, et al. Specific motion processing pathway deficit during eye tracking in schizophrenia: a performance-matched functional magnetic resonance imaging study. Biol Psychiatry 57, 726–732, 2005.
476. Hong SY, Optican LM. New cellular mechanisms for multiple time-scale adaptation in cerebellum. Soc Neurosci Abstr, 933.7, 2005.
477. Honnorat J, Trouillas P, Thivolet C, Aguera M, Belin M. Autoantibodies to glutamate decarboxylase in a patient with cerebellar cortical atrophy, peripheral neuropathy and slow eye movements. Arch Neurol 52, 462–468, 1995.
478. Horita H, Hoashi E, Okuyama Y, Kumagai K, Endo S. The studies of the attacks of abnormal eye movements in a case of infantile spasms. Folia Psychiatrica Neurologica Japonica 31, 393–402, 1977.
479. Horn AKE, Büttner-Enever JA, Gayde M, Messoudi A. Neuroanatomical identification of mesencephalic

premotor neurons coordinating eyelid with upgaze in the monkey and man. J Comp Neurol 420, 19–34, 2000.

480. Horn AKE, Büttner-Ennever JA, Büttner U. Saccadic premotor neurons in the brainstem: functional neuroanatomy and clinical implications. Neuro-ophthalmology 16, 229–240, 1996.
481. Horn AKE, Helmchen C, Wahle P. GABAergic neurons in the rostral mesencephalon of the macaque monkey that control vertical eye movements. Ann N Y Acad Sci 1004, 19–28, 2003.
482. Hornsten G. Wallenberg's syndrome. II Oculomotor and oculostatic disturbances. Acta Neurologica Scand 50, 447–468, 1974.
483. Hotson JR, Langston EB, Langston JW. Saccade responses to dopamine in human MTPT-induced parkinsonism. Ann Neurol 20, 456–463, 1986.
484. Hotson JR, Louis AA, Langston EB, Moreno JA. Vertical saccades in Huntington's disease and nondegenerative choreoathetoid disorders. Neuro-ophthalmology 4, 207–217, 1984.
485. Hotson JR, Sachdev HS. Amitriptyline: another cause of internuclear ophthalmoplegia with coma. Ann Neurol 12, 62, 1982.
486. Hotson JR, Steinke GW. Vertical and horizontal saccades in aging and dementia. Failure to inhibit anticipatory saccades. Neuro-ophthalmology 8, 267–273, 1988.
487. Hoyt CS. Nystagmus and other abnormal ocular movements in children. Ped Clin North Am 34, 1415–1423, 1987.
488. Hoyt CS, Billson FA, Alpins N. The supranuclear disturbances of gaze in kernicterus. Ann Ophthalmol 10, 1487–1492, 1978.
489. Hoyt CS, Mousel DK. Transient supranuclear disturbances of gaze in healthy neonates. Am J Ophthalmol 89, 708–713, 1980.
490. Huebner WP, Leigh RJ, Seidman SH, Billian C. An investigation of horizontal combined eye-head tracking in patients with abnormal vestibular and smooth pursuit eye movements. J Neurol Sci 116, 152–164, 1993.
491. Hunnewell J, Miller NR. Bilateral internuclear ophthalmoplegia related to chronic toluene abuse. J Neuroophthalmol 18, 277–280, 1998.
492. Husain M, Mannan S, Hodgson T, et al. Impaired spatial working memory across saccades contributes to abnormal search in parietal neglect. Brain 124, 941–952, 2001.
493. Husain M, Parton A, Hodgson TL, Mort D, Rees G. Self-control during response conflict by human supplementary eye field. Nat Neurosci 6, 117–118, 2003.
494. Husain M, Stein J. Rezso Balint and his most celebrated case. Arch Neurol 45, 89–93, 1988.
495. Hutton S, Kennard C. Oculomotor abnormalities in schizophrenia—a critical review. Neurology 50, 604–609, 1998.
496. Hutton SB, Crawford TJ, Gibbins H, et al. Short and long term effects of antipsychotic medication on smooth pursuit eye tracking in schizophrenia. Psychopharmacology (Berl) 157, 284–291, 2001.
497. Hutton SB, Huddy V, Barnes TR, et al. The relationship betweem antisaccades smooth pursuit and executive dysfunction in first-episode schizophrenia. Biol Psychiatr 56, 553–559, 2004.
498. Huygen PLM, Verhagen WIM, Hommes OR, Nicolasen MGM. Short vestibulo-ocular reflex time constants associated with oculomotor pathology in multiple sclerosis. Acta Otolaryngol (Stockh) 109, 25–33, 1990.
499. Ishikawa H, Ishikawa S, Mukuno K. Short-cycle periodic (ping-pong) gaze. Neurology 43, 1067–1070, 1993.
500. Israël I, Rivaud S, Gaymard B, Berthoz A, Pierrot-Deseilligny C. Cortical control of vestibular-guided saccades. Brain 118, 1169–1184, 1995.
501. Iwasaki Y, Kinoshita M, Ikeda K, Shiojima T. Palatal myoclonus following Behcet's disease ameliorated by ceruletide a potent analogue of CCK octapeptide. J Neurol Sci 105, 12–13, 1991.
502. Jack ARG, Currie JN, Harvey SK, et al. Perturbations of horizontal saccade velocity profiles in humans as a marker of brainstem dysfunction in Wernicke-Korsakoff syndrome. Soc Neurosci Abstr 23, 864.3, 1997.
503. Jackel RA, Gittinger JW Jr., Smith TW, Passarelli CB. Metastatic adenocarcinoma presenting as a one-and-a-half syndrome. J Clin Neuro-ophthalmol 6, 116–119, 1986.
504. Jacobs L, Heffner RR Jr., Newman RP. Selective paralysis of downward gaze caused by bilateral lesions of the mesencephalic periaqueductal gray matter. Neurology 35, 516–521, 1985.
505. Jacobson DM, Corbett JJ. Downbeat nystagmus associated with dolichoectasia of the vertebrobasilar artery. Arch Neurol 46, 1005–1008, 1989.
506. Jacome DE, FitzGerald R. Monocular ictal nystagmus. Arch Neurol 39, 653–656, 1982.
507. Jammes JL. Bilateral internuclear ophthalmoplegia due to acute cervical hyperextension without head trauma. J Clin Neuro-ophthalmol 9, 112–115, 1989.
508. Jampel RS, Fells P. Monocular elevation paresis caused by a central nervous system lesion. Arch Ophthalmol 80, 45–57, 1968.
509. Jampel RS, Quaglio ND. Eye movements in Tay-Sachs disease. Neurology 14, 1013–1019, 1964.
510. Janssen JC, Larner AJ, Morris H, Bronstein AM, Farmer SF. Upbeat nystagmus: clinicoanatomical correlation. J Neurol Neurosurg Psychiatry 65, 380–381, 1998.
511. Jen J, Kim GW, Baloh RW. Clinical spectrum of episodic ataxia type 2. Neurology 62, 17–22, 2004.
512. Jhee SS, Zarotsky V, Mohaupt SM, Yones CL, Sims SJ. Delayed onset of oculogyric crisis and torticollis with intramuscular haloperidol. Ann Pharmacother 37, 1434–1437, 2003.
513. Jinnah HA, Lewis RF, Visser JE, et al. Ocular motor abnormalities in Lesch-Nyhan disease. Pediatr Neurol 24, 200–204, 2001.
514. Johkura K, Komiyama A, Kuroiwa Y. Eye deviation in patients with one-and-a-half syndrome. Eur Neurol 44, 210–215, 2000.
515. Johkura K, Komiyama A, Kuroiwa Y. Vertical conjugate eye deviation in postresuscitation coma. Ann Neurol 56, 878–881, 2004.
516. Johkura K, Komiyama A, Tobita M, Hasegawa O. Saccadic ping-pong gaze. J Neuroophthalmol 18, 43–46, 1998.
517. Johnston JL, Miller JD, Nath A. Ocular motor dysfunction in HIV-1–infected subjects: A quantitative oculographic analysis. Neurology 46, 451–457, 1996.

518. Johnston JL, Sharpe JA. Sparing of the vestibulo-ocular reflex with lesions of the paramedian pontine reticular formation. Neurology 39, 876, 1989.
519. Johnston JL, Sharpe JA, Morrow MJ. Paresis of contralateral smooth pursuit and normal vestibular smooth eye movements after unilateral brainstem lesions. Ann Neurol 31, 495–502, 1992.
520. Johnston JL, Sharpe JA, Morrow MJ. Spasm of fixation: a quantitative study. J Neurol Sci 107, 166–171, 1992.
521. Johnston JL, Sharpe JA, Ranalli PJ, Morrow MJ. Oblique misdirection and slowing of vertical saccades after unilateral lesions of the pontine tegmentum. Neurology 43, 2238–2244, 1993.
522. Jones A, Friedland RP, Koss B, Stark L, Thompkins-Ober BA. Saccadic intrusions in Alzheimer-type dementia. J Neurol 229, 189–194, 1983.
523. Joseph K, Avallone J, Difazio M. Paroxysmal tonic upgaze and partial tetrasomy of chromosome 15: a novel genetic association. J Child Neurol 20, 165–168, 2005.
524. Josephs KA, Tsuboi Y, Dickson DW. Creutzfeldt-Jakob disease presenting as progressive supranulear palsy. Eur J Neurol 11, 343–346, 2004.
525. Juncos JL, Hirsch EC, Malessa S, et al. Mesencephalic cholinergic nuclei in progressive supranuclear palsy. Neurology 41, 25–30, 1991.
526. Jürgens R, Becker W, Kornhuber H. Natural and drug-induced variations of velocity and duration of human saccadic eye movements: Evidence for a control of the neural pulse generator by local feedback. Biol Cybern 39, 87–96, 1981.
527. Kafil-Hussain NA, Monavari A, Bowell R, et al. Ocular findings in glutaric aciduria type 1. J Pediatr Ophthalmol Strabismus 37, 289–293, 2000.
528. Kameda W, Kawanami T, Kurita K, et al. Lateral and medial medullary infarction: a comparative analysis of 214 patients. Stroke 35, 694–699, 2004.
529. Kaminski HJ, Zee DS, Leigh RJ, Mendez MF. Ocular flutter and ataxia associated with AIDS-related complex. Neuro-ophthalmology 11, 163–167, 1991.
530. Kanayama R, Bronstein AM, Shallo-Hoffmann J, Rudge P, Husain M. Visually and memory guided saccades in a case of cerebellar saccadic dysmetria. J Neurol Neurosurg Psychiatry 57, 1081–1084, 1994.
531. Kandler RH, Davies-Jones GAB. Internuclear ophthalmoplegia in pernicious anemia. Br Med J 297, 1583, 1988.
532. Kaneko CRS. Effect of ibotenic acid lesions of the omnipause neurons on saccadic eye movements in Rhesus macaques. J Neurophysiol 75, 2229–2242, 1996.
533. Kaplan PW. Gaze deviation from contralateral pseudoperiodic lateralized epileptiform discharges (PLEDs). Epilepsia 46, 979, 2005.
534. Kaplan PW, Lesser RP. Vertical and horizontal epileptic gaze deviation and nystagmus. Neurology 39, 1391–1393, 1989.
535. Kaplan PW, Tusa RJ. Neurophysiologic and clinical correlations of epileptic nystagmus. Neurology 43, 2508–2514, 1993.
536. Kaplan PW, Tusa RJ. Epileptic nystagmus—Reply. Neurology 44, 2217–2218, 1994.
537. Karnath H-O, Himmelbach M, Rorden C. The subcortical anatomy of human spatial neglect: putamen caudate nucleus and pulvinar. Brain 125, 350–360, 2002.
538. Kase CS, Maulsby GO, Mohr JP. Partial pontine hematomas. Neurology 30, 652–655, 1980.
539. Kataoka S, Hori A, Shirakawa T, Hirose G. Paramedian pontine infarction. Neurological/topographical correlation. Stroke 28, 809–815, 1997.
540. Kato M, Miyashita N, Hikosaka O, et al. Eye movements in monkeys with local dopamine depletion in the caudate nucleus. 1. Deficits in spontaneous saccades. J Neurosci 15, 912–927, 1995.
541. Kato N, Arai K, Hattori T. Study of the rostral midbrain atrophy in progressive supranuclear palsy. J Neurol Sci 15, 57–60, 2003.
542. Katoh Z. Slowing effects of alcohol on voluntary eye movements. Aviat Space Environ Med 59, 606–610, 1988.
543. Katsarkas A. Positional nystagmus of the "central type" as an early sign of multiple sclerosis. J Otolaryngol 11, 91–93, 1982.
544. Katsuse O, Dickson DW. Inferior olivary hypertrophy is uncommon in progressive supranuclear palsy. Acta Neuropathol (Berl) 108, 143–146, 2004.
545. Kattah JC, Kolsky MP, Luessenhop AJ. Positional vertigo and the cerebellar vermis. Neurology 34, 527–529, 1984.
546. Katz B, Hoyt WF, Townsend J. Ocular bobbing and unilateral pontine hemorrhage. J Clin Neuro-ophthalmol 2, 193–195, 1982.
547. Kaufman SR, Abel LA. The effects of distraction on smooth pursuit in normal subjects. Acta Otolaryngol (Stockh) 102, 57–64, 1986.
548. Kaye SB, Wright N, Ward A, Downgaze paresis following severe head trauma in a child. Dev Med Child Neurol 38, 1046–1052, 1996.
549. Keane JR. Contralateral gaze deviation with supratentorial hemorrhage. Three pathologically verified cases. Arch Neurol 32, 119–122, 1975.
550. Keane JR. Spastic eyelids. Failure of levator inhibition in unconscious states. Arch Neurol 32, 695–698, 1975.
551. Keane JR. Gaze-evoked blepharoclonus. Arch Neurol 3, 243–245, 1978.
552. Keane JR. Sustained upgaze in coma. Ann Neurol 9, 409–412, 1981.
553. Keane JR. Pretectal pseudobobbing. Five patients with 'V'-pattern convergence nystagmus. Arch Neurol 42, 592–594, 1985.
554. Keane JR. Acute bilateral ophthalmoplegia: 60 cases. Neurology 36, 279–281, 1986.
555. Keane JR. Acute vertical ocular myoclonus. Neurology 36, 86–89, 1986.
556. Keane JR. Bilateral ocular motor signs after tentorial herniation in 25 patients. Arch Neurol 43, 806–807, 1986.
557. Keane JR. Traumatic internuclear ophthalmoplegia. J Clin Neuro-ophthalmol 7, 165–166, 1987.
558. Keane JR. Lid-opening apraxia in Wilson's disease. J Clin Neuro-ophthalmol 8, 31–33, 1988.
559. Keane JR. The pretectal syndrome. Neurology 40, 684–690, 1990.
560. Keane JR. Neuro-ophthalmolgic signs in AIDS: 50 patients. Neurology 41, 841–845, 1991.
561. Keane JR. Internuclear ophthalmoplegia. Unusual causes in 114 of 410 patients. Arch Neurol 62, 714–717, 2005.
562. Keane JR, Itabashi HH. Upbeat nystagmus: clinicopathologic study of two patients. Neurology 37, 491–494, 1987.

563. Keane JR, Rawlinson DG, Lu AT. Sustained downgaze deviation. Two cases without structural pretectal lesions. Neurology 26, 594–595, 1976.
564. Kennard C. Scanpaths: the path to understanding abnormal cognitive processing in neurological disease. Ann N Y Acad Sci 956, 242–249, 2002.
565. Kenyon RV, Becker J T, Butters N. Oculomotor function in Wernicke-Korsakoff syndrome. II Smooth pursuit eye movements. Int J Neurosci 25, 67–79, 1984.
566. Kenyon RV, Becker JT, Butters N, Hermann H. Oculomotor function in Wernicke-Korsakoff syndrome. I Saccadic eye movements. Int J Neurosci 25, 53–65, 1984.
566a. Kerber KA, Jen JC, Perlman S, Baloh RW. Late-onset, pure cerebellar ataxia: differentiating those with and without identifiable mutations. J Neurol Sci 238, 41–45, 2005.
567. Kim JS. Pure lateral medullary infarction: clinical-radiological correlation of 130 acute consecutive patients. Brain 126, 1864–1872, 2003.
568. Kim JS. Internuclear ophthalmoplegia as an isolated or predominant symptom of brainstem infarction. Neurology 62, 1491–1496, 2004.
569. Kim JS, Kim HK, Im JH, Lee MC. Oculogyric crisis and abnormal magnetic resonance imaging signals in bilateral lentiform nuclei. Mov Disord 11, 756–758, 1996.
569a. Kim JS, Kim J. Pure midbrain infarction: clinical, radiologic, and pathophysiologic findings. Neurology 64, 1227–1232, 2005.
570. Kimmig H, Haussmann K, Mergner T, Lucking CH. What is pathological with gaze shift fragmentation in Parkinson's disease? J Neurol 249, 683–692, 2002.
571. Kirkham TH, Guitton D, Gans M. Task-dependent variations of ocular lateropulsion in Wallenberg's syndrome. Can J Neurol Sci 8, 21–22, 1981.
572. Kirkham TH, Kamin DF. Slow saccadic eye movements in Wilson's disease. J Neurol Neurosurg Psychiatry 37, 191–194, 1974.
573. Kirkwood SC, Siemers E, Bond C, et al. Confirmation of subtle motor changes among presymptomatic carriers of the Huntington disease gene. Arch Neurol 57, 1040–1044, 2000.
574. Kitagawa M, Fukushima J, Tashiro K. Relationship between antisaccades and the clinical symptoms in Parkinson's disease. Neurology 44, 2285–2289, 1994.
575. Kitthaweesin K, Riley DE, Leigh RJ. Vergence disorders in progressive supranuclear palsy. Ann N Y Acad Sci 956, 504–507, 2002.
576. Klostermann W, Zuhlke C, Heide W, Kompf D, Wessel K. Slow saccades and other eye movement disorders in spinocerebellar atrophy type 1. J Neurol 244, 105–111, 1997.
577. Knight MA, Gardner RJ, Bahlo M, et al. Dominantly inherited ataxia and dysphonia with dentate calcification: spinocerebellar ataxia type 20. Brain 127, 1172–1181, 2004.
578. Knirsch UI, Bachus R, Gosztonyi G, Zschenderlein R, Ludolph AC. Clinicopathological study of atypical motor neuron disease with vertical gaze palsy and ballism. Acta Neuropathol (Berl) 100, 342–346, 2000.
579. Knobler RL, Somasundaram M, Schutta HS. Inverse ocular bobbing. Ann Neurol 9, 194–197, 1981.
580. Knox DL, Green WR, Troncoso JC, et al. Cerebral ocular Whipple's disease: a 62 year-old odyssey from death to diagnosis. Neurology 45, 617–625, 1995.
581. Koeppen AH. The nucleus pontis centralis caudalis in Huntington's disease. J Neurol Sci 91, 129–141, 1989.
582. Koeppen AH, Barron KD, Dentinger MP. Olivary hypertrophy: histochemical demonstration of hydrolytic enzymes. Neurology 30, 471–480, 1980.
583. Kogeorgos J, Scott DF, Swash M. Epileptic dizziness. Br Med J 282, 687–689, 1981.
584. Kohno T, Oohira A, Hori S. Near reflex substituting for acquired horizontal gaze palsy: a case report. Jpn J Ophthalmol 48, 584–586, 2004.
585. Komatsu H, Wurtz RH. Modulation of pursuit eye movements by stimulation of cortical areas MT and MST. J Neurophysiol 62, 31–47, 1989.
586. Komiyama A, Takamatsu K, Johkura K, et al. Internuclear ophthalmoplegia and contralateral exotropia. Nonparalytic pontine exotropia and WEBINO syndrome. Neuro-ophthalmology 19, 33–44, 1998.
587. Kommerell G. Unilateral internuclear ophthalmoplegia. The lack of inhibitory involvement in medial rectus muscle activity. Invest Ophthalmol Vis Sci 21, 592–599, 1981.
588. Kommerell G, Henn V, Bach M, Lucking CH. Unilateral lesion of the paramedian pontine reticular formation. Loss of rapid eye movements with preservation of vestibulo-ocular reflex and pursuit. Neuro-ophthalmology 7, 93–98, 1987.
589. Kommerell G, Hoyt WF. Lateropulsion of saccadic eye movements. Electro-oculographic studies in a patient with Wallenberg's syndrome. Arch Neurol 28, 313–318, 1973.
590. Kömpf D, Gmeiner H-J. Gaze palsy and visual hemineglect in acute hemisphere lesions. Neuro-ophthalmology 9, 49–53, 1989.
591. Kömpf D, Oppermann J. Vertical gaze palsy and thalamic dementia. Syndrome of the posterior thalamosubthalamic paramedian artery. Neuro-ophthalmology 6, 121–124, 1986.
592. Konarski JZ, McIntyre RS, Grupp LA, Kennedy SH. Is the cerebellum relevant in the circuitry of neuropsychiatric disorders? J Psychiatry Neurosci 30, 178–186, 2005.
592a. Kono R, Hasebe S, Ohtsuri H, et al. Impaired vertical phoria adaptation in patients with cerebellar dysfunction. Invest Ophthalmol Vis Sci 43, 673–678, 2002.
593. Kori AA, Das VE, Zivotofsky AZ, Leigh RJ. Memory-guided saccadic eye movements: effects of cerebellar disease. Vision Res 38, 3181–3192, 1998.
594. Kori AA, Robin NH, Jacobs JB, et al. Pendular nystagmus in a peroxisomal assembly disorder. Arch Neurol 55, 554–558, 1998.
595. Kuniyoshi S, Riley DE, Zee DS, et al. Distinguishing progressive supranuclear palsy from other forms of Parkinson's disease: evaluation of new signs. Ann N Y Acad Sci 956, 484–486, 2002.
596. Kupfer C, Cogan DG. Unilateral internuclear ophthalmoplegia: a clinicopathological case report. Arch Ophthalmol 75, 484–489, 1966.
597. Kushner MJ, Parrish M, Burke A, et al. Nystagmus in motor neuron disease: clinicopathological study of two cases. Ann Neurol 16, 71–77, 1984.
598. Lagreze WD, Warner JE, Zamani AA, et al. Mesencephalic clefts with associated eye movement disorders. Arch Ophthalmol 114, 429–432, 1996.

599. Lai MM, Kerrison JB, Miller NR. Reversible bilateral internuclear ophthalmoplegia associated with FK506. J Neurol Neurosurg Psychiatry 75, 776–778, 2004.
600. Lakshminarayanan V, Friedland RP, Muller EC, Koss E, Stark L. The vestibular ocular reflex in Alzheimer's disease. Neuro-ophthalmology 6, 205–208, 1986.
601. Lambert SR, Kriss A, Gresty M, Benton S, Taylor D Joubert syndrome. Arch Ophthalmol 107, 709–713, 1989.
602. Lapresle J. Rhythmic palatal myoclonus and the dentato-olivary pathway. J Neurol 220, 223–230, 1979.
603. Larmande P, Dongmo L, Limodin J, Ruchoux M. Periodic alternating gaze: a case without any hemispheric lesion. Neurosurgery 20, 481–483, 1987.
604. Larmande P, Henin D, Jan M, Elie A, Gouaze A. Abnormal vertical eye movements in the locked-in syndrome. Ann Neurol 11, 100–102, 1982.
605. Larmande P, Limodin J, Henin D, Lapierre F. Ocular bobbing: abnormal eye movement or eye movement's abnormality? Ophthalmologica 187, 161–165, 1983.
606. Larrison-Faucher AL, Matorin AA, Sereno AB. Nicotine reduces antisaccade errors in task impaired schizophrenic subjects. Prog Neuropsychopharmacol Biol Psychiatry 28, 505–516, 2004.
607. Lasker AG, Zee DS. Ocular motor abnormalities in Huntington's disease. Vision Res 37, 3639–3645, 1997.
608. Lasker AG, Zee DS, Hain TC, Folstein SE, Singer HS. Saccades in Huntington's disease: initiation defects and distractability. Neurology 37, 364–370, 1987.
609. Lasker AG, Zee DS, Hain TC, Folstein SE, Singer HS. Saccades in Huntington's disease: slowing and dysmetria. Neurology 38, 427–431, 1988.
610. Lawden MC, Bagelmann H, Crawford TJ, Matthews TD, Kennard C. An effect of structured backgrounds on smooth pursuit eye movements in patients with cerebral lesions. Brain 118, 37–48, 1995.
611. Lawden MC, Bronstein AM, Kennard C. Repetitive paroxysmal nystagmus and vertigo. Neurology 45, 276–280, 1995.
612. Le Ber I, Bouslam N, Rivaud-Pechoux S, et al. Frequency and phenotypic spectrum of ataxia with oculomotor apraxia 2: a clinical and genetic study in 18 patients. Brain 127, 759–767, 2004.
613. Le Ber I, Moreira MC, Rivaud-Pechoux S, et al. Cerebellar ataxia with oculomotor apraxia type 1: clinical and genetic studies. Brain 126, 2761–2772, 2003.
614. Lee H, Ahn BH, Baloh RW. Sudden deafness with vertigo as a sole manifestation of anterior inferior cerebellar artery infarction. J Neurol Sci 222, 105–107, 2004.
615. Lee MS, Kim YD, Lyoo CH. Oculogyric crisis as an initial manifestation of Wilson's disease. Neurology 52, 1714–1715, 1999.
616. Leech J, Gresty M, Hess K, Rudge P. Gaze failure drifting eye movements and centripetal nystagmus in cerebellar disease. Br J Ophthalmol 61, 774–781, 1977.
617. Lees AG. Whipple disease with supranuclear ophthalmoplegia diagnosed by polymerase chain reaction of cerebrospinal fluid. J Neuro-ophthalmol 22, 18–21, 2005.
618. LeHeron CJ, MacAskill MR, Anderson TJ. Memory-guided saccades in Parkinson's disease: long delays can improve performance. Exp Brain Res 161, 293–298, 2005.
619. Leigh RJ. The cortical control of ocular pursuit movements. Rev Neurol (Paris) 145, 605–612, 1989.
620. Leigh RJ, Foley JM, Remler BF, Civil RH. Oculogyric crisis: a syndrome of thought disorder and ocular deviation. Ann Neurol 22, 13–17, 1987.
621. Leigh RJ, Hanley DF, Munschauer FEI, Lasker AG. Eye movements induced by head rotations in unresponsive patients. Ann Neurol 15, 465–473, 1983.
622. Leigh RJ, Hong S, Zee DS, Optican LM. Oculopalatal tremor: clinical and computational study of a disorder of the inferior olive. Soc Neurosci Abstr 933.8, 2005.
623. Leigh RJ, Mapstone T, Weymann C. Eye movements in children with the Dandy-Walker syndrome. Neuroophthalmol 12, 285–288, 1992.
624. Leigh RJ, Newman SA, Folstein S E, Lasker AG, Jensen BA. Abnormal ocular motor control in Huntington's disease. Neurology 33, 1268–1275, 1983.
625. Leigh RJ, Parhad IM, Clark AW, Buettner-Ennever JA, Folstein SE. Brainstem findings in Huntington's disease. J Neurol Sci 71, 247–256, 1985.
626. Leigh RJ, Riley DE. Eye movements in parkinsonism: it's saccadic speed that counts. Neurology 54, 1018–1019, 2000.
627. Leigh RJ, Rottach KG, Das VE. Transforming sensory perceptions into motor commands: evidence from programming of eye movements. Ann N Y Acad Sci 835, 353–362, 1997.
628. Leigh RJ, Seidman SH, Grant MP, Hanna JP. Loss of ipsidirectional quick phases of torsional nystagmus with a unilateral midbrain lesion. J Vestib Res 3, 115–122, 1993.
629. Leigh RJ, Tomsak RL. Syndrome resembling PSP after surgical repair of ascending aorta dissection or aneurysm. Neurology 63, 1141–1142, 2004.
630. Leigh RJ, Tusa RJ. Disturbance of smooth pursuit caused by infarction of occipitoparietal cortex. Ann Neurol 17, 185–187, 1985.
631. Lekwuwa GU, Barnes GR. Cerebral control of eye movements. I The relationship between cerebral lesion sites and smooth pursuit deficits. Brain 119, 473–490, 1996.
632. Lekwuwa GU, Barnes GR. Cerebral control of eye movements. II Timing of anticipatory eye movements predictive pursuit and phase errors in focal cerebral lesions. Brain 119, 491–505, 1996.
633. Lekwuwa GU, Barnes GR, Grealy MA. Effects of prediction on smooth-pursuit eye velocity gain in cerebellar patients and controls. In Findlay JM, Walker R, Kentridge RW (eds). Eye Movement Research: Mechanisms, processes and applications. Elsevier, Amsterdam, pp 119–129.
634. Lempert T, von Brevern M. The eye movements of syncope. Neurology 46, 1086–1088, 1996.
635. Lennox G, Jones R. Gaze distractibility in Wilson's disease. Ann Neurol 25, 415–417, 1989.
636. Leon-Carrion J, van Eeckhout P, Dominguez-Morales MR, Perez-Santamaria FJ. The locked-in syndrome: a syndrome looking for a therapy. Brain Inj 16, 571–582, 2002.
637. Lepore FE, Gulli V, Miller DC. Neuro-ophthalmological findings with neuropathological correlation in bilateral thalamic-mesencephalic infarction. J Clin Neuro-ophthalmol 5, 224–228, 1985.
638. Lepore FE, Nissenblatt MJ. Bilateral internuclear

ophthalmoplegia after intrathecal chemotherapy and cranial irradiation. Am J Ophthalmol 92, 851–853, 1981.
639. Lepore FE, Steele JC, Cox TA, et al. Supranuclear disturbances of ocular motility in Lytico-Bodig. Neurology 38, 1849–1853, 1988.
640. Lessell S, Wolf PA, Chronley D. Prolonged vertical nystagmus after pentobarbital sodium administration. Am J Ophthalmol 80, 151–152, 1975.
641. Lesser RP, Leigh RJ, Dinner DS, et al. Preservation of voluntary saccades after intracarotid injection of barbiturate. Neurology 35, 1108–1112, 1985.
642. Levin S, Jones A, Stark L, Marrin EL, Holzman PS. Identification of abnormal patterns in eye movements of schizophrenic patients. Arch Gen Psychiatry 39, 1125–1130, 1982.
643. Levin S, Luebke A, Zee DS, et al. Smooth pursuit eye movements in schizophrenics. Quantitative measurements with the search-coil technique. J Psychiatr Res 22, 195–206, 1988.
644. Levy DE, Plum F. Outcome prediction in comatose patients: significance of reflex eye movement analysis. J Neurol Neurosurg Psychiatry 51, 318, 1988.
645. Levy DL, Dorus E, Shaughnessy R, et al. Pharmacologic evidence for specificity of pursuit dysfunction to schizophrenia. Lithium carbonate associated with abnormal smooth pursuit. Arch Gen Psychiatry 42, 335–341, 1985.
646. Levy DL, Holzman PS, Matthysse S, Mendell NR. Eye tracking and schizophrenia—a selective review. Schizophrenia Bulletin 20, 47–62, 1995.
647. Levy DL, Lipton RB, Holzman PS. Smooth pursuit eye movements: effects of alcohol and chloral hydrate. J Psychiatr Res 16, 1–11, 1981.
648. Lewis AJ, Gawel MJ. Diffuse Lewy body disease with dementia and oculomotor dysfunction. Mov Disord 5, 143–147, 1990.
649. Lewis AR, Kline LB, Sharpe JA. Acquired esotropia due to Arnold-Chiari I Malformation. J Neuro-ophthalmol 16, 49–54, 1996.
650. Lewis RF, Crawford TO. Ocular motor abnormalities in ataxia telangiectasia. Neurology 50 (Suppl), 1998.
651. Lewis RF, Crawford TO. Slow target-directed eye movements in ataxia-telangiectasia. Invest Ophthalmol Vis Sci 43, 686–691, 2002.
652. Lewis RF, Zee DS. Ocular motor disorders associated with cerebellar lesions: pathophysiology and topical diagnosis. Rev Neurol (Paris) 149, 665–677, 1993.
653. LeWitt PA. Conjugate eye deviations as dyskinesias induced by levodopa in Parkinson's disease. Mov Disord 13, 731–734, 1998.
654. Lisberger SG, Miles FA, Zee DS. Signals used to compute errors in monkey vestibuloocular reflex: possible role of flocculus. J Neurophysiol 52, 1140–1153, 1984.
655. Litman RE, Hommer DW, Clem T, et al. Smooth pursuit eye movements in schizophrenia: effects of neuroleptic treatment and caffeine. Psychopharmacol Bull 25, 473–478, 1989.
656. Litvan I. Progressive supranuclear palsy. In Litvan I (ed). Atypical Parkinsonian Disorders. Clinical and Research Aspects. Humana Press, Totowa NJ, 2005, pp 287–308.
657. Litvan I, Agid Y, Calne D, et al. Accuracy of clinical criteria for the diagnosis of progressive supranuclear palsy (Steele-Richardson-Olszewski syndrome). Neurology 46, 922–930, 1996.
658. Liu GT, Carrazana EJ, Macklis JD, Mikati MA. Delayed oculogyric crises associated with striatocapsular infarction. J Clin Neuro-ophthalmol 11, 198–201, 1991.
659. Lopez L, Ochoa S, Mesropian H, Lacman M, Granillo R. Acute transient upside-down inversion of vision with brainstem-cerebellar infarction. Neuro-ophthalmology 15, 277–280, 1995.
660. Lopez LI, Gresty MA, Bronstein AM, DuBoulay EP, Rudge P. Acquired pendular nystagmus: oculomotor and MRI findings. Acta Oto-Laryngologica 285–287, 1995.
661. Lossos A, Reches A, Gal A, et al. Frontotemporal dementia and parkinsonism with the P301S tau gene mutation in a Jewish family. J Neurol 250, 733–740, 2003.
662. Louis ED, Klataka LA, Liu Y, Fahn S. Comparison of extrapyramidal features in 31 pathologically confirmed cases of diffuse Lewy body disease and 34 pathologically confirmed cases of Parkinson's disease. Neurology 48, 376–380, 1997.
663. Louis ED, Lynch T, Kaufmann P, Fahn S, Odel J. Diagnostic guidelines in central nervous system Whipple's disease. Ann Neurol 40, 561–568, 1996.
664. Lowsky R, Archer GL, Fyles G, et al. Diagnosis of Whipple's disease by molecular analysis of peripheral blood. N Engl J Med 331, 1343–1346, 1994.
665. Luda E. Ocular dipping. Arch Neurol 39, 67, 1982.
666. Lueck CJ, Crawford TJ, Henderson L, et al. Saccadic eye movements in Parkinson's disease: II Remembered saccades—towards a unified hypothesis? Quart J Exp Psychol 45A 211–233, 1992.
667. Lueck CJ, Tanyeri S, Crawford TJ, Henderson L, Kennard C. Antisaccades and remembered saccades in Parkinson's disease. J Neurol Neurosurg Psychiatry 53, 284–288, 1990.
668. Lueck CJ, Tanyeri S, Crawford TJ, Henderson L, Kennard C. Saccadic eye movements in Parkinson's disease: I Delayed saccades. Quart J Exp Psychol 45A 193–210, 1992.
669. Luria A, Pravdine-Vinarskaya E, Yarbus A. Disorders of ocular movement in a case of simultanagnosia. Brain 86, 219–228, 1963.
670. Lutz A. Ueber die Bahnen der Blickwendung und deren Dissoziierung. Klin Monatsble Augenheilkd 70, 213–235, 1923.
671. Lynch JC. Saccade initiation and latency deficits after combined lesions of the frontal and posterior eye fields in monkeys. J Neurophysiol 68, 1913–1916, 1992.
672. Maas EF, Ashe J, Spiegel P, Zee DS, Leigh RJ. Acquired pendular nystagmus in toluene addiction. Neurology 41, 282–285, 1991.
673. MacAskill MR, Anderson TJ, Jones RD. Suppression of displacement in severely slowed saccades. Vision Res 40, 3405–3413, 2000.
674. MacAskill MR, Anderson TJ, Jones RD. Adaptive modification of saccade amplitude in Parkinson's disease. Brain 125, 1570–1582, 2002.
675. MacAvoy MG, Bruce CJ. Comparison of the smooth pursuit eye tracking disorder of schizophrenics with that of nonhuman primates. Int J Neurosci 80, 117–151, 1995.

676. Maccario M, Seelinger D, Snyder R. Thallotoxicosis with coma and abnormal eye movements. Electroencephalogr Clin Neurophysiol 38, 98–99, 1975.
677. MacDonald JT, Sher PK. Ophthalmoplegia as a sign of metabolic disease in the newborn. Neurology 27, 971–973, 1977.
678. Machado L, Rafal RD. Control of fixation and saccades in humans with chronic lesions of oculomotor cortex. Neuropsychology 18, 115–123, 2004.
679. Mackert A, Flechtner K. Saccadic reaction times in acute and remitted schizophrenics. Eur Arch Psychiatry Neurol Sci 239, 33–38, 1989.
680. Magnusson M, Norrving BO. Cerebellar infarctions and 'vestibular neuritis'. Acta Otolaryngol 503, 64–66, 1993.
681. Magnusson M, Padoan S, Ornhagen H. Evaluation of smooth pursuit and voluntary saccades in nitrous oxide induced narcosis. Aviat Space Environ Med 60, 977–982, 1989.
682. Maher ER, Lees AJ. The clinical features and natural history of the Steele-Richardson-Olszewski syndrome (progressive supranuclear palsy). Neurology 36, 1005–1008, 1986.
683. Maiwald M, von Herbay A, Fredricks DN, et al. Cultivation of Tropheryma whipplei from cerebrospinal fluid. J Infect Dis 188, 801–808, 2003.
684. Malessa S, Gaymard B, Rivaud S, et al. Role of pontine nuclei damage in smooth pursuit impairment of progressive supranuclear palsy: a clinical pathologic study. Neurology 44, 716–721, 1994.
685. Malm G, Lying-Tunnell U. Cerebellar dysfunction related to toluene sniffing. Acta Neurol Scand 62, 188–190, 1980.
686. Manoach DS, Lindgren KA, Barton JJ. Deficient saccadic inhibition in Asperger's disorder and the social-emotional processing disorder. J Neurol Neurosurg Psychiatry 75, 1719–1726, 2005.
687. Manto MU. The wide spectrum of spincerebellar ataxia (SCAs). Cerebellum 4, 2–6, 2005.
688. Marchiori PE, Mies S, Scaff M. Cyclosporine A-induced ocular opsoclonus and reversible leukoencephalopathy after orthotopic liver transplantation: brief report. Clin Neuropharmacol 27, 195–197, 2004.
689. Maria BL, Bozorgmanesh A, Kimmel KN, Theriaque D, Quisling RG. Quantitative assessment of brainstem development in Joubert syndrome and Dandy-Walker syndrome. J Child Neurol 16, 751–758, 2001.
690. Maria BL, Hoang KB, Tusa RJ, et al. "Joubert syndrome" revisited: key ocular motor signs with magnetic resonance imaging correlation. J Child Neurol 12, 423–430, 1997.
691. Marti F, Roig C. Oculomotor abnormalities in motor neuron disease. J Neurol 240, 475–478, 1993.
692. Marti S, Palla A, Straumann D. Gravity dependence of ocular drift in patients with cerebellar downbeat nystagmus. Ann Neurol 52, 712–721, 2002.
693. Martidis A, Yee RD, Azzarelli B, Biller J. Neuro-ophthalmic radiographic and pathologic manifestations of adult-onset Alexander disease. Arch Ophthalmol 117, 265–267, 1999.
694. Martyn CN, Kean D. The one-and-a-half syndrome. Clinical correlations with a pontine lesion demonstrated by nuclear magnetic resonance imaging in a case of multiple sclerosis. Br J Ophthalmol 72, 515–517, 1988.
695. Masai H, Kashii S, Kimura H, Fukuyama H. Neuro-Behcet disease presenting with internuclear ophthal moplegia. Am J Ophthalmol 122, 897–898, 1996.
695a. Maschke M, Oehlert G, Xie TD, et al. Clinical feature profile of spinocerebellar ataxia type 1–8 predicts genetically defined subtypes. Mov Disord 20, 1405–1412, 2005.
696. Masdeu JC, Rosenberg M. Midbrain-diencephalic horizontal gaze paresis. J Clin Neuro-ophthalmol 7, 227–234, 1987.
697. Mason WP, Graus F, Lang B, et al. Small-cell lung cancer paraneoplastic cerebellar degeneration and the Lambert-Eaton myasthenic syndrome. Brain 120, 1279–1300, 1997.
698. Mastaglia FL, Grainger KMR. Internuclear ophthalmoplegia in progressive supranuclear palsy. J Neurol Sci 25, 303–308, 1975.
699. Masucci EF, Kurtzke JF. Downbeat nystagmus secondary to multiple sclerosis. Ann Ophthalmol 20, 347–348, 1988.
700. Matthysse S, Holzman PS, Gusella JF, et al. Linkage of eye movement dysfunction to chromosome 6p in schizophrenia: additional evidence. Am J Med Genet B Neuropsychiatr Genet 128B, 30–36, 2004.
701. Maurer C, Mergner T, Lucking CH, Becker W. Adaptive changes of saccadic eye-head coordination resulting from altered head posture in torticollis spasmodicus. Brain 124, 413–426, 2001.
702. Meador KJ, Loring DW, Lee GP, et al. Hemisphere asymmetry for eye gaze mechanisms. Brain 112, 103–111, 1989.
703. Medina L, Figueredo-Cardenas G, Rothstein JD, Reiner A. Differential abundance of glutamate transporter subtypes in amyotrophic lateral sclerosis (ALS)-vulnerable versus ALS-resistent brain stem motor cell groups. Exp Neurol 142, 287–295, 1996.
704. Mehler MF. The clinical spectrum of ocular bobbing and ocular dipping. J Neurol Neurosurg Psychiatry 51, 725–727, 1988.
705. Mehler MF. The neuro-ophthalmologic spectrum of the rostral basilar artery syndrome. Arch Neurol 45, 966–971, 1988.
706. Meienberg O. Clinical examination of saccadic eye movements in hemianopia. Neurology 33, 1311–1315, 1983.
707. Meienberg O, Burgunder J-M. Saccadic eye movement disorder in cephalic tetanus. Eur Neurol 24, 182–190, 1985.
708. Meienberg O, Büttner-Ennever JA, Kraus-Ruppert R. Unilateral paralysis of conjugate gaze due to lesion of the abducens nucleus. Clinico-pathological case report. Neuro-ophthalmol 2, 47–52, 1981.
709. Meienberg O, Mumenthaler M, Karbowski K. Quadriparesis and nuclear oculomotor palsy with total bilateral ptosis mimicking coma. A mesencephalic "locked-in syndrome"? Arch Neurol 36, 708–710, 1979.
710. Meienberg O, Müri R, Rabineau PA. Clinical and oculographic examinations of saccadic eye movements in the diagnosis of multiple sclerosis. Arch Neurol 43, 438–443, 1986.
711. Meienberg O, Rover J, Kommerell G. Prenuclear paresis of homolateral inferior rectus and contralateral superior oblique eye muscles. Arch Neurol 35, 231–233, 1978.
712. Meienberg O, Zangemeister WH, Rosenberg M, Hoyt WF, Stark L. Saccadic eye movement strate-

gies in patients with homonymous hemianopia. Ann Neurol 9, 537–544, 1981.
713. Merril PT, Paige GD, Abrams RA, Jacoby RG, Clifford DB. Ocular motor abnormalities in human immunodeficiency virus infection. Ann Neurol 30, 130–138, 1991.
713a. Meyniel C, Rivaud-Pechoux S, Damier P, Gaymard B. Saccade impairments in patients with fronto-temporal dementia. J Neurol Neurosurg Psychiatry 76, 1581–1584, 2005.
714. Migliaccio AA, Halmagyi GM, McGarvie LA, Cremer PD. Cerebellar ataxia with bilateral vestibulopathy: description of a syndrome and its characteristic clinical sign. Brain 127, 280–293, 2004.
715. Milder DG, Reinecke RD. Phoria adaptation to prisms. A cerebellar dependent process. Arch Neurol 40, 339–342, 1983.
716. Milea D, Lehericy S, Rivaud-Pechoux S, et al. Antisaccade deficit after anterior cingulate cortex resection. Neuroreport 14, 283–287, 2003.
717. Milea D, Napolitano M, Dechy H, et al. Complete bilateral horizontal gaze paralysis disclosing multiple sclerosis. J Neurol Neurosurg Psychiatry 70, 252–255, 2001.
718. Miller JW, Ferrendelli JA. Eyelid twitching seizures and generalized tonic-clonic convulsions: a syndrome of idiopathic generalized epilepsy. Ann Neurol 27, 334–336, 1990.
719. Miller NR, Biousse V, Hwang T, et al. Isolated acquired unilateral horizontal gaze paresis from a putative lesion of the abducens nucleus. J Neuroophthalmol 22, 204–207, 2002.
720. Minagar A, Schatz NJ, Glaser JS. Case report: one-and-a-half-syndrome and tuberculosis of the pons in a patient with AIDS. AIDS Patient Care STDS 14, 461–464, 2000.
721. Minor LB, Haslwanter T, Straumann D, Zee DS. Hyperventilation-induced nystagmus in patients with vestibular schwannoma. Neurology 53, 2158–2168, 1999.
722. Misbah SA, Aslam A, Costello C. Whipple's disease. Lancet 363, 654–656, 2004.
723. Mitra K, Gangopadhaya PK, Das SK. Parkinsonism plus syndrome—a review. Neurol India 51, 183–188, 2003.
724. Miura K, Optican LM. Membrane channel properties of premotor excitatory burst neurons may underlie saccade slowing after lesions of omnipause neurons. Neural Netw, In Press, 2005.
725. Mizutani T, Aki M, Shiozawa R, et al. Development of ophthalmoplegia in amyotrophic lateral sclerosis during long-term use of respirators. J Neurol Sci 99, 311–319, 1990.
726. Mochizuki A, Eto H, Takasu M, Utsunomiya K, Schoji S. Cheiro-oral syndrome with internuclear ophthalmoplegia and cerebellar ataxia following midbrain infarction. European Neurology 34, 286–287, 1994.
727. Mokri B, Ahlskog E, Fulgham JR, Matsumoto JY. Syndrome resembling PSP after surgical repair of ascending aorta dissection or aneurysm. Neurology 62, 971–973, 2005.
728. Morata TC, Nylén P, Johnson A, Dunn DE. Auditory and vestibular functions after single or combined exposure to toluene: a review. Arch Toxicol 69, 431–443, 1995.
729. Moreira MC, Barbot C, Tachi N, et al. The gene mutated in ataxia-ocular apraxia 1 encodes the new HIT/Zn-finger protein aprataxin. Nat Genet 29, 189–193, 2001.
730. Moreira MC, Klur S, Watanabe M, et al. Senataxin the ortholog of a yeast RNA helicase is mutant in ataxia-ocular apraxia 2. Nat Genet 36, 225–227, 2004.
731. Morris AA, Leonard JV, Brown GK, et al. Deficiency of respiratory chain complex I is a common cause of Leigh disease. Ann Neurol 40, 25–30, 1996.
732. Morrow MJ. Epileptic nystagmus. Neurology 44, 2217, 1994.
733. Morrow MJ. Craniotopic defects of smooth pursuit and saccadic eye movement. Neurology 46, 514–521, 1996.
734. Morrow MJ, Sharpe JA. Torsional nystagmus in the lateral medullary syndrome. Ann Neurol 24, 390–398, 1988.
735. Morrow MJ, Sharpe JA. Retinoptic and directional deficits of smooth pursuit initiation after posterior cerebral hemispheric lesions. Neurology 43, 595–603, 1993.
736. Morrow MJ, Sharpe JA. Deficits of smooth-pursuit eye movement after unilateral frontal lobe lesions. Ann Neurol 37, 443–451, 1995.
737. Morrow MJ, Zinn AB, Tucker T, Leigh RJ. Maculopathy in spinocerebellar ataxia type 7. Neurology 53, 244, 1999.
738. Moschner C, Zangemeister WH, Demer JL. Anticipatory smooth eye movements of high velocity triggered by large target steps. Normal performance and effect of erebellar degeneration. Vision Res 36, 1341–1348, 1996.
739. Moschovakis AK, Gregoriou GG, Ugolini G, et al. Oculomotor areas of the primate frontal lobes: a transneuronal transfer of rabies virus and [14C]-2–deoxyglucose functional imaging study. J Neurosci 24, 5726–5740, 2004.
740. Moschovakis AK, Scudder CA, Highstein SM. A structural basis for Hering's law: Projections to extraocular motoneurons. Science 248, 1118–1119, 1990.
741. Moschovakis AK, Scudder CA, Highstein SM. Structure of the primate oculomotor burst generator. I Medium-lead burst neurons with upward on-directions. J Neurophysiol 65, 203–217, 1991.
742. Moschovakis AK, Scudder CA, Highstein SM, Warren JD. Structure of the primate oculomotor burst generator. II Medium-lead burst neurons with downward on-directions. J Neurophysiol 65, 218–229, 1991.
743. Moser A, Kömpf D, Arolt V, Resch T. Quantitative analysis of eye movements in schizophrenia. Neuro-ophthalmology 10, 73–80, 1990.
744. Moser A, Kompf D, Olschinka J. Eye movement dysfunction in dementia of the Alzheimer type. Dementia 6, 264–268, 1995.
745. Moses HI, Zee DS. Multi-infarct PSP. Neurology 37, 1819, 1987.
746. Mosimann UP, Muri RM, Burn DJ, et al. Saccadic eye movement changes in Parkinson's disease dementia and dementia with Lewy bodies. Brain 128, 1267–1276, 2005.
747. Mossman SS, Bronstein AM, Gresty MA, Kendall B, Rudge P. Convergence nystagmus associated with Arnold-Chiari malformation. Arch Neurol 47, 357–359, 1990.

748. Mueller C, Koch S, Toifl K. Transient bilateral internuclear ophthalmoplegia after minor head trauma. Dev Med Child Neurol 35, 163–166, 1993.
749. Mueller-Jensen A, Neunzig H-P, Emskotter T. Outcome prediction in comatose patients: significance of reflex eye movement analysis. J Neurol Neurosurg Psychiatry 50, 389–392, 1987.
750. Mullally WJ. Carbamazepine-induced ophthalmoplegia. Arch Neurol 39, 64, 1982.
751. Muller C, Wenger S, Fertl L, Auff E. Initiation of visual-guided random saccades and remembered saccades in parkinsonian patients with severe motor-fluctuations. J Neural Transm 7, 101–108, 1994.
752. Muni RH, Wennberg R, Mikulis DJ, Wong AM. Bilateral horizontal gaze palsy in presumed paraneoplastic brainstem encephalitis associated with a benign ovarian teratoma. J Neuroophthalmol 24, 114–118, 2004.
753. Munro NA, Gaymard B, Rivaud S, Majdalani A, Pierrot-Deseilligny C. Upbeat nystagmus in a patient with a small medullary infarct. J Neurol Neurosurg Psychiatry 56, 1126–1128, 1993.
754. Müri RM, Chermann JF, Cohen L, Rivaud S, Pierrot-Deseilligny C. Ocular motor consequences of damage to the abducens nucleus area in humans. J Neuro-ophthalmology 16, 191–195, 1996.
755. Müri RM, Meienberg O. The clinical spectrum of internuclear ophthalmoplegia in multiple sclerosis. Arch Neurol 42, 851–855, 1985.
756. Muthukumar N, Veerarajkumar N, Madeswaran K Bilateral internuclear ophthalmoplegia following mild head injury. Childs Nerv Syst 17, 366–369, 2001.
757. Mutschler V, Eber AM, Rumbach L. et al. Internuclear ophthalmoplegia in 14 patients. Clinical and topographic correlation using magnetic resonance imaging. Neuro-ophthalmology 10, 319–325, 1990.
758. Mwanza JC, Nyamabo LK, Tylleskar T, Plant GT. Neuro-ophthalmological disorders in HIV infected subjects with neurological manifestations. Br J Ophthalmol 88, 1455–1459, 2004.
759. Nakada T, Kwee IL, Lee H. Sustained upgaze in coma. J Clin Neuro-ophthalmol 1, 185–189, 1981.
760. Nakamagoe K, Iwamoto Y, Yoshida K. Evidence for brainstem structures participating in oculomotor integration. Science 288, 857–859, 2000.
761. Nakamura T, Bronstein AM, Lueck CJ, Marsden CD, Rudge P. Vestibular, cervical and visual remembered saccades in Parkinson's disease. Brain 117, 1423–1432, 1994.
762. Nakashima H, Terada S, Ishizu H, et al. An autopsied case of dementia with Lewy bodies with supranuclear gaze palsy. Neurol Res 25, 533–537, 2003.
763. Narita AS, Shawkat FS, Lask B, Taylor DS, Harris CM. Eye movement abnormalities in a case of Tourette syndrome. Dev Med Child Neurol 39, 270–273, 1997.
764. Nath U, Ben-Shlomo Y, Thomson R, Lees A, Burn D. Clinical features and natural history of progressive supranuclear palsy. A clinical cohort study. Neurology 60, 910–916, 2003.
765. Nathanson M, Bergman PS, Anderson PJ. Significance of oculocephalic and caloric responses in the unconscious patient. Neurology 7, 829–832, 1957.
766. Nawrot M, Rizzo M. Motion perception deficits from midline cerebellar lesions in human. Vision Res 35, 723–731, 1995.
767. Nayyar M, Strobos RJ, Singh BM, Brown-Wagner M, Pucillo A. Caloric-induced nystagmus with isoelectric electroencephalogram. Ann Neurol 21, 98–100, 1987.
768. Nedzelski JM. Cerebellopontine angle tumors: bilateral flocculus compression as a cause of associated oculomotor abnormalities. Laryngoscope 93, 1251–1260, 1983.
769. Neggers SF, Raemaekers MA, Lampmann EE, Postma A, Ramsey NF. Cortical and subcortical contributions to saccade latency in the human brain. Eur J Neurosci 21, 2853–2863, 2005.
770. Nelson KR, Brenner RP, Carlow TJ. Divergent-convergent eye movements and transient eyelid opening associated with an EEG burst-suppression pattern. J Clin Neuro-ophthalmol 6, 43–46, 1986.
771. Nemeth AH, Bochukova E, Dunne E, et al. Autosomal recessive cerebellar ataxia with oculomotor apraxia (ataxia-telangiectasia-like syndrome) is linked to chromosome 9q34. Am J Hum Genet 67, 1320–1326, 2000.
772. Newman GC. Treatment of progressive supranuclear palsy with tricyclic antidepressants. Neurology 35, 1189–1193, 1985.
773. Newton HB, Miner ME. "One-and-a-half" syndrome after resection of a midline cerebellar astroctyoma: case report and discussion of the literature. Neurosurgery 29, 768–772, 1991.
774. Nezu A. Neurophysiological study in Pelizaeus-Merzbacher diease. Brain Dev 17, 175–181, 1995.
775. Nguyen N, Rimmer S, Katz B. Slowed saccades in the acquired immunodeficiency syndrome. Am J Ophthalmol 107, 356–360, 1989.
776. Nielsen JE, Sorensen S, Hasholt L, Norremolle A. Dentatorubral-pallidoluysian atrophy. Clinical features of a five-generation Danish family. Mov Disord 11, 533–541, 1996.
777. Nielsen JM. Tornado epilepsy simulating Ménière's syndrome. Neurology 9, 794–796, 1959.
778. Nieman DH, Bour LJ, Linszen DH, et al. Neuropsychological and clinical correlates of antisaccade task performance in schizophrenia. Neurology 54, 866–871, 2000.
779. Nishida T, Tychsen L, Corbett JJ. Resolution of saccadic palsy after treatment of brain-stem metastasis. Arch Neurol 43, 1196–1197, 1986.
780. Nishie M, Yoshida Y, Hirata Y, Matsunaga M. Generation of symptomatic palatal tremor is not correlated with inferior olivary hypertrophy. Brain 125, 1348–1357, 2002.
781. Nishizaki T, Tamaki N, Nishida Y, Matsumoto S. Bilateral internuclear ophthalmoplegia due to hydrocephalus. Neurosurgery 17, 822–825, 1985.
782. Noda S, Ide K, Umezaki H, Itoh H, Yamamoto K. Repetitive divergence. Ann Neurol 21, 109–110, 1987.
783. Noda S, Umezaki H. Carbamazepine-induced ophthalmoplegia. Neurology 32, 1320, 1982.
784. Nozaki S, Mukuno K, Ishikawa S. Internuclear ophthalmoplegia associated with ipsilateral downbeat and contralateral incyclorotatory nystagmus. Ophthalmologica 187, 210–216, 1983.
785. Nuti D, Passero S, Di Girolamo S. Bilateral vestibular loss in vertebrobasilar dolichoectasia. J Vestib Res 6, 85–91, 1996.
786. O'Sullivan JD, Maruff P, Tyler P, et al. Unilateral pal-

lidotomy for Parkinson's disease disrupts ocular fixation. J Clin Neurosci 10, 181–185, 2003.
787. Oas J, Baloh RW. Vertigo and the anterior inferior cerebellar artery syndrome. Neurology 42, 2274–2279, 1992.
788. Oba H, Yagishita A, Terada H, et al. New and reliable MRI diagnosis for progressive supranuclear palsy. Neurology 64, 2050–2055, 2005.
789. Ochs AL, Stark L, Hoyt WF, D'Amico D. Opposed adducting saccades in convergence-retraction nystagmus. A patient with sylvian aqueduct syndrome. Brain 102, 479–508, 1979.
790. Ochs R, Gloor P, Quesney F, Ives J, Olivier A. Does head-turning during a seizure have lateralizing or localizing significance? Neurology 34, 884–890, 1984.
791. Ödkvist LM, Bergenius J, Moller C. When and how to use gentamicin in the treatment of Meniere's disease. Acta Otolaryhgol (Stockh) 526, 54–57, 1997.
792. Ödkvist LM, Möller C, Thuomas K. Otoneurologic disturbances caused by solvent pollution. Otolaryngol Head Neck Surg 106, 687–692, 1992.
793. Ogren MP, Mateer CA, Wyler AR. Alterations in visually related eye movements following left pulvinar damage in man. Neuropsychologia 22, 187–196, 1984.
794. Oguro H, Okada K, Suyama N, et al. Decline of vertical gaze and convergence with aging. Gerontology 50, 177–181, 2004.
795. Oh AK, Jacobson KM, Jen JC, Baloh RW. Slowing of voluntary and involuntary saccades: an early sign in spinocerebellar ataxia type 7. Ann Neurol 49, 801–804, 2001.
796. Ohtsuka K, Sawa M, Matsuda S, Uno A, Takeda M. Non-visual eye position control in a patient with ocular lateropulsion. Ophthalmologica 197, 85–89, 1988.
797. Okamoto K, Hirai S, Amari M, et al. Oculomotor nuclear pathology in amyotrophic lateral sclerosis. Acta Neuropathol 85, 458–462, 1993.
798. Okuda B, Yamasaki M, Hashimoto S, Maya K, Imai T. Spinocerebellar degeneration with slow eye movements and abducens nerve palsy. J Clin Neuro-ophthalmol 11, 118–121, 1991.
799. Olincy A, Johnson LL, Ross RG. Differential effects of cigarette smoking on performance of a smooth pursuit and a saccadic eye movement task in schizophrenia. Psychiatry Res 117, 223–236, 2003.
800. Oliveri RL, Bono F, Quattrone A. Pontine lesion of the abducens fasciculus producing so-called posterior internuclear ophthalmoplegia. Eur Neurol 37, 67–69, 1997.
801. Oliverio PJ, Restrepo L, Mitchell SA, Tornatore CS, Frankel SR. Reversible tacrolimus-induced neurotoxicity isolated to the brain stem. AJNR Am J Neuroradiol 21, 1251–1254, 2000.
802. Olson CR, Musil SY, Goldberg ME. Single neurons in posterior cingulate cortex of behaving macaque: eye movement signals. J Neurophysiol 76, 3285–3300, 1996.
803. Onofrj M, Iacono D, Luciano AL, Armellino K, Thomas A. Clinically evidenced unilateral dissociation of saccades and pursuit eye movements. J Neurol Neurosurg Psychiatry 75, 1048–1050, 2004.
804. Oommen KJ, Smith MS, Labadie EL. Pontine hemorrhage causing Fisher one-and-a-half syndrome with facial paralysis. J Clin Neuroophthalmol 2, 129–132, 1982.
805. Optican LM, Robinson DA. Cerebellar-dependent adaptive control of primate saccadic system. J Neurophysiol 44, 1058–1076, 1980.
806. Osenbach RK, Blumenkopf B, McComb B, Huggins MJ. Ocular bobbing with ruptured giant distal posterior inferior cerebellar artery aneurysm. Surg Neurol 25, 149–152, 1986.
807. Osher RH, Corbett JJ, Schatz NJ, Savino PJ, Orr LS. Neuro-ophthalmological complications of enlargement of the third ventricle. Br J Ophthalmol 62, 536–542, 1978.
808. Ouahchi K, Arita M, Kayden H, et al. Ataxia with isolated vitamin E deficiency is caused by mutations in the alpha-tocopherol transfer protein. Nature Genetics 9, 141–145, 1995.
809. Ouvrier R, Billson F. Paroxysmal tonic upgaze of childhood—a review. Brain Dev 27, 185–188, 2005.
810. Ouvrier RA, Billson F. Benign paroxysmal tonic upgaze of childhood. J Child Neurol 3, 177–180, 1988.
811. Oyanagi K, Chen KM, Craig UK, Yamazaki M, Perl DP. Parkinsonism dementia and vertical gaze palsy in a Guamanian with atypical neuroglial degeneration. Acta Neuropathol (Berl) 99, 73–80, 2000.
812. Oyanagi K, Takeda S, Takahashi H, Ohama E, Ikuta F A quantitative investigation of the substantia nigra in Huntington's disease. Ann Neurol 26, 13–19, 1989.
813. Padoan S, Korttila K, Magnusson M, Pyykkö I, Schalén L. Reduction of gain and time constant of vestibulo-ocular reflex in man induced by diazepam and thiopental. J Vestib Res 1, 97–104, 1990.
814. Padoan S, Korttila K, Magnusson M, Pyykkö, I, Schalén L. Effect of intravenous diazepam and thiopental on voluntary saccades and pursuit eye movements. Acta Otolaryngol (Stockh) 112, 579–588, 1992.
815. Page NGR, Leans JS, Sanders MD. Vertical supranuclear gaze palsy with secondary syphilis. J Neurol Neurosurg Psychiatry 45, 86–88, 1982.
816. Pambakian AL, Mannan SK, Hodgson TL, Kennard C. Saccadic visual search training: a treatment for patients with homonymous hemianopia. J Neurol Neurosurg Psychiatry 75, 1443–1448, 2004.
817. Park S, Holzman PS. Schizophrenics show spatial working memory deficits. Arch Gen Psychiatry 49, 975–982, 1992.
818. Partsalis AM, Highstein SM, Moschovakis AK. Lesions of the posterior commissure disable the vertical neural integrator of the primate oculomotor system. J Neurophysiol 71, 2582–2585, 1994.
819. Pasik P, Pasik T, Bender MB. The pretectal syndrome in monkeys. I. Disturbances of gaze and body posture. Brain 92, 521–534, 1969.
820. Pasik T, Pasik P, Bender MB. The superior colliculi and eye movements: An experimental study in the monkey. Arch Neurol 15, -420, 1966.
821. Pasik T, Pasik P, Bender MB. The pretectal syndrome in monkeys. II Spontaneous and induced nystagmus and lightning" eye movements. Brain 92, 871–884, 1969.
822. Patterson MC, Horowitz M, Abel RB. Isolated horizontal supranuclear gaze palsy as a marker of severe systemic involvement in Gaucher's disease. Neurology 43, 1993–1997, 1993.

823. Paulson GW. Overdose of Lioresal. Neurology 26, 1105–1106, 1976.
824. Paviour DC, Lees AJ, Josephs KA, et al. Frontotemporal lobar degeneration with ubiquitin-only-immunoreactive neuronal changes: broadening the clinical picture to include progressive supranuclear palsy. Brain 127, 2441–2451, 2004.
825. Paviour DC, Schott JM, Stevens JM, et al. Pathological substrate for regional distribution of increased atrophy rates in progressive supranuclear palsy. J Neurol Neurosurg Psychiatry 75, 1772–1775, 2004.
826. Pedersen RA, Troost BT, Abel LA, Zorub D. Intermittent downbeat nystagmus and oscillopsia reversed by suboccipital craniectomy. Neurology 30, 1239–1242, 1980.
827. Percheron G. Les artères du thalamus humain. I I Artères et territoires thalamique paramedians de l'artère basilair communicante. Rev Neurol (Paris) 132, 309–324, 1976.
828. Pessin MS, Adelman LS, Prager RJ, Lathi ES, Lange DJ. "Wrong-way eyes" in supratentorial hemorrhage. Ann Neurol 9, 79–81, 1981.
829. Peterson K, Rosenblum MK, Kotanides H, Posner JB. Paraneoplastic cerebellar degeneration. I A clinical analysis of 55 anti-Yo antibody-positive patients. Neurology 42, 1931–1937, 1995.
830. Petit L, Orssaud C, Tzourio N, et al. PET study of voluntary saccadic eye movements in humans: basal ganglia-thalamocortical system and cingulate cortex involvement. J Neurophysiol 69, 1009–1017, 1993.
831. Pfister HW, Einhaupl KM, Büttner U, et al. Dissociated nystagmus as a common sign of ocular motor disorders in HIV-infected patients. Eur Neurol 29, 277–280, 1989.
832. Pieh C, Gottlob I. Arnold-Chiari malformation and nystagmus of skew. J Neurol Neurosurg Psychiatry 69, 124–126, 2000.
833. Pierrot-Deseilligny C. Saccades and smooth-pursuit impairment after cerebral hemispheric lesions. Eur Neurol 34, 121–134, 1994.
834. Pierrot-Deseilligny C, Amarenco P, Roullet E, Marteau R. Vermal infarct with pursuit eye movement disorders. J Neurol Neurosurg Psychiatry 53, 519–521, 1990.
835. Pierrot-Deseilligny CH, Chain F, Gray F, et al. Parinaud's syndrome. Electro-oculographic and anatomical analyses of six vascular cases with deductions about vertical gaze organization in the premotor structures. Brain 105, 667–696, 1982.
836. Pierrot-Deseilligny C, Gautier JC, Loron P. Acquired ocular motor apraxia due to bilateral fronto-parietal infarcts. Ann Neurol 23, 199–202, 1988.
837. Pierrot-Deseilligny C, Gaymard B, Müri R, Rivaud S. Cerebral ocular motor signs. J Neurol 244, 65–70, 1997.
838. Pierrot-Deseilligny C, Goasguen J, Chain F, Lapresle J. Pontine metastasis with dissociated bilateral horizontal gaze paralysis. J Neurol Neurosurg Psychiatry 47, 159–164, 1984.
839. Pierrot-Deseilligny C, Gray F, Brunet P. Infarcts of both inferior parietal lobules with impairment of visually guided eye movements, peripheral visual inattention and optic ataxia. Brain 109, 81–97, 1986.
840. Pierrot-Deseilligny C, Milea D. Vertical nystagmus: vlinical facts and hypotheses. Brain 128, 1237–1246, 2005.
841. Pierrot-Deseilligny C, Milea D, Müri RM. Eye movement control by the cerebral cortex. Curr Opin Neurol 17, 17–25, 2004.
842. Pierrot-Deseilligny C, Müri RM, Ploner CJ, et al. Decisional role of the dorsolateral prefrontal cortex in ocular motor behaviour. Brain 126, 1460–1473, 2003.
843. Pierrot-Deseilligny C, Müri RM, Rivaud-Pechoux S, Gaymard B, Ploner CJ. Cortical control of spatial memory in humans: the visuooculomotor model. Ann Neurol 52, 10–19, 2002.
844. Pierrot-Deseilligny C, Rivaud S, Gaymard B, Agid Y. Cortical control of reflexive visually-guided saccades. Brain 114, 1473–1485, 1991.
845. Pierrot-Deseilligny C, Rivaud S, Gaymard B, Müri RM, Vermersch AI. Cortical control of saccades. Ann Neurol 37, 557–567, 1995.
846. Pierrot-Deseilligny C, Rivaud S, Penet C, Rigolet MH. Latencies of visually guided saccades in unilateral hemispheric cerebral lesions. Ann Neurol 21, 138–148, 1987.
847. Pierrot-Deseilligny C, Rivaud S, Pillon B, Fournier E, Agid Y. Lateral visually-guided saccades in progressive supranuclear palsy. Brain 112, 471–487, 1989.
848. Pierrot-Deseilligny C, Rosa A, Masmoudi K, Rivaud S, Gaymard B. Saccade deficits after a unilateral lesion affecting the superior colliculus. J Neurol Neurosurg Psychiatry 54, 1106–1109, 1991.
849. Pillay N, Gilbert JJ, Ebers GC, Brown JD. Internuclear ophthalmoplegia and "optic neuritis": paraneoplastic effects of bronchial carcinoma. Neurology 34, 788–791, 1984.
850. Pirozzolo FJ, Hansch EC. Oculomotor reaction time in dementia reflects degree of cerebral disturbance. Science 214, 349–351, 1981.
851. Ploner CJ, Gaymard BM, Rivaud-Pechoux S, et al. Lesions affecting the parahippocampal cortex yield spatial memory deficits in humans. Cereb Cortex 10, 1211–1216, 2000.
852. Ploner CJ, Gaymard BM, Rivaud-Pechoux S, Pierrot-Deseilligny C. The prefrontal substrate of reflexive saccade inhibition in humans. Biol Psychiatr 57, 1159–1165, 2005.
853. Ploner C J, Rivaud-Pechoux S, Gaymard BM, Agid Y, Pierrot-Deseilligny C. Errors of memory-guided saccades in humans with lesions of the frontal eye field and the dorsolateral prefrontal cortex. J Neurophysiol 82, 1086–1090, 1999.
854. Plum F, Posner JB. The Diagnosis of Stupor and Coma. FA Davis, Philadelphia, 1981.
855. Poisson M, van Effentere R, Mashaly R. Pituitary apoplexy with retraction nystagmus. Ann Neurol 7, 286, 1980.
856. Posner JB. Neurological complications of cancer. FA Davis, Philadelphia, 1995.
857. Posner M, Walker J, Friedrich F, Rafal R. Effects of parietal injury on covert orienting of attention. J Neurosci 4, 1863–1874, 1984.
858. Press GA, Hesselink JR. MR imaging of cerebellopontine angle and internal auditory canal lesions at 1.5 T Am J Neuroradiol 9, 241–251, 1988.
859. Proudlock FA, Gottlob I, Constantinescu CS. Oscillopsia without nystagmus caused by head titu-

bation in a patient with multiple sclerosis. J Neuro-ophthalmol 22, 88–91, 2002.
860. Prueter C, Schiefer J, Norra C, Podoll K, Sass H. Ping-pong gaze in combined intoxication with tranylcypromine thioridazine and clomipramine. Neuropsychiatry Neuropsychol Behav Neurol 14, 246–247, 2001.
861. Pujol J, Roig C, Capdevila A, et al. Motion of the cerebellar tonsils in Chiari type I malformation studies by cine phase-contrast MRI. Neurology 45, 1746–1753, 1995.
862. Pullicino P, Lincoff N, Truax BT. Abnormal vergence with upper brainstem infarcts: pseudoabducens palsy. Neurology 55, 352–358, 2000.
863. Pullicino PM, Wong EH. Tonic downward and inward ocular deviation ipsilateral to pontine tegmental hemorrhage. Cerebrovasc Dis 10, 327–329, 2000.
864. Pulst S-M, Lombroso CT. External ophthalmoplegia alpha and spindle coma in imipramine overdose: case report and review of the literature. Ann Neurol 14, 587–590, 1983.
865. Quinn N. The "round the houses" sign in progressive supranuclear palsy. Ann Neurol 40, 951, 2003.
866. Quinzii CM, Kattah AG, Naini A, et al. Coenzyme Q deficiency and cerebellar ataxia associated with an aprataxin mutation. Neurology 64, 539–541, 2005.
867. Rabiah PK, Bateman JB, Demer JL, Perlman S. Ophthalmologic findings in patients with cerebellar ataxia. Am J Ophthalmol 123, 108–117, 1997.
868. Racette BA, Gokden MS, Tychsen LS, Perlmutter JS. Convergence insufficiency in idiopathic Parkinson's disease responsive to levodopa. Strabismus 7, 169–174, 1999.
869. Radtke A, Bronstein AM, Gresty MA, et al. Paroxysmal alternating skew deviation and nystagmus after partial destruction of the uvula. J Neurol Neurosurg Psychiatry 70, 790–793, 2001.
870. Rafal R, McGrath M, Machado L, Hindle J. Effects of lesions of the human posterior thalamus on ocular fixation during voluntary and visually triggered saccades. J Neurol Neurosurg Psychiatry 75, 1602–1606, 2004.
871. Rajput AJ, McHattie JD. Ophthalmoplegia and leg myorhythmia in Whipple's disease. Mov Disord 12, 111–114, 1997.
872. Ramat S, Das VE, Somers JT, Leigh RJ. Tests of two hypotheses to account for different-sized saccades during disjunctive gaze shifts. Exp Brain Res 129, 500–510, 1999.
873. Ramat S, Leigh RJ, Zee DS, Optican LM. Ocular oscillations generated by coupling of brainstem excitatory and inhibitory saccadic burst neurons. Exp Brain Res 160, 89–106, 2005.
874. Rambold H, Helmchen C. Spontaneous nystagmus in dorsolateral medullary infarction indicates vestibular semicircular canal imbalance. J Neurol Neurosurg Psychiatry 76, 88–94, 2005.
875. Rambold H, Kompf D, Helmchen C. Convergence retraction nystagmus: a disorder of vergence? Ann Neurol 50, 677–681, 2001.
876. Rambold H, Neumann G, Helmchen C. Vergence deficits in pontine lesions. Neurology 62, 1850–1853, 2004.
877. Rambold H, Sander T, Neumann G, Helmchen C. Palsy of "fast" and "slow" vergence by pontine lesions. Neurology 64, 338–340, 2005.
878. Ramchandran RS, Manoach DS, Cherkasova MV, et al. The relationship of saccadic peak velocity to latency: evidence for a new prosaccadic abnormality in schizophrenia. Exp Brain Res 159, 99–107, 2004.
879. Ramos AE, Shytle RD, Silver AA, Sanberg PR. Ziprasidone-induced oculogyric crisis. J Am Acad Child Adolesc Psychiatry 42, 1013–1014, 2003.
880. Ranalli PJ, Sharpe JA. Contrapulsion of saccades and ipsilateral ataxia: a unilateral disorder of the rostral cerebellum. Ann Neurol 20, 311–316, 1986.
881. Ranalli PJ, Sharpe JA. Upbeat nystagmus and the ventral tegmental pathway of the upward vestibulo-ocular reflex. Neurology 38, 1329–1330, 1988.
882. Ranalli PJ, Sharpe JA. Vertical vestibulo-ocular reflex smooth pursuit and eye-head tracking dysfunction in internuclear ophthalmoplegia. Brain 111, 1299–1317, 1988.
883. Ranalli PJ, Sharpe JA, Fletcher WA. Palsy of upward and downward saccadic pursuit and vestibular movements with a unilateral midbrain lesion: pathophysiologic correlations. Neurology 38, 114–122, 1988.
884. Raps EC, Galetta SL, King JT Jr., Yachnis AT, Flamm ES. Isolated one-and-a-half syndrome with pontine cavernous angioma: successful surgical removal. J Clin Neuro-ophthalmol 10, 287–290, 1990.
885. Rascol O, Clanet M, Montastruc JL, et al. Abnormal ocular movements in Parkinson's disease. Evidence for involvement of dopaminergic systems. Brain 112, 1193–1214, 1989.
886. Rascol O, Hain TC, Brefel C, et al. Antivertigo medications and drug-induced vertigo: a pharmacological review. Drugs 50, 777–791, 1995.
887. Rascol O, Sabatini U, Fabre N, et al. Abnormal vestibuloocular reflex cancellation in multiple system atrophy and progressive supranuclear palsy but not in Parkinson's disease. Mov Disord 10, 163–170, 1995.
888. Rascol O, Sabatini U, Simonetta-Moreau M, et al. Square wave jerks in parkinsonian syndromes. J Neurol Neurosurg Psychiatry 54, 599–602, 1991.
889. Rashbass C. Barbiturate nystagmus and mechanics of visual fixation. Nature 183, 897–898, 1959.
890. Raymond JL, Lisberger SG, Mauk MD. The cerebellum: a neuronal learning machine? Science 272, 1126–1131, 1996.
891. Reichert WH, Doolittle J, McDowell FH. Vestibular dysfunction in Parkinson's disease. Neurology 32, 1133–1138, 1982.
892. Reilly JL, Harris MS, Keshavan MS, Sweeney JA. Abnormalities in visually guided saccades suggest corticofugal dysregulation in never-treated schizophrenia. Biol Psychiatry 57, 145–154, 2005.
893. Remler BF, Leigh RJ, Osorio I, Tomsak RL. The characteristics and mechanisms of visual disturbance associated with anticonvulsant therapy. Neurology 40, 791–796, 1990.
894. Rennie IG, Wright JGC, Wilkinson JL. Iatrogenic internuclear ophthalmoplegia. J Neurol Neurosurg Psychiatry 49, 842, 1986.
895. Repka MX, Claro MC, Loupe DN, Reich S. Ocular motility in Parkinson's disease. Pediatr Ophthalmol Strabismus 33, 144–147, 1996.

896. Reulen JPH, Sander EACM, Jogenhuis LAH. Eye movement abnormalities in multiple sclerosis and optic neuritis. Brain 106, 121–140, 1983.
897. Revesz T, Sangha H, Daniel SE. The nucleus raphe interpositus in the Steele-Richardson-Olszewski syndrome (progressive supranuclear palsy). Brain 119, 1137–1143, 1996.
898. Ridley A, Kennard C, Scholtz CL, et al. Omnipause neurons in two cases of opsoclonus associated with oat cell carcinoma of the lung. Brain 110, 1699–1709, 1987.
899. Riker WK, Downes H, Olsen GD, Smith B. Conjugate lateral gaze nystagmus and free phenytoin concentrations in plasma: lack of correlation. Epilepsia 19, 93–98, 1978.
900. Riley DE, Fogt N, Leigh RJ. The syndrome of 'pure akinesia' and its relationship to progressive supranuclear palsy. Neurology 44, 1025–1029, 1994.
901. Riley DE, Lang AE, Lewis A, et al. Cortical-basal ganglionic degeneration. Neurology 40, 1203–1212, 1990.
902. Rinne JO, Lee MS, Thompson PD, Marsden CD. Corticobasal degeneration: a clinical study of 36 cases. Brain 117, 1183–1196, 1994.
903. Riordan-Eva P, Faldon M, Büttner-Ennever JA, et al. Abnormalities of torsional fast eye movements in unilateral rostral midbrain disease. Neurology 47, 201–207, 1996.
904. Rismondo V, Borchert M. Position-dependent Parinaud's syndrome. Am J Ophthalmol 114, 107–108, 1992.
905. Rivaud S, Müri RM, Gaymard B, Vermersch AI, Pierrot-Deseilligny C. Eye movement disorders after frontal eye field lesions in humans. Exp Brain Res 102, 110–120, 1994.
906. Rivaud-Pechoux S, Durr A, Gaymard B, et al. Eye movement abnormalities correlate with genotype in autosomal dominant cerebellar ataxia type 1. Ann Neurol 43, 297–302, 1998.
907. Rivaud-Pechoux S, Vermersch AI, Gaymard B, et al. Improvement of memory guided saccades in parkinsonian patients by high frequency subthalamic nucleus stimulation. J Neurol Neurosurg Psychiatry 68, 381–384, 2000.
908. Rivaud-Pechoux S, Vidailhet M, Gallouedec G, et al. Longitudinal ocular motor study in corticobasal degeneration and progressive supranuclear palsy. Neurology 54, 1029–1032, 2000.
909. Rizzo M. 'Balint's syndrome' and associated visuospatial disorders. Baillière's Clinical Neurology 2, 415–437, 1993.
910. Rizzo M, Corbett J. Bilateral internuclear ophthalmoplegia reversed by naloxone. Arch Neurol 40, 242–243, 1983.
911. Rizzo M, Hurtig R. The effect of bilateral visual cortex lesions on the development of eye movements and perception. Neurology 39, 406–413, 1989.
912. Robinson FR, Straube A, Fuchs AF. Role of the caudal fastigial nucleus in saccade generation. II Effects of muscimol inactivation. J Neurophysiol 70, 1741–1758, 1993.
913. Robinson FR, Straube A, Fuchs AF. Participation of the caudal fastigial nucleus in smooth-pursuit eye movements. II. Effects of muscimol inactivation. J Neurophysiol 78, 848–859, 1994.
914. Roos Y, de Jongh FE, Crevits L. The effect of smoking on ocular saccadic latency time. Neuroophthalmol 13, 75–79, 1993.
915. Roos Y, de Jongh FE, Crevits L. The effects of smoking on anti-saccades-a study in regular smokers. Neuroophthalmol 15, 3–8, 1995.
916. Ropper AH. Atypical ocular bobbing. Ann Neurol 10, 400, 1981.
917. Ropper AH. Ocular dipping in anoxic coma. Arch Neurol 38, 297–299, 1981.
918. Ropper AH, Miller DC. Acute traumatic midbrain hemorrhage. Ann Neurol 18, 80–86, 1985.
919. Rosa A, Masmoudi K, Mizon JP. Typical and atypical ocular bobbing. Pathology through five case reports. Neuroophthalmol 7, 285–290, 1987.
920. Rosenbaum DA, Siegel M, Rowan AJ. Contraversive seizures in occipital epilepsy: Case report and review of the literature. Neurology 36, 281–284, 1986.
921. Rosenberg DR, Averbach DH, O'Hearn KM, et al. Oculomotor response inhibition abnormalities in pediatric obsessive-compulsive disorder. Arch Gen Psychiatry 54, 831–838, 1997.
922. Rosenberg M, Sharpe J, Hoyt WF. Absent vestibulo-ocular reflexes and supratentorial lesions. J Neurol Neurosurg Psychiatry 38, 6–10, 1975.
923. Rosenberg ML. The eyes in hysterical states of unconsciousness. J Clin Neuro-ophthalmol 2, 259–260, 1982.
924. Rosenberg ML. Spontaneous vertical eye movements in coma. Ann Neurol 20, 635–637, 1986.
925. Rosenberg ML, Calvert PC. Ocular bobbing in association with other signs of midbrain dysfunction. Arch Neurol 43, 314–315, 1986.
926. Ross DE, Thaker GK, Holcomb HH, et al. Abnormal smooth pursuit eye movements in schizophrenic patients are associated with cerebral glucose metabolism in oculomotor regions. Psychiatry Research 58, 53–67, 1995.
927. Ross RG, Olincy A, Mikulich SK, et al. Admixture analysis of smooth pursuit eye movements in probands with schizophrenia and their relatives suggests gain and leading saccades are potential endophenotypes. Psychophysiology 39, 809–819, 2002.
928. Rothenberg SJ, Selkoe D. Specific oculomotor deficit after diazepam. I Saccadic eye movements. Psychopharmacology 74, 232–236, 1981.
929. Rothenberg SJ, Selkoe D. Specific oculomotor deficit after diazepam. II Smooth pursuit eye movements. Psychopharmacology 74, 237–240, 1981.
930. Rothenberg SJ, Shottenfeld S, Gross K, Selkoe D. Specific oculomotor deficit after acute methadone. I Saccadic eye movements. Psychopharmacology 67, 221–227, 1980.
931. Rothenberg SJ, Shottenfeld S, Selkoe D, Gross K. Specific oculomotor deficit after acute methadone. II Smooth pursuit eye movements. Psychopharmacology 67, 229–234, 1980.
932. Rothlind JC, Brandt J, Zee D, Codori AM, Folstein S. Verbal memory and oculomotor control are unimpaired in asymptomatic adults with the genetic marker for Huntington's disease. Arch Neurol 50, 799–802, 1993.
933. Rottach KG, Riley DE, DiScenna AO, Zivotofsky

AZ, Leigh RJ. Dynamic properties of horizontal and vertical eye movements in parkinsonian syndromes. Ann. Neurol 39, 368–377, 1996.
934. Röttach KG, von Maydell RD, Das VE, et al. Evidence for independent feedback control of horizontal and vertical saccades from Niemann-Pick type C disease. Vision Res 37, 3627–3638, 1997.
935. Rüb U, Brunt ER, de Vos RA, et al. Degeneration of the central vestibular system in spinocerebellar ataxia type 3 (SCA3) patients and its possible clinical significance. Neuropathol Appl Neurobiol 30, 402–414, 2004.
936. Rüb U, Brunt ER, Gierga K, et al. The nucleus raphe interpositus in spinocerebellar ataxia type 3 (Machado-Joseph disease). J Chemical Neuroanatomy 12, 115–127, 2003.
937. Rüb U, Burk K, Schols L, et al. Damage to the reticulotegmental nucleus of the pons in spinocerebellar ataxia type 1, 2, and 3. Neurology 63, 1258–1263, 2004.
938. Rüb U, Del TK, Schultz C, Buttner-Ennever JA, Braak H. The premotor region essential for rapid vertical eye movements shows early involvement in Alzheimer's disease-related cytoskeletal pathology. Vision Res 41, 2149–2156, 2001.
939. Rüb U, Gierga K, Brunt ER, et al. Spinocerebellar ataxias types 2 and 3: degeneration of the precerebellar nuclei isolates the three phylogenetically defined regions of the cerebellum. J Neural Transm 112, 1523–1545, 2005
940. Rubin AJ, King WM, Reinbold KA, Shoulson I. Quantitative longitudinal assessment of saccades in Huntington's disease. J Clin Neuro-opthalmol 13, 59–66, 1993.
941. Rubinstein RL, Norman DM, Schindler RA, Kaseff L. Cerebellar infarction—a presentation of vertigo. Laryngoscope 90, 505–514, 1980.
942. Rucker JC, Jen J, Stahl JS, et al. Internuclear ophthalmoparesis in episodic ataxia type 2. Ann N Y Acad Sci 1039, 571–574, 2005.
943. Rucker JC, Shapiro BE, Han YH, et al. Neuro-ophthalmology of late-onset Tay-Sachs disease (LOTS). Neurology 63, 1918–1926, 2004.
944. Rudick R, Satran R, Eskin TA. Ocular bobbing in encephalitis. J Neurol Neurosurg Psychiatry 44, 441–443, 1981.
945. Ruigrok TJ, de Zeeuw CI, Voogd J. Hypertrophy of inferior olivary neurons: a degenerative regenerative or plasticity phenomenon. Eur J Morphol 28, 224–239, 1990.
946. Russo PA, Flynn MF, Veith J. Congenital ocular motor apraxia with torsional oscillations: a case report. Optom Vision Sci 72, 925–930, 1995.
947. Rybakowski JK, Borkowska A, Czerski PM, Dmitrzak-Weglarz M, Hauser J. The study of cytosolic phospholipase A2 gene polymorphism in schizophrenia using eye movement disturbances as an endophenotypic marker. Neuropsychobiology 47, 115–119, 2003.
948. Sacco RL, Freddo L, Bello JA, et al. Wallenberg's lateral medullary syndrome. Clinical-magnetic resonance imaging correlations. Arch Neurol 50, 609–614, 1993.
949. Sachdev P. Tardive and chronically recurrent oculogyric crises. Mov Disord 8, 93–97, 1993.
950. Safran AB, Berney J. Synchronism of reverse ocular bobbing and blinking. Am J Ophthalmol 95, 401–402, 1983.
951. Salman MS, Sharpe JA, Eizenman M, et al. Saccades in children with spina bifida and Chiari type II malformation. Neurology 64, 2098–2101, 2005.
952. Sample JR, Howard FM Jr., Okazaki H. Syringomesencephalia. Report of a case. Arch Neurol 40, 757–759, 1983.
953. Samuel M, Torun N, Tuite P J, Sharpe JA, Lang AE. Progressive ataxia and palatal tremor (PAPT): clinical and MRI assessment with review of palatal tremors. Brain 127, 1252–1268, 2004.
954. Sand JJ, Biller J, Corbett JJ, Adams HP Jr., Dunn V. Partial dorsal mesencephalic hemorrhages: report of three cases. Neurology 36, 529–533, 1986.
955. Sandyk R. Oculogyric crisis induced by lithium carbonate. Eur Neurol 23, 92–94, 1984.
956. Saraiva JM, Baraitser M. Joubert syndrome: a review. Am J Med Genet 43, 726–731, 1992.
957. Sarnat HB, Alcala H. Human cerebellar hypoplasia: a syndrome of diverse causes. Arch Neurol 37, 300–305, 1980.
958. Saver JL, Liu GT, Charness ME. Idiopathic striopallidodentate calcification with prominent supranuclear abnormality of eye movement. J Neuro-ophthalmology 14, 29–33, 1994.
959. Sawaguchi T, Goldman-Rakic PS. The role of D1–dopamine receptor in working memory: local injections of dopamine antagonists into the prefrontal cortex of rhesus monkeys performing an oculomotor-delayed response task. J Neurophysiol 71, 515–528, 1994.
960. Schalen L, Pyykkö, I, Korttila K, Magnusson M, Enbom H. Effects of intravenously given barbiturate and diazepam on eye motor performance in man. Adv Oto-Rhino-Laryngol 42, 260–264, 1988.
961. Scharf D. Opsoclonus-myoclonus following the intranasal usage of cocaine. J Neurol Neurosurg Psychiatry 59, 1447–1448, 1989.
962. Schewe HJ, Uebelhack R, Vohs K. Abnormality in saccadic eye movement in dementia. Eur Psychiatry 14, 52–53, 1999.
963. Schiller PH, True SD, Conway JL. Deficits in eye movements following frontal eye-field and superior colliculus ablations. J Neurophysiol 44, 1175–1189, 1980.
964. Schmid-Burgk W, Becker W, Jürgens R, Kornhuber HH. Saccadic eye movements in psychiatric patients. Neuropsychobiology 10, 193–198, 1983.
965. Schmidtke K, Büttner-Ennever JA. Nervous control of eyelid function. A review of clinical experimental and pathological data. Brain 115, 227–247, 1992.
966. Schneider JA, Mirra SS. Neuropathologic correlate of persistent neurological deficit in lithium intoxication. Ann Neurol 36, 928–931, 1994.
967. Schneider RC, Calhoun HD, Crosby EC. Vertigo and rotational movement in cortical and subcortical lesions. J Neurol Sci 6, 493–516, 1968.
968. Schon F, Hodgson TL, Mort D, Kennard C. Ocular flutter associated with a localized lesion in the paramedian pontine reticular formation. Ann Neurol 50, 413–416, 2001.
969. Schonfeld SM, Golbe LI, Sage JI, Safer JN, Duvoisin RC. Computed tomographic findings in progressive

supranuclear palsy: correlation with clinical grade. Mov Disord 2, 263–278, 1987.
970. Schraeder PL, Cohen MM, Goldman W. Bilateral internuclear ophthalmoplegia associated with fourth ventricular epidermoid tumor. J Neurosurg 54, 403–405, 1981.
971. Schultz W, Romo R, Scarnati E, et al. Saccadic reaction times eye-arm coordination and spontaneous eye movements in normal and MTPT-treated monkeys. Exp Brain Res 78, 253–267, 1989.
972. Schwankhaus JD, Parisi JE, Gulledge WR, Chin L, Currier RD. Hereditary adult-onset Alexander's disease with palatal myoclonus, spastic paraparesis and cerebellar ataxia. Neurology 45, 2266–2271, 1995.
973. Schwartz MA, et al. Oculomasticatory myorhythmia: a unique movement disorder occurring in Whipple's disease. Ann Neurol 20, 677–683, 1986.
974. Seaber JH, Nashold BS. Comparison of ocular motor effects of unilateral stereotactic midbrain lesions in man. Neuro-ophthalmology 1, 95–99, 1980.
975. Sedwick LA, Burde RM, Hodges FJ. Leigh's subacute necrotizing encephalopathy manifesting as spasmus nutans. Arch Ophthalmol 102, 1046–1048, 1984.
976. Seemungal BM, Faldon M, Revesz T, et al. Influence of target size on vertical gaze palsy in a pathologically proven case of progressive supranuclear palsy. Mov Disord 18, 818–822, 2003.
977. Segraves MA, Goldberg ME, Deng SY, et al. The role of striate cortex in the guidance of eye movements in the monkey. J Neurosci 7, 3040–3058, 1987.
978. Selhorst JB, Stark L, Ochs AL, Hoyt WF. Disorders in cerebellar ocular motor control. I Saccadic overshoot dysmetria. An oculographic control system and clinico-anatomic analysis. Brain 99, 497–508, 1976.
979. Selhorst JB, Stark L, Ochs AL, Hoyt WF. Disorders in cerebellar ocular motor control. II Macrosaccadic oscillation. An oculographic control system and clinico-anatomical analysis. Brain 99, 509–522, 1976.
980. Seo SW, Shin HY, Kim SH, et al. Vestibular imbalance associated with a lesion in the nucleus prepositus hypoglossi area. Arch Neurol 61, 1440–1443, 2004.
981. Serra A, Derwenskus J, Downey DL, Leigh RJ. Role of eye movement examination and subjective visual vertical in clinical evaluation of multiple sclerosis. J Neurol 250, 569–575, 2003.
982. Shafiq-Antonacci R, Maruff P, Masters C, Currie J. Spectrum of saccade system function in Alzheimer disease. Arch Neurol 60, 1272–1278, 2003.
983. Shanzer S, April R, Atkin A. Seizures induced by eye deviation. Arch Neurol 13, 621–626, 1965.
984. Sharma S, Sumich PM, Francis IC, Kiernan MC, Spira PJ. Wernicke's encephalopathy presenting with upbeating nystagmus. J Clin Neurosci 9, 476–478, 2002.
985. Sharpe JA. Adaptation to frontal lobe lesions. In Keller EL, Zee DS (eds). Adaptive Processes in Visual and Oculomotor Systems. Pergamon, Oxford, 1986, pp 239–246.
986. Sharpe JA, Bondar RL, Fletcher WA. Contralateral gaze deviation after frontal lobe haemorrhage. J Neurol Neurosurg Psychiatry 48, 86–88, 1985.
987. Sharpe JA, Fletcher WA, Lang AE. Smooth pursuit during dose-related on-off fluctuations in Parkinson's disease. Neurology 37, 1389–1392, 1987.
988. Sharpe JA, Goldberg HJ, Lo AW, Herishanu YO. Visual-vestibular interaction in multiple sclerosis. Neurology 31, 427–433, 1981.
989. Sharpe JA, Herishanu YO, White OB. Cerebral square wave jerks. Neurology 37, 1389–1392, 1982.
990. Sharpe JA, Kim JS. Midbrain disorders of vertical gaze: a quantitative re-evaluation. Ann N Y Acad Sci 956, 143–154, 2002.
991. Sharpe JA, Lo AW. Voluntary and visual control of the vestibuloocular reflex after cerebral hemidecortication. Ann Neurol 10, 164–172, 1981.
992. Sharpe JA, Lo AW, Rabinovitch HE. Control of the saccadic and smooth pursuit systems after cerebral hemidecortication. Brain 102, 387–403, 1979.
993. Sharpe JA, Rosenberg MA, Hoyt WF, Daroff RB. Paralytic pontine exotropia. A sign of acute unilateral pontine gaze palsy and internuclear ophthalmoplegia. Neurology 24, 1076–1081, 1974.
994. Shaunak S, O'Sullivan E, Blunt S, et al. Remembered saccades with variable delay in Parkinson's disease. Mov Disord 14, 80–86, 1999.
995. Shaunak S, Orrell RW, O'Sullivan E, et al. Oculomotor function in amyotrophic lateral sclerosis: evidence for frontal impairment. Ann Neurol 38, 38–44, 1995.
996. Shawkat FS, Harris CM, Jacobs M, Taylor D, Brett EM. Eye movement tics. Brit J Ophthalmol 76, 697–699, 1992.
997. Shimpo T, Fuse S, Yoshizawa A. Retrocollis and oculogyric crisis in association with bilateral putaminal hemorrhages. Rinsho Shinkeigaku 33, 40–44, 1993.
998. Shiozawa M, Fukutani Y, Sasaki K, et al. Corticobasal degeneration: an autopsy case clinically diagnosed as progressive supranuclear palsy. Clin Neuropathol 19, 192–199, 2000.
999. Shipp S, Dejong BM, Zihl J, Frackowiak RS, Zeki S. The brain activity related to residual motion vision in a patient with bilateral lesions of V5. Brain 117, 1023–1038, 1994.
1000. Siatkowski RM, Schatz NJ, Sellitti TP, Galetta SL, Glaser JS. Do thalamic lesions really cause vertical gaze palsies? J Clin Neuro-ophthalmol 13, 190–193, 1993.
1001. Sibony PA, Evinger C, Manning K. Tobacco-induced primary-position upbeat nystagmus. Ann Neurol 21, 53–58, 1987.
1002. Sibony PA, Evinger C, Manning K, Pellegrini JJ. Nicotine and tobacco-induced nystagmus. Ann Neurol 28, 198, 1990.
1003. Sibony PA, Evinger C, Manning KA. The effects of tobacco smoking on smooth pursuit eye movements. Ann Neurol 23, 238–241, 1988.
1004. Simon JE, Morgan SC, Pexman JH, Hill MD, Buchan AM. CT assessment of conjugate eye deviation in acute stroke. Neurology 60, 135–137, 2003.
1005. Simon RP. Forced downward ocular deviation. Occurrence during oculovestibular testing in sedative drug-induced coma. Arch Neurol 35, 456–458, 1978.
1006. Simon RP, Aminoff MJ. Electrographic status epilepticus in fatal anoxic coma. Ann Neurol 20, 351–355, 1986.
1007. Simpson DA, Wishnow R, Gargulinski RB, Pawlak AM. Orofacial-skeletal myorhythmia in central

nervous system Whipple's disease: additional case and review of the literature. Mov Disord 10, 195–200, 1995.

1008. Singh BM, Strobos RJ. Retraction nystagmus elicited by bilateral simultaneous cold caloric stimulation. Ann Neurol 8, 79, 1980.

1009. Sinha KK, Worth PF, Jha DK, et al. Autosomal dominant cerebellar ataxia: SCA2 is the most frequent mutation in eastern India. J Neurol Neurosurg Psychiatry 75, 448–452, 2004.

1010. Slavin ML. A clinicoradiographic correlation of bilateral horizontal gaze palsy with slowed vertical saccades with midline dorsal pontine lesion on magnetic resonance imaging. Am J Ophthalmol 101, 118–120, 1986.

1011. Slyman ML, Kline LB. Dorsal midbrain syndrome in multiple sclerosis. Neurology 31, 196–198, 1981.

1012. Smith BH. Vestibular disturbances in epilepsy. Neurology 10, 465–469, 1960.

1013. Smith DB, Demasters BKK. Demyelinative disease presenting as Wallenberg's syndrome. Stroke 12, 877–878, 1981.

1014. Smith MS, Buchsbaum HW, Masland WS. One and a half syndrome. Occurrence after trauma with computerized tomographic correlation. Arch Neurol 37, 251, 1980.

1015. Smith MS, Laguna JF. Upward gaze paralysis following unilateral pretectal infarction. Arch Neurol 38, 127–129, 1981.

1016. Smith SJ, Kocen RS. A Creutzfeldt-Jakob like syndrome due to lithium toxicity. J Neurol Neurosurg Psychiatry 51, 120–123, 1988.

1017. Soliveri P, Rossi G, Monza D, et al. A case of dementia parkinsonism resembling progressive supranuclear palsy due to mutation in the tau protein gene. Arch Neurol 60, 1454–1456, 2003.

1018. Solms M, Kaplan-Solms K, Saling M, Miller P. Inverted vision after frontal lobe disease. Cortex 24, 499–509, 1988.

1019. Solomon D, Galetta SL, Liu GT. Possible mechanisms for horizontal gaze deviation and lateropulsion in the lateral medullary syndrome. J Neuroophthalmol 15, 26–30, 1995.

1020. Solomon D, Winkelman AC, Zee DS, Gray L, Büttner-Ennever J. Niemann-pick type C disease in two affected sisters: ocular motor recordings and brain-stem neuropathology. Ann N Y Acad. Sci. 1039, 436–445, 2005.

1021. Sommer MA, Tehovnik EJ. Reversible inactivation of macaque frontal eye field. Exp Brain Res 116, 229–249, 1997.

1022. Sommer MA, Wurtz RH. What the brain stem tells the frontal cortex. II Role of the SC-MD-FEF pathway in corollary discharge. J Neurophysiol 91, 1403–1423, 2004.

1023. Specht U, May TW, Rohde M, et al. Cerebellar atrophy decreases the threshold of carbamazepine toxicity in patients with chronic focal epilepsy. Arch Neurol 54, 427–431, 1997.

1024. Spector RH, Schnapper R. Amitriptyline-induced ophthalmoplegia. Neurology 31, 1188–1190, 1981.

1025. Sperling MR, Herrmann J. Syndrome of palatal myoclonus and progressive ataxia: Two cases with magnetic resonance imaging. Neurology 35, 1212–1214, 1985.

1026. Spieker S, Schulz JB, Petersen D, et al. Fixation instability and oculomotor abnormalities in Friedreich's ataxia. J Neurol 242, 517–521, 1995.

1027. Spooner JW, Baloh RW. Arnold-Chiari malformation. Improvement in eye movements after surgical treatment. Brain 104, 51–60, 1981.

1028. Stahl JS, James RA. Neural integrator function in murine CACNA1A mutants. Ann N Y Acad Sci 1039, 580–582, 2005.

1029. Standaert DG, Galetta SL, Atlas SW. Meningovascular syphilis with a gumma of the midbrain. J Clin Neuroophthalmol 11, 139–143, 1991.

1030. Stanford PM, Halliday GM, Brooks WS, et al. Progressive supranuclear palsy pathology caused by a novel silent mutation in exon 10 of the tau gene: expansion of the disease phenotype caused by tau gene mutations. Brain 123, 880–893, 2000.

1031. Starck M, Albrecht H, Straube A, Dieterich M. Drug therapy for acquired pendular nystagmus in multiple sclerosis. J Neurology 244, 9–16, 1997.

1032. Stark SR, Masucci EF, Kurtzke JF. Ocular dipping. Neurology 34, 391–393, 1984.

1033. Steele JC, Richardson JC, Olszewski J. Progressive supranuclear palsy. A heterogeneous degeneration involving the brain stem, basal ganglia and cerebellum with vertical gaze and pseudobulbar palsy nuchal dystonia and dementia. Arch Neurol 10, 333–359, 1964.

1034. Stein RW, Kase CS, Hier DB, Caplan LR, Mohr JP. Caudate hemorrhage. Neurology 34, 1549–1554, 1984.

1035. Steiner I, Melamed E. Conjugate eye deviation after acute hemispheric stroke: Delayed recovery after previous contralateral frontal lobe damage. Ann Neurol 16, 509–511, 1984.

1036. Steinlin MI, Blaser SI, MacGregor DL, Buncic JR. Eye problems in children with multiple sclerosis. Ped Neurol 12, 207–212, 1995.

1037. Stell R, Bronstein AM, Marsden CD. Vestibulo-ocular abnormalites in spasmodic torticollis before and after botulinum toxin injections. J Neurol Neurosurg Psychiatry 52, 57–62, 1989.

1038. Stell R, Bronstein AM, Plant GT, Harding AE. Ataxia telangiectasia: a reappraisal of the ocular motor features and their value in the diagnosis of atypical cases. Mov Disord 4, 320–329, 1989.

1039. Stolz SE, Chatrian G, Spence AM. Epileptic nystagmus. Epilepsia 32, 910–918, 1991.

1040. Straube A, Brandt T. Importance of the visual and vestibular cortex for self-motion perception in man (circularvection). Human Neurobiol 6, 211–218, 1987.

1041. Straube A, Büttner U. Pathophysiology of saccadic contrapulsion in unilateral rostral cerebellar lesions. Neuro-ophthalmology 14, 3–7, 1994.

1042. Straube A, Ditterich J, Oertel W, Kupsch A. Electrical stimulation of the posteroventral pallidum influences internally guided saccades in Parkinson's disease. J Neurol 245, 101–105, 1998.

1043. Straube A, Mennicken JB, Riedel M, Eggert T, Muller N. Saccades in Gilles de la Tourette's syndrome. Mov Disord 12, 536–546, 1997.

1044. Straube A, Scheuerer W, Eggert T. Unilateral cerebellar lesions affect initiation of ipsilateral smooth

pursuit eye movements in humans. Ann Neurol 42, 891–898, 1997.
1045. Straumann D, Müller E Torsional rebound nystagmus in a patient with type I Chiari malformation. Neuro-ophthalmology 14, 79–84, 1994.
1046. Straumann D, Zee DS, Solomon D. Three-dimensional kinematics of ocular drift in humans with cerebellar atrophy. J Neurophysiol 83, 1125–1140, 2000.
1047. Strauss C, Ganslandt O, Huk WJ, Jonas JB. Isolated unilateral internuclear ophthalmoplegia following head injury. Findings in magnetic resonance imaging. Neuroophthalmol 15, 15–19, 1995.
1048. Strominger MB, Mincy EJ, Strominger AI, Strominger NL. Bilateral internuclear ophthalmoplegia with absence of convergence eye movements. Clinico-pathological correlations. J Clin Neuro-ophthalmol 6, 57–65, 1986.
1049. Stroud MH, Newman NM, Keltner JL, Gay AJ. Abducting nystagmus in the medial longitudinal fasciculus (MLF) syndrome—internuclear ophthalmoplegia (INO). Arch Ophthalmol 92, 2–5, 1974.
1050. Stuve TA, et al. The relationship between smooth pursuit performance, motion perception and sustained visual attention in patients with schizophrenia and normal controls. Psychological Medicine 27, 143–152, 1997.
1051. Sullivan HC, Kaminski HJ, Maas EF, Weissman JD, Leigh RJ. Lateral deviation of the eyes on forced lid closure in patients with cerebral lesions. Arch Neurol 48, 310–311, 1991.
1052. Susac JO, Hoyt WF, Daroff RB, Lawrence W. Clinical spectrum of ocular bobbing. J Neurol Neurosurg Psychiatry 33, 771–775, 1970.
1053. Suyama N, Kobayashi S, Isino H, Iijima M, Imaoka K. Progressive supranuclear palsy with palatal myoclonus. Acta Neuropathol (Berl) 94, 290–293, 1997.
1054. Suzuki Y, Büttner-Ennever JA, Straumann D, et al. Deficits in torsional and vertical rapid eye movements and shift of Listing's plane after uni- and bilateral lesions of the rostral interstitial nucleus of the medial longitudinal fasciculus. Exp Brain Res 106, 215–232, 1995.
1055. Swartz BE, Li S, Bespalova I, et al. Pathogenesis of clinical signs in recessive ataxia with saccadic intrusions. Ann Neurol 54, 824–828, 2003.
1056. Sweeney JA, Bauer KS, Keshavan MS, et al. Adverse effects of risperidone on eye movement activity: a comparison of risperidone and haloperidol in anti-psychotic-naive schizophrenic patients. Neuropsychopharmacol 16, 217–228, 1997.
1057. Sweeney JA, Brew BJ, Keilp JG. Pursuit eye movement dysfunction in HIV-1 seropositive individuals. J Psychiatric Neurosci 16, 247–252, 1991.
1058. Sweeney JA, Clementz BA, Haas GL, et al. Eye tracking dysfunction in schizophrenia: characterization of component eye movement abnormalities, diagnostic specificity and the role attention. J Abnormal Psych 103, 222–230, 1994.
1059. Sweeney JA, Haas GL, Li SH, Weiden PJ. Selective effects of antipsychotic medications on eye-tracking performance in schizophrenia. Psychiatry Res 54, 185–198, 1994.
1060. Sweeney JA, Luna B, Haas GL, et al. Pursuit tracking impairments in schizophrenia and mood disorders: step-ramp studies with unmedicated patients. Biol Psychiatry 46, 671–680, 1999.
1061. Swick HM. Pseudointernuclear ophthalmoplegia in acute idiopathic polyneuritis (Fisher's syndrome). Am J Ophthalmol 77, 725–728, 1974.
1062. Takagi M, Zee DS, Tamargo R. Effects of lesions of the oculomotor vermis on eye movements in primate: saccades. J Neurophysiol 80, 1911–1930, 1998.
1063. Takagi M, Tamargo R, Zee DS. Effects of lesions of the cerebellar oculomotor vermis on eye movements in primate: binocular control. Prog Brain Res 142, 19–33, 2003.
1064. Takagi M, Zee DS, Tamargo RJ. Effects of lesions of the oculomotor cerebellar vermis on eye movements in primate: smooth pursuit. J Neurophysiol 83, 2047–2062, 2000.
1065. Takarae Y, Minshew NJ, Luna B, Krisky CM, Sweeney JA. Pursuit eye movements deficits in autism. Brain 127, 2584–2594, 2004.
1066. Takeichi N, Fukushima K, Sasaki H, et al. Dissociation of smooth pursuit and vestibulo-ocular reflex cancellation in SCA-6. Neurology 54, 860–866, 2000.
1067. Tamura EE, Hoyt CS. Oculomotor consequences of intraventricular hemorrhages in premature infants. Arch Ophthalmol 105, 533–535, 1987.
1068. Tanaka H, Arai M, Kubo J, Hirata K. Conjugate eye deviation with head version due to a cortical infarction of the frontal eye field. Stroke 33, 642–643, 2002.
1069. Tanaka M. Involvement of the central thalamus in the control of smooth pursuit eye movements. J Neurosci 25, 5866–5876, 2005.
1070. Taroni F, DiDonato S. Pathways to motor incoordination: The inherited ataxias. Nature Rev Neurosci 5, 641–655, 2004.
1071. Tatu L, Moulin T, Bogousslavsky J, Duvernoy H. Arterial territories of human brain: brainstem and cerebellum. Neurology 47, 1125–1135, 1996.
1072. Taylor JR, Selhorst JB, Houff SA, Martinez AJ. Chlordecone intoxication in man. I Clinical observations. Neurology 28, 626–630, 1978.
1073. Taylor RW, Turnbull DM. Mitochondrial DNA mutations in human disease. Nat Rev Genetics 6, 389–402, 2005.
1074. Tedeschi G, Bittencourt PRM, Smith AT, Richens A. Effect of amphetamine on saccadic and smooth pursuit eye movements. Psychopharmacology 79, 190–192, 1983.
1075. Tedeschi G, Casucci G, Allocca S, et al. Neuroocular side effects of carbamazepine and phenobarbital in epileptic patients as measured by saccadic eye movement analysis. Epilepsia 30, 62–66, 1989.
1076. Tetrud JW, Golbe LI, Forno LS, Farmer PM. Autopsy-proven progressive supranuclear palsy in two siblings. Neurology 46, 931–934, 1996.
1077. Thakare NJ, Pioro EP, Rucker JC, Leigh RJ. Motor neuron disease with dropped hands and downbeat nystagmus: a novel syndrome. BMC Neurology, in press, 2006.
1078. Thaker GK, Ellsberry R, Moran M, Lahti A, Tamminga C. Tobacco smoking increases square-wave jerks during pursuit eye movements. Biol Psychiatry 29, 82–88, 1991.
1079. Thaker GK, Nguyen JA, Tamminga CA. Increased

saccadic distractibility in tardive dyskinesia: functional evidence for subcortical GABA dysfunction. Biol Psychiatry 25, 49–59, 1989.

1080. Thaker GK, Nguyen JA, Tamminga CA. Saccadic distractibility in schizophrenic-patients with tardive-dyskinesia. Arch Gen Psychiatry 46, 755–756, 1989.

1081. Thaker GK, Ross DE, Buchanan RW, et al. Does pursuit abnormality in schizophrenia represent a deficit in the predictive mechanism? Psychiatry Res 59, 221–237, 1996.

1082. Thaker GK, Ross DE, Cassady SL, et al. Saccadic eye movement abnormalities in relatives of patients with schizophrenia. Schizophr Res 45, 235–244, 2000.

1083. Thames PB, Trobe JD, Balinger WE. Upgaze paralysis caused by lesion of the periaqueductal gray matter. Arch Neurol 41, 437–440, 1984.

1084. Thier P, Bachor A, Faiss J, Dichgans J, Koenig E. Selective impairment of smooth-pursuit eye movements due to an ischemic lesion of the basal pons. Ann Neurol 29, 443–448, 1991.

1085. Thömke F, Hopf HC. Abduction paresis with rostral pontine and/or mesencephalic lesions: Pseudoabducens palsy and its relation to the so-called posterior internuclear ophthalmoplegia of Lutz. BMC Neurol 1, 4, 2001.

1086. Thömke F, Hopf HC, Breen LA. Slowed abduction saccades in bilateral internuclear ophthalmoplegia. Neuro-ophthalmology 12, 241–246, 1992.

1087. Thurston SE, Leigh RJ, Abel LA, Dell'Osso LF. Slow saccades and hypometria in anticonvulsant toxicity. Neurology 34, 1593–1596, 1984.

1088. Thurston SE, Leigh RJ, Abel LA, Dell'Osso LF. Hyperactive vestibuloocular reflex in cerebellar degeneration: Pathogenesis and treatment. Neurology 37, 53–57, 1987.

1089. Thurston SE, Leigh RJ, Crawford TJ, Thompson A, Kennard C. Two distinct deficits of visual tracking caused by unilateral lesions of cerebral cortex in humans. Ann Neurol 23, 266–273, 1988.

1090. Thurston SE, Leigh RJ, Osorio I. Epileptic gaze deviation and nystagmus. Neurology 35, 1518–1521, 1985.

1091. Tian JR, Zee DS, Lasker AG, Folstein SE. Saccades in Huntington's disease: predictive tracking and interaction between release of fixation and initiation of saccades. Neurology 41, 875–881, 1991.

1092. Tien AY, Pearlson GD, Machlin SR, Bylsma FW, Hoehn-Saric R. Oculomotor performance in obsessive-compulsive disorder. Am J Psychiatry 149, 641–646, 1992.

1093. Tijssen CC. Contralateral conjugate eye deviation in acute supratentorial lesions. Stroke 25, 1516–1519, 1994.

1094. Tijssen CC, Bastiaensen LA, Voskuil PH. Epileptic eye deviation. Neuro-ophthalmology 13, 39–44, 1993.

1095. Tijssen CC, De Letter MAC J, Op de Coul AAW. Convergence-retraction nystagmus. Neuro-ophthalmology 16, 215–218, 1996.

1096. Tijssen CC, Ter Bruggen JP. Locked-in syndrome associated with ocular bobbing. Acta Neurol Scand 73, 444–446, 1986.

1097. Tijssen CC, Van Gisbergen JA. Conjugate eye deviation after hemispheric stroke—A contralateral saccadic palsy? Neuro-ophthalmology 13, 107–118, 1993.

1098. Tijssen CC, Van Gisbergen JA, Schulte BP. Conjugate eye deviation: side site and size of the hemispheric lesion. Neurology 41, 846–850, 1991.

1099. Tiliket C, Ventre J, Vighetto A, Grochowicki M. Room tilt illusion—a central otolith dysfunction. Arch Neurol 53, 1259–1264, 1996.

1100. Tilikete C, Hermier M, Pelisson D, Vighetto A. Saccadic lateropulsion and upbeat nystagmus: disorders of caudal medulla. Ann Neurol 52, 658–662, 2002.

1101. Tilikete C, Vighetto A, Trouillas P, Honnorat J. Potential role of anti-GAD antibodies in abnormal eye movements. Ann N Y Acad Sci 1039, 446–454, 2005.

1102. Titer E M, Laureno R. Inverse/reverse ocular bobbing. Ann Neurol 23, 103–104, 1988.

1103. Todd L, King J, Darlington CL, Smith PF. Optokinetic reflex dysfunction in multiple sclerosis. Neuroreport 12, 1399–1402, 2001.

1104. Tolosa E, Calandrella D, Gallardo M. Caribbean parkinsonism and other atypical parkinsonian disorders. Parkinsonism Relat Disord 10 Suppl 1, S19–S26, 2004.

1105. Tomsak RL, Volpe BT, Stahl JS, Leigh RJ. Saccadic palsy after cardiac surgery: visual disability and rehabilitation. Ann N Y Acad Sci 956, 430–433, 2002.

1106. Toyoda K, Hasegawa Y, Yonehara T, Oita J, Yamaguchi T. Bilateral medial medullary infarction with oculomotor disorders. Stroke 23, 1657–1659, 1992.

1107. Toyoda K, Imamura T, Saku Y, et al. Medial medullary infarction: analysis of eleven cases. Neurology 47, 1141–1147, 1996.

1108. Traccis S, Puliga MV, Ruiu MC, Marras MA, Rosati G. Unilateral occipital lesion causing hemianopia affects the acoustic saccadic programming. Neurology 41, 1633–1638, 1991.

1109. Tregellas JR, Tanabe JL, Martin LF, Freedman R. FMRI of response to nicotine during a smooth pursuit eye movement task in schizophrenia. Am J Psychiatry 162, 391–393, 2005.

1110. Trend P, Graham E. Internuclear ophthalmoplegia in giant-cell arteritis. J Neurol Neurosurg Psychiatry 53, 532–533, 1990.

1111. Trillenberg P, Heide W, Junghanns K, et al. Target anticipation and impairment of smooth pursuit eye movements in schizophrenia. Exp Brain Res 120, 316–324, 1998.

1112. Trobe JD, Sharpe JA, Hirsh DK, Gebarski SS. Nystagmus of Pelizaeus-Merzbacher disease. Arch Neurol 48, 87–91, 1991.

1113. Troost BT, Daroff RB. The ocular motor defects in progressive supranuclear palsy. Ann Neurol 2, 397–403, 1977.

1114. Troost BT, Daroff RB, Weber RB, Dell'Osso LF. Hemispheric control of eye movements. II Quantitative analysis of smooth pursuit in a hemispherectomy patient. Arch Neurol 27, 449–452, 1972.

1115. Troost BT, Martinez J, Abel LA, Heros RC. Upbeat nystagmus and internuclear ophthalmoplegia with brain stem glioma. Arch Neurol 37, 453–456, 1980.

1116. Troost BT, Weber RB, Daroff RB. Hemispheric control of eye movements. I Quantitative analysis of refixation saccades in a hemispherectomy patient. Arch Neurol 27, 441–448, 1972.

1117. Tusa RJ, Hove MT. Ocular and oculomotor signs in Joubert syndrome. J Child Neurol 14, 621–627, 1999.
1118. Tusa RJ, Kaplan PW, Hain TC, Naidu S. Ipsiversive eye deviation and epileptic nystagmus. Neurology 40, 662–665, 1990.
1119. Tusa RJ, Zee DS, Herdman SJ. Effect of unilateral cerebral cortical lesions on ocular motor behavior in monkeys: saccades and quick phases. J Neurophysiol 56, 1590–1625, 1986.
1120. Uematsu D, Suematsu M, Fukuchi Y, Ebihara S-I, Gotoh F. Midbrain locked-in state with oculomotor subnucleus lesion. J Neurol Neurosurg Psychiatry 48, 952–953, 1985.
1121. Umeda Y, Sakata E. Equilibrium disorder in carbamazepine toxicity. Ann Otol Rhinol Laryngol 86, 318–322, 1977.
1122. Uno A, Mukuno K, Sekiya H, et al. Lateropulsion in Wallenberg's syndrome and contrapulsion in the proximal type of the superior cerebellar artery syndrome. Neuro-ophthalmology 9, 75–80, 1998.
1123. Uyama E, Iwagoe H, Maeda J, et al. Presenile-onset cerebral adrenoleukodystrophy presenting as Balint's syndrome and dementia. Neurology 43, 1249–1251, 1993.
1124. Vahedi K, Rivaud S, Amarenco P, Pierrot-Deseilligny C. Horizontal eye movement disorders after posterior vermis infarctions. J Neurol Neurosurg Psychiatry 58, 91–94, 1995.
1125. Vaina LM, Soloviev S. First-order and second-order motion: neurological evidence for neuroanatomically distinct systems. Prog Brain Res 144, 197–212, 2004.
1126. van Leeuwen TH, Verbaten MN, Koelega HS, et al. Effects of oxazepam on eye movements and performance in vigilance tasks with static and dynamic stimuli. Psychopharmacol 114, 109–118, 1994.
1127. van Steveninck AL, Verver S, Schoemaker HC, et al. Effects of temazepam on saccadic eye movements: concentration-effect relationships in individual volunteers. Clin Pharmacol Ther 52, 402–408, 1992.
1128. van Weerden TW, van Woerkom TC. Ocular dipping. Neurology 35, 135, 1985.
1129. Velazquez-Perez L, Seifried C, Santos-Falcon N, et al. Saccade velocity is controlled by polyglutamine size in spinocerebellar ataxia 2. Ann Neurol 56, 444–447, 2004.
1130. Ventre J, Vighetto A, Bailly G, Prablanc C. Saccade metrics in multiple sclerosis: versional velocity disconjugacy as the best clue? J Neurol Sci 102, 144–149, 1991.
1131. Ventre J, Zee DS, Papageorgiou H, Reich S. Abnormalities of predictive saccades in hemiparkinson's disease. Brain 115, 1147–1165, 1992.
1132. Verhagen WIM, Huygens PLM, Mulleners WM. Lack of optokinetic nystagmus and visual motion perception in acquired cortical blindness. Neuro-ophthalmology 17, 211–216, 1997.
1133. Vermersch AI, Rivaud S, Vidailhet M, et al. Sequences of memory-guided saccades in Parkinson's disease. Ann Neurol 35, 487–490, 1994.
1134. Vermersch AL, Muri RM, Rivaud S, et al. Saccade disturbances after bilateral lentiform nucleus lesions in humans. J Neurol Neurosurg Psychiatry 60, 179–184, 1996.
1135. Verny M, Duyckaerts C, Agid Y, Hauw J. The significance of cortical pathology in progressive supranuclear palsy—clinico-pathological data in 10 cases. Brain 119, 1123–1136, 1996.
1136. Versino M, Beltrami G, Uggetti C, Cosi V. Auditory saccade impairment after central thalamus lesions. J Neurol. Neurosurg. Psychiatry 68, 234–237, 2000.
1137. Versino M, Hurko O, Zee DS. Disorders of binocular control of eye movements in patients with cerebellar dysfunction. Brain 119, 1933–1950, 1996.
1138. Versino M, Zavanone C, Colnaghi S, et al. Binocular control of saccades in idiopathic Parkinson's disease. Ann N Y Acad Sci 1039, 588–592, 2005.
1139. Vidailhet M, Rivaud S, Gouider-Khouja N, et al. Eye movements in parkinsonian syndromes. Ann Neurol 35, 420–426, 1994.
1140. Vignaendra V, Lim CL. Epileptic discharges triggered by eye convergence. Neurology 28, 589–591, 1978.
1141. Vivian AJ, Harris CM, Kriss A, et al. Oculomotor signs in infantile Gaucher disease. Neuro-ophthalmology 13, 151–155, 1993.
1142. von Noorden GK, Tredici TD, Ruttum M. Pseudo-internuclear ophthalmoplegia after surgical paresis of the medial rectus muscle. Am J Ophthalmol 98, 602–608, 1984.
1143. Wadia N, Pang J, Desai J, et al. A clinicogenetic analysis of six Indian spinocerebellar ataxia (SCA2 pedigrees. The significance of slow saccades in diagnosis. Brain 121, 2341–2355, 1998.
1144. Wadia NH, Swami RK. A new form of heredo-familial spinocerebellar degeneration with slow eye movements (nine families). Brain 94, 359–374, 1971.
1145. Waespe W. Deficits of smooth-pursuit eye movements in two patients with a lesion in the (para) floccular or dorsolateral pontine region. Neuro-ophthalmology 12, 91–96, 1992.
1146. Waespe W. Saccadic gain adaptivity in the two eyes in Wallenberg's lateral medullary syndrome. Neuro-ophthalmology 15, 193–201, 1995.
1147. Waespe W. Directional reversal of saccadic dysmetria and gain adaptivity in a patient with a superior cerebellar artery infarction. Neuro-ophthalmology 16, 65–74, 1996.
1148. Waespe W, Baumgartner R. Enduring dysmetria and impaired gain adaptivity of saccadic eye movements in Wallenberg's lateral medullary syndrome. Brain 115, 1125–1146, 1992.
1149. Waespe W, Cohen B, Raphan T. Dynamic modification of the vestibulo-ocular reflex by the nodulus and uvula. Science 228, 199–202, 1985.
1150. Waespe W, Wichmann W. Oculomotor disturbances during visual-vestibular interaction in Wallenberg's lateral medullary syndrome. Brain 113, 821–846, 1990.
1151. Waga S, Okada M, Yamamoto Y. Reversibility of Parinaud's syndrome in thalamic hemorrhage. Neurology 29, 407–409, 1979.
1152. Waitzman DM, Pathmanathan J, Presnell R, Ayers A, DePalma S. Contribution of the superior colliculus and the mesencephalic reticular formation to gaze control. Ann N Y Acad Sci 956, 111–129, 2002.
1153. Waitzman DM, Silakov VL. Effects of reversible lesions of the central mesencephalic reticular for-

mation (cMRF) on primate saccadic eye movements. Soc Neurosci Abstr 20, 1399, 1994.
1154. Waitzman DM, Silakov VL, Palma-Bowles S, Ayers AS. Effects of reversible inactivation of the primate mesencephalic reticular formation. I Hypermetric goal-directed saccades. J Neurophysiol 83, 2260–2284, 2000.
1155. Walker MF, Zee DS. The effect of hyperventilation on downbeat nystagmus in cerebellar dosorders. Neurology 53, 1576–1579, 1999.
1156. Walker R, Findlay JM. Saccadic eye movement programming in unilateral neglect. Neuropsychologia 34, 493–508, 1996.
1157. Wall M, Wray SH. The one-and-a-half syndrome - a unilateral disorder of the pontine tegmentum: a study of 20 cases and review of the literature. Neurology 33, 971–980, 1983.
1158. Wania JH, Walsh FB. Absence of ocular signs with cerebellar ablation in an infant. Arch Ophthalmol 61, 655–656, 1959.
1159. Warren NM, Piggott MA, Perry EK, Burn DJ. Cholinergic systems in progressive supranuclear palsy. Brain 128, 239–249, 2005.
1160. Watanabe K, Negoro T, Matsumoto A, et al. Epileptic nystagmus associated with typical absence seizures. Epilepsia 25, 22–24, 1984.
1161. Waterston JA, Barnes GR, Grealy MA. A quantitative study of eye and head movements during smooth pursuit in patients with cerebellar disease. Brain 115, 1343–1358, 1992.
1162. Waterston JA, Barnes GR, Grealy MA, Collins S. Abnormalities of smooth eye and head movement control in Parkinson's disease. Ann Neurology 39, 749–760, 1996.
1163. Watson P, Barber HO, Deck J, Terbrugge K. Positional vertigo and nystagmus of central origin. Can J Neurol Sci 8, 133–137, 1981.
1164. Watson RT, Rapcsak SZ. Loss of spontaneous blinking in a patient with Balint's syndrome. Ann Neurol 46, 567–570, 1989.
1165. Weber JCP. Beta-adrenoreceptor antagonists and diplopia. Lancet II, 826–827, 1982.
1166. Weiler MA, Thaker GK, Lahti AC, Tamminga CA. Ketamine effects on eye movements. Neuropsychopharmacology 23, 645–653, 2000.
1167. Weisbrod M, Hw K, Lempert T. The significance of vertical gaze palsy in the paramedian thalamic artery syndrome. Neuro-ophthalmology 12, 85–90, 1992.
1168. Weissman BM, DiScenna AO, Leigh RJ. Maturation of the vestibuloocular reflex in normal infants during the first 2 months of life. Neurology 39, 534–538, 1989.
1169. Westheimer G. Amphetamine barbiturates and accommodation. Arch Ophthalmol 70, 830–836, 1963.
1170. White OW, Saint-Cyr JA, Sharpe JA. Ocular motor deficits in Parkinson's disease. I The horizontal vestibulo-ocular reflex and its regulation. Brain 106, 555–570, 1983.
1171. White OW, Saint-Cyr JA, Tomlinson RD, Sharpe JA. Ocular motor deficits in Parkinson's disease. II Control of the saccadic and smooth pursuit systems. Brain 106, 571–587, 1983.
1172. White OW, Saint-Cyr JA, Tomlinson RD, Sharpe JA. Ocular motor deficits in Parkinson's disease. III Coordination of eye and head movements. Brain 111, 115–129, 1988.
1173. Whitehouse PJ, Wamsley JK, Zarbin MA, Price DL, Kuhar MJ. Neurotransmitter receptors in amyotrophic lateral sclerosis: possible relationship to sparing of eye movements. Ann Neurol 17, 518, 1985.
1174. Wiest G, Baumgartner C, Schnider P, et al. Monocular elevation paresis and contralateral downgaze paresis from unilateral mesodiencephalic infarction. J Neurol Neurosurg Psychiatry 60, 579–581, 1996.
1174a. Wiest G, Deecke L, Trattnig S, Mueller C. Abolished tilt suppression of the vestibulo-ocular reflex caused by a selective uvulo-nodular lesion. Neurology 52, 417–419, 1999.
1175. Wiest G, Mueller C, Wessely P, et al. Oculomotor abnormalities in dyssynergia cerebellaris myoclonica. Acta Otolaryhgol (Stockh) 20, 392–394, 1995.
1176. Wiest G, Tian JR, Baloh RW, Crane BT, Demer JL. Otolith function in cerebellar ataxia due to mutations in the calcium channel gene CACNA1 ABrain 124, 2407–2416, 2001.
1177. Williams B. Cough headache due to craniospinal pressure dissociation. Arch Neurol 37, 226–230, 1980.
1178. Williams DP, Troost BT, Rogers J. Lithium-induced down-beat nystagmus. Arch Neurol 45, 1022–1023, 1988.
1179. Williams DR, de Silva R, Paviour DC, et al. Characteristics of two distinct clinical phenotypes in pathologically proven progressive supranuclear palsy: Richardson's syndrome and PSP-parkinsonism. Brain 128, 1247–1258, 2005.
1180. Winkelman MD, Banker BQ, Victor M, Moser HW. Non-infantile neuronopathic Gaucher's disease: a clinicopathologic study. Neurology 33, 992–1008, 1983.
1181. Witt ED, Goldman-Rakic PS. Intermittent thiamine deficiency in the rhesus monkey. I Progression of neurological signs and neuroanatomical lesions. Ann Neurol 13, 376–395, 1983.
1182. Wolin MJ, Trent RG, Lavin PJ, Cornblath WT. Oculopalatal myoclonus after the one-and-a-half syndrome with facial nerve palsy. Ophthalmology 103, 177–180, 1996.
1182a. Wong AM, Sharpe JA. Cerebellar skew deviation and the torsional vestibuloocular reflex. Neurology 65, 412–419, 2005.
1183. Woody RC, Reynolds JD. Association of bilateral internuclear ophthalmoplegia and myelomeningocele with Arnold-Chiari malformation type II. J Clin Neuro-ophthalmol 5, 124–126, 1985.
1184. Worthington JM, Halmagyi GM. Bilateral total ophthalmoplegia due to midbrain hematoma. Neurology 47, 1176–1177, 1996.
1185. Wszolek ZK, Pfeiffer RF, Bhatt MH, et al. Rapidly progressive autosomal dominant parkinsonism and dementia with pallido-ponto-nigral degeneration. Ann Neurol 32, 312–320, 1992.
1186. Wyllie E, Luders H, Morris HH, Lesser RP, Dinner DS. The lateralizing significance of versive head and eye movements during epileptic seizures. Neurology 36, 606–611, 1986.

1187. Wyllie E, Ludders H, Morris HH, et al. Ipsilateral forced head and eye turning at the end of the generalized tonic-clonic phase of versive seizures. Neurology 36, 1212–1217, 1986.
1188. Yachnis AT, Rorke LB. Neuropathology of Joubert syndrome. J Child Neurol 14, 655–659, 1999.
1189. Yagi T, Shimizu M, Sekine S, Kamio T. New neurotological test for detecting cerebellar dysfunction. Vestibulo-ocular reflex changes with horizontal vision-reversing prisms. Ann Otol Rhinol Laryngol 90, 276–280, 1981.
1190. Yanagisawa T, Sugihara H, Shibahara K, et al. Natural course of combined limb and palatal tremor caused by cerebellar-brain stem infarction. Mov Disord 14, 851–854, 1999.
1191. Yee RD, Baloh RW, Honrubia V. Episodic vertical oscillopsia and downbeat nystagmus in a Chiari malformation. Arch Ophthalmol 102, 723–725, 1984.
1192. Yee RD, Baloh RW, Honrubia V, Lau CG, Jenkins HA. Slow build-up of optokinetic nystagmus associated with downbeat nystagmus. Invest Ophthalmol Vis Sci 18, 622–629, 1979.
1193. Yee RD, Cogan DG, Zee DS. Ophthalmoplegia and dissociated nystagmus in abetalipoproteinemia. Arch Ophthalmol 94, 571–575, 1976.
1194. Yee RD, Farlow MR, Suzuki DA, Betelak KF, Ghetti B. Abnormal eye movements in Gerstmann-Sträussler-Scheinker disease. Arch Ophthalmol 110, 68–74, 1992.
1195. Yigit A, Bingöl A, Mutluer N, Tasçilar N. The one-and-a-half syndrome in systemic lupus erythematosus. J Neuroophthalmol 16, 274–276, 1996.
1195a. Ying SH, Choi SI, Lee M, et al. Relative atrophy of the flocculus and ocular motor dysfunction in SCA2 and SCA6. Ann N Y Acad Sci 1039, 430–435, 2005.
1196. Yokota T, Shiojiri T, Gotoda T, et al. Friedreich-like ataxia with retinitis pigmentosa caused by the $His^{101}Gln$ mutation of the α-tocopherol transfer protein gene. Ann Neurol 41, 826–832, 1997.
1197. Yokota T, Tsuchiya K, Yamane M, et al. Geotropic ocular deviation with skew and absence of saccade in Creutzfeldt-Jakob disease. J Neurol Sci 106, 175–178, 1991.
1198. Young GB, Brown JD, Boltin CF, Sibbald WM. Periodic lateralized epileptiform discharges (PLEDs) and nystagmus retractorius. Ann Neurol 2, 61–62, 1977.
1199. Zaccara G, Gangemi PF, Messori A, et al. Smooth-pursuit eye movements: alterations in Alzheimer's disease. J Neurol Sci 112, 81–89, 1992.
1200. Zackon DH, Sharpe JA. Midbrain paresis of horizontal gaze. Ann Neurol 16, 495–504, 1984.
1201. Zangemeister WH, Meienberg O, Stark L, Hoyt WF. Eye-head coordination in homonymous hemianopia. J Neurol 226, 243–254, 1982.
1202. Zangemeister WH, Mueller-Jensen A. The coordination of gaze movements in Huntington's disease. Neuro-ophthalmology 5, 193–206, 1985.
1203. Zauel D, Carlow TJ. Internuclear ophthalmoplegia following cervical manipulation. Ann Neurol 1, 308, 1977.
1204. Zee DS. Ophthalmoscopy in examination of patients with vestibular disorders. Ann Neurol 3, 373–374, 1978.
1205. Zee DS. Considerations on the mechanisms of alternating skew deviation in patients with cerebellar lesions. J Vestib Res 6, 1–7, 1996.
1206. Zee DS, Chu FC, Leigh RJ, et al. Blink-saccade synkinesis. Neurology 33, 1233–1236, 1983.
1207. Zee DS, FitzGibbon EJ, Optican LM. Saccade-vergence interactions in humans. J Neurophysiol 68, 1624–1641, 1992.
1208. Zee DS, Freeman JM, Holtzman NA. Ophthalmoplegia in maple syrup urine disease. J Pediatr 84, 113–115, 1974.
1209. Zee DS, Friendlich AR, Robinson DA. The mechanism of downbeat nystagmus. Arch Neurol 30, 227–237, 1974.
1210. Zee DS, Hain TC, Carl JR. Abduction nystagmus in internuclear ophthalmoplegia. Ann Neurol 21, 383–388, 1987.
1211. Zee DS, Leigh RJ. Mathieu-Millaire F Cerebellar control of ocular gaze stability. Ann Neurol 7, 37–40, 1980.
1212. Zee DS, Optican LM, Cook JD, Robinson DA, Engel WK. Slow saccades in spinocerebellar degeneration. Arch Neurol 33, 243–251, 1976.
1213. Zee DS, Robinson DA. A hypothetical explanation of saccadic oscillations. Ann Neurol 5, 405–414, 1979.
1214. Zee DS, Tusa RJ, Herdman SJ, Butler PH, Gücer G. Effects of occipital lobectomy upon eye movements in primate. J Neurophysiol 58, 883–907, 1987.
1215. Zee DS, Yamazaki A, Butler P H, Gücer G. Effects of ablation of flocculus and paraflocculus on eye movements in primate. J Neurophysiol 46, 878–899, 1981.
1216. Zee DS, Yee RD, Cogan DG, Robinson DA, Engel WK. Ocular motor abnormalities in hereditary cerebellar ataxia. Brain 99, 207–234, 1976.
1217. Zee DS, Yee RD, Singer HS. Congenital ocular motor apraxia. Brain 100, 581–599, 1977.
1218. Zegers de Beyl D, Flament-Durand J, Borenstein S, Brunko E. Ocular bobbing and myoclonus in central pontine myelinolysis. J Neurol Neurosurg Psychiatry 46, 564–565, 1983.
1219. Zeviani M, Bertagnolio B, Uziel G. Neurological presentations of mitchondrial diseases. J Inherit Metab Dis 19, 504–520, 1996.
1220. Ziffer AJ, Rosenbaum AL, Demer J L, Yee RD. Congenital double elevator palsy: Vertical saccadic velocity utilizing the scleral search coil technique. J Pediatr Ophthalmol Strabismus 29, 142–149, 1992.
1221. Zihl J, Hebel N. Patterns of oculomotor scanning in patients with unilateral posterior parietal or frontal lobe damage. Neuropsychologia 35, 893–906, 1997.
1222. Zihl J, Von Crammon D. The contribution of the "second" visual system to directed visual attention in man. Brain 102, 835–856, 1979.
1223. Zimmerman CF, Roach ES, Troost BT. See-saw nystagmus associated with Chiari malformation. Arch Neurol 43, 299–300, 1986.

Appendix A

A Summary Scheme for the Bedside Ocular Motor Examination with Video Examples of Abnormal Responses

Although the order and specific details of testing may be modified according to the nature of the clinical problem, systematic examination of each ocular motor subsystem is worthwhile, particularly in evaluating signs such as nystagmus. Here we outline a scheme for examining eye movements, providing video examples of abnormal findings for certain tests. The technical details of each step in the ocular motor examination are described in the respective chapters. The reader should note that ocular motor signs are rarely diagnostic touchstones; they require interpretation in the context of the history and full examination.

1. General Features
   a. Look for abnormal head postures, such as turns or tilts (see Video Display: Disorders of the Vestibular System), abnormal patterns of eye-head coordination—such as the head thrusts of ocular motor apraxia (see Video Display: Acquired Ocular Motor Apraxia), and head tremors (see Video Display: Congenital Forms of Nystagmus).
   b. Look for abnormalities of the lids including ptosis, retraction, lid nystagmus, lid-opening apraxia after forceful closure (see Video Display: Parkinsonian Disorders), and synkinesis (e.g., due to aberrant regeneration, such as Marcus Gunn phenomenon).
2. Examination of Vision
   a. Measure corrected visual acuity and check confrontation visual fields with each eye viewing.
   b. Check color vision (Hardy-Rand-Rittler or Ishihara plates), to screen for optic neuropathy (e.g., in patients with monocular pendular nystagmus or retinal abnormalities).
   c. Test stereopsis (e.g., Titmus Optical or Randot stimuli), especially when ocular misalignment is thought to be of early onset.
   d. Test pupillary reflexes to light and with convergence.
3. Range of Movement and Alignment of the Visual Axes
   a. Establish range of motion with ductions (one eye viewing) and versions (both eyes viewing) (see Video Display: Diplopia and Strabismus).
   b. Test ocular misalignment (in patients with diplopia or strabismus)
   - Confirm that diplopia is only present during binocular viewing
   - Subjective tests, such as the red glass, and Maddox rod (Fig. 9–11)
   - The cover test (Fig. 9–12) (see Video Display: Diplopia and Strabismus) for tropias
   - The alternate cover test (Fig. 9–13) (see Video Display: Diplopia and

Strabismus) for phorias. Measure deviation at both near and far, and in the nine cardinal positions of gaze.
- Quantify with prisms by nullifying the deviation as measured with alternate cover test (Fig. 9–13) or Maddox rod (Fig. 9–11).
- For vertical deviations, use the Bielschowsky head-tilt test (Fig. 9–14) (see Video Display: Diplopia and Strabismus), to diagnose superior oblique muscle paresis.

4. Fixation (using simple visual inspection, the ophthalmoscope, and Frenzel goggles)
   a. In primary position: Look for extraneous saccades (see Video Display: Saccadic Oscillations and Intrusions) and nystagmus.
   b. In eccentric gaze: Look for gaze-evoked and then rebound nystagmus (see Video Display: Disorders of Gaze Holding).
   c. Determine the position of the eyes under closed lids by noting corrective movements when the patients open their eyes (e.g., steady-state deviation of the eyes toward the side of the lesion in Wallenberg's syndrome) (see Video Display: Medullary Syndromes).
   d. In patients with nystagmus, the time in the cycle when the image of the target is brought to the fovea can be determined during ophthalmoscopy by having the patient fix upon the center of the ophthalmoscope cross hairs,
5. Vestibular
   a. Measure visual acuity (Snellen chart) before and during head shaking (horizontal and vertical) at a frequency of greater than 1 cycle/second.
   b. Look for corrective saccades during sinusoidal head oscillations at about 1 Hz and following brief but high acceleration head impulses, while the patient is required to fix upon a target straight ahead (see Video Display: Disorders of the Vestibular System).
   c. Using Frenzel goggles*, look for nystagmus after 10 to 15 seconds of brisk horizontal head shaking, then after vertical head shaking, (see Video Display: Disorders of the Vestibular System). In cases of suspected bilateral vestibular loss, look for nystagmus following circular head-shaking, in which case it should be absent.
   d. Using the ophthalmoscope, watch for abnormal movement of the retinal vessels or optic nerve head with the head still. Recall that the direction of horizontal or vertical motion of the retina is opposite to that of the front of the eye. For torsional nystagmus, the direction of the movement of the retinal vessels will change with looking to the right or left (it will be vertical) and with looking up or down (it will be horizontal). Alternately cover and uncover the other eye, to see if any drift of the retina is brought out or exacerbated by the removal of fixation. Watch for oscillation of the optic disc during small-amplitude head shaking (horizontal and vertical) at a frequency of greater than 1 cycle/second, to see if the gain of the VOR is correct. If the gain is too high, the disc appears to move with the head, if too low, opposite the head.
   e. Use positional maneuvers to elicit nystagmus. First use the Dix-Hallpike maneuver: the head is turned 45 degrees to the right or left, then the patient is brought to a supine position with the head just below the horizontal (Fig. 11–4); observe any nystagmus, preferably behind Frenzel goggles (see Video Display: Disorders of the Vestibular System). The patient is then brought back to the upright position; look again for nystagmus. The same maneuver is then repeated with the head turned 45 degrees in the opposite direction. Second, put the patient supine, look for nystagmus and then rotate the head to the right ear down, then straight back, then left ear

---

**Frenzel goggles* consist of 10- to 20-diopter spherical convex lenses that defocus the patient's vision (so preventing fixation of objects) and also provide the examiner with a magnified, illuminated view of the patient's eyes. An alternative is +20 diopter lenses mounted in a spectacle frame and fitted with side-blinkers. The room lights should be turned off and either the lights of the goggles or a pen light used to illuminate the eyes.

down positions. Each time wait for 10 to 15 seconds to look for nystagmus.

f. With Frenzel goggles or using the ophthalmoscope to observe for nystagmus, irrigate with small amounts of ice-water (less than 1 ml), always being careful not to allow the catheter to go too far in the external ear canal.

g. Rotate the patient in a swivel chair to elicit per-rotational nystagmus; when the chair stops, look for post-rotational nystagmus. Test responses in each plane of head rotation: horizontal (head upright), vertical (head tilted over 90 degrees, ear-to-shoulder), or torsional (head looking to the ceiling).

h. With Frenzel goggles, use the Valsalva maneuver (first against a closed glottis and then against pinched nostrils), tragal compression, and mastoid vibration to elicit nystagmus (see Video Display: Disorders of the Vestibular System).

i. With Frenzel goggles, look for nystagmus after hyperventilating for 30 seconds (see Video Display: Disorders of the Vestibular System).

6. Saccades
   a. Observe spontaneous saccades, saccades to visual or auditory targets, and saccades to command and rapid self-paced saccades. Note latency, velocity, trajectory, accuracy, and conjugacy (see Video Displays: Disorders of Saccades and Parkinsonian Syndromes).
   b. Assess quick phases induced by vestibular rotation or caloric stimuli, and a hand-held optokinetic drum or tape. During vertical stimulation, with stripes moving down, check for retraction nystagmus (see Video Display: Disorders of Vergence).
7. Smooth Pursuit
   a. Instruct the patient to track a small moving target smoothly, horizontally and vertically. Look for corrective saccades that indicate an inappropriate smooth pursuit gain. If the gain is low, saccades will be catch-up, if the gain is too high, saccades will be back-up (see Video Display: Disorders of Smooth Pursuit).
   b. Use a small optokinetic drum, tape, or mirror to bring out pursuit asymmetries, or "inverted" optokinetic nystagmus, as occurs with congenital nystagmus.
8. Eye-Head Coordination
   a. Assess head and eye movements (latency, accuracy, velocity) during combined, eye-head rapid (saccadic) refixations (see Video Display: Acquired Ocular Motor Apraxia).
   b. Test cancellation of the vestibulo-ocular reflex by asking the patient to fixate a target moving with the head. Look for corrective saccades (see Video Display: Disorders of Smooth Pursuit).
9. Vergence
   a. Test vergence to disparity stimuli (place a prism in front of one eye)
   b. Test vergence to accommodative stimuli: With one eye covered with a semi-opaque Spielmann occluder, the other eye alternately fixes upon the near and distant targets (Fig. 8–1 and Video Display: Disorders of Vergence).
   c. Test vergence to combined disparity and accommodative stimuli by asking the patient to fixate a target brought in along the mid-sagittal plane toward the nose (Video Display: Disorders of Vergence).
   d. Note pupillary changes during vergence movements.

Appendix B

Methods Available for Measuring Eye Movements

Method	Advantages	Disadvantages
Clinical observation, ophthalmoscopy	Simple, no discomfort, resolution of 10 minutes of arc, effective way to assess fixation.[28]	No "record" to analyze. May be difficult to distinguish different types of oscillations or to judge eye velocity.
D.C. Electro-oculography (EOG)	Non-invasive, minimal discomfort; can accurately record a large range of horizontal movement (± 40 degrees); resolution of about 1 degree; applicable to children and poorly cooperative patients. The most widely used clinical method to record eye movements.	Electrical and electromyographic noise, lid artifact; unstable baseline, requiring repeat calibration and adaptation to level of ambient lighting. Unreliable for vertical eye movements. Cost depends mainly on amplifiers selected, but usually not very expensive.
Infrared differential limbus reflection technique	Non-invasive, minimal discomfort; resolution of 0.5 degrees or better; little noise.	Limited range (± 20 degrees horizontally and ± 10 degrees vertically). Intermediate cost.
Purkinje image tracker (lens and cornea)	Non-invasive; resolution of 0.5 degrees or better; little noise.	Lens motion artifact. Subject's head must be immobilized on bite bar. Expensive to buy and maintain.
Video-based systems (tracking pupil or reflected corneal images)	Non-invasive, minimal discomfort; resolution of 0.5 degrees or better; noise depends on camera resolution and digitization rate.	Subject required to wear headgear, which may be bulky; digitization noise of system may limit analysis of slow eye movements.[9] May be expensive.
Magnetic search coil technique using scleral annulus	Sensitive to <1 minute of arc; precise; potential linear range of ± 180 degrees; capable of measuring horizontal, vertical, and torsional rotations of eyes and head.	Subject required to wear scleral annulus on eye; topical anesthetic drops required. Large (2 m) field coils are expensive; scleral annulus for measuring 3-D rotations is expensive.
Ocular electromyography (EMG)[18]	Provides information about extraocular muscle activity; especially useful in problems of anomalous innervation or co-contraction.	Uncomfortable; technically difficult. With a few exceptions (prior to strabismus surgery) probably only justifiable for research.

The table above summarizes techniques currently available to measure rotations of the eyes, each methodology having its strengths and limitations.[4,10,27] At present, the *magnetic search coil technique* (Fig. 1–1) is generally regarded as the most reliable and versatile method, and is used widely to measure eye movements in human and many animal species,[2,6,14,19,23] except for those with very small eyes.[24] It allows measurement of eye rotations around all three axes, with a sensitivity of greater than 5 minutes of arc (the standard deviation of system noise is typically less than 0.02 degree), a potential linear range of 360 degrees, a bandwidth of 0 Hz–500 Hz, minimal drift, insensitivity to translation of the eye, and an unlimited field of view.[3,11] One disadvantage is that the subject must wear a "contact lens" (a silastic annulus in which fine coils of wire are imbedded); this annulus is placed after applying topical anesthetic eye drops. Our experience, based on studying well over 1000 patients, is that the scleral search coil is well tolerated for periods of up to 60 minutes, even by individuals in their tenth decade and those with advanced neurological disease. Most subjects tolerate the procedure well, with little effects on vision and, in those who notice blurring of vision, the effects are transient and usually relieved by frequent and gentle blinking, brief eye closure and application of artificial tears every 15 or 20 minutes.[16,22] A disadvantage is the potential for corneal abrasion, but the incidence in our laboratories is less than 1 in 500. The search coil method is especially valuable for measuring eye movements in patients who cannot reliably point their eyes at calibration targets (e.g., due to nystagmus), since the scleral annulus that the patient wears can be pre-calibrated on a protractor device. Comparison of the search coil technique suggests that saccadic peak velocities may be mildly slow, but also less variable, than with other available methods.[13,25] When using the torsional coil, care must be given to checking that the coil does not slip, and in positioning the wire as it exits from the eye, because it may move during blinks.[3]

Electro-oculography (EOG) is widely used for clinical testing because it allows measurement of a large range of movement, and is relatively inexpensive. However, it suffers from a number of limitations including inability to reliably measure vertical eye movements, low sensitivity (due to muscle artifact and other noise sources), baseline drift, and limited bandwidth due to the filtering required to remove noise from the signal. Computer algorithms have been developed to improve the quality of EOG signals.[8] However, EOG is unreliable for measuring vertical eye movements because of an associated eyelid artifact.[1] A lid artifact also confounds attempts to record eye movements using conventional electroencephalography.[17]

Photoelectric methods that track the limbus (scleral-iris edge) of the eye by measuring the amount of scattered light from infrared sources are generally more sensitive and reliable than EOG, but provide a limited linear range, especially vertically. Their main advantage is that they do not require a contact lens device and are therefore suitable for measurement of eye movements in children. Most photoelectric systems use photodectors that must be mounted close to the eyes, so they may restrict the field of view. Photoelectric methods also suffer from potentially large errors if there is lateral motion of the sensors relative to the eye.

Another approach has been to measure movement of images reflected by the eye as it rotates; a stationary source of infrared light can be used. Because the center of curvature of the corneal bulge differs from the center of rotation of the globe, eye movements cause displacement of the corneal, or first Purkinje, image. Alternatively, the video image of the pupil can be tracked. However, measurement of movement of one such image suffers from the disadvantage that movement of the transducer relative to the subject's head will be interpreted as eye rotation. In systems that measure eye rotation by tracking only corneal reflections, 1 mm of lateral motion of the sensor relative to the eyes introduces errors of approximately 10 degrees. For systems that measure eye rotations by tracking only the center of the pupil, the errors are approximately 5 degrees per 1 mm of lateral motion. Since it is very difficult to eliminate this lateral motion completely, an alternative approach is to measure movement of reflected light from one surface of the eye (e.g., the cornea) in conjunction with another reflected image (e.g., the pupil, or the fourth Purkinje image from the posterior surface of the lens). Such an approach allows measurement of horizontal and vertical eye movements that is insensitive to translation of the eye with respect to the transducer. The latter is the case because the circumferences of rotation of the two images differ, and hence the two images move relative to one another during rotation but not during translation.

One such method that has been used mainly as a research tool is the *double Purkinje image tracker*, which uses the first and fourth Purkinje images.[7] This tracker suffers from disadvantages that limit its usefulness, especially in evaluating patients: failure to detect the rather dim fourth image of certain subjects; the presence of an artifact due to lens movement during saccades; the requirement that the subject's head be fixed on a bite-bar, and substantial expense to purchase and maintain.

An alternative has been to measure the first Purkinje image and the pupil, and this approach, which is technically easier, has been incorporated in a number of recently developed *video-based oculography* systems. The conventional video camera has a bandwidth of 0 Hz–30 Hz (imposed by its frame rate 60 Hz), which suffices for smooth pursuit eye movements but is inadequate to accurately measure saccades. Many new video monitoring devices have recently become available offering frame rates that make measurement of saccadic dynamics reliably.[5,15,26] Some models allow measurement of 3-D eye movements,[12,26,29] and have been used to measure animal eye movements.[21] By also incorporating a head monitor, it is possible to remove artifacts due to movement of the device with respect to the head and even measure microsaccades.[12,20] One disadvantage of video-based systems is that their calibration depends on the ability of the subjects to foveate visual targets at known angular positions; patients with ocular motor palsies or oscillations may not be able to do this reliably.

REFERENCES

1. Barry W, Jones GM. Influence of eye lid movement upon electro-oculographic recording of vertical eye movements. Aerosp Med 36, 855–858, 1965.
2. Beck JC, Gilland E, Baker R, Tank DW. Instrumentation for measuring oculomotor preformance and plasticity in larval organisms. Methods Cell Biol 76, 385–413, 2004.
3. Bergamin O, Ramat S, Straumann D, Zee DS. Influence of orientation of exiting wire of search coil annulus on torsion after saccades. Invest Ophthalmol Vis Sci 45, 131–137, 2004.
4. Carpenter RHS. Movements of the Eyes. Pion, London, 1988.
5. Clarke AH, Ditterich J, Druen K, Schonfeld U, Steineke C. Using high frame rate CMOS sensors for three-dimensional eye tracking. Behav Res Methods Instrum Comput 34, 549–560, 2002.
6. Collewijn H, Van der Steen J, Ferman L, Jansen TC. Human ocular counterroll: assessment of static and dynamic properties from electromagnetic scleral coil recordings. Exp Brain Res 59, 185–196, 1985.
7. Cornsweet TN, Crane HD. Accurate two-dimensional eye tracker using first and fourth Purkinje images. J Opt Soc Am 63, 921–928, 1973.
8. Coughlin MJ, Cutmore TR, Hine TJ. Automated eye tracking system calibration using artificial neural networks. Comput Methods Programs Biomed 76, 207–220, 2004.
9. Das VE, Thomas CW, Zivotofsky AZ, Leigh RJ. Measuring eye movements during locomotion. Filtering techniques for obtaining velocity signals from a video-based eye monitor. J Vestib Res 6, 455–461, 1996.
10. DiScenna AO, Das VE, Zivotofsky AZ, Seidman SH, Leigh RJ. Evaluation of a video tracking device for measurement of horizontal and vertical eye rotations during locomotion. J Neurosci Methods 58, 89–95, 1995.
11. Fetter M, Haslwanter T. 3D eye movements—basics and clinical applications. J Vestib Res 9, 181–187, 1999.
12. Foroozan R, Brodsky MC. Microsaccadic opsoclonus: an idiopathic cause of oscillopsia and episodic blurred vision. Am J Ophthalmol 138, 1053–1054, 2004.
13. Frens MA, van der Geest JN. Scleral search coils influence saccade dynamics. J Neurophysiol 88, 692–698, 2002.
14. Hess BJM. Dual-search coil for measuring 3-dimensional eye movements in experimental animals. Vision Res 30, 597–602, 1990.
15. Imai T, Sekine K, Hattori K, et al. Comparing the accuracy of video-oculography and the scleral search coil system in human eye movement analysis. Auris Nasus Larynx 32, 3–9, 2005.
16. Irving EL, Zacher JE, Allison RS, Callender MG. Effects of scleral search coil wear on visual function. Invest Ophthalmol Vis Sci 44, 1933–1938, 2003.
17. Iwasaki M, Kellinghaus C, Alexopoulos AV, et al. Effects of eyelid closure, blinks, and eye movements on the electroencephalogram. Electroencephalogr Clin Neurophysiol 116, 878–885, 2005.
18. Jampolsky A. What can electromyography do for the ophthalmologist? Invest Ophthalmol Vis Sci 9, 570–579, 1970.
19. Judge SJ, Richmond BJ, Chu FC. Implantation of magnetic search coils for measurement of eye position: an improved method. Vision Res 20, 535–538, 1980.
20. Martinez-Conde S, Macknik SL, Hubel DH. The role of fixational eye movements in visual perception. Nat Rev Neurosci 5, 229–240, 2004.
21. Migliaccio AA, MacDougall HG, Minor LB, Della Santina CC. Inexpensive system for real-time 3-dimensional video-oculography using a fluorescent marker array. J Neurosci Methods 143, 141–150, 2005.

22. Murphy PJ, Duncan AL, Glennie AJ, Knox PC. The effect of scleral search coil lens wear on the eye. Br J Ophthalmol 85, 332–335, 2001.
23. Robinson DA. A method of measuring eye movement using a scleral search coil in a magnetic field. IEEE Trans Biomed Eng 10, 137–145, 1963.
24. Stahl JS, van Alphen AM, De Zeeuw CI. A comparison of video and magnetic search coil recordings of mouse eye movements. J Neurosci Methods 99, 101–110, 2000.
25. Traisk F, Bolzani R, Ygge J. A comparison between the magnetic scleral search coil and infrared reflection methods for saccadic eye movement analysis. Graefes Arch Clin Exp Ophthalmol 243, 791–797, 2005.
26. Yagi T, Koizumi Y, Aoyagi M, Kimura M, Sugizaki K. Three-dimensional analysis of eye movements using four times high-speed video camera. Auris Nasus Larynx 32, 107–112, 2005.
27. Young LR, Sheena D. Eye-movement measurement techniques. Am Psychol 30, 315–330, 1975.
28. Zee DS. Ophthalmoscopy in examination of patients with vestibular disorders. Ann Neurol 3, 373–374, 1978.
29. Zhu D, Moore ST, Raphan T. Robust and real-time torsional eye position calculation using a template-matching technique. Comput Methods Programs Biomed 74, 201–209, 2004.

Index

Note: Page numbers followed by f refer to figures; page numbers followed by t refer to tables.

Instructions for Using the DVD

Included with this edition is a DVD on which the reader can find video clips (MPEG format), all 12 chapters with figures and the appendices (Adobe PDF format), and Video Displays (Adobe PDF format). The video clips show examples of eye movement disorders and can be played using the Windows Media Player or Windows Built-In Player on PC computers, and with Apple QuickTime Player on Macintosh computers. To read the chapters and Video Displays, Adobe Acrobat Reader version 6 or higher is required; this can be downloaded from the Web at no cost.

The video clips are also embedded in Video Displays of clinical syndromes, which also include related figures, some commentary, and references to pertinent pages of the book text. In the Video Displays, a legend describing each video clip is provided in a pop-up window designated by a key icon. The Video Displays are in Adobe Acrobat PDF format; to play the videos on a PC, the option for using the Windows Media Player or Windows Built-In Player should be selected from the Tasks toolbar under Edit → Preferences → Multimedia → Preferred Media Player. Click on the video to start it; escape will stop the video. Macintosh users can play the videos within Adobe Acrobat simply by clicking on the video to start it, clicking on a playing video to pause it, and double-clicking on a paused video to resume playing. (Note: these Video Display documents are viewable in Apple's "Preview" application; however, the videos will not play.)

The chapters of the book contain links to the Video Displays. Thus, as the reader browses the electronic version of the text, it is possible to use the links to jump to the Video Displays and view pertinent video clips with their legends, commentary, and related images. To return to the text, click on the "Back" button in the browser. Also included on the DVD are David A. Robinson's hand-written lecture notes, "Linear Control Systems in the Oculomotor System."

To use the DVD, insert it into the computer's DVD drive; the disc will automatically start up and present a Web-browser screen that lists the contents, which can be accessed with a click of the mouse. It is also possible to explore the DVD using the computer's file access software.

SYSTEM REQUIREMENTS

DVD drive

Internet Explorer (recommended) or other Web browser

Adobe Acrobat Reader version 6 or higher

Movie Viewer: Windows Media Player or Windows Built-In Player or QuickTime Player